INTEGRATIVE ORTHOPEDICS

Third Edition with New Information on Laboratory Interpretation, Iron Overload, and Fibromyalgia

Integrative, Nutritional, Botanical, and Manipulative Therapeutics
with Concepts, Perspectives, Algorithms, and Protocols
for the In-Office Diagnosis and Management of
the Most Common Neuromusculoskeletal Problems

*The art of co-creating wellness
while effectively managing
acute and chronic
musculoskeletal disorders*

DR. ALEX VASQUEZ

- Doctor of Osteopathic Medicine, graduate of University of North Texas Health Science Center, Texas College of Osteopathic Medicine (2010)
- Doctor of Naturopathic Medicine, graduate of Bastyr University (1999)
- Doctor of Chiropractic, graduate of Western States Chiropractic College (1996)
- Director of the Medical Board of Advisors (2011-present), Researcher and Lecturer (2004-2010), Biotics Research Corporation in Rosenberg, Texas
- Adjunct Faculty (2004-2005, 2010-present) and Former Forum Consultant (2003-2007), The Institute for Functional Medicine in Gig Harbor, Washington
- Professor of Pharmacology, University of Western States in Portland, Oregon
- Former Adjunct Professor of Orthopedics (2000) and Rheumatology (2001), Bastyr University in Kenmore, Washington
- Private practice in Seattle, Washington (2000-2001), Houston, Texas (2001-2006), Portland, Oregon (2011-present)
- Author of approximately 90 articles and letters published in *Annals of Pharmacotherapy, The Lancet, Nutritional Perspectives, BMJ (British Medical Journal), Journal of Manipulative and Physiological Therapeutics, JAMA (Journal of the American Medical Association), The Original Internist, Integrative Medicine: A Clinician's Journal, Holistic Primary Care, Nutritional Wellness, Dynamic Chiropractic, Alternative Therapies in Health and Medicine, Journal of the American Osteopathic Association, Evidence-based Complementary and Alternative Medicine, Journal of Clinical Endocrinology and Metabolism,* and *Arthritis & Rheumatism*: Official Journal of the American College of Rheumatology

OPTIMALHEALTHRESEARCH.COM

Vasquez A. <u>Integrative Orthopedics Third Edition</u>. Portland, Oregon; Integrative and Biological Medicine Research and Consulting, LLC.

The intended audiences for this book are health science students and doctorate-level clinicians. This book has been written with every intention to make it as accurate as possible, and each section has undergone peer-review by an interdisciplinary group of clinicians. In view of the possibility of human error and as well as ongoing discoveries in the biomedical sciences, neither the author nor any party associated in any way with this text warrants that this text is perfect, accurate, or complete in every way, and we disclaim responsibility for harm or loss associated with the application of the material herein. Information and treatments applicable to a specific *condition* may not be appropriate for or applicable to a specific *patient*; this is especially true for patients with multiple comorbidities and those taking pharmaceutical medications with multiple adverse effects and drug/nutrient/herb interactions. Given that this book is available on an open market, lay persons who read this material should discuss the information with a licensed healthcare provider before implementing the treatments and interventions described herein.

See website for updated information: www.OptimalHealthResearch.com

Dedications: I dedicate this book to the following people in appreciation for their works, their direct and indirect support of this work, and for their contributions to the advancement of true healthcare.

- **To the students and practitioners of chiropractic and naturopathic medicine**, those who continue to learn so that they can provide the best possible care to their patients.
- **To the researchers** whose works are cited in this text.
- **To Drs Alan Gaby, Jeffrey Bland, Ronald LeFebvre, Robert Richard, and Gilbert Manso,** my most memorable and influential professors and mentors.
- **To Dr Bruce Ames**[1] **and the late Dr Roger Williams**[2], for helping us to view our individuality as biochemically unique.
- **To Dr Chester Wilk**[3,4] **and important others** for documenting and resisting the organized oppression of natural, non-pharmaceutical, non-surgical healthcare.[5,6,7]
- **To Jorge Strunz and Ardeshir Farah,** for artistic inspiration

Acknowledgments for Peer and Editorial Review: Acknowledgement here does not imply that the reviewer fully agrees with or endorses the material in this text but rather that they were willing to review specific sections of the book for clinical applicability and clarity and to make suggestions to their own level of satisfaction. Credit for improvements and refinements to this text are due in part to these reviewers; responsibility for oversights remains that of the author.

- 2012 Edition of Migraine Headaches, Hypothyroidism, and Fibromyalgia: Holly Furlong DC
- 2011 Edition of *Integrative Chiropractic Management of High Blood Pressure and Chronic Hypertension*: Barry Morgan MD, Holly Furlong DC, Kris Young DC, Erika Mennerick DC, and Bill Beakey DOM
- 2011 Edition of *Integrative Medicine and Functional Medicine for Chronic Hypertension*: Erika Mennerick DC, Holly Furlong DC, JoAnn Fawcett DC, Ileana Bourland MSOM LAc, James Bogash DC, Bill Beakey
- 2010 Edition of *Chiropractic Management of Chronic Hypertension*: Joseph Paun MS DC, Joe Brimhall DC, David Candelario OMS4 (TCOM c/o 2010), James Bogash DC, Bill Beakey DOM, Robert Richard DO
- 2009 Edition of *Chiropractic and Naturopathic Mastery of Common Clinical Disorders*: Heather Kahn MD, Robert Richard DO, James Leiber DO, David Candelario (UNT-HSC TCOM DO4)
- 2007 Edition of *Integrative Orthopedics*: Barry Morgan MD, Dennis Harris DC, Richard Brown DC (DACBI candidate), Ron Mariotti ND, Patrick Makarewich MBA, Reena Singh (SCNM ND4), Zachary Watkins DC, Charles Novak MS DC, Marnie Loomis ND, James Bogash DC, Sara Croteau DC, Kris Young DC, Joshua Levitt ND, Jack Powell III MD, Chad Kessler MD, Amy Neuzil ND
- 2006 Edition of *Integrative Rheumatology*: Amy Neuzil ND, Cathryn Harbor MD, Julian Vickers DC, Tamara Sachs MD, Bob Sager BSc MD DABFM (Clinical Instructor in the Department of Family Medicine, University of Kansas), Ron Mariotti ND, Titus Chiu (DC4), Zachary Watkins (DC4), Gilbert Manso MD, Bruce Milliman ND, William Groskopp DC, Robert Silverman DC, Matthew Breske (DC4), Dean Neary ND, Thomas Walton DC, Fraser Smith ND, Ladd Carlston DC, David Jones MD, Joshua Levitt ND
- 2004 Edition of *Integrative Orthopedics*: Peter Knight ND, Kent Littleton ND MS, Barry Morgan MD, Ron Hobbs ND, Joshua Levitt ND, John Neustadt (Bastyr ND4), Allison Gandre BS (Bastyr ND4), Peter Kimble ND, Jack Powell III MD, Chad Kessler MD, Mike Gruber MD, Deirdre O'Neill ND, Mary Webb ND, Leslie Charles ND, Amy Neuzil ND

Format and Layout: The format and layout of this book is designed to efficiently take the reader though the clinically relevant spectrum of considerations for each condition that is detailed. Important topics are given their own section within each chapter, while other less important or less common conditions are only described briefly in terms of the four "clinical essentials" of 1) definition/pathophysiology, 2) clinical presentation, 3)

[1] Ames BN, Elson-Schwab I, Silver EA. High-dose vitamin therapy stimulates variant enzymes with decreased coenzyme binding affinity (increased K(m)): relevance to genetic disease and polymorphisms. *Am J Clin Nutr*. 2002 Apr;75(4):616-58 http://www.ajcn.org/cgi/content/full/75/4/616
[2] Williams RJ. Biochemical Individuality: The Basis for the Genetotrophic Concept. Austin and London: University of Texas Press; 1956
[3] Wilk CA. Medicine, Monopolies, and Malice: How the Medical Establishment Tried to Destroy Chiropractic. Garden City Park: Avery, 1996
[4] Getzendanner S. Permanent injunction order against AMA. *JAMA*. 1988 Jan 1;259(1):81-2 http://optimalhealthresearch.com/archives/wilk.html
[5] Carter JP. Racketeering in Medicine: The Suppression of Alternatives. Norfolk: Hampton Roads Pub; 1993
[6] Morley J, Rosner AL, Redwood D. A case study of misrepresentation of the scientific literature: recent reviews of chiropractic. *J Altern Complement Med*. 2001 Feb;7(1):65-78
[7] Terrett AG. Misuse of the literature by medical authors in discussing spinal manipulative therapy injury. *J Manipulative Physiol Ther*. 1995 May;18(4):203-10

assessment/diagnosis, and 4) treatment/management. Each expanded section which details the more important/common conditions maintains a consistent format, taking the reader through the spectrum of primary clinical considerations: definition/pathophysiology, clinical presentations, differential diagnoses, assessments (physical examination, laboratory, imaging), complications, management, and treatment. As my books have progressed, I am increasingly using an article-by-article review format (especially in the sections on management and treatment) so that readers have more direct access to the information so as to understand and *incorporate* more deeply what the research actually states; the goal and general approach here is to use a *representative sampling* of the research literature.

References and Citations: Citations to articles, abstracts, texts, and personal communications are footnoted throughout the text to provide supporting information and to provide interested readers the resources to find additional information. Many of the cited articles are available on-line for free, and when possible I have included the website addresses so that readers can access the complete article.

Peer-review and Quality Control: Peer-review is essential to help ensure accuracy and clinical applicability of health-related information. Consistent with the importance of our goals, I have employed several "checks and balances" to increase the accuracy and applicability of the information within my textbooks:

- Reliance upon authoritative references: Nearly all important statements are referenced to peer-reviewed biomedical journals or authoritative texts, such as *The Merck Manual* and *Current Medical Diagnosis and Treatment*. Each citation is provided by a footnote at the bottom of each page so that readers will know quickly and easily exactly from where the information was obtained.
- Extensive cross-referencing: Readers will notice, if not be overwhelmed by, the number of references and citations. Many important statements have several references. Many references (especially textbooks) are referenced several times even on the same page. The purpose of this extensive referencing is three-fold: 1) to guide you to additional information, 2) to help me (as writer) stay organized, and 3) to help you and me (the practicing physicians) employ this information with confidence.
- Periodic revision: All of my books will be updated and revised on an *as-needed* basis. New information is added; superfluous information removed. Inspired by the popular text *Current Medical Diagnosis and Treatment* which is updated every year, I want my books to be accurate, timely, and in pace with the ever-growing literature on natural medicine. Any significant errors that are discovered will be posted at OptimalHealthResearch.com/updates; please check this page periodically to ensure that you are working with the most accurate information of which I am aware.
- Peer-review: The peer-review process for my books takes several forms. First, colleagues and students are invited to review new and revised sections of the text before publication; every section of the book that you are holding has been independently reviewed by health science students and/or practicing clinicians from various backgrounds: allopathic, chiropractic, osteopathic, naturopathic. Second, you - the reader - are invited to provide feedback about the information in the book, typographical errors, syntax, case reports, new research, etc. If your ideas truly change the nature of the material, I will be glad to acknowledge you in the text (with your permission, of course). If your contribution is hugely significant, such as reviewing three or more chapters or helping in some important way, I will be glad to not only acknowledge you, but to also send you the next edition at a discount or courtesy when your ideas take effect. Third, I keep abreast of new literature by constantly perusing new research and advancements in the health sciences. Having been successful in three separate doctoral programs in the health sciences, I have learned not only to master large amounts of material but to also separate and integrate different viewpoints as appropriate. I also "field test" my protocols with patients in the various clinical arenas in which I work and also with professionals and academicians via presentations and critical dialogue. By implementing these quality control steps, I hope to create a useful text and advance our professions and our practices by improving the quality of care that we deliver to our patients. Readers with suggestions or corrections can email via the website: http://OptimalHealthResearch.com/corrections.

How to Use This Book Safely and Most Effectively: Ideally, these books should be read cover-to-cover within a context of coursework that is supervised by an experienced professor. For post-graduate professionals, they might consider forming a local "book club" and meeting for weekly or monthly discussions to check their understandings and share their clinical experiences to refine the application of clinical knowledge, perceptions, and skills. Virtual groups and internet forums—specifically the forum hosted by the Institute for Functional Medicine at www.FunctionalMedicine.org—can provide access to an assembly of international professional peers wherein sharing of clinical questions and experiences are synergistic. Throughout this book, references are amply provided and are often footnoted with hyperlinks providing full-text access. This book is intended for licensed doctorate-level healthcare professionals with graduate and post-graduate training.

Notice: The intention and scope of this text are to provide doctorate-level clinicians with useful information and a familiarity with available research and resources pertinent to the management of patients in an integrative primary care setting. Specifically, the information in this book is intended to be used by licensed healthcare professionals who have received hands-on clinical training and supervision at accredited health science colleges. Additionally, information in this book should be used in conjunction with other resources, texts, and in combination with the clinician's best judgment and intention to *"first, do no harm"* and second to provide effective healthcare. Information and treatments applicable to a specific *condition* may not be appropriate for or applicable to a specific *patient* in your office; this is especially true for patients with multiple comorbidities and those taking pharmaceutical medications with multiple adverse effects and drug/nutrient/herb interactions. Throughout this text, I describe treatments—manual, dietary, nutritional, botanical, pharmacologic, and occasionally surgical—and their research support for the clinical condition being discussed; each practitioner must determine appropriateness of these treatments for his/her individual patient and with consideration of the doctor's scope of practice, education, training, skill, and the appropriateness of "off label" use of medications and treatments. This book has been carefully written and checked for accuracy by the author and professional colleagues. However, in view of the possibility of human error and new discoveries in the biomedical sciences, neither the author nor any party associated in any way with this text warrants that this text is perfect, accurate, or complete in every way, and we disclaim responsibility for harm or loss associated with the application of the material herein. With all conditions/treatments described herein, each physician must be sure to consider the balance between what is best for the patient and the physician's own level of ability, expertise, and experience. When in doubt, or if the physician is not a specialist in the treatment of a given severe condition, referral is appropriate. These notes are written with the routine "outpatient" in mind and are not tailored to severely injured patients or "playing field" or "emergency response" situations. Consult your First Aid and Emergency Response texts and course materials for appropriate information. These notes represent the author's perspective based on academic education, experience, and post-graduate continuing education and are not inclusive of every fact that a clinician may need to know. This is not an "entry level" book except when used in an academic setting with a knowledgeable professor who can explain the concepts, tests, physical exam procedures, and treatments; this book requires a certain level of knowledge from the reader and familiarity with clinical concepts, laboratory assessments, and physical examination procedures.

Updates, Corrections, and Newsletter: When and if omissions, errata, and the need for important updates become clear, I will post these at the website: OptimalHealthResearch.com/updates. A reader might access this page periodically to ensure staying informed of any corrections that might have clinical relevance. This book consists not only of the text in the printed pages you are holding, but also the footnotes and any updates at the website. Be alerted to new integrative clinical research and updates to this textbook by signing-up for the free newsletter at www.OptimalHealthResearch.com/newsletter.

Language, Semantics, and Perspective: As a diligent student who previously aspired to be an English professor, I have written this text with great (though inevitably imperfect) attention to detail. Individual words were chosen with care. I confess to knowing, pushing, and creatively breaking several rules of grammar and punctuation. With regard to the he/she and him/her debacle of the English language, I've mixed singular and plural pronouns for the sake of being efficient and so that the images remain gender-neutral to the extent reasonable. The subtitle

The art of creating wellness while effectively managing acute and chronic musculoskeletal/health disorders was chosen to emphasize the intentional creation of wellness rather than a limited focus on disease treatment and symptom suppression. For the 2009 printing of *Chiropractic and Naturopathic Mastery of Common Clinical Disorders*, this subtitle was slightly modified from "creating" to "co-creating" to emphasize the **team effort** required between physician and patient. *Managing* was chosen to emphasize the importance of treating-monitoring-referring-reassessing, rather than merely *treating*. *Disorders* was chosen to reflect the fact that a distinguishing characteristic of *life* is the ability to habitually create *organized structure* and *higher order* from chaos and *disorder*. For example, plants organize the randomly moving molecules of air and water into the organized structure of biomolecules which eventually take shape as plant structure—fiber, leaves, flowers, petals. Similarly, the human body creates organized structure of increased complexity from consumed plants and other foods; molecules ingested and inhaled from the environment are organized into specific biochemicals and tissue structures with distinct characteristics and definite functions. Injury and disease *result in* or *result from* a lack of order, hence my use of the word "disorders" to characterize human illness and disease. A motor vehicle accident that results in bodily injury, for example, is an example of an external chaotic force, which, when imparted upon human body tissues, results in a disruption (disorder) of the normal structure and organization that previously defined and characterized the now-damaged tissues of the body. Likewise, an autoimmune disease process that results in tissue destruction is an *anti-evolutionary* process that takes molecules of higher complexity and reverts them to simpler, fragmented, and non-functional forms. From the perspective of "health" as *organized structure and meaningful function* and "disease" as *the reversion to chaos, destruction of structure, and the loss of function*, the task of healthcare providers is essentially to restore order, and to acutely reduce and proactively prevent/eliminate clinical-biochemical-biomechanical-emotional chaos insofar as it adversely affects the patient's life experience as an individual and our collective experience as an interdependent society. What is required of clinicians then is the ability first to create conceptual order from what appears to be chaotic phenomena, and then second to materialize that conceptual order into our physical world; this is our task, and no small task it is.

Integrity and Creativity: I have endeavored to accurately represent the facts as they have been presented in texts and research, and to specifically resist any temptation to embellish or misrepresent data as others have done.[8,9] Conversely, I have not endeavored to make this book appeal to the "average" student or reader; my goal is to write and teach to the students at the top of the class, thereby affirming them and pulling the other students forward and upward. While I offer *explanations*, I intentionally resist *simplifications*, except when one simplification might facilitate the comprehension of a more complex phenomenon, or when such a simplification might facilitation the conveyance of information from clinician to patient. I have allowed this text to be unique in format, content, and style, so that the personality of this text can be contrasted with that of the instructor and reader, thus enabling the learner to at least benefit from an intentionally different – and intentionally honest – perspective and approach. Students using this text with the guidance of a qualified professor will benefit from the experience of "two teachers" rather than just one.

Linearity, Nonlinearity, Redundancy, Asynchronicity: Although the overall flow of the text is highly linear and sequential, occasionally I place a conclusion before its introduction for the sake of foreshadowing and therefore for preparing the reader for what is to come. The purpose of this is not simply one of preparation for the sake of allowing the reader to know what is already lying ahead on the path, but more to begin creating new "shelf space" in the reader's intellectual-neuronal "library" so that when the new—particularly if *neoparadigmatic*—information is encountered, a space will already exist for it; it other words: the intent is to make learning easier. Likewise, for the sake of *information retention*—or what is better understood as synaptogenesis—important points are presented more than once, either identically or variantly. Given that *"No one ever reads the same book twice"*[10] (because the "person who starts" the reading of a meaningful book is changed into the "person who finishes" the

---

[8] **Vasquez A**. Zinc treatment for reduction of hyperplasia of prostate. *Townsend Letter for Doctors and Patients* 1996; January: 100

[9] Broad W, Wade N. *Betrayers of the Truth: Fraud and Deceit in the Halls of Science*. New York: Simon and Schuster; 1982

[10] Davies R. *Reading and Writing*. Salt Lake City: University of Utah Press; 1992, page 23

reading of that book (assuming proper intentionality and application of one's "self"), the person reading these words might consider a second glace after the first.

Preface to the 2009 Edition of ***Chiropractic and Naturopathic Mastery of Common Clinical Disorders***: *Chiropractic and Naturopathic Mastery of Common Clinical Disorders* steps beyond the obviously musculoskeletal focus of my first three textbooks *Integrative Orthopedics*, *Integrative Rheumatology*, and *Musculoskeletal Pain: Expanded Clinical Strategies* to provide students and clinicians an evidence-based foundational approach to treating common clinical disorders such as Asthma, Hypertension, Diabetes Mellitus Type-2 and Metabolic Syndrome, and Disorders of Mood and Behavior—a section that emphasizes adult depression and anxiety. Readers of these sections and the works derived from them (e.g., the chapter on hypertension was expanded into the book *Chiropractic Management of Chronic Hypertension* and later *Integrative Medicine and Functional Medicine for Chronic Hypertension*) will note that they differ in format from the other chapters with regard to a stronger emphasis on presenting an article-by-article review in the effort to strengthen the evidence-based nature of the clinical protocols. As with my previous books and all other clinical resources, clinicians should still consult other sources and texts for additional information, updated guidelines, and changes to standards of care. The goal of *Chiropractic and Naturopathic Mastery of Common Clinical Disorders* has been to further bridge the gap that continues to exist between so-called "complementary and alternative medicine" (CAM) and so-called "conventional" medicine.[11]

The Functional Medicine Matrix (version presented in 2003): In the 2009 edition of *Chiropractic and Naturopathic Mastery of Common Clinical Disorders*, I reintroduced the Functional Medicine Matrix that I originally diagramed for the Institute for Functional Medicine (IFM) in 2003; the diagram used is updated from the original, and readers should appreciate that IFM has changed the Matrix since this version was made. My perspective is that functional medicine, naturopathic medicine, and *authentic* holistic medicine share much in common in their fundamental models of health and disease. The functional medicine matrix—designed and owned by the Institute for Functional Medicine (FunctionalMedicine.org)—is unique to the discipline of functional medicine and provides a conceptual framework for understanding the complexity of health and disease.

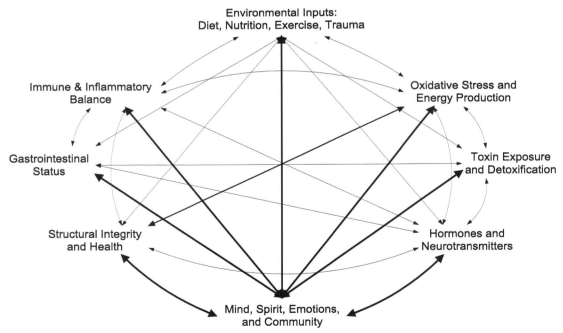

2003 Version of the Functional Medicine Matrix: Updated from the original diagram by Vasquez in 2003 for the Institute for Functional Medicine (IFM). See www.FunctionalMedicine.org for updated information and additional training.

---

[11] MacIntosh A. Understanding the Differences between Conventional, Alternative, Complementary, Integrative and Natural Medicine. *Townsend Letter*, July 1999. http://www.tldp.com/medicine.htm Accessed March 2011

<u>Distinguishing "Integrative Medicine" from "Functional Medicine"—the author's perspective</u>[12]: The distinction of integrative medicine from functional medicine is that of *quantity* from *quality*. Integrative medicine can be understood as a quantitative extension of other already-existing healthcare models, to which additional perspectives and treatments are added; in this way, various conceptual models are "integrated" and used together in a more holistic and comprehensive approach. In contrast, functional medicine is a distinct model of health and disease that has developed an identity beyond mere integration of various models and treatments. Functional medicine is qualitatively distinct in its viewpoint of disease causation and treatment by the unique combination of emphases placed on ❶ patient-centered care (in contrast to the disease-centered care of allopathic medicine and most osteopathic medicine), ❷ detailed appreciation of the importance of the web-like interconnected nature of various organ systems[13] and psychological, physiological, and pathological processes (to a greater extent than allopathic, osteopathic, chiropractic and naturopathic medicine), ❸ its rigorous evidence-based standards, and ❹ its willingness to eagerly-yet-appropriately include *all* therapeutic options, ranging from (for example) surgical to meditative, dietary to pharmaceutical, manipulative to botanical, and antidysbiotic to psychological. In short, functional medicine can be described as an ***antiparadigmatic patient-centered discipline***, hence its therapeutic flexibility, broad applicability, and enhanced efficacy; it is antiparadigmatic due to its lack of adherence to a specific and limited set of tools (most professional disciplines are quite limited in their expertise and scope) and due to the emphasis placed on patient-centered healthcare, which first and always foremost seeks to determine the most efficient path for patient empowerment and healing.

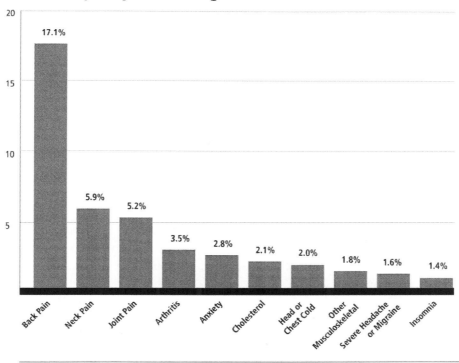

Diseases/Conditions for Which CAM Is Most Frequently Used Among Adults - 2007

Source: Barnes PM, Bloom B, Nahin R. *CDC National Health Statistics Report #12*. Complementary and Alternative Medicine Use Among Adults and Children: United States, 2007. December 2008.

<u>Health problems for which patients most often seek so-called CAM treatment</u>: Illustration from National Center for Complementary and Alternative Medicine, NIH, DHHS (http://nccam.nih.gov/news/camstats/2007/graphics.htm).

---

[12] Dr Vasquez's perspective: I have trained in functional medicine since 1994, first as a student of Jeffrey Bland PhD *et al* and later as Forum Consultant and Faculty (2003 – present in 2011) for the Institute of Functional Medicine, and I wrote three chapters in *Textbook of Functional Medicine* published by Institute of Functional Medicine. My opinions here are not necessarily currently representative of the Institute of Functional Medicine in this context.

[13] **Vasquez A**. Web-like Interconnections of Physiological Factors. *Integrative Medicine: A Clinician's Journal* 2006, April/May, 32-37

The table on this page provides a listing—in order of percentage—of the most common conditions seen in a general family practice of medicine, with hypertension and diabetes mellitus—two conditions highly amenable to integrative therapeutics—clearly dominating the clinical landscape.

Top diagnoses	Notes and comments
1. Hypertension	5.9% of family medicine diagnoses; nearly 11 million patient visits per year.
2. Diabetes mellitus	4.1% of family medicine diagnoses; more than 7.6 million patient visits per year.
3. Acute upper respiratory infection	3.2% of family medicine diagnoses; more than 10 million patient visits per year. Most of these are caused by viral infections for which there is no direct medical treatment.
4. Sinusitis	2.5% of family medicine diagnoses; more than 10 million patient visits per year.
5. Acute pharyngitis	2.3% of family medicine diagnoses; more than 4 million patient visits per year.
6. Otitis media	2.3% of family medicine diagnoses; > 4 million patient visits per year.
7. Bronchitis	1.9% of family medicine diagnoses; > 3 million patient visits per year.
8. Back problems	1.8% of family medicine diagnoses; > 3 million patient visits per year. This is a diverse group of conditions ranging from post-traumatic to benign to developmental problems such as scoliosis. Note that back pain is listed separately below.
9. Hyperlipidemia	1.7% of family medicine diagnoses; > 3 million patient visits per year. This mostly includes the lifestyle-generated dyslipidemia epidemic, with comparably fewer cases of genotropic disorders requiring pharmacotherapy.
10. Urinary tract disorders	1.6% of family medicine diagnoses; almost 3 million patient visits per year. This can include a diverse group of problems ranging from simple and self-limited urinary tract infections to sexually transmitted diseases.
11. Allergic rhinitis	1.2% of family medicine diagnoses; > 2 million patient visits per year. A general approach to allergy treatment is included in this text.
12. Back pain	1.2% of family medicine diagnoses; > 2 million patient visits per year.
13. Abdominal or pelvic symptoms	1.1% of family medicine diagnoses; > 2 million patient visits per year. This can include a wide range of diagnoses ranging from appendicitis to dysmenorrhea. Due to the breadth and complexity, these are not covered in this text.
14. Joint pain	1.1% of family medicine diagnoses; > 2 million patient visits per year.
15. Depression or anxiety	1.1% of family medicine diagnoses; > 2 million patient visits per year.
16. Asthma	1.1% of family medicine diagnoses; almost 2 million patient visits per year. An approach to allergy treatment is included in this text, with a section on asthma.
17. Chest pain or shortness of breath	1.1% of family medicine diagnoses; almost 2 million patient visits per year. Some of these are benign musculoskeletal pain or gastroesophageal reflux while others turn out to be life-threatening conditions such as myocardial infarction, pneumothorax, pneumonia, or—rarely—aortic dissection. These are not directly covered in this text.
18. Soft tissue problems	1% of family medicine diagnoses; 1.8 million patient visits per year.
19. Acute bronchitis and bronchiolitis	1% of family medicine diagnoses; 1.8 million patient visits per year. These include bacterial and viral infections, ranging from mild to life-threatening, especially in patients with cardiopulmonary disease.
20. Skin problems	1% of family medicine diagnoses; 1.8 million patient visits per year.
21. Tendonitis	1% of family medicine diagnoses; 1.7 million patient visits per year.

Data from *Essentials of Family Medicine, 5th edition* edited by Sloane PD, Slatt LM, Ebell MH, Jacques LB, Smith MA published by Lippincott Williams & Wilkins (April 1, 2007)

<u>**Bon Voyage**</u>: All artists and scientists—regardless of genre—grapple with the divergent goals of perfecting their work and presenting their work; the former is impossible, while the latter is the only means by which the effort can create the desired effect in the world, whether that is pleasure, progress, or both. At some point, we must all agree that it is "good enough" and that it contains the essence of what needs to be communicated. While neither this nor any future edition of this book is likely to be "perfect", I am content with the literature reviewed, presented, and the new conclusions and implications which are described—many for the first time ever—in this text. Particularly for *Integrative Rheumatology* and *Chiropractic and Naturopathic Mastery*, each chapter aims to achieve a paradigm shift which distances us further from the simplistic pharmacocentric model and toward one which authentically empowers both practitioners and patients. With time, I will make future editions more complete and perhaps less polemical—but not less passionate. I hope you are able to implement these conclusions and research findings *into your own life* and into the treatment plans for your patients. In short time, I believe that we will see many of these concepts more broadly implemented. Hopefully this work's value and veracity will promote patients' vitality via the vigilant and virtuous clinicians viewing this volume. To the more attentive and thoroughgoing reader, more is revealed.

Authentic learning is life integration
"Ultimately, no one can extract from things—*books included*—more than he already knows. What one has no access to through experience, one has no ear for."
Friedrich Nietzsche [translated by RJ Hollingdale]. *Ecce Homo: How One Becomes What One Is*. New York & London: Penguin Books; 1979, page 70

Thank you, and I wish you and your patients the best of success and health.

[signature]

Alex Vasquez, D.C., N.D., D.O.
December 26, 2011

Work as love
"You work that you may keep pace with the earth and the soul of the earth. For to be idle is to become a stranger unto the seasons, and to step out of life's procession. ... Work is love made visible."
Kahlil Gibran (1883-1930). *The Prophet*. Publisher Alfred A. Knopf, 1973

Newsletter & Updates
Be alerted to new integrative clinical research and updates to this textbook by signing-up for the free newsletter, sent several times per year as needed. Join at: www.OptimalHealthResearch.com/newsletter

Examples of commonly used abbreviations:

- **25-OH-D** = serum 25-hydroxy-vitamin D(3)
- **ACEi** = angiotensin-2 converting enzyme inhibitor
- **Alpha-blocker** = alpha-adrenergic antagonist
- **ARB** = angiotensin-2 receptor blocker/antagonist
- **ARF** = acute renal failure
- **BB** = beta blocker or beta-adrenergic antagonist
- **BMP** = basic metabolic panel, includes serum Na, K, Cl, CO2, BUN, creatinine, and glucose
- **BP** = blood pressure, **HBP** = high blood pressure
- **BUN** = blood urea nitrogen
- **C&S** = culture and sensitivity
- **CAD** = coronary artery disease
- **CBC** = complete blood count
- **CCB** = calcium channel blocker/antagonist
- **CE** = cardiac enzymes, generally including creatine kinase (CK), creatine kinase myocardial band (CKMB), and troponin-1, with the latter being the most specific serologic marker for acute myocardial injury; for the evaluation of acute MI, these are generally tested 2-3 times at 6-hour intervals with ECG performed at least as often.
- **CHF** = congestive heart failure
- **CHO** = carbohydrate
- **CK** = creatine kinase, historically named creatine phosphokinase (CPK)
- **CKD** = chronic kidney disease, generally stratified into five stages based on GFR of roughly <90, 90-60, 60-30, 30-15, and >15, respectively
- **CMP** = comprehensive metabolic panel, also called a chemistry panel, includes the BMP along with markers of hepatic status albumin, protein, ALT, AST, may also include alkaline phosphatase and rarely GGT; panels vary per laboratory and hospital
- **CNS** = central nervous system
- **COPD** = chronic obstructive pulmonary disease
- **CRF**, **CRI** = chronic renal failure/insufficiency
- **CRP** = c-reactive protein, **hsCRP** = high-sensitivity c-reactive protein
- **CT** = computed tomography
- **CVD** = cardiovascular disease
- **CXR** = chest X-ray
- **DM** = diabetes mellitus
- **ECG** or **EKG** = electrocardiograph
- **Echo** = echocardiography
- **GFR** = glomerular filtration rate
- **HDL** = high density lipoprotein cholesterol
- **HTN** = hypertension
- **Ig** = immune globulin = antibodies of the G, A, M, E, or D classes.
- **IHD** = ischemic heart disease
- **IV** = intravenous
- **MCV** = mean cell volume
- **MI** = myocardial infarction
- **MRI** = magnetic resonance imaging, **MRI** = magnetic resonance angiography
- **PRN** = from the Latin "pro re nata" meaning "on occasion" or "when necessary"
- **PTH** = parathyroid hormone, **iPTH** = intact parathyroid hormone
- **PVD** = peripheral vascular disease
- **RA** = rheumatoid arthritis
- **RAD** = reactive airway disease, similar to asthma
- **SLE** = systemic lupus erythematosus
- **TRIG(s)** = serum triglycerides
- **UA** = urinalysis
- **US** = ultrasound

Dosing shorthand (mostly Latin abbreviations): q = each; qd = each day; bid = twice daily; tid = thrice daily; qid = four times per day; po = per os = by mouth; prn = as needed.

Chapter 1:
Review of Clinical Assessments and Concepts

Clinical Assessments and Concepts:

This review is included for students and for graduates desiring a concise overview of basic and advanced clinical concepts. Many clinical pearls are included.

Reviewed herein are the three essential components of patient assessment: history, physical examination, and laboratory assessment. Additional concepts and perspectives are provided that will help facilitate risk management and optimal patinet care.

<u>Topics:</u>

- **Core Competencies**
- **Moving past disease- and drug-centered medicine toward patient-centered health optimization: the goal is *wellness***
- **Acute Care and Musculoskeletal Care as Opportunities for Health Optimization**
- **Clinical Assessments**
  - History taking & physical examination
  - Orthopedic/musculoskeletal examination: Concepts and goals
  - Neurologic assessment: Review
  - Laboratory assessments: General considerations of commonly used tests
    i. *Routine tests*: Chemistry/metabolic panel, lipid panel, CBC, 25(OH)-vitamin D, ferritin, thyroid stimulating hormone, CRP, ESR,
    ii. *Rheumatology/inflammation*: ANA (antinuclear antibodies), ANCA (antineutrophilic cytoplasmic antibodies), RF (rheumatoid factor), CCP (cyclic citrullinated protein antibodies), complement proteins, HLA-B27
    iii. *Functional assessments*: Lactulose-mannitol assay, comprehensive stool analysis and comprehensive parasitology
- **High-Risk Pain Patients**
- **Clinical Concepts**
  - Not all injury-related problems are injury-related problems
  - Safe patient + safe treatment = safe outcome
  - Four clues to underlying problems
  - Special considerations in the evaluation of children
  - No errors allowed: Differences between primary healthcare and spectator sports
  - "Disease treatment" is different from "patient management"
  - Clinical practice involves much more than "diagnosis and treatment"
  - Risk management: A note especially to students and recent licensees
- **Musculoskeletal Emergencies**
  - Acute compartment syndrome
  - Acute red eye, including acute iritis and scleritis
  - Atlantoaxial subluxation and instability
  - Cauda equina syndrome
  - Giant cell arteritis, temporal arteritis
  - Myelopathy, spinal cord compression
  - Neuropsychiatric lupus
  - Osteomyelitis
  - Septic arthritis, acute nontraumatic monoarthritis
- **Brief Overview of Integrative Healthcare Disciplines**
  - Chiropractic
  - Naturopathic Medicine
  - Osteopathic Medicine
  - Functional Medicine

Moving past "disease and drug"-centered medicine toward patient-centered health optimization: the goal is *wellness*

Written for students and experienced clinicians, this chapter introduces and reviews many new and common terms, procedures, and concepts relevant to the management of patients with musculoskeletal disorders. Especially for students, the reading of this chapter is essential to understanding the extensive material in this book and will facilitate the clinical assessment and management of patients with various clinical presentations.

Healthcare is currently in a time of significant fluctuation and is ready for changes in the balance of power and the paradigms which direct our therapeutic interventions. For nearly a century, allopathic medicine has hailed itself as "the gold standard", and other professions have either submitted to or been crushed by their ongoing political/scientific manipulations and their continual proclamation of intellectual and therapeutic superiority[1,2,3,4,5,6,7,8,9,10,11,12,13] despite 180,000-220,000 iatrogenic *medically-induced* deaths per year (500-600 iatrogenic deaths per day)[14,15] and consistent documentation that most medical/allopathic physicians are unable to provide accurate musculoskeletal diagnoses due to pervasive inadequacies in medical training.[16,17,18,19] Increasing disenchantment with allopathic *heroic medicine* and its adverse outcomes of inefficacy, exorbitant expenses, and unnecessary death are fostering change, such that allopathic medicine has been dethroned as the leading paradigm among American patients, who spend the majority of their discretionary healthcare dollars on consultations and treatments provided by "alternative" healthcare providers.[20,21] With the ever-increasing utilization of chiropractic, naturopathic, and osteopathic medical services, we must see that our paradigms and interventions keep pace with the evolving research literature and our increasing professional responsibilities so that we can deliver the highest possible quality of care.

> **Medical iatrogenesis kills 493 Americans per day**
> "Recent estimates suggest that each year more than 1 million patients are injured while in the hospital and approximately 180,000 die because of these injuries. Furthermore, drug-related morbidity and mortality are common and are estimated to cost more than $136 billion a year."
>
> Holland EG, Degruy FV. Drug-induced disorders. *Am Fam Physician*. 1997;56(7):1781-8, 1791-2

While we all readily acknowledge the importance of emergency care for emergency situations, those of us who advocate and practice a more complete approach to healthcare and life readily see the shortcomings of a limited and mechanical approach to healthcare, and we aspire to do more than simply fix problems. The

[1] Wilk CA. Medicine, Monopolies, and Malice: How the Medical Establishment Tried to Destroy Chiropractic. Garden City Park: Avery, 1996

[2] Getzendanner S. Permanent injunction order against AMA. *JAMA*. 1988 Jan 1;259(1):81-2 http://optimalhealthresearch.com/archives/wilk.html

[3] Carter JP. Racketeering in Medicine: The Suppression of Alternatives. Norfolk: Hampton Roads Pub; 1993

[4] Morley J, Rosner AL, Redwood D. A case study of misrepresentation of the scientific literature: recent reviews of chiropractic. *J Altern Complement Med*. 2001 Feb;7:65-78

[5] Terrett AG. Misuse of the literature by medical authors in discussing spinal manipulative therapy injury. *J Manipulative Physiol Ther*. 1995;18(4):203-10

[6] National Alliance of Professional Psychology Providers. AMA Seeks To Control and Restrict Psychologist's Scope of Practice. http://www.nappp.org/scope.pdf Accessed November 25, 2006

[7] "In an effort to marshal the medical community's resources against the growing threat of expanding scope of practice for allied health professionals, the AMA has formed a national partnership to confront such initiatives nationwide… The committee will use $25,000..." Daly R, American Psychiatric Association. AMA Forms Coalition to Thwart Non-M.D. Practice Expansion. *Psychiatric News* 2006 March; 41: 17 http://pn.psychiatryonline.org/cgi/content/full/41/5/17-a?eaf Accessed November 25, 2006

[8] Spivak JL. The Medical Trust Unmasked. Louis S. Siegfried Publishers; New York: 1961

[9] Trever W. In the Public Interest. Los Angeles; Scriptures Unlimited; 1972. This is probably the most authoritative documentation of the illegal actions of the AMA up to 1972; contains numerous photocopies of actual AMA documents and minutes of official meetings with overt intentionality of destroying Americans' healthcare options so that the AMA and related organizations would have a monopoly in national healthcare.

[10] Wenban AB. Inappropriate use of the title 'chiropractor' and term 'chiropractic manipulation' in the peer-reviewed biomedical literature. *Chiropr Osteopat*. 2006;14:16 http://chiroandosteo.com/content/14/1/16

[11] Orme-Johnson DW, Herron RE. An innovative approach to reducing medical care utilization and expenditures. *Am J Manag Care*. 1997 Jan;3:135-44 http://www.ajmc.com/Article.cfm?Menu=1&ID=2154

[12] van der Steen WJ, Ho VK. Drugs versus diets: disillusions with Dutch health care. *Acta Biotheor*. 2001;49(2):125-40

[13] Texas Medical Association. Physicians Ask Court to Protect Patients From Illegal Chiropractic Activities. http://www.texmed.org/Template.aspx?id=5259 Accessed February 20, 2007

[14] Starfield B. Is US health really the best in the world? *JAMA*. 2000 Jul 26;284(4):483-5

[15] "Recent estimates suggest that each year more than 1 million patients are injured while in the hospital and approximately 180,000 die because of these injuries. Furthermore, drug-related morbidity and mortality are common and are estimated to cost more than $136 billion a year." Holland EG, Degruy FV. Drug-induced disorders. *Am Fam Physician*. 1997;56(7):1781-8, 1791-2

[16] Freedman KB, Bernstein J. The adequacy of medical school education in musculoskeletal medicine. *J Bone Joint Surg Am*. 1998;80(10):1421-7

[17] Freedman KB, Bernstein J. Educational deficiencies in musculoskeletal medicine. *J Bone Joint Surg Am*. 2002;84-A(4):604-8

[18] Matzkin E, Smith ME, Freccero CD, Richardson AB. Adequacy of education in musculoskeletal medicine. *J Bone Joint Surg Am*. 2005;87-A(2):310-4

[19] Schmale GA. More evidence of educational inadequacies in musculoskeletal medicine. *Clin Orthop Relat Res*. 2005 Aug;(437):251-9

[20] "...Americans made an estimated 425 million visits to providers of unconventional therapy. This number exceeds the number of visits to all U.S. primary care physicians (388 million)." Eisenberg DM, Kessler RC, Foster C, Norlock FE, Calkins DR, Delbanco TL. Unconventional medicine in the United States. Prevalence, costs, and patterns of use. *N Engl J Med*. 1993 Jan 28;328(4):246-52

[21] "Estimated expenditures for alternative medicine professional services increased 45.2% between 1990 and 1997 and were conservatively estimated at $21.2 billion in 1997, with at least $12.2 billion paid out-of-pocket. This exceeds the 1997 out-of-pocket expenditures for all US hospitalizations." Eisenberg DM, Davis RB, Ettner SL, Appel S, Wilkey S, Van Rompay M, Kessler RC. Trends in alternative medicine use in the United States, 1990-1997: results of a follow-up national survey. *JAMA*. 1998 Nov 11;280(18):1569-75

implementation of *multidimensional* (i.e., *comprehensive* and *multifaceted*) treatment plans that address many aspects of pathophysiologic phenomena is a huge step forward in creating improved health and preventing future illness in the patients who seek our professional assistance. However, even complete multidimensional treatment plans still fall short of the goal of creating wellness, if for no other reasons than 1) they are still disease- and problem-oriented, rather than health-oriented, 2) they are prescribed from outside ("The doctor told me to do it.") rather than originating internally and spontaneously by the patient's own direction and affirmation ("I *do* this because I *am* this."), and, finally and most difficult to relay, 3) they are mechanistic rather than organic, they can do no better than the sum of their parts, they flow exclusively from the mind ("do") and not also from the body-soul ("am"). The art of creating wellness takes time to understand, longer to implement clinically, and even longer to apply to one's own life. Wellness is a state of being rather than a checklist of activities in a "preventive health program." The subtle differences that distinguish "wellness" from any "program" or "prescription" are the differences between *leading* versus *following* and *flowing* versus *performing*. **Wellness is multidimensional self-actualization, full integration of one's life—present, past, and future; physical, mental, emotional, spiritual, biochemical—one's shadow[22], work[23], feelings, thoughts, and goals into a cohesive living whole – "a wheel rolling from its own center."[24]**

Ever-increasing popularity of nonallopathic medicine

"...Americans made an estimated 425 million visits to providers of unconventional therapy. This number exceeds the number of visits to all U.S. primary care physicians (388 million)."

Eisenberg DM, et al. Unconventional medicine in the United States. Prevalence, costs, and patterns of use. *N Engl J Med* 1993;328:246-52

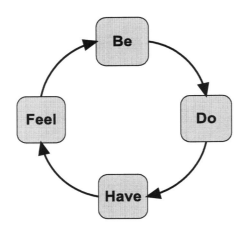

[22] Robert Bly. The Human Shadow. Sound Horizons 1991 [ISBN: 1879323001] and Bly R. A Little Book on the Human Shadow.[ISBN: 0062548476]

[23] Rick Jarow. Creating the Work You Love: Courage, Commitment and Career; Inner Traditions Intl Ltd; (December 1995) [ISBN: 0892815426]

[24] Walter Kaufmann (Translator), Friedrich Wilhelm Nietzsche. Thus Spoke Zarathustra: A Book for None and All. Penguin USA; 1978, page 27

<u>Acute Care and Musculoskeletal Care: Opportunities for Health Optimization</u>

Clinicians should appreciate that every patient encounter is an opportunity for comprehensive care, disease prevention, and health optimization. This is true whether the presenting complaint is acne, psoriasis, a respiratory infection, or musculoskeletal pain. Given the relatively high frequency of musculoskeletal complaints in clinical practice in general and chiropractic and osteopathic practices in particular, the following section will emphasize the clinical presentation of musculoskeletal complaints as an underappreciated opportunity for wellness care.

Since **approximately 1 of every 7 (14% of total) visits to a primary healthcare provider is for the treatment of musculoskeletal pain or dysfunction**[25], every healthcare provider needs to have 1) knowledge of important concepts related to musculoskeletal medicine, 2) the ability to recognize urgent and emergency conditions, 3) the ability to competently perform orthopedic examination procedures and interpret laboratory assessments, and 4) the knowledge and ability to design and implement effective treatment plans and to coordinate patient management.

In pharmacosurgical allopathic medicine, the goal of musculoskeletal treatment is to address the patient's injury or disorder by alleviating pain with the use of drugs, preventing further injury, and returning the patient to his/her previous status and activities. The most commonly employed interventions are 1) rest and "watchful waiting", 2) non-steroidal anti-inflammatory drugs (NSAIDS) and cyclooxygenase-2-inhibitors (COX-2 inhibitors, or "coxibs"), and 3) surgery. The more action-oriented approaches used by many chiropractic, naturopathic, and osteopathic physicians differs from the allopathic approach because, although avoidance of and "rest" from damaging activities is reasonable and valuable, too much rest without an emphasis on active preventive rehabilitation ❶ encourages patient passivity and ❷ the assumption of the sick role, and it ❸ fails to actively promote tissue healing and ❹ fails to address the underlying proprioceptive deficits that are common in patients with chronic musculoskeletal pain and recurrent injuries.[26,27,28] **NSAIDs are considered "first line" therapy for musculoskeletal disorders by allopaths** despite the data showing that "**There is no evidence that widely used NSAIDs have any long-term benefit on osteoarthritis.**"[29] What is worse than this lack of efficacy is the evidence showing that NSAIDs *exacerbate* musculoskeletal disease (rather than *cure* it). **NSAIDs are known to inhibit cartilage formation and to promote bone necrosis and joint degradation with long-term use**[30,31,32,33] and **NSAIDs are responsible for more than 16,000 gastrohemorrhagic deaths and 100,000 hospitalizations each year.**[34] The "coxibs" were supposed to provide anti-inflammatory benefits with an enhanced safety profile, but the gastrocentric focus of the drug developers failed to appreciate

> **Allopathic medicine has been sold to the public under the banner of "scientific" from a time when this was not the case**
>
> "…only about 15% of medical interventions are supported by solid scientific evidence…"
>
> Smith R. Where is the wisdom…? The poverty of medical evidence. *BMJ*. 1991 Oct 5;303:798-9

that COX-2 is necessary for the formation of prostacyclin, a prostaglandin created from arachidonic acid via COX-2 that plays an important role in vasodilation and antithrombosis; not surprisingly therefore, use of COX-2-inhibiting drugs has consistently been associated with increased risk for adverse cardiovascular effects including

---

[25] American College of Rheumatology Ad Hoc Committee on Clinical Guidelines. Guidelines for the initial evaluation of the adult patient with acute musculoskeletal symptoms. *Arthritis Rheum*. 1996 Jan;39(1):1-8 See also: **Vasquez A**. Musculoskeletal disorders and iron overload disease: comment on the American College of Rheumatology guidelines. *Arthritis Rheum* 1996;39: 1767-8

[26] McPartland JM, Brodeur RR, Hallgren RC. Chronic neck pain, standing balance, and suboccipital muscle atrophy--a pilot study. *J Manipulative Physiol Ther*. 1997;20:24-9

[27] Bullock-Saxton JE, Janda V, Bullock MI. Reflex activation of gluteal muscles in walking. An approach to restoration of muscle function for patients with low-back pain. *Spine* 1993 May;18(6):704-8

[28] Sinaki M, Brey RH, Hughes CA, Larson DR, Kaufman KR. Significant reduction in risk of falls and back pain in osteoporotic-kyphotic women through a Spinal Proprioceptive Extension Exercise Dynamic (SPEED) program. *Mayo Clin Proc*. 2005 Jul;80(7):849-55

[29] Beers MH, Berkow R (eds). <u>The Merck Manual. 17th Edition</u>. Whitehouse Station; Merck Research Laboratories 1999 page 451

[30] "At…concentrations comparable to those… in the synovial fluid of patients treated with the drug, several NSAIDs suppress proteoglycan synthesis… These NSAID-related effects on chondrocyte metabolism … are much more profound in osteoarthritic cartilage than in normal cartilage, due to enhanced uptake of NSAIDs by the osteoarthritic cartilage." Brandt KD. Effects of nonsteroidal anti-inflammatory drugs on chondrocyte metabolism in vitro and in vivo. *Am J Med*. 1987 Nov 20; 83(5A): 29-34

[31] "The case of a young healthy man, who developed avascular necrosis of head of femur after prolonged administration of indomethacin, is reported here." Prathapkumar KR, Smith I, Attara GA. Indomethacin induced avascular necrosis of head of femur. *Postgrad Med J*. 2000 Sep; 76(899): 574-5

[32] "This highly significant association between NSAID use and acetabular destruction gives cause for concern, not least because of the difficulty in achieving satisfactory hip replacements in patients with severely damaged acetabula." Newman NM, Ling RS. Acetabular bone destruction related to non-steroidal anti-inflammatory drugs. *Lancet*. 1985 Jul 6; 2(8445): 11-4

[33] Vidal y Plana RR, Bizzarri D, Rovati AL. Articular cartilage pharmacology: I. In vitro studies on glucosamine and non steroidal antiinflammatory drugs. *Pharmacol Res Commun*. 1978 Jun;10(6):557-69

[34] Singh G. Recent considerations in nonsteroidal anti-inflammatory drug gastropathy. *Am J Med*. 1998;105(1B):31S-38S

myocardial infarction, unstable angina, cardiac thrombus, resuscitated cardiac arrest, sudden or unexplained death, ischemic stroke, and transient ischemic attacks.[35] Additionally, the use of a COX-2 inhibiting treatment in patients who overconsume arachidonic acid (i.e., most people in America and other industrialized nations[36]) would be expected to shunt bioavailable arachidonate into the formation of leukotrienes, a group of inflammatory mediators now known to contribute directly to atherogenesis.[37] Thus, the outcome was entirely predictable: overuse of COX-2 inhibitors should have been expected to create a catastrophe of iatrogenic cardiovascular death, and this is exactly what was allowed to occur—clearly indicating independent but synergistic failures on the part of pharmaceutical companies, the FDA, and the medical profession.[38,39,40,41] According to statements by David J. Graham, MD, MPH, (Associate Director for Science, Office of Drug Safety, FDA) in 2005, an estimated 139,000 Americans who took Vioxx suffered serious complications including stroke or myocardial infarction; between 26,000 and 55,000 Americans died as a result of their doctors' prescribing Vioxx.[42] Additionally, the surgical procedures employed by allopaths for the treatment of musculoskeletal pain do not consistently show evidence of efficacy, safety, or cost-effectiveness. Arthroscopic surgery for osteoarthritis of the knee, for example, costs thousands of dollars to each individual and billions of dollars to the American healthcare system but is no more effective than placebo.[43,44,45] In a review which also noted that only 15% of medical procedures are supported by literature references and that only 1% of such references are deemed scientifically valid, Rosner[46] showed that the risks of serious injury (i.e., cauda equina syndrome or vertebral artery dissection) associated with spinal manipulation are "*400 times lower* than the death rates observed from gastrointestinal bleeding due to the use of nonsteroidal anti-inflammatory drugs and *700 times lower* than the overall mortality rate for spinal surgery."

In chiropractic, osteopathic, and naturopathic medicine, the goal and means of musculoskeletal treatment is to address the patient's injury or disorder by simultaneously alleviating pain with the use of natural, noninvasive, low-cost, and low-risk interventions while improving the patient's overall health, preventing future health problems, and "upgrading" the patient's overall paradigm of health maintenance and disease prevention from one that is passive and reactive to one that is empowered and pro-active. Commonly employed therapeutics include spinal manipulation[47,48,49], exercise[50] and the use of nutritional supplements and botanical medicines[51,52] which have been demonstrated in peer-reviewed clinical trials to be safe and effective for the alleviation of musculoskeletal pain. More specifically, chiropractic and naturopathic physicians are particularly well-versed in the clinical utilization of such treatments as niacinamide[53], glucosamine and chondroitin sulfates[54], vitamin D[55],

[35] Mukherjee D, Nissen SE, Topol EJ. Risk of cardiovascular events associated with selective COX-2 inhibitors. *JAMA*. 2001 Aug 22-29;286(8):954-9

[36] Seaman DR. The diet-induced proinflammatory state: a cause of chronic pain and other degenerative diseases? *J Manipulative Physiol Ther*. 2002;25(3):168-79

[37] Dwyer JH, Allayee H, Dwyer KM, Fan J, Wu H, Mar R, Lusis AJ, Mehrabian M. Arachidonate 5-lipoxygenase promoter genotype, dietary arachidonic acid, and atherosclerosis. *N Engl J Med*. 2004 Jan 1;350(1):29-37

[38] Topol EJ. Arthritis medicines and cardiovascular events--"house of coxibs". *JAMA*. 2005 Jan 19;293(3):366-8. Epub 2004 Dec 28

[39] Ray WA, Griffin MR, Stein CM. Cardiovascular toxicity of valdecoxib. *N Engl J Med*. 2004 Dec 23;351(26):2767. Epub 2004 Dec 17

[40] Topol EJ. Failing the public health--rofecoxib, Merck, and the FDA. *N Engl J Med*. 2004 Oct 21;351(17):1707-9

[41] Horton R. Vioxx, the implosion of Merck, and aftershocks at the FDA. *Lancet*. 2004 Dec 4-10;364(9450):1995-6

[42] David J. Graham, MD, MPH, (Associate Director for Science, Office of Drug Safety, US FDA) estimated that 139,000 Americans who took Vioxx suffered serious side effects; he estimated that the drug killed between 26,000 and 55,000 people. http://www.commondreams.org/views05/0223-35.htm http://www.fda.gov/cder/drug/infopage/vioxx/vioxxgraham.pdf Accessed November 25, 2006

[43] Gina Kolata. A Knee Surgery for Arthritis Is Called Sham. *The New York Times*, July 11, 2002

[44] Moseley JB, O'Malley K, Petersen NJ, Menke TJ, Brody BA, Kuykendall DH, Hollingsworth JC, Ashton CM, Wray NP. A controlled trial of arthroscopic surgery for osteoarthritis of the knee. *N Engl J Med*. 2002;347:81-8

[45] Bernstein J, Quach T. A perspective on the study of Moseley et al: questioning the value of arthroscopic knee surgery for osteoarthritis. *Cleve Clin J Med*. 2003;70(5):401, 405-6, 408-10

[46] Rosner AL. Evidence-based clinical guidelines for the management of acute low-back pain: response to the guidelines prepared for the Australian Medical Health and Research Council. *J Manipulative Physiol Ther*. 2001;24(3):214-20

[47] Manga P, Angus D, Papadopoulos C, et al. The Effectiveness and Cost-Effectiveness of Chiropractic Management of Low-Back Pain. Richmond Hill, Ontario: Kenilworth Publishing; 1993

[48] Meade TW, Dyer S, Browne W, Townsend J, Frank AO. Low-back pain of mechanical origin: randomised comparison of chiropractic and hospital outpatient treatment. *BMJ*. 1990;300(6737):1431-7

[49] Meade TW, Dyer S, Browne W, Frank AO. Randomised comparison of chiropractic and hospital outpatient management for low-back pain: results from extended follow up. *BMJ*. 1995;311(7001):349-5

[50] Harold Elrick, MD. Exercise is Medicine. *The Physician and Sportsmedicine* - Volume 24 - No. 2 - February 1996

[51] **Vasquez A**. Revisiting the Five-Part Nutritional Wellness Protocol: The Supplemented Paleo-Mediterranean Diet. *Nutritional Perspectives* 2011 January http://optimalhealthresearch.com/part8

[52] **Vasquez A**. Reducing pain and inflammation naturally - Part 3: Improving overall health while safely and effectively treating musculoskeletal pain. *Nutritional Perspectives* 2005; 28: 34-38, 40-42 http://optimalhealthresearch.com/part3

[53] Kaufman W. Niacinamide therapy for joint mobility. Therapeutic reversal of a common clinical manifestation of the "normal" aging process. *Conn State Med J* 1953;17:584-591

[54] Reginster JY, Deroisy R, Rovati LC, Lee RL, Lejeune E, Bruyere O, Giacovelli G, Henrotin Y, Dacre JE, Gossett C. Long-term effects of glucosamine sulphate on osteoarthritis progression: a randomised, placebo-controlled clinical trial. *Lancet*. 2001;357(9252):251-6

[55] **Vasquez A**, Manso G, Cannell J. The clinical importance of vitamin D: a paradigm shift with implications for all healthcare providers. *Altern Ther Health Med* 2004;10:28-36 http://optimalhealthresearch.com/monograph04

vitamin B-12[56], balanced and complete fatty acid therapy[57,58], anti-inflammatory diets[59,60,61], proteolytic/pancreatic enzymes[62], and botanical medicines such as *Boswellia*[63], *Harpagophytum*[64], *Uncaria*, and willow bark[65,66]—each of these interventions has been validated in peer-reviewed research for safety and effectiveness.[67] Furthermore, from the perspective of integrative chiropractic and naturopathic medicine, aiming for such a limited accomplishment as mere "returning the patient to previous status and activities" would be considered substandard, since the patient's overall health was neither addressed nor improved and since returning the patient to his/her previous status and activities would be a direct invitation for the problem to recur indefinitely. Chiropractic and naturopathic physicians appreciate that, especially regarding chronic health problems, any treatment plan that allows the patient to resume his/her previous lifestyle is by definition doomed to fail because a return to the patient's previous lifestyle and activities that allowed the onset of the disease/disorder in the first place will most certainly result in the perpetuation and recurrence of the illness or disorder. **Stated more directly: for *healing* to truly be effective, the comprehensive treatment plan must generally result in a permanent and profound change in the patient's lifestyle and emotional climate, which are the primary modifiable determinants of either health or disease.**

---

[56] Mauro GL, Martorana U, Cataldo P, Brancato G, Letizia G. Vitamin B12 in low back pain: a randomised, double-blind, placebo-controlled study. *Eur Rev Med Pharmacol Sci.* 2000 May-Jun;4(3):53-8

[57] **Vasquez A**. Reducing Pain and Inflammation Naturally. Part 1: New Insights into Fatty Acid Biochemistry and the Influence of Diet. *Nutritional Perspectives* 2004; Oct: 5, 7-10,12,14 http://optimalhealthresearch.com/part1

[58] **Vasquez A**. Reducing Pain and Inflammation Naturally. Part 2: New Insights into Fatty Acid Supplementation and Its Effect on Eicosanoid Production and Genetic Expression. *Nutritional Perspectives* 2005; January: 5-16 http://optimalhealthresearch.com/part2

[59] Seaman DR. The diet-induced proinflammatory state: a cause of chronic pain and other degenerative diseases? *J Manipulative Physiol Ther.* 2002 Mar-Apr;25(3):168-7

[60] **Vasquez A**. *Integrative Orthopedics. Second Edition 2007*. http://optimalhealthresearch.com/orthopedics.html

[61] **Vasquez A**. Reducing Pain and Inflammation Naturally. Part 1: New Insights into Fatty Acid Biochemistry and the Influence of Diet. *Nutritional Perspectives* 2004; October: 5, 7-10, 12, 14

[62] Trickett P. Proteolytic enzymes in treatment of athletic injuries. *Appl Ther.* 1964;30:647-52

[63] Kimmatkar N, Thawani V, Hingorani L, Khiyani R. Efficacy and tolerability of Boswellia serrata extract in treatment of osteoarthritis of knee--a randomized double blind placebo controlled trial. *Phytomedicine.* 2003 Jan;10(1):3-7

[64] Chrubasik S, Junck H, Breitschwerdt H, Conradt C, Zappe H. Effectiveness of Harpagophytum extract WS 1531 in the treatment of exacerbation of low-back pain: a randomized, placebo-controlled, double-blind study. *Eur J Anaesthesiol* 1999 Feb;16(2):118-29

[65] Chrubasik S, Eisenberg E, Balan E, Weinberger T, Luzzati R, Conradt C. Treatment of low-back pain exacerbations with willow bark extract: a randomized double-blind study. *Am J Med.* 2000;109:9-14

[66] **Vasquez A**, Muanza DN. Comment: Evaluation of Presence of Aspirin-Related Warnings with Willow Bark. *Ann Pharmacotherapy* 2005 Oct;39(10):1763

[67] **Vasquez A**. Reducing pain and inflammation naturally. Part 3: Improving overall health while safely and effectively treating musculoskeletal pain. *Nutritional Perspectives* 2005;28:34-42 http://optimalhealthresearch.com/part3

Clinical Assessments

The clinical assessments reviewed in the following sections are history-taking, orthopedic/musculoskeletal, and neurologic examinations, and commonly used laboratory tests. **History taking is the art of conducting an *informative* and *collaborative* patient interview.**

The role of the doctor during the interview process is not merely that of a data-collecting machine, spewing out questions and receiving responses. Patient interviews can be a creative, enjoyable, comforting opportunity to build rapport and to establish meaningful connection with another human being. Patients are not simply people with health problems – they are first and foremost our fellow human beings, not so dissimilar from ourselves perhaps, and always full of complexity. Our task is not to fully understand their complexity nor to solve all of their mysteries, but rather to help orchestrate these dynamics into a coordinated if not unified direction that promotes health and healing.

Beyond its diagnostic value, the interview process also provides a key opportunity to gain insight into the patient's psychoepistimology—the patient's operating system for interacting with data and the world and internalizing and metabolizing external inputs in such a way as to merge these with internal experiences (ie, emotions, feelings, preferences, responses). Epistemology is the branch of philosophy concerned with the nature and scope of knowledge. Per Rand[68], psychoepistimology is a person's "method of awareness"; a person's psychoepistimology creates a "corollary view of existence" and in turn, "A man's method of using his consciousness determines his method of survival." By understanding how the patient views him/herself in the world, understanding his/her goals, and—in essence—what "drives" the patient and what "makes him/her tick", clinicians can shape the nuances of the conversation and the treatment plan to promote the desired congnitive-conceptual-behavioral changes in behavior that are prerequisite for the attainment of optimized health outcomes.

History & Assessment

History of the primary complaint: "D.O.P.P. Q.R.S.T."
- Description/location
- Onset
- Provocation: exacerbates
- Palliation: alleviates
- Quality
- Radiation of pain
- Severity
- Timing

Associated complaints
- Additional manifestations
- Concomitant diseases

Review of systems
- Head-to-toe inventory of health status, associated health problems, and complications

Past health history
- Surgeries
- Hospitalizations
- Traumas
- Vaccinations and medications
- Successful and failed treatments for the current complaint(s)

Family health history
- Genotropic illnesses and predispositions
- Lifestyle patterns
- Emotional expectations

Social history
- Hobbies, work, exposures
- Relationships and emotional experiences
- Interpersonal support
- Malpractice litigation

Health Habits
- Diet: appropriate intake of protein, fruits, vegetables, fats, sugars
- Sleep
- Stress management
- Exercise / Sedentary Lifestyle
- Spirituality / Centeredness
- Caffeine and tobacco
- Ethanol and recreational drugs

Medication and supplements
- Reason, doses, duration, cost
- Side-effects
- Interactions

Responsibility and Compliance
- Ability and willingness to comply with prescribed treatment plan and to incorporate the necessary diet-exercise-relationship-emotional-lifestyle modifications
- *Internal* versus *external* locus of control

---

[68] Rand A. For the New Intellectual. New York; Signet:1961, 16

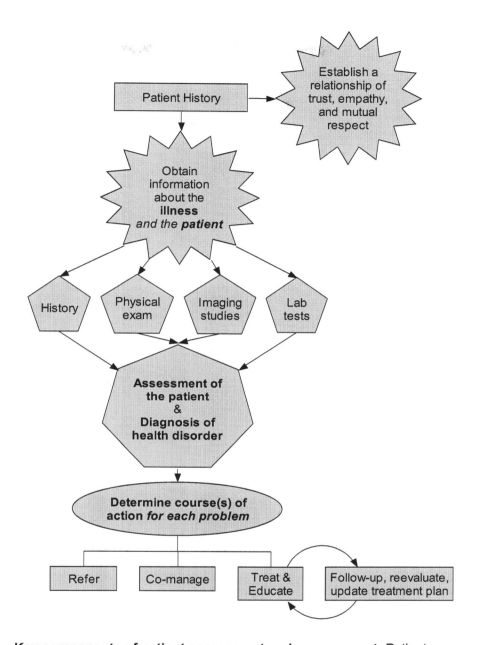

Key components of patient assessment and management: Patient assessment and management is an on-going process that begins with the initial history taken at the first clinical encounter and continues through the physical examination and laboratory assessments and thereafter by monitoring the patient's implementation of and response to the treatment plan. The plan is complete when the desired outcome of health optimization is achieved and sustained.

Components of a Complete Patient History: "D.O.P.P. Q.R.S.T."

Category	Patient history questions and implications
Description, Location: Always start with open-ended questions	• *What is it like for you?* • *What do you experience?* • *What are you feeling?* • *Where is the pain/sensation/problem)?* • Ask about specifics: **Pain, numbness, weakness, tingling,** fatigue, recent or chronic infections, burning, aching, dull, sharp, cramping, stretching, pins and needles, weakness, changes in function (i.e., bowel and bladder continence).
Onset	• *When did it begin? Have you ever had anything like this before?* • *Was there a specific event associated with the onset of the problem, such as an injury or an illness, or did the problem start gradually or insidiously?* • *How has it changed over time?* • *Prior injuries to site?* • *Why are you seeking care for this now (rather than last week or last month)?* • *What has changed? How is the pain/problem developing over time—getting worse or getting better?*
Palliation	• *How have you tried treating it? Does anything make it go away?* • *What makes it better? What relieves the pain?* • Ask about prior and current treatments, radiographs, medications, supplements (herbs, vitamins, minerals), injections, surgery, massage, manipulation, counseling. • Knowing response/resistance to previous treatments can provide clinical insight.
Provocation	• *Are your symptoms constant, or does the problem come and go?* • *What makes it worse? What makes the pain worse?* • *When during the day/week/month/year are your symptoms the worst?*
Quality	• *Can you describe the pain to me?* • *What does it feel like?* • *What do you experience?* • Get a clear understanding of the type of sensation(s): stabbing, shooting pain, pins and needles, sharp pain, electric sensation, numbness, burning, aching, throbbing, weakness, tingling, gel phenomenon (stiffness worsened by inactivity), dizziness, confusion, fatigue, shortness of breath.
Radiation	• *Does the pain stay localized or does it move to your arm/leg/head/face?* • *Do you feel pain in other areas of your body?*
Severity	• *How bad is it? How would you rate it on a scale of one to ten if one were almost no pain and ten was the worst pain you could imagine?* Use the validated VAS—visual analog scale—to quantify the level of pain and impairment. • *Does this problem prevent you from engaging in your daily activities, such as work, exercise, or hobbies?* This is a very important question for determining functional impairment and internal consistency; if the patient is "too injured to work" yet is still able to fully participate in recreational activities that are physically challenging, then malingering is likely.
Timing	• *When do you notice this problem?* • *Is it constant, or does it come and go? Where are you when you notice it the most?* • *Is it worse in the morning, or worse in the evening?* • *Does anyone else in your [home/office/worksite] have this same problem?* • *What times of the day or what days of the week is it the worst?*

Components of a Complete Patient History: "D.O.P.P. Q.R.S.T."—*continued*

Category	Patient history questions and implications
Associated manifestations and constitutional symptoms	• *Have you noticed any other problems associated with this problem?* • **Fatigue?** • **Fever?** • **Weight loss?** *Weight gain?* • *Night sweats?* • **Diarrhea? Constipation?** • **Weakness?** • *Nausea?* • *Bowel or bladder difficulties or changes? Difficulty with sexual function?* These could be related to hormonal imbalances, drug side-effects, relationship problems, nutritional deficiencies, nerve compression, and/or depression. • *Change in sensation near your anus/genitals?* Cauda equina syndrome is an important consideration in patients with low-back pain. • *Loss of appetite?* • *Difficulty sleeping?* • *Skin rash or change in pigmentation?*
ROS: review of systems	• <u>**General constitution**</u>: fatigue, malaise, fever, chills, weight gain/loss… • *"Now we are going to conduct a head-to-toe inventory just to make sure that we have covered everything."* • <u>**Head**</u>: headaches, head pain, pressure inside head, difficulty concentrating, difficulty remembering, mental function • <u>**Ears**</u>: ringing in ears, dizziness, hearing loss, hypersensitivity to noise, ear pain, discharge from ear, pressure in ears • <u>**Eyes**</u>: eye pain, loss of vision or decreased vision or ability to focus, redness or irritation, seeing flashing lights or spots, double vision • <u>**Nose**</u>: sinus problems, chronically stuffy nose, difficulty smelling things, nose bleeds, change or decrease in sense of smell or taste • <u>**Mouth**</u>, teeth, TMJ, pain or sores in mouth, difficulty chewing, sensitive teeth, bleeding gums, pain in jaw joint, change or decrease in sense of taste • <u>**Neck**</u>: pain at the base of skull, pain in neck, stiffness • <u>**Throat**</u>: difficulty swallowing, pain in throat, feeling like things get stuck in throat, change in voice, difficulty getting air or food in or out • <u>**Chest and breasts**</u>: any chest pain, difficult breathing, wheezing, coughing, pain, lumps, or discharge from nipple • <u>**Shoulders**</u>: pain or aching in your shoulders, restricted motion or stiffness • <u>**Arms, elbows, hands**</u>: pain or problems with your arms, elbows, hands, …in the joints or the muscles…, numbness, tingling, weakness, swelling, changes in fingernails, cold hands? • <u>**Stomach, abdomen, pelvis, genitals, urinary tract, rectum,**</u> : pain in stomach or abdomen, difficulty with digestion, gas, bloating, regurgitation, ulcer, any problems lower down in your abdomen—near your lower intestines? Pain, lumps, swelling, difficulty passing stool, pain or itching near your anus, genitalia; any genital pain, burning, discharge, redness, irritation, sexual dysfunction or impotence, loss of bowel or bladder control? Diarrhea or constipation? How often do you have a bowel movement? • <u>**Hips, legs, knees, ankles, feet**</u>: numbness, weakness, pain or tingling in the hips, knees, ankles, or feet; pain in calves with walking, swelling of ankles, cold feet • *Is there anything else that you think I should know in order to help you?*

Components of a Complete Patient History: "D.O.P.P. Q.R.S.T." —*continued*

Category	Patient history questions and implications

Medical history	• *Are you taking any* **medications**? *What medications have you taken in the past few years?* Finding out that your new patient recently discontinued his 20-year regimen of valproic acid, lithium, and risperidone may significantly change your interpretation of the clinical interview
	• *Have you been* **treated for any medical conditions** *or health problems?*
	• *Have you ever been* **hospitalized**?
	• *Have you ever had* **surgery**?
	• *Have you ever been* **diagnosed with any health problems** *such as high blood pressure or diabetes?*
	• Investigate for specific problems in the past health history that would be a major oversight to miss:
	    o Current or past diseases: Cancer, Diabetes, Mental illness
	    o Hypertension or high cholesterol
	    o Medications, especially corticosteroids
	    o Surgeries & Hospitalizations
	    o Infections, Immune disorders
	    o Trauma or previous injuries

Social history	• **Work**—*What do you do for work? Are you exposed to chemicals or fumes at your workplace?* • **Hobbies**—*What do you do for recreation or hobbies? Are you exposed to chemicals or fumes at home or with your hobbies (e.g., painting, gardening)?* • **Eat**—*Tell me about your breakfast, lunch, dinner, snacks… Do you consume foods or drinks that contain aspartame* (linked to increased incidence of brain tumors[69]) *or carrageenan* (possibly linked to increased risk of breast cancer and inflammatory bowel disease[70,71])? • **Exercise**—*What do you do for exercise or physical activity?* • **Drink**—*Do you* **drink alcohol**? *Coffee/caffeine? Water?* • **Drugs**—*Do you use recreational* **drugs**? **Now or in the past?** • **Smoke**—*Do you* **smoke**? • **Sex**—*Are you* **sexually active**? *If so, do you practice safer sex practices? For all women: Is there any chance you could be pregnant right now? A "yes" reply may contraindicate radiographic assessment and the use of certain nutrients, botanicals, and/or drugs.* • **Emotional support** • **Family contact and relationships**
Family health history	• *Does anyone in your family have any health problems, especially your parents and siblings?* • *Do you have any children? Do they have any health problems?* • *Do any diseases "run in the family" such as cancer, diabetes, arthritis, heart disease?*
Additional questions	• *Do you have any other information for me? Is there anything that I did not ask?* • *What is your opinion as to why you are having this health problem?* • *Are you in litigation for your illness or injuries?*

---

[69] "In the past two decades brain tumor rates have risen in several industrialized countries, including the United States... Compared to other environmental factors putatively linked to brain tumors, the artificial sweetener aspartame is a promising candidate to explain the recent increase in incidence and degree of malignancy of brain tumors." Olney JW, Farber NB, Spitznagel E, Robins LN. Increasing brain tumor rates: is there a link to aspartame? *J Neuropathol Exp Neurol* 1996 Nov;55(11):1115-23
[70] Tobacman JK. Review of harmful gastrointestinal effects of carrageenan in animal experiments. *Environ Health Perspect.* 2001 Oct;109(10):983-94
[71] "However, the gum carrageenan which is comprised of linked, sulfated galactose residues has potent biological activity and undergoes acid hydrolysis to poligeenan, an acknowledged carcinogen." Tobacman JK, Wallace RB, Zimmerman MB. Consumption of carrageenan and other water-soluble polymers used as food additives and incidence of mammary carcinoma. *Med Hypotheses.* 2001 May;56(5):589-98

Physical Examination

<u>**Goals and purpose of the orthopedic/musculoskeletal examination**</u>:
1. **To establish an accurate diagnosis (or diagnoses),**
2. **To assess the patient's functional status and current condition,**
3. **To assess for concomitant and/or underlying and preexisting problems,**
4. **To rule out emergency situations**
- *Example*: If your patient presents with low back and leg pain, and you determine that his fall off a horse resulted in ischial bursitis, have you also excluded a lumbar compression fracture? You can send the patient home with anti-inflammatory treatments and icepacks for the bursitis; but if you missed the spinal fracture, your patient could suffer neurologic injury resultant from your "failure to diagnose." **Don't assume that the patient has only one problem until you have proven with your history and examination that other likely problems do not exist.**

<u>**Functional assessment**</u>: When working with patients with acute injuries and systemic diseases, **take a wider view of the patient than simply diagnosing the problem.**
- *Will she be able to return to work?*
- *Will he be able to drive home safely?*
- *Will she need help with activities of daily living?*
- *Is there an occult disease, infection, malignancy, or toxic exposure that is causing these problems?*
- *Is this an acute presentation of a new problem, or an acute exacerbation of a chronic problem?*

<u>**Neurologic examination**</u>: One of the most important areas to assess when a patient presents with a musculoskeletal complaint is the neurologic system, especially if the complaint is related to a recent traumatic injury. Blood circulation is essential for life; but lack of circulation is only a major consideration in a small number of injuries, and it is usually readily apparent when severe because the problem will become acute quickly. Nerve injuries, however, can be subtle. All patients with spine (neck, thoracic, low back) pain must be questioned thoroughly for evidence of neurologic compromise. **Neurologic insults—such as cauda equina syndrome and transverse myelitis—can be painless**, can progress rapidly, and can lead to permanent functional disability from muscle weakness or paralysis. **Every patient with pain, weakness, or recent trauma must be evaluated for neurologic deficits before the patient is treated and released from care.** Neurologic examinations are briefly reviewed in the pages that follow; citations can be used for sources of additional information.

<u>**Resources for students on neurologic assessment**</u>:
- Goldberg S. <u>The Four-Minute Neurologic Exam</u>. Medmaster http://www.medmaster.net/
- http://www.neuroexam.com/neuroexam/ Information and free videos of a neurologic exam.
- http://rad.usuhs.mil/rad/eye_simulator/eyesimulator.html Excellent interactive simulation of assessment of extraocular muscles in a neurologic examination.
- http://emedicine.medscape.com/article/1147993-overview Excellent review, noteworthy for its description of a "+5" level of reflex grading denoting sustained clonus.

Orthopedic Musculoskeletal Examination: Concepts and Goals

Orthopedic tests are detailed or reviewed in each respective chapter of *Integrative Orthopedics*[72] (i.e., shoulder exams are in the chapter on shoulders, knee exams in the chapter on knees). This section reviews the concepts and goals that provide the rationale for performing these tests. **Orthopedic tests are designed to place particular types of stress on specific body tissues.** Types of stress include tension/distraction, compression/pressure, shear force, vibration, friction, and percussion. Each type of stress is applied to elicit specific information about the exact tissue or structure that is being tested. *If you understand the reason for the type of stress that you are applying, and you are aware of the tissue/structure that you are testing, then you will find it much easier to perform the dozens of tests that are required in clinical practice.* If you understand the "how" and the "why" then you won't be overwhelmed with named tests that otherwise appear illogical or superfluous.

The tests that are described in *Integrative Orthopedics* meet at least one of the following two criteria: 1) it is a common test that all doctors know and which is needed for the sake of communication and for passing academic and licensing examinations, or 2) it is going to be a useful test in clinical practice.

Always remember that abnormalities found during the physical examination—particularly the neurologic examination—are often indicative of an underlying *nonmusculoskeletal* problem that must be identified or—at the very least—considered and then excluded by additional testing. For example, a patient **shoulder pain** and neurologic deficits found during the neuromusculoskeletal portion of your examination could have a **herniated cervical disc** as the underlying cause; but the cause could also be **syringomyelia**, or an **apical lung tumor** that is invading local bone and destroying the nerves of the brachial plexus.[73]

Types of stress applied during the physical examination for specific purposes
• **Tension, traction**: To provoke pain from injured/compromised tissues: tendons, muscles, ligaments, and nerves
• **Compression, pressure**: To provoke pain from inflamed tissues; also used to assess for swelling and fluid accumulation in subcutaneous tissue, bursa, and joint spaces such as the knee
• **Shearing force**: To test the integrity of ligaments and intervertebral discs
• **Vibration (using ultrasound or 128 Hz tuning fork)**: To assess vibration sense (neurologic: peripheral nerves and dorsal columns) and screen for broken bones (orthopedic)
• **Friction, grinding**: To elicit pain from injured tissues (cross-fiber friction) and articular surfaces (grinding tests)
• **Percussion, over bone and discs**: To assess for bone fractures, bone infections, and acute disc injuries
• **Percussion, over peripheral nerves**: To assess hypesthesia/tingling suggesting reduced threshold for depolarization secondary to nerve irritation or compression, i.e., Tinel's sign
• **Fulcrum tests**: To assess for bone fractures: commonly the doctor's arm or a firm object is placed centrally under the bone in question and increasingly firm downward stress is applied to both ends of the bone to test for occult fracture
• **Torque, twisting**: To test joint integrity (restriction or laxity) or for occult bone fracture (particularly of the digits)

As a clinician, the successful management and treatment of your patients depends in large part on the following: ❶ **knowledge**: your ability to conceptualize broadly and to consider many *functional* and *pathologic* causes of your patient's complaints, ❷ **tact**: the efficiency and accuracy with which you assess, accept, and exclude the various differential diagnoses into your final working diagnosis from which your treatment, management, referral, and co-management decisions are made, ❸ **art**: your ability to create the changes in your patient's outlook, lifestyle, biochemistry, biomechanics/anatomy, and physiology to effect the desired outcome.

Neurologic Assessment

Clinical neurology is a complex area of study. However, for most doctors, knowledge of clinical neurology hinges on answering three questions:

- **Is this patient's presentation normal or abnormal?**
- **If it is abnormal, does it indicate a specific disease or lesion?**
- **Does this condition require referral to a specialist or emergency care?**

---

[72] **Vasquez A**. Integrative Orthopedics: Concepts, Algorithms, and Therapeutics. www.OptimalHealthResearch.com

[73] "Pancoast tumor has long been implicated as a cause of brachial plexopathy...The possibility of Pancoast lesion should be considered not only in the presence of brachial plexopathy, but also when C8 or T1 radiculopathy is found." Vargo MM, Flood KM. Pancoast tumor presenting as cervical radiculopathy. *Arch Phys Med Rehabil*. 1990 Jul;71(8):606-9

Every clinician needs thorough training in anatomy and clinical neurology to be competent in the management of patients, because even common problems such as "pain" and "fatigue" and "headache" may herald devastating neurologic illness that must be assessed accurately and managed skillfully. While a complete review of clinical neurology is beyond the scope of this text, the following section provides a basic review of the clinical essentials. Clinicians needing an refresher course in clinical neurology are encouraged to read the concise reviews by Goldberg.[74,75]

<u>Reliable indicators of organic neurologic disease</u>: These cannot be feigned and must be assumed to reveal organic neurologic illness that **must be evaluated by a neurologist**:
- **Significant asymmetry of pupillary light reflex,**
- **Ocular divergence,**
- **Papilledema,**
- **Marked nystagmus,**
- **Muscle atrophy and fasciculation,**
- **Muscle weakness with neurologic deficit**; upper motor neuron lesions (UMNL) indicate a central nervous system (CNS) lesion and need to be fully evaluated by a specialist; the need for referral is less necessary in cases of peripheral neuropathy of known cause.

<u>Purpose of Neurologic Examination and *Principle of Neurologic Localization*</u>:
The purpose of the neurologic examination is to qualify ("yes" or "no") the presence of a neurologic deficit, and—if present—to localize the lesion so that it can be further assessed with the proper laboratory, imaging, electrodiagnostic, or biopsy techniques. The following 9-point summary of localized lesions does not supplant independent studies of neurology and neuroanatomy but is useful for a quick clinically-relevant review:
1. **<u>Cerebral cortex and internal capsule</u>**: Neurologic deficit depends on location of lesion but is typically a combination of sensory/motor deficit and impaired higher neurologic function such as comprehension (superior temporal gyrus) or socially appropriate behavior (frontal lobe, ventral frontal gyri).
2. **<u>Basal ganglia and striatal system</u>**: Athetosis (lentiform nucleus: putamen and globus pallidus), (hemi)ballism (subthalamic nucleus), chorea (putamen), akinesia, bradykinesia, hypokinesia (lack of nigrostriatal dopamine).
3. **<u>Cerebellum</u>**: Ataxia, awkward clumsy execution of *intentional* motions; may have nystagmus, hypotonia.
4. **<u>Brainstem</u>**: Cranial nerve deficit(s) with contralateral distal sensory and/or UMN motor deficits.
5. **<u>Spinal cord</u>**: Cranial nerves and higher cortical functions are intact; lesion can be a combination of sensory and motor (UMN and LMN) deficits and the pattern distal to lesion may be a complete or incomplete pattern of sensory and motor deficits on one or both sides of body depending on area of spinal cord affected.
6. **<u>Nerve root</u>**: Segmental unilateral motor deficit; dermatomal distribution pain or sensory disturbance.
7. **<u>Peripheral nerve</u>**: Localized combination of sensory and motor deficits; may be bilateral or unilateral.
8. **<u>Neuromuscular junction</u>**: Painless weakness and "fatigable weakness": weakness that *worsens* with repeated testing; typically involves cranial nerves first in myasthenia gravis; also consider Lambert-Eaton Syndrome (LES: autoimmune neuromuscular junction disorder associated with occult malignancy; contrasts with myasthenia gravis in that in LES strength *increases* with repeated testing).
9. **<u>Muscle disease</u>**: Painless weakness, typically involving proximal hip/shoulder muscles first; test for elevated serum aldolase and (phospho)creatine kinase.

[74] Goldberg S. <u>Clinical Neuroanatomy Made Ridiculously Simple</u>. Miami, Medimaster, Inc, 1990. Now in a third edition with interactive CD.
[75] Goldberg S. <u>The Four-Minute Neurologic Exam</u>. Miami, Medimaster, Inc, 1992

Clinical assessments of neurologic function and structures

Cortex	Cerebellum
<ul><li>Orientation: Person, place, time, situation.</li><li>Mood and cooperation</li><li>Level of consciousness: Alert, lethargic, stupor, coma (indirect assessment of reticular system in brainstem)</li><li>Memory: Remember objects or numbers; *recent* memory is most commonly affected by brain lesions: *What day of the month is it? How did you get here?*</li><li>Mentation: *Count backward from 100 by 7's.*</li><li>Spelling: *Spell the word "hand" backwards.*</li><li>Stereognosis: Identify by touch a familiar object such as a key or coin.</li><li>Hoffman's reflex: Doctor rapidly extends distal joint of patient's middle finger and watches for patient's hand to perform grasp reflex; this test is performed for motor tract lesions involving the cerebral cortex, cerebellum, and upper motor neurons of the spinal cord.</li><li>Pronator drift: Supinated hands and arms outstretched forward for 30 seconds; doctor taps on palms; falling of hands and arms into pronation suggests UMNL.</li><li>Babinski reflex: Scraping the bottom of the foot results in splaying and flexing of the toes and extension (dorsiflexion) of the big toe; normal in infants.</li></ul>	<ul><li>Gait (lesion: ataxia)</li><li>Heel-to-toe walk</li><li>Tandem gait</li><li>Hand flip, foot tap (lesion: dysdiadochokinesia)</li><li>Finger-to-nose: Patient reaches out to doctor's finger, then patient touches patient nose, then back to new location of doctor's finger.</li><li>Heel-to-shin: Slide heel along shin.</li><li>Walk in circle around chair</li><li>Move eyes in a rapid "figure 8": Technique for provoking latent nystagmus</li><li>Rhomberg's test: Patient stands with feet close together and eyes closed; tests proprioception (peripheral nerves, dorsal columns, spinocerebellar tracts); vision (eyes open tests optic righting reflex) and coordinated motor activity (cerebellum).</li></ul>

Several of the above '"cerebral" deficits may also result from intoxicative, nutritional, or metabolic disorders rather than an organic irreversible physical lesion. Likewise "cerebellar" deficits may also result from lesion of the brainstem tracts/nuclei and cerebellar peduncles, rather than the cerebellum itself.

Brainstem and Cranial Nerves	Spinal Cord, Roots, Nerves
1. Olfactory: **smell** <ul><li>Smell: Test with strong and common odors such as coffee; do not use ammonia or other irritants which are perceived via trigeminal nerve (cranial nerve 5)</li><li>This is a worthwhile test in patients with recent head trauma (direct or indirect) such as from motor vehicle accidents (MVA); any violent motion of the head may result in injury to the olfactory fibers passing through the cribiform plate; patients may have associated anosmia or altered sense of flavor; frontal lobe disorders such as altered social behavior may be noted in lesioned patients</li></ul> 2. Ophthalmic: **reading, peripheral vision, fundoscopic** <ul><li>Snellen chart for far vision, Rosenbaum card for near vision</li><li>Peripheral vision</li><li>Fundoscopic examination</li></ul> 3. Oculomotor: **move eyes and constrict pupils** <ul><li>Eye motion in cardinal fields of gaze</li><li>Pupil contraction to light</li><li>Pupil contraction to accommodation</li></ul> 4. Trochlear: **motor to superior oblique** <ul><li>Look "down and in" toward nose</li></ul> 5. Trigeminal: **bite, sensory to face and eyes** <ul><li>Bite (motor to muscles of mastication)</li><li>Feel (sensory to face, eyes, and tongue)</li></ul> 6. Abducens: **motor to lateral rectus** <ul><li>Looks laterally to the ear</li></ul> 7. Facial: **face muscles and taste to anterior tongue** <ul><li>Furrow forehead, close eyes forcefully, smile and frown</li><li>Taste to anterior tongue</li></ul> 8. Vestibulocochlear: **hearing and balance** <ul><li>Hearing, Rinne-Weber tests[76]</li><li>Balance: observe gait and Romberg test</li></ul> 9. Glossopharyngeal: **swallowing, and gag reflex** <ul><li>Swallow</li><li>Gag reflex (sensory component)</li></ul> 10. Vagus: **motor to palate** <ul><li>Say "ahh" to raise uvula</li><li>Gag reflex (motor component)</li></ul> 11. Spinal accessory: **motor to SCM and trapezius** <ul><li>Raise your shoulders (against resistance)</li><li>Turn your head (against resistance)</li></ul> 12. Hypoglossal: **motor to tongue** <ul><li>Stick out tongue to front</li></ul>	Motor and reflex <ul><li>Strength: Specific muscles are tested and rated 0-5</li><li>Plantar (Babinski) reflex: Signifies UMNL</li><li>Abdominal reflexes: "Present" or "absent" (not rated 0-4); superficial reflexes are lost (rather than hyperactive) with UMNL<ul><li>Upper abdominal: T8-10</li><li>Lower abdominal: T10-12</li></ul></li><li>Anal reflex: Cauda equina and sacral nerve roots</li><li>Reflexes: Rate 0-4; asymmetric reflexes are more significant than finding absent or hyperactive (+3) reflexes; +4 reflex with sustained clonus is almost always pathologic and requires neurologist referral. Deep tendon reflexes with main spinal root levels are as follows:<ul><li>Biceps: C5</li><li>Brachioradialis: C6</li><li>Triceps: C7</li><li>Patellar: L3-L4</li><li>Hamstring: L5</li><li>Achilles: S1</li></ul></li></ul> Sensory <ul><li>Light touch</li><li>Two-point discrimination</li><li>Vibration (use 128 Hz tuning fork)</li><li>Joint position sense and proprioception (eyes closed, locate position of joint)</li><li>Sharp and dull</li><li>Hot and cold</li><li>Sensory loss mapping (if deficits are found)</li><li>Romberg (peripheral nerves, dorsal columns, vestibular, cerebellar)</li><li>Nerve root tension tests such as straight leg raising</li><li>**Subjective pain and discomfort can be indicated on pain diagrams and VAS (visual analog scale) as shown on the following page**</li></ul>

---

[76] "The Rinne and Weber tuning fork tests are the most important tools in distinguishing between conductive and sensorineural hearing loss." Ruckenstein MJ. Hearing loss. A plan for individualized management. *Postgrad Med.* 1995 Oct;98(4):197-200, 203, 206

Deep tendon reflexes are summarized below and on the following page. Hyperreflexia is noted with upper motor neuron lesions (UMNL) in the cortex, subcortical nuclei, brainstem, or corticospinal tracts of the spinal cord, whereas hyporeflexia can result from lesions of lower motor neurons (LMNL) in spinal cord, peripheral nerves, as well as from sensory/afferent defects including diabetic neuropathy, vitamin B-12 deficiency, and Guillain-Barre disorder. Muscle strength should always be "five over five" to be considered normal, whereas in the testing of reflexes, symmetry/asymmetry is generally more important than the grade of response (except with sustained clonus). **Asymmetry of reflex or strength (especially when seen together) is never normal and requires clinical correlation and investigation.** Reflexes and strength are evaluated as follows in the following table.

Deep tendon reflexes	Muscle strength
+5 <u>Hyperreflexia with sustained clonus</u>: Sustained clonus strongly suggests UMNL and requires investigation; most textbooks use a 0-4 scale, yet this 0-5 scale facilitates clear communication of observed lesions.[77]	5/5 <u>Normal</u>: **Full strength: able to withstand gravity and full resistance.**
+4 <u>Marked hyperreflexia</u>: Up to 4 beats of unsustained clonus may be normal[78]; suggests UMNL but may be caused by medications, electrolyte disturbances, etc.	4/5 <u>Partial strength</u>: Able to withstand gravity and partial resistance.
+3 <u>Hyperreflexia</u>: More than normal.	3/5 <u>Partial strength</u>: Only able to resist gravity.
+2 <u>Normal</u>: **Neither hyporeflexia nor hyperreflexia.**	2/5 <u>Partial strength</u>: Able to contract muscle but unable to resist gravity.
+1 <u>Hyporeflexia</u>: Less than normal	1/5 <u>Slight flicker of muscle contraction</u>: Does not result in joint movement.
0 <u>No reflex</u>: Requires clinical correlation for lesion of sensory receptors, peripheral nerve, spinal cord, anterior horn, or neuromuscular junction; this is a common finding in normal individuals.	0/5 <u>No clinically detectable contraction</u>: Correlate with lesion of peripheral nerve, cord, cerebrum, anterior horn, or neuromuscular junction.

---

[77] Oommen K, edited by Berman SA, et al. Neurological History and Physical Examination. Last Updated: October 4, 2006. *eMedicine* http://www.emedicine.com/neuro/topic632.htm

[78] "…three to four beats of clonus can be elicited at the ankles in some normal individuals." Waxman SG. <u>Clinical Neuroanatomy 25th Edition</u>. McGraw Hill Medical, New York, 2003, p 325

Patients can be asked to <u>localize</u> and <u>describe</u> their pain/discomfort on drawings such as these.
Examples of descriptions:

- Numb
- Hypersensitive
- Tingling

- Shooting pain
- Electrical pain
- Stabbing pain

- Burning pain
- Dull ache
- Muscle weakness

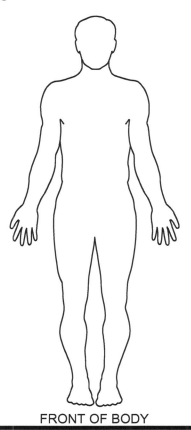

FRONT OF BODY

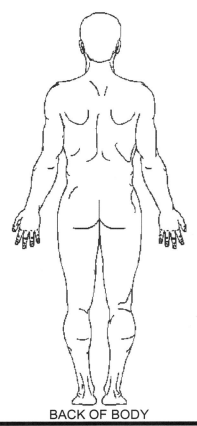

BACK OF BODY

On the lines below, indicate which pain/discomfort you are referring to and then quantify it by placing an "X" on the line.

Location of pain:_____

No pain at all   Worst pain imaginable

Location of pain:_____

No pain at all   Worst pain imaginable

Laboratory Assessments: General Considerations of Commonly Used Tests

"The laboratory evaluation of patients with rheumatic disease is often informative but rarely definitive."[79]

Laboratory tests are immensely important in evaluating patients with musculoskeletal pain, as these tests allow the clinician to 1) assess for infection (e.g., subacute osteomyelitis), 2) quantify the degree of inflammation (i.e., with CRP or ESR), 3) assess or exclude other disease processes that may be the cause of pain or dysfunction, and 4) assess for concomitant diseases (e.g., septic arthritis complicating rheumatoid arthritis). Additionally, 5) these tests open the door to more complete patient care and holistic management of the whole person because they allow for a more comprehensive and complete understanding of the patient's underlying physiology. **The recommended routine is to use the following panel of tests when assessing patients with musculoskeletal pain: 1) CBC, 2) CRP, 3) chemistry/metabolic panel, and preferably also 4) ferritin, 5) 25(OH)-vitamin D, and 6) thyroid assessment, minimally including TSH** and optimally including free T4, total T3, reverse T3 and anti-thyroid antibodies. The use of a screening evaluation on a routine basis helps identify patients with occult diseases and also allows for more comprehensive management of the patient's overall health. Other tests are indicated in specific situations. *Orthopedics* relies heavily upon physical examination and imaging, whereas *Rheumatology* relies more heavily upon laboratory analysis. In Orthopedics, laboratory tests are used mainly for the purposes of discovering or excluding rheumatic and systemic diseases. In Rheumatology, lab tests are used to specifically identify the type of illness, quantify the severity of the condition, and to assess for concomitant illnesses and complications.

Essential Tests: These Tests are <u>Required</u> for <u>Basic</u> Patient Assessment

Test	Purpose	Clinical application
CRP (or ESR)	Screening for **infection, inflammation**, and possibly **cancer**; if inflammation is present, then these tests allow for a generalized quantification of severity.	**Useful in all new patients** for helping to differentiate systemic/inflammatory disorders from those which are noninflammatory and mechanical. Also very helpful as a general "barometer" of health since higher values correlate with increased risk for diabetes mellitus and cardiovascular disease; thus this test helps bridge the gap between acute care and wellness promotion.
CBC	Screening for **anemia, infection,** certain cancers (namely **leukemia**).	Useful in any patient with **nontraumatic musculoskeletal pain** or **systemic manifestations**, especially **fever or weight loss;** occasionally detects occult B-12 and folate deficiencies.
Chemistry panel	Screening for **diabetes, liver disease, kidney failure,** bone lesions (alkaline phosphatase), **electrolyte disturbances,** adrenal insufficiency (hyponatremia with hyperkalemia), **hyperparathyroidism, hypercalcemia.**	Use this panel in any patient with **nontraumatic musculoskeletal pain** or **systemic manifestations;** all patients with **hypertension, diabetes,** or who use **medications** that cause **hepatotoxicity, nephrotoxicity,** etc.
Thyroid assessments	Hypothyroidism is a common problem and is an often overlooked cause of musculoskeletal pain.[80]	This is a reasonable test panel for any patient with fatigue, cold extremities, depression, "arthritis", muscle pain, hypercholesterolemia, or other manifestations of hypothyroidism.

---

[79] Klippel JH (ed). <u>Primer on the Rheumatic Diseases. 11th Edition</u>. Atlanta: Arthritis Foundation. 1997 page 94
[80] "Hypothyroidism is frequently accompanied by musculoskeletal manifestations ranging from myalgias and arthralgias to true myopathy and arthritis." McLean RM, Podell DN. Bone and joint manifestations of hypothyroidism. *Semin Arthritis Rheum.* 1995 Feb;24(4):282-90

<u>Overview of Important Tests</u>: **Common Components of Routine Evaluation**

Test	*Purpose*	*Clinical Application*
Ferritin *For more details on the treatment of iron overload and iron deficiency, see the guidelines on the website.*[81]	Important for assessing for **iron overload** (e.g., hemochromatoic polyarthropathy), and **iron deficiency** (e.g., low back pain due to colon cancer metastasis). Ferritin values less than 20 in adults (e.g., iron deficiency) or greater than 200 in women and 300 in men (e.g., iron overload) necessitate evaluation and effective treatment.	*Ferritin is the ideal test for both iron overload and iron deficiency.* All patients should be screened for hemochromatosis and other hereditary forms of iron overload regardless of age, gender, or ethnicity.[82] Iron deficiency—particularly in adults—may be the first clue to gastric/colon cancer and generally necessitates referral to gastroenterologist.
Serum 25-hydroxy-vitamin D, 25(OH)D	**Vitamin D deficiency is a common cause of musculoskeletal pain and inflammation**[83,84], and vitamin D deficiency is a significant risk factor for cancer and other serious health problems.[85,86,87]	Measurement of serum 25(OH) vitamin D (or empiric treatment with 2,000 – 4,000 IU vitamin D3 per day for adults) is indicated in patients with chronic musculoskeletal pain.[88,89] Optimal vitamin D status correlates with serum 25(OH)D levels of 50 – 100 ng/mL.[90]
Antinuclear antibodies (ANA)	Sensitive (but not specific) for the detection of several autoimmune diseases, especially systemic lupus erythematosus (SLE).	This test is particularly valuable for assessing patients with polyarthropathy, facial rash, and/or fatigue.
Rheumatoid factor (RF)	The primary value of this test is in supporting a diagnosis of rheumatoid arthritis; specificity is low.	RF may be positive in normal health, iron overload, chronic infections, hepatitis, sarcoidosis, and bacterial endocarditis.
Cyclic citrullinated protein (CCP) antibodies	Cyclic citrullinated protein (CCP) antibodies are currently the single best laboratory test for rheumatoid arthritis (RA) and have largely replaced RF.	Citrullinated protein antibodies are rapidly becoming *the test* for diagnosing and confirming RA; used with RF for highly specific "conjugate seropositivity."
Lactulose-mannitol assay	Assesses for malabsorption and excess intestinal permeability—"leaky gut."	Diagnostic test for intestinal damage; excellent nonspecific screening test for pathology or pathophysiology such as celiac and Crohns.
Comprehensive parasitology, stool analysis	Identification and quantification of intestinal yeast, bacteria, and other microbes.	Extremely valuable test when working with patients with chronic fatigue syndromes, fibromyalgia, or autoimmunity; see chapter 4 of *Integrative Rheumatology*.

---

[81] Excerpt from **Vasquez A**. <u>Integrative Rheumatology</u> on iron overload http://optimalhealthresearch.com/hemochromatosis.html

[82] **Vasquez A**. Musculoskeletal disorders and iron overload disease: comment on the American College of Rheumatology guidelines for the initial evaluation of the adult patient with acute musculoskeletal symptoms. *Arthritis Rheum* 1996;39: 1767-8

[83] Masood H, Narang AP, Bhat IA, Shah GN. Persistent limb pain and raised serum alkaline phosphatase the earliest markers of subclinical hypovitaminosis D in Kashmir. *Indian J Physiol Pharmacol.* 1989 Oct-Dec;33(4):259-61

[84] Al Faraj S, Al Mutairi K. Vitamin D deficiency and chronic low back pain in Saudi Arabia. *Spine.* 2003 Jan 15;28(2):177-9

[85] Grant WB. An estimate of premature cancer mortality in the U.S. due to inadequate doses of solar ultraviolet-B radiation. *Cancer.* 2002;94(6):1867-75

[86] Zittermannn A. Vitamin D in preventive medicine: are we ignoring the evidence? *Br J Nutr.* 2003 May;89(5):552-72

[87] Holick MF. Vitamin D: importance in the prevention of cancers, type 1 diabetes, heart disease, and osteoporosis. *Am J Clin Nutr.* 2004;79(3):362-71

[88] Plotnikoff GA, Quigley JM. Prevalence of severe hypovitaminosis D in patients with persistent, nonspecific musculoskeletal pain. *Mayo Clin Proc.* 2003 Dec;78(12):1463-70

[89] Al Faraj S, Al Mutairi K. Vitamin D deficiency and chronic low back pain in Saudi Arabia. *Spine.* 2003 Jan 15;28(2):177-9

[90] **Vasquez A**, Manso G, Cannell J. The Clinical Importance of Vitamin D (Cholecalciferol): A Paradigm Shift with Implications for All Healthcare Providers. *Alternative Therapies in Health and Medicine* 2004;10:28-37 and *Integrative Medicine* 2004;3:44-54 optimalhealthresearch.com/monograph04

Chemistry/metabolic panel	
Overview and interpretation:	▪ Accurate interpretation requires knowledge and pattern-recognition by the doctor to translate numbers into differential diagnoses that are correlated with the clinical presentation, examination, and imaging findings to arrive at probable diagnoses. ▪ Variation exists in the components and ranges offered by different laboratories.
Advantages:	▪ Inexpensive and easy to perform—venipuncture + serum separator tube. ▪ Provides a quick screen for diabetes, hepatitis, renal insufficiency, suggestions of alcohol abuse, hyperparathyroidism, electrolyte imbalances, etc.
Limitation and considerations:	▪ Individual tests and the most common clinical considerations for low and high values are listed in the following section. These values and considerations are provided with the routine adult outpatient in mind and are not inclusive of every possible differential diagnosis and therapeutic consideration. Consult your laboratory texts and reference manuals as needed per patient. ▪ Abnormal laboratory results are always due to one of four problems: 1. Technical error: Error with the laboratory analysis, improper patient identification correlating with the sample, alteration of the sample before delivery to the laboratory (e.g., too much time, too much heat, lysis of cells). Given the importance of laboratory accuracy and the life-and-death decisions that are based upon such reports, this type of error is inexcusable, however, it does occur, occasionally producing results that defy physiologic possibility or which contradict the clinical picture. Repeating the test is appropriate. *Example:* Hypercalcemia (elevated serum calcium) may be reported in error by the laboratory due to problems with the analyzing machinery. 2. Drug effect: An otherwise healthy patient may develop a laboratory abnormality due to a drug effect. *Example:* Hypercalcemia can be secondary to the effect of a calcium-sparing diuretic, such as hydrochlorothiazide (HCTZ). 3. Pathology: The patient has a diagnosable disease causing the laboratory abnormality. *Example:* Hypercalcemia can be secondary to a parathyroid adenoma which secretes abnormally high amounts of parathyroid hormone; hypercalcemia can also be a presentation of malignancy such as breast cancer or prostate cancer, or from a granulomatous disease such as sarcoidosis. 4. Physiologic abnormality: The patient has a physiologic abnormality causing the laboratory abnormality. *Example:* Hypercalcemia can be secondary to excess intake of vitamin D. In practice, hypercalcemia from hypervitaminosis D is very rare because vitamin D has a wide safety margin; but for the sake of this discussion, vitamin D toxicity will be listed as a possible cause of hypercalcemia.
Comments:	▪ All abnormalities require follow-up—repeat test within 2-4 weeks as part of routine follow-up along with additional investigation and clinical re-assessment. Extraordinary abnormalities and those with life-threatening implications should of course be retested immediately; often, the laboratory will hold the blood sample for 7 days and the repeat analysis can be performed on the same blood sample to exclude technical error. ▪ Many ill patients (such as those with chronic fatigue syndrome, fibromyalgia, etc) will have normal results with the metabolic panel and other basic routine laboratory assessments. Therefore, normal results do not ensure that the patient is healthy nor without life-threatening illness. ▪ Generally, laboratory tests are performed in the morning under fasting conditions; such is the standard but is not necessarily required depending on the nature of the test, convenience, and the clinical situation.

Practical overview of common abnormalities on the chemistry/metabolic panel —*continued*

Low values—considerations	Analyte[91]	High values—considerations
Technical error due to faulty processing of sample (i.e., hemolysis); insulinoma, exogenous insulin administration (test serum C-peptide), overdose of anti-hyperglycemic drugs, hypopituitarism and adrenal insufficiency.	**Glucose:** 65-99 mg/dL *Clinical pearl*: *Fasting glucose levels can miss mild type-2 diabetes mellitus; a better test for long-term glucose status is hemoglobin A1c.*	Postprandial sample, diabetes mellitus type-1 or type-2, Cushing disease or syndrome, acromegally, pheochromocytoma, glucagonoma, hyperthyroidism. If glucose is >300 mg/dL and patient is unstable (e.g., tachypnic or stuporous), evaluate for diabetic ketoacidosis or hyperosmolar state. Optimal fasting serum glucose is in the range of 70-75 up to 85 mg/dL, since levels >85 mg/dL have been associated with increased mortality.
Hyponatremia is potentially fatal and is also a cause of permanent neurologic injury (e.g., pontine myelinolysis). Clinicians should be particularly concerned when the sodium level drops below 125 mmol/L. Symptomatic hyponatremia is worthy of treatment in hospital setting; mild cases due to a recent event such as excess diaphoresis (e.g., prolonged sweating and exercise) or excess fluid intake (e.g., beer potomania [i.e., binge drinking], overhydration with unmineralized water) might be managed with sodium replacement and water restriction. Older patients, patients with pulmonary disease, and patients taking certain drugs such as serotonin-reuptake inhibitors may develop a chronic and relatively benign mild hyponatremia associated with "reset osmostat syndrome." Sodium levels can be altered downward by conditions that introduce osmotically active substances into the serum, such as immunoglobulins (e.g., multiple myeloma), hyperglycemia, and hypertriglyceridemia; corrective equations are available for such situations. For additional information see on-line reviews by Goh[92] and Decaux and Musch.[93]	**Sodium:** 136 to 144 mEq/L (mmol/L)	Hypernatremia in outpatients is rare; assess for drug effect and dehydration with hemoconcentration. Some clinicians will determine the free water deficit, while others will treat with oral or IV hydration with plain water or half-normal saline, respectively. Electrolyte abnormalities—particularly involving sodium—should generally be corrected slowly and with close supervision.

---

[91] The reference range for this table and some provisional information was derived from Medline Plus provided by the U.S. Department of Health and Human Services and National Institutes of Health. http://www.nlm.nih.gov/medlineplus/ency/article/003468.htm Accessed June 28, 2011. However, the majority of the information in this table comes from the author's (Dr Vasquez's) clinical training and experience. Editorial and peer reviews were provided by colleagues Barry Morgan MD (emergency medicine), Holly Furlong DC, Kris Young DC, Erika Mennerick DC, and Bill Beakey DOM of Professional Co-op Services, Inc. professionalco-op.com.
[92] Goh KP. Management of hyponatremia. *Am Fam Physician*. 2004;69:2387-94 http://www.aafp.org/afp/2004/0515/p2387.html Accessed June 2011.
[93] Decaux G, Musch W. Clinical laboratory evaluation of the syndrome of inappropriate secretion of antidiuretic hormone. *Clin J Am Soc Nephrol*. 2008 Jul;3(4):1175-84 http://cjasn.asnjournals.org/content/3/4/1175.full.pdf Accessed June 29, 2011.

Practical overview of common abnormalities on the chemistry/metabolic panel — *continued*

Low values — considerations	Analyte	High values — considerations
Hypokalemia can cause fatal cardiac arrhythmias and needs to be taken seriously. Replacement is generally via oral administration of potassium-rich foods, juices, or supplements such as potassium citrate (best option) or potassium chloride (KCl, inexpensive and therefore commonly used in medical settings even though KCl is clearly not optimal therapy due to the acidifying effect of the chloride anion). Recalcitrant hypokalemia is often a sign of magnesium depletion.[94] Causes of hypokalemia include diarrhea, vomiting, diuretics, Cushing disease/syndrome, dietary insufficiency, overhydration with mineral-free fluids, hyperaldosteronism and renal artery stenosis. Acute metabolic acidosis should cause relative or absolute elevations in serum K; the finding of normal or low serum K in a patient with acidosis (e.g., diabetic ketoacidosis) indicates (severe) potassium depletion.	**Potassium**: 3.6 to 5.2 mEq/L (mmol/L)	**Hyperkalemia is defined as a potassium level greater than 5.5 mmol/L. Severe hyperkalemia (>7 mmol/L) can be fatal and needs to be taken seriously.** In severe hyperkalemia, treatment and emergency management should be implemented before a complete evaluation and differential diagnosis are performed.[95] ❶ Ensure that blood sample was not hemolyzed. Repeat test if patient is stable and time allows. ❷ If hyperkalemia is severe or patient is symptomatic or has electrocardiographic changes, treat hyperkalemia with intravenous calcium, beta-adrenergic agonists (e.g., albuterol), bicarbonate, insulin and glucose; magnesium sulfate may also help alleviate arrhythmias; oral sodium polystyrene sulfonate (SPS, also known as Kayexalate) is a frequently used potassium-binding agent. ❸ DDX includes adrenal insufficiency, potassium-sparing diuretics, ACE-inhibitors and ARBs, NSAIDs, rhabdomyolysis, renal failure, massive cell necrosis such as with tumor lysis syndrome.
Evaluate hypocalcemia clinically with Chvostek's sign (~30% sensitive) and Trousseau sign (~90% sensitive) which may also be present in hypomagnesemia; evaluate clinically for arrhythmia, muscle spasm/hypertonicity, and hyperreflexia. Measure serum albumin and perform equation for "corrected calcium" if albumin is low. DDX includes renal failure, hypoparathyroidism, malabsorption, and drug effect (e.g., rarely a loop diuretic such as furosemide). Chronic mild hypocalcemia is treated with oral vitamin D and calcium supplementation; subacute symptomatic hypocalcemia can be treated with intravenous calcium gluconate especially if cardiac arrhythmias are present.	**Calcium**: 8.6 to 10.2 mg/dL	Outpatient hypercalcemia is potentially serious and needs to be evaluated in a stepwise manner: ❶ repeat the test to rule out lab error unless you are confident in the performance of the laboratory and stability of the submitted sample, ❷ review drug list for adverse effect, such as from hydrochlorothiazide (HCTZ) or rarely from excess cholecalciferol intake, ❸ test intact parathyroid hormone (iPTH) to evaluate for hyperparathyroidism, ❹ evaluate for possible granulomatous disease such as sarcoidosis, tuberculosis, Crohns disease, and possible leukemia or lymphoma, ❺ consider metabolic bone disease such as Paget disease of bone or metastatic bone disease, ❻ evaluate for cancer, ❼ test urine calcium for familial hypocalciuric hypercalcemia, ❽ refer to specialist such as internist or endocrinologist if hypercalcemia persists and answer is not forthcoming.

Corrected calcium (cCa) equations: Used when both serum calcium and albumin are low
<u>American units</u>: cCa (mg/dL) = serum Ca (mg/dL) + 0.8 (4.0 - serum albumin [g/dL])
<u>International units</u>: cCa (mmol/L) = measured total Ca (mmol/L) + 0.02 (40 - serum albumin [g/L])

---

[94] "Herein is reviewed literature suggesting that magnesium deficiency exacerbates potassium wasting by increasing distal potassium secretion." Huang CL, Kuo E. Mechanism of hypokalemia in magnesium deficiency. *J Am Soc Nephrol*. 2007;18:2649-52 jasn.asnjournals.org/content/18/10/2649
[95] "If the hyperkalemia is severe (potassium >7.0 mEq/L) or if the patient is symptomatic, begin treatment before diagnostic investigation of the underlying cause." Garth D. Hyperkalemia in emergency medicine treatment and management. *Medscape Reference* http://emedicine.medscape.com/article/766479-treatment#a1126 Accessed June 2011

Practical overview of common abnormalities on the chemistry/metabolic panel —*continued*

Low values—considerations	*Analyte*	*High values—considerations*
Clinically meaningful hypochloremia is rare among outpatients. Hypochloremic metabolic alkalosis is commonly seen after persistent vomiting. Consider syndrome of inappropriate diuretic hormone (SIADH) secretion, cardiopulmonary disease, and adrenal insufficiency.	**Chloride**: 97 to 111 mmol/L	Hyperchloremia in outpatients is rare; assess for drug effect and dehydration with hemoconcentration; assess for acid-base disturbance, especially acidosis.
Reduced CO_2 correlates with hyperventilation; consider acid-base disturbance, salicylate overdose, asthma. Slight decrements in healthy outpatients are probably due to anxious hyperventilation at time of venipuncture.	**CO2 (carbon dioxide)**: 20 - 30 mmol/L	Elevated CO_2 can suggest cardiopulmonary compromise and/or acid-base disturbance; assess clinically. Slight elevations in otherwise healthy outpatients are probably due to breath-holding at time of venipuncture.
Reduced total protein with normal albumin suggests hypogammaglobulinemia; evaluate for nephrotic syndrome, liver disease, protein deficiency and malabsorption/enteropathy, immunosuppressive syndromes and consider intravenous gammaglobulin therapy.	**Total protein (albumin + globulins)**: 6.3 - 8.0 g/dL	Elevated total protein with normal albumin suggests hypergammaglobulinemia, such as due to infection or plasma cell dyscrasia (e.g., multiple myeloma and Waldenstrom's disease). Evaluate within the clinical context; order serum protein electrophoresis if cause remains elusive, especially if patient has immune complex disease, neuropathy, or nephropathy.
Assess for liver disease, nephrotic syndrome, protein deficiency, malabsorption (consider celiac disease).	**Albumin**: 3.9 - 5.0 g/dL	Assess for dehydration/hemoconcentration.
Loss of hepatic mass due to cirrhosis, possible pyridoxine deficiency.	**ALT (alanine aminotransferase)**: 10 - 40 IU/L	Hepatocellular liver injury due to chemical toxicity, viral hepatitis, hemochromatosis, metastatic or infectious disease, muscle injury. ALT is preferentially elevated over AST in viral hepatitis.
Loss of hepatic mass due to cirrhosis, possible pyridoxine deficiency.	**AST (aspartate aminotransferase)**: 10 - 40 IU/L	Hepatocellular liver injury due to chemical toxicity, viral hepatitis, hemochromatosis, metastatic or infectious liver disease, myocardial infarct, muscle injury. AST is preferentially elevated over ALT in alcoholic hepatitis and rhabdomyolysis.
Consider zinc deficiency, malnutrition.	**Alkaline phosphatase**: 44 - 147 IU/L	Metabolic bone disease, metastatic bone disease, vitamin D deficiency, congestive liver disease. Test isoenzymes to differentiate bone versus hepatic origin if cause of elevation remains unclear.

Practical overview of common abnormalities on the chemistry/metabolic panel—*continued*

Low values—considerations	*Analyte*	*High values—considerations*
Low values are rare but might be noted with severe chronic anemia.	**Total bilirubin**: 0.2 to 1.5 mg/dL Direct (conjugated) bilirubin: 0 to 0.3 mg/dL Indirect (unconjugated) bilirubin: Determined by subtracting the *direct* from the *total* bilirubin.	Indirect/unconjugated bilirubin is elevated with hemolysis (e.g., hemolytic anemia) and impaired enzymatic conjugation (e.g., Gilbert's syndrome) or both (e.g., neonates). Direct/conjugated bilirubin has been enzymatically conjugated with glucuronic acid but is blocked from hepatobiliary excretion; consider performing liver and gall bladder sonogram (or CT or MRI) to evaluate for causes of biliary obstruction in addition to a careful abdominal exam. In patients with advanced liver disease, perform the Model for End-Stage Liver Disease (MELD) score and/or the MELD-Na score to predict 3-month mortality.[96] Fluoridated water inhibits glucuronidation in some patients with Gilbert's syndrome; biochemical improvement follows avoidance of fluoridated water.[97]
Liver disease, nephrotic syndrome, protein deficiency and malabsorption. **BUN-to-creatinine ratio (normal = 10)** >10-20: Renal underperfusion, post-renal obstruction ≤10: Suggests intrinsic renal disease	**BUN (blood urea nitrogen)**: 7 to 20 mg/dL	Consider renal underperfusion (e.g., due to heart failure, GI bleeding, renal artery stenosis, dehydration), intrinsic renal failure, post-renal urinary tract obstruction. When renal disease is initially considered, order a urinalysis with microscopic analysis—see following section on urinalysis (UA).
Sarcopenia (insufficient muscle mass), protein deficiency and malabsorption. **Methods for estimating creatinine clearance, glomerular filtration rate (GFR)** 1. Modification of Diet in Renal Disease (MDRD) equation*, 2. 24-hour urine creatinine measurement, 3. Serum cystatin-C measurement, 4. Cockcroft-Gault equation (below): $$GFR = \frac{(140 - age\ years) \times wt\ kg \times (0.85\ if\ female)}{72 \times serum\ creatinine\ in\ mg/dL}$$ Clinical pearls for managing the chronic kidney disease (CKD) patient with declining renal function: • When the GFR ≤ 60 (CKD stage 3): Modify dosages or withdraw certain drugs. Treat the causative problem and/or begin specialist co-management. • When the GFR ≤ 30 (CKD stage 4): The patient needs to consult a nephrologist. • When the GFR ≤ 15 (CKD stage 5): The patient needs a transplant or dialysis. *National Institute of Diabetes and Digestive and Kidney Diseases (NIDDK). GFR MDRD Calculator for Adults (Conventional units). Accessed June 2011 nkdep.nih.gov/professionals/gfr_calculators/idms_con.htm	**Creatinine**: 0.8 to 1.3 mg/dL	Excess dietary protein, creatine supplementation, renal hypoperfusion; the most important consideration is intrinsic renal failure. Creatinine production (from arginine and creatine) is proportional to muscle mass. A rise in creatinine does not become evident until renal function (measured by glomerular filtration rate [GFR]) has fallen by approximately 50%. Creatinine levels indicative of impaired renal function to such an extent that modifications in diet, medications, and co-management become relevant are 1.4 mg/dL in women and 1.5 mg/dL in men. In the evaluation of renal function, the patient's age is a crucial determinant of how the serum creatinine is interpreted for the estimation of renal function (via GFR—see the Cockcroft-Gault equation). Cystatin C is more sensitive than are singular or conjugate interpretations of BUN and creatinine. If drug-induced nephritis is suspected, test urine eosinophils.

---

[96] MELD calculations are best performed electronically, such as with http://www.mayoclinic.org/meld/mayomodel8.html or other medical calculator.
[97] Lee J. Gilbert's disease and fluoride intake. *Fluoride* 1983; 16: 139-45

<u>69yo female presenting for routine outpatient health assessment with no acute complaints</u>: Review the following labs and outline your treatment plan before reading the discussion below.

PATIENT NAME	PATIENT ID	ROOM NUMBER	AGE	SEX	PHYSICIAN
			69 Y 1941	F	*Vasquez*

REQUISITION NO	ACCESSION NO	ID.NO.	COLLECTION DATE & TIME	LOG-IN-DATE	REPORT DATE & TIME
			09/22/10 08:00 AM	09/22/10 06:37 PM	09/23/10 03:36AM

NOTES:
   PT FASTING

TEST	RESULTS OUT OF RANGE	RESULTS WITHIN RANGE	UNITS	EXPECTED RANGE	LAB
BASIC METABOLIC PROFILE					
GLUCOSE		98	MG/DL	65-100	
BUN		19	MG/DL	8-25	
CREATININE		1.2	MG/DL	0.6-1.3	
EGFR AFRICAN AMER.	54		ML/MIN/1.73	>60	
EGFR NON-AFRICAN AMER.	45		ML/MIN/1.73	>60	
SODIUM		136	MEQ/L	133-146	
POTASSIUM	8.5		MEQ/L	3.5-5.3	

RESULTS RECHECKED AND VERIFIED
NOTE: NO VISIBLE HEMOLYSIS OBSERVED.

CHLORIDE		100	MEQ/L	97-110	
CARBON DIOXIDE		27	MEQ/L	18-30	
CALCIUM		10.0	MG/DL	8.5-10.5	
LIPID PANEL					
CHOLESTEROL		193	MG/DL	<200	
TRIGLYCERIDES		129	MG/DL	<150	
HDL CHOLESTEROL		52	MG/DL	>39	
CALCULATED LDL CHOL	115		MG/DL	<100	
RISK RATIO LDL/HDL		2.22	RATIO	<3.22	
HEMOGLOBIN A1C	7.0		%	4.0-5.6	

AMERICAN DIABETES ASSOCIATION GUIDELINES FOR HGB A1C:
   GLYCEMIC GOAL IN DIABETES . . . . . . <7.0%
   DIAGNOSIS OF DIABETES . . . . >/=6.5%
      CONFIRMED ON REPEAT ANALYSIS OR
      WITH APPROPRIATE SYMPTOMS.
   INCREASED RISK FOR DIABETES 5.7-6.4%

TSH	10.6		UIU/ML	0.3-5.1	

PERFORMING LAB(S) LEGEND:

> **Chemistry/metabolic panels should be performed on all new patients prior to the initiation of treatment and periodically on all established patients to monitor for disease emergence, disease progression, and response to treatment**
>
> Treating this diabetic patient with a potassium-rich diet emphasizing low-carbohydrate fruits and vegetables would exacerbate her already life-threatening hyperkalemia. Note also that her hypothyroidism would be expected to contribute to her obesity which is exacerbating her diabetes and that (somewhat theoretically since we don't have her vital signs here) hypothyroid bradycardia could also reduce renal perfusion and contribute to her low GFR and hyperkalemia.

Assessments and plan: ❶ <u>Life-threatening hyperkalemia</u>: The clinician must focus on the emergency issue(s). Many books quote a potassium of 6 mEq/L as a panic value; note that the laboratory already excluded technical error and checked for hemolysis, which are the two most common causes of spurious hyperkalemia. This patient should be called at home and advised to immediately seek transportation by a secondary driver (e.g., taxi, ambulance, friend, neighbor, or relative) to the nearest hospital. If the patient is demented or otherwise incompetent, the clinician should contact the patient's caretaker or call directly for an ambulance. Attention must be given to the reliability of the driver, the urgency of the situation, and the speed by which the driver can get the patient to the hospital; failure by the clinician to ensure proper patient care—which in this case and most situations is best ensured by enrolling the ambulance service—could easily result in medicolegal complications. Hospital treatment for hyperkalemia will include assessment for electrocardiographic changes and treatment of hyperkalemia with intravenous calcium to stabilize cardioelectroconductivity, beta-adrenergic agonists, bicarbonate, diuretics, insulin and glucose; magnesium may also help alleviate arrhythmias; oral sodium polystyrene sulfonate (Kayexalate) is a potassium-binding agent. ❷ <u>Diabetes mellitus</u>: Notice that this patient's fasting glucose level is "normal" and yet the patient is clearly diabetic per the hemoglobin A1c value >6.5%. This patient needs a comprehensive nutritional plan for diabetes management. Promoting dependence on drugs at this early point should be considered inappropriate. ❸ <u>Hypothyroidism</u>: The TSH >10 indicates primary hypothyroidism by any standard; in all probability, unless major contraindications exist (of which very few exist), this patient should be started on a thyroid hormone combination as discussed in the section on thyroid assessment. ❹ <u>Renal insufficiency</u>: This patient has stage-3 chronic kidney disease and should begin a renoprotective and renorestorative program—beyond the basics of hypertension and hyperglycemia control—as discussed in *Chiropractic and Naturopathic Mastery of Common Clinical Disorders*. Use of ACE-inhibitor or ARB is contraindicated due to hyperkalemia. ❺ <u>Dyslipidemia</u>: The elevated LDL cholesterol and triglycerides should both be below 100 mg/dL. Diet is key, followed by fatty acid therapy, niacin, berberine.

Lipid panel:	
Overview and interpretation:	• "High cholesterol" was a buzz phrase many years ago indicating an unfavorable lipid profile causally associated with accelerated atherogenesis and the resultant CVD in its myriad forms. The next step was to identify low-density lipoprotein (LDL) cholesterol as the most obvious kingpin of vascular villains. Advances over the past decade include: 1. Appreciation that other non-lipid molecules such as homocysteine and c-reactive protein are important contributors to the atherogenic process, 2. Renewed interest in the beneficial effects of high-density lipoprotein (HDL) cholesterol in mediating vasculoprotection, and 3. Additional appreciation that the "non-standard" lipid mediators such as very-low-density lipoprotein (VLDL), β-VLDL, intermediate-density lipoprotein (IDL) cholesterol and lipoprotein-a (Lp-a) are also clinically important. For the sake of this introductory section on the basics of laboratory interpretation, the discussion will be limited to the components of the standard lipid panel; additional tests and details are provided in the disease-specific chapters on metabolic and inflammatory disorders.

Lipids: Goals	*Clinical notes:*
Total cholesterol: < 200 mg/dL	• Higher cholesterol levels correlate with increased risk for CVD. Except in very rare cases of genotropic disease, the vast majority of humans should be able to achieve a total cholesterol <200 mg/dL via nutritional optimization, exercise, and proper endocrine (especially thyroid) status. The so-called "statin" drugs which block HMG-CoA reductase (3-hydroxy-3-methyl-glutaryl-CoA reductase, the rate-limiting enzyme for the endogenous production of cholesterol) would and should be *orphan drugs*. Reducing serum levels of insulin—the primary inducer of HMG-CoA reductase—is the most rational means by which to reduce total cholesterol levels. Thyroid hormone downregulates HMG-CoA reductase; this explains the well-established association of hypothyroidism with dyslipidemia and hypercholesterolemia.
LDL: <100 mg/dL	• O'Keefe and Cordain and colleagues[98] have noted that optimal LDL is 50-70 mg/dl and that lower is better and is physiologically normal for humans who eat appropriate diets and who are physically active.
HDL: >50-60 mg/dL	• Per the American Heart Association[99], "An HDL of 60 mg/dL and above is considered protective against heart disease." Of note, a recent report linked accumulation of persistent organic pollutants (POP) with elevated HDL levels.[100]
Triglycerides: <100 mg/dL	• Elevated serum triglycerides—except in rare cases of genotropic disease—are indicators of dietary carbohydrate excess and/or alcohol excess and/or insulin resistance. Hypertriglyceridemia is associated with increased CVD risk, higher body mass index (BMI), vitamin D deficiency, and increased risks of breast cancer and prostate cancer. Extreme hypertriglyceridemia (500 mg/dL or more) can cause pancreatitis; administration of omega-3 fatty acids from fish oil is protective.
Advantages	• Allows for the monitoring of established cardiovascular risk factors and a surrogate marker for dietary compliance and lifestyle optimization.
Limitations:	• Other non-lipid risk factors should also be monitored and optimized.
Comments:	• Important panel for overall patient management and disease prevention.

---

[98] O'Keefe JH Jr, Cordain L, Harris WH, Moe RM, Vogel R. Optimal low-density lipoprotein is 50 to 70 mg/dl: lower is better and physiologically normal. *J Am Coll Cardiol*. 2004 Jun 2;43(11):2142-6

[99] American Heart Association. heart.org/HEARTORG/Conditions/What-Your-Cholesterol-Levels-Mean_UCM_305562_Article.jsp Accessed June 2011

[100] "However, unlike the findings with p,p'-DDE, after the initial decrease of HDL-cholesterol from the 1st to 2nd quartile, HDL-cholesterol increased from the 2nd to 4th quartile of these PCBs." Lee DH, Steffes MW, Sjödin A, Jones RS, Needham LL, Jacobs DR Jr. Low dose organochlorine pesticides and polychlorinated biphenyls predict obesity, dyslipidemia, and insulin resistance among people free of diabetes. *PLoS One*. 2011 Jan 26;6(1):e15977

CBC: complete blood count

Overview and interpretation:	This test measures numbers and indices of white and red blood cells and platelets. A routine "CBC with differential" is affordable, practical, and thus preferred for the vast majority of situations (step 1); the next step when the clinical picture remains unclear is—generally—to order a peripheral blood smear (step 2) before proceeding to a hematologist referral (step 3). Additional tests—more components of step 2—are listed below per topic. If all three blood cell populations are reduced (pancytopenia) consider nutritional anemia, hypersplenism (especially secondary to hepatic cirrhosis), autoimmunity (especially systemic lupus erythematosus), or bone marrow disorder such as myelofibrosis or aplastic anemia.

- WBC (white blood cells): The three most commonly encountered disorders that cause an abnormal WBC count are ❶ bone marrow suppression (causing low WBC count) and conditions associated with elevated WBC count including ❷ leukemia/lymphoma and ❸ response to infection. An elevated WBC count suggests the possibility of infection (especially bacterial infection) or leukemia/lymphoma and therefore requires the clinician's attention. However, relying on the WBC count for the assessment of serious infection is potentially misleading, particularly since, for example, it is elevated in less than 50% of patients with acute and chronic musculoskeletal infections; per Shaw et al[101] "Therefore, it [the WBC count] is helpful when it is high, but potentially misleading when it is normal." Clinicians can gain additional information by assessing percentage and quantitative indices of neutrophils, lymphocytes, and eosinophils, elevations of which may suggest bacterial infections, viral infections, or allergic or parasitic conditions, respectively. Primary care clinicians may also choose to perform lymphocyte immunophenotyping by flow cytometry in patients with unexplained lymphocytosis prior to hematologist consult.

  - Neutropenia: Severe suppression of WBC count resulting in neutropenia can occur in liver disease, viral infections (including but not limited to HIV), autoimmune disorders, bone marrow infiltration/failure, and toxin/alcohol exposure. For severe neutropenia, hospitalization, isolation precautions, prophylactic antibiotics, and marrow-stimulating agents are often indicated. Neutropenia is defined by an absolute neutrophil count (ANC) less than 1500 neutrophilic cells per mm3. Neutropenia is most commonly due to use of anti-cancer cytotoxic agents; other drugs that can cause neutropenia include anticonvulsants (e.g., carbamazepine, valproic acid, diphenylhydantoin), thyroid inhibitors (carbimazole, methimazole, propylthiouracil), antibacterial drugs (penicillins, cephalosporins, sulfonamides, chloramphenicol, vancomycin, trimethoprim-sulfamethoxazole), antipsychotic drugs (clozapine), antiarrhythmics (procainamide), antirheumatic drugs (penicillamine, gold salts, hydroxychloroquine), and NSAIDs.[102] The ANC is calculated with "segs" (segmented neutrophils) and "bands" (band neutrophils) reported on CBC with differential: ANC = Total WBC x (% Segs + % Bands).

> **Absolute neutrophil count (ANC) = Total WBC x (% "Segs" + % "Bands")**
> - Normal value: ≥ 1500 cells/mm3,
> - Mild neutropenia: 1000-1500/mm3,
> - Moderate neutropenia: 500-1000/mm3,
> - Severe neutropenia: ≤ 500/mm3; hospitalization is generally advised

---

[101] Shaw BA, Gerardi JA, Hennrikus WL. How to avoid orthopedic pitfalls in children. *Patient Care* 1999; Feb 28: 95-116

[102] Tefferi A, Hanson CA, Inwards DJ. How to interpret and pursue an abnormal complete blood cell count in adults. *Mayo Clin Proc.* 2005 Jul;80(7):923-36 www.mayoclinicproceedings.com/content/80/7/923.long This article serves as the main review for this section on CBC interpretation.

Overview and interpretation —continued:	▪ RBC (red blood cells and associated indices): Since polycythemia is relatively rare, in most situations the clinician is looking for anemia, most often related to the categories in the subsections that follow this paragraph. The first step is to classify the anemia based on the mean corpuscular volume (MCV) as microcytic (MCV, <80 fL), normocytic (MCV, 80-95 fL), or macrocytic (MCV, >95 fL)—details on following page.

▪ Clinical notes on the most common anemias:

- o Nutritional deficiency of B-12 or folate: My approach is to critique the mean corpuscular volume (MCV) and to interpret MCV values greater than 90 with an increased suspicion for folate and/or B-12 deficiency. Clinical experience has shown that MCV values greater than 95 correlate with increased homocysteine levels, and a clinical response (improvement in mood, energy, and a reduction in MCV) is commonly seen following three months of nutritional supplementation. Deficiency of vitamin B-12 can easily be treated with oral administration of 2,000 mcg per day of vitamin B-12.[103] I generally use 5 mg (rarely up to 20 mg) per day of oral folate for the treatment of probable or documented folic acid deficiency; this is safe for most patients, excluding those on antiepileptic drugs.[104] Vitamin B-12 and folic acid *function together* and should be *administered together*. Cyanocobalamin should be avoided due to the cyanide.

- o Iron deficiency (confirmed with assessment of serum ferritin): While inadequate intake, malabsorption, or menstrual bleeding may cause iron deficiency, **adult patients with iron deficiency are at higher probability for gastrointestinal pathology and should therefore be evaluated with endoscopy or other comprehensive assessment** *beyond fecal occult-blood testing* **to rule out gastrointestinal disease.**[105,106] **The standard of care for all healthcare professionals is that adult patients with inexplicable iron deficiency are referred for gastroenterscopic evaluation to assess for occult gastrointestinal pathology; the major concerns are gastric/colon carcinoma, but malabsorptive conditions and bleeding noncancerous polyps are also worthy of diagnosis.** Iron supplementation should be administered and can reasonably be withheld during acute viral and bacterial infections as it promotes bacterial and viral replication and pathogenicity.

- o The anemia of chronic disease: Generally associated with a corresponding disease history such as long-term RA or renal insufficiency and often associated with increased ESR, CRP, and ferritin. **Do not assume that an anemic patient has iron deficiency until proven with measurement of serum ferritin.** Anemia of chronic kidney disease (CKD) is associated with reduced renal production of erythropoietin, thereby resulting in understimulation of bone marrow.

- o Anemia caused by hemolysis or splenic sequestration: Autoimmune hemolytic anemia most commonly occurs in patients with systemic lupus erythematosus (SLE). Pancytopenia—reduced numbers of RBC, WBC, and platelets—is seen with chronic liver disease that has progressed to cirrhosis and has resulted in hemolysis and splenic sequestration of blood cells; such patients are at risk for esophageal varicies, encephalopathy, and ascites with spontaneous bacterial peritonitis and should be screened and treated appropriately.

[103] Kuzminski AM, et al. Effective treatment of cobalamin deficiency with oral cobalamin. *Blood* 1998 Aug 15;92(4):1191-8

[104] "PGA administered in doses up to 1,000 mg orally a day... The folate was well absorbed, as reflected by marked increases in the serum and erythrocyte folate concentrations... There was no evidence of clinical or laboratory toxicity at these high doses of folate." Boss GR, Ragsdale RA, Zettner A, Seegmiller JE. Failure of folic acid (pteroylglutamic acid) to affect hyperuricemia. *J Lab Clin Med* 1980 Nov;96(5):783-9

[105] Rockey DC, Cello JP. Evaluation of the gastrointestinal tract in patients with iron-deficiency anemia. *N Engl J Med.* 1993;329(23):1691-5

[106] "Endoscopy revealed a clinically important lesion in 23 (12%) of 186 patients. ... CONCLUSIONS: Endoscopy yields important findings in premenopausal women with iron deficiency anemia, which should not be attributed solely to menstrual blood loss." Bini EJ, Micale PL, Weinshel EH. Evaluation of the gastrointestinal tract in premenopausal women with iron deficiency anemia. *Am J Med.* 1998 Oct;105(4):281-6

Anemia—the most common considerations in outpatient practice: Always assess patient for tachycardia, hypovolemia, orthostasis, and adequate perfusion; always test serum ferritin during the initial evaluation then perform peripheral blood smear (PBS) if diagnosis remains unclear

- Microcytic anemia:
  - Iron deficiency anemia (IDA)—Test serum ferritin. The confirmation of iron deficiency in adults generally requires gastroenterologic consultation to assess for occult gastrointestinal blood loss; this is especially true for all men and post-menopausal women but also applies to premenopausal women.* Testing for celiac disease and hematuria is advised.**
  - Thalassemia—Check for polycythemia, test Hgb electrophoresis; because the diagnosis of the various thalassemias can be complex, consider consulting a hematologist,
  - Anemia of chronic disease (ACD)—Assess patient, inflammatory markers, and renal function. The most common causes of ACD are temporal (giant cell) arteritis and polymyalgia rheumatica, rheumatoid arthritis, chronic infection, Hodgkin lymphoma, renal cell carcinoma, myelofibrosis, and Castleman disease (a noncancerous lymphoproliferative disorder).
- Normocytic anemia:
  - Nutritional anemia: Iron deficiency and vitamin B-12 deficiency can both cause normocytic anemia.
  - Bleeding—Assess patient for tachycardia, hypovolemia, and shock; consider transfusion and/or volume repletion as needed. Assess serum ferritin and the reticulocyte count.
  - Chronic renal failure (CRF): Anemia associated with elevated BUN and creatinine.
  - Hypersplenism: Assess for chronic hepatitis and cirrhosis. Cirrhotic patients are at increased risk for gastroesophageal hemorrhage and ascites with spontaneous bacterial peritonitis.
  - Hemolysis: Expect to see elevated reticulocytes (chronic) and lactate dehydrogenase (acute); expect high indirect bilirubin and low serum haptoglobin with intravascular hemolysis; assess for autoimmunity (ANA, direct Coombs test [direct antiglobulin test]), glucose-6-phosphate dehydrogenase (G6PD) deficiency, drug-induced hemolysis, and other causes as case warrants.
  - Bone marrow disorder: Correlate lab findings with patient presentation; consult hematologist if solution is not forthcoming.
- Macrocytosis:
  - Induced by toxins, drugs, alcohol—Assess per patient history and other findings; the most notorious offenders are hydroxyurea, zidovudine, and alcohol.
  - Vitamin B-12 and/or folate deficiency: Consider testing serum methylmalonate and homocysteine followed by empiric supplementation with B-12 at 2,000 or more micrograms per day and folate at 1-5 milligrams per day; determine cause of problem and strongly consider autoimmune gastritis, bacterial overgrowth, celiac disease. Test serum ferritin because nutritional deficiencies commonly occur together. Administration of vitamin B-12 is advised in all patients suspected of having B-12 deficiency.*** Regarding the clinical presentation of vitamin B-12 deficiency, clinicians should remember the adage that one-third of patients will present with anemia, one-third with peripheral neuropathy, and one-third with central neurologic problems such as depression, psychosis, and/or other disturbances of mood, memory, or personality. Failure to diagnose and treat vitamin B-12 deficiency in a timely manner will result in permanent neurologic damage.
  - Hypothyroidism: Measure TSH and free T4 at a minimum; assess basal body temperature, and speed of Achilles reflex return.

* "A gastrointestinal source of chronic blood loss was identified in a substantial proportion of premenopausal women with iron deficiency anemia." Green BT, Rockey DC. Gastrointestinal endoscopic evaluation of premenopausal women with iron deficiency anemia. *J Clin Gastroenterol.* 2004 Feb;38(2):104-9

** Goddard AF, James MW, McIntyre AS, Scott BB; on behalf of the British Society of Gastroenterology. Guidelines for the management of iron deficiency anaemia. *Gut.* 2011 Jun 6. [Epub ahead of print] http://www.epocrates.com/dacc/1106/irondefbmj1106.pdf

*** "Thus, therapeutic trials of Cbl are warranted when clinical findings consistent with Cbl deficiency are present..." Solomon LR. Cobalamin-responsive disorders in the ambulatory care setting: unreliability of cobalamin, methylmalonic acid, and homocysteine testing. *Blood.* 2005 Feb 1;105(3):978-85 http://bloodjournal.hematologylibrary.org/content/105/3/978.full.pdf

CBC: complete blood count—*continued*	
Overview and interpretation —continued:	▪ <u>Platelets:</u> Elevated platelet count (thrombocytosis) can be due to malignant primary thrombocytosis, iron-deficiency anemia, hemolysis, asplenia, and reactive thrombocytosis due to cancer, infection, or chronic inflammation. Low platelet count (thrombocytopenia, fewer than 150,000 platelets per microliter) increases risk for spontaneous bleeding and can—rarely but importantly—be associated with serious and potentially life-threatening disorders such as thrombotic thrombocytopenic purpura/hemolytic uremic syndrome (TTP/HUS) and disseminated intravascular coagulation (DIC). In relatively asymptomatic and nonacute outpatients, the most common causes of thrombocytopenia are hypersplenism due to liver cirrhosis, idiopathic thrombocytopenic purpura (ITP), and drug reaction, most notoriously secondary to trimethoprim-sulfamethoxazole ("Bactrim"), cardiac medications (e.g., quinidine, procainamide, thiazide diuretics), antirheumatic drugs (gold salts [rarely used these days]), and heparin. Heparin-induced thrombocytopenia (HIT, type-2) is potentially fatal and requires immediate cessation of heparin administration. Patients with unexplained persistent thrombocytopenia should be tested for HIV, autoimmunity (ANA), and lymphoproliferative disorders (PBS, immunophenotyping, serum protein electrophoresis and serum immunofixation). Isolated mild to moderate thrombocytopenia (75,000 – 150,000 platelets per microliter) during pregnancy generally is considered nonpathologic.
Advantages:	▪ The **CBC with differential** is inexpensive and easy to perform and is appropriate for asymptomatic patients. The "CBC with diff" is an appropriate first test for patients who are symptomatic (e.g., fatigue, fever) or have an ongoing history of health problems. In certain healthcare settings where cost containment is a major priority, CBC *without* differential is commonly ordered; however, in outpatient private practice, the additional expenditure of $2 for the CBC *with* differential is the preferred evaluation. It provides a quick screen for anemia, leukemia, infection, and for provisional evidence of B-12/folate and iron deficiencies. The CBC can also identify more complex conditions such as pancytopenia and thereby promote comprehensive patient management; for example, pancytopenia may unmask hepatic cirrhosis which may necessitate use of nadolol for prophylaxis against gastroesophageal variceal hemorrhage as well as use of prophylactic antibiotics against spontaneous bacterial peritonitis. ▪ The **peripheral blood smear (PBS)** is used to further evaluate leukocytosis, anemias, and other abnormalities. In the investigation of persistent leukocytosis, the PBS is of limited value and therefore, while the PBS should certainly be performed, it is generally followed by **immunophenotyping by flow cytometry** if not a direct referral to a hematologist. An excellent review by Tefferi et al[107] concluded, "In general, it is prudent to perform a PBS in most instances of abnormal CBC, along with basic tests that are dictated by the type of CBC abnormalities. The latter may include, for example, serum ferritin in patients with microcytic anemia or lymphocyte immunophenotyping by flow cytometry in patients with lymphocytosis..."
Limitations:	▪ WBC count may be normal even in patients with serious infections. ▪ RBC indices may be normal in people with severe iron deficiency. ○ **Dr Vasquez's experience**—*Many outpatients with no evidence of anemia on the CBC will be grossly iron deficient with ferritin values less than 6 mcg/L, clearly indicating iron deficiency. Nonanemic iron deficiency contributes to fatigue, depression, and attention deficit.*
Comments:	▪ The **CBC** is a foundational part of the assessment for all new patients. Generally, "CBC *with* differential" should be ordered.

---

[107] Tefferi A, Hanson CA, Inwards DJ. How to interpret and pursue an abnormal complete blood cell count in adults. *Mayo Clin Proc* 2005;80(7):923-3

Case of classic iron insufficiency in a healthy 32yo athletic female: This limited laboratory report is from a 32yo athletic female whose primary complaint is that of "less endurance than expected" given her healthy lifestyle and frequent participation in physical exercise of various types such as running, biking, hiking, and kayaking. Her TSH is on the low end of normal consistent with her taking 17 mcg daily of liothyroinine (T3); note however that the total T3 level remains on the low end of the normal range, suggesting that she may benefit from additional T3 supplementation. The RBC parameters Hgb and Hct are on the low end of the normal range consistent with recent menstruation; the response of the bone marrow to recent blood loss is noted with the RDW being toward the high end of normal, refecting increased marrow production of reticulocytes. Ferritin is suboptimal at 25 ng/mL, given that the optimal range is approximately 40-70 ng/mL.[108] Altough various iron supplements are available on the market and high-iron foods such as beef and blackstrap molasis can be used, typical treatment is with iron 18 mg per day often provided as ferrous sulfate 90 mg; note that 5 mg ferrous sulfate = 1 mg elemental iron. Other forms of iron such as ferrous aspartate may be better tolerated. Daily iron supplementation for 2-3 months should elevate the ferritin level and improve the feeling of energy not simply by ❶ improving oxygen delivery to tissues but also by ❷ improving function of the electron transport chain where iron is a required cofactor, ❸ improving the conversion of thyroid hormone (T4) into the active form of T3, and by ❹ improving the production of dopamine and norepinephrine, since iron is a required cofactor for the enzyme tyrosine hydroxylase which converts the amino acid tyrosine into L-DOPA which is converted to dopamine and then partially to norepinephrine. Given that this patient menstruates monthly and has no significant medical history and—specifically—no gastrointestinal complaints; the probability is high that her state of iron insufficiency is due to physiologic blood loss; however, a case could be made for endoscopic evaluation[109], and in the event that the patient suffered from an diagnosed intestinal lesion such as colon cancer, the practitioner who did not refer for gastroenterologic evaluation would be challenged to produce effective medicolegal defense. Guidelines[110] published in 2011 support testing for celiac disease, *H. pylori* infection, and hematuria while reserving endoscopy in premenopausal women to those aged 50 years or older, or with symptoms of gastrointestinal disease, or those with a strong family history of colorectal cancer.

Reported: 07/07/2011 / 06:02 CDT

Test Name	In Range	Out Of Range	Reference Range
TSH, 3RD GENERATION	0.54		mIU/L
Reference Range			
> or = 20 Years 0.40-4.50			
Pregnancy Ranges			
First trimester 0.20-4.70			
Second trimester 0.30-4.10			
Third trimester 0.40-2.70			
T3, TOTAL	97		76-181 ng/dL
CBC (INCLUDES DIFF/PLT)			
WHITE BLOOD CELL COUNT	7.1		3.8-10.8 Thousand/uL
RED BLOOD CELL COUNT	4.28		3.80-5.10 Million/uL
HEMOGLOBIN	12.1		11.7-15.5 g/dL
HEMATOCRIT	36.2		35.0-45.0 %
MCV	84.5		80.0-100.0 fL
MCH	28.4		27.0-33.0 pg
MCHC	33.6		32.0-36.0 g/dL
RDW	14.8		11.0-15.0 %
PLATELET COUNT	248		140-400 Thousand/uL
ABSOLUTE NEUTROPHILS	3586		1500-7800 cells/uL
ABSOLUTE LYMPHOCYTES	2854		850-3900 cells/uL
ABSOLUTE MONOCYTES	525		200-950 cells/uL
ABSOLUTE EOSINOPHILS	107		15-500 cells/uL
ABSOLUTE BASOPHILS	28		0-200 cells/uL
NEUTROPHILS	50.5		%
LYMPHOCYTES	40.2		%
MONOCYTES	7.4		%
EOSINOPHILS	1.5		%
BASOPHILS	0.4		%
FERRITIN	25		10-154 ng/mL

[108] See excerpt from Vasquez A. *Integrative Rheumatology*. http://optimalhealthresearch.com/hemochromatosis.html
[109] "A gastrointestinal source of chronic blood loss was identified in a substantial proportion of premenopausal women with iron deficiency anemia." Green BT, Rockey DC. Gastrointestinal endoscopic evaluation of premenopausal women with iron deficiency anemia. *J Clin Gastroenterol*. 2004 Feb;38(2):104-9
[110] Goddard AF, James MW, McIntyre AS, Scott BB; on behalf of the British Society of Gastroenterology. Guidelines for the management of iron deficiency anaemia. *Gut*. 2011 Jun 6. [Epub ahead of print] http://www.epocrates.com/dacc/1106/irondefbmj1106.pdf

Clinical consequences of vitamin B-12 deficiency with or without hematologic abnormality: case report and discussion: This elderly patient shows no signs of anemia; note also that the MCV is perfectly normal. Given that the psychiatric literature supports a minimal serum vitamin B-12 level of 600 pg/ml, the advocation by medical reference laboratories of a lower "normal" limit of 200 pg/ml is scientifically absurd and ethically indefensible; this is yet another example of the importance of clinicians' knowledge of the literature overriding the laboratory's reference range. The consistent documentation of the rapid reversibility of severe neuropsychiatric illness with vitamin B-12 therapy as the only intervention[111,112] provides additional justification for empiric vitamin B-12 administration in patients with clinical symptoms consistent with vitamin B-12 deficiency regardless of hematologic and serologic findings.[113] Vitamin B-12 deficiency is very serious because it can lead to permanent brain damage, resulting in personality changes, memory impairment, and overt psychotic disorders, including catatonia; mechanisms of neurologic injury may include homocysteine toxicity, autoimmune neuronal demyelinization, and axonal degeneration and nerve-sheath demyelination especially in the median forebrain bundle area.[114]

HEMATOLOGY

----- CBC - WBC STUDIES -----

	WBC 10E3
Procedure:	WBC 10E3
Reference:	[4.50-11.00]
Units:	/CMM
07DEC06 0926 THU	7.32

----- CBC - RBC STUDIES -----

	RBC 10E6	HEMOGLOBIN	HEMATOCRIT	MCV	MCH	MCHC	RDW-CV
Procedure:	RBC 10E6	HEMOGLOBIN	HEMATOCRIT	MCV	MCH	MCHC	RDW-CV
Reference:	[4.50-5.90]	[13.5-17.5]	[41.0-53.0]	[80.0-94.0]	[27.0-31.0]	[32.0-36.0]	[11.0-16.0]
Units:	/CMM	G/DL	%	FL	PG	%	%
07DEC06 0926 THU	5.16	15.7	46.3	89.7	30.4	33.9	14.1

----- CBC - PLATELET STUDIES -----

	PLATELET 10E3	MPV
Procedure:	PLATELET 10E3	MPV
Reference:	[150-500]	[9.0-13.0]
Units:	/CMM	FL
07DEC06 0926 THU	308	11.2

CHEMISTRY PROFILES

----- ROUTINE CHEMISTRY PROFILES -----

	SODIUM	POTASSIUM	CHLORIDE	CO2	GLUCOSE	BUN	CREATININE	CALCIUM
Procedure:	SODIUM	POTASSIUM	CHLORIDE	CO2	GLUCOSE	BUN	CREATININE	CALCIUM
Reference:	[133-145]	[3.5-5.3]	[100-110]	[22.0-29.0]	[70-110]	[5-25]	[0.5-1.4]	[8.3-10.3]
Units:	MMOL/L	MEQ/L	MMOL/L	MMOL/L	MG/DL	MG/DL	MG/DL	MG/DL
07DEC06 0926 THU	137	4.3	101	27.0	90	16	0.9	9.9

	ANION GAP	OSMOLARITY	BUN/CREAT
Procedure:	ANION GAP	OSMOLARITY	BUN/CREAT
Reference:	[6-14]	[272-305]	
Units:	MEQ/L	MOSM/K	MG/DL
07DEC06 0926 THU	13	275	17.8

SPECIAL CHEMISTRY

----- CHEMISTRY SPECIAL/MISCELLANEOUS -----

	FOLATE	VITAMIN B-12
Procedure:	FOLATE	VITAMIN B-12
Reference:	[2.0-18.0]	[193-982]
Units:	NG/ML	PG/ML
07DEC06 0926 THU	14.7	182 L

[111] Berry N, Sagar R, Tripathi BM. Catatonia and other psychiatric symptoms with vitamin B12 deficiency. *Acta Psychiatr Scand.* 2003 ;108(2):156-9
[112] Newbold HL. Vitamin B-12: placebo or neglected therapeutic tool? *Med Hypotheses.* 1989 Mar;28(3):155-64
[113] Solomon LR. Cobalamin-responsive disorders in the ambulatory care setting: unreliability of cobalamin, methylmalonic acid, and homocysteine testing. *Blood.* 2005 Feb 1;105(3):978-85
[114] Catalano G, Catalano MC, Rosenberg EI, Embi PJ, Embi CS. Catatonia. Another neuropsychiatric presentation of vitamin B12 deficiency? *Psychosomatics.* 1998 Sep-Oct;39(5):456-60 http://psy.psychiatryonline.org/cgi/reprint/39/5/456

Nutritional deficiency, diet-responsive disorders, and the allopathic medical paradigm: Review and commentary with emphases on diabetes mellitus and vitamins D and B-12

Consequences of vitamin B-12 deficiency:

Initially the manifestations are mild and reversible, but over time they become more severe and strongly refractory to treatment to the point that permanent damage (particularly in the CNS) is anticipated:

- "Bipolar disorder"—a condition indistinguishable from a bipolar disorder,
- Organic brain syndrome, delirium, confusion, poor memory, impaired cognition,
- Dementia and erroneous diagnosis of "Alzheimer's disease",
- Mood disorders, depression, catatonia, paranoia, paranoid psychosis, violent behavior,
- Peripheral neuropathy, "combined degeneration" of anterior and posterior columns of the spinal cord,
- As a result of the above problems, patients who are mismanaged by doctors unknowledgeable about basic nutrition often suffer directly from these effects but also suffer from the medical management from these problems. Mood disorders and psychosis may result from B-12 deficiency, and the medical management of mood disorders and psychosis includes medicalization, electroconvulsive therapy (ECT), and institutionalization.

The medical profession's failure to train its students and doctors in nutrition is widely and consistently documented; given that such a profession-wide policy can do nothing other than result in patient harm and/or drug dependency under the guise of "healthcare", it is—borrowing a phrase from Nietzsche—"the highest of all conceivable corruptions."

- Nutritional deficiencies and the medical paradigm (*J Clin Endocrinol Metab* 2003 Nov): "But public health measures in the first half of the 20th century eradicated the most extreme of the vitamin deficiencies in the industrialized nations, and the physician's actual experience of [obvious] deficiency disease dropped to near zero. Perhaps as a result, the medical profession's approach to nutrition today is still dominated by the external agent paradigm, as witnessed in the national campaigns for cholesterol, saturated fat, and salt. Those who think more seriously in terms of the continuing importance of deficiency per se are often derogated or relegated to the quackery fringe. The result, at the very least, is inattention to the real deficiencies that may masquerade as other disorders, or that may simply be ignored altogether."
- Failure of surgical treatment for low-back pain caused by vitamin D deficiency (*J Am Board Fam Med* 2009 Jan): The author of this case series describes six cases of chronic debilitating back pain—three of which "required surgery"—which were greatly relieved or completely cured by correction of vitamin D deficiency. The author notes, "Chronic low back pain and failed back surgery may improve with repletion of vitamin D from a state of deficiency/insufficiency to sufficiency. Vitamin D insufficiency is common; repletion of vitamin D to normal levels in patients who have chronic low back pain or have had failed back surgery may improve quality of life or, in some cases, result in complete resolution of symptoms."

That nutritional deficiencies can cause mood disorders and mental disease is well-known; in contrast to what patients actually need, the general allopathic approach to these clinical presentations is founded upon the administration of drugs, followed by ECT, institutionalization, and psychosurgery and—lately, instead of scalpel-induced brain damage—radiofrequency heating (thermocapsulotomy) or gamma radiation (radiosurgery, gammacapsulotomy) for the destruction of brain structures, and the surgical implantation of brain electrostimulators. Meanwhile, thousands of these psychiatrically-labeled patients simply need nutritional supplementation. Minor exceptions noted, the medical profession as a whole chooses to remain blind to the value of nutrition so that the pharmacosurgical paradigm can remain dominant by continuing to *appear* omnipotent. The dual illusions that are maintained are "Drugs and surgery are the answers to all major health problems" and "If no drug exists for a condition, then it is idiopathic and no curative treatment is available."

As an example, type-2 diabetes mellitus (T2DM) has burgeoned into an epidemic under the dominance of the allopathic disease model, and patients are told that the condition is genetic, progressive and incurable; a review published in the May 2011 issue of *Journal of the American Osteopathic Association* admonished physicians to (mis)educate their patients as follows, with Dr Vasquez's comments in brackets: "Be absolutely clear that T2DM is a lifelong disease [false statement] that will require lifelong treatment [false statement fostering dependency]. Success in controlling the disease and preventing future complications will depend on the patient and physician working together [creation of dependency under the guise of "working together"]. There is often a fatalistic attitude in patients with T2DM [perhaps because they have been lied to and disempowered], so it is important to establish a relationship that on one hand offers hope [creating the illusion of hope while enforcing drug dependency] and on the other does not suggest that the disease will be cured [although the diseases is generally curable with appropriate nutritional intervention]. Be up front with the patient from the first visit and make it clear that T2DM is a chronic illness [enforce drug dependency starting a the first visit]..." This babble was published in a peer-reviewed medical journal despite clear multi-decade evidence showing that T2DM is reversible with nutritional intervention. Recent examples of the safety and efficacy of diet intervention for T2DM are provided here with many more examples and details in *Nutritional, Integrative and Functional Medicine Mastery of Common Clinical Disorders*.

- T2DM is rapidly reversible with diet (*Diabetologia* 2011 Jun): "Normalization of both beta cell function and hepatic insulin sensitivity in type 2 diabetes was achieved by dietary energy restriction alone. This was associated with decreased pancreatic and liver triacylglycerol stores. **The abnormalities underlying type 2 diabetes are reversible by reducing dietary energy intake.**"
- Diet therapy effective, safe, and is at least as effective as injected insulin for reducing chronic hyperglycemia in T2DM (*Nutr Metab* 2009 May): "The number of patients on sulfonylureas decreased from 7 at baseline to 2 at 6 months. No patient required inpatient care or insulin therapy. In summary, the 30%-carbohydrate diet over 6 months led to a remarkable reduction in HbA1c levels, even among outpatients with severe type 2 diabetes, without any insulin therapy, hospital care or increase in sulfonylureas. **The effectiveness of the [low-carbohydrate] diet may be comparable to that of insulin therapy.**"

Ironically (or not), the first-line drug for T2DM—metformin—causes vitamin B-12 (cobalamin, Cbl) deficiency and exacerbation of the often debilitating peripheral neuropathy of T2DM which is often treated with the drugs gabapentin/Neurontin or pregabalin/Lyrica, which exacerbates obesity and T2DM, thereby promoting a vicious cycle.

- Pregabalin/Lyrica and gabapentin/Neurontin promote fat-weight gain, thereby exacerbating T2DM (*Prescrire Int* 2005 Dec): "Pregabalin, like gabapentin, can lead to weight gain and peripheral edema especially in elderly patients."
- Metformin causes vitamin B-12 deficiency and exacerbates diabetic peripheral neuropathy (*Diabetes Care* 2010 Jan): "Metformin-treated patients had depressed Cbl levels and elevated fasting MMA and Hcy levels. Clinical and electrophysiological measures identified more severe peripheral neuropathy in these patients; the cumulative metformin dose correlated strongly with these clinical and paraclinical group differences. CONCLUSIONS: Metformin exposure may be an iatrogenic cause for exacerbation of peripheral neuropathy in patients with type 2 diabetes."
- Vitamin B-12 deficiency secondary to metformin prescription (*Rev Assoc Med Bras* 2011 Jan): "The present findings suggest a high prevalence of vitamin B12 deficiency in metformin-treated diabetic patients [n=144]. Older patients, patients in long term treatment with metformin and low vitamin B12 intake are probably more prone to this deficiency."
- Metformin-induced vitamin B12 deficiency presenting as a peripheral neuropathy (*South Med J* 2010 Mar): "Chronic metformin use results in vitamin B12 deficiency in 30% of patients. ... **Vitamin B12 deficiency, which may present without anemia and as a peripheral neuropathy, is often misdiagnosed as diabetic neuropathy, although the clinical findings are usually different. Failure to diagnose the cause of the neuropathy will result in progression of central and/or peripheral neuronal damage which can be arrested but not reversed with vitamin B12 replacement.**"
- Low vitamin B-12 status correlates with expedited brain atrophy (*Neurology* 2008 Sep): "The decrease in brain volume was greater among those with lower vitamin B(12) and holoTC levels and higher plasma tHcy and MMA levels at baseline. ... Using the upper (for the vitamins) or lower tertile (for the metabolites) as reference in logistic regression analysis and adjusting for the above covariates, vitamin B(12) in the bottom tertile (<308 pmol/L) was associated with increased rate of brain volume loss (odds ratio 6.17, 95% CI 1.25-30.47)."

Consequences for the clinician:
Given that the evidence in favor of early and empiric treatment for possible vitamin B-12 deficiency is stronger than evidence in favor of allowing vitamin B-12 deficiency or dependency to persist with potentially catastrophic outcomes, no scientific argument can be made in favor of failing to diagnose and treat vitamin B-12 deficiency/dependency. However, since, in general, the allopathic and osteopathic medical professions have failed to educate their students and doctors about nutrition, these professions have established ignorance as their defense and therefore no standard of care exists for the treatment or failure of treatment of chronic nutritional deficiencies. Ethically, the results are failure to achieve beneficence via failure to diagnose and treat, and the widespread implementation of malfeasance via diagnostic/therapeutic failure complicated by the unnecessary expenses and adverse effects of drugs/surgeries/interventions used in place of nutritional

Nutritional deficiency, diet-responsive disorders, and the allopathic medical paradigm: Review and commentary with emphases on diabetes mellitus and vitamins D and B-12

supplementation. The enforcement of a standard of care is meaningless when nutritional incompetence is the standard. Fortunately for patients, the biomedical literature uses increasingly strong language in favor of mandating standards for nutritional evaluation and treatment:

- Nutritional deficiencies and the medical paradigm (*J Clin Endocrinol Metab* 2003 Nov): "J. Cannell (submitted for publication) has written that measures such as this editorial will not change the situation, and that only tort litigation will work. One can only hope that he is wrong. Either way, something needs to change"
- Physicians should routinely use vitamin supplementation as treatment for patients (*JAMA* 2002 Jun): "Physicians should make specific efforts to ensure that patients are taking vitamins they should..."
- Testing and treating for vitamin D deficiency among patients with chronic nonspecific musculoskeletal pain should be the standard of care (*Mayo Clin Proc* 2003 Dec): "Because osteomalacia is a known cause of persistent, nonspecific musculoskeletal pain, screening all outpatients with such pain for hypovitaminosis D should be standard practice in clinical care."
- Testing and treating for vitamin D deficiency among patients with chronic low-back pain should be the standard of care (*Spine* 2003 Jan): "Screening for vitamin D deficiency and treatment with supplements should be mandatory in this setting."

Citations for this section:
1. Catalano G, Catalano MC, Rosenberg EI, Embi PJ, Embi CS. Catatonia. Another neuropsychiatric presentation of vitamin B12 deficiency? *Psychosomatics*. 1998 Sep-Oct;39(5):456-60
2. Newbold HL. Vitamin B-12: placebo or neglected therapeutic tool? *Med Hypotheses*. 1989 Mar;28(3):155-64
3. Solomon LR. Cobalamin-responsive disorders in the ambulatory care setting: unreliability of cobalamin, methylmalonic acid, and homocysteine testing. *Blood*. 2005 Feb 1;105(3):978-85
4. Christmas D, Eljamel MS, Butler S, et al. Long term outcome of thermal anterior capsulotomy for chronic, treatment refractory depression. *J Neurol Neurosurg Psychiatry*. 2011 Jun;82(6):594-600
5. Malone DA Jr. Use of deep brain stimulation in treatment-resistant depression. *Cleve Clin J Med*. 2010 Jul;77 Suppl 3:S77-80
6. Heaney RP. Vitamin D, nutritional deficiency, and the medical paradigm. *J Clin Endocrinol Metab*. 2003;88:5107-8
7. Schwalfenberg G. Improvement of chronic back pain or failed back surgery with vitamin D repletion: a case series. *J Am Board Fam Med*. 2009 Jan-Feb;22(1):69-74
8. Gavin JR 3rd, Freeman JS, Shubrook JH Jr, Lavernia F. Type 2 diabetes mellitus: practical approaches for primary care physicians. *J Am Osteopath Assoc*. 2011 May;111(5 Suppl 4):S3-S12
9. Lim EL, Hollingsworth KG, Aribisala BS, et al. Reversal of type 2 diabetes: normalisation of beta cell function in association with decreased pancreas and liver triacylglycerol. *Diabetologia*. 2011 Jun 9. Published on-line.
10. Haimoto H, Sasakabe T, Wakai K, Umegaki H. Effects of a low-carbohydrate diet on glycemic control in outpatients with severe type 2 diabetes. *Nutr Metab* 2009:6;21
11. Gabapentin/Neurontin causes "Gains of up to 15 kg (33lbs) during 3 months of treatment." http://pacmedweightloss.com/docs/medications_that_cause_weight_gain.pdf Accessed July 2011.
12. Vogiatzoglou A, Refsum H, Johnston C, Smith SM, Bradley KM, de Jager C, Budge MM, Smith AD. Vitamin B12 status and rate of brain volume loss in community-dwelling elderly. *Neurology*. 2008 Sep 9;71(11):826-32
13. Wile DJ, Toth C. Association of metformin, elevated homocysteine, and methylmalonic acid levels and clinically worsened diabetic peripheral neuropathy. *Diabetes Care*. 2010 Jan;33(1):156-61
14. Nervo M, Lubini A, Raimundo FV, Faulhaber GA, Leite C, Fischer LM, Furlanetto TW. Vitamin B12 in metformin-treated diabetic patients: a cross-sectional study in Brazil. *Rev Assoc Med Bras*. 2011 Jan-Feb;57(1):46-9
15. Bell DS. Metformin-induced vitamin B12 deficiency presenting as a peripheral neuropathy. *South Med J*. 2010 Mar;103(3):265-7
16. [No authors listed] Pregabalin: new drug. Very similar to gabapentin. *Prescrire Int*. 2005 Dec;14(80):203-6
17. Fletcher RH, Fairfield KM. Harvard Medical School. Vitamins for chronic disease prevention in adults: clinical applications. *JAMA*. 2002;287:3127-9
18. Plotnikoff GA, Quigley JM. Prevalence of severe hypovitaminosis D in patients with persistent, nonspecific musculoskeletal pain. *Mayo Clin Proc*. 2003;78:1463-70
19. Al Faraj S, Al Mutairi K. Vitamin D deficiency and chronic low back pain in Saudi Arabia. *Spine* 2003 ;28:177-9

UA: Urinalysis	

Overview and interpretation:	▪ <u>Collection</u>: Unless catheterized, patients are advised to pass approximately one-third of their available urine into the toilet, then pass approximately the middle-third of their urine into the specimen container. Use of an antiseptic to clean the urethral meatus was once advocated to avoid/reduce specimen contamination, but this step is ineffective and therefore unnecessary because contamination rates remain similar at 32% and 29% whether or not, respectively, urethral meatus cleansing is performed.[115]
	
	▪ <u>Analysis</u>: Analysis should be performed on fresh urine, preferably within 1-2 hours; in outpatient clinical practice this two-hour timeframe is consistently possible only if the clinician performs in-office dipstick analysis (and perhaps microscopic visualization). Samples that cannot be analyzed within 1-2 hours or those which are destined for a reference laboratory should be refrigerated. Dipstick UA can be performed in office and is simple, inexpensive, and—when performed and interpreted with a modicum of competence— sufficiently accurate. Per Klatt[116], "The color change occurring on each segment of the strip is compared to a color chart to obtain results. However, a careless doctor, nurse, or assistant is entirely capable of misreading or misinterpreting the results." Urine samples can be sent to a reference laboratory for more accurate chemical analysis as well as microscopic analysis, culture and sensitivity. Whether infection is clinically suspected or not, clinicians might chose to order "UA with reflex to microscopy and culture" to ensure that urine samples are appropriately processed if the laboratory finds suspicion of UTI upon dipstick analysis.
	
	▪ <u>Scope of this review</u>: The purpose of this brief review is to concisely refresh clinicians' appreciation of the components of the routine urinalysis, one that is generally performed in-office with a dipstick reagent stick or that is performed by a reference laboratory. This is not an exhaustive review, and microscopic findings have not been detailed here because most clinicians do not perform microscopy in their offices; additional details on UA and microscopic assessment is available in articles such as the excellent review by Simerville, Maxted, and Pahira published in *American Family Physician* 2005 and available on-line at http://www.aafp.org/afp/2005/0315/p1153.html as of July 2011.
	
	▪ <u>Components of routine urinalysis</u>:
	
	   o <u>Visual inspection</u>: Urine should be clear with a color ranging from faint yellow (well hydrated, dilute urine) to bright yellow (especially with B-vitamin supplementation). An amber-brown hue might be due to dehydration or a pathologic process resulting in myoglobinuria (i.e., rhabdomyolysis) or the presence of bile pigments (i.e., biliary tract obstruction). A red color to urine suggests hematuria, recent beet consumption, or use of certain drugs or food dyes; the antibiotic rifampin/rifampicin is notorious for adding a red-orange color to the urine (and to a lesser extent to sweat and tears). The urine of patients with porphyria cutanea tarda will be red-brown in natural light and pink-red in fluorescent light.[117] Cloudy urine is due to pyruia (infection), proteinuria, or precipitated phosphate crystals in alkaline urine.
	
	   o <u>Strong odor</u>: Odiferous or malodorous urine suggests infection, recent ingestion of foods such as asparagus or nutritional supplements such as lipoic acid, certain medications, concentrated urine due to dehydration or underperfusion of the kidneys.
	
	   o <u>Specific gravity</u>: Specific gravity is a measure of solute concentration and thus is proportional to urine osmolality; as such it reflects renal perfusion, hydration, and the ability of the kidneys to perform their critical function of concentrating filtrate. Dilute urine has a specific gravity <1.010 and is seen with adequate/excessive hydration, diuretic use, diabetes insipidus, adrenal insufficiency, hyperaldosteronism, and impaired renal function (i.e., failure of the kidneys to concentrate urine). Concentrated urine has a

[115] Simerville JA, Maxted WC, Pahira JJ. Urinalysis: a comprehensive review. *Am Fam Physician*. 2005 Mar 15;71(6):1153-62 http://www.aafp.org/afp/2005/0315/p1153.html
[116] Klatt EC. WebPath. Savannah, Georgia, USA. http://library.med.utah.edu/WebPath/tutorial/urine/urine.html Accessed July 1, 2011
[117] Rich MW. Porphyria cutanea tarda. Don't forget to look at the urine. *Postgrad Med*. 1999 Apr;105(4):208-10, 213-4

UA: Urinalysis

specific gravity >1.020 and correlates with dehydration, renal artery stenosis, hypoperfusion/shock, glucosuria, and syndrome of inappropriate anti-diuretic hormone secretion (SIADH), which is often associated with hyponatremia.

o **pH**: Urine pH may range from 4.5 (very acidic) to as high as 8.5 (very alkaline). Urine pH correlates with serum pH except in patients with renal tubular acidosis (RTA type-1, a condition associated with chronically alkaline urine). Therefore, urine pH can be used to screen for various conditions of systemic alkalosis and acidosis. The Western diet—also called the standard American diet or S.A.D.—causes mild diet-induced metabolic acidosis[118] which promotes degenerative diseases; in contrast, a diet rich in fruits and vegetables such as the Paleo-Mediterranean diet[119] promotes mild systemic and urinary alkalinization.[120] From a wellness perspective, urine pH should be 7.5 up to 8.0 because urinary alkalinization facilitates xenobiotic excretion[121], promotes urinary retention of minerals such as potassium, magnesium, and calcium, and causes a reduction in serum cortisol.[122] Urine pH—like urine sodium:potassium ratio—can be used as a marker of compliance for intake of fruits, vegetables, and alkalinizing supplements such as potassium citrate. For some patients (mostly female), urine alkalinization may encourage urinary tract infection, especially if gastrointestinal dysbiosis[123] is present; in such situations, the often causative GI dysbiosis should be treated, and consistent or transient urinary acidification can be achieved with oral ascorbic acid. Urea-splitting bacteria can cause the urine to be alkaline, and such bacteria can also promote development of magnesium-ammonium phosphate crystals and so-called staghorn nephrolithiasis. Acidic urine promotes development of uric acid nephrolithiasis; therapeutic urinary alkalinization such as by use of supplemental potassium citrate or an alkalinizing diet is preventive and therapeutic. On this topic, Cicerello et al[124] wrote, "In conclusion urinary alkalization with maintaining continuously high urinary pH values, could be the treatment of choice for stone dissolution and prevention of uric acid stones."

o <u>Bilirubin in urine</u>: If present, bilirubin in urine is of the direct/conjugated fraction (rather than indirect/unconjugated, which is nonhydrosoluble) and indicates the need to evaluate for biliary tract obstruction.

o <u>Urobilinogen</u>: Urobilinogen is (direct) bilirubin that has been conjugated in the liver, passed through the biliary system into the intestine, partially metabolized by bacteria, then reabsorbed via the portal circulation and filtered by the kidney. Elevated urobilinogen is associated with liver disease and hemolytic diseases.

o <u>Ketones</u>: UA dipsticks detect acetic acid; other products of fatty acid metabolism found in urine include acetone and beta-hydroxybutyric acid. Ketonuria indicates either metabolic disturbance such as diabetes mellitus or normal physiology in the fasting or lipolytic state. Many clinicians—particularly medical students and physicians[(note 125)]—have been

---

[118] "The modern Western-type diet is deficient in fruits and vegetables and contains excessive animal products, generating the accumulation of non-metabolizable anions and a lifespan state of overlooked metabolic acidosis, whose magnitude increases progressively with aging due to the physiological decline in kidney function." Adeva MM, Souto G. Diet-induced metabolic acidosis. *Clin Nutr*. 2011 Aug;30(4):416-21. Epub 2011 Apr 9.

[119] **Vasquez A**. Revisiting the Five-Part Nutritional Wellness Protocol: The Supplemented Paleo-Mediterranean Diet. *Nutritional Perspectives* 2011 January This article is available at http://optimalhealthresearch.com/part8 and is also included in this textbook.

[120] Cordain L, Eaton SB, Sebastian A, Mann N, Lindeberg S, Watkins BA, O'Keefe JH, Brand-Miller J. Origins and evolution of the Western diet: health implications for the 21st century. *Am J Clin Nutr*. 2005 Feb;81(2):341-54

[121] Proudfoot AT, Krenzelok EP, Vale JA. Position Paper on urine alkalinization. *J Toxicol Clin Toxicol*. 2004;42(1):1-26

[122] Maurer M, Riesen W, Muser J, Hulter HN, Krapf R. Neutralization of Western diet inhibits bone resorption independently of K intake and reduces cortisol secretion in humans. *Am J Physiol Renal Physiol*. 2003 Jan;284(1):F32-40

[123] **Vasquez A**. Reducing Pain and Inflammation Naturally - Part 6: Nutritional and Botanical Treatments Against "Silent Infections" and Gastrointestinal Dysbiosis, Commonly Overlooked Causes of Neuromusculoskeletal Inflammation and Chronic Health Problems. *Nutritional Perspectives* 2006; January. For a more extensive review, see the most recent edition of <u>Integrative Rheumatology</u>: http://optimalhealthresearch.com/rheumatology.html

[124] Cicerello E, Merlo F, Maccatrozzo L. Urinary alkalization for the treatment of uric acid nephrolithiasis. *Arch Ital Urol Androl*. 2010 Sep;82(3):145-8

[125] One of the arguments most commonly leveled against the ketogenic diet—in particular the Atkins diet—is that the induction of ketosis, as measured by ketonuria, is a potentially problematic state that should be avoided. This is an example of selective medical ignorance since mild ketosis is physiologically normal is clinically advantageous for weight loss and seizure control. In our osteopathic medical school, one lecturer advised our student body of 170 that ketosis was evidence of the "danger from diet therapies." On the contrary, given that most of my medical school professors were obese, they should have more carefully considered the benefits of rational dietary therapy, including low-

taught to view ketonuria as synonymous with ketoacidosis; this is obviously inaccurate since lipolysis and the resulting ketonuria are normal *and quite desirable* physiologic states. Ketonuria can be measured with ketone-specific dipsticks as a marker of weight-loss efficacy and compliance with diet and exercise programs.

o Glucose: Glucose is found in the urine when the serum glucose exceeds approximately 190 mg/dL and overwhelms the reabsorptive capacity of the proximal tubule. Glucose in the urine is presumptive evidence supporting the diagnosis of diabetes mellitus. Rare non-diabetic causes of glucosuria/glycosuria include liver disease, pancreatic disease, and Fanconi's syndrome (characterized by a failure of the proximal renal tubules to reabsorb glucose, amino acids, uric acid, phosphate and bicarbonate).

o Protein: Urine should not contain measurable protein on routine urinalysis. Any finding of protein in the urine—even a "trace" amount—requires follow-up; specifically, the test should be repeated within 2-4 weeks and consistently positive results require more detailed testing including serum BUN and creatinine. Urine protein can also be measured in 24-hour urine collections and should not exceed 150 mg/day; greater than this amount is diagnostic of proteinuria, while ≥ 3.5 gm/day is consistent with nephrotic syndrome, mandating a much more comprehensive *and urgent* patient evaluation. Testing for "protein" with a routine urinalysis will not detect all forms of clinically relevant proteinuria; specifically and classically, routine UA is insensitive for the microalbuminuria of diabetes mellitus (detected with the urinary albumin:creatinine ratio) and also the Bence-Jones proteinuria seen with multiple myeloma.

Evaluation of persistent proteinuria
1. Comprehensive evaluation of patient history, physical exam, and overall clinical impression,
2. Measurement of serum BUN, creatinine, albumin, and lipids; consider measuring cystatin c,
3. Microscopic examination of urinary sediment,
4. Assessment for conditions that commonly cause proteinuria, especially hypertension (sphygmomanometry), diabetes (hemoglobin A1c), autoimmune conditions (screen with ANA);
5. Measurement of 24-hour urinary creatinine excretion (or spot urinary albumin-creatinine ratio),
6. Urinary protein electrophoresis,
7. If the above measures are pathoetiologically unfruitful, refer to an internist or nephrologist.

carbohydrate versions of the Paleo-Mediterranean diet (described in this text) which can produce mild ketosis en route to alleviating diabetes mellitus and hypertension. Examples of selective medical ignorance and bias against low-carbohydrate ketogenic diets abound from allopathic institutions. "One diet that has raised safety concerns among the scientific community is the low-carbohydrate, high-protein diet." Tapper-Gardzina Y, Cotugna N, Vickery CE. Should you recommend a low-carb, high-protein diet? *Nurse Pract.* 2002 Apr;27(4):52-3, 55-6, 58-9. "High Protein / Low Carb (Carbohydrate) Diets. Long term, these fad diets can be harmful. Many of the health claims about these diets are not based on scientific proof. Low carb diets are still just that – a diet. Most people find maintaining a low carb diet difficult if not impossible long term. Even if weight is lost, 90% of fad dieters gain all or most of the weight back in five years." Ohio State University. http://medicalcenter.osu.edu/PatientEd/Materials/PDFDocs/nut-diet/nut-other/high-pro.pdf Accessed July 2011.

UA: Urinalysis—*continued*	
Overview and interpretation:	o **Nitrite:** Urinary nitrite is most often the result of bacterial action on excreted urinary nitrate; students and clinicians can remember this by recalling that nitr*a*te is consumed in foods via the *a*limentary tract, while nitr*i*te in the urine generally indicates urinary tract *i*nfection (UTI). A small amount of nitrate is naturally present in some foods, including tap water, beer, some cheese products, cured meats and bacon. Additional environmental sources of nitrate include the nitrates that are intentionally added to foods as preservatives, those which are contaminants from nitrate-containing fertilizers, and those which are present in our polluted environment from pesticides and the manufacture of rubber and latex. Not all bacteria can convert nitrate to nitrite; generally, this reaction indicates the presence of Gram-negative rods such as *Escherichia coli*, the causative agent in the vast majority of UTIs in both men and women. Much less commonly, Gram-positive bacteria may also cause nitrite-positive UTI. A negative urine nitrite does not exclude UTI as it may be due to either a low-nitrate diet, diuretic use, or infection with bacteria that are incapable of reducing nitrate to nitrite.

> **UTI management**
> Finding evidence of a UTI requires the clinician to determine the nature of that UTI—urethritis, prostatitis/vaginitis, cystitis, pyelonephritis—and to evaluate the severity of the infection in the context of the patient's age and comorbitidies.

o **Leukocyte esterase:** Leukocyte esterase—as its name suggests—is an enzyme produced by white blood cells and is therefore associated with urinary tract infection. Up to five minutes is required for the enzyme to fully react with the dipstick reagent. Obviously, a positive dipstick leukocyte esterase does not itself distinguish between benign infectious cystitis and life-threatening pyelonephritis.

o **Red blood cells (RBC):** On a dipstick urinalysis (in contrast to a legitimate microscopic exam), "RBC" are reported not because of the presence of cells but because of the peroxidase activity of erythrocytes, which is also noted with myoglobinuria or hemoglobinuria. Thus, a dipstick analysis "positive for RBC" could indicate legitimate hematuria, or the presence of hemoglobin or myoglobin such as from marked intravascular hemolysis or rhabdomyolysis, respectively. Red blood cells in urine are not "normal" per se, but are not necessarily pathologic. Microhematuria can be induced by many benign events, including sexual

> **Overt hematuria and cancer**
> "Up to 20 percent of patients with gross hematuria have urinary tract malignancy; a full work-up with cystoscopy and upper-tract imaging is indicated in patients with this condition."
>
> Simerville JA, Maxted WC, Pahira JJ. Urinalysis: a comprehensive review. *Am Fam Physician.* 2005 Mar 15;71(6):1153-62 aafp.org/afp/2005/0315/p1153.html

intercourse, exercise, and sample contamination from menstruation. Conversely, pathologic causes of hematuria include urinary tract infections, glomerulonephritis, IgA nephropathy, and nephrolithiasis; overt hematuria is often the first sign of renal or bladder carcinoma. Thus, when consistently present over 2-3 samples, overt or microscopic hematuria—just like any degree of proteinuria—always requires the clinician's attention.

Advantages:	▪ Allows point-of-care testing and thereby facilitates assessment and treatment.
Limitations:	▪ Noted above, e.g., insensitivity to microalbuminuria and mild Bence-Jones proteinuria
Comments:	▪ For additional information, please see any of several excellent clinically-oriented reviews such as Simerville JA, Maxted WC, Pahira JJ. Urinalysis: a comprehensive review. *Am Fam Physician* 2005 Mar http://www.aafp.org/afp/2005/0315/p1153.html

Routine lab evaluation in an asymptomatic elderly female—part 1: Whereas a healthy young adult might be treated nonpharmacologically such as with fluid loading and cranberry juice for a routine UTI, clinicians should appreciate several nuances of this case that add to the complexity of appropriate management. This female patient presented for a routine annual examination. Note the patient's date of birth and the date of examination in the lower right-hand corner of the report. Because of the patient's advanced age, additional considerations are warranted. This patient was also noted to be vitamin D deficient and diabetic at the time of the exam—how does this change the overall management? Clinicians must appreciate that elderly patients are less likely to mount a symptomatic and febrile response to advanced urinary tract infections; therefore consideration to the possiblity of pyelonephritis (life-threatening) in contrast to a simple cystitis (benign) must be considered. If the patient has dementia or clinically significant forgetfulness (both of which are easily tested during the office visit), compliance with treatment is much less likely, particularly if the patient does not have access to home nursing and/or does not have a spouse, relative, friend or neighbor who can aid with the supervision of care. Urinary tract infections tend to be more aggressive in elderly patients, especially those who are diabetic, especially those with micronutrient deficiencies.

Questions:
1. What additional assessments are warranted?
2. Would fluid-loading and use of cranberry juice be appropriate treatment for this patient's UTI?
3. What follow-up is recommended?

```
URINALYSIS              01/06/10
                        11:21
U COLOR                 YELLOW
U CLARITY               CLOUDY**
U GLUCOSE               NEGATIVE
U BILE                  NEGATIVE
U KETONES               NEGATIVE
U SPEC GRAVITY          1.012
U BLOOD                 NEGATIVE
U PH                    6.0
                        (NOTE06)
U PROTEIN QUAL          20**
U UROBILINOGEN          0.2
U NITRITE               NEGATIVE
U LEUK ESTERASE         MODERATE**
U WBC                   53*H
U WBCC                  RARE**
U RBC                   5*H
U SQUAM EPITH           13
U HYALINE CAST          2
U MUCOUS                RARE
(NOTE06)
URINE SAMPLES SUBMITTED FOR TESTING MORE THAN 2 HOURS AFTER COLLECTION MAY
YIELD UNRELIABLE RESULTS WHICH INCLUDE INCREASED pH, INCREASED CRYSTAL
FORMATION AND BACTERIAL CONTENT, AND DEGRADATION OF CELLULAR ELEMENTS.
- - - - - - - - - - - - - - - - - - - - - - - - - - - - - - - - - - - - - - - - - - -
                                BDATE: 03/20/1926 SEX: F RACE:
                                13:59 01/29/10
```

Answers:
1. Assessments: Clinical examination should include cardiac auscultatory exam, careful pulmonary auscultation for basilar crackles, distal extremity examination for edema and peripheral vascular disease, assessment for tenderness of the flanks, abdomen, and back. Vital signs must be assessed: ❶ temperature, ❷ pulse, ❸ blood pressure, ❹ respiratory rate, and ❺ pain. A chemistry panel, CBC with differential, and CRP or ESR should be performed. The urinalysis is sent for microbial culture and sensitivity. Review patient's current drug regimen. If WBC casts were noted on the microscopic exam, then suspected pyelonephritis would warrant hospitalization.
2. Treatments: Fluid-loading would not be appropriate in an elderly patient who might have cardiopulmonary failure, renal insufficiency, or plasma electrolyte imbalance. Cranberry juice is not universally effective and is generally used for UTIs in younger patients who have evidence of *E coli* infection as evidenced by positive urinary nitrite; because this patient's nitrite is negative, a more likely probability exists that the UTI is due to Gram-positive bacteria and thus cranberry juice is less likely to be effective. A clinician could reasonably label this a complicated UTI due to the patient's advanced age and diabetes; thus, either an extended course of Bactrim DS (po b.i.d. for 7-10 days), or Ciprofloxacin (250-500 mg po b.i.d. for 3 days), or Nitrofurantoin (50-100 mg po q6h x7 days or 100 mg ER po q12h x7 days; give w/ food) would be considered. Drug choice depends on patient's tolerance, recent exposure, renal status, drugs, and results of culture and sensitivity.
3. Follow-up: Review laboratory results as soon as possible; if this visit is occurring at the end of the week, the lab should be alerted to phone the clinician with results over the weekend because concomitant leukocytosis or severe acute phase response (suggesting possible pyelonephritis or urosepsis) would change the management on an urgent basis. Patient should return to the office within 24-48 hours for reassessment and repeat UA. Patient is advised to return to office or go to hospital if symptoms develop— especially fever, chills, dizziness, or persistent nausea. Patient requires treatment of vitamin D deficiency and diabetes with appropriate monitoring.

Routine laboratory evaluation in an asymptomatic elderly female—part 2: Readers should review the lab report in the left side of the page before reading the discussion on the right side of the page. *Write the appropriate interpretation and intervention before looking at the answers in the column on the right.* Normal ranges were not provided with the original report.

```
CBC                      01/06/10
                         11:21
 WBC 10E3                  7.50
 NRBC %                     0.0
 NRBC 10E3                 0.00
 RBC 10E6                 4.08*L
 HGB                      11.7*L
 HCT                      35.1*L
 MCV                       86.0
 MCH                       28.7
 MCHC                      33.3
 RDW-CV                    13.7
 RDW-SD                    43.1
 PLATELET 10E3             175
 MPV                       12.3
-----------------------------------
CHEM PANEL               01/06/10
                         11:21
 SODIUM                    140
 POTASSIUM                 4.2
 CHLORIDE                  102
 CO2 VENOUS               27.0
 GLUCOSE                  248*H
 BUN                       22
 SER CREATININE           1.2
 CALCIUM                   9.5
 GLOBULIN                  3.2
 TOTAL PROTEIN            7.3
 ALBUMIN TOT              4.1
 BILI TOTAL               0.5
 ALKALINE PHOSPHA          63
 SGOT (AST)                15
 CHOLESTEROL              186
                        (NOTE01)
 TRIGLYCERIDES            122
 SGPT (ALT)                11
 ANION GAP                 11
 OSMOLRTY CALC            291
 BUN/CREAT                18.3
 ALB/GLOB RATIO           1.30
 HDL                       31
                        (NOTE02)
 LDL CALC                 131*H
                        (NOTE03)
(NOTE01)
BORDERLINE HIGH RISK = 200-239
HIGH RISK = 240 AND ABOVE.
(NOTE02)
12-16 HR FASTING:
(NOTE03)
NORMAL = LESS THAN 130 MG/DL
130-159 BORDERLINE/HIGH RISK
>/= 160 HIGH RISK
-----------------------------------
CHEM SPECIAL             01/06/10
                         11:21
 HEMOGLOBIN A1C           7.6*H
                        (NOTE04)
 25-OHD TOTAL              29
-----------------------------------
BDATE: 03/20/1926 SEX: F
13:59 01/29/10 FROM E585
```

This patient is anemic. The anemia is not of a severity that would be expected to cause cardiopulmonary/perfusion deficits, but the patient should be assessed, particularly if he/she has history of heart failure or lung disease such as emphysema. The MCV is not elevated, nor is it low. This could be due to combined B-12/folate and iron deficiencies; the patient should be tested and treated appropriately. Assuming that the ferritin is low, what is the next mandatory step in the management of this patient? [Answer: Treat the iron deficiency with iron supplementation but be sure to refer the patient for gastrointestinal endoscopy because of the increased probability of intestinal lesion, especially colon cancer.]

This patient is diagnosed with diabetes mellitus because the glucose is above 200. Cardioprotective measures must be implemented, ophthalmologist eye exam initiated, and foot exam performed. An integrative anti-diabetes plan[126] should be implemented.

Clinicians must appreciate the importance of the MDRD equation in this case. The answer is provided below. Perform the Cockcroft-Gault equation on paper (with use of a calculator if necessary), then perform the MDRD equation. Does this change the management of this patient's UTI? Does this change the overall management of this patient? [Answer: This patient has renal insufficiency (GFR 48-55 if African-American and 42-45 if "other race") and therefore some drugs are now contraindicated. Patient is at increased risk of hyperkalemia, especially if taking ACEi or ARB medications. The wise clinician would consider referral to an internist or nephrologist in order to ensure that the patient receives proper monitoring; for example, if the diabetes and renal insufficiency progress, the patient may require dialysis and—possibly—renal transplant, although transplant is unlikely in a patient of this advanced age.][Note 127]

Triglycerides and LDL are higher than optimal. Diet therapy and combination fatty acid supplementation (described later in this text) is indicated. Berberine might be considered as an adjunct.

HgbA1c greater than 6.5% diagnoses diabetes mellitus.

The vitamin D level is low and should be supported with oral administration of 2,000 - 10,000 IU/d and retested at 2-6 months. Serum calcium should be tested after 2-4 weeks of therapy—sooner if the patient is taking a calcium-sparing drug such as hydrochlorothiazide—and again at about 6 and 12 months.

---

[126] Vasquez A. *Chiropractic and Naturopathic Mastery of Common Clinical Disorders*. http://optimalhealthresearch.com/clinical_mastery.html
[127] Review of this case by Dr Barry Morgan (MD, emergency medicine) is acknowledged and appreciated.

A 45yo HLA-B27+ woman with recurrent UTIs and a 7-year history of ankylosing spondylitis treated with anti-TNF drugs: Positive urine culture and positive stool culture demonstrating bacteria (*Escherichia coli* and *Klebsiella pneumoniae*) known to share molecular mimicry and cross-reactivity with HLA-B27: The Gram-negative bacterium *E. coli* produces a protein named "hypothetical protein 168" (Protein Identification Resource [PIR] data bank access code #jp0612) which shares the amino acid sequence "**RRYLE**" with HLA-B27, which contains the sequence "EWL**RRYLE**IGKETLQRVDP."[128] Per the same citation, *Klebsiella pneumoniae*'s protein (PIR s01840) nitrogenase (reductase) molybdenum-iron protein NifN contains the sequence "EWLRR." This amino acid homology confers validation to the phenomenon of molecular mimicry and thus that immune system components such as immunoglobulins and activated T-cells can cross-react between microbial peptides and human tissue antigens.[129] This patient was treated with the combination pharmaceutical antibiotic trimethoprim and sulfamethoxazole commonly referred to as "Bactrim DS" in addition to dietary optimization, hormonal optimization, and nutritional supplementation. Antimicrobial treatment with amoxicillin-clavulanate would have been reasonable, too, except for this patient's prior allergic reaction to the drug.

```
Urine Culture, Routine
  Urine Culture, Routine          Final Report
  Result 1
      Escherichia coli
      50,000-100,000 colony forming units per mL
  Antimicrobial Susceptibility
      ***** S = Susceptible; I = Intermediate; R = Resistant *****
                   P = Positive; N = Negative
          MICS are expressed in micrograms per mL
```

Antibiotic	RSLT#1
Amoxicillin/Clavulanic Acid	S
Ampicillin	S
Cefazolin	S
Cefepime	S
Ceftriaxone	S
Cefuroxime	S
Cephalothin	I
Ciprofloxacin	R
ESBL	N
Ertapenem	S
Gentamicin	S
Imipenem	S
Levofloxacin	R
Nitrofurantoin	S
Piperacillin	S
Tetracycline	S
Tobramycin	S
Trimethoprim/Sulfa	S

Comprehensive Stool Analysis / Parasitology x3

BACTERIOLOGY CULTURE		
Expected/Beneficial flora	**Commensal (Imbalanced) flora**	**Dysbiotic flora**
4+ Bacteroides fragilis group	3+ Alpha hemolytic strep	3+ Klebsiella pneumoniae ssp pneumoniae
3+ Bifidobacterium spp.		
4+ Escherichia coli		
3+ Lactobacillus spp.		
NG Enterococcus spp.		
2+ Clostridium spp.		
NG = No Growth		

PRESCRIPTIVE AGENTS

	Resistant	Intermediate	Susceptible
Amoxicillin-Clavulanic Acid			S
Ampicillin	R		
Cefazolin			S
Ceftazidime			S
Ciprofloxacin			S
Trimeth-sulfa			S

Susceptible results imply that an infection due to the bacteria may be appropriately treated when the recommended dosage of the tested antimicrobial agent is used.
Intermediate results imply that response rates may be lower than for susceptible bacteria when the tested antimicrobial agent is used.
Resistant results imply that the bacteria will not be inhibited by normal dosage levels of the tested antimicrobial agent.

---

[128] Scofield RH, Warren WL, Koelsch G, Harley JB. A hypothesis for the HLA-B27 immune dysregulation in spondyloarthropathy: contributions from enteric organisms, B27 structure, peptides bound by B27, and convergent evolution. *Proc Natl Acad Sci U S A*. 1993 Oct 15;90(20):9330-4
[129] Rashid T, Ebringer A. Ankylosing spondylitis is linked to Klebsiella--the evidence. *Clin Rheumatol*. 2007 Jun;26(6):858-64

CRP: C-reactive protein	
Overview and interpretation:	<ul><li>CRP is a protein made by the liver in response to the immunologic activation characteristic of infectious and inflammatory conditions. Generally, any tissue injury or inflammatory process especially that involves the immune system's increased production of IL-6 will result in increased production of CRP.[130] High sensitivity CRP (hsCRP) is preferred over regular CRP due to its greater sensitivity and use in assessing cardiovascular risk.</li><li>Elevated values are seen with:<ul><li>Infections: Bacterial, fungal, parasitic, viral diseases; some patients with dysbiosis[131] will have mildly-moderately elevated CRP,</li><li>Inflammatory bowel disease: Crohn's disease and ulcerative colitis (higher in CD than UC),</li><li>Autoimmune disease: Rheumatoid arthritis, polymyalgia rheumatica, giant cell arteritis, polyarteritis nodosa, (not always SLE),</li><li>Acute myocardial infarction or other tissue ischemia</li><li>Organ transplant rejection: Renal, (not cardiac),</li><li>Trauma: Burns, surgery,</li><li>Obesity: Leads to modest elevations in CRP.</li></ul></li></ul>
Advantages:	<ul><li>This is an excellent screening test for differentiating "serious problems" (e.g., inflammatory and infectious arthropathy) from "benign problems" such as osteoarthritis.</li><li>Since higher values of CRP are a well-recognized risk factor for cardiovascular disease, screening "musculoskeletal patients" with hsCRP provides data for cardiovascular risk assessment and a more comprehensive and holistic treatment approach, thus bridging the gap between acute care and preventive care.</li></ul>
Limitations:	<ul><li>Elevations in CRP are completely nonspecific, requiring clinical investigation to determine the underlying cause of the immune activation.</li><li>CRP may be normal in some patients with severe systemic diseases (such as lupus or cancer), and therefore a normal CRP does not entirely exclude the presence of significant illness.</li></ul>
Comments:	<ul><li>Writing in *The New England Journal of Medicine*, authors Gabay and Kushner[132] note that measurements of plasma or serum **C-reactive protein can help differentiate inflammatory from non-inflammatory conditions and are useful in managing the patient's disease, since "the concentration often reflects the response to and the need for therapeutic intervention."** Additionally, they note, "Most normal subjects have plasma C-reactive protein concentrations of 2 mg per liter or less, but some have concentrations as high as 10 mg per liter." Deodhar[133] noted that **"Any clinical disease characterized by tissue injury and/or inflammation is accompanied by significant elevation of serum CRP…"** and that **CRP should replace ESR as a method of laboratory evaluation.** Deodhar also noted that **some patients with severe SLE will have normal CRP levels.**</li></ul>

---

[130] Deodhar SD. C-reactive protein: the best laboratory indicator available for monitoring disease activity. *Cleve Clin J Med* 1989 Mar-Apr;56(2):126-30

[131] See chapter 4 of *Integrative Rheumatology* and Vasquez A. Reducing Pain and Inflammation Naturally. Part 6: Nutritional and Botanical Treatments Against "Silent Infections" and Gastrointestinal Dysbiosis, Commonly Overlooked Causes of Neuromusculoskeletal Inflammation and Chronic Health Problems. *Nutr Perspect* 2006; Jan http://optimalhealthresearch.com/part6

[132] Gabay C, Kushner I. Acute-phase proteins and other systemic responses to inflammation. *N Engl J Med*. 1999 Feb 11;340(6):448-54

[133] Deodhar SD. C-reactive protein: the best laboratory indicator available for monitoring disease activity. *Cleve Clin J Med* 1989 Mar-Apr;56(2):126-30

Elevated hsCRP (high-sensitivity c-reactive protein) in a male patient with metabolic syndrome and rheumatoid arthritis—response to treatment protocol in _Integrative Rheumatology_: This 52-year-old male patient presented with a 4-year history of rheumatoid arthritis which was unresponsive to prednisone and anti-TNF (tumor necrosis factor alpha) drugs, ie, "biologics." As expected, the prednisone exacerbated the patient's insulin resistance and hypertension; the drug failed to produce an anti-inflammatory benefit for this patient. At a cost of several thousand dollars per treatment, the anti-TNF "biologic" drugs failed to provide any benefit. At the intial visit in July 2005, the hsCRP level was 124 mg/L (normal range 0-3 mg/L), as shown in these lab results.

DATE OF SPECIMEN	TIME	DATE RECEIVED	DATE REPORTED	TIME		Houston		TX	77036-0000
7/08/2005	16:19	7/08/2005	7/11/2005	7:38	419	ACCOUNT NUMBER:	42407150		

TEST	RESULT	LIMITS	LAB
C-Reactive Protein, Cardiac			
> C-Reactive Protein, Cardiac	124.00H mg/L	0.00 - 3.00	HD

Relative Risk for Future Cardiovascular Event
Low   <1.00
Average   1.00 - 3.00
High   >3.00

The patient was treated with the protocol outlined in Chapter 4 of _Integrative Rheumatology_.[134] Stool testing showed _Citrobacter freundii_ (renamed _Citrobacter rodentium_) which was addressed with botanical medicines; the insufficiency dysbiosis was also corrected per the five-part protocol. Slightly low testosterone and slightly elevated estradiol was optimized with a pharmaceutical aromatase inhibitor (Arimidex) given twice weekly. The five-part nutritional wellness protocol (supplemented Paleo-Mediterranean diet [SPMD]) was implemented.[135]

Comprehensive Parasitology, stool, x2

MICROBIOLOGY

Bacteriology Culture

Beneficial flora		Imbalances		Dysbiotic flora	
Bifidobacter	0+	Gamma strep	1+	Citrobacter freundii	1+
E. coli	2+	Enterobacter sp.	1+		
Lactobacillus	0+				

Mycology (Yeast) Culture

Normal flora	Dysbiotic flora
No yeast isolated	

PARASITOLOGY

	Sample 1		Sample 2
No	Ova or Parasites	No	Ova or Parasites

No anti-inflammatory drugs or botanicals were used. Within five weeks of treatment, the patient's hsCRP dropped from 124 mg/L to 7.58 mg/L—a reduction of approximately 95%—far superior to any previoius response to corticosteroid and biologic drugs. Patient experienced significant alleviation of pain and improved mobility.

8/17/2005	11:06	8/18/2005	8/18/2005	12:32	708	ACCOUNT NUMBER:	42407150	

TEST	RESULT	LIMITS	LAB
C-Reactive Protein, Cardiac			
C-Reactive Protein, Cardiac	7.58H mg/L	0.00 - 3.00	HD

---

[134] Vasquez A. _Integrative Rheumatology_. http://optimalhealthresearch.com/textbooks/rheumatology.html
[135] Vasquez A. Revisiting the Five-Part Nutritional Wellness Protocol. _Nutritional Perspectives_ 2011 January http://optimalhealthresearch.com/spmd

ESR: erythrocyte sedimentation rate	

Overview and interpretation:	▪ Values may be elevated even when no pathology is present because ESR increases with anemia and with age.
	
	▪ Much more sensitive than WBC count when screening for infection.[136]
	
	▪ May be normal in about 10% of patients who have pathology such as **giant cell arteritis** and **polymyalgia rheumatica** (conditions where it is generally the only lab abnormality, besides anemia); may also be normal in several other diseases.
	
	▪ **May be normal in patients with septic arthritis and patients with crystal-induced arthritis: joint aspiration for synovial fluid analysis is indicated if septic arthritis is suspected.**[137]
	
	▪ Increased with age, anemia, inflammation; higher in women than men. Age-adjusted normal ranges: any value over 25 is considered high in young people, or 40 in elderly women.
	
	▪ Age-related adjustments for men and women are as follows:
	  1. Men: age divided by 2
	  2. Women: (age + 10) divided by 2

Advantages:	▪ Inexpensive and easy to perform—use the same lavender-topped tube that you use for CBC. ▪ Provides a quick screen for infection, inflammation, and multiple myeloma—the most common primary bone tumor in adults. ▪ In patients with elevated levels, ESR can be used to monitor progression of disease and response to treatment.[138] However, a negative/normal test result does not exclude the presence of significant disease; some noteworthy examples include the following: 1) elderly—due to diminished ability to mount an inflammatory response, 2) patients taking anti-inflammatory drugs and immunosuppressants, 3) a significant proportion of patients with lupus will have normal ESR despite aggressive disease, and 4) some cancer patients with clinically significant tumor burden will not show signs of systemic inflammation. ▪ **ESR may be more reliable than CRP for multiple myeloma.**[139]
Limitations:	▪ ESR may be normal in a subset of patients with clinically significant infection or inflammation. ▪ Values are elevated in the elderly and patients with anemia and are thus not necessarily indicative of disease in these populations.
Comments:	▪ **This test is generally considered *outdated* and has been replaced in most circumstances by CRP for the evaluation of inflammation and infection.** ▪ **The only time I use this test clinically is when I am highly suspicious of inflammation and the CRP is normal. Further, this test may be preferred when assessing for temporal arteritis and for multiple myeloma, two conditions which are classically associated with elevated ESR.**

---

[136] Shaw BA, Gerardi JA, Hennrikus WL. How to avoid orthopedic pitfalls in children. *Patient Care* 1999; Feb 28: 95-116

[137] Klippel JH (ed). <u>Primer on the Rheumatic Diseases. 11th Edition</u>. Atlanta: Arthritis Foundation. 1997 page 94

[138] Shojania K. Rheumatology: 2. What laboratory tests are needed? *CMAJ*. 2000 Apr 18;162(8):1157-63 http://www.cmaj.ca/cgi/content/full/162/8/1157

[139] "We conclude that ESR, a simple and easily performed marker, was found to be an independent prognostic factor for survival in patients with multiple myeloma." Alexandrakis MG, Passam FH, Ganotakis ES, Sfiridaki K, Xilouri I, Perisinakis K, Kyriakou DS. The clinical and prognostic significance of erythrocyte sedimentation rate (ESR), serum interleukin-6 (IL-6) and acute phase protein levels in multiple myeloma. *Clin Lab Haematol.* 2003;25:41-6

Ferritin	
Overview and interpretation:	▪ Ferritin levels are directly proportional to body iron stores, except in patients with inflammation, infection, hepatitis, or cancer. Therefore, measuring ferritin allows assessment for iron deficiency (a cause of fatigue, or early manifestation of GI cancer) and allows for assessment of iron overload (as a cause of joint pain and arthropathy). This test should be performed in all African Americans[140,141], white men over age 30 years[142], diabetics[143], and patients with peripheral arthropathy[144], and exercise-associated joint pain[145,146] The research also justifies testing children[147], women[148], young adults[149] and the general asymptomatic public.[150] ▪ <u>Low ferritin = iron deficiency</u> ▪ <u>High ferritin = iron overload, cancer, inflammation, infection, and/or hepatitis (viral, alcoholic, or toxic)</u>
Advantages:	▪ Reliable screening test for iron overload when used in conjunction with patient assessment and evidence (e.g., normal CRP) of no infection or acute phase response. ▪ This is the blood test of choice for iron deficiency *and* iron overload.
Limitations:	▪ Iron-deficient patients with an acute phase response may have a falsely normal level of ferritin since ferritin is an acute phase reactant and will be elevated *disproportionate to iron status* during inflammation. ▪ Elevations of ferritin (i.e., >200 mcg/L in women and >300 mcg/L in men) need to be retested along with CRP (to rule out false elevation due to excessive inflammation) before making the presumptive diagnosis of iron overload. **In the absence of significant inflammation, ferritin values >200 mcg/L in women and >300 mcg/L in men indicate iron overload and the need for treatment regardless of the absence of symptoms or end-stage complications.**[151]
Comments:	▪ Note that since ferritin is an acute-phase reactant, a high level of serum ferritin by itself does not allow differentiation between iron overload, infection, and the inflammation associated with tissue injury or metastatic disease. Ferritin must be evaluated within the context of the patient's clinical condition and the assessment of at least one other marker for inflammation such as CRP. If the patient is not acutely ill or has not recently suffered tissue injury (e.g., myocardial infarction) and the CRP is normal, then an elevated ferritin value indicates iron overload until proven otherwise with diagnostic phlebotomy, which is safer and less expensive than liver biopsy or MRI. Transferrin saturation can also be measured when the interpretation of ferritin is unclear. By itself, serum iron is unreliable.

[140] Barton JC, Edwards CQ, Bertoli LF, Shroyer TW, Hudson SL. Iron overload in African Americans. *Am J Med*. 1995 Dec;99(6):616-23

[141] Wurapa RK, Gordeuk VR, Brittenham GM, et al. Primary iron overload in African Americans. *Am J Med*. 1996;101(1):9-18

[142] Baer DM, Simons JL, et al. Hemochromatosis screening in asymptomatic ambulatory men 30 years of age and older. *Am J Med*. 1995 May;98:464-8

[143] Phelps G, Chapman I, Hall P, Braund W, Mackinnon M. Prevalence of genetic haemochromatosis among diabetic patients. *Lancet* 1989; 2: 233-4

[144] Olynyk J, Hall P, Ahern M, KwiatekR, MackinnonM. Screening for hemochromatosis in a rheumatology clinic. *Aust NZ J Med* 1994; 24: 22-5

[145] McCurdie I, Perry JD. Haemochromatosis and exercise related joint pains. *BMJ*. 1999 Feb 13;318(7181):449-5

[146] "RESULTS: Our findings indicate a high prevalence of HFE gene mutations in this population (49.2%) compared with sedentary controls (33.5%). No association was detected in the athletes between mutations and blood iron markers. CONCLUSIONS: The findings support the need to assess regularly iron stores in elite endurance athletes." Chicharro JL, Hoyos J, Gomez-Gallego F, Villa JG, Bandres F, Celaya P, Jimenez F, Alonso JM, Cordova A, Lucia A. Mutations in the hereditary haemochromatosis gene HFE in professional endurance athletes. *Br J Sports Med*. 2004 Aug;38(4):418-21. Erratum in: *Br J Sports Med*. 2004 Dec;38(6):793 http://bjsm.bmjjournals.com/cgi/content/full/38/4/418 Accessed September 12, 2005

[147] Kaikov Y, Wadsworth LD, Hassall E, Dimmick JE, Rogers PCJ. Primary hemochromatosis in children: report of three newly diagnosed cases and review of the pediatric literature. *Pediatrics* 1992; 90: 37-42

[148] Edwards CQ, Kushner JP. Screening for hemochromatosis. *N Engl J Med* 1993; 328: 1616-20

[149] Gushusrt TP, Triest WE. Diagnosis and management of precirrhotic hemochromatosis. *W Virginia Med J* 1990; 86: 91-5

[150] Balan V, et al. Screening for hemochromatosis: a cost-effectiveness study based on 12, 258 patients. *Gastroenterology* 1994; 107: 453-9

[151] **Barton JC, McDonnell SM, Adams PC, Brissot P, Powell LW, Edwards CQ, Cook JD, Kowdley KV. Management of hemochromatosis. Hemochromatosis Management Working Group.** *Ann Intern Med*. **1998 Dec 1;129(11):932-9—one of the best papers ever written on this topic.**

Ferritin — *Interpretation of serum levels*

Ferritin	Categorization and management
≥ 800 mcg/L	<u>Practically diagnostic of iron overload</u>[152]: Repeat tests; rule out inflammation or occult pathology. Initiate phlebotomy and consider liver biopsy or MRI.
≥ 300 mcg/L	<u>Probable iron overload</u>[153]: Repeat tests; rule out inflammation or occult pathology. In men, initiate phlebotomy and consider liver biopsy or MRI.[154]
≥ 200 mcg/L	*In women*: <u>Suggestive of iron overload</u>[155]: Repeat tests, rule out inflammation or occult pathology. In women, initiate phlebotomy and consider liver biopsy or MRI.[156] *In men*: <u>High-normal *unhealthy* iron status with increased risk of myocardial infarction</u>[157]: Rule out inflammation or occult pathology. No follow-up is mandated, yet blood donation and/or abstention from dietary iron are recommended preventative healthcare measures.
≥ 160 mcg/L	*In women*: <u>Abnormal iron status</u>[158]: Repeat tests, rule out inflammation or occult pathology. Consider phlebotomy and liver biopsy or MRI.
≥80-120 mcg/L	<u>High-normal unhealthy iron status</u>[159,160]: No follow-up is mandated; blood donation and abstention from dietary iron are suggested preventative healthcare measures.
40-70 mcg/L	**<u>Optimal iron status for most people</u>[161,162]**
< 20 mcg/L	<u>Iron deficiency</u>: Search for occult gastrointestinal blood loss with endoscopy or imaging assessments in adults; refer to gastroenterologist.[163,164]

Ferritin is an acute-phase reactant, which means that its production is increased during the acute phase of inflammatory and/or infectious disorders. Therefore the numeric value and hence its clinical meaning can be interpreted only within a context that also includes assessment of the patient's inflammatory status, which is best assessed with either ESR or CRP. If CRP/ESR is high, then the physician might assume that the ferritin value is "falsely elevated" — disproportionately elevated with respect to body iron stores. *Common clinical examples requiring use and skillful interpretation of ferritin*:

- **<u>Elderly or arthritic patient with iron deficiency despite normal serum ferritin</u>**: An elderly patient with normal ferritin and elevated CRP/ESR is probably iron deficient; retesting of ferritin and measurement of transferrin saturation and CBC should be performed promptly. If iron deficiency is confirmed or cannot be excluded, referral for endoscopic examination must be implemented. In a patient with known inflammatory arthropathy, the ferritin may appear normal even though the patient is iron deficient and in need of supplementation and endoscopy.

- **<u>Non-anemic iron deficiency</u>**: A middle-aged patient (commonly a premenopausal woman) presents with fatigue and during the course of evaluation is found to have a normal CBC. **Do not let a normal CBC prevent you from assessing ferritin; many of these patients are completely iron deficient with ferritin values of 2-6 mcg/L and are in need of iron replacement as well as evaluation for celiac disease, *H. pylori* infection, hematuria, and — as is often warranted — gastrointestinal bleeding/lesions.**

[152] Milman N, Albeck MJ. Distinction between homozygous and heterozygous subjects with hemochromatosis using iron status markers and receiver operating characteristic (ROC) analysis. *Eur J Clin Biochem* 1995; 33: 95-8. See also Milman N. Iron status markers in hereditary hemochromatosis: distinction between individuals being homozygous and heterozygous for the hemochromatosis allele. *Eur J Haematol* 1991;47:292-8

[153] Olynyk JK, Bacon BR. Hereditary hemochromatosis: detecting and correcting iron overload. *Postgrad Med* 1994;96: 151-65

[154] "Therapeutic phlebotomy is used to remove excess iron and maintain low normal body iron stores, … initiated in men with serum ferritin levels of 300 microg/L or more and in women with serum ferritin levels of 200 microg/L or more, regardless of the presence or absence of symptoms." Barton JC, McDonnell SM, Adams PC, Brissot P, Powell LW, Edwards CQ, Cook JD, Kowdley KV. Management of hemochromatosis. Hemochromatosis Management Working Group. *Ann Intern Med.* 1998 Dec 1;129(11):932-9

[155] Barton JC, Edwards CQ, Bertoli LF, Shroyer TW, Hudson SL. Iron overload in African Americans. *Am J Med* 1995; 99: 616-23

[156] Barton JC, McDonnell SM, Adams PC, et al. Management of hemochromatosis. *Ann Intern Med.* 1998 Dec 1;129(11):932-9

[157] Salonen JT, Nyyssonen K, Korpela H, Tuomilehto J, Seppanen R, Salonen R. High stored iron levels are associated with excess risk of myocardial infarction in eastern Finnish men. *Circulation* 1992; 86: 803-11

[158] Nicoll D. Therapeutic drug monitoring and laboratory reference ranges. In: Tierney LM, McPhee SJ, Papadakis MA. *Current Medical Diagnosis and Treatment 1996 (35th Edition)*. Stamford: Appleton and Lange, 1996: 1442

[159] Lauffer, RB. *Iron and Your Heart*. New York: St. Martin's Press, 1991: 79-8, 83-88, 162

[160] Sullivan JL. Iron and the sex difference in heart disease risk. *Lancet.* 1981 Jun 13;1(8233):1293-4

[161] Lauffer, RB. *Iron and Your Heart*. New York: St. Martin's Press, 1991: 79-8, 83-88, 162

[162] **Vasquez A**. High body iron stores: causes, effects, diagnosis, and treatment. *Nutritional Perspectives* 1994; 17: 13, 15-7, 19, 21, 28 and **Vasquez A**. Men's Health: Iron in men: why men store this nutrient in their bodies and the harm that it does. *MEN Magazine* 1997; Jan:11,21-23 vix.com/menmag/alexiron.htm

[163] Rockey DC, Cello JP. Evaluation of the gastrointestinal tract in patients with iron-deficiency anemia. *N Engl J Med.* 1993;329(23):1691-5

[164] "Endoscopy revealed a clinically important lesion in 23 (12%) of 186 patients. … CONCLUSIONS: Endoscopy yields important findings in premenopausal women with iron deficiency anemia, which should not be attributed solely to menstrual blood loss." Bini EJ, Micale PL, Weinshel EH. Evaluation of the gastrointestinal tract in premenopausal women with iron deficiency anemia. *Am J Med.* 1998 Oct;105(4):281-6

Arthritis & Rheumatism

Official Journal of the American College of Rheumatology

VOLUME 39   OCTOBER 1996   NO. 10

1767   1768

Musculoskeletal disorders and iron overload disease: comment on the American College of Rheumatology guidelines for the initial evaluation of the adult patient with acute musculoskeletal symptoms

To the Editor:

The recent clinical guidelines for the initial evaluation of the adult patient with acute musculoskeletal symptoms, proposed by the American College of Rheumatology (1), provide useful information and a good review for clinicians. However, there is one important omission in these guidelines. Nowhere in the guidelines is hemochromatosis mentioned. Such a prevalent and potentially life-threatening disease certainly deserves to be considered in the evaluation of patients with musculoskeletal disorders.

Hereditary hemochromatosis is now thought to be the most common genetic disorder in the white population (2). Approximately 1 in 250 persons is homozygous for this disorder and will develop the characteristic clinical manifestations such as diabetes, cardiomyopathy, liver disease, endocrine dysfunction, and, most notable for this discussion, arthropathy or other musculoskeletal disorders (2). Although hereditary iron overload disorders have traditionally been thought of as occurring exclusively in whites, recent research by Barton et al (3) indicates that approximately 1 in 67 African-Americans is affected by an etiologically distinct and severe form of iron overload. Hereditary iron overload disorders have been detected in persons of every ethnic background.

Arthropathy affects up to 80% of iron-overloaded patients and is often the only manifestation of this disease (4). Joint pain is a common and early symptom of iron overload, and "bone pain" has also been described as a common initial complaint (5). Clinically and radiographically, hemochromatoic arthropathy can resemble osteoarthritis, calcium pyrophosphate dihydrate deposition disease, pseudogout, rheumatoid arthritis, ankylosing spondylitis, or generalized osteopenia with osteoporotic fractures (4,6,7). Since iron overload can cause such a wide array of musculoskeletal manifestations and because definitive clinical differentiation of iron overload from other arthropathies is very difficult, patients with peripheral arthropathy should be screened for iron overload. Indeed, recent research by Olynyk et al (8) indicates that the prevalence of iron overload is 5 times higher in patients with peripheral arthropathy than in the general population. Therefore, screening of patients with peripheral arthropathy for the possible presence of iron overload is justified.

Thus, since iron overload affects such a large portion of the population and arthropathy is a common manifestation of this disorder, patients with musculoskeletal symptoms should be screened for iron overload (4,8). The current literature suggests that everyone should be screened for iron overload even if there are no symptoms (8–10).

Alex Vasquez, DC
Seattle, WA

1. American College of Rheumatology Ad Hoc Committee on Clinical Guidelines: Guidelines for the initial evaluation of the adult patient with acute musculoskeletal symptoms. Arthritis Rheum 39:1–8, 1996
2. Olynyk JK, Bacon BR: Hereditary hemochromatosis: detecting and correcting iron overload. Postgrad Med 96:151–165, 1994
3. Barton JC, Edwards CQ, Bertoli LF, Shroyer TW, Hudson SL: Iron overload in African Americans. Am J Med 99:616–623, 1995
4. Faraawi R, Harth M, Kertesz A, Bell D: Arthritis in hemochromatosis. J Rheumatol 20:448–452, 1993
5. Adams PC, Kertesz AE, Valberg LS: Clinical presentation of hemochromatosis: a changing scene. Am J Med 90:445–449, 1991
6. Bywaters EGL, Hamilton EBD, Williams R: The spine in idiopathic hemochromatosis. Ann Rheum Dis 30:453–465, 1971
7. Eyres KS, McCloskey EV, Fern ED, Rogers S, Beneton M, Aaron JE, Kanis JA: Osteoporotic fractures: an unusual presentation of hemochromatosis. Bone 13:431–433, 1992
8. Olynyk J, Hall P, Ahern M, Kwiatek R, Mackinnon M: Screening for hemochromatosis in a rheumatology clinic. Aust N Z J Med 24:22–25, 1994
9. Baer DM, Simmons JL, Staples RL, Runmore GJ, Morton CJ: Hemochromatosis screening in asymptomatic ambulatory men 30 years of age and older. Am J Med 98:464–468, 1995
10. Adams PC, Gregor JC, Kertesz AE, Valberg LS: Screening blood donors for hereditary hemochromatosis: decision analysis model based on a 30-year database. Gastroenterology 109:177–188, 1995

Vasquez A. Musculoskeletal disorders and iron overload disease: comment on the American College of Rheumatology guidelines for the initial evaluation of the adult patient with acute musculoskeletal symptoms. *Arthritis Rheum.* 1996 Oct;39(10):1767-8 http://www.ncbi.nlm.nih.gov/pubmed/8843875

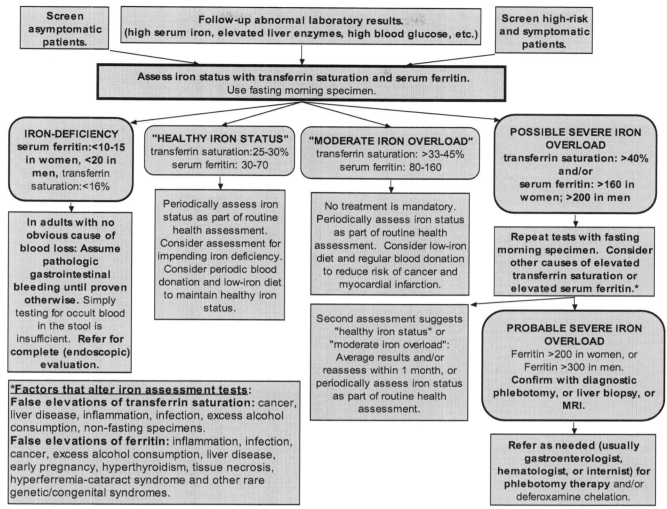

| Screen asymptomatic patients. | Follow-up abnormal laboratory results. (high serum iron, elevated liver enzymes, high blood glucose, etc.) | Screen high-risk and symptomatic patients. |

Assess iron status with transferrin saturation and serum ferritin.
Use fasting morning specimen.

IRON-DEFICIENCY
serum ferritin:<10-15 in women, <20 in men, transferrin saturation:<16%

"HEALTHY IRON STATUS"
transferrin saturation:25-30%
serum ferritin: 30-70

"MODERATE IRON OVERLOAD"
transferrin saturation: >33-45%
serum ferritin: 80-160

POSSIBLE SEVERE IRON OVERLOAD
transferrin saturation: >40% and/or
serum ferritin: >160 in women; >200 in men

In adults with no obvious cause of blood loss: Assume pathologic gastrointestinal bleeding until proven otherwise. Simply testing for occult blood in the stool is insufficient. **Refer for complete (endoscopic) evaluation.**

Periodically assess iron status as part of routine health assessment. Consider assessment for impending iron deficiency. Consider periodic blood donation and low-iron diet to maintain healthy iron status.

No treatment is mandatory. Periodically assess iron status as part of routine health assessment. Consider low-iron diet and regular blood donation to reduce risk of cancer and myocardial infarction.

Repeat tests with fasting morning specimen. Consider other causes of elevated transferrin saturation or elevated serum ferritin.*

Second assessment suggests "healthy iron status" or "moderate iron overload": Average results and/or reassess within 1 month, or periodically assess iron status as part of routine health assessment.

PROBABLE SEVERE IRON OVERLOAD
Ferritin >200 in women, or Ferritin >300 in men.
Confirm with diagnostic phlebotomy, or liver biopsy, or MRI.

*Factors that alter iron assessment tests:
False elevations of transferrin saturation: cancer, liver disease, inflammation, infection, excess alcohol consumption, non-fasting specimens.
False elevations of ferritin: inflammation, infection, cancer, excess alcohol consumption, liver disease, early pregnancy, hyperthyroidism, tissue necrosis, hyperferremia-cataract syndrome and other rare genetic/congenital syndromes.

Refer as needed (usually gastroenterologist, hematologist, or internist) for phlebotomy therapy and/or deferoxamine chelation.

Algorithm for the comprehensive management of iron status: The above flow-chart delineates the management of high-moderate-healthy-low iron status.

Basic treatments for severe iron overload:
- **Iron-removal therapy is mandatory:** Phlebotomy therapy is generally performed weekly or twice-weekly; deferoxamine chelation is reserved for patients who do not withstand phlebotomy (due to cardiomyopathy, severe anemia, or hypoproteinemia) or may be used concurrently with phlebotomy in some patients. Periodically assess hematologic and iron indexes. Continue with weekly iron removal therapy until patient reaches mild iron-deficiency anemia, then decrease frequency and continue phlebotomy as needed (e.g., 4 times per year).
- **Laboratory tests and physical examination:** Assess general physical condition and hepatic, cardiac, endocrine, and general health status.
- **Confirm diagnosis:** Liver biopsy ("gold standard") or diagnostic phlebotomy; perhaps MRI.
- **Assess liver status:** Liver biopsy ("gold standard") or perhaps MRI. Cirrhosis indicates increased risk of hepatocellular carcinoma and reduced life expectancy. Consider liver ultrasound, serum liver enzyme measurement, and serum alpha-fetoprotein to screen for hepatocellular carcinoma every 6 months. Hepatoma surveillance is mandatory in cirrhotic patients.
- **Implement dietary modifications and nutritional therapies:** Avoid iron supplements, multivitamin supplements with iron, iron-fortified foods, liver, beef, pork, alcohol, and excess vitamin C. Ensure adequate protein intake to replace protein lost during phlebotomy. Diet modifications are not substitutes for iron removal therapy. Consider antioxidant therapy.
- **Screen all blood relatives of patients with primary iron overload**. *Mandatory!*
- **Monitor patient condition, and compliance** with lifelong phlebotomy therapy
- **Assess and address psychoemotional issues/concerns**

25(OH)D: serum 25(OH) vitamin D	
Overview and interpretation:	▪ **Vitamin D deficiency is a common cause of musculoskeletal pain**[165,166,167], and vitamin D deficiency is a significant risk factor for cancer and other serious health problems.[168,169,170] ▪ Measurement of serum 25(OH) vitamin D (or empiric treatment with 2,000 – 10,000 IU vitamin D3 per day for adults) is indicated in patients with chronic musculoskeletal pain, particularly low-back pain.[171] Optimal vitamin D status correlates with serum 25(OH)D levels of 50 – 100 ng/mL (125 - 250 nmol/L)—see our review article for more details[172]; levels greater than 100 ng/mL are unnecessary and increase the risk of hypercalcemia. 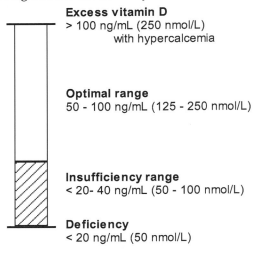 **Interpretation of serum 25(OH) vitamin D levels**. Modified from Vasquez et al, *Alternative Therapies in Health and Medicine* 2004 and Vasquez A. *Musculoskeletal Pain: Expanded Clinical Strategies* (Institute for Functional Medicine) 2008.
Advantages:	▪ Accurate assessment of vitamin D status.
Limitations:	▪ Patients with certain granulomatous conditions such as sarcoidosis or Crohn's disease and patients taking certain drugs such as thiazide diuretics (hydrochlorothiazide) can develop hypercalcemia due to "vitamin D hypersensitivity" or drug side effects—these patients require frequent monitoring of serum calcium while taking vitamin D supplements.
Comments:	▪ **Routine measurement and/or empiric treatment with vitamin D3 needs to become a routine component of patient care.**[173] ▪ Periodic assessment of 25(OH)D and serum calcium are required to ensure effectiveness and safety of treatment, respectively.

[165] Masood H, Narang AP, Bhat IA, Shah GN. Persistent limb pain and raised serum alkaline phosphatase the earliest markers of subclinical hypovitaminosis D in Kashmir. *Indian J Physiol Pharmacol.* 1989 Oct-Dec;33(4):259-61

[166] Al Faraj S, Al Mutairi K. Vitamin D deficiency and chronic low back pain in Saudi Arabia. *Spine.* 2003 Jan 15;28(2):177-9

[167] Plotnikoff GA, Quigley JM. Prevalence of severe hypovitaminosis D in patients with persistent, nonspecific musculoskeletal pain. *Mayo Clin Proc.* 2003 Dec;78(12):1463-70

[168] Grant WB. An estimate of premature cancer mortality in the U.S. due to inadequate doses of solar ultraviolet-B radiation. *Cancer* 2002;94(6):1867-75

[169] Zittermannn A. Vitamin D in preventive medicine: are we ignoring the evidence? *Br J Nutr.* 2003 May;89(5):552-72

[170] Holick MF. Vitamin D: importance in the prevention of cancers, type 1 diabetes, heart disease, and osteoporosis. *Am J Clin Nutr.* 2004;79(3):362-71

[171] Al Faraj S, Al Mutairi K. Vitamin D deficiency and chronic low back pain in Saudi Arabia. *Spine.* 2003 Jan 15;28(2):177-9

[172] Vasquez A, Manso G, Cannell J. The Clinical Importance of Vitamin D (Cholecalciferol): A Paradigm Shift with Implications for All Healthcare Providers. *Alternative Therapies in Health and Medicine* 2004; 10: 28-37 http://optimalhealthresearch.com/cholecalciferol.html

[173] Heaney RP. Vitamin D, nutritional deficiency, and the medical paradigm. *J Clin Endocrinol Metab.* 2003;88:5107-8 http://jcem.endojournals.org/cgi/content/full/88/11/5107

ELSEVIER

THE LANCET.com

May 6, 2005

Subphysiologic Doses of Vitamin D are Subtherapeutic: Comment on the Study by The Record Trial Group

Dear Editor,
Based on recently published research, it is clear that the study by The Record Trial Group [1] on vitamin D and calcium in the prevention of fractures suffered from at least four important shortcomings which negatively skewed their results.

First, and most important, the dose of vitamin D used in their study (800 IU/d) is subphysiologic and would therefore not be expected to produce a clinically meaningful effect. The physiologic requirement for vitamin D was determined scientifically in a recent study by Heaney and colleagues [2], who showed that healthy men utilize 3,000 to 5,000 IU of cholecalciferol per day, and several recent clinical trials have been published documenting the safety and effectiveness of administering vitamin D in physiologic doses of at least 4,000 IU per day.[3-5] In fact, studies have shown a dose-response relationship with vitamin D supplementation [6], and low doses (e.g., 600 IU) are clearly less effective than higher doses in the physiologic range (e.g., 4,000 IU).[5] It is important to note that the commonly used dose of vitamin D at 800 IU per day was not determined scientifically; rather this amount was determined arbitrarily before sufficient scientific methodology was available.[2,7] Given that the commonly recommended daily intake of vitamin D in the range of 200-800 IU is not sufficient for maintaining adequate serum levels of vitamin D [8], it is therefore incumbent upon modern researchers and clinicians to use doses of vitamin D that are consistent with the physiologic requirement as established in current research.

Second, the authors recognize that patient compliance in their study population was quite poor. This poor compliance obviously contributed to the purported lack of treatment efficacy.

Third, and consistent with recent data published elsewhere [8], virtually all of their patients were still vitamin D deficient at the end of one year of treatment, thereby affirming the inadequacy of the treatment dose. Vitamin D deficiency is common in industrialized nations, particularly those of northern latitudes [9-11], including the UK, where this study was performed. By modern criteria for serum vitamin D levels [12], virtually all of the patients in this study were vitamin D deficient at the beginning of the study, and the insufficient treatment dose of 800 IU/d failed to correct this deficiency even after 1 year of treatment. Given that vitamin D levels must be raised to approximately 40 ng/mL (100 nmol/L) in order to maximally reduce parathyroid hormone levels and bone resorption [13,14], supplementation that does not accomplish the goal of raising serum vitamin D levels into the optimal physiologic range cannot be considered adequate therapy.[12]

Fourth, and finally, there is reason to question the bioavailability of their vitamin D3 supplement, as the authors note that their dose-response was generally lower than that seen in other studies. Bioavailability is a prerequisite for treatment efficacy, and the elderly have higher likeliness of comorbid conditions that impair digestion and absorption of nutrients. Specifically, it is well documented that vitamin D absorption is decreased in elderly patients compared to younger controls [15,16], and this is complicated by an age-related reduction in renal calcitriol production [17,18] and intestinal vitamin D receptors [19], thereby further impairing vitamin D metabolism and calcium absorption. Since emulsification of fat soluble vitamins is required for their absorption [20], and since pre-emulsification of nutrients has been shown to increase absorption and dose-responsiveness of the fat-soluble nutrient coenzyme Q [21, 22], it seems apparent that attention to the form (not merely the dose) of nutrient supplementation is clinically important, particularly when working with elderly patients.

These shortcomings, when combined, could have lead to an additive or synergistic reduction in treatment potency that skewed their results toward a conclusion of inefficacy. In order to produce more meaningful results in clinical trials, our group published guidelines [12] recommending that future studies 1) ensure patient compliance, 2) use physiologic doses of vitamin D (e.g., 4,000 IU per day), and 3) ensure that serum levels are raised to a minimum of 40 ng/mL (100 nmol/L), since levels below this threshold are associated with increased parathyroid hormone levels, increased bone resorption, and recalcitrance to bone-building interventions.[23,24]

Alex Vasquez
Biotics Research Corporation
Rosenberg, Texas, USA 77471

Competing Interests: Dr. Vasquez is a researcher at Biotics Research Corporation, an FDA-licensed drug manufacturing facility in the USA.

References:
1. Record Trial Group. Oral vitamin D3 and calcium for secondary prevention of low-trauma fractures in elderly people (Randomised Evaluation of Calcium Or vitamin D, RECORD): a randomised placebo-controlled trial. *Lancet* (Early Online Publication), 28 April 2005
2. Heaney RP, Davies KM, Chen TC, Holick MF, Barger-Lux MJ. Human serum 25-hydroxycholecalciferol response to extended oral dosing with cholecalciferol. *Am J Clin Nutr* 2003;77:204-10
3. Vieth R, Chan PC, MacFarlane GD. Efficacy and safety of vitamin D3 intake exceeding the lowest observed adverse effect level. *Am J Clin Nutr.* 2001;73:288-94
4. Al Faraj S, Al Mutairi K. Vitamin D deficiency and chronic low back pain in Saudi Arabia. *Spine.* 2003;28:177-9
5. Vieth R, Kimball S, Hu A, Walfish PG. Randomized comparison of the effects of the vitamin D3 adequate intake versus 100 mcg (4000 IU) per day on biochemical responses and the wellbeing of patients. *Nutr J.* 2004 Jul 19;3(1):8 http://www.nutritionj.com/content/pdf/1475-2891-3-8.pdf
6. Van den Berghe G, Van Roosbroeck D, Vanhove P, Wouters PJ, De Pourcq L, Bouillon R. Bone turnover in prolonged critical illness: effect of vitamin D. *J Clin Endocrinol Metab.* 2003;88:4623-32
7. Vieth R. Vitamin D supplementation, 25-hydroxyvitamin D concentrations, and safety. *Am J Clin Nutr.* 1999;69:842-56 http://www.ajcn.org/cgi/reprint/69/5/842.pdf
8. Glerup H, Mikkelsen K, Poulsen L, Hass E, Overbeck S, Thomsen J, Charles P, Eriksen EF. Commonly recommended daily intake of vitamin D is not sufficient if sunlight exposure is limited. *J Intern Med.* 2000;247:260-8
9. Thomas MK, Lloyd-Jones DM, Thadhani RI, Shaw AC, Deraska DJ, Kitch BT, Vamvakas EC, Dick IM, Prince RL, Finkelstein JS. Hypovitaminosis D in medical inpatients. *N Engl J Med* 1998;338:777-83
10. Dubbelman R, Jonxis JH, Muskiet FA, Saleh AE. Age-dependent vitamin D status and vertebral condition of white women living in Curacao (The Netherlands Antilles) as compared with their counterparts in The Netherlands. *Am J Clin Nutr* 1993;58:106-9
11. Kauppinen-Makelin R, Tahtela R, Loyttyniemi E, Karkkainen J, Valimaki MJ. A high prevalence of hypovitaminosis D in Finnish medical in- and outpatients. *J Intern Med.* 2001;249:559-63
12. Vasquez A, Manso G, Cannell J. The clinical importance of vitamin D (cholecalciferol): a paradigm shift with implications for all healthcare providers. *Altern Ther Health Med.* 2004;10:28-36; quiz 37, 94
13. Kinyamu HK, Gallagher JC, Rafferty KA, Balhorn KE. Dietary calcium and vitamin D intake in elderly women: effect on serum parathyroid hormone and vitamin D metabolites. *Am J Clin Nutr* 1998;67:342-8
14. Dawson-Hughes B, Harris SS, Dallal GE. Plasma calcidiol, season, and serum parathyroid hormone concentrations in healthy elderly men and women. *Am J Clin Nutr* 1997;65:67-71
15. Harris SS, Dawson-Hughes B, Perrone GA. Plasma 25-hydroxyvitamin D responses of younger and older men to three weeks of supplementation with 1800 IU/day of vitamin D. *J Am Coll Nutr.* 1999;18:470-4
16. Barragry JM, France MW, Corless D, Gupta SP, Switala S, Boucher BJ, Cohen RD. Intestinal cholecalciferol absorption in the elderly and in younger adults. *Clin Sci Mol Med.* 1978;55:213-20
17. Tsai KS, Heath H 3rd, Kumar R, Riggs BL. Impaired vitamin D metabolism with aging in women. Possible role in pathogenesis of senile osteoporosis. *J Clin Invest.* 1984;73:1668-72
18. Gallagher JC, Riggs BL, Eisman J, Hamstra A, Arnaud SB, DeLuca HF. Intestinal calcium absorption and serum vitamin D metabolites in normal subjects and osteoporotic patients: effect of age and dietary calcium. *J Clin Invest.* 1979;64:729-36
19. Ebeling PR, Sandgren ME, DiMagno EP, Lane AW, DeLuca HF, Riggs BL. Evidence of an age-related decrease in intestinal responsiveness to vitamin D: relationship between serum 1,25-dihydroxyvitamin D3 and intestinal vitamin D receptor concentrations in normal women. *J Clin Endocrinol Metab.* 1992;75:176-82
20. Gallo-Torres HE. Obligatory role of bile for the intestinal absorption of vitamin E. *Lipids.* 1970;5:379-84
21. Bucci LR, Pillors M, Medlin R, Henderson R, Stiles JC, Robol HJ, Sparks WS. Enhanced uptake in humans of coenzyme Q10 from an emulsified form. *Third International Congress of Biomedical Gerontology*; Acapulco, Mexico: June 1989
22. Bucci LR, Pillors M, Medlin R, Klenda B, Robol H, Stiles JC, Sparks WS. Enhanced blood levels of coenzyme Q-10 from an emulsified oral form. In Faruqui SR and Ansari MS (editors). *Second Symposium on Nutrition and Chiropractic Proceedings*. April 15-16, 1989 in Davenport, Iowa
23. Stepan JJ, Burckhardt P, Hana V. The effects of three-month intravenous ibandronate on bone mineral density and bone remodeling in Klinefelter's syndrome: the influence of vitamin D deficiency and hormonal status. *Bone* 2003;33:589-596
24. Vasquez A. Health care for our bones: a practical nutritional approach to preventing osteoporosis. [letter] *J Manipulative* Physiol Ther. 2005;28:213

Citation: Vasquez A. Subphysiologic Doses of Vitamin D are Subtherapeutic: Comment on the Study by The Record Trial Group. *Lancet* 2005 published online May 6

Internet: Originally posted at http://www.thelancet.com/journals/lancet/article/PIIS0140673605630139/comments and now available at http://optimalhealthresearch.com/cholecalciferol.html

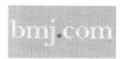

Calcium and vitamin D in preventing fractures

Data are not sufficient to show inefficacy

EDITOR—The study by Porthouse et al had two major design flaws.[1] Firstly, the dose of vitamin D (800 IU per day) is subphysiological and therefore subtherapeutic. Secondly, their use of "self report" as a measure of compliance is unreliable.

The dose of vitamin D at 800 IU daily was not determined scientifically but determined arbitrarily before sufficient scientific methodology was available.[2-4] Heaney et al determined the physiological requirement of vitamin D by showing that healthy men use 4000 IU cholecalciferol daily,[2] an amount that is safely attainable with supplementation[3] and often exceeded with exposure of the total body to equatorial sun.[4]

We provided six guidelines for interventional studies with vitamin D.[5] Dosages of vitamin D must reflect physiological requirements and natural endogenous production and should therefore be in the range of 3000-10 000 IU daily. Vitamin D supplementation must be continued for at least five to nine months. The form of vitamin D should be D_3 rather than D_2. Supplements should be assayed for potency. Effectiveness of supplementation must include measurement of serum 25-hydroxyvitamin D. Serum 25(OH)D concentrations must enter the optimal range, which is 40-65 ng/ml (100-160 nmol/l).

Since the study by Porthouse et al met only the second and third of these six criteria, their data cannot be viewed as reliable for documenting the inefficacy of vitamin D supplementation.

Alex Vasquez, *researcher*

Biotics Research Corporation, 6801 Biotics Research Drive, Rosenberg, TX 77471, USA avasquez@bioticsresearch.com

John Cannell, *president*

Vitamin D Council, 9100 San Gregorio Road, Atascadero, CA 93422, USA

Competing interests: AV is a researcher at Biotics Research Corporation, a drug manufacturing facility in the United States that has approval from the Food and Drug Administration.

References

1. Porthouse J, Cockayne S, King C, Saxon L, Steele E, Aspray T, et al. Randomised controlled trial of calcium and supplementation with cholecalciferol (vitamin D3) for prevention of fractures in primary care. *BMJ* 2005;330: 1003. (30 April.)[Abstract/Free Full Text]
2. Heaney RP, Davies KM, Chen TC, Holick MF, Barger-Lux MJ. Human serum 25-hydroxycholecalciferol response to extended oral dosing with cholecalciferol. *Am J Clin Nutr* 2003;77: 204-10.[Abstract/Free Full Text]
3. Vieth R, Chan PC, MacFarlane GD. Efficacy and safety of vitamin D3 intake exceeding the lowest observed adverse effect level. *Am J Clin Nutr* 2001;73: 288-94.[Abstract/Free Full Text]
4. Vieth R. Vitamin D supplementation, 25-hydroxyvitamin D concentrations, and safety. *Am J Clin Nutr* 1999;69: 842-56.[Abstract/Free Full Text]
5. Vasquez A, Manso G, Cannell J. The clinical importance of vitamin D (cholecalciferol): a paradigm shift with implications for all healthcare providers. *Altern Ther Health Med* 2004;10: 28-36.[ISI][Medline]

Related Article

Randomised controlled trial of calcium and supplementation with cholecalciferol (vitamin D₃) for prevention of fractures in primary care
Jill Porthouse, Sarah Cockayne, Christine King, Lucy Saxon, Elizabeth Steele, Terry Aspray, Mike Baverstock, Yvonne Birks, Jo Dumville, Roger Francis, Cynthia Iglesias, Suezann Puffer, Anne Sutcliffe, Ian Watt, and David J Torgerson
BMJ 2005 330: 1003. [Abstract] [Full Text]

Vasquez A, Cannell J. Calcium and vitamin D in preventing fractures: data are not sufficient to show inefficacy. *BMJ*. 2005 Jul 9;331(7508):108-9 http://www.ncbi.nlm.nih.gov/pubmed/16002891

Thyroid status—laboratory assessments	
Overview and interpretation:	• <u>Context</u>: Thyroid disorders are common in clinical practice and thus all clinicians need to have a clear understanding of the clinical presentations and laboratory assessments. Although various aspects of thyroid dysfunction, laboratory tests and clinical presentations will be reviewed here, the primary emphasis will be upon hypothyroidism, which is the most common and *unnecessarily* enigmatic of the thyroid disorders. • <u>Controversy</u>: In the allopathic medical paradigm, much confusion exists regarding a common but "mysterious" and "enigmatic" condition known as hypothyroidism—low thyroid function. Its converse—**hyper**thyroidism and Graves disease—is well understood, easily diagnosed, and readily treated. Because the medical treatment for **hyper**thyroidism often leaves patients in a **hypo**thyroid state, affected patients thus transition from *clarity* (hyperthyroidism) wherein they feel ill due to the disease process into *"mystery"* (hypothyroidism) wherein they feel ill due to incomplete/inaccurate treatment. The basis for the confusion within the allopathic medical community about hypothyroidism is primarily two-fold: ❶ first, they rely on the wrong test (TSH) as the main basis for laboratory assessment, ❷ second, they use incomplete treatment (T4 without T3) which defies the known physiology of the thyroid gland, which makes at least two hormones rather than one. One might get the impression that perpetual confusion is at times the goal of the medical profession; we certainly see this with the management of hypertension, depression, diabetes mellitus, psoriasis and other inflammatory/autoimmune conditions. For people who seek clarity, it is available. • <u>Basic physiology</u>: The hypothalamus produces thyrotropin-releasing hormone (TRH) which stimulates the anterior pituitary gland to make thyroid-stimulating hormone (TSH), which stimulates the thyroid gland to produce thyroxine (T4, approximately 85% of thyroid gland hormone production) and triiodothyronine (T3, approximately 15% of thyroid gland hormone production). In the periphery, the prohormone T4 is converted to active T3 by deiodinase enzymes. Stress, glucagon, and environmental toxins (halogenated phenolics, plastic monomers, flame retardants[174]) impair production of T3 and/or increase production of reverse T3, which is either inert or inhibitory to the action of T3. If the thyroid gland begins to fail, then TSH levels increase as the body attempts to stimulate production of thyroid hormones from a failing gland, which typically fails due to autoimmune attack (Hashimoto's thyroiditis); hence the association of elevated blood TSH levels with "primary hypothyroidism." Thyroid hormones have many different functions in the body, and one of the chief effects is contributing to maintenance of the basal metabolic rate, or the speed of reactions within and the temperature of the body. An insufficiency of thyroid hormone adversely effects numerous biochemical reactions and body/organ functions; hence the myriad of clinical presentations reflecting variations in biochemical and physiologic individuality. Conversely yet similarly, excess thyroid hormone (whether endogenously produced or exogenously administered) also affects numerous body systems. • <u>Clinical presentation of *hyper*thyroidism</u>: The clinical pattern of thyroid excess is more narrowly-focused and thus more predictable and consistent than is the presentation of low thyroid function. The clinical manifestations of hyperthyroidism generally fall into three categories: hyper-adrenergic, hypermetabolic, and ophthalmologic/ocular. ❶ <u>hyper-adrenergic</u>: tachycardia, tremor, diaphoresis, insomnia and a feeling of nervousness and psychomotor agitation due to upregulation of adrenergic tone and generally some degree of relative or absolute hyperthermia; increased dopaminergic and noradrenergic tone in the brain accounts for the neuropsychiatric manifestations, such as mania, psychosis, and hypersexuality, ❷ <u>hyper-metabolic</u>: fecal frequency often described as "diarrhea" due to

---

[174] "All studied contaminants inhibited DI activity in a dose-response manner… This study suggests that some halogenated phenolics, including current use compounds such as plastic monomers, flame retardants and their metabolites, may disrupt thyroid hormone homeostasis through the inhibition of DI activity in vivo." Butt CM, Wang D, Stapleton HM. Halogenated Phenolic Contaminants Inhibit the In Vitro Activity of the Thyroid Regulating Deiodinases in Human Liver. *Toxicol Sci.* 2011 May 11. [Epub ahead of print]

Thyroid status—laboratory assessments	
	expedited intestinal transit, elevated temperature, and weight loss due to increased overall metabolic rate, ❸ <u>ophthalmologic/ocular</u>: in chronic cases particularly of the autoimmune variety, exophthalmos develops secondary to retro-orbital connective tissue proliferation and autoimmunity directed toward the extraocular muscles; the histologic abnormalities are chiefly characterized by increased accumulation of collagen (behind the eye and within the extraocular muscles, leading to muscle weakness), accumulation of glycosaminoglycans (GAGs), and the attendant edema.

- <u>Clinical presentation of *hypo*thyroidism</u>: In his classic book <u>*Biochemical Individuality*</u>, Williams[175] noted that "a wide variation in thyroid activity exists among 'normal' human beings." Clearly, some patients do not make enough thyroid hormone to function optimally[176]; or, perhaps more precisely, they make enough thyroid hormone (T4) but do not efficiently convert it to the active form (T3) in the periphery. Further complicating the picture is that some patients make appropriate amounts of TSH, T4, and T3 but they make excess of inactive reverse T3 (rT3) which puts them into a physiologic state of hypothyroidism despite adequate glandular function. Patients may have one or more of the following: fatigue, depression, **cold hands and feet** (excluding Raynaud's syndrome, peripheral vascular disease)**,** dry skin, menstrual irregularities, infertility, premenstrual syndrome (PMS), uterine fibroids, excess menstrual bleeding, **low basal body temperature,** weak fingernails, sleep apnea and increased need for sleep (hypersomnia), slow heart rate (relative or absolute **bradycardia**), easy weight gain and difficult weight loss (thus, predisposition to overweight and obesity), hypercholesterolemia, slow healing, decreased memory and concentration, frog-like husky voice, low libido, recurrent infections, hypertension especially diastolic hypertension, poor digestion (due to insufficient gastric production of hydrochloric acid), **delayed Achilles return** (due to delayed muscle relaxation), carotenodermia, vitamin A deficiency, and gastroesophageal acid reflux, constipation, and predisposition to small intestine bacterial overgrowth (SIBO) due to slow intestinal transit. Of these manifestations, cold hands and feet, low basal body temperature, bradycardia, and delayed Achilles return are the most specific; some very competent physicians will—following proper patient evaluation—treat with thyroid hormone based on the clinical presentation of the patient and *with proper consideration of* and *without dependency upon* laboratory findings.

- <u>Overview of thyroid tests</u>:
  - <u>Thyrotropin-releasing hormone (TRH)</u>: The hypothalamus releases TRH to stimulate pituitary production of TSH. TRH is not routinely tested in clinical practice, although abnormalities of TRH secretion are noted in patients with mental "depression."
  - <u>Thyroid-stimulating hormone (TSH: 0.4 - 5.0 mIU/L [milli-international units per liter])</u>: TSH is the most commonly performed test for evaluating thyroid status; its frequent (over)use owes more to habit and inexpensiveness than to aspirations for clinical excellence. TSH values greater than 2 mIU/L represent a disturbance of the thyroid-pituitary axis and an increased risk for future thyroid problems[177], and the American Association of Clinical Endocrinologists states, "The target TSH level should be between 0.3 and 3.0 µIU/mL."[178] Clinical rationale is available to support implementation of a therapeutic trial of thyroid hormone treatment in patients who are clinically hypothyroid even if they are biochemically euthyroid (per TSH) provided

---

[175] Williams RJ. <u>*Biochemical Individuality: The Basis for the Genetotrophic Concept*</u>. Austin and London: University of Texas Press, 1956 page 82

[176] Broda Barnes MD, Lawrence Galton, <u>*Hypothyroidism: The Unsuspected Illness*</u>. Ty Crowell Co; 1976

[177] Weetman AP. Fortnightly review: Hypothyroidism: screening and subclinical disease. *BMJ: British Medical Journal* 1997;314: 1175

[178] American Association of Clinical Endocrinologists. "The target TSH level should be between 0.3 and 3.0 µIU/mL." AACE Medical Guidelines for Clinical Practice for Evaluation and Treatment of Hyperthyroidism and Hypothyroidism. 2002, 2006 Amended Version. https://www.aace.com/sites/default/files/hypo_hyper.pdf Accessed August 2011

that treatment is implemented cautiously, in appropriately selected patients, and patients are appropriately informed.[179,180] If the clinical world were as perfect as it is portrayed in basic physiology textbooks, then a clinician might fancifully rely on TSH to perform the diagnosis *prima facie*, with reduced TSH values correlating with glandular overperformance and negative feedback suppressing TSH secretion, whilst an underperforming gland would require greater stimulation with elevated TSH levels; however, TSH has never been thus vested with infallible reliability, which explains in part why doctors need brains of their own and why better clinicians have developed the capacity for independent thought.

o Free thyroxine (free T4: 4.5 - 11.2 mcg/dL): Unbound T4 is tested to provide evidence of glandular production of thyroid hormone(s). Because T4 is the major thyroid hormone produced by the thyroid gland it serves as an excellent marker for glandular productivity but it reveals nothing about peripheral conversion of T4 to the active thyroid hormone triiodothyronine (T3); in the practice of medicine, conversion of T4 to the active T3 is assumed to reliably occur unabated despite evidence to the contrary, especially among symptomatic patients.

o Triiodothyronine (T3: 100 - 200 ng/dL[181]): In textbook-perfect physiology, T4 is converted by deiodinase enzymes type-1 and type-2 to the active thyroid hormone T3; in reality, this is only part of the story. Because T3 is the active form of the hormone responsible for the physiologic functions of thyroid physiology, a clinician desiring to assess a patient's thyroid status might reasonably ask the proper question by performing the proper test. T3 is tested as "total T3" or "free T3" in large part based on the clinician's preference; the current author prefers total T3 because it can be compared to the total level of reverse T3 (rT3) in a ratio, the optimal range of which is generally considered to be 10-14 as originally presented by McDaniel[182] and reviewed in the following pages. Patients with psychiatric depression have lower levels of T3 than do healthy controls and have been described as having "low T3 syndrome"[183]; very obviously—whether cause or effect—the low T3 levels in these patients would serve to promote and perpetuate their state of mental depression. Although the focus of this review within the subject of laboratory evaluation is not to describe the implementation of thyroid hormone treatment, clinicians should be aware that T3 administration increases hepatic production of sex hormone binding globulin (SHBG) and that therefore T3 administration can reduce cellular bioavailability of protein-bound hormones. Many authoritative and clinically-experienced sources recommend using a time-released (e.g., sustained-release) form of T3 due to its shorter half-life compared with T4. However, obtaining time-released T3 via a compounding pharmacy can be cumbersome and expensive for the patient; clearly some patients respond to once daily dosing of *non*-time-released preparations with good effects and without adverse effects. Some patients can divide the immediate-release dose into two servings per day for enhanced effect and lessened physiologic fluctuations, if necessary. Per Drugs.com[184] in August 2011, "Since liothyronine sodium (T3) is not firmly bound to serum protein, it is readily available to body tissues. The onset of activity of liothyronine sodium is rapid, occurring within a few hours. Maximum pharmacologic

[179] Skinner GR, Thomas R, Taylor M, Sellarajah M, Bolt S, Krett S, Wright A. Thyroxine should be tried in clinically hypothyroid but biochemically euthyroid patients. *BMJ: British Medical Journal* 1997 Jun 14; 314(7096): 1764

[180] McLaren EH, Kelly CJ, Pollack MA. Trial of thyroxine treatment for biochemically euthyroid patients has been approved. *BMJ* 1997; 315: 1463

[181] U.S. National Library of Medicine (NLM) and National Institutes of Health (NIH) http://www.nlm.nih.gov/medlineplus/ency/article/003687.htm Accessed August 2011

[182] McDaniel AB. Thyroid Assessment: Controversies and Conundrums. Institute for Functional Medicine Fourteenth International Symposium. Tucson, Arizona. May 23-26, 2007

[183] "Out of 250 subjects with major psychiatric depression, 6.4% exhibited low T3 syndrome (mean serum T3 concentration 0.94 nmol/l vs normal mean serum concentration of 1.77 nmol/l)." Premachandra BN, Kabir MA, Williams IK. Low T3 syndrome in psychiatric depression. *J Endocrinol Invest.* 2006 Jun;29(6):568-72

[184] http://www.drugs.com/pro/cytomel.html Accessed August 2011.

Thyroid status—laboratory assessments

response occurs within 2 or 3 days, providing early clinical response. The biological half-life is about 2.5 days." Very clearly, a significant portion of hypothyroid patients respond to T3 alone (either time-released, divided-dosing, or once-daily dosing) or a combination of T4 and T3 when other treatments have failed.[185,186]

○ Reverse triiodothyronine (rT3: 90 - 320 pg/mL[187]): T4 is converted by deiodinase enzymes type-1 and type-3 to the inactive thyroid hormone rT3; per a standard endocrinology textbook, "Approximately 70–80% of released T4 is converted by deiodinases to the biologically active T3, the remainder to reverse-T3 (rT3) which has no significant biological activity."[188] Clinicians must know that, "The prohormone T4 must be converted to T3 in the body before it can exert biological effects. **During periods of illness or stress, this conversion is often inhibited and can be diverted to the inactive reverse T3 (rT3) moiety.**"[189] Furthermore and very importantly, clinicians should appreciate that rT3 is not simply inactive but that it may actually impair production/utilization of normal T3; "T4-T3 and T4-rT3 conversion are provoked by different enzymes. The **elevation of rT3** might be a cause of the observed decrease in **peripheral T3 generation** in old [elderly] subjects, acting by an **inhibition of the T4-T3 conversion**."[190] During times of psychologic/physiologic stress and specific types of pharmacologic stress (e.g., propanolol[191] and corticosteroids), T4 metabolism is preferentially shunted away from T3 toward rT3; an anthropocentric explanation holds that by making less of the active T3 and more of the inactive rT3, the body is better able to conserve energy during times of stress by reducing overall metabolic rate, particularly resting energy expenditure and protein utilization. For example, caloric restriction and fasting result in a decrease in resting metabolic rate (RMR), and the reduced RMR persists for months after the fasting has ended and a normal diet is resumed.[192] This author (AV) terms this stress-induced impairment of thyroid hormone conversion "**metabolic hypothyroidism**" or "**functional hypothyroidism**" because the defect is in the metabolism (not the production) of thyroid hormone into its most active form; "**peripheral hypothyroidism**" might also be used to distinguish the fact that the defect is in the peripheral metabolism rather than located more centrally, within the thyroid gland itself. Because psychologic stress and certain pharmacologic exposures—as well as the thyro-metabolic stress of fasting and caloric restriction in which the counterregulatory hormone glucagon appears to trigger enhanced rT3 production—reduce T3 while simultaneously increasing rT3 levels, clinicians can appreciate that calculation of the T3/rT3 ratio will be more significantly altered (and thus a more sensitive indicator of metabolic disruption) than will be the isolated measurements of T3 or rT3 alone. Functional medicine clinicians[193] note the importance of the ratio of

---

[185] Bunevicius R, Kazanavicius G, Zalinkevicius R, Prange AJ Jr. Effects of thyroxine as compared with thyroxine plus triiodothyronine in patients with hypothyroidism. *N Engl J Med.* 1999 Feb 11;340(6):424-9

[186] Kelly T, Lieberman DZ. The use of triiodothyronine as an augmentation agent in treatment-resistant bipolar II and bipolar disorder NOS. *J Affect Disord.* 2009 Aug;116(3):222-6

[187] The reference range provided here for rT3 is a compilation from the laboratory reference ranges from the sample reports on the following pages, each of which is performed by either Quest Diagnostics or LabCorp, the two largest medical laboratories in the United States.

[188] Nussey S, Whitehead S. *Endocrinology: An Integrated Approach*. Oxford: BIOS Scientific Publishers; 2001. See also Box 3.29 Metabolism of thyroid hormones. http://www.ncbi.nlm.nih.gov/books/NBK28/box/A270/?report=objectonly Accessed July 2011

[189] *1998 Mosby's GenRX. Sixth Edition*. St. Louis Missouri; Mosby-Year Book, Inc., 1998

[190] Szabolcs I, Weber M, Kovács Z, Irsy G, Góth M, Halász T, Szilágyi G. The possible reason for serum 3,3'5'-(reverse) triiodothyronine increase in old people. *Acta Med Acad Sci Hung.* 1982;39(1-2):11-7

[191] "Propranolol administration (40 mg t.i.d. for a week) caused a similar rT3 elevation in old persons (n = 18) as in 12 young ones." Szabolcs I, Weber M, Kovács Z, Irsy G, Góth M, Halász T, Szilágyi G. The possible reason for serum 3,3'5'-(reverse) triiodothyronine increase in old people. *Acta Med Acad Sci Hung.* 1982;39(1-2):11-7

[192] Elliot DL, Goldberg L, Kuehl KS, Bennett WM. Sustained depression of the resting metabolic rate after massive weight loss. *Am J Clin Nutr* 1989 Jan;49(1):93-96

[193] The conclusion of this paragraph is derived from **Vasquez A**. *Musculoskeletal Pain: Expanded Clinical Strategies*. Published 2008 by The Institute for Functional Medicine. http://www.functionalmedicine.org/ifm_ecommerce/ProductDetails.aspx?ProductID=127

total T3 to reverse T3 (tT3:rT3 ratio) and consider the optimal range to be 10-14 with lower ratios indicating impaired formation or T3 and/or excess production of rT3.[194] Contrary to the previous view which held that rT3 was simply inactive, we now appreciate that rT3 actually impairs normal thyroid hormone metabolism thus functioning as an thyrometabolic monkeywrench or "brake" on normal metabolism. Elevated rT3 levels predict mortality among critically ill patients.[195] Aberrancies in thyroid hormone levels may reflect organic disease, psychoemotional stress, or nutritional deficiency[196], and therefore such serologic abnormalities warrant consideration of underlying problems and direct treatment when possible. If no underlying cause is apparent, then a trial of thyroid hormone/hormones is reasonable in appropriately selected patients. Beyond stress reduction, allergen/gluten avoidance, and nutritional supplementation with iodine, selenium, and zinc (as indicated per patient), correction of overt, subclinical, and functional hypothyroidism generally centers on the administration of natural or synthetic thyroid hormones in the form of T4 and T3. Correction of functional hypothyroidism (relatively reduced total T3 and increased rT3) is accomplished with either time-released or twice-daily dosing of T3 *without T4* to suppress endogenous T4 conversion to T3, thereby allowing rT3 levels to fall precipitously. T3 administration allows temporary downregulation of transforming enzymes so that rT3 production is reduced following withdrawal of T3 replacement; thus, short-term and/or periodic T3 administration helps normalize or "reset" peripheral thyroid metabolism so that, following withdrawal of T3 administration, T4 can be converted to T3 without excess production of rT3. The safety and effectiveness of this approach — using T3 administration (often twice daily or in a sustained-release compounded tablet or capsule) to recalibrate peripheral thyroid hormone metabolism — has documented safety and effectiveness.[197] Alleviation of symptoms, restoration of morning body temperature to 98.6° F (oral or axillary) and other clinical objective improvements achieved by the judicious and safe administration of T3 are the criteria of success; physiologic improvement following T3 administration retrospectively confirms the diagnosis.

o <u>Antithyroid antibodies — antithyroglobulin (anti-TG) and anti-thyroid peroxidase (anti-TPO)</u>: Autoimmune thyroiditis (also called Hashimoto's disease or chronic lymphocytic thyroiditis) or is the most common cause of overt primary hypothyroidism. The diagnosis of autoimmune thyroiditis can be made clinically (i.e., without biopsy) upon detection of elevated blood levels of antibodies against thyroglobulin (anti-thyroglobulin antibodies) and anti-thyroid peroxidase (anti-TPO) antibodies. Autoimmune thyroiditis may present asymptomatically and with normal thyroid hormone levels; classically, patients may have a slightly hyperthyroid presentation as the inflamed gland releases extra thyroid hormone before becoming atrophic and hypofunctional.

Advantages:	▪ Thyroid disorders are quite common in general practice and are often undiagnosed, undertreated, or inappropriately treated.
	▪ Consistent with the principle of beneficence, patients and doctors benefit when thyroid disorders are diagnosed and treated appropriately.

[194] McDaniel AB. Thyroid Assessment: Controversies and Conundrums. Institute for Functional Medicine Fourteenth International Symposium. Tucson, Arizona. May 23-26, 2007

[195] Peeters RP, Wouters PJ, van Toor H, Kaptein E, Visser TJ, Van den Berghe G. Serum 3,3',5'-triiodothyronine (rT3) and 3,5,3'-triiodothyronine/rT3 are prognostic markers in critically ill patients and are associated with postmortem tissue deiodinase activities. J Clin Endocrinol Metab. 2005 Aug;90(8):4559-65

[196] Kelly GS. Peripheral metabolism of thyroid hormones: a review. Altern Med Rev. 2000 Aug;5(4):306-33

[197] Friedman M, Miranda-Massari JR, Gonzalez MJ. Supraphysiological cyclic dosing of sustained release T3 in order to reset low basal body temperature. *P R Health Sci J.* 2006 Mar;25(1):23-9

Thyroid status—laboratory assessments	
Limitations:	▪ A properly interpreted TSH may overlook problems of T4 production or conversion to active T3. Additionally, in some patients, all of these tests are normal but they may have thyroid autoimmunity (i.e., thyroid peroxidase antibodies, anti-TPO) and should receive treatment with thyroid hormone[198] or some other corrective treatment (e.g., selenium supplementation[199,200] and a gluten-free diet[201]) to normalize thyroid status.
Comments:	▪ Comprehensive thyroid laboratory testing including ❶ TSH, ❷ free T4, ❸ total T3, ❹ rT3, ❺ antithyroid antibodies, should be evaluated alongside the ❻ heart rate, ❼ cold extremities, ❽ basal body temperature, ❾ Achilles' return rate, and ❿ overall symptoms and clinical picture. ▪ The combination of T3 and T4 (as in the prescription Liotrix/Thyrolar or Armour thyroid) appears to have similar safety to T4 alone (Levothyroxine, Synthroid) and may result in greater improvements in mood and neuropsychological function.[202] ▪ Glandular thyroid supplements and Armour thyroid generally should *not* be used in patients with thyroid autoimmunity (Hashimoto's thyroiditis) because the bovine/porcine antigens will exacerbate the anti-thyroid immune response as evidenced by increased anti-TPO antibodies.

Optimal thyroid status

Concept by Dr Vasquez: Optimal thyroid status is not defined by basic laboratory testing with TSH and free T4. It is defined *per patient* based on the levels and ratios of all major thyroid-related hormones and antibodies—in association with other hormonal, psychologic, dysbiotic, nutritional and environmental factors— that work best for that particular unique biochemically-individual patient.

Laboratory interpretation by Dr McDaniel: "Optimal hormone balance is debatable. My observations: A few "well" people and patients treated successfully with T4 and T3 seem best with:

- TSH around 0.7–0.9µIU/mL
- fT4 around 0.7–0.8ng/dL
- fT3 optimally 3.4–3.8pg/mL
- **Total T3-RT3 ratio 12 +/-2**"

McDaniel AB. Thyroid Assessment: Controversies and Conundrums. Institute for Functional Medicine Fourteenth International Symposium. Tucson, Arizona. May 23-26, 2007

---

[198] Beers MH, Berkow R (eds). The Merck Manual. 17th Edition. Whitehouse Station; Merck Research Laboratories 1999 page 96

[199] Duntas LH, Mantzou E, Koutras DA. Effects of a six month treatment with selenomethionine in patients with autoimmune thyroiditis. *Eur J Endocrinol*. 2003 Apr;148(4):389-93 http://eje-online.org/cgi/reprint/148/4/389

[200] Gartner R, Gasnier BC. Selenium in the treatment of autoimmune thyroiditis. *Biofactors*. 2003;19(3-4):165-70

[201] Sategna-Guidetti C, Volta U, Ciacci C, Usai P, Carlino A, De Franceschi L, Camera A, Pelli A, Brossa C. Prevalence of thyroid disorders in untreated adult celiac disease patients and effect of gluten withdrawal: an Italian multicenter study. *Am J Gastroenterol*. 2001 Mar;96(3):751-7

[202] "CONCLUSIONS: In patients with hypothyroidism, partial substitution of triiodothyronine for thyroxine may improve mood and neuropsychological function; this finding suggests a specific effect of the triiodothyronine normally secreted by the thyroid gland." Bunevicius R, Kazanavicius G, Zalinkevicius R, Prange AJ Jr. Effects of thyroxine as compared with thyroxine plus triiodothyronine in patients with hypothyroidism. *N Engl J Med*. 1999 Feb 11;340(6):424-9

Presentation: 38yo male under extreme psychological stress with a complaint of constantly cold extremities—testing performed in February 2010 by LabCorp: Review the following labs and outline your treatment plan before reading the discussion below.

Date and Time Collected	Date Entered	Date and Time Reported	Physician Name	NPI	Ph
02/04/10 11:41	02/04/10	02/09/10 04:06E	3AN		190

Tests Ordered

Triiodothyronine (T3);Reverse T3;Triiodothyronine,Free,Serum

General Comments

PID: 8282293

TESTS	RESULT	FLAG	UNITS	REFERENCE INTERV
Triiodothyronine (T3)				
Triiodothyronine (T3)	57	Low	ng/dL	71-180
Reverse T3				
Reverse T3	312		pg/mL	90-350
Triiodothyronine,Free,Serum				
Triiodothyronine,Free,Serum	2.5		pg/mL	2.0-4.4

Discussion: In this case, because the T3 level is low, *prima facie* justification for administration of T3 is provided, assuming that the clinical picture is compatible and that no contraindications to treatment are present. To calculate the total T3/rT3 ratio, equilibrate the units (multiply total T3 in ng/dL x 10 to convert to pg/mL; 1 pg = 0.001 ng (1 ng = 1,000 pg); 1 dl = 100 ml). The total T3/rT3 ratio should be >10-14 (per McDaniel[203]), but in this patient's case 570/312 = 1.8. Remember, more T3 than rT3 is better; hence, the higher ratio is better. On-line calculators for this conversion have been developed[204] and surely more will be available in the future. This athletic and otherwise healthy 220-lb (100 kg) patient responded very well to T3 (liothyronine/Cytomel) with a starting dose of 150 mcg which was eventually tapered to 25 mcg and then to 12.5 mcg; in this patient's case, the initial high dose of T3 was well-tolerated because of the initially low level of T3, the elevated rT3 which appears to block T3 function, and the patient's overall excellent cardiovascular fitness. A reasonable dosage range for liothyronine/Cytomel supplementation is 12.5-50 mcg for most patients tapered to the constellation of patient tolerance, patient preference, heart rate, basal body temperature optimization to 98.6° F, suppression of TSH and T4, resolution of symptoms and objective markers, and clinician's impression and experience.

Step-by-step conversion from ng/dL to pg/mL—end result is multiply by 10 (i.e., 10x)

Original units	Convert ng to pg[205]	Convert dL to mL	Simplify the fraction
1 ng / 1 dL	1,000 pg/ 1 dL	1,000 pg/ 100 mL	10 pg/ 1 ml
57 ng/ 1 dL	57,000 pg / 1 dL	57,000 pg / 100 mL	570 pg / 1 mL

Contraindications to T3, liothyronine, Cytomel

Absolute contraindications:
- Anaphylaxis or severe hypersensitivity,
- Acute (current) myocardial infarction,
- Hyperthyroidism,
- Untreated adrenal insufficiency.

Relative contraindications and cautions:
- CAD, angina pectoris, or cardiac arrhythmia,
- Elderly patients—start with low dose and titrate as tolerated.

Reference: Epocrates.com August 2011

---

[203] McDaniel AB. Thyroid Assessment: Controversies and Conundrums. Institute for Functional Medicine Fourteenth International Symposium. Tucson, AZ. May 23-26, 2007
[204] http://www.stopthethyroidmadness.com/rt3-ratio/ Accessed—but not necessarily endorsed—August 2011
[205] Double-checked with http://www.unitconversion.org/weight/nanograms-to-picograms-conversion.html July 2011

Presentation: A 42yo male with fatigue—testing performed by Quest Diagnostics in January 2010: Review the following labs and outline your treatment plan before reading the discussion below. Note that the "optimal ratio" provided by the laboratory in this example was performed using free T3 rather than total T3 and without converting to equal units.

```
FREE T3/REVERSE T3 RATIO
    FREE T3/REVERSE T3 RATIO                    0.93 L          1.05-1.91**
    FREE T3                        325                          230-420 pg/dL
    REVERSE T3                                  350 H           100-340*** pg/mL
            **Ratio= Free T3 in pg/dL : reverse T3 in pg/mL. Ratio for reference
            range is calculated by dividing the lower and upper end of free T3
            with the mean of reverse T3 (220 pg/mL).

            ***Observed reference range is reported for reverse T3 per client
            request.

            This test was performed using a kit that has not been approved or
            cleared by the FDA. The analytical performance characteristics of this
            test have been determined by Quest Diagnostics Nichols Institute, San
            Juan Capistrano. This test should not be used for diagnosis without
            confirmation by other medically established means.
```

Discussion: Note that if the T3 had been tested without rT3 the results would have been reported as "normal" and that a "depressed" patient so assessed would have likely been given an "antidepressant" medication and a diagnosis of depression rather than the proper treatment with T3 and a diagnosis of functional hypothyroidism. Luckily for this patient, his clinician tested rT3 and upon finding it impressively elevated treated with patient with T3 to suppress rT3 production by temporarily suppressing T4 production. The ratio calculation is provided and interpreted by the laboratory; notice that the "ideal ratio" for **total T3/rT3 (>10)** differs from that of **free T3/rT3 (>1.05)** *and that per the ratio provided by the labotatory does not equilibriate the measurement units.* This method is acceptable but is not the preferred method for determining functional thyroid status. The preferred method is the one presented by McDaniel[206] at the Institute for Functional Medicine's 14th International Symposium in 2007 wherein he advocated using total T3 (not free T3) in comparison with rT3 interpreted by an optimal ratio of 10-14.

Step-by-step conversion from pg/dL to pg/mL—end result is divide by 100 (i.e., 0.01x): Provided for the sake of completeness even though the conversion is not necessary per the laboratory interpretation provided above.

Original units	Convert dL to mL	Simplify the fraction
1 pg / 1 dL	1 pg/ 100 mL	0.01 pg/ 1 mL
325 pg/ 1 dL	325 pg / 100 mL	3.25 pg / 1 mL

---

[206] McDaniel AB. Thyroid Assessment: Controversies and Conundrums. Institute for Functional Medicine Fourteenth International Symposium. Tucson, Arizona. May 23-26, 2007

Presentation: 31yo female with fatigue, a recent history of extreme emotional stress (death of first-degree family member), maternal history of Hashimotos thyroiditis, and a personal history of presumed gluten intolerance—testing performed in May 2010 by Quest Diagnostics: Outline your treatment plan before reading discussion.

Test Name	In Range	Out of Range	Reference Range
THYROGLOBULIN ANTIBODIES	<20		<20 IU/mL
THYROID PEROXIDASE ANTIBODIES		38 H	<35 IU/mL
T3, TOTAL	89		76-181 ng/dL
T3 UPTAKE		37 H	22-35 %
T4, FREE	1.6		0.8-1.8 ng/dL
T4 (THYROXINE), TOTAL			
T4 (THYROXINE), TOTAL	10.9		4.5-12.5 mcg/dL
FREE T4 INDEX (T7)		4.0 H	1.4-3.8
TSH, 3RD GENERATION	0.82		mIU/L

Reference Range

> or = 20 Years   0.40-4.50

       Pregnancy Ranges
First trimester   0.20-4.70
Second trimester   0.30-4.10
Third trimester   0.40-2.70

Test Name	In Range	Out of Range	Reference Range
T3, FREE	318		230-420 pg/dL
T3, REVERSE		43 H	11-32 ng/dL

This test was performed using a kit that has not been approved or cleared by the FDA. The analytical performance characteristics of this test have been determined by Quest Diagnostics Nichols Institute, San Juan Capistrano. This test should not be used for diagnosis without confirmation by other medically established means.

Discussion: Note that the TSH is completely normal and thus would give the impression of normalcy and "health" if the clinician had not ordered the additional tests. Thyroid peroxidase antibodies are minimally elevated; this is consistent with thyroid autoimmunity but titers this low are of limited clinical importance. Note that the rT3 level is abnormally elevated. Note that because the units provided for total T3 (89 ng/dL) and rT3 (43 ng/dL) are identical, no unit conversion is required, thereby making the calculation of the ideal ratio (range: 10-14) very simple. In this patient's case, the ratio comes to 2.06 which is obviously significantly lower than the proposed optimal of 10-14; the patient responded well to liothyronine/Cytomel supplementation with 15 mcg/d. Patients with thyroid autoimmunity often benefit from a gluten-free diet[207] and supplementation with selenium 200 mcg/d.[208] Finally, note that the reference range for total T3 provided by this laboratory is 76-181 ng/dL which contrasts significantly from the range recommended by the US National Institutes of Health (NIH) 100 to 200 ng/dL[209]; using the NIH's reference range, this patient's T3 production is inadequate.

[207] "Hypothyroidism, diagnosed in 31 patients (12.9%) and nine controls (4.2%), was subclinical in 29 patients and of nonautoimmune origin in 21. ... In most patients who strictly followed a 1-yr gluten withdrawal (as confirmed by intestinal mucosa recovery), there was a normalization of subclinical hypothyroidism. The greater frequency of thyroid disease among celiac disease patients justifies a thyroid functional assessment. In distinct cases, gluten withdrawal may single-handedly reverse the abnormality." Sategna-Guidetti C, Volta U, Ciacci C, et al. Prevalence of thyroid disorders in untreated adult celiac disease patients and effect of gluten withdrawal: an Italian multicenter study. *Am J Gastroenterol.* 2001 Mar;96(3):751-7

[208] "Patients with HT assigned to Se supplementation for 3 months demonstrated significantly lower thyroid peroxidase autoantibodies (TPOab) titers (four studies, random effects weighted mean difference: −271.09, 95% confidence interval: −421.98 to −120.19, p< 10⁻⁴) and a significantly higher chance of reporting an improvement in well-being and/or mood (three studies, random effects risk ratio: 2.79, 95% confidence interval: 1.21-6.47, p= 0.016) when compared with controls. .. On the basis of the best available evidence, Se supplementation is associated with a significant decrease in TPOab titers at 3 months and with improvement in mood and/or general well-being."Toulis KA, Anastasilakis AD, Tzellos TG, Goulis DG, Kouvelas D. Selenium supplementation in the treatment of Hashimoto's thyroiditis: a systematic review and a meta-analysis. *Thyroid.* 2010 Oct;20(10):1163-73

[209] U.S. National Library of Medicine and NIH www.nlm.nih.gov/medlineplus/ency/article/003687.htm Accessed Aug 2011

Toxic metal testing—emphasis on lead and mercury	
Overview and application:	• <u>Introduction</u>: Per the US Department of Labor's Occupational Safety and Health Administration (OSHA)[210], toxic metals, including "heavy metals", are individual metals and metal compounds that negatively affect people's health. While lists of toxic metals can vary per source, OSHA names the following: arsenic, beryllium, cadmium, hexavalent chromium, lead, and mercury; of these, lead and mercury are the most commonly observed problematic toxic metals in outpatient practice. The three most important clinical concepts with regard to testing for "heavy metals" or "toxic metals" are as follows: 1. <u>Heavy metal toxicity/accumulation is not uncommon in clinical practice</u>: Toxic/heavy metal accumulation is clinically important due both to its frequency and its pathophysiologic consequences. An article published in *Journal of the American Medical Association (JAMA)*[211] showed that approximately 8% of [1,709 American] women had [blood mercury] concentrations higher than the US Environmental Protection Agency's recommended reference dose (5.8 µg/L), below which exposures are considered to be without adverse effects; **stated more plainly, 8% of American women have (potentially) toxic levels of mercury** *even when evaluated by the least sensitive of laboratory methods—blood mercury,* **which represents only 5% of total body mercury.** Another study, also published in *JAMA*[212], showed a positive relationship between blood lead levels and hypertension, even at blood lead levels considered within the normal range; the authors wrote, "At levels well below the current US occupational exposure limit guidelines (40 µg/dL), **blood lead level is positively associated with both systolic and diastolic blood pressure and risks of both systolic and diastolic hypertension among women aged 40 to 59 years.**" 2. <u>The clinical presentation of heavy metal toxicity/accumulation is generally diverse and nonspecific</u>: Clinical presentations due to or associated with toxic metal accumulation can include dyscognition, fatigue, anemia, chronic pain from myalgia or neuropathy, hypertension, autism, and immune disorders including autoimmunity and allergy. In particular, autism[213,214,215] and hypertension[216,217] are noteworthy for their consistent associations with mercury and with mercury and lead, respectively. 3. <u>(Therefore), clinicians should test for and treat toxic metal accumulation</u>: When problems are clinically significant and not extremely unlikely, clinicians have an obligation to test for and treat such problems for the benefit of the patient. Therefore, because toxic metal accumulation is common, clinically significant, and because it is a reversible cause of numerous symptoms, syndromes, and a contributing factor to many other diagnosable conditions (e.g., hypertension, immune disorders, mood disorders), clinicians have an obligation to consider and test for toxic metals among their patients. • <u>Additional details—mercury</u>: Mercury is an established neurotoxin, immunotoxin, and

[210] http://www.osha.gov/SLTC/metalsheavy/index.html Accessed July 2011.

[211] Schober SE, Sinks TH, Jones RL, Bolger PM, McDowell M, Osterloh J, Garrett ES, Canady RA, Dillon CF, Sun Y, Joseph CB, Mahaffey KR. Blood mercury levels in US children and women of childbearing age, 1999-2000. *JAMA* 2003;289:1667-74 http://jama.ama-assn.org/content/289/13/1667.long

[212] Nash D, Magder L, Lustberg M, Sherwin RW, Rubin RJ, Kaufmann RB, Silbergeld EK. Blood lead, blood pressure, and hypertension in perimenopausal and postmenopausal women. *JAMA*. 2003 Mar 26;289(12):1523-32. See also Muntner P, He J, Vupputuri S, Coresh J, Batuman V. Blood lead and chronic kidney disease in the general United States population: results from NHANES III. *Kidney Int.* 2003 Mar;63(3):1044-50 http://www.nature.com/ki/journal/v63/n3/pdf/4493526a.pdf

[213] Stamova B, Green PG, Tian Y, Hertz-Picciotto I, Pessah IN, Hansen R, Yang X, Teng J, Gregg JP, Ashwood P, Van de Water J, Sharp FR. Correlations between gene expression and mercury levels in blood of boys with and without autism. *Neurotox Res.* 2011;19:31-48. Epub 2009 Nov 24.

[214] "The results of the study indicated that the participants' overall ATEC scores and their scores on each of the ATEC subscales (Speech/Language, Sociability, Sensory/Cognitive Awareness, and Health/Physical/Behavior) were linearly related to urinary porphyrins associated with mercury toxicity. The results show an association between the apparent level of mercury toxicity as measured by recognized urinary porphyrin biomarkers of mercury toxicity and the magnitude of the specific hallmark features of autism as assessed by ATEC." Kern JK, Geier DA, Adams JB, Geier MR. A biomarker of mercury body-burden correlated with diagnostic domain specific clinical symptoms of autism spectrum disorder. *Biometals.* 2010 Dec;23(6):1043-51

[215] Kempuraj D, Asadi S, Zhang B, Manola A, Hogan J, Peterson E, Theoharides TC. Mercury induces inflammatory mediator release from human mast cells. *J Neuroinflammation.* 2010 Mar 11;7:20 http://www.jneuroinflammation.com/content/7/1/20

[216] Schober SE, Sinks TH, Jones RL, Bolger PM, McDowell M, Osterloh J, Garrett ES, Canady RA, Dillon CF, Sun Y, Joseph CB, Mahaffey KR. Blood mercury levels in US children and women of childbearing age, 1999-2000. *JAMA* 2003;289:1667-74 http://jama.ama-assn.org/content/289/13/1667.long

[217] Nash D, Magder L, Lustberg M, Sherwin RW, Rubin RJ, Kaufmann RB, Silbergeld EK. Blood lead, blood pressure, and hypertension in perimenopausal and postmenopausal women. *JAMA.* 2003 Mar 26;289(12):1523-32

nephrotoxin. Because pathophysiologic effects are noted even with very small doses of exposure, one could reasonably argue that no safe amount exists and therefore that any detected mercury is an indication for therapeutic intervention to remove this toxicant. According to an article by Schober et al[218] published in *JAMA—Journal of the American Medical Association* in 2003, "Approximately 8% of [1,709 American] women had [blood mercury] concentrations higher than the US Environmental Protection Agency's recommended reference dose (5.8 µg/L), below which exposures are considered to be without adverse effects." Sources of exposure include dental amalgams, vaccinations, airborne pollution, deepwater fish such as tuna, some cosmetics[219], and selected herbicides, fungicides, and germicides; recently, high-fructose corn syrup was shown to contain mercury in clinically meaningful amounts.[220] Mercury impairs catecholamine degradation and can thereby cause a clinical syndrome that can include hypertension, tremor, tachycardia, diaphoresis, and neurocognitive changes.[221] Per Shih and Gartner[222], "Mercury combines with the sulfhydryl group of S-adenosylmethionine, which is a cofactor for catecholamine-O-methyltransferase (COMT), and this inhibition of COMT allows accumulation of norepinephrine, epinephrine, and dopamine." The clinical presentation of mercury toxicity can include any of the following: diffuse erythematosus rash, dermatitis (acrodynia), anorexia, malaise, **fatigue**, **muscle pain**, proximal and/or distal muscle weakness, tremor, weight loss, **insomnia**, night sweats, burning peripheral neuropathy (axonal neuropathy), renal insufficiency/failure, **inattention**, neurocognitive compromise, personality changes, **depression**, diaphoresis, tachycardia, and **hypertension**. Mercury poisoning/accumulation can occur in humans as a result of consumption of contaminated foods—especially seafood such as shark, swordfish, king mackerel, tilefish, and albacore ("white") tuna.[223] The immunologic effects of organic and/or inorganic mercury include immunosuppression, immunostimulation, formation of antinucleolar antibodies targeting fibrillarin, and formation and deposition of immune-complexes, resulting in a syndrome called "mercury-induced autoimmunity" which can be induced by exposure of susceptible animals to mercury.[224] Mercury/"silver" amalgam dental fillings rank highly among the most significant source of mercury exposure in humans, and implantation of mercury-silver dental amalgams in susceptible animals causes chronic stimulation of the immune system with induction of systemic autoimmunity.[225] Besides being a neurotoxin with no safe exposure limit[226], mercury is known to modify/antigenize/haptenize endogenous proteins to promote autoimmunity[227], and mercury may also promote

[218] Schober SE, Sinks TH, Jones RL, et al. Blood mercury levels in US children and women of childbearing age, 1999-2000. *JAMA*. 2003 Apr 2;289(13):1667-74 http://jama.ama-assn.org/content/289/13/1667.long
[219] "Most makeup manufacturers have phased out the use of mercury, but it's still added legally to some eye products as a preservative and germ-killer, said John Bailey, chief scientist with the Personal Care Products Council in Washington." Associated Press. Minnesota Bans Adding Mercury To Cosmetics. February 11, 2009. http://www.cbsnews.com/stories/2007/12/14/health/main3618048.shtml Accessed August 2011
[220] "Average daily consumption of high fructose corn syrup is about 50 grams per person in the United States. With respect to total mercury exposure, it may be necessary to account for this source of mercury in the diet of children and sensitive populations." Dufault R, LeBlanc B, Schnoll R, Cornett C, Schweitzer L, Wallinga D, Hightower J, Patrick L, Lukiw WJ. Mercury from chlor-alkali plants: measured concentrations in food product sugar. *Environ Health*. 2009 Jan 26;8:2. See also: "High fructose corn syrup has been shown to contain trace amounts of mercury as a result of some manufacturing processes, and its consumption can also lead to zinc loss." Dufault R, Schnoll R, Lukiw WJ, Leblanc B, Cornett C, Patrick L, Wallinga D, Gilbert SG, Crider R. Mercury exposure, nutritional deficiencies and metabolic disruptions may affect learning in children. *Behav Brain Funct*. 2009 Oct 27;5:44.
[221] Wössmann W, Kohl M, Grüning G, Bucsky P. Mercury intoxication presenting with hypertension and tachycardia. *Arch Dis Child*. 1999 Jun;80(6):556-7 http://www.ncbi.nlm.nih.gov/pmc/articles/PMC1717944/pdf/v080p00556.pdf
[222] Shih H, Gartner JC Jr. Weight loss, hypertension, weakness, and limb pain in an 11-year-old boy. *J Pediatr*. 2001 Apr;138(4):566-9
[223] See http://www.fda.gov/Food/FoodSafety/Product-SpecificInformation/Seafood/FoodbornePathogensContaminants/Methylmercury/ucm115662.htm for the white-washed version; see http://www.ewg.org/news/bamboozled-fish for a more accurate and complete perspective.
[224] Havarinasab S, Hultman P. Organic mercury compounds and autoimmunity. *Autoimmun Rev*. 2005;4(5):270-5 www.generationrescue.org/pdf/havarinasab.pdf Accessed December 27, 2005
[225] "We hypothesize that under appropriate conditions of genetic susceptibility and adequate body burden, heavy metal exposure from dental amalgam may contribute to immunological aberrations, which could lead to overt autoimmunity." Hultman P, Johansson U, Turley SJ, Lindh U, Enestrom S, Pollard KM. Adverse immunological effects and autoimmunity induced by dental amalgam and alloy in mice. *FASEB J*. 1994 Nov;8(14):1183-90
[226] University of Calgary Faculty of Medicine. How Mercury Causes Brain Neuron Degeneration. http://commons.ucalgary.ca/mercury/ Current Aug 2011
[227] Havarinasab S, Hultman P. Organic mercury compounds and autoimmunity. *Autoimmun Rev*. 2005 Jun;4(5):270-5. Full-text available at www.generationrescue.org/pdf/havarinasab.pdf on December 27, 2005

Toxic metal testing—emphasis on lead and mercury

autoimmunity by contributing to a pro-inflammatory environment that awakens quiescent autoreactive immunocytes via bystander activation.[228] For example, administration of mercury to "susceptible" mice induces autoimmunity via modification of the nucleolar protein *fibrillarin*[229]; noteworthy in this regard is the fact that antifibrillarin antibodies are characteristic of the human autoimmune disease scleroderma.[230] The mercury-based preservative thimerosol is a type-IV (delayed hypersensitivity) sensitizing agent[231], and recent research implicates mercury as a contributor to autism[232,233] and eczema.[234] A review and clinical report published by Bains et al[235], stated, "Eczematous eruptions may be produced through topical contact with mercury and by systemic absorption in mercury sensitive individuals. Mercury…may cause hypersensitivity leading to contact dermatitis or Coomb's Type IV hypersensitivity reactions. The typical manifestation is an urticarial or erythematous rash, and pruritus on the face and flexural aspects of limbs, followed by progression to dermatitis." Thus, this survey of the literature supports the notions that mercury toxicity—i.e., a level of mercury in human patients sufficient to cause adverse health effects—is ❶ common (e.g., 8% of American women), ❷ problematic via causation of or contribution to various health problems commonly encountered in clinical practice, ❸ diagnosable via laboratory testing followed by monitoring response to treatment, and ❹ treatable, most notably with DMSA but also to a lesser extent with potassium citrate, selenium, and phytochelatins.

- Additional details—lead: The International Agency for Research on Cancer (IARC, part of the World Health Organization [WHO]) classified lead as a "possible human carcinogen" in 1987. A 2003 review published in *British Medical Bulletin* by Järup[236] noted that lead exposure (which comes equally from air and food, particularly food served via lead-contaminated ceramics) should be avoided as much as possible because physiologic toxicity occurs with low-level exposure; "Blood levels in children should be reduced below the levels so far considered acceptable, recent data indicating that there may be neurotoxic effects of lead at lower levels of exposure than previously anticipated." Occupational exposure to lead occurs in mines, smelting plants, glass-manufacturing facilities, battery plants, and among workers who weld metals already painted with lead-containing paints; air emissions near such facilities and activities may also contaminate nonworkers. Air contamination frequently leads to water contamination, threatening wildlife and humans who are exposed to contaminated water. Children are particularly vulnerable to lead exposure due to very efficient (compared with adults) gastrointestinal absorption and a more permeable ("leaky") blood-brain barrier. Organic lead compounds such as tetramethyl lead and tetraethyl lead easily penetrate skin and blood-brain barrier of children as well as adults. Classic, large-dose, acute and subacute lead poisoning manifests as anemia, renal tubular damage, and dark blue line of lead sulphide at the gingival margin; clinicians awaiting this classic presentation prior to considering lead

[228] "It is therefore theoretically possible that compounds present in vaccines such as thiomersal or aluminium hydroxyde can trigger autoimmune reactions through bystander effects." Fournie GJ, Mas M, Cautain B, et al. Induction of autoimmunity through bystander effects. Lessons from immunological disorders induced by heavy metals. *J Autoimmun*. 2001 May;16(3):319-26

[229] Nielsen JB, Hultman P. Mercury-induced autoimmunity in mice. *Environ Health Perspect*. 2002 Oct;110 Suppl 5:877-81 http://ehp.niehs.nih.gov/docs/2002/suppl-5/877-881nielsen/abstract.html

[230] "Since anti-fibrillarin antibodies are specific markers of scleroderma, the present animal model may be valuable for studies of the immunological aberrations which are likely to induce this autoimmune response." Hultman P, Enestrom S, Pollard KM, Tan EM. Anti-fibrillarin autoantibodies in mercury-treated mice. *Clin Exp Immunol*. 1989;78(3):470-7

[231] "Thimerosal is an important preservative in vaccines and ophthalmologic preparations. The substance is known to be a type IV sensitizing agent. High sensitization rates were observed in contact-allergic patients and in health care workers who had been exposed to thimerosal-preserved vaccines." Westphal GA, Schnuch A, Schulz TG, Reich K, Aberer W, Brasch J, Koch P, Wessbecher R, Szliska C, Bauer A, Hallier E. Homozygous gene deletions of the glutathione S-transferases M1 and T1 are associated with thimerosal sensitization. *Int Arch Occup Environ Health*. 2000 Aug;73(6):384-8

[232] Vojdani A, Pangborn JB, Vojdani E, Cooper EL. Infections, toxic chemicals and dietary peptides binding to lymphocyte receptors and tissue enzymes are major instigators of autoimmunity in autism. *Int J Immunopathol Pharmacol*. 2003 Sep-Dec;16(3):189-99

[233] Geier DA, Geier MR. A comparative evaluation of the effects of MMR immunization and mercury doses from thimerosal-containing childhood vaccines on the population prevalence of autism. *Med Sci Monit*. 2004 Mar;10(3):PI33-9. http://www.medscimonit.com/pub/vol_10/no_3/3986.pdf

[234] Weidinger S, Kramer U, Dunemann L, Mohrenschlager M, Ring J, Behrendt H. Body burden of mercury is associated with acute atopic eczema and total IgE in children from southern Germany. *J Allergy Clin Immunol*. 2004 Aug;114(2):457-9

[235] Bains VK, Loomba K, Loomba A, Bains R. Mercury sensitisation: review, relevance and a clinical report. *Br Dent J*. 2008 Oct 11;205(7):373-8 http://www.intolsante.com/documents/publications/-mercury-sensitisation-review-relevance-and-clinical-report-22.pdf Accessed August 2011

[236] Järup L. Hazards of heavy metal contamination. *Br Med Bull*. 2003;68:167-82

	toxicity should fortify their knowledge of and reconsider their perspective on this topic. Other symptoms of acute lead poisoning are headache, irritability, abdominal pain and various neurologic-psychiatric symptoms generally referred to as "lead encephalopathy" characterized by sleeplessness, restlessness, confusion/dyscognition, behavioral disturbances, particularly learning and concentration difficulties in children; more extreme manifestations can include acute psychosis and stupor. Per the previously cited review by Järup, "Individuals [chronically exposed to lead] with average blood lead levels under 3 μmol/l may show signs of peripheral nerve symptoms with reduced nerve conduction velocity and reduced dermal sensibility."
Overview and application:	▪ No universally accepted consensus exists for the most accurate testing methodology. However, from the science-based perspectives that **toxic metals have been proven to cause harm at levels previously believed to be "acceptable" and that—very importantly—toxic metals are exponentially more toxic when in combination than when present alone**, reasonable clinicians can therefore conclude that the best test for clinical use is the one that is most sensitive, along with being reasonably convenient for the patient as well as affordable. For these reasons, the current author and many other clinicians chose DMSA-provoked urine toxic metal testing. Hair and nails can also be tested for chronic exposure, as can blood which is generally only useful for recent and relatively high-level exposure. Our clinical concern in general outpatient practice is not with recent and relatively high-level exposure, and therefore blood is not necessarily optimal. Our clinical concern in general outpatient practice is with chronic low-level exposure which leads to adverse cellular effects despite the failure to "spike" the serum level into the detectable toxic range. Arguments in favor of allowing symptomatic patients to persist untreated in a state of toxic metal accumulation would be difficult to justify scientifically and ethically.
Advantages:	▪ Toxic metal accumulation is ❶ <u>sufficiently common to warrant testing in selected patients,</u> ❷ <u>problematic</u> via causation of or contribution to various health problems commonly encountered in clinical practice, ❸ <u>diagnosable</u> via laboratory testing followed by monitoring response to treatment, and ❹ <u>treatable</u>. Therefore, clinicians should establish pathways for the assessment and treatment of metal toxicity.
Limitations:	▪ Patients with toxic metal accumulation frequently have accumulation of chemical xenobiotics as well; thus testing for and treating toxicity due to metals only relieves one type of toxicity.
Comments:	▪ Clinicians should establish pathways for the assessment and treatment of toxic metal accumulation.

Presentation: Widespread musculoskeletal pain (resembling fibromyalgia) secondary to lead and mercury accumulation: This 54yo athletic female with healthy diet, lifestyle, and supportive relationship presented with chronic diffuse musculoskeletal pain. Health history was sigificant for decades of environmental illness/intolerance (EI) also known as multiple chemical sensitivity (MCS). Family history was positive for maternal temporal (giant cell) arteritis. Physical examination revealed numerous tender points consistent with fibromyalgia; yet the history and stool analysis with comprehensive bacteriology and parasitology were unsupportive of gastrointestinal dysbiosis, particularly of the subtype small intestine bacterial overgrowth, which is causal for fibromyalgia.[237] Laboratory investigations revealed normal results for hsCRP (high-sensitity c-reactive protein), CK (creatine kinase, a marker of muscle damage and myositis), ANA (anti-nuclear antibodies), vitamin D, calcium, phosphorus, and comprehensive thyroid evaluation. The patient was then (defensively) referred to an osteopathic internist who diagnosed fibromyalgia.

Date Completed: 10/22/2005

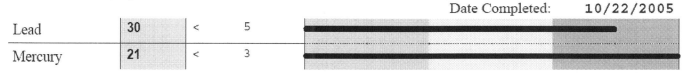

| Lead | 30 | < | 5 |
| Mercury | 21 | < | 3 |

Discussion: The patient, unsatisfied with the diagnosis of fibromyalgia, returned to the current author, who then performed urine heavy metal testing provoked with 10 mg per kilogram of dimercaptosuccinic acid (DMSA). Results revealed the highest levels of lead and mercury encountered in the author's practice at that time. As shown above, lead levels were 6x above the reference range and mercury levels were 7x above the reference range. The patient was commenced on DMSA 10 mg/kg/d on alternating weeks to avoid toxicity in general and bone marrow toxicity (neutropenia) in particular, selenium 800 mcg/d to promote excretion of toxic metals and to support renal and antoxidant protection, vegetable juices to provide potassium and citrate for urinary alkalinization and enhanced excretion of xenobiotics[238], and a proprietary phytochelatin (metal-binding peptides from plants[239]) concetrate to bind toxic metals in the gut and thereby promote their fecal excretion by blocking enterohepatic recirculation. The use of DMSA for children and adults is supported by peer-reviewed literature[240,241,242,243,244] and has been reviewed in more detail by this author in *Integrative Rheumatology*[245] and to a lesser extent in *Musculoskeletal Pain: Expanded Clinical Strategies*.[246] DMSA chelation is approved by the US Food and Drug Administration (FDA) for the treatment of lead toxicity in children.[247] After approximately 8 months of treatment, the patient was completely free of pain, and the clinical improvement was associated with a reduction in both lead and mercury of approximately 50% as demonstrated by follow-up laboratory testing. Testing was performed by Doctors Data. This case was published in peer-reviewed literature for continuing education credits.[248]

Date Completed: 6/30/2006

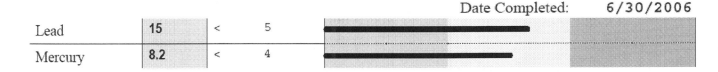

| Lead | 15 | < | 5 |
| Mercury | 8.2 | < | 4 |

[237] **Vasquez A**. Musculoskeletal Pain: Expanded Clinical Strategies. Institute for Functional Medicine. 2008

[238] Crinnion WJ. Environmental medicine, part three: long-term effects of chronic low-dose mercury exposure. *Altern Med Rev*. 2000 Jun;5(3):209-23 http://www.thorne.com/altmedrev/.fulltext/5/3/209.pdf

[239] Cobbett CS. Phytochelatins and their roles in heavy metal detoxification. *Plant Physiol*. 2000;123:825-32 plantphysiol.org/content/123/3/825

[240] Bradstreet J, Geier DA, Kartzinel JJ, Adams JB, Geier MR. A case-control study of mercury burden in children with autistic spectrum disorders. *Journal of American Physicians and Surgeons* 2003; 8: 76-79 http://www.jpands.org/vol8no3/geier.pdf

[241] Crinnion WJ. Environmental medicine, part three: long-term effects of chronic low-dose mercury exposure. *Altern Med Rev*. 2000 Jun;5(3):209-23

[242] Forman J, Moline J, Cernichiari E, Sayegh S, Torres JC, Landrigan MM, Hudson J, Adel HN, Landrigan PJ. A cluster of pediatric metallic mercury exposure cases treated with meso-2,3-dimercaptosuccinic acid (DMSA). *Environ Health Perspect*. 2000 Jun;108(6):575-7 http://ehp.niehs.nih.gov/docs/2000/108p575-577forman/abstract.html

[243] Miller AL. Dimercaptosuccinic acid (DMSA), a non-toxic, water-soluble treatment for heavy metal toxicity. *Altern Med Rev*. 1998 Jun;3(3):199-207 http://www.thorne.com/altmedrev/.fulltext/3/3/199.pdf

[244] DMSA. *Altern Med Rev*. 2000 Jun;5(3):264-7 http://thorne.com/altmedrev/.fulltext/5/3/264.pdf

[245] **Vasquez A**. Integrative Rheumatology. IBMRC 2006, 2007 and all future editions. http://optimalhealthresearch.com/rheumatology.html

[246] **Vasquez A**. Musculoskeletal Pain: Expanded Clinical Strategies. Institute for Functional Medicine. 2008

[247] "The Food and Drug Administration has recently licensed the drug DMSA (succimer) for reduction of blood lead levels >/= 45 micrograms/dl. This decision was based on the demonstrated ability of DMSA to reduce blood lead levels. An advantage of this drug is that it can be given orally." Goyer RA, Cherian MG, Jones MM, Reigart JR. Role of chelating agents for prevention, intervention, and treatment of exposures to toxic metals. *Environ Health Perspect*. 1995 Nov;103(11):1048-52 Http://ehp.niehs.nih.gov/docs/1995/103-11/meetingreport.html

[248] **Vasquez A**. Musculoskeletal Pain: Expanded Clinical Strategies. Institute for Functional Medicine. 2008

Presentation: Chronic "idiopathic" hypertension associated with lead and mercury accumulation (per DMSA-provoked urine testing): This 43yo male presents with recalcitrant stage-1 hypertension. His cardiologist prescribed drugs to "treat" (some would say "mask") his elevated blood pressure. Since hypertension always has an underlying cause, the ethical and appropriate course of action is to determine the cause of the problem rather than silencing the alarm that is alerting to an underlying dysfunction. While this case is currently in progress at the time of this writing (the patient's medical records arrived in July 2011), it does offer a model case for clinical decision-making. Clinicians should be aware that, per animal studies, the toxicity of lead and mercury are greatly enhanced when both toxins are present at the same time.

Date Collected: 6/3/2010

| Lead | 8.5 | < | 2 | |
| Mercury | 17 | < | 3 | |

Mercury and hypertension: Mercury is an established neurotoxin, immunotoxin, and nephrotoxin. Because pathophysiologic effects are noted even with very small doses of exposure, one could reasonably argue that no safe amount exists and therefore that any detected mercury is an indication for therapeutic intervention to remove this toxicant. Sources of exposure include dental amalgams, vaccinations, airborne pollution, and fish; recently, high-fructose corn syrup was shown to contain mercury.[249] Mercury impairs catecholamine degradation and can thereby cause a clinical syndrome that can include hypertension, tremor, tachycardia, diaphoresis, and neurocognitive changes.[250] Per Shih and Gartner[251], "Mercury combines with the sulfhydryl group of S-adenosylmethionine, which is a cofactor for catecholamine-O-methyltransferase (COMT), and this inhibition of COMT allows accumulation of norepinephrine, epinephrine, and dopamine."

Lead and hypertension: In the United States, a consistent correlation has been found between body burden of lead and HTN, even when blood lead levels are well below the current US occupational exposure limit guidelines (40 microg/dl).[252] Harlan et al[253] analyzed data from the second National Health and Nutrition Examination Survey (1976-1980) and thereby found a direct relationship between blood lead levels and systolic and diastolic pressures for men and women and for white and black persons aged 12 to 74 years; they concluded, "Blood lead levels were significantly higher in younger men and women (aged 21 to 55 years) with high blood pressure, but not in older men or women (aged 56 to 74 years)." Schwartz and Stewart[254] found that blood lead was the assessment that most strongly correlated with HTN; they concluded, "Systolic blood pressure was elevated by blood lead levels as low as 5 microg/dl." Thus, clinicians might first measure blood lead levels, which do not measure total body burden but rather the lead that is mobile or *in transit* within the body and which appears to have the best correlation with HTN; the finding of normal blood lead results could then be followed with the more sensitive DMSA-provoked heavy metal testing before concluding that heavy metals are noncontributory to that particular patient's HTN. For heavy metal testing in various clinical scenarios, this author's preference is to use DMSA-provoked measurement of urine toxic metals. After a minimal test dose of DMSA (e.g., in the range of 50-100 mg) to screen for hypersensitivity, patients take oral DMSA 10 mg/kg as a single oral dose in the morning on an empty stomach after emptying the bladder and send a sample from the next urination for laboratory analysis; follow laboratory protocol if different from these instructions. Use of DMSA for lead and mercury chelation/detoxification and for diagnostic purposes is generally safe and effective[255,256,257]; detoxification procedures are reviewed in much greater detail in *Integrative Rheumatology*.[258]

[249] "Average daily consumption of high fructose corn syrup is about 50 grams per person in the United States. With respect to total mercury exposure, it may be necessary to account for this source of mercury in the diet of children and sensitive populations." Dufault R, LeBlanc B, Schnoll R, Cornett C, Schweitzer L, Wallinga D, Hightower J, Patrick L, Lukiw WJ. Mercury from chlor-alkali plants: measured concentrations in food product sugar. *Environ Health*. 2009 Jan 26;8:2. See also: "High fructose corn syrup has been shown to contain trace amounts of mercury as a result of some manufacturing processes, and its consumption can also lead to zinc loss." Dufault R, Schnoll R, Lukiw WJ, Leblanc B, Cornett C, Patrick L, Wallinga D, Gilbert SG, Crider R. Mercury exposure, nutritional deficiencies and metabolic disruptions may affect learning in children. *Behav Brain Funct*. 2009 Oct 27;5:44.
[250] Wössmann W, Kohl M, Grüning G, Bucsky P. Mercury intoxication presenting with hypertension and tachycardia. *Arch Dis Child*. 1999 Jun;80(6):556-7 http://www.ncbi.nlm.nih.gov/pmc/articles/PMC1717944/pdf/v080p00556.pdf
[251] Shih H, Gartner JC Jr. Weight loss, hypertension, weakness, and limb pain in an 11-year-old boy. *J Pediatr*. 2001 Apr;138(4):566-9
[252] Nash D, Magder L, Lustberg M, Sherwin RW, Rubin RJ, Kaufmann RB, Silbergeld EK. Blood lead, blood pressure, and hypertension in perimenopausal and postmenopausal women. *JAMA*. 2003 Mar 26;289(12):1523-32 http://jama.ama-assn.org/cgi/content/full/289/12/1523
[253] Harlan WR, Landis JR, Schmouder RL, Goldstein NG, Harlan LC. Blood lead and blood pressure. Relationship in the adolescent and adult US population. *JAMA*. 1985 Jan 25;253(4):530-4
[254] "Systolic blood pressure was elevated by blood lead levels as low as 5 microg/dl." Schwartz BS, Stewart WF. Different associations of blood lead, meso 2,3-dimercaptosuccinic acid (DMSA)-chelatable lead, and tibial lead levels with blood pressure in 543 former organolead manufacturing workers. *Arch Environ Health*. 2000 Mar-Apr;55(2):85-92
[255] Bradstreet J, Geier DA, Kartzinel JJ, Adams JB, Geier MR. A case-control study of mercury burden in children with autistic spectrum disorders. *Journal of American Physicians and Surgeons* 2003; 8: 76-79 http://www.jpands.org/vol8no3/geier.pdf
[256] Miller AL. Dimercaptosuccinic acid (DMSA), a non-toxic, water-soluble treatment for heavy metal toxicity. *Altern Med Rev*. 1998 Jun;3(3):199-207
[257] DMSA. *Altern Med Rev*. 2000 Jun;5(3):264-7 http://thorne.com/altmedrev/.fulltext/5/3/264.pdf
[258] Vasquez A. Integrative Rheumatology. IBMRC 2006, 2007 and all future editions. http://optimalhealthresearch.com/rheumatology.html

Antinuclear antibody: ANA	
Overview and interpretation:	• **Good screening test for autoimmune conditions**: SLE, Sjogren's syndrome, and various other connective tissue diseases. • Good and "highly sensitive" for initial assessment of SLE; positive in 95-98% of SLE patients; negative result strongly suggests against diagnosis of SLE.[259] Only 2% of patients with SLE have a negative ANA test—these patients may be identified by testing with anti-RO antibodies and CH50 (complement levels). • This test measures for the presence of antibodies that react to nucleoproteins. Some labs report titers of 1:20 or 1:40 as "positive"; however, low levels of ANA are common (5-15%) in the general population. Thus, ANA is not specific for any one disease; may be positive in SLE, RA, scleroderma, Sjogren's, also seen with elderly, infected patients, cancer, and certain medications. Titers less than 1:160 should be interpreted cautiously as they may not indicate the presence of *clinical* autoimmunity.[260] **Titers greater than 1:320 are considered indicative of clinically significant autoimmunity.** • Methodologies (indirect immunofluorescence is most popular), subtypes, and patterns reported for ANA results may be irrelevant or clinically meaningful; the most common descriptors are provided in the table below.

ANA patterns and descriptions[261,262]	*Clinical correlation*
Homogeneous, diffuse nuclear staining	Nonspecific
Speckled	Least specific
Rim or **peripheral staining**	Suggests SLE and warrants assessment for anti-dsDNA, which is specific for lupus
Anti-centromere: selective staining of the centromeres of nuclei in metaphase	Highly specific for the limited scleroderma subtype associated with CREST syndrome
Nucleolar	Correlated with diffuse scleroderma (systemic sclerosis)
FANA: fluorescent ANA	The standard ANA test in the US
Anti-Sm: anti-Smith[263]	Virtually diagnostic of SLE: Highly specific for SLE; insensitive: positive in 20-30% of SLE patients
Anti-dsDNA: anti-double stranded DNA	Virtually diagnostic of SLE: Highly specific for SLE and indicative of an increased likelihood of poor prognosis with major organ involvement[264] especially active renal disease
Anti-Ro (anti-SS-A)	Correlates with SLE, Sjögren's syndrome, and neonatal SLE
Anti-La (anti-SS-B)	Sjögren's syndrome or low risk of SLE nephritis
Anti-RNP	SLE and/or mixed connective tissue disease (MCTD)
Anti-Jo-1	Specific but not sensitive for polymyositis/dermatomyositis
Antihistone	SLE and especially drug-induced SLE
Antitopoisomerase (Scl-70)	Correlates with diffuse scleroderma, especially with interstitial lung disease

[259] Shojania K. Rheumatology: 2. What laboratory tests are needed? *CMAJ.* 2000 Apr 18;162(8):1157-63 http://www.cmaj.ca/cgi/content/full/162/8/1157
[260] Hardin JG, Waterman J, Labson LH. Rheumatic disease: Which diagnostic tests are useful? *Patient Care* 1999; March 15: 83-102
[261] Shojania K. Rheumatology: 2. What laboratory tests are needed? *CMAJ.* 2000 Apr 18;162(8):1157-63 http://www.cmaj.ca/cgi/content/full/162/8/1157
[262] Ward MM. Laboratory testing for systemic rheumatic diseases. *Postgrad Med.* 1998 Feb;103(2):93-100.
[263] Lane SK, Gravel JW Jr. Clinical utility of common serum rheumatologic tests. *Am Fam Physician.* 2002;65:1073-80 http://www.aafp.org/afp/20020315/1073.html
[264] Shojania K. Rheumatology: 2. What laboratory tests are needed? *CMAJ.* 2000 Apr 18;162(8):1157-63 http://www.cmaj.ca/cgi/content/full/162/8/1157

Antinuclear antibody: ANA—*continued*	
Advantages:	▪ ANA has 98% sensitivity and 90% specificity for SLE in an unselected population. ▪ The negative predictive value in an unselected population is greater than 99%. ANA is therefore an excellent test for *excluding* the diagnosis of SLE.
Limitations:	▪ The positive predictive value in an unselected population is about 30%; **only 30% of unselected people with a positive result will have SLE**—this fact underscores the importance of patient selection and judicious interpretation of this test. ▪ Positive ANA is seen in patients with conditions other than SLE, including rheumatoid arthritis, Sjogren's syndrome, scleroderma, polymyositis, vasculitis, juvenile rheumatoid arthritis (JRA), and infectious diseases.
Comments:	▪ ANA is most often used to support the diagnosis of SLE in a patient with multisystemic illness and a clinical picture compatible with SLE. Nearly all patients with SLE will have positive ANA. **A positive ANA does not mean that the patient necessarily has SLE; be weary of paraneoplastic syndromes and viral hepatitis as underlying causative processes in patients with an unclear clinical picture.** ▪ I view any "positive ANA" as an indicator of poor health in general and immune dysfunction in particular. The goal, then, is to restore health. I have seen ANA show a trend toward normalization or completely normalize with effective health restoration as detailed in *Integrative Rheumatology* (chapter 4). I realize that my experience in this regard contrasts sharply with the allopathic view that serial measurements of ANA are worthless because the result never normalizes once a patient is ANA-positive[265]; I consider this evidence of the effectiveness of my integrative-functional approach and the comparable failure of the allopathic approach.

Antineutrophilic cytoplasmic antibodies: ANCA	
Overview:	▪ ANCA are autoantibodies to the cytoplasmic constituents of granulocytes and are characteristically found in vasculitic syndromes and also in (Chinese) patients with inflammatory bowel disease[266] and nearly all patients with hepatic amebiasis due to *Entamoeba histolytica*.[267] <u>Two types:</u> ▪ <u>Cytoplasmic ANCA (C-ANCA)</u>: classically seen in **Wegener's granulomatosis**; also seen in some types of glomerulonephritis and vasculitis; this test is highly sensitive and specific for these conditions. In fact, a positive C-ANCA result can replace biopsy in a patient with a clinical picture of **Wegener's granulomatosis.**[268] ▪ <u>Perinuclear ANCA (P-ANCA)</u>: considered a nonspecific finding[269] that correlates with SLE, drug induced lupus, and some types of glomerulonephritis and vasculitis. Shojania[270] stated that this test must be confirmed with antimyeloperoxidase antibodies to evaluate for Churg–Strauss syndrome, crescentic glomerulonephritis, and microscopic polyarteritis.
Advantages, limitations, and comments	▪ Not to be used as a screening test, except in patients with idiopathic vasculitis or glomerulonephritis. ▪ The fact that hepatic amebiasis due to *Entamoeba histolytica* induces production of C-ANCA antibodies in nearly 100% of infected patients may support the hypothesis that autoimmunity can be induced or exacerbated by parasitic infections.

[265] Shojania K. Rheumatology: 2. What laboratory tests are needed? *CMAJ*. 2000 Apr 18;162(8):1157-63 http://www.cmaj.ca/cgi/content/full/162/8/1157
[266] "Fourteen patients (73.5%) were positive, of which six (31.5%) showed a perinuclear staining pattern and eight (42%) demonstrated a cytoplasmic pattern." Sung JY, Chan KL, Hsu R, Liew CT, Lawton JW. Ulcerative colitis and antineutrophil cytoplasmic antibodies in Hong Kong Chinese. *Am J Gastroenterol*. 1993 Jun;88(6):864-9
[267] "ANCA was detected in 97.4% of amoebic sera; the pattern of staining was cytoplasmic, homogeneous, without central accentuation (C-ANCA)." Pudifin DJ, Duursma J, Gathiram V, Jackson TF. Invasive amoebiasis is associated with the development of anti-neutrophil cytoplasmic antibody. *Clin Exp Immunol*. 1994 Jul;97(1):48-5
[268] Shojania K. Rheumatology: 2. What laboratory tests are needed? *CMAJ*. 2000 Apr 18;162(8):1157-63 http://www.cmaj.ca/cgi/content/full/162/8/1157
[269] Shojania K. Rheumatology: 2. What laboratory tests are needed? *CMAJ*. 2000 Apr 18;162(8):1157-63 http://www.cmaj.ca/cgi/content/full/162/8/1157
[270] Shojania K. Rheumatology: 2. What laboratory tests are needed? *CMAJ*. 2000 Apr 18;162(8):1157-63 http://www.cmaj.ca/cgi/content/full/162/8/1157

RF: Rheumatoid Factor	
Overview and application:	▪ Rheumatoid factor—"anti-IgG antibodies"—are antibodies directed to the Fc portion of the patient's own IgG. Rheumatoid factors are anti-immunoglobulin antibodies, classically anti-IgG IgM. RF are found in low levels in most patients, and despite the "rheumatoid" name, RF is not specific for rheumatoid arthritis.[271] Current tests (latex fixation or nephelometry) detect IgM anti-immunoglobulin antibodies; however Ig<u>A</u>-RF appears to have clinical superiority over other forms of RF because it correlates more strongly with clinical status.[272] ▪ This test is most commonly used to support the diagnosis of rheumatoid arthritis in a patient with a compelling clinical picture: peripheral polyarthritis lasting >6 weeks.[273] A negative result with a compelling clinical presentation of RA is termed "seronegative rheumatoid arthritis" by allopathic textbooks whereas a more appropriate term might be oligoarthritis, a condition described as "idiopathic" by allopathic text books despite the clear evidence that the majority of patients have one or more subsets of dysbiosis.[274] ▪ **Titers (latex fixation) of 1:160 are considered clinically significant, favoring the diagnosis of RA.**[275] However the positive predictive value is low—only 20-34% of people in an unselected population with a positive test result actually have RA.[276,277]
Advantages:	▪ Supports the diagnosis of rheumatoid arthritis: about 60-85% positive/sensitive in patients with rheumatoid arthritis (RA).[278,279] Quantitative titers of RF correlate with prognosis: a very high RF value portends a poor prognosis.
Limitations:	▪ **Positive findings are common in the following conditions: rheumatoid arthritis, viral hepatitis, Sjögren's syndrome, endocarditis, scleroderma, mycobacteria diseases, polymyositis and dermatomyositis, syphilis, systemic lupus erythematosus, old age, mixed connective tissue disease, sarcoidosis;** positive results may also been noted in: **cryoglobulinemia, parasitic infection, interstitial lung disease, asymptomatic relatives of people with autoimmune diseases.** ▪ Febrile patients with arthralgia are more likely to have endocarditis than RA.[280] ▪ Patients with iron overload present with a similar clinical picture (i.e., polyarthropathy with systemic complaints) and may have a positive RF. Thus, patients with positive RF and polyarthropathy should be tested for iron overload; use serum ferritin.[281,282]
Comments:	▪ This test should only be used to confirm the diagnosis of rheumatoid arthritis in patients with a compelling clinical picture of the disease: inflammatory peripheral polyarthropathy with systemic complaints for > 6 weeks. A negative result does not mean that the patient *does not* have rheumatoid arthritis; a positive result does not mean that the patient *does* have rheumatoid arthritis.[283] ▪ CCP (cyclic citrullinated protein) antibodies appear to be more specific and sensitive for RA and is becoming the test of choice for RA as described on the following page.

[271] Shojania K. Rheumatology: 2. What laboratory tests are needed? *CMAJ*. 2000 Apr 18;162(8):1157-63 http://www.cmaj.ca/cgi/content/full/162/8/1157
[272] Jonsson T, Valdimarsson H. What about IgA rheumatoid factor in rheumatoid arthritis? *Ann Rheum Dis*. 1998 Jan;57(1):63-4
[273] Shojania K. Rheumatology: 2. What laboratory tests are needed? *CMAJ*. 2000 Apr 18;162(8):1157-63 http://www.cmaj.ca/cgi/content/full/162/8/1157
[274] See chapter 4 of *Integrative Rheumatology* and Vasquez A. Reducing Pain and Inflammation Naturally. Part 6: Nutritional and Botanical Treatments Against "Silent Infections" and Gastrointestinal Dysbiosis, Commonly Overlooked Causes of Neuromusculoskeletal Inflammation and Chronic Health Problems. *Nutr Perspect* 2006; Jan http://optimalhealthresearch.com/part6
[275] Beers MH, Berkow R (eds). The Merck Manual. Seventeenth Edition. Whitehouse Station; Merck Research Laboratories 1999 Page 417
[276] Ward MM. Laboratory testing for systemic rheumatic diseases. *Postgrad Med*. 1998 Feb;103(2):93-100.
[277] Shojania K. Rheumatology: 2. What laboratory tests are needed? *CMAJ*. 2000 Apr 18;162(8):1157-63 http://www.cmaj.ca/cgi/content/full/162/8/1157
[278] Tierney ML. McPhee SJ, Papadakis MA (eds). Current Medical Diagnosis and Treatment 2002, 41st Edition. New York: Lange Medical, 2002 p854
[279] Shojania K. Rheumatology: 2. What laboratory tests are needed? *CMAJ*. 2000 Apr 18;162(8):1157-63 http://www.cmaj.ca/cgi/content/full/162/8/1157
[280] Klippel JH (ed). Primer on the Rheumatic Diseases. 11th Edition. Atlanta: Arthritis Foundation. 1997 page 96
[281] Bensen WG, Laskin CA, Little HA, Fam AG. Hemochromatoic arthropathy mimicking rheumatoid arthritis. A case with subcutaneous nodules, tenosynovitis, and bursitis. *Arthritis Rheum* 1978; 21: 844-8
[282] **Vasquez A**. Musculoskeletal disorders and iron overload disease: comment on the American College of Rheumatology guidelines for the initial evaluation of the adult patient with acute musculoskeletal symptoms. *Arthritis Rheum* 1996;39: 1767-8
[283] Shojania K. Rheumatology: 2. What laboratory tests are needed? *CMAJ*. 2000 Apr 18;162(8):1157-63 http://www.cmaj.ca/cgi/content/full/162/8/1157

CCP: Cyclic citrullinated protein antibody; Citrullinated protein antibodies (CPA); anti-CCP antibodies: anticyclic citrullinated peptide antibody	
Overview and use:	• CCP—cyclic citrullinated protein antibodies; anticitrullinated protein antibodies: this is a relatively new auto-antibody marker that shows great promise and specificity for the early diagnosis of rheumatoid arthritis (RA). The test often becomes positive/present in asymptomatic patients years before the onset of clinical manifestations of RA. • As of the first inclusion of this information in my books in December 2006, the information on anti-CCP antibodies is so new that it is not even included in most 2006-edition medical and rheumatology reference textbooks; nonetheless, doctors nationwide are already starting to use this test for the early diagnosis of RA. This may be particularly important because some research has shown that *early* and *aggressive* treatment of RA has an important impact on long-term prognosis[284]; however, the importance of early intervention is debatable.[285] • Anti-CCP antibodies are directed toward several native proteins (e.g., filaggrin, fibrinogen, and vimentin) that have become posttranslationally modified by a uncharged citrulline in contrast to the normal positively charged arginine. This "citrullination" is catalyzed by a calcium-dependent enzyme, **peptidylarginine deiminase (PAD).** These changes in protein charge and sequence make the native protein a target of auto-antibody attack by IgG antibodies in RA.[286] However, this does not necessarily imply that citrullination of native proteins is "the cause" of RA because citrullination of native proteins can also occur *de novo* in inflamed joints, which are then further targeted for inflammatory destruction. Until more information is available, we should withhold final judgment as to the ultimate role and origin of anti-CCP antibodies and in the meanwhile view them as a very strong and sensitive association with RA that facilitates the early diagnosis of this disease.
Advantages:	• Anti-CCP antibodies have 98% specificity for RA[287] and is likely to become the future laboratory standard in the diagnosis and prognosis of RA.[288] Anti-CCP antibodies with a positive rheumatoid factor (RF) is termed "composite seropositivity" and appears to be more specific than isolated anti-CCP antibodies or RF.[289]
Limitations:	• **The best current data indicates that anti-CCP antibodies are sensitive and specific for RA[290], and clinicians should use this test to diagnose and confirm RA.**
Comments:	• Healthy people do not generally have anti-CCP antibodies. Asymptomatic patients with anti-CCP antibodies are at increased risk for clinical RA and are probably *en route* to the manifestation of clinical autoimmunity—RA, Sjogren's disease, or SLE. *Holistically intervene.* • I hypothesize that PAD may become upregulated in synovial joints exposed to allergens, xenobiotics, bacterial debris/toxins/lipopolysaccharides and that the subsequent citrullination of joint proteins may lead to an autoimmune arthropathy that persists, perhaps despite removal of the inciting immunogen. More obviously, given that PAD is calcium-dependent, it may be upregulated secondary to intracellular hypercalcinosis secondary to vitamin D deficiency, magnesium deficiency, or fatty acid imbalance.[291]

---

[284] "CONCLUSION: An initial 6-month cycle of intensive combination treatment that includes high-dose corticosteroids results in sustained suppression of the rate of radiologic progression in patients with early RA, independent of subsequent antirheumatic therapy." Landewe RB, et al. COBRA combination therapy in patients with early rheumatoid arthritis: long-term structural benefits of a brief intervention. *Arthritis Rheum.* 2002 Feb;46:347-56

[285] "By 5 years patients receiving early DMARDs had similar disease activity and comparable health assessment questionnaire scores to patients who received DMARDs later in their disease course." Scott DL. Evidence for early disease-modifying drugs in rheumatoid arthritis. *Arthritis Res Ther.* 2004;6(1):15-18 http://arthritis-research.com/content/6/1/15

[286] Hill J, Cairns E, Bell DA. The joy of citrulline. *J Rheumatol.* 2004 Aug;31(8):1471-3 http://www.jrheum.com/subscribers/04/08/1471.html

[287] Hill J, Cairns E, Bell DA. The joy of citrulline. *J Rheumatol.* 2004 Aug;31(8):1471-3

[288] "We conclude that, at present, the antibody response directed to citrullinated antigens has the most valuable diagnostic and prognostic potential for RA." van Boekel MA, Vossenaar ER, van den Hoogen FH, van Venrooij WJ. Autoantibody systems in rheumatoid arthritis: specificity, sensitivity and diagnostic value. *Arthritis Res.* 2002;4(2):87-93 http://arthritis-research.com/content/4/2/87

[289] "…our findings suggest that a positive anti-CCP antibody result does not necessarily exclude SLE in African American patients presenting with inflammatory arthritis. In such patients, the additional assessment of IgA-RF or IgM-RF isotypes may be of added value since composite seropositivity appears to be nearly exclusive to patients with RA." Mikuls TR, Holers VM, Parrish L, et al. Anti-cyclic citrullinated peptide antibody and rheumatoid factor isotypes in African Americans with early rheumatoid arthritis. *Arthritis Rheum.* 2006 Sep;54(9):3057-9

[290] "Serum antibodies reactive with citrullinated proteins/peptides are a very sensitive and specific marker for rheumatoid arthritis." Migliorini P, Pratesi F, Tommasi C, Anzilotti C. The immune response to citrullinated antigens in autoimmune diseases. *Autoimmun Rev.* 2005 Nov;4(8):561-4

[291] See optimalhealthresearch.com/archives/intracellular-hypercalcinosis and naturopathydigest.com/archives/2006/sep/vasquez.php for discussion

HLA-B27: Human leukocyte antigen B-27	

Overview and interpretation:	▪ A common (5-10% of general population) genetic marker strongly associated with seronegative* spondyloarthropathy (all of which occur more commonly in men[292]):
	    1. Ankylosing spondylitis (90-95% of 'whites' and 50% of 'blacks')[293]
	    2. Reiter's syndrome (85%)
	    3. Enteropathic spondyloarthropathy
	    4. Psoriatic spondylitis (<60%)
	* Recall that "seronegative" in this context implies that the *rheumatoid factor is negative,* even though *the HLA-B27 may be positive.*

Advantages: *Limitations:* *Comments:*	▪ *From a diagnostic perspective*: The clinical application and significance of this test is of limited value. All of the above-listed conditions are better assessed with the combination of clinical assessment and radiographs. In a patient with early and mild disease, this test may add evidence either supporting or refuting the diagnosis; but the test itself is not diagnostic of anything other than a genetic/histologic marker associated with various types of infection-induced arthropathy and autoimmunity (dysbiotic arthropathy[294]). ▪ *From an integrative/functional medicine perspective*: This test can be of some value if the result is positive and the patient has evidence of a systemic inflammatory/autoimmune disorder since it therefore more strongly suggests that a dysbiotic locus is the cause of disease.[295] A consistent theme in the rheumatology literature is that of "molecular mimicry"—the phenomenon by which structural similarities between human and microbial structures lead to targeting of human tissues by immune responses aimed at microbial antigens. This topic is explored in considerable detail in the section on multifocal dysbiosis in *Integrative Rheumatology*. The important link between microbe-induced autoimmunity and HLA-B27 is that many dysbiotic bacteria produce an HLA-B27-like molecule that appears to trigger an immune response which then erroneously affects human tissues, leading to the clinical picture of autoimmune inflammation. Many of these HLA-B27-producing bacteria colonize the gastrointestinal and genitourinary tracts, promoting musculoskeletal inflammation via molecular mimicry and other mechanisms.[296,297] A strong and growing body of research shows that HLA-B27 is a risk factor for microbe-induced autoimmunity. "Autoimmune" patients positive for HLA-B27 are presumed to have an occult infection—especially gastrointestinal, genitourinary, or sinorespiratory—until proven otherwise. ▪ **Keep in mind that HLA-B27 itself is not a disease** and therefore a "positive" result merely means that the patient has this particular human leukocyte antigen; this test is not and will never be diagnostic of a specific disease—it simply correlates with increased propensity toward dysbiotic arthropathy and suggests the need for dysbiosis testing and the (re)establishment of eubiosis.[298]

[292] "The major diseases associated with HLA-B27 (Reiter's disease, ankylosing spondylitis, acute anterior uveitis, and psoriatic arthritis) all occur much more commonly in men." James WH. Sex ratios and hormones in HLA related rheumatic diseases. *Ann Rheum Dis*. 1991 Jun;50(6):401-4

[293] Shojania K. Rheumatology: 2. What laboratory tests are needed? *CMAJ*. 2000 Apr 18;162(8):1157-63 http://www.cmaj.ca/cgi/content/full/162/8/1157

[294] See chapter 4 of *Integrative Rheumatology* and **Vasquez A**. Reducing Pain and Inflammation Naturally. Part 6: Nutritional and Botanical Treatments Against "Silent Infections" and Gastrointestinal Dysbiosis, Commonly Overlooked Causes of Neuromusculoskeletal Inflammation and Chronic Health Problems. *Nutr Perspect* 2006; Jan http://optimalhealthresearch.com/part6

[295] "The association between HLA-B27 and reactive arthritis (ReA) has also been well established... In a similar way, microbiological and immunological studies have revealed an association between Klebsiella pneumoniae in AS and Proteus mirabilis in RA." Ebringer A, Wilson C. HLA molecules, bacteria and autoimmunity. *J Med Microbiol*. 2000 Apr;49(4):305-11

[296] **Inman RD. Antigens, the gastrointestinal tract, and arthritis. *Rheum Dis Clin North Am*. 1991 May;17(2):309-21**

[297] **Hunter JO. Food allergy--or enterometabolic disorder? *Lancet*. 1991 Aug 24;338(8765):495-6**

[298] Dysbiotic arthropathy—joint inflammation and destruction as a result of a neuroimmune inflammatory response to microorganisms. Phrase coined by Alex Vasquez on December 15, 2005. No matching term on Medline or Google search. See chapter 4 of *Integrative Rheumatology* and **Vasquez A**. Reducing Pain and Inflammation Naturally. Part 6: Nutritional and Botanical Treatments Against "Silent Infections" and Gastrointestinal Dysbiosis, Commonly Overlooked Causes of Neuromusculoskeletal Inflammation and Chronic Health Problems. *Nutr Perspect* 2006; Jan http://optimalhealthresearch.com/part6

Complement C3 and C4	
Overview and interpretation:	• Complement proteins are consumed in the complement cascades (typically activated by immune complexes) and thus low levels of complement proteins provide indirect evidence of extensive consumption due to immune complex-mediated inflammation. **Low levels of complement are seen with immune complex disorders (such as SLE, vasculitis, mixed cryoglobulinemia, rheumatoid vasculitis, glomerulonephritis) and inherited complement deficiencies.** • 10%–15% of Caucasian patients with SLE have an inherited complement deficiency.[299]
Advantages:	• Low complement levels provide indirect evidence of immune complex-mediated inflammation. • Elevated levels of complement are seen in conditions of infection or inflammation.
Limitations:	• Some patients have a hereditary absence of complement proteins and thus their levels are always abnormally low; obviously the test cannot be used in these patients for monitoring inflammatory disease.

CIC: Circulating immune complexes	
Overview and interpretation:	• Antibodies/immunoglobulins are produced in several different "classes": IgG, IgA, IgM, IgE, IgD. IgA antibodies are produced mostly in response to mucosal infections, such as from gastrointestinal dysbiosis or overt infections. When antibodies (in the shape of the letter "Y" with 2 antigen-binding sites on one end and the immuno-reactive site on the other) combine with the target antigen (depicted here in the shape of an oval, such as a bacteria or globular protein), "immune complexes" are formed which are chain-like links of antigens and antibodies. 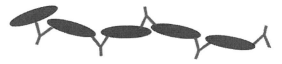 • Although formed in small amounts in healthy persons, in certain disease states, immune complexes may accumulate and initiate complement-dependent injury in various organs and tissues. This activation of complement may begin a series of potentially destructive events in the host, including anaphylatoxin production, cell lysis, leukocyte stimulation, and activation of macrophages and other cells. When immune complexes become fixed to vessel walls, destruction of normal tissue can occur, as in some types of glomerulonephritis and vasculitis. Predisposed to deposition in joints, vessels, and kidneys, immune complexes contribute directly to tissue injury in several autoimmune-inflammatory diseases.[300] **Immune Complexes, (Raji Cell), Quantitative** • Reference Range: (Enzyme immunoassay [EIA]; cost $130) • Normal: ≤15.0 µg Eq/mL • Equivocal: 15.1-19.9 µg Eq/mL • **Positive: ≥20.0 µg Eq/mL**
Advantages:	• This test allows for direct quantification of immune-complex production.
Limitations:	• This test has only recently become available to practicing clinicians; however, it is very well supported by many publications in peer-reviewed research.[301]

---

[299] Shojania K. Rheumatology: 2. What laboratory tests are needed? *CMAJ*. 2000 Apr 18;162(8):1157-63 http://www.cmaj.ca/cgi/content/full/162/8/1157
[300] Jancar S, Sánchez Crespo M. Immune complex-mediated tissue injury: a multistep paradigm. *Trends Immunol*. 2005 Jan;26(1):48-55
[301] Davies KA,etal. Immune complex processing in patients with systemic lupus erythematosus.*JClinInvest*1992;90:2075-83 jci.org/articles/view/116090

Lactulose-mannitol assay: assessment for intestinal hyperpermeability and malabsorption	
Overview and interpretation:	▪ The lactulose-mannitol assay is a highly validated assessment for the accurate determination of small intestine permeability. This test is used to diagnose "leaky gut", which is a common problem and contributor to systemic inflammation in patients with inflammation and immune dysfunction—see chapter 4 of *Integrative Rheumatology*. Intestinal hyperpermeability reflects inflammation of and damage to the small intestine mucosa and is seen in patients with parasite infections, food allergies, celiac disease, malnutrition, bacterial infections, systemic ischemia or inflammation, ankylosing spondylitis, Crohn's disease, eczema, psoriasis, and those who consume enterotoxins such as NSAIDs and excess ethanol.[302] ▪ Elevations of **lactulose** indicate increased **paracellular** permeability caused by intestinal damage and are diagnostic of "leaky gut." *Clinical pearl*: remember that the "L" in *lactulose* rhymes with *leaky*. ▪ Decrements in **mannitol** suggest impaired **transcellular** absorption and suggest malabsorption in general and villous atrophy in particular. *Clinical pearl*: remember that the "M" in *mannitol* rhymes with *malabsorption*. ▪ Classically, in patients with damaged intestinal mucosa, we generally see a combined *increase in paracellular permeability* (measured with lactulose) and a *reduction in transcellular transport* (measured with mannitol); these divergent effects result in an increased lactulose-to-mannitol ratio.
Advantages:	▪ This test is safe and affordable for the assessment of small intestine mucosal integrity. Abnormal results—"leaky gut" and/or malabsorption—generally indicate one or more of following: 1. <u>Malnutrition</u>: may be due to poor intake, catabolism, or malabsorption. 2. <u>Enterotoxins</u>: generally NSAIDs or ethanol 3. <u>Food allergies</u>: including celiac disease 4. <u>"Parasites"</u>: including yeast, bacteria, protozoa, amebas, worms, etc. [303] 5. <u>Systemic inflammation</u>: tissue hypoxia, trauma, recent surgery, etc. 6. <u>Genetic predisposition toward enteropathy</u>: check family history for IBD.
Limitations:	▪ Abnormalities and the identification of "leaky gut" are nonspecific and do not point to a specific or single diagnosis or treatment.
Comments:	▪ The value of this test is two-fold: 1) as a screening test for the above-mentioned disorders, and 2) as a method for determining the efficacy of treatment once the cause of the problem has been putatively identified and treated. ▪ This test can be used to promote compliance and to encourage the use of additional testing in patients who are otherwise prone to noncompliance or who resist other tests, such as stool testing. In other words, the clinician can gain an advantage by showing the patient an objective abnormality which then validates the need for treatment and additional testing. ▪ I only use this test on rare occasions because I more commonly either assume that a patient has leaky gut if he/she has one of the aforementioned conditions or we move directly to stool testing and comprehensive parasitology—clearly one of the most valuable tests in the management and treatment of systemic inflammation and immune dysfunction—otherwise known as "autoimmunity" and "allergy."

---

[302] Miller AL. The Pathogenesis, Clinical Implications, and Treatment of Intestinal Hyperpermeability. *Alt Med Rev 1997*:2(5):330-345 http://www.thorne.com/pdf/journal/2-5/intestinalhyperpermiability.pdf
[303] See chapter 4 of *Integrative Rheumatology* and **Vasquez A**. Reducing Pain and Inflammation Naturally. Part 6: Nutritional and Botanical Treatments Against "Silent Infections" and Gastrointestinal Dysbiosis, Commonly Overlooked Causes of Neuromusculoskeletal Inflammation and Chronic Health Problems. *Nutr Perspect* 2006; Jan http://optimalhealthresearch.com/part6

Presentation: Highly abnormal lactulose-mannitol ratio in a patient with idiopathic peripheral neuropathy prior to comprehensive stool analysis and parasitology showing intestinal dysbiosis: Patient presented with a multiyear history of periodic febrile exacerbations of peripheral neuropathy that would cause severe paresthesias and motor deficits. Patient had been evaluated by several board-certified medical neurologists to no avail. Laboratory, imaging, electrodiagnostic studies, and cerebrospinal fluid (CSF) analysis revealed nonspecific abnormalities that did not lead to an established diagnosis. From an integrative naturopathic and functional medicine perspective, food allergy and intestinal dysbiosis are the most obvious probable etiologies; these clinical suspicions were confirmed with laboratory testing showing increased intestinal permeability and dysbiosis.

Patient:

Age: 40
Sex: M
MRN:

Order Number: 40220637
Completed: April 24, 2003
Received: April 22, 2003
Collected: April 21, 2003

HOUSTON OPTIMAL HEALTH
ALEX VASQUEZ DC ND

Houston, TX 77098

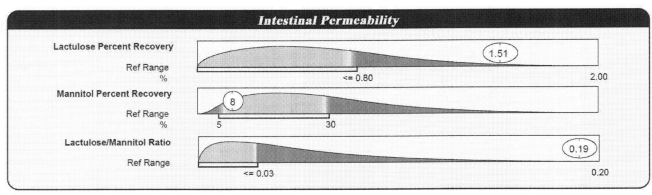

As expected, comprehensive parasitology showed intestinal dysbiosis, including insufficiency of *Lactobacillus* and presence of *Psuedomonas* and abnormal yeast species. Of particular note, *Psuedomonas aeruginosa* shows cross-reactivity with human neuronal tissues.[304,305] Eradication of the dysbiotic condition with a combination of dietary improvement, nutritional supplementation, hormonal optimization, and antimicrobial drugs and herbs lead to rapid and sustained remission of this "idiopathic peripheral neuropathy" which had defied standard medical diagnosis and treatment for many years.

Comprehensive Stool Analysis / Parasitology x3

MICROBIOLOGY

Bacteriology Culture

Beneficial flora		Imbalances		Dysbiotic flora	
Bifidobacter	4+	Haemolytic E. coli	4+	Pseudomonas sp.	4+
E. coli	4+	Gamma strep	2+		
Lactobacillus	2+				

Mycology (Yeast) Culture

Normal flora		Dysbiotic flora	
Candida glabrata	1+		
Rhodotorula sp.	1+		

[304] Hughes LE, Bonell S, Natt RS, et al. Antibody responses to Acinetobacter spp. and Pseudomonas aeruginosa in multiple sclerosis: prospects for diagnosis using the myelin-acinetobacter-neurofilament antibody index. *Clin Diagn Lab* Immunol. 2001 Nov;8(6):1181-8 http://cvi.asm.org/content/8/6/1181.full.pdf

[305] Hughes LE, Smith PA, Bonell S, Natt RS, Wilson C, Rashid T, Amor S, Thompson EJ, Croker J, Ebringer A. Cross-reactivity between related sequences found in Acinetobacter sp., Pseudomonas aeruginosa, myelin basic protein and myelin oligodendrocyte glycoprotein in multiple sclerosis. *J Neuroimmunol*. 2003 Nov;144(1-2):105-15

Comprehensive stool analysis and comprehensive parasitology	
Overview and interpretation:	▪ **This is clearly one of the most valuable tests in clinical practice when working with patients with chronic fatigue, systemic inflammation, and autoimmunity. Second only to routine laboratory assessments such as CBC, chemistry panel, and CRP, the importance of stool testing and comprehensive parasitology assessments must be appreciated by progressive clinicians of all disciplines.** ▪ Stool testing must be performed by a specialty laboratory because the quality of testing provided by most standard "medical labs" and hospitals is completely inadequate. Initial samples should be collected on three separate occasions by the patient and each sample should be analyzed separately by the laboratory. ▪ Important qualitative and quantitative markers include the following: 1. **Beneficial bacteria (" probiotics")**: Microbiological testing should quantify and identify various beneficial bacteria, which should be present at "+4" levels on a 0-4 scale. 2. **Harmful and potentially harmful bacteria, protozoans, amebas, etc.**: Questionable or harmful microbes should be eradicated even if they are not identified as true pathogens in the paleo-classic Pasteurian/Kochian sense.[306] 3. **Yeast and mycology**: At least two tests must be performed for a complete assessment: 1) yeast culture, and 2) microscopic examination for yeast elements. Both tests are necessary because some patients—perhaps those with the most severe symptomatology and the most favorable response to anti-yeast treatment—will have a negative yeast culture and positive findings on the microscopic examination. In other words, these patients have intestinal yeast that contributes to their disease/symptomatology but which does not grow on culture despite being clearly visible with microscopy; a similar pattern (using a swab of the rectal mucosa rather than microscopy) is referred to as "negative culture with positive smear."[307] 4. **Microbial sensitivity testing**: An important component to parasitology testing is the determination of which anti-microbial agents (natural and synthetic) the microbe is sensitive to. This helps to guide and enhance the effectiveness of anti-microbial therapy. 5. **Secretory IgA**: SIgA levels are elevated in patients who are having an immune response to either food or microbial antigens.[308] Thus, in a patient with minimal dysbiosis, say for example with *Candida albicans*, an elevated sIgA can indicate that the patient is having a hypersensitivity reaction to an otherwise benign microbe—in this case, eradication of the microbe is warranted and may result in a positive clinical response. Low sIgA suggests either primary or secondary immune defect such as selective sIgA deficiency[309] or malnutrition, stress, prednisone/corticosteroids, or possibly mycotoxicosis (immunosuppression due to fungal immunotoxins). In addition to addressing any systemic causative factors, a low sIgA may be addressed with the administration of bovine colostrum, glutamine, vitamin A, and *Saccharomyces boulardii*; the following doses may be considered for use in adults with proportionately smaller doses for children: ▪ Bovine colostrum: 2.4 – 3.6 grams per day in divided doses for adults. No drug interactions are known. Side effects may include increased energy, insomnia, and

---

[306] **Vasquez A.** Reducing Pain and Inflammation Naturally. Part 6: Nutritional and Botanical Treatments Against "Silent Infections" and Gastrointestinal Dysbiosis, Commonly Overlooked Causes of Neuromusculoskeletal Inflammation and Chronic Health Problems. *Nutr Perspect* 2006; Jan http://optimalhealthresearch.com/part6.html

[307] "According to Galland, the best predictor of who will respond to anticandida medication is a negative stool culture combined with a positive smear of the rectal mucosa (for the identification of intracellular hyphal forms of the organism); however, even that test is not 100% reliable." Gaby AR. Before you order that lab test: part 2. *Townsend Letter for Doctors and Patients*. 2004; January findarticles.com/p/articles/mi_m0ISW/is_246/ai_112728028

[308] Quig DW, Higley M. Noninvasive assessment of intestinal inflammation: inflammatory bowel disease vs. irritable bowel syndrome. *Townsend Letter for Doctors and Patients* 2006;Jan:74-5

[309] "Selective IgA deficiency is the most common form of immunodeficiency. Certain select populations, including allergic individuals, patients with autoimmune and gastrointestinal tract disease and patients with recurrent upper respiratory tract illnesses, have an increased incidence of this disorder." Burks AW Jr, Steele RW. Selective IgA deficiency. *Ann Allergy*. 1986;57:3-13

stimulation. One study in particular used very large doses of 10 grams per day for four days in children and found no adverse effects[310]; another case report of a child involved the use of 50 grams per day for at least two weeks and showed no adverse effects.[311]

- Glutamine: 6 grams 3 times per day (18 grams per day) is a common dosage with significant literature support.
- Vitamin A: Correction of subclinical vitamin A deficiency improves mucosal integrity and increases sIgA production in humans.[312] Common doses used by integrative clinicians are in the range of 200,000 IU to 300,000 for a limited amount of time, generally 1-4 weeks; thereafter the dose is tapered. Patients are educated as to manifestations of toxicity (see the chapter on *Therapeutics* toward the end of this book) and the importance of limited duration of treatment.
- *Saccharomyces boulardii*: Common dose for adults is 250 mg thrice daily; ability of this treatment to increase sIgA levels and its anti-infective efficacy have been documented in human and animal studies.

6. **Short-chain fatty acids**: These are produced by intestinal bacteria. Quantitative excess indicates bacterial overgrowth of the intestines, while insufficiency indicates a lack of probiotics or an insufficiency of dietary substrate, i.e., soluble fiber. Abnormal patterns of individual short-chain fatty acids indicate qualitative/quantitative abnormalities in gastrointestinal microflora, particularly anaerobic bacteria that cannot be identified with routine bacterial cultures.

7. **Beta-glucuronidase**: This is an enzyme produced by several different intestinal bacteria. High levels of beta-glucuronidase in the intestinal lumen serve to nullify the benefits of detoxification (specifically glucuronidation) by cleaving the toxicant from its glucuronide conjugate. This can result in re-absorption of the toxicant through the intestinal mucosa which then re-exposes the patient to the toxin that was previously detoxified ("enterohepatic recirculation" or "enterohepatic recycling"[313]). This is an exemplary aspect of "auto-intoxication" that results in chronic fatigue and upregulation of Phase 1 detoxification systems (chapter 4 of *Integrative Rheumatology*).

8. **Lactoferrin**: The iron-binding glycoprotein lactoferrin is an inflammatory marker that helps distinguish functional disorders (i.e., IBS) from more serious diseases (i.e., IBD). Approximate values are as follows:
   - Healthy and IBS: 2 mcg/ml
   - Severe dysbiosis: up to 120 mcg/ml
   - Inactive IBD: 60-250 mcg/ml
   - Active IBD: > 400 mcg/ml.

9. **Lysozyme**: Elevated in proportion to intestinal inflammation in dysbiosis and IBD.

10. **Other markers**: Other markers of digestion, inflammation, and absorption are reported with the more comprehensive panels performed on stool samples. These tests are not always necessary, but such additional information is always helpful when working with complex patients. These markers are relatively self-explanatory

[310] "In this double blind placebo-controlled trial, 80 children with rotavirus diarrhea were randomly assigned to receive orally either 10 g of IIBC (containing 3.6 g of antirotavirus antibodies) daily for 4 days or the same amount of a placebo preparation." Sarker SA, Casswall TH, Mahalanabis D, Alam NH, Albert MJ, Brussow H, Fuchs GJ, Hammerstrom L. Successful treatment of rotavirus diarrhea in children with immunoglobulin from immunized bovine colostrum. *Pediatr Infect Dis J*. 1998 Dec;17(12):1149-54

[311] Lactobin-R is a commercial hyperimmune bovine colostrum with some specificity for cryptosporidiosis; administration to a 4 year old child with AIDS and severe diarrhea resulted in significant clinical improvement in the diarrhea and "permanent elimination of the parasite from the gut as assessed through serial jejunal biopsy and stool specimens." Shield J, Melville C, Novelli V, Anderson G, Scheimberg I, Gibb D, Milla P. Bovine colostrum immunoglobulin concentrate for cryptosporidiosis in AIDS. *Arch Dis Child*. 1993 Oct;69(4):451-3

[312] "It can increase resistance to infection by increasing mucosal integrity, increasing surface immunoglobulin A (sIgA) and enhancing adequate neutrophil function. If infection occurs, vitamin A can act as an immune enhancer, increasing the adequacy of natural killer (NK) cells and increasing antibody production." Faisel H, Pittrof R. Vitamin A and causes of maternal mortality: association and biological plausibility. *Public Health Nutr*. 2000 Sep;3(3):321-7

[313] Parker RJ, Hirom PC, Millburn P.Enterohepatic recycling of phenolphthalein, morphine, lysergic acid diethylamide (LSD) and diphenylacetic acid in the rat. Hydrolysis of glucuronic acid conjugates in the gut lumen. *Xenobiotica*. 1980 Sep;10(9):689-70

Comprehensive stool analysis and comprehensive parasitology	
	and/or are described on the results of the test by the laboratory.
Advantages:	▪ **Stool analysis in general and parasitology assessments in particular provide supremely valuable information in the comprehensive assessment and treatment of patients with complex illnesses such as chronic fatigue, irritable bowel syndrome, fibromyalgia, and all of the autoimmune/rheumatic diseases.**
Limitations:	▪ Tests vary in price from about $250-$400. ▪ Anaerobic bacteria are difficult to culture. ▪ Specialty examinations, such as for *Helicobacter pylori* antigen and enterohemorrhagic *E. coli* cytotoxin, must be requested specifically at additional cost.
Comments:	▪ I have found stool testing to be the single most powerful diagnostic tool for helping chronically ill patients to attain improved health. Insights from stool/parasitology testing can be used to implement powerfully effective treatments. The value of this test in the treatment of patients with rheumatic disease must be appreciated and is extensively detailed in chapter 4 of ***Integrative Rheumatology***.

Concept: Not all "Injury-related Problems" are "Injury-related Problems"

In the case of most acute injuries, the underlying problem is often the injury itself. However, the physician must conduct a thorough history and examination to assess for possible underling pathologies that cause or contribute to the problem that "appears" to be injury-related. Congenital anomalies, underlying pathology, previous injury, occult infections, and psychoemotional disorders may have been present *before* the "injury." Just because the patient reports a problem such as pain following an injury does not mean that the injury is the

> **"Pediatric infections and neoplasms are notorious for masquerading as sport injuries."**
>
> "...Take the relevant history directly from the patient, and keep tumors and infections high on your list of differential diagnoses... For example, about 15% of children with leukemia present with musculoskeletal complaints..."
>
> Shaw BA, Gerardi JA, Hennrikus WL. How to avoid orthopedic pitfalls in children. *Patient Care* 1999; Feb 28: 95-116

sole cause of the pain. *Do not let a biased history lead you down the wrong path.* **In children and young adults, 5% of "sports-related" injuries are associated with preexisting infection, anomalies, or other conditions.** In adult women, "...between 9% and 20% of women with breast cancer attribute their symptoms to previous trauma to the breast. In these cases, the association of the breast mass with a traumatic event resulted in a delay in diagnosis ranging from four months to one year."[314]

When treating children, be very careful to get an accurate history—this is difficult since your two sources of information are not very reliable: parents often think that they already have the problem figured out, and so their history will be biased toward convincing you of what they think is the problem and solution; children are often not good historians and can form illogical relationships between events that can be misleading.

A group of German physicians describe a man who presented with a soft-tissue pain following a soccer game; he was later diagnosed with a malignant tumor—synovial sarcoma.[315] Similarly, Wakeshima and Ellen[316] describe a young athletic woman who presented with chronic hip pain. The woman's history was significant for ulcerative colitis, but otherwise her radiographs were normal and her history and examination lead to a diagnosis of trochanteric bursitis. However, the patient's condition did not respond to routine treatment, and additional investigation over several

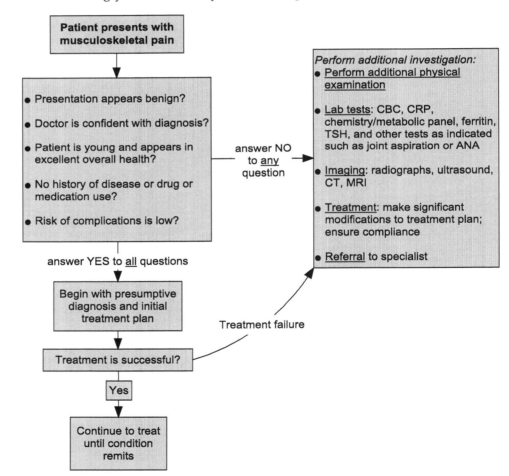

Inconsistencies between the history, exams, and response to treatment suggest the need for additional investigation and additional diagnostic considerations.

---

[314] Seifert S. Medical Illness Simulating Trauma (MIST) syndrome: case reports and discussion of syndrome. *Fam Med* 1993 Apr;25(4):273-6

[315] Engel C, Kelm J, Olinger A. Blunt trauma in soccer. The initial manifestation of synovial sarcoma. [Article in German] *Zentralbl Chir* 2001 Jan;126(1):68-71

[316] Wakeshima Y, Ellen MI. Atypical hip pain origin in a young athletic woman: a case report of giant cell carcinoma. *Arch Phys Med Rehabil* 2001 Oct;82(10):1472-5

months lead to a diagnosis of giant cell carcinoma. The authors concluded, "This case shows **the importance of repeat radiographic studies in patients whose joint pain does not respond or responds slowly to conservative therapy, despite initial normal findings."**

What you expect to find and hear when taking a trauma-related history is that **1) a healthy patient** with no previous health concerns was **2) exposed to a traumatic event**, the history and consequences of which perfectly coincide with the injury you are assessing in your office, and that **3) your physical examination findings are all consistent** and lead to a specific diagnosis, which then **4) responds to your treatment. If you find discrepancies between the history of the injury and your physical examination findings (e.g., fever after a "sports-related" injury), if the patient appears unhealthy in disproportion to the presenting complaint, or if the patient does not respond to your treatment, then you must consider the possibility of preexisting or concomitant disease.**

Astute doctors search for and rule out preexisting and underlying pathology before ascribing the problem to the "obvious cause." Always assess for consistency between the history, examination findings, and response to treatment—inconsistencies suggest the need for additional investigation.

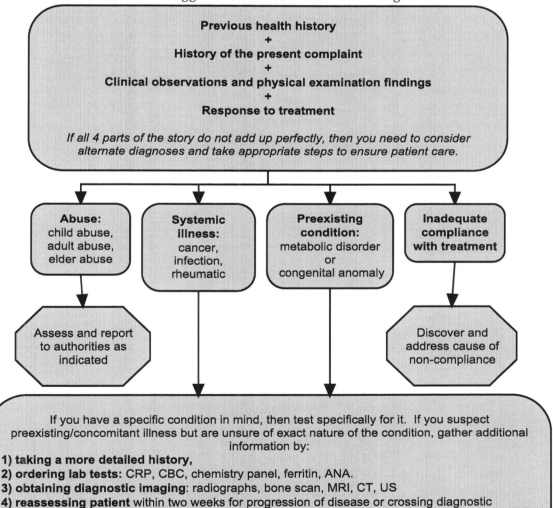

Inconsistencies between the history, exams, and response to treatment suggest the need for additional investigation and additional diagnostic considerations.

High-Risk Pain Patients

When a patient has musculoskeletal pain and any of the following characteristics, radiographs should be considered as an appropriate component of comprehensive evaluation. These considerations are particularly—though not exclusively—relevant for spine and low-back pain.[317]

1. **More than 50 years of age**
2. **Physical trauma** (accident, fall, etc.)
3. **Pain at night**
4. **Back pain not relieved by lying supine**
5. **Neurologic deficits** (motor or sensory)
6. **Unexplained weight loss**
7. **Documentation or suspicion of inflammatory arthropathy**[318]
   - **Ankylosing spondylitis**
   - **Lupus**
   - **Rheumatoid arthritis**
   - **Juvenile rheumatoid arthritis**
   - **Psoriatic arthritis**
8. **Drug or alcohol abuse** (increased risk of infection, nutritional deficiencies, anesthesia)
9. **History of cancer**
10. **Intravenous drug use**
11. **Immunosuppression, due to illness** (e.g., HIV) **or medications** (e.g., steroids or cyclosporine)
12. **History of corticosteroid use** (causes osteoporosis and increased risk for infection)
13. **Fever above 100° F or suspicion of septic arthritis or osteomyelitis**
14. **Diabetes** (increased risk of infection, nutritional deficiencies, anesthesia)
15. **Hypertension** (abdominal aneurysm: low back pain, nausea, pulsatile abdominal mass)
16. **Recent visit for same problem and not improved**
17. **Patient seeking compensation for pain/ injury** (increased need for documentation)
18. **Skin lesion** (psoriasis, melanoma, dermatomyositis, the butterfly rash of lupus, scars from previous surgery, accident, etc....)
19. **Deformity or immobility**
20. **Lymphadenopathy** (suggests cancer or infection)
21. **Elevated ESR/CRP** (cancer, infection, inflammatory disorder)
22. **Elevated WBC count**
23. **Elevated alkaline phosphatase** (bone lesions, metabolic bone disease, hepatopathy, vitamin D deficiency)
24. **Elevated acid phosphatase** (occasionally used to monitor prostate cancer)
25. **Positive rheumatoid factor and/or CCP—cyclic citrullinated protein antibodies**
26. **Positive HLA-B27** (propensity for inflammatory arthropathies)
27. **Serum gammopathy** (multiple myeloma is the most common primary bone tumor)
28. **"High-risk for disease"** *examples:*
    - Long-term heavy smoking of cigarettes
    - Long-term exposure to radiation
    - Obesity
29. **Strong family history of inflammatory, musculoskeletal, or malignant disease**

---

[317] Remember that metastasis often travel first from the primary site to bone, therefore bone pain may be an early manifestation of occult cancer. Most of the above are from "Table 1: The high-risk patient: clinical indications for radiography in low back pain patients." J Taylor, DC, DACBR, D Resnick, MD. Imaging decisions in the management of low back pain. Advances in Chiropractic. Mosby Year Book. 1994; 1-28

[318] Radiographs are often essential for diagnosis or to rule out complications of the disease. For example, in patients with inflammatory arthropathies such as these, spontaneous rupture of the transverse ligament (at the odontoid process) has been reported; although rare, this complication could be life-threatening if mismanaged or undiagnosed.

Concept: Safe Patient + Safe Treatment = Safe Outcome

The purpose of performing the history and physical examination on a new *or established* patient is to determine their current health status—including their mental and emotional health and their physical health, particularly as this relates to important and life-threatening possibilities such as cancer, infections, fractures, systemic diseases, and neurologic compromise. The questions that lead this investigation are: "**What is this patient's current status?**" "**Does this patient have a serious disease, neurologic injury, or are they at high risk for developing a serious complication in the near future that can be prevented with appropriate care** *now*?"

"Is this patient safe?"
- ◆ The question to ask yourself is, "Is this patient's health problem or current complaint/exacerbation a manifestation of an underlying condition that could result in a negative outcome?
- ◆ If a patient comes to you with a headache, and you neglect to find that their blood pressure is 230/130, then you missed the opportunity to help them avoid the stroke that they could have after leaving your office.
- ◆ If a patient comes to you with a complaint of low back pain, and you neglect to perform a neurologic examination to find that *the patient already has a neurologic deficit even before you treated them*, then you have lost the opportunity to defend yourself in court when the patient later claims that *your* treatment and *your* management of their case is the reason that they now have a permanent neurologic deficit.

Is your treatment safe?: Have you been perfectly clear with the patient about the risks and benefits of your treatment plan? **Have you obtained informed consent?** Have you charted **"PAR-B"** to indicate that you have discussed the <u>P</u>rocedures, <u>A</u>lternatives, <u>R</u>isks, and <u>B</u>enefits of your treatment plan? Have you been clear about the duration of treatment and the need for appropriate follow-up? If you are prescribing nutrition or botanical medicines, have you informed the patient about the duration of treatment? **Have you looked for contraindications to your otherwise brilliant treatment plan?** What about the fact that this patient was on corticosteroids for the past 15 years and only discontinued prednisone 2 months before arriving at your office? *The patient may have steroid-induced osteoporosis even though he is no longer on prednisone.* When you recommend that your patient take 100,000 IU of vitamin A to treat her throat infection, what happens when she presents to your office 8 months later with signs of vitamin A toxicity because she continued her treatment plan indefinitely

> Double-check to ensure that your patient is safe (no forthcoming complications or predictable emergencies) and that your treatment is safe (appropriate, effective, clearly communicated, and time-limited with instructions to return for office visit).

rather than using it only for 7 days as you had intended? *Be sure to put a time limit on your treatment plans.* Every treatment plan should be 1) given to the patient in legible print and clear statements, 2) be copied for the chart, 3) include "what to do if things get worse" in the event of adverse treatment effect or exacerbation of problem, and 4) include patient's responsibility for returning to office/clinic for follow-up and reassessment.

Informed consent: From a legal standpoint, doctors can only treat a patient after the patient has given *consent to treatment*. Patients can only authoritatively consent to treatment after they have been fully educated about the treatment—thus they can provide *informed consent*. Full disclosure about the treatment plan includes informing the patient of the Procedures—what will take place; Alternatives—what options are available; Risks—what risks are involved, and (optionally) Benefits—what benefits can be expected. This is commonly charted as "**PAR—no questions**" or "**PAR—questions answered**" once the patient gives consent to treatment.

Concept: Four Clues to Discovering Underlying Problems

When I taught Orthopedics at Bastyr University I encouraged students to search for specific **sets of clues** when evaluating patients. These clues—often insignificant in isolation but meaningful in combination—were often the "red flags" that could help make the difference between an accurate diagnosis and a missed diagnosis. These four categories can be recalled with the mnemonic "*S.C.I.N.*" or "*S.C.I.M.*" These four areas of assessment/safety emphasis differ from the "vindicates" mnemonic which is used for differential diagnosis.

Vindicates: a popular mnemonic for differential diagnosis	
V	Vascular
	Visceral referral
I	Infectious
	Inflammatory
	Immunologic
N	Neurologic
	Nutritional
	New growth: neoplasia or pregnancy
D	Deficiency
	Degenerative
I	Iatrogenic (drug related)
	Intoxication
	Idiosyncratic
C	Congenital
	Cardiac or circulatory
A	Allergy / Autoimmune
	Abuse: drugs, alcohol, physical
T	Trauma
	Toxicity
E	Endocrine
	Exposure
S	Subluxation
	Somatic dysfunction
	Structural
	Stress
	Secondary gain

- **Systemic symptoms and signs**: Ask about systemic signs and symptoms such as fever, weight loss, lymphadenopathy, or skin rash in patients who present with pain because these "whole body" manifestations might indicate an underlying or concomitant disease that deserves attention, either independently from the musculoskeletal pain, or as a cause of the musculoskeletal pain. For example, "headache" may appear benign, whereas "headache with fever and skin rash" suggests meningitis—a medical emergency. "Low-back pain" is a common occurrence; yet "low-back pain with weight loss and fever" might suggest occult malignancy, osteomyelitis, or other systemic disease.

- **Complications:** We ask about and look for already existing complications, such as "numbness, weakness, tingling in the arms or hands, legs or feet" to rapidly screen for neurologic deficits and we follow this up with screening assessments such as "squat and rise", toe walk, heel walk, and reflexes for spinal cord and lower extremity neuromuscular integrity. Additionally, when dealing with patients with spine-related complaints or injuries, we also ask about changes or loss of function in bowel and bladder control and numbness near the anus or genitals, which may be the *only* clinical clues to cauda equina syndrome—a medical emergency. Ask about effects of the condition on ADL (activities of daily living) to attain a more comprehensive view of the condition and to ensure that the patient's story is consistent.

- **Indicators from the history**: We look for specific "red flags" and "yellow flags" such as trauma, risk factors (such as smoking, prednisone, alcohol), or a positive history of chronic infections or cancer. Nonmechanical musculoskeletal pain in a patient with a history of or high risk for cancer is highly suspicious and mandates thorough investigation.

- **Non-Mechanical pain**: Non-mechanical pain suggests a pathologic etiology rather than simple joint dysfunction. Pain at night, pain that occurs without an inciting injury, pain that is not strongly affected by motion and is not powerfully provoked by your physical examination assessments suggests the possibility of underlying disorder such as cancer, neuropathy, or infection. However, the ability to elicit an exacerbation of pain with "mechanical" maneuvers does not indicate that the pain is "mechanical" and therefore "non-pathologic." Mechanical pain can still be pathologic pain, such as the exquisite pain felt by patients with spinal fractures—they may be neurologically intact, they do have pain worse with motion, but they are not safe to manipulate, and they require appropriate treatment and referral on an urgent basis.

> Keeping these four assessment categories in mind can serve as a useful "checkpoint" to ensure that your patient is safe, and that your treatment is appropriate and therefore safe, too.

Concept: Special Considerations in the Evaluation of Children

"Pediatric infections and neoplasms are notorious for masquerading as sport injuries. ... There is only one way to avoid this trap: Take the relevant history directly from the patient, and keep tumors and infections high on your list of differential diagnoses."[319]

- **Consider the possibility of child abuse when a child presents with an injury:** As a non-naïve physician, you always have to consider the possibility of child abuse when a child presents with an injury. Be detailed in your history taking, and be sure to search for discrepancies between 1) the child's version of the incident, 2) the adult's version of the incident, and 3) what is realistic (based on your practical life experience and clinical training). As a primary care physician, you are obligated to report your *suspicion* of child abuse to law enforcement agencies and/or child protective services.
- **Children heal quickly:** This rapid healing is good as long as tissues are approximated. But if a fractured bone is displaced and not correctly replaced, then problematic malunion deformities may result *within **days***.
- **Children are more susceptible to rapidly progressing infections than are adults:** Soft tissue, joint, and bone infections need to be diagnosed expeditiously and treated aggressively.
- **Children are radiographically different from adults:** Make sure that your radiographs are interpreted by a competent radiologist with experience in the interpretation of *pediatric radiographs*. Radiographic considerations specific to children include:
  - **Epiphyseal growth plates**
  - **Secondary ossification centers**
  - **Variants in trabecular patterns and bone densities**
  - **Specific conditions that happen only in children, such as slipped capital femoral epiphysis**
  - **Congenital anomalies**
  - **Difficulty following directions with positioning** (applies to some adults, too!)
  - **Bone scans can be difficult to interpret in children:** Bone scans derive their value from the demonstration of a focal increase in uptake of radioactive isotopes, which demonstrates and localizes an area of increased metabolic activity. In adults, this increased and localized activity generally indicates pathology, especially malignant disease in bone (primary or metastatic) and recent fracture. In children, however, since their bones are already highly metabolically active due to the normal growth process, bone scans are difficult to interpret and are not highly reliable for the demonstration of focal lesions.

> Always consider the possibility of abuse, cancer, infection, or congenital anomaly as a cause of musculoskeletal pain in children, even if the injury appears to be related to injury or trauma. Strongly consider lab tests, as well as radiographs (interpreted by a pediatric radiologist). When in doubt, refer for second opinion. If you suspect abuse, you have a legal and ethical obligation to report your *suspicion*.

---

[319] Shaw BA, Gerardi JA, Hennrikus WL. How to avoid orthopedic pitfalls in children. *Patient Care* 1999; Feb 28: 95-116

Concept: Differences between Primary Healthcare and Spectator Sports

In baseball, "errors" have been defined as "a defensive mistake that allows a batter to stay at the plate or reach first base, or that advances a base runner."[320] In baseball, a few errors can make the difference between winning and losing a particular game or season. However, a few errors in a game are to be expected, and ultimately the team can start over at the next game or season and try to do better.

Healthcare, however, is not a game, and even relatively minor errors such as the doctor's forgetting to ask a particular question or perform a specific test can result in a patient's catastrophic injury or death. In healthcare, when we are dealing with serious injuries and illnesses, even a single "error" is not allowed. "Failure to diagnose" is one of the biggest reasons for malpractice claims against doctors; such judgments often result in loss of licensure and awards of hundreds of thousands of dollars. "Failure to treat" results when the patient is injured because the doctor failed to

> While your compassion for human suffering and your love of nutrition and exercise may have directed you into healthcare, your professional success and survival will depend in large part on your ability to manage the technical and defensive aspects of clinical practice.
>
> Neuromusculoskeletal disorders and autoimmune diseases are "big league" clinical problems, and they need to be taken seriously.

effectively treat the patient or when the doctor failed to provide the appropriate referral to a specialist in a timely manner. Such failures are not only capable of destroying a physician's career and forcing the liquidation of his/her possessions, but such cases can also greatly damage the integrity of whole professions, especially the naturopathic and chiropractic professions which are generally guilty until proven innocent due to the double standards imposed by those adherent to the "always right" dogma of the medical paradigm.[321] Stated differently, **if the doctor does not ask the right questions and perform the right tests, then the doctor may miss an emergency diagnosis. Missing an emergency diagnosis can result in patient death. Patient death may result in litigation, loss of license for the doctor, and irreparable harm to the profession.** The upcoming section on **Musculoskeletal Emergencies** represents *core competencies* that every clinician must keep present in his/her mind during each interaction with a patient with musculoskeletal complaints, especially patients who are elderly, on medications such as prednisone, and those with known autoimmune or immunosuppressive disorders.

Concept: "Disease Treatment" is Different from "Patient Management"

> "The key to successful intervention for orthopedic problems in a primary care practice is to know what conditions to refer and when and to whom to refer the refractory patient."[322]

Treating a problem is one thing, managing a patient is something different. "Problems" such as "low back pain" are abstract concepts, and we automatically form mental lists of treatments for problems that are irrespective of the patient who has the condition. However this list may be of only very limited applicability to the individual patient with whom you are working. Management of patients includes ❶ assessing and reassessing the differential diagnoses, ❷ monitoring compliance with treatments, including the treatments of other healthcare providers, ❸ co-treating with other healthcare providers, ❹ assessing for contraindications, ❺ monitoring patient status and effectiveness of treatments, and also ❻ the office-related tasks of charting, documentation, billing, and correspondence. The management of emergency conditions often involves transport to the nearest hospital. In some situations, the patient will be able to drive himself/herself without difficulty. In other situations, the patient should be driven by friend, family, or taxi. In the most extreme, the patient should be transported by ambulance. When in doubt about the mode of transport, do not hesitate to call 911 for an ambulance. If the taxi driver gets lost on the way to the hospital, or your patient goes into shock while being driven by a friend, the liability will come back to haunt the *doctor*, not the *friend* or the *taxi driver*.

---

[320] http://www.nocryinginbaseball.com/glossary/glossary.html Accessed November 11, 2006
[321] Micozzi MS. Double standards and double jeopardy for CAM research. *J Altern Complement Med.* 2001 Feb;7(1):13-4
[322] Brier S. Primary Care Orthopedics. St. Louis: Mosby, 1999 page ix

Concept: Clinical Practice Involves Much More than "Diagnosis and Treatment"

Emergency room and hospital-based physicians are appropriately able to focus solely on diagnosis and treatment as their primary spheres of activity and interaction with patients. However, those of us in private practice learn that *healthcare* involves much more than simply being a "good doctor." From an integrative perspective we have to go beyond diagnosis and treatment *for each health disorder* with each patient. Beyond *diagnosis* and *treatment* are *understanding* and *integration*. Orchestrating all of this into a treatment plan that the patient can actually implement requires creativity, resourcefulness, and the ability to enroll patients in the process of *redesigning*—often *rebuilding*—their lives.

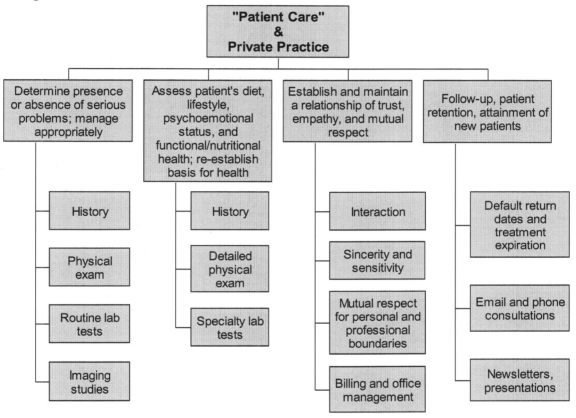

Recall that **28% of malpractice claims involve mistakes made by medical office staff**; this includes unreturned phone calls which can culminate in malpractice by way of "patient abandonment." Similarly, inability to get a timely consultation may result in sufficient "sense of harm" that a patient may decide to sue; this is a factor in 10% of malpractice cases.[323]

---

[323] James R. Hall, Ph.D., L.Psych., FABMP, FGICPP. Departments of Internal Medicine and Psychology, UNT Health Science Center at Fort Worth. "Communication and Medico-Legal Issues." October 19, 2006

Risk Management: A Note Especially to Students and Recent Licensees

Even if you are a board-certified rheumatologist and an assertive and astute clinician with years of experience, the consideration of these guidelines may help protect **you** from malpractice liability and **your patient** from harm. Practicing "good medicine" is inherently defensive and in the best interests of the patient and the doctor.

1. **Document the specifics of your treatment plan and the rationale behind it**.
2. **Do not tell your patient to discontinue their anti-rheumatic drugs unless these drugs are in your scope of practice** *and* **discontinuing such drugs is therapeutically appropriate.**
3. **Give your patient written instructions, and specifically delineate time parameters for the next visit to monitor for therapeutic effectiveness, adverse effects, and disease progression/regression.**
4. **Always have an internist or rheumatologist (or appropriate specialist) on-board as part of the clinical team in case the patient experiences an exacerbation and needs to be hospitalized or acutely immunosuppressed.**
5. **When working with patients that have potentially serious diseases such as most of the autoimmune diseases, you should have a back-up plan integrated into your treatment plan from day one.** You might consider having patients sign a consent form that includes language consistent with the following:
   - *"Due to the uniqueness of each disease and each individual, including his or her willingness and ability to implement the treatment plan, no guarantees of successful treatment can be offered."*
   - *"Dr.___ may not be available on a 24-hour basis at all times. If you have a serious health problem that requires immediate attention, you should call your other doctors(s), call 911, or have someone take you to the nearest hospital emergency room. If you notice an adverse effect from one of the components of your health plan, you should discontinue it then call Dr.__ and inform him/her of what occurred."*
   - *"Treatments with other physicians or healthcare providers are not necessarily to be discontinued. Please let Dr.__ know if you are being treated by other healthcare providers (physicians, counselors, therapists, etc.). Consult your prescribing doctor before discontinuing medications."*
6. **Test responsibly.**
7. **Treat responsibly.**
8. **Re-test to document effectiveness of your intervention.**
9. **When in doubt, refer the patient for co-management.** If you are working with a serious life-threatening disease, and *your plan* or *the patient's implementation of it* is unable to produce *documentable results*, then you should refer the patient for allopathic/osteopathic/specialist co-management for the sake of protecting the patient from harm and for protecting yourself from undue liability.
10. **Practice defensively.** You will thereby safeguard your patient and your livelihood.

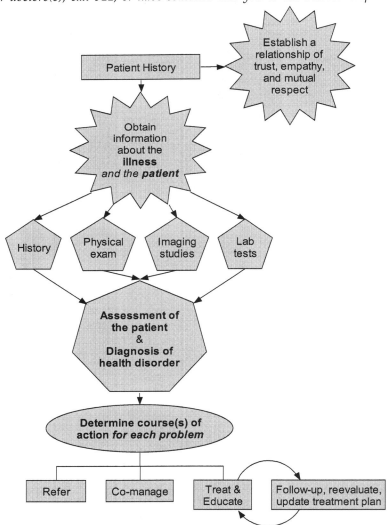

Musculoskeletal Emergencies

These are some of the "core competencies" that clinicians can never afford to miss, and these are pertinent to patients with musculoskeletal disorders, whether structural/orthopedic or metabolic/rheumatic. With these conditions, clinicians are wise to err on the side of caution— *"When in doubt, refer out"*—and implement the appropriate referral on an expedient basis. These are organized in a clinical/logical manner rather than listed alphabetically.

Neurovascular Disorders

Problem	*Presentation*	*Assessment*	*Management*
Neuropsychiatric lupus	▪ Psychosis ▪ Seizures ▪ Transient ischemic attacks ▪ Severe depression ▪ Delirium, confusion	▪ Neuropsychiatric manifestations with history of lupus	▪ Emergency or prompt referral as indicated
Giant cell arteritis, Temporal arteritis: Considered a medical emergency since it may rapidly progress to blindness due to associated involvement of the ophthalmic artery: *"Loss of vision is the most feared manifestation and occurs quite commonly."*[324]	Presentation typically includes the following: ▪ Headache, scalp tenderness ▪ Jaw claudication ▪ Changes in vision ▪ Systemic manifestations of rheumatic disease: fever, weight loss, muscle aches	▪ Palpation of the temporal artery may reveal a "cord-like" artery ▪ Elevated ESR ▪ CBC may show anemia ▪ Temporal artery biopsy is diagnostic	▪ Standard medical treatment is with immediate prednisone ▪ Implement treatment that is immediately effective or refer patient for medical treatment
Acute red eye: General term including acute iritis and scleritis; despite the name of this condition, redness may actually be rather minimal, and it is typically accompanied by cloudy changes in region of the iris and lens	▪ Eye pain and redness ▪ May have facial pain ▪ May be the presenting manifestation of rheumatic disease	▪ Red eye ▪ Photophobia ▪ Reduced vision ▪ May have fixed pupil ▪ Differential diagnosis includes acute glaucoma, bacterial/amebic/ viral conjunctivitis or keratitis, allergy, and irritation due to contact lens	▪ "The **acute** onset of a **painful, red** eye, even in the absence of visual upset, should be regarded primarily as an ophthalmological emergency."[325] ▪ **Granulomatous uveitis** occurs in 15% of patients with sarcoidosis and can result in bilateral blindness—this must be managed as a medically urgent condition

[324] Tierney ML. McPhee SJ, Papadakis MA (eds). <u>Current Medical Diagnosis and Treatment, 41st Edition</u>. New York: Lange Medical ; 2002. P999-1005
[325] McInnes I, Sturrock R. Rheumatological emergencies. *Practitioner.* 1994 Mar;238(1536):220-4

Neural canal compression

Problem	Presentation	Assessment	Management
Atlantoaxial instability: Excess mobility between the atlas and axis (commonly due to lesion of the dens or transverse ligament) makes the spinal cord vulnerable to compressive injury when the atlas translates anteriorly on the axis especially during cervical flexion; may progress to neurologic compromise including respiratory and somatic paralysis	• Post-traumatic neck injury • Down's syndrome • May present spontaneously (without trauma) in patients with inflammatory rheumatic disease, especially rheumatoid arthritis and ankylosing spondylitis • May have gradual or sudden onset of myelopathy: upper motor neuron lesion (UMNL) signs (e.g., spastic weakness), changes in bowel-bladder function, numbness	• Clinical suspicion is followed by lateral cervical and APOM (anteroposterior open mouth) radiographs to assess ADI (atlantodental interval) and dens • MRI should be performed in patients with suspected myelopathy • Neurologic examination of the upper and lower extremities • Do not force neck flexion; do not perform the Soto Hall test	• **Urgent neurosurgical consultation is recommended; stabilizing surgery is the best option for the prevention of neurologic catastrophes**[326] • Onset of myelopathy mandates referral to ER and/or neurosurgeon; immobilize with spine board or hard cervical collar and transport appropriately • Asymptomatic and mild increases in ADI (< 5mm) might be managed conservatively with activity restriction, exercises, and bracing/collars) • PAR discussion and referral for surgical consultation is necessary for informed consent and safe management
Myelopathy, spinal cord compression or lesion: May occur due to infection, edema, tumor, spinal fracture, stenosis, or inflammatory disease	• **Spastic weakness** • Bowel-bladder dysfunction • Numbness • Problems are distal to cord lesion	• Hyperreflexia • Rigidity • Muscle weakness • MRI (with and without contrast) should be performed in patients with suspected myelopathy; CT may also be indicated	• Obtain MRI to confirm diagnosis • Immobilize spine and transport if necessary • Acute myelopathy is a medical emergency that can result in rapid-onset paralysis
Cauda equina syndrome: Compression of the sacral nerve roots due to lumbar disc herniation **Cauda equina syndrome is a surgical emergency.**	• History of sciatic low back pain • Urinary retention, perineal numbness, and fecal incontinence are common • May have lower extremity weakness	• Assess for bladder distention • Assess anal sphincter strength with rectal exam • Lower extremity neurologic examination	• Urgent referral for CT/MRI to confirm diagnosis • If diagnosis is confirmed or strongly suspected clinically, urgent referral for surgical decompression is mandatory

---

[326] "When atlantoaxial stability is lost...it is thought that surgical stabilisation of the atlantoaxial joint is more reasonable and beneficial than conservative management. Minimal trauma of an unstable atlantoaxial joint can lead to serious neurological injury." Moon MS, Choi WT, Moon YW, Moon JL, Kim SS. Brooks' posterior stabilization surgery for atlantoaxial instability: review of 54 cases. *J Orthop Surg* (Hong Kong). 2002 Dec;10(2):160-4. http://www.josonline.org/PDF/v10i2p160.pdf

Acute peripheral nerve compression

Problem	Presentation	Assessment	Management
Acute compartment syndrome: acute onset of *potentially irreversible* muscle and/or nerve compression injury due to inflammation, swelling, or bleeding within a fascial compartment **Acute compartment syndrome is a surgical emergency.**	▪ Most commonly occurs in the anterior leg; may also occur in the posterior leg as well as forearm—these are the areas most notable anatomically for the investment of muscle in tight and resilient fascial sheaths ▪ Onset generally follows strenuous exercise that leads to reactive hyperemia and secondary edema ▪ May occur following trauma or fracture	Assess for: ▪ Pulselessness ▪ Palor ▪ Painful passive stretch ▪ Weakness ▪ **Numbness** ▪ Assessment and treatment should be performed on an emergency basis since irreversible nerve damage begins within 6 hours of intracompartmental hypertension	▪ Decompressive fasciotomy is the standard treatment for acute compartment syndrome that could result in permanent muscle necrosis and/or permanent nerve death ▪ Acute compartment syndrome can be fatal if rhabdomyolysis precipitates renal failure[327]

Musculoskeletal infections

Problem	Presentation	Assessment	Management
Septic arthritis: intraarticular bacterial infection; complications of septic arthritis are 1) articular destruction and 2) **death in 5-10% of patients**[328] **Septic arthritis is a medical emergency**	▪ **Febrile** patient has **acute/subacute mono/oligo-arthritis** ▪ Some patients may not have fever ▪ Other possible findings: Immuno-suppression due to medications, concomitant disease (RA, DM), elderly ▪ In some patients with concomitant disease or medications, the clinical picture can be blurred.	▪ **Warm, swollen, tender joint** ▪ Clinical assessment with **immediate referral for joint aspiration**, which reveals manifestations of infection such as WBC's and bacteria ▪ Differential diagnosis includes trauma, gout, CPPD, hemochromatosis	▪ **Immediate referral for joint aspiration** ▪ **An aggressive and prolonged course of IV and oral antimicrobials** ▪ "Immune support" such as vitamin A and glutamine and general measures to improve health and prevent recurrence
Osteomyelitis, infectious discitis: considered a medical emergency[329] **Osteomyelitis—especially vertebral osteomyelitis—is a medical emergency**	▪ Febrile patient with bone pain ▪ Assess for constitutional manifestations such as weight loss, night sweats, and malaise	▪ Exacerbation of bone pain when stress/percussion is applied to the bone ▪ Lab: CRP & WBC may be elevated ▪ MRI is more sensitive than CT, bone scan, or radiography[330]	▪ Emergency referral for vertebral osteomyelitis, since **up to 15% of patients will develop nerve lesions or cord compression**[331] ▪ Urgent referral for other types of osteomyelitis

[327] Paula R. Compartment Syndrome, Extremity. *eMedicine* June 22, 2006 http://www.emedicine.com/emerg/topic739.htm Accessed November 26, 2006

[328] Tierney ML. McPhee SJ, Papadakis MA. Current Medical Diagnosis and Treatment. 35th edition. Stamford: Appleton & Lange, 1996 page 759

[329] American College of Rheumatology Ad Hoc Committee on Clinical Guidelines. Guidelines for the initial evaluation of the adult patient with acute musculoskeletal symptoms. *Arthritis Rheum.* 1996;39(1):1-8

[330] Tierney ML. McPhee SJ, Papadakis MA (eds). Current Medical Diagnosis and Treatment 2002, 41st Edition. New York: Lange Medical; 2002. p 883

[331] King RW, Johnson D. Osteomyelitis. Updated July 13, 2006. *eMedicine* http://www.emedicine.com/emerg/topic349.htm Accessed Dec 24, 2006

Acute Nontraumatic Monoarthritis and Septic Arthritis

- "Acute monoarthritis is a potential medical emergency that must be investigated and treated promptly."[332]
- "Monoarthropathies should initially be investigated to exclude sepsis. ... Diagnostic joint aspiration ... should be carried out immediately."[333]
- "In acute monoarthritis, it is essential that infection of a joint be diagnosed or excluded, and this can only be done by joint aspiration and synovial fluid culture."[334]
- "Acute monoarthritis should be considered infectious until proven otherwise."[335]

Clinical presentations:

- Patient presents with acute joint pain in one joint (occasionally more than one joint may be involved).
- May or may not have fever and other systemic manifestations of infection.

> **Clinical Pearl**
>
> The primary goal of this section is to solidify your awareness of septic arthritis, its differential diagnoses, and the method and importance of assertive diagnosis and management.
>
> Septic arthritis is a medical emergency, and some authoritative textbooks report a mortality rate of 5-10%.
>
> Septic arthritis must be diagnosed urgently with joint aspiration, and it must be treated with antibiotics in order to preserve the joint and prevent spread of the infection.

Major Differential Diagnoses for Nontraumatic Monoarthritis

Problem	Presentation	Assessment & Management
Septic arthritis: intraarticular bacterial infection; complications of septic arthritis are 1) articular destruction and 2) **death in 5-10% of patients**[336]	▪ **Febrile** patient has **acute/subacute mono/oligo-arthritis** ▪ **Onset over hours or days** Other possible findings: ▪ Immuno-suppression due to medications, concomitant disease (RA, DM), elderly ▪ Some patients may not have fever ▪ In some patients with a previous or concomitant disease process, the clinical picture can be blurred	▪ **Warm, swollen, red, painful joint** ▪ Clinical assessment with **immediate referral for joint aspiration**, which reveals characteristic manifestations of infection such as WBCs and bacteria ▪ **Immediate joint aspiration** ▪ An aggressive and prolonged course of IV and oral antimicrobials ▪ "Immune support" and general measures to improve health and prevent recurrence **"Septic arthritis is still a life-threatening disease with a mortality of 2–5% and high morbidity."** Zacher J, Gursche A. Regional musculoskeletal conditions: 'hip' pain. *Best Practice & Research Clinical Rheumatology*. 2003 Feb;17:71-85

---

[332] Cibere J. Rheumatology: 4. Acute monoarthritis. CMAJ (*Canadian Medical Association Journal*). 2000;162(11):1577-83 http://www.cmaj.ca/cgi/content/full/162/11/1577 January 24, 2004

[333] McInnes I, Sturrock R. Rheumatological emergencies. Practitioner. 1994 Mar;238(1536):220-4

[334] American College of Rheumatology Ad Hoc Committee on Clinical Guidelines. Guidelines for the initial evaluation of the adult patient with acute musculoskeletal symptoms. *Arthritis Rheum*. 1996 Jan;39(1):1-8

[335] Cibere J. Rheumatology: 4. Acute monoarthritis. CMAJ (*Canadian Medical Association Journal*). 2000;162(11):1577-83 http://www.cmaj.ca/cgi/content/full/162/11/1577 January 24, 2004

[336] Tierney ML. McPhee SJ, Papadakis MA. Current Medical Diagnosis and Treatment. 35th edition. Stamford: Appleton and Lange, 1996 page 759

Major differential diagnoses for non-traumatic monoarthritis—*continued*

Problem	Presentation	Assessment & Management
Osteochondritis dissecans: A disorder of unclear etiology (trauma and/or avascular necrosis) which results in the death and subsequent fragmentation of subchondral bone[337]	▪ Primarily affects ages 10-30 years ▪ **Most common in the knees and elbows** ▪ Locking and crepitus due to intraarticular loose bodies ("joint mice") ▪ Some patients are almost asymptomatic, while others have acute pain ▪ Swelling of the affected joint	▪ Radiographs—consider to assess both knees as the condition is bilateral in 30% ▪ MRI is used to assess severity and need for surgical intervention ▪ Stable and nondisplaced lesions may be managed nonsurgically; larger and displaced fragments require surgical repair to reduce long-term complications[338]
Transient synovitis, irritable hip: Non-specific short-term inflammation and effusion of the hip joint	▪ Acute onset of painful hip and limp ▪ Decreased pain with hip in flexion and abduction ▪ Considered the most common cause of hip pain in children[339] ▪ More common in boys, age 3-6 years and generally younger than 10 years ▪ May have recent history of viral infection, and some children (1.5-10%) eventually manifest RA or AVN[340]	▪ May have slight elevation of ESR ▪ Normal WBC ▪ <u>No</u> fever; the child appears healthy ▪ "…radiography is indicated to exclude osseous pathological conditions…"[341] ▪ **Joint aspiration is indicated if septic arthritis is suspected**[342] ▪ Conservative treatment, restricted exertion and weight-bearing for several weeks
Legg-Calve-Perthe's disease: Idiopathic ischemic necrosis of the femoral head occurring in children **Avascular necrosis (AVN) of the femoral head, osteonecrosis**: Ischemic necrosis of the femoral head	Perthe's disease: ▪ 80% occur in children generally between ages of 4-9 years; more common in boys; may present with hip pain or knee pain AVN: ▪ Ages 20-40 years ▪ Unilateral hip pain ▪ May have knee pain ▪ History of trauma is common AVN associations: ▪ Steroid use, prednisone ▪ Hyperlipidemia ▪ Alcoholism ▪ Pancreatitis ▪ Hemoglobinopathies ▪ Smoking ▪ Fatty liver disease: "fat globules from the liver"[343]	▪ Limited ROM ▪ **Radiographs**; if normal and clinical suspicion is high order MRI or bone scan ▪ **Crutches** ▪ **Orthopedic referral is recommended** although not all patients will require surgery and some may be managed conservatively[344]

[337] Tatum R. Osteochondritis dissecans of the knee: a radiology case report. *J Manipulative Physiol Ther* 2000 Jun;23(5):347-51

[338] Browne RF, Murphy SM, Torreggiani WC, Munk PL, Marchinkow LO. Radiology for the surgeon: musculoskeletal case 30. Osteochondritis dissecans of the medial femoral condyle. *Can J Surg.* 2003;46(5):361-3 cma.ca/multimedia/staticContent/HTML/N0/l2/cjs/vol-46/issue-5/pdf/pg361.pdf

[339] Maroo S. Diagnosis of hip pain in children. *Hosp Med* 1999 Nov;60(11):788-93

[340] Souza TA. <u>Differential Diagnosis for the Chiropractor: Protocols and Algorithms</u>. Gaithersberg, Maryland: Aspen Publications. 1997 page 265

[341] Maroo S. Diagnosis of hip pain in children. *Hosp Med* 1999 Nov;60(11):788-93

[342] Maroo S. Diagnosis of hip pain in children. *Hosp Med* 1999 Nov;60(11):788-93

Major differential diagnoses for non-traumatic monoarthritis—*continued*

Problem	Presentation	Assessment & Management
Gout	• **Febrile** patient has **acute/subacute mono/oligo-arthritis** • **Onset over hours or days** • "A history of discreet attacks, usually affecting one joint, that precede the onset of fixed symmetric arthritis is the major clue."[345] • May have fever, chills, tachycardia, leukocytosis—just like septic arthritis	• Clinical presentation may be sufficient for DX; however septic arthritis should be excluded • Serum uric acid is generally meaningless for the diagnosis of gout since many gout patients will have normal serum uric acid • Medical treatment is rest, NSAID's, and allopurinol • Fluid loading: >3 liters per day; monitor for electrolyte imbalances and hyponatremia as needed • Integrative assessment and treatment for insulin resistance, hormonal imbalances, and nutritional deficiencies
CPPD: Calcium pyrophosphate dihydrate deposition disease	• Idiopathic • May be caused by iron overload in some patients • Presentation may be acute or subacute	• Medical diagnosis is by synovial biopsy • Radiographs reveal chondrocalcinosis • Allopathic treatment is NSAIDs; phytonutritional anti-inflammatory treatments may also be used (see chapter 3 of *Integrative Orthopedics/Rheumatology*) • Oral colchicine 0.5 to 1.5 mg per day prevents attacks[346]
Hemarthrosis: Generally associated with trauma, anticoagulation (i.e., coumadin), leukemia, hemophilia	• Monoarthralgia with limited motion • May follow direct trauma • Nontraumatic hemarthrosis may be due to anticoagulation, leukemia, hemophilia	• Synovial fluid analysis reveals blood • Treatment of underlying disorder; refer as indicated
Slipped capital femoral epiphysis (SCFE): The most common cause of hip pain in adolescents[347]	• Seen in adolescents generally 8-17 years of age • Classic presentation is a tall overweight boy with **hip pain**, knee pain, and/or a painful limp: *"Slipped femoral capital epiphysis is a developmental injury that must be considered in any adolescent who presents with hip pain."*[348]	• **Radiographs** of both hips (bilateral SCFE in 40%): "**AP and frog lateral views are recommended in all children over age of 9 years with hip pain.**"[349] • Orthopedic referral—*"...the patient should be referred immediately to an orthopedist for surgical stabilization."* [350]

[343] Skinner HB, Scherger JE. Identifying structural hip and knee problems. Patient age, history, and limited examination may be all that's needed. *Postgrad Med* 1999;106(7):51-2, 55-6, 61-4

[344] Souza TA. Differential Diagnosis for the Chiropractor: Protocols and Algorithms. Gaithersberg, Maryland: Aspen Publications. 1997 page 263

[345] Hardin JG, Waterman J, Labson LH. Rheumatic disease: Which diagnostic tests are useful? *Patient Care* 1999; March 15: 83-102

[346] Beers MH, Berkow R (eds). The Merck Manual. Seventeenth Edition. Whitehouse Station; Merck Research Laboratories 1999 Page

[347] Maroo S. Diagnosis of hip pain in children. *Hosp Med* 1999 Nov;60(11):788-93

[348] O'Kane JW. Anterior hip pain. *Am Fam Physician* 1999 Oct 15;60(6):1687-96

[349] Maroo S. Diagnosis of hip pain in children. *Hosp Med* 1999 Nov;60(11):788-93

[350] O'Kane JW. Anterior hip pain. *Am Fam Physician* 1999 Oct 15;60(6):1687-96

<u>Clinical assessment</u>:
- History and orthopedic assessment of the joint
- Laboratory tests must be performed if you have a suspicion of infection

<u>History/subjective</u>:
- Acute or subacute joint pain with or without systemic manifestations and fever.
- History or may not be significant; other than the obvious risk factor of immunosuppression, septic arthritis can occur with impressive spontaneity and randomness

<u>Differential physical examination and objective findings</u>:
- **Septic arthritis**: pain and limitation of motion, swelling, redness; patient may have systemic symptoms of fever and malaise
- **Gout**: pain and limitation of motion, swelling, redness; patient may have systemic symptoms of fever and malaise
- **Pseudogout and calcium pyrophosphate dihydrate deposition disease (CPDD/CPPD)**: pain and limitation of motion, swelling, redness; patient may have systemic symptoms of fever and malaise
- **Ischemic necrosis**: pain and limitation of motion; swelling, redness and systemic symptoms are less likely.
- **Hemarthrosis**: pain and limitation of motion; often associated with trauma, use of anticoagulant medications[351], or hemophilia and other hematologic abnormalities[352]
- **Tumor**: assess with history, imaging, and biopsy if possible
- **Injury**: Meniscal injury, fracture, ligament injury; physical examination procedures are described in the chapters that follow

<u>Imaging and laboratory assessments</u>:
- **Septic arthritis**: joint aspiration; STAT CBC (for WBC count) and CRP
- **Gout**: joint aspiration; CBC (for WBC count) and CRP
- **Pseudogout and PPDD**: rule out septic arthritis with joint aspiration, CBC, and CRP; radiographs often show chondrocalcinosis
- **Ischemic necrosis**: radiographs are diagnostic
- **Hemarthrosis**: joint aspiration and assessment for underlying disease or medication, especially if the condition was not trauma-induced
- **Tumor**: assess with radiographs
- **Injury**: rule out infection; consider imaging with radiography or MRI.

<u>Establishing the diagnosis</u>:
- The aforementioned examinations and lab assessments should establish the exact diagnosis. **The priorities are 1) first exclude life-threatening illness (i.e., septic arthritis), then 2) to exclude serious injury or illness,** and finally 3) to help manage the exact problem.

<u>Complications</u>:
- **Septic arthritis can result in death 5-10% of patients. "Five to 10 percent of patients with an infected joint die, chiefly from respiratory complications of sepsis. The mortality rate is 30% for patients with polyarticular sepsis. Bony ankylosis and articular destruction commonly also occur if the treatment is delayed or inadequate."[353]** Complications vary per location, infecting organism, severity, and patient.

[351] Riley SA, Spencer GE. Destructive monarticular arthritis secondary to anticoagulant therapy. *Clin Orthop*. 1987 Oct;(223):247-51
[352] Jean-Baptiste G, De Ceulaer K. Osteoarticular disorders of haematological origin. *Baillieres Best Pract Res Clin Rheumatol*. 2000 Jun;14(2):307-23
[353] Tierney ML. McPhee SJ, Papadakis MA. <u>Current Medical Diagnosis and Treatment. 35th edition</u>. Stamford: Appleton & Lange, 1996 page 759

Clinical management:

- **Suspected septic arthritis requires referral for joint aspiration and antimicrobial drugs.**
- Referral if clinical outcome is unsatisfactory or if serious complications are evident.
- Treatment of other conditions that cause acute monoarthritis (such as gout and calcium pyrophosphate dihydrate deposition disease) is based on the problem and individual patient.

Treatments:

- **Septic arthritis requires IV/oral antimicrobial drugs**: Intravenous antibiotics are generally started before culture results are available. After results and culture from synovial fluid analysis have been considered, the dose, combination, and administration of antibiotics can be fine-tuned. Frequently, antibiotics are administered intravenously for at least 3-4 weeks. Surgical/endoscopic drainage/debridement and immobilization during the acute phase may also be implemented.[354]
- **Immunonutrition considerations:** Immunonutritional considerations are listed below; doses listed are for adults. Although studies have not been performed specifically in patients with bone/joint infections, general benefits derived from the use of immunonutrition are reductions in severity/frequency/duration of major infections, abbreviated hospitalization (i.e., early discharge due to expedited healing and recovery), reductions in the need for medications, significant improvements in survival, and hospital savings.[355,356,357,358,359,360,361]
    - Paleo-Mediterranean diet: as detailed later in this text and elsewhere[362,363]
    - Vitamin and mineral supplementation: anti-infective benefits shown in elderly diabetics[364]
    - High-dose vitamin A: Vitamin A shows potent immunosupportive benefits, and vitamin A stores are depleted by the stress of infection and injury. Consider 200,000-300,000 IU per day of retinol palmitate for 1-4 weeks, then taper; reduce dose or discontinue with onset of toxicity symptoms such as skin problems (dry skin, flaking skin, chapped or split lips, red skin rash, hair loss), joint pain, bone pain, headaches, anorexia (loss of appetite), edema (water retention, weight gain, swollen ankles, difficulty breathing), fatigue, and/or liver damage.
    - Arginine: Dose for adults is in the range of 5-10 grams daily

---

[354] Brusch JL. Septic Arthritis (Last Updated: October 18, 2005). *eMedicine*. http://www.emedicine.com/med/topic3394.htm Accessed Nov 25, 2006

[355] "To evaluate the metabolic and immune effects of dietary arginine, glutamine and omega-3 fatty acids (fish oil) supplementation, we performed a prospective study... CONCLUSIONS: The feeding of Neomune in critically injured patients was well tolerated as Traumacal and significant improvement was observed in serum protein. Shorten ICU stay and wean-off respirator day may benefit from using the immunonutrient formula." Chuntrasakul C, Siltham S, Sarasombath S, Sittapairochana C, Leowattana W, Chockvivatavanit S, Bunnak A. Comparison of a immunonutrition formula enriched arginine, glutamine and omega-3 fatty acid, with a currently high-enriched enteral nutrition for trauma patients. *J Med Assoc Thai*. 2003 Jun;86(6):552-6

[356] "CONCLUSIONS: In conclusion, arginine-enhanced formula improves fistula rates in postoperative head and neck cancer patients and decreases length of stay." de Luis DA, Izaola O, Cuellar L, Terroba MC, Aller R. Randomized clinical trial with an enteral arginine-enhanced formula in early postsurgical head and neck cancer patients. *Eur J Clin Nutr*. 2004;58(11):1505-8

[357] "In this prospective, randomised, double-blind, placebo-controlled study, we randomly assigned 50 patients who were scheduled to undergo coronary artery bypass to receive either an oral immune-enhancing nutritional supplement containing L-arginine, omega3 polyunsaturated fatty acids, and yeast RNA (n=25), or a control (n=25) for a minimum of 5 days... Intake of an oral immune-enhancing nutritional supplement for a minimum of 5 days before surgery can improve outlook in high-risk patients who are undergoing elective cardiac surgery." Tepaske R, Velthuis H, Oudemans-van Straaten HM, Heisterkamp SH, van Deventer SJ, Ince C, Eysman L, Kesecioglu J. Effect of preoperative oral immune-enhancing nutritional supplement on patients at high risk of infection after cardiac surgery: a randomised placebo-controlled trial. *Lancet*. 2001 Sep 1;358(9283):696-701

[358] "The feeding of IMMUNE FORMULA was well tolerated and significant improvement was observed in nutritional and immunologic parameters as in other immunoenhancing diets. Further clinical trials of prospective double-blind randomized design are necessary to address the so that the necessity of using immunonutrition in critically ill patients will be clarified." Chuntrasakul C, Siltharm S, Sarasombath S, Sittapairochana C, Leowattana W, Chockvivatavanit S, Bunnak A. Metabolic and immune effects of dietary arginine, glutamine and omega-3 fatty acids supplementation in immunocompromised patients. *J Med Assoc Thai*. 1998 May;81(5):334-43

[359] "enteral diet supplemented with arginine, dietary nucleotides, and omega-3 fatty acids (IMPACT, Sandoz Nutrition, Bern, Switzerland)" Senkal M, Mumme A, Eickhoff U, Geier B, Spath G, Wulfert D, Joosten U, Frei A, Kemen M. Early postoperative enteral immunonutrition: clinical outcome and cost-comparison analysis in surgical patients. *Crit Care Med* 1997;25(9):1489-96

[360] "supplemented diet with glutamine, arginine and omega-3-fatty acids... It was clearly established in this trial that early postoperative enteral feeding is safe in patients who have undergone major operations for gastrointestinal cancer. Supplementation of enteral nutrition with glutamine, arginine, and omega-3-fatty acids positively modulated postsurgical immunosuppressive and inflammatory responses." Wu GH, Zhang YW, Wu ZH. Modulation of postoperative immune and inflammatory response by immune-enhancing enteral diet in gastrointestinal cancer patients. *World J Gastroenterol*. 2001 Jun;7(3):357-62 http://www.wjgnet.com/1007-9327/7/357.pdf

[361] "using a formula supplemented with arginine, mRNA, and omega-3 fatty acids from fish oil (Impact)... CONCLUSIONS: Immune-enhancing enteral nutrition resulted in a significant reduction in the mortality rate and infection rate in septic patients admitted to the ICU. These reductions were greater for patients with less severe illness." Galban C, Montejo JC, Mesejo A, Marco P, Celaya S, Sanchez-Segura JM, Farre M, Bryg DJ. An immune-enhancing enteral diet reduces mortality rate and episodes of bacteremia in septic intensive care unit patients. *Crit Care Med*. 2000 Mar;28(3):643-8

[362] **Vasquez A**. A Five-Part Nutritional Protocol that Produces Consistently Positive Results. *Nutritional Wellness* 2005 September http://optimalhealthresearch.com/protocol

[363] **Vasquez A**. Implementing the Five-Part Nutritional Wellness Protocol for the Treatment of Various Health Problems. *Nutritional Wellness* 2005 November. http://optimalhealthresearch.com/protocol

[364] "CONCLUSIONS: A multivitamin and mineral supplement reduced the incidence of participant-reported infection and related absenteeism in a sample of participants with type 2 diabetes mellitus and a high prevalence of subclinical micronutrient deficiency." Barringer TA, Kirk JK, Santaniello AC, Foley KL, Michielutte R. Effect of a multivitamin and mineral supplement on infection and quality of life. A randomized, double-blind, placebo-controlled trial. *Ann Intern Med*. 2003 Mar 4;138(5):365-71 http://www.annals.org/cgi/reprint/138/5/365

o <u>Fatty acid supplementation</u>: In contrast to the higher doses used to provide an anti-inflammatory effect in patients with autoimmune/inflammatory disorders, doses used for immunosupportive treatments should be kept rather modest to avoid the *relative* immunosuppression that has been controversially reported in patients treated with EPA and DHA. Reasonable doses are in the following ranges for adults: EPA+DHA: 500-1,500, and GLA: 300-500 mg.

o <u>Glutamine</u>: Glutamine enhances bacterial killing by neutrophils[365], and administration of 18 grams per day in divided doses to patients in intensive care units was shown to improve survival, expedite hospital discharge, and reduce total healthcare costs.[366] Another study using glutamine 12-18 grams per day showed no benefit in overall mortality but significant benefits in terms of reduced healthcare costs (-30%) and significantly reduced need for medical interventions.[367] After administering glutamine 26 grams/d to severely burned patients, Garrel et al[368] concluded that glutamine reduced the risk of infection by 3-fold and that oral glutamine "may be a life-saving intervention" in patients with severe burns. A dose of 30 grams/d was used in a recent clinical trial showing hemodynamic benefit in patients with sickle cell anemia.[369] The highest glutamine dose that the current author is aware of is the study by Scheltinga et al[370] who used 0.57 gm/kg/day in cancer patients following chemotherapy administration; for a 220-lb-pt, this would be approximately 57 grams of glutamine per day.

o <u>Melatonin</u>: 20-40 mg hs (*hora somni*—Latin: sleep time). Immunostimulatory anti-infective action of melatonin was demonstrated in a small clinical trial wherein septic newborns administered 20 mg melatonin showed significantly increased survival over nontreated controls.[371]

---

[365] Furukawa S, Saito H, Fukatsu K, Hashiguchi Y, Inaba T, Lin MT, Inoue T, Han I, Matsuda T, Muto T. Glutamine-enhanced bacterial killing by neutrophils from postoperative patients. *Nutrition* 1997;13(10):863-9. *In vitro* study.
[366] Griffiths RD, Jones C, Palmer TE. Six-month outcome of critically ill patients given glutamine-supplemented parenteral nutrition. *Nutrition* 1997;13(4):295-302
[367] "There was no mortality difference between those patients receiving glutamine-containing enteral feed and the controls. However, there was a significant reduction in the median postintervention ICU and hospital patient costs in the glutamine recipients $23 000 versus $30 900 in the control patients." Jones C, Palmer TE, Griffiths RD. Randomized clinical outcome study of critically ill patients given glutamine-supplemented enteral nutrition. *Nutrition*. 1999 Feb;15(2):108-15
[368] The glutamine dose in this study was "a total of 26 g/day" administered in four divided doses. CONCLUSION: "The results of this prospective randomized clinical trial show that enteral G reduces blood culture positivity, particularly with P. aeruginosa, in adults with severe burns and may be a life-saving intervention." Garrel D, Patenaude J, Nedelec B, et al. Decreased mortality and infectious morbidity in adult burn patients given enteral glutamine supplements: a prospective, controlled, randomized clinical trial. *Crit Care Med*. 2003 Oct;31(10):2444-9
[369] Niihara Y, Matsui NM, Shen YM, et al. L-glutamine therapy reduces endothelial adhesion of sickle red blood cells to human umbilical vein endothelial cells. *BMC Blood Disord*. 2005 Jul 25;5:4 http://www.biomedcentral.com.proxy.hsc.unt.edu/1471-2326/5/4
[370] "Subjects with hematologic malignancies in remission underwent a standard treatment of high-dose chemotherapy and total body irradiation before bone marrow transplantation. After completion of this regimen, they were randomized to receive either standard parenteral nutrition (STD, n = 10) or an isocaloric, isonitrogenous nutrient solution enriched with crystalline L-glutamine (0.57 g/kg/day, GLN, n = 10)." Scheltinga MR, Young LS, Benfell K, Bye RL, Ziegler TR, Santos AA, Antin JH, Schloerb PR, Wilmore DW. Glutamine-enriched intravenous feedings attenuate extracellular fluid expansion after a standard stress. *Ann Surg*. 1991 Oct;214(4):385-93; discussion 393-5 pubmedcentral.nih.gov/articlerender.fcgi?tool=pubmed&pubmedid=1953094 For additional review, see Ziegler TR. Glutamine supplementation in cancer patients receiving bone marrow transplantation and high dose chemotherapy. J Nutr. 2001 Sep;131(9 Suppl):2578S-84S http://jn.nutrition.org/cgi/content/full/131/9/2578S
[371] Gitto E, et al. Effects of melatonin treatment in septic newborns. *Pediatr Res*. 2001;50:756-60 pedresearch.org/cgi/content/full/50/6/756

Brief Overview of Integrative Healthcare Disciplines

Chiropractic

"Doctors of Chiropractic are physicians who consider man as an integrated being and give special attention to the physiological and biochemical aspects including structural, spinal, musculoskeletal, neurological, vascular, nutritional, emotional and environmental relationships." *American Chiropractic Association, 2004*[372]

"The human body represents the actions of three laws—spiritual, mechanical, and chemical—united as one triune. As long as there is perfect union of these three, there is health." *Daniel David Palmer, founder of the modern chiropractic profession*[373]

The basic philosophical model which is taught in many chiropractic colleges is to envision health, disease, and patient care from a conceptual model named the "triad of health" which gives its attention to the three fundamental foundations for well-being: namely, the physical/structural, mental/emotional, and biochemical/nutritional aspects of health. Revolutionary at the time of its inception in the early 1900's, this model now forms the foundation for the increasingly dominant and very popular paradigm of "holistic medicine." It remains a powerful contrast and an attractive alternative to the reductionistic allopathic approach, which generally approaches the human body as if it were simply a conglomerate of independent organ systems that have little or no functional relationship to each other.[374]

Using the state of the sciences before the year 1910, chiropractic was founded with a profound appreciation of the integrated nature of health, and the therapeutic focus was on spinal

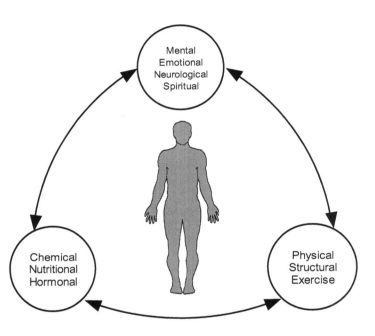

The chiropractic "triad of health"

manipulation. In describing the chiropractic model of health, DD Palmer[375] wrote, "The human body represents the actions of three laws—spiritual, mechanical, and chemical—united as one triune. As long as there is perfect union of these three, there is health." While the therapeutic focus of the profession has been spinal manipulation, from its inception the chiropractic profession has emphasized a holistic, integrative model of therapeutic intervention, health, and disease, and chiropractic was the first healthcare profession in America to specifically claim that the optimization of health requires attention to spiritual-emotional-psychological, mechanical-physical-structural, and biochemical-nutritional-hormonal-chemical considerations. Accordingly, these cornerstones are fundamental to the 2005 definition of the chiropractic profession articulated by the American Chiropractic Association[376]: "Doctors of Chiropractic are physicians who consider man as an integrated being and give special attention to the physiological and biochemical aspects including structural, spinal, musculoskeletal, neurological, vascular, nutritional, emotional, and environmental relationships."

[372] American Chiropractic Association. http://www.amerchiro.org/media/whatis/ Accessed March 13, 2004
[373] Palmer DD. The Science, Art, and Phiosophy, of Chiropractic. Portland, OR; Portland Printing House Company, 1910: 107
[374] Beckman JF, Fernandez CE, Coulter ID. A systems model of health care: a proposal. *J Manipulative Physiol Ther*. 1996 Mar-Apr; 19(3): 208-15
[375] Palmer DD. The Science, Art, and Phiosophy, of Chiropractic. Portland, OR; Portland Printing House Company, 1910: 107
[376] American Chiropractic Association. What is Chiropractic? http://amerchiro.org/media/whatis/ Accessed January 9, 2005

From its inception, chiropractic was a philosophy of healing that considered the entire health of the patient by addressing the interconnected aspects of our chemical-spiritual-physical being. Later, intraprofessional factions polarized between holistic and vitalistic paradigms; the latter has been presumed to be the philosophy of the entire profession by organizations such as the American Medical Association[377] that have sought to contain and eliminate chiropractic and other forms of natural healthcare[378] by falsifying research[379,380], intentionally misleading the public and manipulating politicians[381,382,383], arriving at illogical conclusions which support the medical paradigm and refute the value of manual therapies[384], and exploiting weaknesses within the profession for its own financial profitability and political advantage.[385] Intentional misrepresentation and defamation of chiropractic continues to occur today, as documented by the 2006 review by Wenban.[386]

Chiropractic Training and Clinical Benefits: In addition to the basic sciences and foundational skills of laboratory and clinical diagnosis, chiropractic physicians receive extensive training in manual physical manipulation, rehabilitation, therapeutic exercise, and clinical nutrition.

An irony exists in the observation that chiropractic education emphasizes anatomy, musculoskeletal therapeutics, and nutrition while these are the very topics that are neglected in allopathic and osteopathic education; the majority medical students and medical physicians who have graduated from allopathic and osteopathic medical schools lack competence in their knowledge of clinical anatomy and musculoskeletal medicine[387,388,389,390,391,392] as well as diet and nutrition.[393,394,395] In contrast to this replicable data showing that osteopathic and allopathic students and graduates generally fail to demonstrate competence in musculoskeletal medicine and nutrition, one study with 123 chiropractic students and 10 chiropractic doctors showed that chiropractic training in musculoskeletal medicine is significantly superior to allopathic and osteopathic musculoskeletal training.[396]

In accord with the comprehensive chiropractic training in musculoskeletal management, numerous sources of evidence demonstrate that chiropractic management of the most common spinal pain syndromes is

---

[377] American Medical Association. Report 12 of the Council on Scientific Affairs (A-97) Full Text. http://www.ama-assn.org/ama/pub/category/13638.html Accessed September 10, 2005.

[378] Getzendanner S. Permanent injunction order against AMA. *JAMA*. 1988 Jan 1;259(1):81-2

[379] Terrett AG. Misuse of the literature by medical authors in discussing spinal manipulative therapy injury. *J Manipulative Physiol Ther*. 1995 May;18(4):203-10

[380] Morley J, Rosner AL, Redwood D. A case study of misrepresentation of the scientific literature: recent reviews of chiropractic. *J Altern Complement Med*. 2001 Feb;7(1):65-78

[381] Spivak JL. The Medical Trust Unmasked. Louis S. Siegfried Publishers; New York: 1961

[382] Trever W. In the Public Interest. Los Angeles; Scriptures Unlimited; 1972. This is probably the most authoritative documentation of the illegal actions of the AMA up to 1972; contains numerous photocopies of actual AMA documents and minutes of official meetings with overt intentionality of destroying Americans' healthcare options so that the AMA and related organizations would have a monopoly in healthcare.

[383] Wolinsky H, Brune T. The Serpent on the Staff: The Unhealthy Politics of the American Medical Association. GP Putnam and Sons, New York, 1994

[384] Mein EA, Greenman PE, McMillin DL, Richards DG, Nelson CD. Manual medicine diversity: research pitfalls and the emerging medical paradigm. *J Am Osteopath Assoc*. 2001 Aug;101(8):441-4

[385] Wilk CA. Medicine, Monopolies, and Malice: How the Medical Establishment Tried to Destroy Chiropractic. Garden City Park: Avery, 1996

[386] Wenban AB. Inappropriate use of the title 'chiropractor' and term 'chiropractic manipulation' in the peer-reviewed biomedical literature. *Chiropr Osteopat*. 2006;14:16 http://chiroandosteo.com/content/14/1/16

[387] "In summary, seventy (82 per cent) of eighty-five medical school graduates failed a valid musculoskeletal competency examination. We therefore believe that medical school preparation in musculoskeletal medicine is inadequate." Freedman KB, Bernstein J. The adequacy of medical school education in musculoskeletal medicine. *J Bone Joint Surg Am*. 1998;80(10):1421-7

[388] "CONCLUSIONS: According to the standard suggested by the program directors of internal medicine residency departments, a large majority of the examinees once again failed to demonstrate basic competency in musculoskeletal medicine on the examination. It is therefore reasonable to conclude that medical school preparation in musculoskeletal medicine is inadequate." Freedman KB, Bernstein J. Educational deficiencies in musculoskeletal medicine. *J Bone Joint Surg Am*. 2002;84-A(4):604-8

[389] Joy EA, Hala SV. Musculoskeletal Curricula in Medical Education: Filling In the Missing Pieces. *The Physician and Sportsmedicine* 2004; 32: 42-45

[390] "CONCLUSIONS: Seventy-nine percent of the participants failed the basic musculoskeletal cognitive examination. This suggests that training in musculoskeletal medicine is inadequate in both medical school and nonorthopaedic residency training programs." Matzkin E, Smith ME, Freccero CD, Richardson AB. Adequacy of education in musculoskeletal medicine. *J Bone Joint Surg Am*. 2005 Feb;87-A(2):310-4

[391] "Despite generally improved levels of competency with each year at medical school, less than 50% of fourth-year students showed competency. ... These results suggested that the curricular approach toward teaching musculoskeletal medicine at this medical school was insufficient and that competency increased when learning was reinforced during the clinical years." Schmale GA. More evidence of educational inadequacies in musculoskeletal medicine. *Clin Orthop Relat Res*. 2005 Aug;(437):251-9

[392] "RESULTS: When the minimum passing level as determined by orthopedic program directors was applied to the results of these examinations, 70.4% of graduating COM students (n=54) and 82% of allopathic graduates (n=85) failed to demonstrate basic competency in musculoskeletal medicine." Stockard AR, Allen TW. Competence levels in musculoskeletal medicine: comparison of osteopathic and allopathic medical graduates. *J Am Osteopath Assoc*. 2006 Jun;106(6):350-5

[393] "CONCLUSIONS: Internal medicine interns' perceive nutrition counseling as a priority, but lack the confidence and knowledge to effectively provide adequate nutrition education." Vetter ML, Herring SJ, Sood M, Shah NR, Kalet AL. What do resident physicians know about nutrition? An evaluation of attitudes, self-perceived proficiency and knowledge. *J Am Coll Nutr*. 2008 Apr;27(2):287-98

[394] "CONCLUSIONS: The amount of nutrition education that medical students receive continues to be inadequate." Adams KM, Kohlmeier M, Zeisel SH. Nutrition education in U.S. medical schools: latest update of a national survey. *Acad Med*. 2010 Sep;85(9):1537-42

[395] CONCLUSIONS: This survey suggests that multiple barriers exist that prevent the primary care practitioner from providing dietary counseling. A multifaceted approach will be needed to change physician counseling behavior." Kushner RF. Barriers to providing nutrition counseling by physicians: a survey of primary care practitioners. *Prev Med*. 1995 Nov;24(6):546-52

[396] Humphreys BK, Sulkowski A, McIntyre K, Kasiban M, Patrick AN. An examination of musculoskeletal cognitive competency in chiropractic interns. *J Manipulative Physiol Ther*. 2007;30(1):44-9

safer and less expensive than allopathic medical treatment, particularly for the treatment of low-back pain. In their extensive review of the literature, Manga et al[397] published in 1993 that chiropractic management of low-back pain is superior to allopathic medical management in terms of greater safety, greater effectiveness, and reduced cost; they concluded, "There is an overwhelming body of evidence indicating that chiropractic management of low-back pain is more cost-effective than medical management" and "There would be highly significant cost savings if more management of LBP [low-back pain] was transferred from medical physicians to chiropractors." In a randomized trial involving 741 patients, Meade et al[398] showed, "Chiropractic treatment was more effective than hospital outpatient management, mainly for patients with chronic or severe back pain... The benefit of chiropractic treatment became more evident throughout the follow up period. Secondary outcome measures also showed that chiropractic was more beneficial." A 3-year follow-up study by these same authors[399] in 1995 showed, "At three years the results confirm the findings of an earlier report that when chiropractic or hospital therapists treat patients with low-back pain as they would in day to day practice, those treated by chiropractic derive more benefit and long term satisfaction than those treated by hospitals." More recently, in 2004 Legorreta et al[400] reported that the availability of chiropractic care was associated with significant cost savings among 700,000 patients with chiropractic coverage compared to 1 million patients whose insurance coverage was limited to allopathic medical treatments. Simple extrapolation of the average savings per patient in this study ($208 annual savings associated with chiropractic coverage) to the US population (295 million citizens in 2005[401]) suggests that, if fully implemented in a nation-wide basis, America could save $61,360,000,000 (more than $61 billion per year) in annual healthcare expenses by ensuring chiropractic for all citizens in contrast to failing to provide such coverage; obviously extrapolations such as this should consider other variables, such as the relatively higher prevalence of injury and death among patients treated with drugs and surgery.[402,403] Furthermore, whether the cost savings associated with chiropractic availability are due to 1) improved overall health and reduced need for pharmacosurgical intervention, 2) greater safety and lower cost of chiropractic treatment versus pharmacosurgical treatment, and/or 3) self-selection by wellness-oriented, perhaps healthier, and higher-income patients, remains to be determined.

A literature review by Dabbs and Lauretti[404] showed that spinal manipulation is safer than the use of NSAIDs in the treatment of neck pain. Contrasting the rates of manipulation-associated cerebrovascular accidents to the dangers of medical and surgical treatments for spinal disorders, Rosner[405] noted, "These rates are 400 times lower than the death rates observed from gastrointestinal bleeding due to the use of nonsteroidal anti-inflammatory drugs and 700 times lower than the overall mortality rate for spinal surgery." Similarly, in his review of the literature comparing the safety of chiropractic manipulation in patients with low-back pain associated with lumbar disc herniation, Oliphant[406] showed that, "The apparent safety of spinal manipulation, especially when compared with other [medically] accepted treatments for [lumbar disk herniation], should stimulate its use in the conservative treatment plan of [lumbar disk herniation]."

The clinical benefits and cost-effectiveness of chiropractic management of musculoskeletal conditions is extensively documented, and that spinal manipulation generally shows superior safety to drug and surgical treatment of back and neck pain is also well established.[407,408,409,410,411,412,413] Adjunctive therapies such as post-

[397] Manga P, Angus D, Papadopoulos C, et al. The Effectiveness and Cost-Effectiveness of Chiropractic Management of Low-Back Pain. Richmond Hill, Ontario: Kenilworth Publishing; 1993
[398] Meade TW, Dyer S, Browne W, Townsend J, Frank AO. Low-back pain of mechanical origin: randomised comparison of chiropractic and hospital outpatient treatment. *BMJ*. 1990;300(6737):1431-7
[399] Meade TW, Dyer S, Browne W, Frank AO. Randomised comparison of chiropractic and hospital outpatient management for low-back pain: results from extended follow up. *BMJ*. 1995;311(7001):349-5
[400] Legorreta AP, Metz RD, Nelson CF, Ray S, Chernicoff HO, Dinubile NA. Comparative analysis of individuals with and without chiropractic coverage: patient characteristics, utilization, and costs. *Arch Intern Med*. 2004;164:1985-92
[401] US Census Bureau http://factfinder.census.gov/home/saff/main.html?_lang=en Accessed January 12, 2005
[402] Rosner AL. Evidence-based clinical guidelines for the management of acute low-back pain: response to the guidelines prepared for the Australian Medical Health and Research Council. *J Manipulative Physiol Ther*. 2001;24(3):214-20
[403] Topol EJ. Failing the public health--rofecoxib, Merck, and the FDA. *N Engl J Med*. 2004 Oct 21;351(17):1707-9
[404] Dabbs V, Lauretti WJ. A risk assessment of cervical manipulation vs. NSAIDs for the treatment of neck pain. *J Manipulative Physiol Ther*. 1995;18:530-6
[405] Rosner AL. Evidence-based clinical guidelines for the management of acute low-back pain: response to the guidelines prepared for the Australian Medical Health and Research Council. *J Manipulative Physiol Ther*. 2001;24(3):214-20
[406] Oliphant D. Safety of spinal manipulation in the treatment of lumbar disk herniations: a systematic review and risk assessment. *J Manipulative Physiol Ther*. 2004;27:197-210
[407] Dabbs V, Lauretti WJ. A risk assessment of cervical manipulation vs. NSAIDs for the treatment of neck pain. *J Manipulative Physiol Ther*. 1995;18:530-6
[408] Rosner AL. Evidence-based clinical guidelines for the management of acute low-back pain: response to the guidelines prepared for the Australian Medical Health and Research Council. *J Manipulative Physiol Ther*. 2001 Mar-Apr;24(3):214-20
[409] Oliphant D. Safety of spinal manipulation in the treatment of lumbar disk herniations: a systematic review and risk assessment. *J Manipulative Physiol Ther*. 2004;27:197-210
[410] Meade TW, Dyer S, Browne W, Townsend J, Frank AO. Low-back pain of mechanical origin: randomised comparison of chiropractic and hospital outpatient treatment. *BMJ*. 1990;300(6737):1431-7

isometric relaxation[414] and correction of myofascial dysfunction[415] can lead to tremendous and rapid reductions in musculoskeletal pain without the hazards and expense associated with pharmaceutical drugs. Nonmusculoskeletal benefits of musculoskeletal/spinal manipulation include improved pulmonary function and/or quality of life in patients with asthma[416,417,418,419] and—according to a series of cases published by an osteopathic ophthalmologist—improvement or restoration of vision in patients with post-traumatic and acute-onset visual loss.[420,421,422,423,424,425,426,427] More research is required to quantify the potential benefits of spinal manipulation in patients with wide-ranging conditions such as epilepsy[428,429], attention-deficit hyperactivity disorder[430,431], and Parkinson's disease.[432] Given that most pharmaceutical drugs work on single biochemical pathways, spinal manipulation is discordant with the medical/drug paradigm because its effects are numerous (rather than singular) and physical and physiological (rather than biochemical). Thus, when viewed through the allopathic/pharmaceutical lens, spinal manipulation (like acupuncture and other physical modalities) "does not make sense" and will be viewed as "unscientific" simply because it is based in physiology rather than pharmacology. In this case, the fault lies with the viewer and the lens, not with the object.

Research documenting the systemic and "nonmusculoskeletal" benefits of spinal manipulation mandates that our concept of "musculoskeletal" must be expanded to appreciate that **musculoskeletal interventions benefit nonmusculoskeletal body systems and physiologic processes**. This conceptual expansion applies also to soft tissue therapeutics such as massage, which can reduce adolescent aggression[433], improve outcome in preterm infants[434], alleviate premenstrual syndrome[435], and increase serotonin and dopamine levels in patients with low-back pain.[436]

[411] Meade TW, Dyer S, Browne W, Frank AO. Randomised comparison of chiropractic and hospital outpatient management for low-back pain: results from extended follow up. *BMJ*. 1995;311(7001):349-5

[412] Manga P, Angus D, Papadopoulos C, et al. The Effectiveness and Cost-Effectiveness of Chiropractic Management of Low-Back Pain. Richmond Hill, Ontario: Kenilworth Publishing; 1993

[413] Legorreta AP, Metz RD, Nelson CF, Ray S, Chernicoff HO, Dinubile NA. Comparative analysis of individuals with and without chiropractic coverage: patient characteristics, utilization, and costs. *Arch Intern Med*. 2004;164:1985-92

[414] Lewit K, Simons DG. Myofascial pain: relief by post-isometric relaxation. *Arch Phys Med Rehabil*. 1984;65(8):452-6

[415] Ingber RS. Iliopsoas myofascial dysfunction: a treatable cause of "failed" low-back syndrome. *Arch Phys Med Rehabil*. 1989 May;70(5):382-6

[416] Nielson NH, Bronfort G, Bendix T, Madsen F, Wecke B. Chronic asthma and chiropractic spinal manipulation: a randomized clinical trial. *Clin Exp Allergy* 1995;25:80-8

[417] Mein EA, Greenman PE, McMillin DL, Richards DG, Nelson CD. Manual medicine diversity: research pitfalls and the emerging medical paradigm. *J Am Osteopath Assoc*. 2001 Aug;101(8):441-4

[418] "There were small increases (7 to 12 liters per minute) in peak expiratory flow in the morning and the evening in both treatment groups,... Symptoms of asthma and use of beta-agonists decreased and the quality of life increased in both groups, with no significant differences between the groups." Balon J, Aker PD, Crowther ER, Danielson C, Cox PG, O'Shaughnessy D, Walker C, Goldsmith CH, Duku E, Sears MR. A comparison of active and simulated chiropractic manipulation as adjunctive treatment for childhood asthma. *N Engl J Med*. 1998 Oct 8;339(15):1013-20

[419] Bronfort G, Evans RL, Kubic P, Filkin P. Chronic pediatric asthma and chiropractic spinal manipulation: a prospective clinical series and randomized clinical pilot study. *J Manipulative Physiol Ther*. 2001 Jul-Aug;24(6):369-77

[420] Stephens D, Pollard H, Bilton D, Thomson P, Gorman F. Bilateral simultaneous optic nerve dysfunction after periorbital trauma: recovery of vision in association with chiropractic spinal manipulation therapy. *J Manipulative Physiol Ther*. 1999 Nov-Dec;22(9):615-21

[421] Stephens D, Gorman F, Bilton D. The step phenomenon in the recovery of vision with spinal manipulation: a report on two 13-yr-olds treated together. *J Manipulative Physiol Ther*. 1997;20(9):628-33

[422] Stephens D, Gorman R. The association between visual incompetence and spinal derangement: an instructive case history. *J Manipulative Physiol Ther*. 1997 Jun;20(5):343-50.

[423] Stephens D, Gorman RF. Does 'normal' vision improve with spinal manipulation? *J Manipulative Physiol Ther*. 1996 Jul-Aug;19(5):415-8

[424] Gorman RF. Monocular scotomata and spinal manipulation: the step phenomenon. *J Manipulative Physiol Ther*. 1996 Jun;19(5):344-9

[425] Gorman RF. Monocular visual loss after closed head trauma: immediate resolution associated with spinal manipulation. *J Manipulative Physiol Ther*. 1995 Jun;18(5):308-14

[426] Gorman RF. The treatment of presumptive optic nerve ischemia by spinal manipulation. *J Manipulative Physiol Ther*. 1995;18(3):172-7

[427] Gorman RF. Automated static perimetry in chiropractic. *J Manipulative Physiol Ther*. 1993 Sep;16(7):481-7

[428] Elster EL. Treatment of bipolar, seizure, and sleep disorders and migraine headaches utilizing a chiropractic technique. *J Manipulative Physiol Ther*. 2004 Mar-Apr;27(3):E5

[429] Alcantara J, Heschong R, Plaugher G, Alcantara J. Chiropractic management of a patient with subluxations, low-back pain and epileptic seizures. *J Manipulative Physiol Ther*. 1998;21(6):410-8

[430] Giesen JM, Center DB, Leach RA. An evaluation of chiropractic manipulation as a treatment of hyperactivity in children. *J Manipulative Physiol Ther*. 1989 Oct;12(5):353-63

[431] Bastecki AV, Harrison DE, Haas JW. Cervical kyphosis is a possible link to attention-deficit/hyperactivity disorder. *J Manipulative Physiol Ther*. 2004 Oct;27(8):e14

[432] Elster EL. Upper cervical chiropractic management of a patient with Parkinson's disease: a case report. *J Manipulative Physiol Ther*. 2000 Oct;23(8):573-7

[433] Diego MA, Field T, Hernandez-Reif M, Shaw JA, Rothe EM, Castellanos D, Mesner L. Aggressive adolescents benefit from massage therapy. *Adolescence* 2002 Fall;37(147):597-607

[434] Mainous RO. Infant massage as a component of developmental care: past, present, and future. *Holist Nurs Pract* 2002 Oct;16(5):1-7

[435] **Hernandez-Reif M, Martinez A, Field T, Quintero O, Hart S, Burman I. Premenstrual symptoms are relieved by massage therapy.** *J Psychosom Obstet Gynaecol* 2000 Mar;21(1):9-15

[436] "RESULTS: By the end of the study, the massage therapy group, as compared to the relaxation group, reported experiencing less pain, depression, anxiety and improved sleep. They also showed improved trunk and pain flexion performance, and their serotonin and dopamine levels were higher." Hernandez-Reif M, Field T, Krasnegor J, Theakston H. Lower back pain is reduced and range of motion increased after massage therapy. *Int J Neurosci* 2001;106(3-4):131-45

Spinal Manipulation: Mechanistic Considerations: Applied to either the spine or peripheral joints, high-velocity low-amplitude (HVLA) joint manipulation appears to have numerous physical and physiological effects, including but not limited to the following:

1. Releasing entrapped intraarticular menisci and synovial folds,
2. Acutely reducing intradiscal pressure, thus promoting replacement of decentralized disc material,
3. Stretching of deep periarticular muscles to break the cycle of chronic autonomous muscle contraction by lengthening the muscles and thereby releasing excessive actin-myosin binding,
4. Promoting restoration of proper kinesthesia and proprioception,
5. Promoting relaxation of paraspinal muscles by stretching facet joint capsules,
6. Promoting relaxation of paraspinal muscles via "postactivation depression", which is the temporary depletion of contractile neurotransmitters,
7. Temporarily elevating plasma beta-endorphin,
8. Temporarily enhancing phagocytic ability of neutrophils and monocytes,
9. Activation of the diffuse descending pain inhibitory system located in the periaqueductal gray matter—this is an important aspect of nociceptive inhibition by intense sensory/mechanoreceptor stimulation, which will be discussed in a following section for its relevance to neurogenic inflammation, and
10. Improving neurotransmitter balance and reducing pain (soft-tissue manipulation).[437]

While the above list of mechanisms-of-action is certainly not complete, for purposes of this paper it is sufficient for the establishment that—indeed—joint manipulation in general and spinal manipulation in particular have objective mechanistic effects that correlate with their clinical benefits. Additional details are provided in numerous published reviews and primary research[438,439,440,441,442,443,444] and by Leach[445], whose extensive description of the mechanisms of action of spinal manipulative therapy is unsurpassed. Given such a wide base of experimental and clinical support published in peer-reviewed journals and widely-available textbooks, denigrations directed toward spinal manipulation on the grounds that it is "unscientific" or "unsupported by research" are unfounded and are indicative of selective ignorance.

Mechanoreceptor-Mediated Inhibition of Neurogenic Inflammation: A Possible Mechanism of Action of Spinal Manipulation: Neurogenic inflammation causes catabolism of articular structures and thus promotes joint destruction[446,447], a phenomena that the current author has termed "neurogenic chondrolysis."[448] The biologic and scientific basis for this concept rests on the following sequence of events which ultimately form a self-perpetuating and multisystem cycle:

1. Using joint pain as an example, we know that acute or chronic joint injury results in the release of inflammatory mediators in local tissues as **immunogenic inflammation**.

[437] "RESULTS: By the end of the study, the massage therapy group, as compared to the relaxation group, reported experiencing less pain, depression, anxiety and improved sleep. They also showed improved trunk and pain flexion performance, and their serotonin and dopamine levels were higher." Hernandez-Reif M, Field T, Krasnegor J, Theakston H. Lower back pain is reduced and range of motion increased after massage therapy. *Int J Neurosci* 2001;106(3-4):131-45

[438] Maigne JY, Vautravers P. Mechanism of action of spinal manipulative therapy. *Joint Bone Spine*. 2003;70(5):336-41

[439] Brennan PC, Triano JJ, McGregor M, Kokjohn K, Hondras MA, Brennan DC. Enhanced neutrophil respiratory burst as a biological marker for manipulation forces: duration of the effect and association with substance P and tumor necrosis factor. *J Manipulative Physiol Ther*. 1992 Feb;15(2):83-9

[440] Brennan PC, Kokjohn K, Kaltinger CJ, Lohr GE, Glendening C, Hondras MA, McGregor M, Triano JJ. Enhanced phagocytic cell respiratory burst induced by spinal manipulation: potential role of substance P. *J Manipulative Physiol Ther*. 1991 Sep;14(7):399-408

[441] Heikkila H, Johansson M, Wenngren BI. Effects of acupuncture, cervical manipulation and NSAID therapy on dizziness and impaired head repositioning of suspected cervical origin: a pilot study. *Man Ther*. 2000 Aug;5(3):151-7

[442] Rogers RG. The effects of spinal manipulation on cervical kinesthesia in patients with chronic neck pain: a pilot study. *J Manipulative Physiol Ther*. 1997;20(2):80-5

[443] Bergman, Peterson, Lawrence. Chiropractic Technique. New York: Churchill Livingstone 1993. An updated edition is now availabe from Mosby.

[444] Herzog WH. Mechanical and physiological responses to spinal manipulative treatments. *JNMS: J Neuromusculoskeltal System* 1995; 3: 1-9

[445] Leach RA. (ed). The Chiropractic Theories: A Textbook of Scientific Research. Fourth Edition. Baltimore: Lippincott, Williams & Wilkins, 2004

[446] Gouze-Decaris E, Philippe L, Minn A, Haouzi P, Gillet P, Netter P, Terlain B. Neurophysiological basis for neurogenic-mediated articular cartilage anabolism alteration. *Am J Physiol Regul Integr Comp Physiol*. 2001;280(1):R115-22

[447] Decaris E, Guingamp C, Chat M, Philippe L, Grillasca JP, Abid A, Minn A, Gillet P, Netter P, Terlain B. Evidence for neurogenic transmission inducing degenerative cartilage damage distant from local inflammation. *Arthritis Rheum*. 1999;42(9):1951-60

[448] Vasquez A. *Integrative Orthopedics: Exploring the Structural Aspect of the Matrix*. Applying Functional Medicine in Clinical Practice. Tampa, Florida November 29-December 4, 2004. Hosted by the Institute for Functional Medicine: www.FunctionalMedicine.org

2. Nociceptive input is received centrally and results in release of inflammatory mediators *from sensory neurons* termed **neurogenic inflammation**[449] and results in a neurologically-mediated catabolic effect in articular cartilage[450,451] termed here as **neurogenic chondrolysis**.

3. As immunogenic and neurogenic inflammation synergize to promote joint destruction, pain from degenerating joints further increases nociceptive afferent transmission to further increase neurogenic and thus immunogenic inflammation. Thus, a *positive feedback* vicious cycle of immunogenic and neurogenic inflammation promotes and perpetuates joint destruction.

4. Further complicating this *regional* cycle of neurogenic-immunogenic inflammation and tissue destruction would be any pain or inflammation *in distant parts of the body*, since pain in one part of the body can exacerbate neurogenic inflammation in another part of the body via **neurogenic switching**[452,453] and immunologic reactivity such as allergy or autoimmunity in one part of the body may be transmitted *via the nervous system* to cause immunogenic inflammation in another part of the body via **immunogenic switching.**[454]

The clinical relevance of neurogenic inflammation and immunogenic switching is that when combined they provide a means *beyond biochemistry* by which to understand how and why inflammation ❶ is *transmitted and perpetuated by the nervous system* and ❷ must be treated with a body-wide *holistic* approach.

The current author is the first to propose the concept of **mechanoreceptor-mediated inhibition of neurogenic inflammation.**[455] Since neurogenic chondrolysis is inhibited by interference with C-fiber (type IV) mediated afferent transmission[456] and since chiropractic high-velocity low-amplitude (HVLA) manipulation appears to inhibit C-fiber mediated nociception[457,458], then chiropractic-type HVLA manipulation may reduce neurogenic inflammation and may promote articular integrity by inhibiting neurogenic chondrolysis. Further, mechanoreceptor-mediated inhibition of neurogenic inflammation would, for example, help explain the benefits of spinal manipulation in the treatment of asthma[459,460,461], since asthma is known to be mediated in large part by neurogenic inflammation.[462,463] Thus, spinal manipulation appears to provide a means—*in addition to the use of other anti-inflammatory interventions such as diet, lifestyle and phytonutritional interventions*—by which pain and inflammation can be treated naturally, without drugs and surgery.

A science-based comprehensive protocol can be implemented against pain and inflammation by using ❶ an anti-inflammatory diet, ❷ frequent exercise, ❸ lifestyle and bodyweight optimization, ❹ nutritional supplementation, ❺ botanical supplementation[464,465], ❻ spinal manipulation (with its kinesthetic, analgesic,

[449] Meggs WJ. Mechanisms of allergy and chemical sensitivity. *Toxicol Ind Health.* 1999 Apr-Jun;15(3-4):331-8

[450] Gouze-Decaris E, Philippe L, Minn A, Haouzi P, Gillet P, Netter P, Terlain B. Neurophysiological basis for neurogenic-mediated articular cartilage anabolism alteration. *Am J Physiol Regul Integr Comp Physiol.* 2001;280(1):R115-22

[451] Decaris E, Guingamp C, Chat M, Philippe L, Grillasca JP, Abid A, Minn A, Gillet P, Netter P, Terlain B. Evidence for neurogenic transmission inducing degenerative cartilage damage distant from local inflammation. *Arthritis Rheum.* 1999;42(9):1951-60

[452] Meggs WJ. Neurogenic Switching: A Hypothesis for a Mechanism for Shifting the Site of Inflammation in Allergy and Chemical Sensitivity. *Environ Health Perspect* 1995; 103:54-56

[453] Meggs WJ. Mechanisms of allergy and chemical sensitivity. *Toxicol Ind Health.* 1999 Apr-Jun;15(3-4):331-8

[454] "...—immunogenic switching—... In this scenario, the afferent stimulation from the cranial vasculature, which is inflamed during a migraine because of neurogenic processes, is rerouted by the CNS to produce immunogenic inflammation at the nose and sinuses." Cady RK, Schreiber CP. Sinus headache or migraine? Considerations in making a differential diagnosis. *Neurology.* 2002;58(9 Suppl 6):S10-4

[455] Vasquez A. *Integrative Orthopedics: Exploring the Structural Aspect of the Matrix.* Applying Functional Medicine in Clinical Practice. Tampa, Florida November 29-December 4, 2004. Hosted by the Institute for Functional Medicine: www.FunctionalMedicine.org

[456] Gouze-Decaris E, Philippe L, Minn A, Haouzi P, Gillet P, Netter P, Terlain B. Neurophysiological basis for neurogenic-mediated articular cartilage anabolism alteration. *Am J Physiol Regul Integr Comp Physiol.* 2001;280(1):R115-22

[457] Gillette R. A speculative argument for the coactivation of diverse somatic receptor populations by forceful chiropractic adjustments. *Man Med* 1987; 3:1-14

[458] Boal RW, Gillette RG. Central neuronal plasticity, low-back pain and spinal manipulative therapy. *J Manipulative Physiol Ther.* 2004;27(5):314-26

[459] Nielson NH, Bronfort G, Bendix T, Madsen F, Wecke B. Chronic asthma and chiropractic spinal manipulation: a randomized clinical trial. *Clin Exp Allergy* 1995;25:80-8

[460] "There were small increases (7 to 12 liters per minute) in peak expiratory flow in the morning and the evening in both treatment groups,... Symptoms of asthma and use of beta-agonists decreased and the quality of life increased in both groups, with no significant differences between the groups." Balon J, Aker PD, Crowther ER, Danielson C, Cox PG, O'Shaughnessy D, Walker C, Goldsmith CH, Duku E, Sears MR. A comparison of active and simulated chiropractic manipulation as adjunctive treatment for childhood asthma. *N Engl J Med.* 1998 Oct 8;339(15):1013-20

[461] Bronfort G, Evans RL, Kubic P, Filkin P. Chronic pediatric asthma and chiropractic spinal manipulation: a prospective clinical series and randomized clinical pilot study. *J Manipulative Physiol Ther.* 2001 Jul-Aug;24(6):369-77

[462] Renz H. Neurotrophins in bronchial asthma. *Respir Res.* 2001;2(5):265-8

[463] Groneberg DA, Quarcoo D, Frossard N, Fischer A. Neurogenic mechanisms in bronchial inflammatory diseases. *Allergy.* 2004 Nov; 59(11): 1139-52

[464] Jancso N, Jancso-Gabor A, Szolcsanyi J. Direct evidence for neurogenic inflammation and its prevention by denervation and by pretreatment with capsaicin. *Br J Pharmacol.* 1967 Sep;31(1):138-51

[465] Miller MJ, Vergnolle N, McKnight W, Musah RA, Davison CA, Trentacosti AM, Thompson JH, Sandoval M, Wallace JL. Inhibition of neurogenic inflammation by the Amazonian herbal medicine sangre de grado. *J Invest Dermatol.* 2001;117(3):725-30

directly and *indirectly* anti-inflammatory, and *probably* piezoelectric benefits[466]), ❼ stress reduction[467,468], ❽ anti-dysbiosis protocols[469], ❾ hormonal correction ("orthoendocrinology"), and ❿ ancillary treatments such as acupuncture.[470,471] Additional details and citations for these interventions are provided in chapter 3 of *Integrative Orthopedics*[472] and chapter 4 of *Integrative Rheumatology*.[473] Pain and inflammation are self-perpetuating vicious cycles, well suited to intervention with comprehensive and multicomponent treatment plans as profiled above.

Wilk vs American Medical Association

The following two pages provide the transcript of the judgement in 1987 that supposedly ended the American Medical Association's antitrust violations and attempt to destroy the chiropractic profession.

---

[466] Lipinski B. Biological significance of piezoelectricity in relation to acupuncture, Hatha Yoga, osteopathic medicine and action of air ions. *Med Hypotheses*. 1977;3(1):9-12 See also: Athenstaedt H. Pyroelectric and piezoelectric properties of vertebrates. *Ann N Y Acad Sci*. 1974;238:68-94 See also: Athenstaedt H. "Functional polarity" of the spinal cord caused by its longitudinal electric dipole moment. *Am J Physiol*. 1984;247(3 Pt 2):R482-7

[467] Lutgendorf S, Logan H, Kirchner HL, Rothrock N, Svengalis S, Iverson K, Lubaroff D. Effects of relaxation and stress on the capsaicin-induced local inflammatory response. *Psychosom Med*. 2000;62:524-34

[468] "Couples who demonstrated consistently higher levels of hostile behaviors across both their interactions healed at 60% of the rate of low-hostile couples. High-hostile couples also produced relatively larger increases in plasma IL-6 and tumor necrosis factor alpha..." Kiecolt-Glaser JK, Loving TJ, Stowell JR, Malarkey WB, Lemeshow S, Dickinson SL, Glaser R. Hostile marital interactions, proinflammatory cytokine production, and wound healing. *Arch Gen Psychiatry*. 2005 Dec;62(12):1377-84

[469] Chapter 4 of Integrative Rheumatology and Vasquez A. Reducing Pain and Inflammation Naturally. Part 6: Nutritional and Botanical Treatments Against "Silent Infections" and Gastrointestinal Dysbiosis, Commonly Overlooked Causes of Neuromusculoskeletal Inflammation and Chronic Health Problems. *Nutr Perspect* 2006; Jan http://optimalhealthresearch.com/part6

[470] Joos S, Brinkhaus B, Maluche C, Maupai N, Kohnen R, Kraehmer N, Hahn EG, Schuppan D. Acupuncture and moxibustion in the treatment of active Crohn's disease: a randomized controlled study. *Digestion*. 2004;69(3):131-9

[471] "These results demonstrate an unorthodox new type of neurohumoral regulatory mechanism of sensory fibres and provide a possible mode of action for the anti-inflammatory effect of counter-irritation and acupuncture." Pinter E, Szolcsanyi J. Systemic anti-inflammatory effect induced by antidromic stimulation of the dorsal roots in the rat. *Neurosci Lett*. 1996;212(1):33-6

[472] Vasquez A. *Integrative Orthopedics: Second Edition*. Fort Worth, Texas; Integrative and Biological Medicine Research and Consulting, 2007 OptimalHealthResearch.com

[473] Vasquez A. *Integrative Rheumatology: Second Edition*. Fort Worth, Texas; Integrative and Biological Medicine Research and Consulting, 2007 OptimalHealthResearch.com

Special Communication

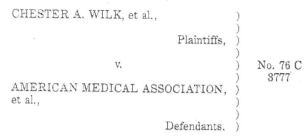

IN THE UNITED STATES DISTRICT COURT
FOR THE NORTHERN DISTRICT OF ILLINOIS
EASTERN DIVISION

CHESTER A. WILK, et al.,)
)
               Plaintiffs,)
)
       v.   ) No. 76 C
) 3777
AMERICAN MEDICAL ASSOCIATION,)
et al.,)
)
               Defendants.)

PERMANENT INJUNCTION ORDER AGAINST AMA

Susan Getzendanner, District Judge

The court conducted a lengthy trial of this case in May and June of 1987 and on August 27, 1987, issued a 101 page opinion finding that the American Medical Association ("AMA") and its members participated in a conspiracy against chiropractors in violation of the nation's antitrust laws. Thereafter an opinion dated September 25, 1987 was substituted for the August 27, 1987 opinion. The question now before the court is the form of injunctive relief that the court will order.

See also p 83.

As part of the injunctive relief to be ordered by the court against the AMA, the AMA shall be required to send a copy of this Permanent Injunction Order to each of its current members. The members of the AMA are bound by the terms of the Permanent Injunction Order if they act in concert with the AMA to violate the terms of the order. Accordingly, it is important that the AMA members understand the order and the reasons why the order has been entered.

The AMA's Boycott and Conspiracy

In the early 1960s, the AMA decided to contain and eliminate chiropractic as a profession. In 1963 the AMA's Committee on Quackery was formed. The committee worked aggressively—both overtly and covertly—to eliminate chiropractic. One of the principal means used by the AMA to achieve its goal was to make it unethical for medical physicians to professionally associate with chiropractors. Under Principle 3 of the AMA's Principles of Medical Ethics, it was unethical for a physician to associate with an "unscientific practitioner," and in 1966 the AMA's House of Delegates passed a resolution calling chiropractic an unscientific cult. To complete the circle, in 1967 the AMA's Judicial Council issued an opinion under Principle 3 holding that it was unethical for a physician to associate professionally with chiropractors.

The AMA's purpose was to prevent medical physicians from referring patients to chiropractors and accepting referrals of patients from chiropractors, to prevent chiropractors from obtaining access to hospital diagnostic services and membership on hospital medical staffs, to prevent medical physicians from teaching at chiropractic colleges or engaging in any joint research, and to prevent any cooperation between the two groups in the delivery of health care services.

Published by order of Susan Getzendanner, US District Judge, Sept 25, 1987.

The AMA believed that the boycott worked—that chiropractic would have achieved greater gains in the absence of the boycott. Since no medical physician would want to be considered unethical by his peers, the success of the boycott is not surprising. However, chiropractic achieved licensing in all 50 states during the existence of the Committee on Quackery.

The Committee on Quackery was disbanded in 1975 and some of the committee's activities became publicly known. . Several lawsuits were filed by or on behalf of chiropractors and this case was filed in 1976.

Change in AMA's Position on Chiropractic

In 1977, the AMA began to change its position on chiropractic. The AMA's Judicial Council adopted new opinions under which medical physicians could refer patients to chiropractors, but there was still the proviso that the medical physician should be confident that the services to be provided on referral would be performed in accordance with accepted scientific standards. In 1979, the AMA's House of Delegates adopted Report UU which said that not everything that a chiropractor may do is without therapeutic value, but it stopped short of saying that such things were based on scientific standards. It was not until 1980 that the AMA revised its Principles of Medical Ethics to eliminate Principle 3. Until Principle 3 was formally eliminated, there was considerable ambiguity about the AMA's position. The ethics code adopted in 1980 provided that a medical physician "shall be free to choose whom to serve, with whom to associate, and the environment in which to provide medical services."

The AMA settled three chiropractic lawsuits by stipulating and agreeing that under the current opinions of the Judicial Council a physician may, without fear of discipline or sanction by the AMA, refer a patient to a duly licensed chiropractor when he believes that referral may benefit the patient. The AMA confirmed that a physician may also choose to accept or to decline patients sent to him by a duly licensed chiropractor. Finally, the AMA confirmed that a physician may teach at a chiropractic college or seminar. These settlements were entered into in 1978, 1980, and 1986.

The AMA's present position on chiropractic, as stated to the court, is that it is ethical for a medical physician to professionally associate with chiropractors provided the physician believes that such association is in the best interests of his patient. This position has not previously been communicated by the AMA to its members.

Antitrust Laws

Under the Sherman Act, every combination or conspiracy in restraint of trade is illegal. The court has held that the conduct of the AMA and its members constituted a conspiracy in restraint of trade based on the following facts: the purpose of the boycott was to eliminate chiropractic; chiropractors are in competition with some medical physicians; the boycott had substantial anti-competitive effects; there were no pro-competitive effects of the boycott; and the plaintiffs were injured as a result of the conduct. These facts add up to a violation of the Sherman Act.

In this case, however, the court allowed the defendants the opportunity to establish a "patient care defense" which has the following elements:

(1) that they genuinely entertained a concern for what they perceive as scientific method in the care of each person with whom they have entered into a doctor-patient relationship; (2) that this concern is objectively reasonable; (3) that this concern has been the dominant motivating factor in defendants' promulgation of Principle 3 and in the

conduct intended to implement it; and (4) that this concern for scientific method in patient care could not have been adequately satisfied in a manner less restrictive of competition.

The court concluded that the AMA had a genuine concern for scientific methods in patient care, and that this concern was the dominant factor in motivating the AMA's conduct. However, the AMA failed to establish that throughout the entire period of the boycott, from 1966 to 1980, this concern was objectively reasonable. The court reached that conclusion on the basis of extensive testimony from both witnesses for the plaintiffs and the AMA that some forms of chiropractic treatment are effective and the fact that the AMA recognized that chiropractic began to change in the early 1970s. Since the boycott was not formally over until Principle 3 was eliminated in 1980, the court found that the AMA was unable to establish that during the entire period of the conspiracy its position was objectively reasonable. Finally, the court ruled that the AMA's concern for scientific method in patient care could have been adequately satisfied in a manner less restrictive of competition and that a nationwide conspiracy to eliminate a licensed profession was not justified by the concern for scientific method. On the basis of these findings, the court concluded that the AMA had failed to establish the patient care defense.

None of the court's findings constituted a judicial endorsement of chiropractic. All of the parties to the case, including the plaintiffs and the AMA, agreed that chiropractic treatment of diseases such as diabetes, high blood pressure, cancer, heart disease and infectious disease is not proper, and that the historic theory of chiropractic, that there is a single cause and cure of disease is wrong. There was disagreement between the parties as to whether chiropractors should engage in diagnosis. There was evidence that the chiropractic theory of subluxations was unscientific, and evidence that some chiropractors engaged in unscientific practices. The court did not reach the question of whether chiropractic theory was in fact scientific. However, the evidence in the case was that some forms of chiropractic manipulation of the spine and joints was therapeutic. AMA witnesses, including the present Chairman of the Board of Trustees of the AMA, testified that some forms of treatment by chiropractors, including manipulation, can be therapeutic in the treatment of conditions such as back pain syndrome.

Need for Injunctive Relief

Although the conspiracy ended in 1980, there are lingering effects of the illegal boycott and conspiracy which require an injunction. Some medical physicians' individual decisions on whether or not to professionally associate with chiropractors are still affected by the boycott. The injury to chiropractors' reputations which resulted from the boycott has not been repaired. Chiropractors suffer current economic injury as a result of the boycott. The AMA has never affirmatively acknowledged that there are and should be no collective impediments to professional association and cooperation between chiropractors and medical physicians, except as provided by law. Instead, the AMA has consistently argued that its conduct has not violated the antitrust laws.

Most importantly, the court believes that it is important that the AMA members be made aware of the present AMA position that it is ethical for a medical physician to professionally associate with a chiropractor if the physician believes it is in the best interests of his patient, so that the lingering effects of the illegal group boycott against chiropractors finally can be dissipated.

Under the law, every medical physician, institution, and hospital has the right to make an individual decision as to whether or not that physician, institution, or hospital shall associate professionally with chiropractors. Individual choice by a medical physician voluntarily to associate professionally with chiropractors should be governed only by restrictions under state law, if any, and by the individual medical physician's personal judgment as to what is in the best interest of a patient or patients. Professional association includes referrals, consultations, group practice in partnerships, Health Maintenance Organizations, Preferred Provider Organizations, and other alternative health care delivery systems; the provision of treatment privileges and diagnostic services (including radiological and other laboratory facilities) in or through hospital facilities; association and cooperation in educational programs for students in chiropractic colleges; and cooperation in research, health care seminars, and continuing education programs.

An injunction is necessary to assure that the AMA does not interfere with the right of a physician, hospital, or other institution to make an individual decision on the question of professional association.

Form of Injunction

1. The AMA, its officers, agents and employees, and all persons who act in active concert with any of them and who receive actual notice of this order are hereby permanently enjoined from restricting, regulating or impeding, or aiding and abetting others from restricting, regulating or impeding, the freedom of any AMA member or any institution or hospital to make an individual decision as to whether or not that AMA member, institution, or hospital shall professionally associate with chiropractors, chiropractic students, or chiropractic institutions.

2. This Permanent Injunction does not and shall not be construed to restrict or otherwise interfere with the AMA's right to take positions on any issue, including chiropractic, and to express or publicize those positions, either alone or in conjunction with others. Nor does this Permanent Injunction restrict or otherwise interfere with the AMA's right to petition or testify before any public body on any legislative or regulatory measure or to join or cooperate with any other entity in so petitioning or testifying. The AMA's membership in a recognized accrediting association or society shall not constitute a violation of this Permanent Injunction.

3. The AMA is directed to send a copy of this order to each AMA member and employee, first class mail, postage prepaid, within thirty days of the entry of this order. In the alternative, the AMA shall provide the Clerk of the Court with mailing labels so that the court may send this order to AMA members and employees.

4. The AMA shall cause the publication of this order in JAMA and the indexing of the order under "Chiropractic" so that persons desiring to find the order in the future will be able to do so.

5. The AMA shall prepare a statement of the AMA's present position on chiropractic for inclusion in the current reports and opinions of the Judicial Council with an appropriate heading that refers to professional association between medical physicians and chiropractors, and indexed in the same manner that other reports and opinions are indexed. The court imposes no restrictions on the AMA's statement but only requires that it be consistent with the AMA's statements of its present position to the court.

6. The AMA shall file a report with the court evidencing compliance with this order on or before January 10, 1988.

It is so ordered.

Susan Getzendanner
United States District Judge

Naturopathic Medicine

"The work of the naturopathic physician is to elicit healing by helping patients to create or recreate conditions for health to exist within them. Health will occur where the conditions for health exist. Disease is the product of conditions which allow for it." *Jared Zeff, ND*[474]

The diagram on this page is derived from the review by Zeff published in 1997 in *Journal of Naturopathic Medicine* entitled "The process of healing: a unifying theory of naturopathic medicine." By my interpretation, the diagram is important for at least three reasons.

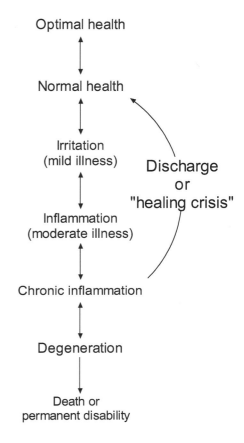

First, whereas the allopathic profession describes the genesis of most diseases as *idiopathic* and therefore [somehow] exclusively serviceable by drugs and surgery, the naturopathic profession describes disease processes as *multifactorial* and *logical* and therefore treatable by the skilled discovery and treatment of the underlying causes. Such underlying causes, which nearly always occur as a plurality, may vary mildly or significantly even within a group of patients with the same diagnosis.

Second, the diagram shows that the development of disease and the restoration of health are both *processes*. The restoration and retention of health requires *intentionality* and *tenacity* in lieu of the simplistic *miracle medicines* and *passive treatments* proffered by the pharmaceutical industry. Generally, disease does not arrive from outside; it is the result of one or more internal imbalances. Chronic illness is generally the result of manifold internal imbalances that culminate in numerous physiologic insults which compromise essential functions to the point that one or more organ systems begin to fail; we as patients and doctors generally label this as some specific "disease" or other, and the general—often erroneous—assumption has been that each *specific disease* (i.e., label, ...abstraction, ...conceptual entity) requires a *specific treatment* rather than a generalized health-restorative approach. Health is restored through a progressive and stepwise program that addresses as many facets of the illness as possible while vigorously supporting optimal physiologic function.

Third, the fact that Zeff considered the discharge or "healing crisis" so important that it merited inclusion in this diagram shows, indirectly, the naturopathic emphasis on detoxification and the eradication of dysbiosis. Both in the treatment of toxic metal/chemical exposure and in the treatment of chronic infections, patients often go through an acute or subacute phase of feeling ill before experiencing a dramatic alleviation of symptoms; the fact that symptoms may temporarily "get worse before getting better" has been referred to as the "healing crisis." This can occur for at least three reasons. First, in the elimination of chemicals and metals from the body, they must first be released from the tissues; the transition from tissues to blood is similar to a subacute re-exposure which triggers symptoms of toxicity until the toxin is excreted via sweat, urine, bile, or breath. Similarly, improvement in nutritional status—a cornerstone of all naturopathic interventions—expedites/facilitates/restores physiologic processes that have been relatively dormant due to lack of enzymatic cofactors such as vitamins and minerals[475]; optimization of nutritional status provides an opportunity for these pathways (such as detoxification of stored xenobiotics) to function again at which time they must "catch up" on work that has not been performed during the time of nutritional deficiency. The activation of these pathways is an essential step toward health restoration but results in an initial upregulation of hepatic phase-1/oxidative biotransformation which often results in the formation of reactive intermediates that temporarily impair physiologic processes and cause an

---

[474] Zeff JL. The process of healing: a unifying theory of naturopathic medicine. *Journal of Naturopathic Medicine* 1997; 7: 122-5
[475] Ames BN. The metabolic tune-up: metabolic harmony and disease prevention. *J Nutr.* 2003 May;133(5 Suppl 1):1544S-8S

initial exacerbation of symptoms. Third, whether through immunorestoration or the use of botanical/pharmacologic antimicrobial agents, the symptom-exacerbating "die off" reaction—classically called the Jarisch-Herxheimer reaction in the context of treating syphilis—is a result of increased (endo)toxin production/release by bacteria/microbes in response effective antimicrobial processes, whether physiologic or pharmacologic.

Modern naturopathic medicine has grown from deeply rooted European healing traditions reaching back several centuries. Naturopathic physicians have unwaveringly demonstrated respect, love, and appreciation for the healing powers of nature and the process of life itself.[476] Following their coursework in the basic biomedical sciences, naturopathic physicians are trained in urology, oncology, neurology, pediatrics, obstetrics and gynecology, urology, manual physical manipulation (including spinal manipulation), minor surgery, medical procedures, professional ethics, therapeutic diets, clinical and interventional nutrition, botanical medicines, psychological counseling, environmental medicine, and other modalities. Licensed naturopathic physicians commonly practice as generalists and family doctors.[477,478,479,480]

Naturopathic Principles, Concepts, & the _Vis Medicatrix Naturae_

"The healing power of nature is the inherent self-organizing and healing process of living systems… It is the naturopathic physician's role to support, facilitate and augment this process by identifying and removing obstacles to health and recovery, and by supporting the creation of a healthy internal and external environment."[481]

1. **First, Do No Harm _(Primum Non Nocere)_:** Naturopathic physicians use good judgment and compassion to ensure that the treatment does not cause harm to the patient. This contrasts with the effects of allopathic treatment, which collectively kill more than 180,000-220,000 patients per year, at least 493 American patients per day.[482]
2. **Identify and Treat the Causes _(Tolle Causam)_:** _"Illness does not occur without cause."_ Naturopathic physicians focus on identifying and addressing the underlying deficiency, toxicity, impairment, or imbalance that is the cause of the health problem or disease.
3. **Treat the Whole Person:** _"The multifactorial nature of health and disease requires a personalized and comprehensive approach to diagnosis and treatment."_ On some occasions the illness does take precedence over the person who has it—such in emergency situations like septic arthritis, acute ischemia, and pulmonary edema. In these cases, the situation must be managed appropriately, and these situations are not immediately amenable to long-term lifestyle changes—they require immediate treatment. However, the vast majority of cases in routine outpatient clinical practice will require detailed and bipartite attention to the facets of both **the disease process** and **the person who has the illness**. Our focus as naturopathic physicians on the individual patient is what sets our healing profession apart from others that focus exclusively on the disease and do not consider the manifold intricacies of the individual patient.
4. **The Healing Power of Nature: _Vis Medicatrix Naturae_:** Naturopathic medicine recognizes an inherent self-healing process in the person that is ordered and intelligent. The body has many highly efficient mechanisms for sustaining and regaining health. These mechanisms have their specific and necessary components (e.g., nutrients) and means by which they can be impaired (e.g., xenobiotic immunosuppression). Poor health and disease can result from impairment of these self-healing processes

[476] Kirchfeld F, Boyle W. Nature Doctors: Pioneers in Naturopathic Medicine. Portland, Oregon; Medicina Biologica (Buckeye Naturopathic Press, East Palestine, Ohio), 1994
[477] Boon HS, Cherkin DC, Erro J, Sherman KJ, Milliman B, Booker J, Cramer EH, Smith MJ, Deyo RA, Eisenberg DM. Practice patterns of naturopathic physicians: results from a random survey of licensed practitioners in two US States. _BMC Complement Altern Med._ 2004;4(1):14
[478] Smith MJ, Logan AC. Naturopathy. _Med Clin North Am._ 2002 Jan;86(1):173-84
[479] Cherkin DC, Deyo RA, Sherman KJ, et al. Characteristics of visits to licensed acupuncturists, chiropractors, massage therapists, and naturopathic physicians. _J Am Board Fam Pract._ 2002 Nov-Dec;15(6):463-72
[480] Cherkin DC, Deyo RA, Sherman KJ, et al. Characteristics of licensed acupuncturists, chiropractors, massage therapists, and naturopathic physicians. _J Am Board Fam Pract._ 2002 Sep-Oct;15(5):378-90
[481] Quoted from the American Association of Naturopathic Physicians website http://aanp.net/Basics/h.naturo.philo.html on February 4, 2001. Other italicized quotes in this section are from the same source. This website has since been replaced by http://naturopathic.org/
[482] "Recent estimates suggest that each year more than 1 million patients are injured while in the hospital and approximately 180,000 die because of these injuries. Furthermore, drug-related morbidity and mortality are common and are estimated to cost more than $136 billion a year." Holland EG, Degruy FV. Drug-induced disorders. _Am Fam Physician._ 1997;56(7):1781-8, 1791-2

and biologic mechanisms, and thus the body's inherent, natural, self-healing mechanisms—the "healing power of nature"—can be diminished to the state of ineffectiveness or harm (e.g., autoimmunity). Recognizing that the body has this inherent goal of and movement toward self-healing, naturopathic physicians start by identifying and removing "obstacles to cure" rather than ignoring these factors and masking the manifestations of dysfunction with symptom-suppressing drugs.

5. **Prevention**: Healthy lifestyle, proper nutrition, and emotional hygiene go a long way toward preventing (and treating) most conditions. Specific conditions have specific risk factors and causes that have to be considered per patient and condition.

6. **Doctor As Teacher** *(Docere)*: Naturopathic physicians explain the situation and the proposed solution to the patient so that the patient is empowered with understanding and with the comfort of knowing what has happened, what is happening, and the proposed course of upcoming events. Naturopathic physicians strive to let their own lives serve as a models for our patients. This does not mean that naturopathic doctors have to feign perfection; the task is to live the best and most conscious life that we can, to be present with our emotions, qualities, and faults and to treat ourselves with respect and acceptance. We can exemplify health (rather than perfection) to our patients by being who we authentically are and by so doing we can facilitate their own acceptance of their current health situation, which is a prerequisite to self-initiated change.

> **"Physician, heal thyself.**
> Thus you help your patient, too.
> Let this be his best medicine that he
> beholds with his eyes: the doctor who
> heals himself."
>
> Nietzsche FW. <u>Thus Spoke Zarathustra (1892)</u>.
> [Kaufmann W, translator]. Viking Penguin: 1954,
> page 77

7. **Re-Establish the Foundation for Health**: An overview of this important naturopathic concept is provided throughout this chapter.

8. **Removing "obstacles to cure"**: *examples*

Obstacle to the optimization of health	Example of possible intervention
o Toxic exposures, medication side-effects	▪ Reduce drug use and dependency
o Toxic relationships, emotional obstacles, past events, unfulfilling occupation,	▪ Improve self-esteem, develop conflict resolution skills, determine life goals and values and a plan for their pursuit
o Social isolation: the typical American has only two friends no-one in whom to confide[483]	▪ Encourage social interaction
o Diet with excess fat, arachidonate, sugar, additives, colorants, and insufficiency of protein, fiber, phytonutrients, and health-promoting fatty acids: ALA, GLA, EPA, DHA, and oleic acid	▪ Diet improvement and nutritional supplementation
o Sedentary lifestyle, lack of exercise	▪ Encourage exercise
o Weight gain/loss as necessary for weight optimization	▪ Encourage self-valuing
o Epidemic exposure to mercury, lead, and xenobiotics	▪ Support detoxification process as a lifestyle

Hierarchy of Therapeutics: This naturopathic concept articulates the importance of addressing *the underlying cause* rather than simply focusing on *the presenting problem*, which is the *symptom of the cause*. Further, interventions are **prioritized**, *for example*:

- Patient-implemented *before* doctor-implemented.

---

[483] McPherson M, Smith-Lovin L, Brashears ME. Social Isolation in America: Changes in Core Discussion Networks over Two Decades. *American Sociological Review* 2006; 71: 353-75 http://www.asanet.org/galleries/default-file/June06ASRFeature.pdf

- Removal of harming agent *before* addition of a therapeutic agent: e.g., stop smoking *before* investing in respiratory therapy; implement healthy diet and exercise before higher-risk and higher-cost drugs for hypertension and hypercholesterolemia.
- Low-force interventions *before* high-force interventions.
- Diet *before* nutritional supplements; nutrients *before* botanicals; botanicals *before* drugs; modulatory drugs *before* suppressive/inhibitory drugs; integrative care *before* surgery.
- *See examples below.*

Hierarchy of Therapeutics (specifically sequential)	Example of possible intervention
1. <u>Reestablishing the foundation for health</u>	<ul><li>Mental/emotional/spiritual health</li><li>Meditation, freeze-frame, "time out"</li><li>Relaxation</li><li>Positive visualization, positive expectation, affirmation</li><li>Counseling, social contact, group work[484]</li><li>Family contact and resolution</li><li>Dietary intake and nutritional health which addresses the patient's biochemical individuality[485] and correction of deficiencies or excesses</li><li>Identification and elimination of food allergies and food sensitivities</li><li>Reduce toxin exposure, promote detoxification</li><li>Identification and elimination of exposure to gastrointestinal and inhalant xenobiotics</li><li>Remove or reduce specific "obstacles to cure"</li></ul>
2. <u>Stimulation of the "healing power of nature" and the "vital force"</u>	<ul><li>Constitutional hydrotherapy</li><li>Homeopathy</li><li>Exercise</li><li>Acupuncture, Spinal manipulation</li><li>Meditation, rest</li><li>Tai Chi, Qigong: "energy-cultivation"</li><li>Botanical adaptogens</li></ul>
3. <u>Tonification of weakened systems:</u>	<ul><li>Botanical medicines and other supplements to help restore normal tissue function</li><li>Spinal manipulation to address the primary somatovisceral dysfunction and/or secondary musculoskeletal disorders</li><li>Hormonal supplementation</li><li>Nutritional supplementation</li><li>Exercise</li><li>Physiotherapy</li></ul>
4. <u>Correction of structural integrity:</u>	<ul><li>Spinal manipulation, deep tissue massage, visceral manipulation, lymphatic pump to promote immune surveillance[486]</li><li>Stretching, balancing, muscle strengthening, and proprioceptive retraining</li><li>Surgery, as a last resort</li></ul>

[484] See http://www.mkp.org and www.WomanWithin.org for examples.
[485] Williams RJ. Biochemical Individuality: The Basis for the Genetotrophic Concept. Austin and London: University of Texas Press, 1956
[486] "Lymph flow in the thoracic duct increased from 1.57±0.20 mL·min-1 to a peak TDF of 4.80±1.73 mL·min-1 during abdominal pump, and from 1.20±0.41 mL·min-1 to 3.45±1.61 mL·min-1 during thoracic pump." Knott EM, Tune JD, Stoll ST, Downey HF. Increased lymphatic flow in the thoracic duct during manipulative intervention. *J Am Osteopath Assoc.* 2005 Oct;105(10):447-56 http://www.jaoa.org/cgi/content/full/105/10/447

Osteopathic Medicine

Osteopathic medicine and chiropractic are American-born healthcare professions and paradigms that started at nearly the same time in history and from many of the same foundational principles. Both professions were started in the late 1800's and early 1900's and were founded upon the philosophical premise that the body functioned as a whole and that therefore medicine in general and therapeutic interventions in particular needed to be comprehensive in scope and multifaceted in their application. Further, both professions emphasized the importance of structural integrity as a foundational component of health and thus embraced manual manipulative therapy and spinal manipulation.

From their common origins, subtle differences and chance historic events shaped and further separated these professions from each other. Osteopathy was founded by Andrew Taylor Still, a medical doctor who sought to reform what was then called the "Heroic" paradigm of medicine, which embraced bloodletting and the administration of leeches, purgatives, emetics, and poisons such as mercury as means for "rebalancing" what were perceived to be internal causes of disease, namely the "four humours" of the body which were thought to be blood, phlegm, black bile, and yellow bile. In part because of his training within and identification with the medical profession, Still sought to *reform* rather than *directly oppose* the "mainstream medicine" of his day; in contrast, chiropractic's founder Daniel David Palmer was more strongly opposed to the horrific medicine of his time and thus was more *revolutionary* than *evolutionary* in his approach to forging a new paradigm of health and healthcare. Still's willingness to align with the medical profession and the increasingly powerful and influential pharmaceutical industry unquestionably helped his fledgling profession survive the extinction that otherwise would have been swift at the hands of allopathic groups such as **the American Medical Association (AMA), which labeled osteopathic physicians as "cultists" and systematically restricted inclusion of the osteopathic profession into mainstream healthcare by proclamation in 1953 that "…all voluntary associations with osteopaths are unethical." When osteopathic resistance mounted, the AMA and its co-conspirators, who were later found guilty of violating the nation's antitrust laws by illegally suppressing competition and attempting to build a medical monopoly**[487], acquiesced and accepted osteopaths into its ranks — a strategy which the medical profession believed would eventually destroy the osteopathic profession by forcing it to resign its ideals and identity. In his review of osteopathic history, Gevitz[488] writes, **"…the M.D.'s gradually came to believe that the only way to destroy osteopathy was through the absorption of D.O.'s, much as the homeopaths and eclectics [naturopaths] had been swallowed up early in the century."** Even recently, the AMA has listed osteopathic medicine under "alternative medicine"[489] although several osteopathic medical colleges have consistently provided training that is superior to most "conventional" allopathic medical schools.[490] Today, osteopathic physicians practice in most ways similarly to allopaths — i.e., with unlimited scope of practice in all 50 states, full access to the use of drugs and surgery, and with a very pharmacosurgical paradigm of disease and healthcare. Osteopathic medicine is one of the fastest growing healthcare professions in America.

Osteopathic Manipulative Medicine:

Osteopathic manipulative medicine (OMM) is similar to and yet distinct from chiropractic manipulation; the naturopathic profession — true to its eclectic roots — incorporates techniques from all professions. In contrast to chiropractic, OMM terminology and therapeutics focus much more on soft tissues, and the osteopathic lesion — "somatic dysfunction" — is clearly originated from soft tissues in contrast to the chiropractic lesion — the "vertebral subluxation" — which obviously originates from spinal articulations. Whereas the chiropractic intent of correcting or "adjusting" the "subluxation" was historically to improve function of the nervous system, the osteopathic lesion is addressed to more fully improve not only function of the nervous system but also of the vascular,

---

[487] Getzendanner S. Permanent injunction order against AMA. *JAMA.* 1988 Jan 1;259(1):81-2
[488] Gevitz N. The D.O.'s: Osteopathic Medicine in America. Johns Hopkins University Press; 1991; pages 100-103
[489] American Medical Association. Report 12 of the Council on Scientific Affairs (A-97) Full Text http://www.ama-assn.org/ama/pub/category/13638.html Accessed November 23, 2006
[490] Special report. America's best graduate schools. Schools of Medicine. The top schools: primary care. *US News World Rep.* 2004 Apr 12;136(12):74

lymphatic, and myofascial systems, too.[491] With regard to the latter, the osteopathic profession has always emphasized the importance of fascia in the genesis of "somatic dysfunction." Indeed, fascia appears to play an important and dynamic (not passive) role in neuromusculoskeletal health, particularly as it is a major contributor to proprioception and may also have a more direct effect through the recently described ability of fascia to actively contract in a smooth-muscle-like manner.[492]

From this author's perspective, an unfortunate consequence of the broadness of osteopathic manipulative conceptualizations/techniques (i.e., vertebral, skeletal, vascular, lymphatic, myofascial,...) is the relative lack (compared to chiropractic) of modernization and sophistication and development of its terminology and training textbooks; two of the most widely used osteopathic texts—*Osteopathic Principles in Practice* (1994) by Kuchera and Kuchera[493], and *Outline of Osteopathic Manipulative Procedures* (2006) by Kimberly[494]—both leave very much to be desired with respect to their clarity, terminology, clinical applicability, and referencing to the scientific literature. *Manipulation of the Spine, Thorax and Pelvis: An Osteopathic Perspective* (2006) by Gibbons and Tehan[495] is much more accessible and clinically applicable; however the text focuses exclusively on high-velocity low-amplitude (HVLA) techniques and therefore does not provide sufficient background and training for students in the very techniques that distinguish osteopathic from chiropractic techniques, namely heightened attention to the myofascial dysfunction that (appropriately) underlies the osteopathic lesion.

> ### Osteopathic Interventions need to be Consistent with Osteopathic Philosophy
>
> "In contrast to the description of the osteopathic medical profession by the American Osteopathic Association, namely, "doctors of osteopathic medicine, or D.O.s, apply the philosophy of treating the whole person to the prevention, diagnosis and treatment of illness, disease and injury," [the authors of the article in question] essentially reviewed only pharmacologic treatment.
>
> …
>
> It is hoped that future reviews in this journal can include a more balanced survey of the literature, inclusive of non-pharmacologic and "holistic" interventions that are consistent with osteopathic philosophy."
>
> **Vasquez A**. Interventions Need to be Consistent With Osteopathic Philosophy. [Letter] *JAOA: Journal of the American Osteopathic Association* 2006 Sep;106(9):528-9 http://www.jaoa.org/cgi/content/full/106/9/528

Ironically, the very growth and "allopathicization" of the profession that has threatened the profession's adherence to its holistic tenets has caused a reflexive re-affirmation of these tenets, and the profession has responded with a well-funded and intentional directive to scientifically investigate the mechanisms and efficacy of osteopathic manipulative medicine.[496,497] Recent findings include improved function and reduced pain in patients treated with a comprehensive manipulative technique for the shoulder[498], as well as the significant efficacy of ankle manipulation for patients with recent ankle injuries.[499] Further, OMM treatment of patients medicated for depression was found to triple the effectiveness of drug monotherapy.[500] Other studies have shown benefit of OMM in the treatment of geriatric pneumonia[501], pediatric asthma[502], pediatric dysfunctional voiding[503],

---

[491] Williams N. Managing back pain in general practice--is osteopathy the new paradigm? *Br J Gen Pract*. 1997 Oct;47(423):653-5 http://www.pubmedcentral.nih.gov/articlerender.fcgi?tool=pubmed&pubmedid=9474832

[492] "...the existence of active fascial contractility could have interesting implications for the understanding of musculoskeletal pathologies with an increased or decreased myofascial tonus. It may also offer new insights and a deeper understanding of treatments directed at fascia, such as manual myofascial release therapies or acupuncture." Schleip R, Klingler W, Lehmann-Horn F. Active fascial contractility: Fascia may be able to contract in a smooth muscle-like manner and thereby influence musculoskeletal dynamics. *Med Hypotheses*. 2005;65(2):273-7

[493] Kuchera WA, Kuchera ML. *Osteopathic Principles In Practice, revised second edition*. Kirksville, MO, KCOM Press; 1994

[494] Kimberly PE. *Outline of Osteopathic Manipulative Procedures. The Kimberly Manual 2006*. Kirksville College of Osteopathic Medicine. Walsworth Publishing Company Marceline, Mo

[495] Gibbons P, Tehan P. *Manipulation of the Spine, Thorax and Pelvis: An Osteopathic Perspective*. Churchill Livingstone; 2006. Isbn: 044310039X

[496] Wisnioski SW 3rd. "Circle Turns Round" to "Allopathic Osteopathy." *J Am Osteopath Assoc* 2006; 106: 423-4 http://www.jaoa.org/cgi/content/full/106/7/423

[497] Teitelbaum HS, Bunn WE 2nd, Brown SA, Burchett AW. Osteopathic medical education: renaissance or rhetoric? *J Am Osteopath Assoc*. 2003 Oct;103(10):489-90 http://www.jaoa.org/cgi/reprint/103/10/489

[498] The "seven stages of Spencer" is an organized technique of range-of-motion exercises and post-isometric stretching to improve functionality of the shoulder. This clinical trial showed improved shoulder function in a group of elderly patients treated with this technique. Knebl JA, Shores JH, Gamber RG, Gray WT, Herron KM. Improving functional ability in the elderly via the Spencer technique, an osteopathic manipulative treatment: a randomized, controlled trial. *J Am Osteopath Assoc*. 2002 Jul;102(7):387-96 http://www.jaoa.org/cgi/reprint/102/7/387 See also "CONCLUSION: Manipulative therapy for the shoulder girdle in addition to usual medical care accelerates recovery of shoulder symptoms." Bergman GJ, Winters JC, Groenier KH, Pool JJ, Meyboom-de Jong B, Postema K, van der Heijden GJ. Manipulative therapy in addition to usual medical care for patients with shoulder dysfunction and pain: a randomized, controlled trial. *Ann Intern Med*. 2004 Sep 21;141(6):432-9 http://www.annals.org/cgi/reprint/141/6/432.pdf

[499] This study shows the rapid onset and benefit of manipulative medicine for the treatment of acute ankle sprains: Eisenhart AW, Gaeta TJ, Yens DP. Osteopathic manipulative treatment in the emergency department for patients with acute ankle injuries. *J Am Osteopath Assoc*. 2003 Sep;103(9):417-21 http://www.jaoa.org/cgi/reprint/103/9/417

[500] This study impressively showed that musculoskeletal manipulation improved treatment effectiveness for depression from 33% to 100%. "After 8 weeks, 100% of the OMT treatment group and 33% of the control group tested normal by psychometric evaluation. ... The findings of this pilot study indicate that OMT may be a useful adjunctive treatment for alleviating depression in women." Plotkin BJ, Rodos JJ, Kappler R, Schrage M, Freydl K, Hasegawa S, Hennegan E, Hilchie-Schmidt C, Hines D, Iwata J, Mok C, Raffaelli D. Adjunctive osteopathic manipulative treatment in women with depression: a pilot study. *J Am Osteopath Assoc*. 2001 Sep;101(9):517-23 http://www.jaoa.org/cgi/reprint/101/9/517

[501] This study showed improved clinical outcomes and reduced antibiotic use in elderly patients with pneumonia when treated with manipulative medicine: "The treatment group had a significantly shorter duration of intravenous antibiotic treatment and a shorter hospital stay." Noll DR, Shores JH, Gamber RG, Herron KM, Swift J Jr. Benefits of osteopathic manipulative treatment for hospitalized elderly patients with pneumonia. *J Am Osteopath Assoc*. 2000 Dec;100(12):776-82 http://www.jaoa.org/cgi/reprint/100/12/776

[502] Osteopathic manipulation improved pulmonary function in pediatric patients with asthma: "With a confidence level of 95%, results for the OMT group showed a statistically significant improvement of 7 L per minute to 9 L per minute for peak expiratory flow rates. These results suggest that OMT has a therapeutic effect among this patient population."

carpal tunnel syndrome[504], low-back pain[505], and recovery from cardiac bypass surgery.[506] Replication and validation of these studies—many of which are small or of nonrigorous design (e.g., open clinical trials with no control group)—is important to further define and establish the value of osteopathic manipulation in clinical care.

Guiney PA, Chou R, Vianna A, Lovenheim J. Effects of osteopathic manipulative treatment on pediatric patients with asthma: a randomized controlled trial. *J Am Osteopath Assoc.* 2005 Jan;105(1):7-12 http://www.jaoa.org/cgi/content/full/105/1/7

[503] "RESULTS: The treatment group exhibited greater improvement in DV symptoms than did the control group (Z=-2.63, p=0.008, Mann-Whitney U-test). Improved or resolution of vesicoureteral reflux and elimination of post-void urine residuals were more prominent in the treatment group." Nemett DR, Fivush BA, Mathews R, Camirand N, Eldridge MA, Finney K, Gerson AC. A randomized controlled trial of the effectiveness of osteopathy-based manual physical therapy in treating pediatric dysfunctional voiding. *J Pediatr Urol.* 2008 Apr;4(2):100-6

[504] Sucher BM, Hinrichs RN, Welcher RL, Quiroz LD, St Laurent BF, Morrison BJ. Manipulative treatment of carpal tunnel syndrome: biomechanical and osteopathic intervention to increase the length of the transverse carpal ligament: part 2. Effect of sex differences and manipulative "priming". *J Am Osteopath Assoc.* 2005 Mar;105(3):135-43. Erratum in: J Am Osteopath Assoc. 2005 May;105(5):238 http://www.jaoa.org/cgi/content/full/105/3/135

[505] "CONCLUSION: OMT significantly reduces low back pain. The level of pain reduction is greater than expected from placebo effects alone and persists for at least three months." Licciardone JC, Brimhall AK, King LN. Osteopathic manipulative treatment for low back pain: a systematic review and meta-analysis of randomized controlled trials. *BMC Musculoskelet Disord.* 2005 Aug 4;6:43 http://www.biomedcentral.com/1471-2474/6/43

[506] This study showed benefit from osteopathic manipulation administered immediately after coronary artery bypass graft surgery: "The observed changes in cardiac function and perfusion indicated that OMT had a beneficial effect on the recovery of patients after CABG surgery. The authors conclude that OMT has immediate, beneficial hemodynamic effects after CABG surgery when administered while the patient is sedated and pharmacologically paralyzed." O-Yurvati AH, Carnes MS, Clearfield MB, Stoll ST, McConathy WJ. Hemodynamic effects of osteopathic manipulative treatment immediately after coronary artery bypass graft surgery. *J Am Osteopath Assoc.* 2005 Oct;105(10):475-81 http://www.jaoa.org/cgi/content/full/105/10/475

Functional Medicine

Note: This section is from the final pre-edited draft which introduces functional medicine in *Vasquez A. Musculoskeletal Pain: Expanded Clinical Strategies* (2008), published by the Institute for Functional Medicine; used here with permission. Slight modifications were made to this section during revisions in 2011.

Introduction: The purpose of this monograph is to provide healthcare professionals with an overview of the "functional medicine" assessment and management strategies that are applicable to painful neuromusculoskeletal disorders. A comprehensive description of functional medicine from the Institute for Functional Medicine (IFM) is provided later in this section, while a more comprehensive explication is provided in *The Textbook of Functional Medicine*.[507] In recognition of the diversity of this document's readership (inclusive of students, recent graduates, experienced professionals, academicians, and policymakers) and the pervasive deficiencies in musculoskeletal knowledge among healthcare providers[508,509,510,511,512,513], this monograph on pain will necessarily review some basic concepts; however, this document alone cannot replace professional training in musculoskeletal medicine nor does it include protocols for

A Functional Medicine Monograph

MUSCULOSKELETAL PAIN:
Expanded Clinical Strategies

Alex Vasquez, DC, ND

THE INSTITUTE FOR FUNCTIONAL MEDICINE

The information in this section on functional medicine is derived from the final pre-edited draft of chapter 1 from Vasquez A. *Musculoskeletal Pain: Expanded Clinical Strategies*, published by the Institute for Functional Medicine in 2008 and available from www.FunctionalMedicine.org

patient management and differential diagnosis for each of the neuromusculoskeletal problems seen in clinical practice. This text should be used in conjunction with the reader's professional training and other reference texts. Clinicians utilizing a functional medicine approach to patient care must be knowledgeable in the details of integrative physiology and nutritional biochemistry and must also posses the clinical acumen necessary to ensure safe and expedient patient care. These traits and skills are of particular necessity when a serious condition is presented. Life-threatening and limb-threatening neuromusculoskeletal problems are notorious for presenting under the guise of an apparently benign complaint such as fatigue, headache, or simple joint pain.

Since approximately 1 of every 7 (14% of total) visits to a primary healthcare provider is for the treatment of musculoskeletal pain or dysfunction[514], every healthcare provider needs to have: 1) knowledge of important concepts related to musculoskeletal medicine, 2) the ability to recognize urgent and emergency conditions, 3) the ability to competently perform orthopedic examination procedures and interpret laboratory assessments, and 4) the knowledge and ability to design and implement effective treatment plans and to coordinate patient management. While this monograph will be thorough in its review of topics discussed, like any other textbook it cannot contain every nuance and examination procedure that clinicians should have in their clinical toolkits. This text should be used in conjunction with the clinician's previous professional training, other textbooks, and best judgment for the delivery of personalized care for each individual patient, including those who present with similar or identical diagnoses. Supportive texts include *Current Medical Diagnosis and Treatment* edited by Tierney

---

[507] Jones DS (Editor-in-Chief). *Textbook of Functional Medicine*. Institute for Functional Medicine, Gig Harbor, WA 2005

[508] Freedman KB, Bernstein J. The adequacy of medical school education in musculoskeletal medicine. *J Bone Joint Surg Am*. 1998;80(10):1421-7

[509] Freedman KB, Bernstein J. Educational deficiencies in musculoskeletal medicine. *J Bone Joint Surg Am*. 2002;84-A(4):604-8

[510] Joy EA, Hala SV. Musculoskeletal Curricula in Medical Education: Filling In the Missing Pieces. *The Physician and Sportsmedicine*. 2004; 32: 42-45

[511] Matzkin E, Smith ME, Freccero CD, Richardson AB. Adequacy of education in musculoskeletal medicine. *J Bone Joint Surg Am*. 2005 Feb;87-A(2):310-4

[512] Schmale GA. More evidence of educational inadequacies in musculoskeletal medicine. *Clin Orthop Relat Res*. 2005 Aug;(437):251-9

[513] Stockard AR, Allen TW. Competence levels in musculoskeletal medicine: comparison of osteopathic and allopathic medical graduates. *J Am Osteopath Assoc*. 2006 Jun;106(6):350-5

[514] American College of Rheumatology Ad Hoc Committee on Clinical Guidelines. Guidelines for the initial evaluation of the adult patient with acute musculoskeletal symptoms. *Arthritis Rheum*. 1996 Jan;39(1):1-8 See also: Vasquez A. Musculoskeletal disorders and iron overload disease: comment on the American College of Rheumatology guidelines. *Arthritis Rheum* 1996;39: 1767-8

et al[515], *Orthopedic Physical Assessment* by Magee[516], and *Integrative Orthopedics* and *Integrative Rheumatology* by Vasquez.[517,518] Further, clinicians can note that this monograph is written primarily for routine outpatient management rather than emergency department management or "playing field" situations.

Musculoskeletal disorders are extremely prevalent and represent a major cause of human suffering, healthcare expenses, and lost productivity. Additionally, many standard medical interventions show high rates of inefficacy and iatrogenesis in addition to their high costs.[519,520,521] The vast majority of painful neuromusculoskeletal disorders can be alleviated and often effectively treated with nutritional interventions, but physicians trained only in standard medicine receive little to no training in nutrition and are therefore generally unable or unwilling to use these science-based interventions to help their patients.[522,523] Further, distain toward nutritional and other nonsurgical and nonpharmacologic interventions is represented in many standard medical textbooks despite proof of efficacy shown in replicable high-quality clinical trials published in top-tier medical journals. For example, despite the more than 800 articles documenting the role of nutritional interventions in the direct or adjunctive treatment of rheumatoid arthritis, the seventeenth edition of *The Merck Manual* published in 1999 wrote that, "Food and diet quackery is common and should be discouraged."[524] Combining these factors with the aforementioned pervasive lack of competence in musculoskeletal knowledge among healthcare providers (exceptions noted[525]), we see that patients with musculoskeletal disorders often face a series of difficult and insurmountable obstacles between their present condition of suffering and the relief that they seek and deserve. Clearly, the field of musculoskeletal medicine is in need of pervasive paradigm shifts in both physician training and patient management to improve patient care.

Background: Historically, prevailing views of disorders of pain and inflammation were conceptually similar to those of most other diseases and premodern accounts of life in general. Our clinical predecessors did the best they could to understand, describe, and treat the health problems with which their patients presented, and the paradigm from which these clinical entities were viewed and addressed was shaped by the social, religious, and scientific views and limitations of their time. Lacking a molecular and physiologic understanding of disease origination, and restrained by metaphysical and simplistic models of "cause and effect", premodern clinicians devised models for the understanding and treatment of disease that generally appear unsatisfactory today in light of the advances in our understanding in disparate yet interrelated fields such as psychoneuroimmunology, molecular biology, nutrigenomics, environmental medicine and toxicology. Despite these advances, we as a human society and as healthcare providers still carry many of these previous conceptualizations and misconceptualizations with us as we move forward toward a future wherein our views and interventions will be much more precise and "objective" in contrast to the generalized and phenomenalistic approaches that typified premodern medicine and which still permeate certain aspects of clinical care today. For example, we still use the term "stroke" to describe acute cerebrovascular insufficiency, although the term originated from the view that affected patients had been "struck" by the gods or fates perhaps as a form of punishment for some ethical or religious transgression. Even today, patients and clinicians commonly interpret disease as some form of punishment or as an extension of spiritual or intrapersonal shortcoming. Advancing science allows us to disassemble complex events that were previously experienced as *phenomena*, that is, as undecipherable and enigmatic events that overwhelmed comprehension. The **Functional Medicine Matrix** provides an extremely useful tool for helping clinicians grasp a multidimensional decipherable view of disease and its corresponding

[515] Tierney ML. McPhee SJ, Papadakis MA (eds). <u>Current Medical Diagnosis and Treatment</u>. New York: Lange Medical Books. Updated annually
[516] Magee DJ. <u>Orthopedic Physical Assessment. Third edition</u>. Philadelphia: WB Saunders, 1997. Newer editions have been published.
[517] Vasquez A. *Integrative Orthopedics: Second Edition*. Fort Worth, Texas; Integrative and Biological Medicine Research and Consulting, 2007 OptimalHealthResearch.com
[518] Vasquez A. *Integrative Rheumatology: Second Edition*. Fort Worth, Texas; Integrative and Biological Medicine Research and Consulting, 2007 OptimalHealthResearch.com
[519] Moseley JB, O'Malley K, Petersen NJ, Menke TJ, Brody BA, Kuykendall DH, Hollingsworth JC, Ashton CM, Wray NP. A controlled trial of arthroscopic surgery for osteoarthritis of the knee. *N Engl J Med* 2002 Jul 11;347(2):81-8
[520] Kolata G. A Knee Surgery for Arthritis Is Called Sham. *The New York Times*, July 11, 2002
[521] Rosner AL. Evidence-based clinical guidelines for the management of acute low-back pain: response to the guidelines prepared for the Australian Medical Health and Research Council. *J Manipulative Physiol Ther*. 2001;24(3):214-20
[522] Lo C. Integrating nutrition as a theme throughout the medical school curriculum. *Am J Clin Nutr*. 2000 Sep;72(3 Suppl):882S-9S
[523] Adams KM, Lindell KC, Kohlmeier M, Zeisel SH. Status of nutrition education in medical schools. *Am J Clin Nutr*. 2006 Apr;83(4):941S-944S
[524] Beers MH, Berkow R (eds). <u>The Merck Manual. Seventeenth Edition</u>. Whitehouse Station; Merck Research Laboratories: 1999, page 419
[525] Humphreys BK, Sulkowski A, McIntyre K, Kasiban M, Patrick AN. An examination of musculoskeletal cognitive competency in chiropractic interns. *J Manipulative Physiol Ther*. 2007;30(1):44-9

treatment which facilitates the achievement of higher clinical efficacy, improved patient outcomes, and more favorable safety and cost-effectiveness profiles.

Whereas the advancement of our scientific knowledge often leads us to discard previous models and interventions, occasionally modern science helps us to understand and revisit previous interventions that may have been prematurely or unduly discarded. For example, Hippocrates' admonition to "Let thy food be thy medicine, and thy medicine be thy food" experienced decades of devaluation when dietary, nutritional, and other natural interventions were misbranded as "quackery." On the contrary to these premature and unsubstantiated condemnations, simple natural interventions such as therapeutic fasting and augmentation of vitamin D3 status (via nutritional supplementation or exposure to ultraviolet-B radiation) have shown remarkable safety and efficacy in the mitigation of chronic hypertension, musculoskeletal pain, and autoimmunity.[526,527,528,529,530,531,532,533,534] Furthermore, the appropriate use of vitamin supplements helps prevent chronic disease by numerous mechanisms including modulation of gene transcription, enhancement of DNA repair and stability, and enhancement of metabolic efficiency.[535,536,537] This document will provide a representative survey of current research in the use of dietary, nutritional, and integrative therapeutics commonly utilized in the clinical management of disorders characterized by pain and inflammation.

State of the Evidence: The bulk of information in this monograph is derived from and referenced to peer-reviewed publications indexed in the database known as Medline/Pubmed provided by the U.S. National Library of Medicine and the National Institutes of Health. For the sake of practicality and publishability, not all statements carry citations, but the most important ones do; citations are always provided when referenced to a particular intervention of importance so that clinicians can access the primary source when refining their clinical decisions. A "blanket statement" to cover all the different assessments and interventions described herein would be necessarily inaccurate and therefore each intervention will be considered on the merits of its own rationale, safety, effectiveness, and cost-effectiveness. Again, however, these considerations must ultimately be viewed within the context of the individual patient's condition and the overall cohesion and comprehensiveness of the treatment plan.

While all clinicians can appreciate the importance of protocols and clinical practice guidelines, we must also perpetually ratify the preeminence of patient individuality and therefore the importance of tailoring treatment to the patient's unique combination of biochemical individuality, comorbid conditions, drug use, personal goals, and willingness to participate in a health-promoting lifestyle. Standardized protocols and practice guidelines are founded on the fallacy of disease homogeneity and the irrelevance of physiologic, psychosocial, and biochemical individuality. As the advancement of biomedical science provides the means for and underscores the importance of customized treatments for each patient, so too has the standard of care begun to shift in the direction of requiring the consideration of these variables before and during the implementation of treatment. Failure to utilize nutritional interventions when such interventions are clinically indicated is inconsistent with the delivery of quality healthcare and may be considered malpractice.[538,539,540,541]

A clinician who is unaware of the political forces that shape healthcare policy and research is analogous to a captain of an oceangoing ship not knowing how to use a compass, sextant, or coastline map. Medical science

[526] Goldhamer A, et al. Medically supervised water-only fasting in the treatment of hypertension. *J Manipulative Physiol Ther* 2001 Jun;24(5):335-9
[527] Goldhamer AC, et al. Medically supervised water-only fasting in the treatment of borderline hypertension. *J Altern Complement Med*. 2002 Oct;8(5):643-50
[528] Goldhamer AC. Initial cost of care results in medically supervised water-only fasting for treating high blood pressure and diabetes. *J Altern Complement Med*. 2002 Dec;8(6):696-7
[529] Krause R, Bühring M, Hopfenmüller W, Holick MF, Sharma AM. Ultraviolet B and blood pressure. *Lancet*. 1998 Aug 29;352(9129):709-10
[530] Pfeifer M, Begerow B, Minne HW, Nachtigall D, Hansen C. Effects of a short-term vitamin D(3) and calcium supplementation on blood pressure and parathyroid hormone levels in elderly women. *J Clin Endocrinol Metab*. 2001 Apr;86(4):1633-7
[531] McCarty MF. A preliminary fast may potentiate response to a subsequent low-salt, low-fat vegan diet in the management of hypertension - fasting as a strategy for breaking metabolic vicious cycles. *Med Hypotheses*. 2003 May;60(5):624-33
[532] Hyppönen E, Läärä E, Reunanen A, Järvelin MR, Virtanen SM. Intake of vitamin D and risk of type 1 diabetes: a birth-cohort study. *Lancet*. 2001 Nov 3;358(9292):1500-3
[533] Fuhrman J, Sarter B, Calabro DJ. Brief case reports of medically supervised, water-only fasting associated with remission of autoimmune disease. *Altern Ther Health Med*. 2002 Jul-Aug;8(4):112, 110-1
[534] Holick MF. Vitamin D deficiency: what a pain it is. *Mayo Clin Proc*. 2003 Dec;78(12):1457-9
[535] Fletcher RH, Fairfield KM. Vitamins for chronic disease prevention in adults: clinical applications. *JAMA*. 2002 Jun 19;287(23):3127-9
[536] Heaney RP. Long-latency deficiency disease: insights from calcium and vitamin D. *Am J Clin Nutr*. 2003 Nov;78(5):912-9
[537] Ames BN. The metabolic tune-up: metabolic harmony and disease prevention. *J Nutr*. 2003 May;133(5 Suppl 1):1544S-8S
[538] Heaney RP. Vitamin D, nutritional deficiency, and the medical paradigm. *J Clin Endocrinol Metab*. 2003 Nov;88(11):5107-8
[539] Fletcher RH, Fairfield KM. Vitamins for chronic disease prevention in adults: clinical applications. *JAMA*. 2002 Jun 19;287(23):3127-9
[540] Berg A. Sliding toward nutrition malpractice: time to reconsider and redeploy. *Am J Clin Nutr*. 1993 Jan;57(1):3-7
[541] Cobb DK, Warner D. Avoiding malpractice: the role of proper nutrition and wound management. *J Am Med Dir Assoc*. 2004 Jul-Aug;5(4 Sup):H11-6

and healthcare policy are influenced by a myriad of powerful private interests which are motivated by their own goals, at times different from the stated goals of medicine, which purports to hold paramount the patient's welfare. Scientific objectivity and the guiding ethical principles of informed consent, beneficence, autonomy, and non-malfeasance are subject to different interpretations depending upon the lens through which a dilemma is viewed. When this "dilemma" is the whole of healthcare, what first appears as order and structure now appears as the disarrayed tug-of-war between factions and private interests, with paradigmatic victory often being awarded to those with the best marketing campaigns and political influence with less importance given to safety, efficacy, and the economic burden to consumers.[542,543,544,545,546,547,548,549,550,551,552,553,554,555,556,557,558,559,560,561,562,563,564,565,566,567,568,569,570,571,572,573] To be ignorant of such considerations is to be blind to the nature of research, policy, and our own biased inclinations for and against particular paradigms, assessments, and interventions. Research articles and sources of authority must be approached with an artist's delicacy, and with a willingness to receive new information as worthy of preeminence over deeply rooted and well ensconced institutionalized fallacies.

<u>Understanding the Multifaceted Nature of Disease Pathogenesis: The Functional Medicine Matrix as Paradigm and Clinical Tool</u>: At its simplest and most practical level, the Functional Medicine Matrix is a teaching tool and clinical method that facilitates consideration of the different contributions of major intrinsic systems and

[542] Editorial. Drug-company influence on medical education in USA. *Lancet.* 2000 Sep 2;356(9232):781

[543] Horton R. Lotronex and the FDA: a fatal erosion of integrity. *Lancet.* 2001 May 19;357(9268):1544-5

[544] Editorial. Politics trumps science at the FDA. *Lancet.* 2005 Nov 26;366(9500):1827

[545] Topol EJ. Failing the public health--rofecoxib, Merck, and the FDA. *N Engl J Med.* 2004 Oct 21;351(17):1707-9

[546] Wolinsky H, Brune T. <u>The Serpent on the Staff: The Unhealthy Politics of the American Medical Association</u>. GP Putnam and Sons, New York, 1994

[547] Wilk CA. <u>Medicine, Monopolies, and Malice: How the Medical Establishment Tried to Destroy Chiropractic</u>. Garden City Park: Avery, 1996

[548] Carter JP. <u>Racketeering in Medicine: The Suppression of Alternatives</u>. Norfolk: Hampton Roads Pub; 1993

[549] National Alliance of Professional Psychology Providers. AMA Seeks To Control and Restrict Psychologist's Scope of Practice. http://www.nappp.org/scope.pdf Accessed November 25, 2006

[550] Daly R, American Psychiatric Association. AMA Forms Coalition to Thwart Non-M.D. Practice Expansion. *Psychiatric News* 2006 March; 41: 17

[551] Angell M. <u>The Truth About the Drug Companies: How They Deceive Us and What to Do About it</u>. Random House; August 2004

[552] Terrett AG. Misuse of the literature by medical authors in discussing spinal manipulative therapy injury. *J Manipulative Physiol Ther.* 1995 May;18(4):203-10

[553] Morley J, Rosner AL, Redwood D. A case study of misrepresentation of the scientific literature: recent reviews of chiropractic. *J Altern Complement Med.* 2001 Feb;7(1):65-78

[554] Wenban AB. Inappropriate use of the title 'chiropractor' and term 'chiropractic manipulation' in the peer-reviewed biomedical literature. *Chiropr Osteopat.* 2006 Aug 22;14:16

[555] Spivak JL. <u>The Medical Trust Unmasked</u>. Louis S. Siegfried Publishers; New York: 1961

[556] Trever W. <u>In the Public Interest</u>. Los Angeles; Scriptures Unlimited; 1972. This is probably the most authoritative documentation of the illegal actions of the AMA up to 1972; contains numerous photocopies of actual AMA documents and minutes of official meetings with overt intentionality of destroying Americans' healthcare options so that the AMA and related organizations would have a monopoly in healthcare.

[557] Getzendanner S. Permanent injunction order against AMA. *JAMA.* 1988 Jan 1;259(1):81-2

[558] "A national study released today reports 20 million American families — or one in seven families — faced hardships paying medical bills last year, which forced many to choose between getting medical attention or paying rent or buying food..." Freeman, Liz. 'Working poor' struggle to afford health care. *Naples Daily News.* Published in Naples, Florida and online at http://www.naplesnews.com/npdn/news/article/0,2071,NPDN_14940_3000546,00.html Accessed July 28, 2004

[559] "The USA's 5.8 million small companies... Health care costs are rising about 15% this year for those with fewer than 200 workers vs. 13.5% for those with 500 or more... But many small employers cite increases of 20% or more. That's made insurance the No. 1 small business problem..." Jim Hopkins. Health care tops taxes as small business cost drain. *USA TODAY.* http://www.usatoday.com/news/health/2003-04-20-small-business-costs_x.htm. Accessed July 28, 2004

[560] "Though the U.S. has slightly fewer doctors per capita than the typical developed nation, we have almost twice as many MRI machines and perform vastly more angioplasties. ...at least 31 percent of all the incremental income we'll earn between 1999 and 2010 will go to health care." Pat Regnier, *Money Magazine.* Healthcare myth: We spend too much. October 13, 2003: 11:29 AM EDT http://money.cnn.com/2003/10/08/pf/health_myths_1/ Accessed Monday, July 12, 2004

[561] "Although they spend more on health care than patients in any other industrialized nation, Americans receive the right treatment less than 60 percent of the time, resulting in unnecessary pain, expense and even death..." Ceci Connolly. U.S. Patients Spend More but Don't Get More, Study Finds: Even in Advantaged Areas, Americans Often Receive Inadequate Health Care. *Washington Post,* May 5, 2004; Page A15. On-line at http://www.washingtonpost.com/ac2/wp-dyn/A1875-2004May4 accessed on July 28, 2004

[562] McGlynn EA, Asch SM, Adams J, Keesey J, Hicks J, DeCristofaro A, Kerr EA. The quality of health care delivered to adults in the United States. *N Engl J Med.* 2003 Jun 26;348(26):2635-45

[563] Brennan TA, Leape LL, Laird NM, Hebert L, Localio AR, Lawthers AG, Newhouse JP, Weiler PC, Hiatt HH. Incidence of adverse events and negligence in hospitalized patients: results of the Harvard Medical Practice Study I. 1991. *Qual Saf Health Care.* 2004 Apr;13(2):145-51; discuss 151-2

[564] "Basically, you die earlier and spend more time disabled if you're an American rather than a member of most other advanced countries." Christopher Murray MD PhD, Director of World Health Organization's Global Program on Evidence for Health Policy http://www.who.int/inf-pr-2000/en/pr2000-life.html Accessed July 12, 2004

[565] Shi L. Health care spending, delivery, and outcome in developed countries: a cross-national comparison. *Am J Med Qual* 1997;12(2):83-93

[566] Holland EG, Degruy FV. Drug-induced disorders. *Am Fam Physician.* 1997 Nov 1;56(7):1781-8, 1791-2

[567] Brennan TA, Leape LL, Laird NM, Hebert L, Localio AR, Lawthers AG, Newhouse JP, Weiler PC, Hiatt HH. Incidence of adverse events and negligence in hospitalized patients: results of the Harvard Medical Practice Study I. 1991. *Qual Saf Health Care.* 2004 Apr;13(2):145-51; discuss 151-2

[568] Whitaker R. The case against antipsychotic drugs: a 50-year record of doing more harm than good. *Med Hypotheses.* 2004;62(1):5-13

[569] The relevance of these citations is to show that the misuse of horse estrogens in humans as "hormone replacement therapy" exemplified the application of a strong carcinogen to millions of unsuspecting women: **Zhang F, Chen Y, Pisha E, Shen L, Xiong Y, van Breemen RB, Bolton JL. The major metabolite of equilin, 4-hydroxyequilin, autoxidizes to an o-quinone which isomerizes to the potent cytotoxin 4-hydroxyequilenin-o-quinone. Chem Res Toxicol. 1999 Feb;12(2):204-13; Pisha E, Lui X, Constantinou AI, Bolton JL. Evidence that a metabolite of equine estrogens, 4-hydroxyequilenin, induces cellular transformation in vitro. Chem Res Toxicol. 2001;14(1):82-90; Zhang F, Swanson SM, van Breemen RB, Liu X, Yang Y, Gu C, Bolton JL. Equine estrogen metabolite 4-hydroxyequilenin induces DNA damage in the rat mammary tissues: formation of single-strand breaks, apurinic sites, stable adducts, and oxidized bases. Chem Res Toxicol. 2001 Dec;14(12):1654-9**

[570] Newman NM, Ling RS. Acetabular bone destruction related to non-steroidal anti-inflammatory drugs. *Lancet.* 1985 Jul 6; 2(8445): 11-4

[571] "In 1983, 2876 people died from medication errors. ... By 1993, this number had risen to 7,391 - a 2.57-fold increase." Phillips DP, Christenfeld N, Glynn LM. Increase in US medication-error deaths between 1983 and 1993. *Lancet.* 1998 Feb 28;351(9103):643-4

[572] Smith R. Medical journals are an extension of the marketing arm of pharmaceutical companies. *PLoS Med.* 2005 May;2(5):e138

[573] van der Steen WJ, Ho VK. Drugs versus diets: disillusions with Dutch health care. *Acta Biotheor.* 2001;49(2):125-40

extrinsic influences that are at play in a given disease process or individual patient. When viewed as a diagram, the web of influences can be appreciated to reveal the interconnected nature of influences and body systems and how imbalance or disruption in one area can lead to problems in another. Once homeostatic reserves and compensatory mechanisms are depleted, the patient experiences progressively worsening health (which may be asymptomatic) and the eventual manifestation of clinical disease.

Over the course of many years and discussions and reconsiderations, the faculty at IFM has elucidated eight preeminent systems or loci ("core clinical imbalances") for clinicians to consider when working with any chronic health disorder. These will be listed and described below with particular consideration of the topic of this monograph, which is neuromusculoskeletal pain and inflammation. Interested readers are directed to IFM's monograph series on topics such as "Depression" and "The Role of Gastrointestinal Inflammation in Systemic Disease" to see how this model is applied to disease states in different organ systems.

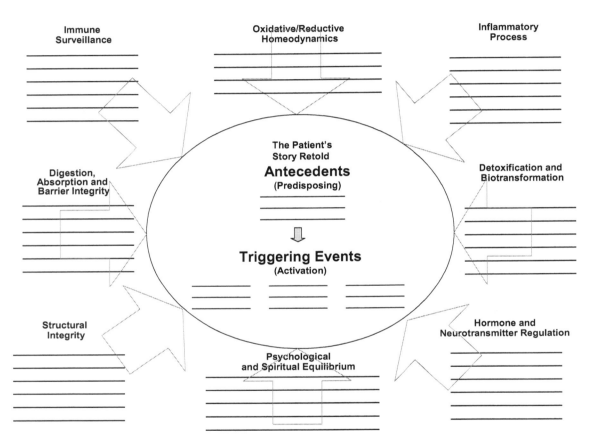

2008 rendering of The Functional Medicine Matrix: A concept, model, and clinical tool for evidence-based clinical care. Copyright Institute for Functional Medicine.

Exploring the Different Aspects of the Functional Medicine Matrix

1. Hormonal and neurotransmitter imbalances: While most clinicians are aware that neurotransmitters can either transmit pain signals or dampen their reception, many clinicians are not aware that neurotransmitter status is somewhat malleable and can be modulated with nutritional supplementation and botanical medicines. The examples that will be considered here are the tryptophan-serotonin-melatonin and the phenylalanine-tyrosine-dopamine-norepinephrine-epinephrine and enkephalin pathways.

   - Tryptophan and 5-hydroxytryptophan (5HTP) are prescription and nonprescription nutritional supplements that are the amino acid precursors for the formation of the neurotransmitter serotonin and, subsequently, the pineal hormone melatonin. Biochemically, these conversions are linear as follows: tryptophan → 5HTP → serotonin → melatonin. Tryptophan depletion and low levels of serotonin are consistently associated with depression, anxiety, exacerbation of eating disorders, and increased sensitivity to acute and chronic pain. Serotonergic pathways are impaired by chronic stress due to increased utilization of serotonin (e.g., serotonin-dependent cortisol release) and increased hepatic degradation of tryptophan by cortisol-stimulated tryptophan pyrrolase.[574] Therapeutically, supplementation with 5HTP augments serotonin and melatonin synthesis and has specific applicability in the alleviation of depression and pain syndromes such as fibromyalgia and headache, including migraine, tension headaches, and juvenile headaches.[575,576] Certainly part of the benefit from 5HTP supplementation is derived from the increased formation of melatonin, as the biological effects of melatonin extend beyond its sleep-promoting role to include powerful antioxidation, anti-infective immunostimulation[577], and preservation of mitochondrial function, a benefit which is of particular relevance to the treatment of fibromyalgia.[578]

- The conditionally essential fatty acids found in fish oil modulate serotonergic and adrenergic activity in the human brain[579], and given the role of serotonin and norepinephrine in the central processing of pain perception[580], a reasonable hypothesis holds that the pain-relieving activity of fish oil supplementation[581] is partly due to central modulation of pain perception and is not wholly due to modulation of eicosanoid production and inflammatory mediator transcription as previously believed.

- Vitamin D3 supplementation may also augment serotonergic activity[582], and this mechanism may partly explain the mood-enhancing and pain-relieving benefits of vitamin D3 supplementation. Attentive readers will note that this brief discussion has already begun to bridge the gaps between nutritional status, neurotransmitter synthesis, pain sensitivity, immune function, and mitochondrial bioenergetics.

- Supplementation with DL-phenylalanine (DLPA; racemic mixture of D- and L-forms of the amino acid phenylalanine derived from synthetic production) has long been used in the treatment of pain and depression.[583] The nutritional L-isomer is converted from phenylalanine to tyrosine to L-dopa to dopamine to norepinephrine and epinephrine. Augmentation of this pathway promotes resistance to fatigue, depression, and pain. The synthetic D-isomer augments pain-relieving enkephalin function by inhibiting enkephalin degradation by the enzyme carboxypeptidase A (enkephalinase); the resultant augmentation of enkephalin levels is generally believed to underlie the analgesic and mood-enhancing benefits of DLPA supplementation.

- Therapeutic massage is yet another means to modulate neurotransmitter synthesis for the alleviation of pain. In a study of patients with chronic back pain, massage increased serotonin and dopamine levels (measured in urine).[584]

Hormonal imbalances are particularly relevant to the discussion of chronic pain caused by inflammation characteristic of autoimmune diseases such as rheumatoid arthritis (RA). Often clinically subtle but nonetheless of extreme importance, these hormonal influences on painful inflammation are worthy of their own detailed discussion and thus will be reviewed later in this monograph in the context of the prototypic inflammatory disease RA. Generally speaking and with a few noted exceptions (such as Sjogren's syndrome), the research literature points to a specific pattern of hormonal imbalances among

[574] Sandyk R. Tryptophan availability and the susceptibility to stress in multiple sclerosis: a hypothesis. *Int J Neurosci*. 1996 Jul;86(1-2):47-53

[575] Turner EH, Loftis JM, Blackwell AD. Serotonin a la carte: supplementation with the serotonin precursor 5-hydroxytryptophan. *Pharmacol Ther*. 2006 Mar;109(3):325-38

[576] Birdsall TC. 5-Hydroxytryptophan: a clinically-effective serotonin precursor. *Altern Med Rev*. 1998 Aug;3(4):271-80

[577] Gitto E, Karbownik M, Reiter RJ, Tan DX, Cuzzocrea S, Chiurazzi P, Cordaro S, Corona G, Trimarchi G, Barberi I. Effects of melatonin treatment in septic newborns. *Pediatr Res*. 2001 Dec;50(6):756-60

[578] Acuna-Castroviejo D, Escames G, Reiter RJ. Melatonin therapy in fibromyalgia. *J Pineal Res*. 2006 Jan;40(1):98-9

[579] Hibbeln JR, Ferguson TA, Blasbalg TL. Omega-3 fatty acid deficiencies in neurodevelopment, aggression and autonomic dysregulation: opportunities for intervention. *Int Rev Psychiatry*. 2006 Apr;18(2):107-18

[580] Wise TN, Fishbain DA, Holder-Perkins V. Painful physical symptoms in depression: a clinical challenge. *Pain Med*. 2007 Sep;8 Suppl 2:S75-82

[581] Goldberg RJ, Katz J. A meta-analysis of the analgesic effects of omega-3 polyunsaturated fatty acid supplementation for inflammatory joint pain. *Pain*. 2007 May;129(1-2):210-23

[582] Lansdowne AT, Provost SC. Vitamin D3 enhances mood in healthy subjects during winter. *Psychopharmacology* (Berl). 1998 Feb;135(4):319-23

[583] Russell AL, McCarty MF. DL-phenylalanine markedly potentiates opiate analgesia - an example of nutrient/pharmaceutical up-regulation of the endogenous analgesia system. *Med Hypotheses*. 2000 Oct;55(4):283-8

[584] Hernandez-Reif M, Field T, Krasnegor J, Theakston H. Lower back pain is reduced and range of motion increased after massage therapy. *Int J Neurosci* 2001;106(3-4):131-45

patients with autoimmunity, and this pattern is consistent with the proinflammatory and immunodysregulatory effects of estrogens and prolactin and the anti-inflammatory and immunomodulatory effects of cortisol, dehydroepiandrosterone (DHEA), and testosterone. Patients with autoimmune neuromusculoskeletal inflammation generally display a complete or partial pattern of hormonal disturbances typified by elevated estrogen and prolactin and lowered testosterone, DHEA, and cortisol; appropriate therapeutic correction of these imbalances can safely result in disease amelioration. Rectification of endocrinologic imbalances ("orthoendocrinology") will be discussed in the section on RA and has been detailed with broader clinical applicability elsewhere by this author.[585]

2. <u>Oxidation-reduction imbalances and mitochondropathy</u>: Oxidative stress results from the chronic systemic inflammation seen in painful inflammatory disorders such as RA, and oxidative stress contributes to the perpetuation and exacerbation of inflammatory diseases via expedited tissue destruction and alterations in gene transcription and resultant enhancement of inflammatory mediator production.[586] Immune activation increases production of reactive oxygen species (ROS; "free radicals"), and oxidant stress increases activation of pro-inflammatory transcription factors (such as nuclear factor KappaB, NFkB) and also increases spontaneous oxidative modification of endogenous proteins such as cartilage matrix which then undergoes expedited degradation or immunologic attack; thus a vicious cycle of oxidation and inflammation exacerbates and perpetuates various inflammation-associated diseases, resulting in therapeutic recalcitrance and autonomous disease progression.[587,588] A rational clinical approach to breaking this vicious pathogenic cycle can include simultaneous antioxidation and immunomodulation, the former with diet optimization and nutritional supplementation and the latter with allergen avoidance, hormonal correction, xenobiotic detoxification, and specific phytonutritional modulation of pro-inflammatory pathways. Severe and acute inflammation can and often should be suppressed pharmacologically, but sole reliance on pharmacologic immunosuppression leaves the patient vulnerable to iatrogenic immunosuppression and the well-known increased risk for cardiovascular disease, infection, and clinical malignancy while failing to address the underlying biochemical and immunologic imbalances which lie at the bottom of all chronic inflammatory and autoimmune diseases. The contribution of mitochondrial dysfunction to chronic recurrent or persistent pain is most plainly demonstrated in migraine and fibromyalgia (discussed later in this monograph). An important characteristic of migraine is mitochondrial dysfunction, the severity of which correlates positively with the severity of the headache syndrome.[589] In fibromyalgia, numerous abnormalities in cellular bioenergetics are noted, which correlate clinically with the lowered lactate threshold, persistent muscle pain, reduced functional capacity, and the subjective fatigue that characterize the disorder.[590] Nutritional preservation and enhancement of mitochondrial function was termed "mitochondrial resuscitation" by Jeffrey Bland PhD in the 1990s, and clinical implementation of such an approach generally includes, in addition to diet and lifestyle modification, supplementation with coenzyme Q-10, niacin, riboflavin, thiamin, lipoic acid, magnesium, and other nutrients and botanical medicines which enhance production of adenosine triphosphate (ATP).[591]

3. <u>Detoxification and biotransformational imbalances</u>: As our environment becomes increasingly polluted and as researchers and clinicians mature and expand their appreciation and knowledge of the adverse effects of xenobiotics (toxic metals and chemicals), healthcare providers will need to attend to their patients' detoxification capacity and xenobiotic load as a component of the prevention and treatment of disease. By now, senior students and practicing clinicians should be aware of the association of xenobiotics in prototypic diseases such as Parkinson's disease[592,593], adult-onset diabetes mellitus[594,595,596,597],

[585] Vasquez A. *Integrative Rheumatology*. Fort Worth, Texas; Integrative & Biological Medicine Research & Consulting, 2007 OptimalHealthResearch.com
[586] Hitchon CA, El-Gabalawy HS. Oxidation in rheumatoid arthritis. *Arthritis Res Ther*. 2004;6(6):265-78
[587] Tak PP, Zvaifler NJ, Green DR, Firestein GS. Rheumatoid arthritis and p53: how oxidative stress might alter the course of inflammatory diseases. *Immunol Today*. 2000 Feb;21(2):78-82
[588] Kurien BT, Hensley K, Bachmann M, Scofield RH. Oxidatively modified autoantigens in autoimmune diseases. *Free Radic Biol Med*. 2006 Aug 15;41(4):549-56
[589] Lodi R, Kemp GJ, Montagna P, Pierangeli G, Cortelli P, Iotti S, Radda GK, Barbiroli B. Quantitative analysis of skeletal muscle bioenergetics and proton efflux in migraine and cluster headache. *J Neurol Sci*. 1997 Feb 27;146(1):73-80
[590] Park JH, Phothimat P, Oates CT, Hernanz-Schulman M, Olsen NJ. Use of P-31 magnetic resonance spectroscopy to detect metabolic abnormalities in muscles of patients with fibromyalgia. *Arthritis Rheum*. 1998 Mar;41(3):406-13
[591] Pieczenik SR, Neustadt J. Mitochondrial dysfunction and molecular pathways of disease. *Exp Mol Pathol*. 2007 Aug;83(1):84-92
[592] Corrigan FM, Wienburg CL, Shore RF, Daniel SE, Mann D. Organochlorine insecticides in substantia nigra in Parkinson's disease. *J Toxicol Environ Health A*. 2000 Feb 25;59(4):229-34

and attention-deficit hyperactivity disorder.[598,599,600] The role of xenobiotic exposure and impaired detoxification in neuromusculoskeletal pain and inflammatory disorders is more subtle and is generally mediated through the resultant immunotoxicity that manifests as autoimmunity. Occasionally, clinicians will encounter patients with musculoskeletal symptomatology that defies standard diagnosis and treatment but which responds remarkably and permanently to empiric clinical detoxification treatment; such a case will be presented in the Case Reports later in this monograph. The numerous roles of xenobiotic exposure in the genesis and perpetuation of chronic health problems and the role of clinical detoxification in the treatment of such problems has been detailed elsewhere by Crinnion[601,602,603,604,605], Rea[606], Bland[607,608], Vasquez[609,610], and others.[611,612]

4. <u>Immune imbalances</u>: Immune imbalances have an obvious role in musculoskeletal inflammation when discussed in the context of autoimmune diseases such as rheumatoid arthritis, ankylosing spondylitis, and systemic lupus erythematosus. While the standard medical approach to this pathophysiology has focused almost exclusively on the pharmacologic suppression of resultant inflammation and tissue destruction, other disciplines such as naturopathic medicine and functional medicine have emphasized the importance of determining and addressing the underlying causes of such immune imbalance. While clinicians of all disciplines must appreciate the important role of pharmacologic immunosuppression in the treatment of inflammatory exacerbations as seen with giant cell arteritis or neuropsychiatric lupus, they should also appreciate that sole reliance on immunosuppression for long-term management of inflammatory disorders is destined to therapeutic failure insofar as it does not correct the underlying cause of the disease and creates dependency upon perpetual immunosuppression with its attendant costs (not uncommonly in the range of $20,000 - 50,000 per year) and adverse effects including infection and increased risk for cancer. Rather than presuming that immune dysfunction and the resultant inflammation and autoimmunity are results of spontaneous generation, astute clinicians seek to identify and correct the causes of these immune imbalances. By identifying and correcting the underlying causes of immune imbalance (when possible), clinicians can lessen or obviate the need for chronic polypharmaceutical treatment with anti-inflammatory and immunosuppressive agents. Vasquez[613] proposed that secondary immune imbalances (distinguished from primary congenital disorders) generally arise from one or more of five main problems: ❶ habitual consumption of a pro-inflammatory diet, ❷ food allergies and intolerances, ❸ microbial dysbiosis, including multifocal polydysbiosis, ❹ hormonal imbalances, and ❺ xenobiotic exposure and accumulation resulting in immunotoxicity via bystander activation and enhanced processing of autoantigens as well as haptenization and neoantigen formation. These influences may act singularly or when combined may be additive and synergistic. While

[593] Fleming L, Mann JB, Bean J, Briggle T, Sanchez-Ramos JR. Parkinson's disease and brain levels of organochlorine pesticides. *Ann Neurol*. 1994 Jul;36(1):100-3

[594] Fujiyoshi PT, Michalek JE, Matsumura F. Molecular epidemiologic evidence for diabetogenic effects of dioxin exposure in U.S. Air force veterans of the Vietnam war. *Environ Health Perspect*, 2006 Nov;114(11):1677-83

[595] Lee DH, Lee IK, Song K, Steffes M, Toscano W, Baker BA, Jacobs DR Jr. A strong dose-response relation between serum concentrations of persistent organic pollutants and diabetes: results from the National Health and Examination Survey 1999-2002. *Diabetes Care* 2006 Jul;29(7):1638-44

[596] Lee DH, Lee IK, Jin SH, Steffes M, Jacobs DR Jr. Association between serum concentrations of persistent organic pollutants and insulin resistance among nondiabetic adults: results from the National Health and Nutrition Examination Survey 1999-2002. *Diabetes Care*, 2007 Mar;30(3):622-8

[597] Remillard RB, Bunce NJ. Linking dioxins to diabetes: epidemiology and biologic plausibility. *Environ Health Perspect*, 2002 Sep;110(9):853-8

[598] Rauh VA, Garfinkel R, Perera FP, Andrews HF, Hoepner L, Barr DB, Whitehead R, Tang D, Whyatt RW. Impact of prenatal chlorpyrifos exposure on neurodevelopment in the first 3 years of life among inner-city children. *Pediatrics*. 2006 Dec;118(6):e1845-59

[599] Cheuk DK, Wong V. Attention-deficit hyperactivity disorder and blood mercury level: a case-control study in Chinese children. *Neuropediatrics*. 2006 Aug;37(4):234-40

[600] Nigg JT, Knottnerus GM, Martel MM, Nikolas M, Cavanagh K, Karmaus W, Rappley MD. Low blood lead levels associated with clinically diagnosed attention-deficit/hyperactivity disorder and mediated by weak cognitive control. *Biol Psychiatry*. 2008 Feb 1;63(3):325-31

[601] Crinnion W. Results of a Decade of Naturopathic Treatment for Environmental Illnesses: A Review of Clinical Records. *J Naturopathic Medicine* vol. 7; 2, 21-27

[602] Crinnion WJ. Environmental medicine, part 1: the human burden of environmental toxins and their common health effects. *Altern Med Rev*. 2000 Feb;5(1):52-63

[603] Crinnion WJ. Environmental medicine, part 2 - health effects of and protection from ubiquitous airborne solvent exposure. *Altern Med Rev*. 2000 Apr;5(2):133-43

[604] Crinnion WJ. Environmental medicine, part 3: long-term effects of chronic low-dose mercury exposure. *Altern Med Rev*. 2000 Jun;5(3):209-23

[605] Crinnion WJ. Environmental medicine, part 4: pesticides - biologically persistent and ubiquitous toxins. *Altern Med Rev*. 2000 Oct;5(5):432-47

[606] Rea WJ, Pan Y, Johnson AR. Clearing of toxic volatile hydrocarbons from humans. *Bol Asoc Med P R*. 1991 Jul;83(7):321-4

[607] Bland JS, Barrager E, Reedy RG, Bland K. A Medical Food-Supplemented Detoxification Program in the Management of Chronic Health Problems. *Altern Ther Health Med*. 1995 Nov 1;1(5):62-71

[608] Minich DM, Bland JS. Acid-alkaline balance: role in chronic disease and detoxification. *Altern Ther Health Med*. 2007 Jul-Aug;13(4):62-5

[609] Vasquez A. <u>Integrative Rheumatology: Second Edition</u>. Fort Worth, Texas; Integrative and Biological Medicine Research and Consulting, 2007 OptimalHealthResearch.com

[610] Vasquez A. Diabetes: Are Toxins to Blame? *Naturopathy Digest* 2007; April

[611] Kilburn KH, Warsaw RH, Shields MG. Neurobehavioral dysfunction in firemen exposed to polychlorinated biphenyls (PCBs): possible improvement after detoxification. *Arch Environ Health*. 1989 Nov-Dec;44(6):345-50

[612] Cecchini M, LoPresti V. Drug residues store in the body following cessation of use: impacts on neuroendocrine balance and behavior--use of the Hubbard sauna regimen to remove toxins and restore health. *Med Hypotheses*. 2007;68(4):868-79

[613] **Vasquez A.** <u>Integrative Rheumatology: Second Edition</u>. Fort Worth, Texas; Integrative and Biological Medicine Research and Consulting, 2007 OptimalHealthResearch.com

it is beyond the scope of this monograph to detail each of these here, they will be sufficiently reviewed in later sections dealing with assessment and interventions as well as in the clinical focus subsections, particularly the section on rheumatoid arthritis.

5. <u>Inflammatory imbalances</u>: Inflammatory imbalances may be distinguished from immune imbalances insofar as inflammatory imbalances connote disorders of inflammatory mediator production in the absence of the immunodysfunction that typifies allergy, autoimmunity, or immunosuppression. Here again, long-term consumption of a pro-inflammatory diet[614] is a primary consideration because such a diet typically oversupplies inflammatory precursors such as arachidonate and undersupplies anti-inflammatory phytonutrients such as vitamin D, zinc, selenium, and the numerous phytochemicals that reduce activation of inflammatory pathways.[615,616,617,618] Three of the best examples of correctable inflammatory imbalances are those due to vitamin D deficiency, fatty acid imbalances, and overconsumption of simple sugars and saturated fats. Vitamin D deficiency is a widespread and serious health problem that spans nearly all geographic regions and socioeconomic strata with several important adverse effects. Vitamin D deficiency results in systemic inflammation[619] and chronic musculoskeletal pain[620] which both resolve quickly upon correction of the nutritional deficiency. Similarly and consistent with the Western/American pattern of dietary intake, overconsumption of alpha-linoleic acid and arachidonate along with underconsumption of alpha-linolenic acid (ALA), gamma-linolenic acid (GLA), eicosapentaenoic acid (EPA), docosahexaenoic acid (DHA), and oleic acid subtly yet powerfully shift nutrigenomic tendency and precursor availability in favor of enhanced systemic inflammation. Correction of this imbalance such as with reduced consumption of arachidonate and increased consumption of EPA and DHA has consistently proven to be of significant clinical value in the management of chronic inflammatory disorders.[621,622] Measurable increases in systemic inflammation and oxidative stress follow glucose challenge[623], consumption of saturated fatty acids as found in cream[624], and consumption of a "fast food" breakfast, which triggers the prototypic inflammatory activator NF-kappaB for enhanced production of inflammatory mediators.[625] This triad (vitamin D deficiency, fatty acid imbalance, and overconsumption of sugars and saturated fats) is typical of the Western/American pattern of dietary intake, and the molecular means and clinical consequences of such dietary choices is quite clear, evidenced by burgeoning epidemics of metabolic and inflammatory diseases.

6. <u>Digestive, absorptive, and microbiological imbalances</u>: The grouping of digestive and absorptive considerations suggests that the alimentary tract and its accessory organs of the liver, gall bladder and pancreas will be the focus of these core clinical imbalances, and the addition of microbiological imbalances should remind current clinicians that gastrointestinal dysbiosis is an important and frequent clinical consideration. Impaired digestion begins neither in the stomach nor in the mouth, but it stems rather from any socioeconomic milieu which deprives people of the means to prepare wholesome health-promoting meals and the time to consume those meals in a relaxed parasympathetic-dominant mode, preferably among good company, stimulating conversation, and appropriate ambiance. Poor dentition, xerostomia, hypochlorhydria, cholestasis or cholecystectomy, pancreatic insufficiency, mucosal atrophy,

[614] Seaman DR. The diet-induced proinflammatory state: a cause of chronic pain and other degenerative diseases? *J Manipulative Physiol Ther*. 2002 Mar-Apr;25(3):168-79

[615] **Vasquez A**. Reducing Pain and Inflammation Naturally. Part 1: New Insights into Fatty Acid Biochemistry and the Influence of Diet. *Nutritional Perspectives* 2004; October: 5, 7-10, 12, 14

[616] **Vasquez A**. Reducing Pain and Inflammation Naturally. Part 2: New Insights into Fatty Acid Supplementation and Its Effect on Eicosanoid Production and Genetic Expression. *Nutritional Perspectives* 2005; January: 5-16

[617] **Vasquez A**. Reducing pain and inflammation naturally - Part 3: Improving overall health while safely and effectively treating musculoskeletal pain. *Nutritional Perspectives* 2005; 28: 34-38, 40-42

[618] **Vasquez A**. Reducing pain and inflammation naturally - Part 4: Nutritional and Botanical Inhibition of NF-kappaB, the Major Intracellular Amplifier of the Inflammatory Cascade. A Practical Clinical Strategy Exemplifying Anti-Inflammatory Nutrigenomics. *Nutritional Perspectives* 2005;July: 5-12

[619] Timms PM, Mannan N, Hitman GA, Noonan K, Mills PG, Syndercombe-Court D, Aganna E, Price CP, Boucher BJ. Circulating MMP9, vitamin D and variation in the TIMP-1 response with VDR genotype: mechanisms for inflammatory damage in chronic disorders? *QJM*. 2002 Dec;95(12):787-96

[620] Al Faraj S, Al Mutairi K. Vitamin D deficiency and chronic low back pain in Saudi Arabia. *Spine*. 2003 Jan 15;28(2):177-9

[621] James MJ, Gibson RA, Cleland LG. Dietary polyunsaturated fatty acids and inflammatory mediator production. *Am J Clin Nutr*. 2000 Jan;71(1 Suppl):343S-8S

[622] James MJ, Proudman SM, Cleland LG. Dietary n-3 fats as adjunctive therapy in a prototypic inflammatory disease: issues and obstacles for use in rheumatoid arthritis. Prostaglandins *Leukot Essent Fatty Acids*. 2003 Jun;68(6):399-405

[623] Mohanty P, Hamouda W, Garg R, Aljada A, Ghanim H, Dandona P. Glucose challenge stimulates reactive oxygen species (ROS) generation by leucocytes. *J Clin Endocrinol Metab*. 2000 Aug;85(8):2970-3

[624] Mohanty P, Ghanim H, Hamouda W, Aljada A, Garg R, Dandona P. Both lipid and protein intakes stimulate increased generation of reactive oxygen species by polymorphonuclear leukocytes and mononuclear cells. *Am J Clin Nutr*. 2002 Apr;75(4):767-72

[625] Aljada A, Mohanty P, Ghanim H, Abdo T, Tripathy D, Chaudhuri A, Dandona P. Increase in intranuclear nuclear factor kappaB and decrease in inhibitor kappaB in mononuclear cells after a mixed meal: evidence for a proinflammatory effect. *Am J Clin Nutr*. 2004 Apr;79(4):682-90

altered gut motility, and bacterial overgrowth of the small bowel are important and common contributors to impaired digestion and absorption; clinicians should consider these frequently and implement treatment with a low threshold for intervention. The relevance of these problems to pain and the musculoskeletal system is generally that of malnutrition and its macro- and micronutrient consequences. Sunlight-deprived individuals must rely on dietary sources of vitamin D, which are hardly adequate for the prevention of overt deficiency; any impairment in digestion, emulsification, or absorption of this fat-soluble vitamin can readily lead to hypovitaminosis D and its resultant musculoskeletal consequences of osteomalacia and unremitting pain.[626] Consumption of foods to which the individual is sensitized ("food allergies") can trigger migraine and other chronic headaches[627,628] as well as generalized musculoskeletal pain and arthritis.[629,630,631.] Avoidance of the offending foods often results in amelioration or complete remission of the painful syndrome at low cost and high efficacy without reliance on expensive or potentially harmful or addictive pain-relieving drugs. Occasionally, gluten enteropathy (celiac disease) presents with arthritic pain and chronic synovitis; the pain and inflammation remit on a gluten-free diet.[632] Alterations in intestinal microbial balance or an individual's unique response to endogenous bacteria (i.e., dysbiosis) can lead to systemic inflammation, arthritis, vasculitis, and musculoskeletal pain; clinical nuances and molecular mechanisms of gastrointestinal dysbiosis will be surveyed later in this monograph based on a previous review by Vasquez.[633] Clinicians should appreciate that dysbiosis can occur at sites other than the gastrointestinal tract, most importantly the nasopharynx and genitourinary tracts. Eradication of the occult infection or mucosal colonization often results in marked reductions in systemic inflammation and its clinical complications. Interested readers are directed to the excellent review by Noah[634] on the relevance of dysbiosis and its treatment relative to psoriasis; additional citations and clinical applications will be discussed later in this monograph.

7. <u>Structural imbalances from cellular membrane function to the musculoskeletal system</u>: Molecular structural imbalances lie at the heart of the concept of "biochemical individuality" originated by Roger J. Williams[635] in 1956, and this concept was soon thereafter expanded into the theory and practice of "orthomolecular medicine" pioneered by Linus Pauling and colleagues.[636,637] Pauling is considered by many authorities to be the original source of the concept of molecular medicine because he coined the phrase "molecular disease" after his team's discovery in 1949 that sickle cell anemia resulted from a single amino acid substitution that caused physical deformation of the hemoglobin molecule in hypoxic conditions.[638] (One of Pauling's students, Jeffery Bland, continued this legacy with the organization of "functional medicine" which now lives on as the Institute for Functional Medicine.[639]) Single nucleotide polymorphisms (SNP; pronounced "snip") are DNA sequence variations that can result in amino acid substitutions that render the final protein (e.g., structural protein or enzyme) abnormal in structure and therefore function. This aberrancy may or may not cause clinical disease (depending on the severity and importance of the variation), and consequences of the dysfunction may be occult, subtle, or obvious. One of the most powerful and effective means for treating diseases resultant from SNPs that result in enzyme defects is the use of high-dose vitamin supplementation, and this forms the scientific basis for "mega-vitamin therapy" as elegantly and authoritatively reviewed by Bruce Ames, et al.[640] SNP-induced

[626] Basha B, Rao DS, Han ZH, Parfitt AM. Osteomalacia due to vitamin D depletion: a neglected consequence of intestinal malabsorption. *Am J Med*. 2000 Mar;108(4):296-300

[627] Grant EC. Food allergies and migraine. *Lancet*. 1979 May 5;1(8123):966-9

[628] Millichap JG, Yee MM. The diet factor in pediatric and adolescent migraine. *Pediatr Neurol*. 2003 Jan;28(1):9-15

[629] van de Laar MA, Aalbers M, Bruins FG, et al. Food intolerance in rheumatoid arthritis. II. Clinical and histological aspects. *Ann Rheum Dis*. 1992 ;51(3):303-6

[630] Golding DN. Is there an allergic synovitis? *J R Soc Med*. 1990 May;83(5):312-4

[631] Hvatum M, Kanerud L, Hällgren R, Brandtzaeg P. The gut-joint axis: cross reactive food antibodies in rheumatoid arthritis. *Gut*. 2006 Sep;55:1240-7

[632] Bourne JT, Kumar P, Huskisson EC, Mageed R, Unsworth DJ, Wojtulewski JA. Arthritis and coeliac disease. *Ann Rheum Dis*. 1985 Sep;44(9):592-8

[633] **Vasquez A**. Reducing Pain and Inflammation Naturally. Part 6: Nutritional and Botanical Treatments Against "Silent Infections" and Gastrointestinal Dysbiosis, Commonly Overlooked Causes of Neuromusculoskeletal Inflammation and Chronic Health Problems. *Nutr Perspect* 2006; Jan: 5-21

[634] Noah PW. The role of microorganisms in psoriasis. *Semin Dermatol*. 1990 Dec;9(4):269-76

[635] Williams RJ. <u>Biochemical Individuality : The Basis for the Genetotrophic Concept</u>. Austin and London: University of Texas Press, 1956. Page x

[636] Pauling L. On the Orthomolecular Environment of the Mind: Orthomolecular Theory. In: Williams RJ, Kalita DK. <u>A Physician's Handbook on Orthomolecular Medicine</u>. New Cannan; Keats Publishing: 1977. Page 76

[637] Pauling L, Robinson AB, Teranishi R, Cary P. Quantitative analysis of urine vapor and breath by gas-liquid partition chromatography. *Proc Natl Acad Sci U S A*. 1971 Oct;68(10):2374-6

[638] Pauling L, Itano HA, Singer SJ, Wells IC. Sickle cell anemia, a molecular disease. *Science*. 1949 Nov 25;110(2865):543-8

[639] Bland JS. Jeffrey S. Bland, PhD, FACN, CNS: functional medicine pioneer. *Altern Ther Health Med*. 2004 Sep-Oct;10(5):74-81

[640] Ames BN, Elson-Schwab I, Silver EA. High-dose vitamin therapy stimulates variant enzymes with decreased coenzyme binding affinity (increased K(m)): relevance to genetic disease and polymorphisms. *Am J Clin Nutr*. 2002 Apr;75(4):616-58

alterations in enzyme structure reduce affinity for vitamin-derived coenzyme binding; this reduced affinity can be "overpowered" by administration of high doses of the required vitamin cofactor to increase tissue concentrations of the nutrient to promote binding of the enzyme with its ligand for the performance of enzymatic function. Thus, the scientific rationale for nutritional therapy is derived in part from the recognition that altered enzymatic function due to altered enzyme structure can often be corrected by administration of supradietary doses of nutrients. Relatedly, the structure and function of cell membranes is determined by their composition, which is influenced by dietary intake of fatty acids, and which influences production prostaglandins and leukotrienes. This is an important aspect of the scientific rationale for the use of specific fatty acid supplements in the prevention and treatment of painful inflammatory musculoskeletal disease. Cell membrane structure and function can also be altered by systemic oxidative stress; the concomitant alterations in intracellular ions (e.g., calcium) and receptor function along with activation of transcription factors such as NF-kappaB contribute to widespread physiologic impairment which creates a vicious cycle of inflammation, metabolic disturbance, and additional free radical generation.[641,642] Somatic dysfunction, musculoskeletal disorders, and inefficient biomechanics contribute to pain, increased production of inflammatory mediators, and the expedited degeneration of tissues such as collagen and cartilage matrix. Physicians trained in clinical biomechanics and physical medicine appreciate the subtle nuances of musculoskeletal structure-function relationships and address these problems directly with physical and manual means rather than ignoring the physical problem and only treating its biochemical sequelae. While biomechanics, palpatory diagnosis, and manual therapeutics takes years of diligent study for the achievement of proficiency, some of these concepts will be reviewed later in this monograph, particularly in the section on chronic low back pain.

8. <u>Psychological and Spiritual Equilibrium</u>: The connections between physical pain and psychoemotional status and events is worthy of thorough discussion and not merely for the sake of improving upon outdated clinical practices which have typically marginalized these ethereal considerations or considered them only long enough to substantiate psychopharmaceutical intervention. A survey of the literature makes clear the interconnected nature of pain, inflammation, psychoemotional stress, depression, social isolation, and nutritional status; due to space limitations in this monograph, a brief overview must necessarily suffice for the exemplification of representative concepts. Stressful and depressive life events promote the development, persistence, and exacerbation of disorders of pain and inflammation through nutritional, hormonal, immunologic, oxidative, and microbiologic mechanisms. Stated most simply, the perception of stressful events and the resultant neurohormonal cascade results in expedited metabolic utilization and increased urinary excretion of nutrients (e.g., tryptophan , and zinc, magnesium, retinol, respectively) which sum to effect nutritional imbalances and depletion, particularly when the stress response is severe and prolonged.[643,644,645] Specific to the consideration of pain, the depletion of tryptophan (and thus serotonin and melatonin) leaves the patient vulnerable to increased pain from lack of antinociceptive serotonin and to increased inflammation due to impaired endogenous production of anti-inflammatory cortisol, the adrenal release of which requires serotonin-dependent stimulation.[646] Severe stress, inflammation, and drugs used to suppress immune-mediated tissue damage (e.g., cyclosporine) increase urinary excretion of magnesium[647], and the eventual magnesium depletion renders the patient more vulnerable to hyperalgesia, depression, and other central nervous system and psychiatric disorders.[648,649] Furthermore, experimental and clinical data have shown that magnesium deficiency leads to a systemic pro-inflammatory state associated with oxidative stress and increased levels of the

[641] Evans JL, Maddux BA, Goldfine ID. The molecular basis for oxidative stress-induced insulin resistance. *Antioxid Redox Signal*. 2005 Jul-Aug;7(7-8):1040-52

[642] Joseph JA, Denisova N, Fisher D, Shukitt-Hale B, Bickford P, Prior R, Cao G. Membrane and receptor modifications of oxidative stress vulnerability in aging. Nutritional considerations. *Ann N Y Acad Sci*. 1998 Nov 20;854:268-76

[643] Stephensen CB, Alvarez JO, Kohatsu J, Hardmeier R, Kennedy JI Jr, Gammon RB Jr. Vitamin A is excreted in the urine during acute infection. *Am J Clin Nutr*. 1994 Sep;60(3):388-92

[644] Ingenbleek Y, Bernstein L. The stressful condition as a nutritionally dependent adaptive dichotomy. *Nutrition*. 1999 Apr;15(4):305-20

[645] Henrotte JG, Plouin PF, Lévy-Leboyer C, Moser G, Sidoroff-Girault N, Franck G, Santarromana M, Pineau M. Blood and urinary magnesium, zinc, calcium, free fatty acids, and catecholamines in type A and type B subjects. *J Am Coll Nutr*. 1985;4(2):165-72

[646] Sandyk R. Tryptophan availability and the susceptibility to stress in multiple sclerosis: a hypothesis. *Int J Neurosci*. 1996 Jul;86(1-2):47-53

[647] DiPalma JR. Magnesium replacement therapy. *Am Fam Physician*. 1990 Jul;42(1):173-6

[648] Murck H. Magnesium and affective disorders. *Nutr Neurosci*. 2002 Dec;5(6):375-89

[649] Hashizume N, Mori M. An analysis of hypermagnesemia and hypomagnesemia. *Jpn J Med*. 1990 Jul-Aug;29(4):368-72

nociceptive and proinflammatory neurotransmitter substance P.[650] Stress increases secretion of prolactin, a hormone which plays an important pathogenic role in chronic inflammation and autoimmunity.[651,652] An abundance of experimental and clinical research supports the model that chronic psychoemotional stress reduces mucosal immunity, increases intestinal permeability, and allows for increased intestinal colonization by microbes that then stimulate immune responses that cross-react with musculoskeletal tissues and result in the clinical manifestation of autoimmunity and painful rheumatic syndromes which appear clinically as variants of acute and chronic reactive arthritis (formerly Reiter' syndrome[653]) in susceptible patients.[654,655,656,657,658,659,660,661] Very interestingly, certain intestinal bacteria can sense when their human host is stressed, and they take advantage of the situation by becoming more virulent whereas previously these same bacteria may have been incapable of causing disease.[662,663] Psychoemotional stress also reduces mucosal immunity and increases colonization in locations other than the gastrointestinal tract. Microbial colonization of the genitourinary tract ("genitourinary dysbiosis"[664]) appears highly relevant in the genesis and perpetuation of rheumatoid arthritis.[665,666,667,668] Stressful life events also lower testosterone in men and the resultant lack of hormonal immunomodulation can increase the frequency and severity of exacerbations of rheumatoid arthritis[669]; resultant inflammation further suppresses testosterone production and bioavailability[670] leading to a self-perpetuating cycle of hypogonadism and inflammation. Thus, by numerous routes and mechanisms, psychoemotional stress increases the prevalence, persistence, and severity of musculoskeletal inflammation and pain.

Psychiatric codiagnoses are common among patients with painful neuromusculoskeletal disorders, and when the prevailing medical logic cannot solve the musculoskeletal riddle, the disorder is often ascribed to its accompanying mental disorder. The "appropriate" treatment from this perspective is the prescription of psychoactive drugs, generally of the "antidepressant" class. Science-based explanations are needed to expand clinicians' consideration of new possibilities which may someday prevail over commonplace suppositions that leave both clinician and patient trapped within a paradigm of futilely cyclical reasoning and its resultant simplistic symptom-targeting interventions. The following subsections provide alternatives to the "idiopathic pain is caused by its associated depression and both should be treated with antidepressant drugs" hypothesis.

    a. <u>Pain, inflammation, and mental depression are final common pathways for nutritional deficiencies and imbalances</u>: As a scientific community we now know that the epidemic problem

[650] Weglicki W, Quamme G, Tucker K, Haigney M, Resnick L. Potassium, magnesium, and electrolyte imbalance and complications in disease management. *Clin Exp Hypertens.* 2005 Jan;27(1):95-112

[651] Imrich R. The role of neuroendocrine system in the pathogenesis of rheumatic diseases (minireview). *Endocr Regul.* 2002 Jun;36(2):95-106

[652] Orbach H, Shoenfeld Y. Hyperprolactinemia and autoimmune diseases. Autoimmun Rev. 2007 Sep;6(8):537-42

[653] Panush RS, Wallace DJ, Dorff RE, Engleman EP. Retraction of the suggestion to use the term "Reiter's syndrome" sixty-five years later: the legacy of Reiter, a war criminal, should not be eponymic honor but rather condemnation. *Arthritis Rheum.* 2007 Feb;56(2):693-4

[654] Tlaskalová-Hogenová H, Stepánková R, Hudcovic T, Tucková L, Cukrowska B, Lodinová-Zádníková R, Kozáková H, Rossmann P, Bártová J, Sokol D, Funda DP, Borovská D, Reháková Z, Sinkora J, Hofman J, Drastich P, Kokesová A. Commensal bacteria (normal microflora), mucosal immunity and chronic inflammatory and autoimmune diseases. *Immunol Lett.* 2004 May 15;93(2-3):97-108

[655] Collins SM. Stress and the Gastrointestinal Tract IV. Modulation of intestinal inflammation by stress: basic mechanisms and clinical relevance. *Am J Physiol Gastrointest Liver Physiol.* 2001 Mar;280(3):G315-8

[656] Hart A, Kamm MA. Review article: mechanisms of initiation and perpetuation of gut inflammation by stress. *Aliment Pharmacol Ther.* 2002 Dec;16(12):2017-28

[657] Farhadi A, Fields JZ, Keshavarzian A. Mucosal mast cells are pivotal elements in inflammatory bowel disease that connect the dots: stress, intestinal hyperpermeability and inflammation. *World J Gastroenterol.* 2007 Jun 14;13(22):3027-30

[658] Yang PC, Jury J, Söderholm JD, Sherman PM, McKay DM, Perdue MH. Chronic psychological stress in rats induces intestinal sensitization to luminal antigens. *Am J Pathol.* 2006 Jan;168(1):104-14

[659] Rashid T, Ebringer A. Ankylosing spondylitis is linked to Klebsiella--the evidence. *Clin Rheumatol.* 2007 Jun;26(6):858-64

[660] Vasquez A. *Integrative Rheumatology.* Fort Worth, Texas; Integrative and Biological Medicine Research and Consulting, 2007 OptimalHealthResearch.com

[661] Samarkos M, Vaiopoulos G. The role of infections in the pathogenesis of autoimmune diseases. *Curr Drug Targets Inflamm Allergy.* 2005 Feb;4(1):99-103

[662] Alverdy J, Holbrook C, Rocha F, Seiden L, Wu RL, Musch M, Chang E, Ohman D, Suh S. Gut-derived sepsis occurs when the right pathogen with the right virulence genes meets the right host: evidence for in vivo virulence expression in Pseudomonas aeruginosa. *Ann Surg.* 2000 Oct;232(4):480-9

[663] Wu L, Holbrook C, Zaborina O, Ploplys E, Rocha F, Pelham D, Chang E, Musch M, Alverdy J. Pseudomonas aeruginosa expresses a lethal virulence determinant, the PA-I lectin/adhesin, in the intestinal tract of a stressed host: the role of epithelia cell contact and molecules of the Quorum Sensing Signaling System. *Ann Surg.* 2003;238(5):754-64

[664] **Vasquez A.** *Integrative Rheumatology: Second Edition.* Fort Worth, Texas; Integrative and Biological Medicine Research and Consulting, 2007 OptimalHealthResearch.com

[665] Ebringer A, Rashid T. Rheumatoid arthritis is an autoimmune disease triggered by Proteus urinary tract infection. *Clin Dev Immunol.* 2006 Mar;13(1):41-8

[666] Erlacher L, Wintersberger W, Menschik M, Benke-Studnicka A, Machold K, Stanek G, Söltz-Szöts J, Smolen J, Graninger W. Reactive arthritis: urogenital swab culture is the only useful diagnostic method for the detection of the arthritogenic infection in extra-articularly asymptomatic patients with undifferentiated oligoarthritis. *Br J Rheumatol.* 1995 Sep;34(9):838-42

[667] Rashid T, Ebringer A. Rheumatoid arthritis is linked to Proteus--the evidence. *Clin Rheumatol.* 2007 Jul;26(7):1036-43

[668] Ebringer A, Rashid T, Wilson C. Rheumatoid arthritis: proposal for the use of anti-microbial therapy in early cases. *Scand J Rheumatol.* 2003;32:2-11

[669] James WH. Further evidence that low androgen values are a cause of rheumatoid arthritis: the response of rheumatoid arthritis to seriously stressful life events. *Ann Rheum Dis* 1997;56:566

[670] Karagiannis A, Harsoulis F. Gonadal dysfunction in systemic diseases. *Eur J Endocrinol.* 2005 Apr;152(4):501-13

of vitamin D deficiency leads to both musculoskeletal pain[671] as well as depression[672], and that supplementation with physiologic doses of vitamin D results in an enhanced sense of well-being[673] and high-efficacy alleviation of musculoskeletal pain and depression while providing other major collateral benefits.[674] Since the existence of vitamin D deficiency is more probable than that of antidepressant deficiency, the appropriate intervention for the former is more scientific and rational than that of the latter. Relatedly, research in various fields has shown that Western/American lifestyle and diet patterns diverge radically from human physiologic expectations and human nutritional requirements.[675] With regard to fatty acid intake and the resultant effects on inflammation and neurotransmission, modernized diets are a "set up" for musculoskeletal pain and mental depression, which frequently occur concomitantly and which are both alleviated by corrective fatty acid intervention such as fish oil supplementation as a source of EPA and DHA.[676,677] Correction of fatty acid imbalance is therefore more rational in the comanagement of pain and depression than is sole reliance on antidepressant and anti-inflammatory drugs; the latter have their place in treatment but neither addresses the primary cause of the problem and both drug classes have important adverse effects and significant cost in contrast to the safety, affordability, and collateral benefits derived from fatty acid supplementation. Also relevant to this discussion of chronic pain triggered and perpetuated by nutritional imbalances are the pro-inflammatory nature of the Western/American diet[678] and the pain-sensitizing effects of epidemic magnesium deficiency.[679] Therefore, correction of nutritional deficiencies and optimization of nutritional status might supersede the prescription of drugs in patients with concomitant depression and pain.

b. <u>Pain, inflammation, and depression are final common pathways of physical inactivity</u>: Exercising muscle elaborates cytokines ("myokines") with anti-inflammatory activity; a sedentary lifestyle fails to stimulate this endogenous anti-inflammation and is therefore relatively pro-inflammatory.[680] Further, exercise has antidepressant benefits mediated by positive influences on neurotransmission, growth factor elaboration, endocrinologic function, self-image, and social contact.[681] Patients with musculoskeletal pain should be encouraged to exercise to the extent possible given the individual's capacity and type of injury and/or degree of disability. Thus, a prescription for exercise might supersede the prescription of drugs in patients with concomitant depression and pain. Exercise prescriptions must consider frequency, duration, intensity, variety, safety, enjoyment, accountability and objective measures of compliance and progress, as well as appropriate combinations of components which emphasize aerobic fitness, strengthening, flexibility, muscle balancing, and coordination.

c. <u>Pain and depression are final common pathways of inflammation</u>: Several pro-inflammatory cytokines are psychoactive and cause depression, social withdrawal, impaired cognition, and sickness behavior.[682] As an alternative to the use of antidepressant drugs, correction of the underlying inflammatory disorder by natural, pharmacologic, or integrative means may subsequently promote restoration of normal affect and cognitive function.

[671] Plotnikoff GA, Quigley JM. Prevalence of severe hypovitaminosis D in patients with persistent, nonspecific musculoskeletal pain. *Mayo Clin Proc.* 2003 Dec;78(12):1463-70
[672] Wilkins CH, Sheline YI, Roe CM, Birge SJ, Morris JC. Vitamin D deficiency is associated with low mood and worse cognitive performance in older adults. *Am J Geriatr Psychiatry.* 2006 Dec;14(12):1032-40
[673] Vieth R, Kimball S, Hu A, Walfish PG. Randomized comparison of the effects of the vitamin D3 adequate intake versus 100 mcg (4000 IU) per day on biochemical responses and the wellbeing of patients. *Nutr J.* 2004 Jul 19;3:8
[674] **Vasquez A**, Manso G, Cannell J. The clinical importance of vitamin D (cholecalciferol): a paradigm shift with implications for all healthcare providers. *Altern Ther Health Med.* 2004 Sep-Oct;10(5):28-36
[675] O'Keefe JH Jr, Cordain L. Cardiovascular disease resulting from a diet and lifestyle at odds with our Paleolithic genome: how to become a 21st-century hunter-gatherer. *Mayo Clin Proc.* 2004 Jan;79(1):101-8
[676] Kiecolt-Glaser JK, Belury MA, Porter K, Beversdorf DQ, Lemeshow S, Glaser R. Depressive symptoms, omega-6:omega-3 fatty acids, and inflammation in older adults. *Psychosom Med.* 2007 Apr;69(3):217-24
[677] Simopoulos AP. Omega-3 fatty acids in inflammation and autoimmune diseases. *J Am Coll Nutr.* 2002 Dec;21(6):495-505
[678] Aljada A, Mohanty P, Ghanim H, Abdo T, Tripathy D, Chaudhuri A, Dandona P. Increase in intranuclear nuclear factor kappaB and decrease in inhibitor kappaB in mononuclear cells after a mixed meal: evidence for a proinflammatory effect. *Am J Clin Nutr.* 2004 Apr;79(4):682-90
[679] Park JH, Niermann KJ, Olsen N. Evidence for metabolic abnormalities in the muscles of patients with fibromyalgia. *Curr Rheumatol Rep.* 2000 Apr;2(2):131-40
[680] Petersen AM, Pedersen BK. The anti-inflammatory effect of exercise. *J Appl Physiol.* 2005 Apr;98(4):1154-62
[681] Cotman CW, Berchtold NC, Christie LA. Exercise builds brain health: key roles of growth factor cascades and inflammation. *Trends Neurosci.* 2007 Sep;30(9):464-72
[682] Wilson CJ, Finch CE, Cohen HJ. Cytokines and cognition--the case for a head-to-toe inflammatory paradigm. *J Am Geriatr Soc.* 2002 Dec;50(12):2041-56

d.   <u>Pain, inflammation, and mental depression are final common pathways for hormonal deficiencies and imbalances</u>: Deficiencies of thyroid hormones, estrogen (insufficiency or excess), testosterone, cortisol, and DHEA can cause depression and impaired neuroemotional status. Hormonal aberrations are common in patients with chronic musculoskeletal pain, particularly of the inflammatory and autoimmune types. Clinical trials have shown that administration of thyroid hormones, testosterone, DHEA, cortisol and suppression prolactin can each provide anti-inflammatory, analgesic, and antidepressant benefits among appropriately selected patients. Thus, identification and correction of hormonal imbalances might supersede the prescription of antidepressant drugs in patients with concomitant depression, inflammation, and pain.

Our cultural and scientific advancements in the knowledge of how the brain and mind function have been paradoxically paralleled by social trends showing increasing depression and social isolation; the typical American has only two friends and no one in whom to confide.[683] In the United States, violent injuries are epidemic, and the level of firearm morbidity and mortality in the US is far higher than anywhere else in the industrialized world.[684] This does to some extent beg the question of the value of "scientific knowledge" of the brain and mind within a social structure that is increasingly violent and fragmented. Further, the mental depression resultant from pandemic social isolation would be better served by physicians' admonition for increased social contact than by the continued overuse of drugs which inhibit neurotransmitter reuptake.

Conclusions: The clinical employment of the functional medicine approach to chronic disease management and health promotion rests upon a foundation of competent patient management and then extends to consider the well documented contributions of the causative *core clinical imbalances* that have allowed the genesis and perpetuation of the problem(s) under consideration. The attainment of wellness, the success of preventive medicine, and the optimization of socioemotional health cannot be attained by pharmacological suppression of the manifestations of dysfunction that result from nutritional and neuroendocrine imbalances, xenobiotic accumulation, sedentary lifestyles, social isolation, and mucosal microbial colonization. Rather, these problems are addressed directly, and these and other causative considerations must remain foremost in the mind of the physician committed to the successful, ethical, and cost-effective long-term prevention and management of chronic health disturbances, particularly those characterized by inflammation and pain.

---

[683] McPherson M, Smith-Lovin L, Brashears ME. Social Isolation in America: Changes in Core Discussion Networks over Two Decades. *American Sociological Review* 2006; 71: 353-75
[684] Preventing firearm violence: a public health imperative. *American College of Physicians. Ann Intern Med.* 1995 Feb 15;122(4):311-3

Functional medicine is a science-based field of health care that is grounded in the following principles:

- **Biochemical individuality** describes the importance of individual variations in metabolic function that derive from genetic and environmental differences among individuals.
- **Patient-centered** medicine emphasizes "patient care" rather than "disease care," following Sir William Osler's admonition that "It is more important to know what patient has the disease than to know what disease the patient has."
- **Dynamic balance** of internal and external factors.
- **Web-like interconnections** of physiological factors – an abundance of research now supports the view that the human body functions as an orchestrated network of interconnected systems, rather than individual systems functioning autonomously and without effect on each other. For example, we now know that immunological dysfunctions can promote cardiovascular disease, that dietary imbalances can cause hormonal disturbances, and that environmental exposures can precipitate neurologic syndromes such as Parkinson's disease.
- **Health as a positive vitality** – not merely the absence of disease.
- **Promotion of organ reserve** as the means to enhance health span.

Functional medicine is anchored by an examination of the core clinical imbalances that underlie various disease conditions. Those imbalances arise as **environmental inputs** such as diet, nutrients (including air and water), exercise, and trauma **are processed** by one's body, mind, and spirit through a unique set of genetic predispositions, attitudes, and beliefs. The **fundamental physiological** processes include communication, both outside and inside the cell; bioenergetics, or the transformation of food into energy; replication, repair, and maintenance of structural integrity, from the cellular to the whole body level; elimination of waste; protection and defense; and transport and circulation. The **core clinical imbalances** that arise from malfunctions within this complex system include:

- **Hormonal and neurotransmitter imbalances**
- **Oxidation-reduction imbalances and mitochondropathy**
- **Detoxification and biotransformational imbalances**
- **Immune imbalances**
- **Inflammatory imbalances**
- **Digestive, absorptive, and microbiological imbalances**
- **Structural imbalances** from cellular membrane function to the musculoskeletal system

Imbalances such as these are the precursors to the signs and symptoms by which we detect and label (diagnose) organ system disease. Improving balance – in the patient's environmental inputs and in the body's fundamental physiological processes – is the precursor to restoring health and it involves much more than treating the symptoms. Functional medicine is dedicated to improving the management of complex, chronic disease by intervening at multiple levels to address these core clinical imbalances and to restore each patient's functionality and health. Functional medicine is not a unique and separate body of knowledge. It is grounded in scientific principles and information widely available in medicine today, combining research from various disciplines into highly detailed yet clinically relevant models of disease pathogenesis and effective clinical management.

Functional medicine emphasizes a definable and teachable **process** of integrating multiple knowledge bases within a pragmatic intellectual matrix that focuses on functionality at many levels, rather than a single treatment for a single diagnosis. Functional medicine uses the patient's story as a key tool for integrating diagnosis, signs and symptoms, and evidence of clinical imbalances into a comprehensive approach to improve both the patient's environmental inputs and his or her physiological function. It is a clinician's discipline, and it directly addresses the need to transform the practice of primary care.

Newsletter & Updates

Be alerted to new integrative clinical research and updates to this textbook by registering for the free newsletter, sent 4-6 times per year. Subscribe via
www.OptimalHealthResearch.com/newsletter.html

Also, check for updates to all books at **http://optimalhealthresearch.com/updates**.html

Chapter 2:
Wellness Promotion
&
Re-Establishing the Foundation for Health

Introduction to Lifestyle Optimization, Wellness Promotion, and Disease Prevention
This section details the lifestyle modifications that support a wellness-promoting whole-health program.
Among the four major primary healthcare professions in the United States—chiropractic, osteopathy, naturopathy, and allopathy—the naturopathic profession stands preeminent in its emphasis upon wellness promotion and lifestyle optimization. This chapter reviews wellness promotion from the current author's perspective and experience—both personal and professional—which is consistent with but not officially representative of the naturopathic profession's concepts "re-establish the foundation of health" and "hierarchy of therapeutics."
This chapter originated many years ago as a handout for patients wherein it explained and described basic concepts that are foundational to health restoration, preservation, and optimization. Over the years that this handout has evolved into a chapter for my books, it has become more detailed and more relevant for clinicians treating patients. In essence, this chapter is a blueprint for the construction of a healthy lifestyle. While it may not cover every consideration, it covers the basics in sufficient detail so as to allow patients to change tracks from the downward descent of the disease-promoting lifestyle to the upward ascent of the health-promoting lifestyle.
Replacing the passive and disempowering drug-surgery paradigm with an active and empowering integrative/functional model of healthcare is one goal of this section.
This section can be thought of as a collection of essays. The review and consideration of a wide range of topics—which might otherwise appear random and nontopical to a reader accustomed to a more limited scope of discussion—is necessary due to the multifaceted nature of human experience and the widely ranging influences on health and disease outcomes.

<u>Topics</u>:

- **Re-establishing the Foundation for Health**
  - o **Healthcare, Health, and Wellness**
  - o **Daily living**
    - Lifestyle habits
    - Motivation: background and clinical applications
    - Exceptional living: the key to exceptional results
    - Recognize and affirm individual uniqueness
    - Individuation & conscious living: alternatives to common paradigms
    - Quality and quantity of sleep: concepts and clinical applications
    - Exercise, obesity, BMI, and proinflammatory activity of adipose tissue
  - o **Diet is a powerful tool for the prevention and treatment of disease**
    - Make "whole foods" the foundation of the diet
    - Increase consumption of fruits and vegetables
    - Phytochemicals: food-derived anti-inflammatory nutrients
    - Eat the right amount of protein
    - Reducing consumption of sugars: exceptions for supercompensation
    - Avoiding artificial sweeteners, colors, and other additives, reducing caffeine
    - To the extent possible, eat "organic" foods
    - Recognize the importance of avoiding food allergens
    - Supplement your healthy diet with vitamins, minerals, and fatty acids
    - General guidelines for the safe use of nutritional supplements
  - o **Advanced concepts in nutrition**
    - "Biochemical Individuality" and "Orthomolecular Medicine"
    - Nutrigenomics: Nutritional genomics
    - Putting it all together: *the supplemented Paleo-Mediterranean diet*
  - o **Emotional, mental, and social health**
    - Stress management and authentic living
    - Stress always has a biochemical/physiologic component
    - The body functions as a whole
    - Healing past experiences
    - Autonomization, intradependence, emotional literacy, corrective experience
  - o **Environmental health**
    - Environmental exposures and the importance of detoxification
    - Avoid unnecessary chemical medications and medical procedures
    - Intestinal health, bowel function, and introduction to dysbiosis
- **Natural holistic healthcare contrasted to standard medical treatment**
- **Opposite influences of health promotion vs. disease promotion**
- **Brief Overview of Integrative Primary Healthcare Disciplines**: Chiropractic, Naturopathic Medicine, Osteopathic Medicine, Functional Medicine
- **Previously published essays**
  - o Five-Part Nutritional Wellness Protocol That Produces Consistently Positive Results
  - o Implementing the Five-Part Nutritional Wellness Protocol for the Treatment of Various Health Problems
  - o Common Oversights and Shortcomings in the Study and Implementation of Nutritional Supplementation
  - o Revisiting the Five-Part Nutritional Wellness Protocol: The Supplemented Paleo-Mediterranean Diet

Introduction to Wellness Promotion: Re-Establishing the Foundation for Health

> "The work of the naturopathic physician is to elicit healing by helping patients to create or recreate conditions for health to exist within them.
> **Health will occur where the conditions for health exist.**
> **Disease is the product of conditions which allow for it."**   *Jared Zeff, N.D.*[1]

One of the most important concepts within the philosophy and practice of naturopathic medicine is that of "re-establishing the foundation for health." This means that instead of first looking to a specific treatment or "magic bullet" to solve a health problem, we first look at the environment in which the problem arose to determine if the patient's environment has initiated or perpetuated the problem. The term *environment* as used here means much more than the patient's immediate surroundings at home and work; it includes all modifiable factors that may have an effect on the patient's health, such as lifestyle, diet, exercise, supplementation, chronic and situational stress, medications with positive and negative effects, exposure to toxicants and microbes, nutritionally-modifiable genetic factors[2], emotions, feelings, and unconscious assumptions[3], and many other considerations. Although the genes that we and our patients have inherited cannot be changed, we can very often modulate the expression of those genes (e.g., via nutrigenomics, described later) by modifying the biochemical, microbial, toxicologic, and neurohormonal milieu that bathes our cells and thus our genes; this concept was expressed in a statement by the US Centers for Disease Control and Prevention in its "Gene-Environment Interaction Fact Sheet" available on-line.[4]

> **Environment—lifestyle, diet, stresses, microbes, toxins—influences genetic expression and the manifestation of health or disease**
>
> "Virtually all human diseases result from the interaction of genetic susceptibility factors and modifiable environmental factors, broadly defined to include infectious, chemical, physical, nutritional, and behavioral factors. ...
>
> "Even so-called single-gene disorders actually develop from the interaction of both genetic and environmental factors. ...
>
> "We do not inherit a disease state per se. Instead, we inherit a set of a susceptibility factors to certain effects of environmental factors and therefore inherit a higher risk for certain diseases."
>
> Gene-Environment Interaction Fact Sheet by the Centers for Disease Control and Prevention, August 2000

"Optimal health" does not and never will come in a pill or tonic—the human body and the interactions that we each have between our genes, outlooks, environments, and lifestyles are far too complex to ever be addressed wholly and completely by a simplistic paradigm or single treatment. Even a superficial observation of the complexity of human physiology and the complexity of our environments (including noise, toxins such as benzene and mercury, chemicals such as formaldehyde from building materials, work stress and multitasking, radiation exposure, microwaves, etc) shows that **our modern lifestyles subject the human body to many more "stressors" than ever before in the history of human existence.** Each of these stressors depletes our psychic and physiologic reserves, such that daily replenishment and protection are necessary.

Research in nutrition and physiology is revealing the mechanisms by which "simple" lifestyle practices and dietary interventions exert their powerful benefits. For example, whole foods such as fruits and vegetables contain over 8,000 phytochemicals with different physiologic effects[5], and simple practices such as meditation and massage can significantly alter hormone and neurotransmitter levels.[6,7] On the surface, a simple practice such as consumption of fruits and vegetables and a multivitamin/multimineral supplement may seem to be a way to

---

[1] Zeff JL. The process of healing: a unifying theory of naturopathic medicine. *Journal of Naturopathic Medicine* 1997; 7: 122-5
[2] Kaput J, Rodriguez LR. Nutritional genomics: the next frontier in the postgenomic era. *Physiol Genomics* 16: 166–177 http://physiolgenomics.physiology.org/cgi/content/full/16/2/166
[3] Miller A. The truth will set you free: overcoming emotional blindness and finding your true adult self. New York: Basic Books; 2001
[4] Gene-Environment Interaction Fact Sheet by the Centers for Disease Control and Prevention, August 2000 http://www.ashg.org/pdf/CDC%20Gene-Environment%20Interaction%20Fact%20Sheet.pdf
[5] "We propose that the additive and synergistic effects of phytochemicals in fruit and vegetables are responsible for their potent antioxidant and anticancer activities, and that the benefit of a diet rich in fruit and vegetables is attributed to the complex mixture of phytochemicals present in whole foods." Liu RH. Health benefits of fruit and vegetables are from additive and synergistic combinations of phytochemicals. *Am J Clin Nutr.* 2003 Sep;78(3 Suppl):517S-520S
[6] "The significant decrease of the catecholamine metabolite VMA (vanillic-mandelic acid) in meditators, that is associated with a reciprocal increase of 5-HIAA supports as a feedback necessity the "rest and fulfillment response" versus "fight and flight"." Bujatti M, Riederer P. Serotonin, noradrenaline, dopamine metabolites in transcendental meditation-technique. *J Neural Transm.* 1976;39(3):257-67
[7] "By the end of the study, the massage therapy group, as compared to the relaxation group, reported experiencing less pain, depression, anxiety and improved sleep. They also showed improved trunk and pain flexion performance, and their serotonin and dopamine levels were higher." Hernandez-Reif M, Field T, Krasnegor J, Theakston H. Lower back pain is reduced and range of motion increased after massage therapy. *Int J Neurosci* 2001;106(3-4):131-45

provide merely "good nutrition"; however the clinical effects can include antidepressant[8] and anti-inflammatory benefits[9] by enhancing the efficiency of biochemical reactions[10] and by reducing excess activity of NF-kappaB[11], respectively. The power of interventional nutrition utilizing high-doses and/or synergistic formulations of nutraceuticals and phytonutraceuticals becomes much more clinically apparent when patients first (re)establish a healthy foundation of diet and lifestyle practices upon which these treatments can be added; **I estimate that the effectiveness of treatments for complex illness such as inflammatory diseases and cancer is** *at least* **doubled when patients implement these lifestyle changes in addition to specific treatments rather than relying on specific treatments alone without a healthy supportive lifestyle.** In other words, *"foundation for health* + specific treatments" is much more effective than *"unhealthy lifestyle* + specific treatments." This explains, in part, the discrepancy between the relatively lackluster response seen in *single-intervention* clinical trials* compared to the better results that we attain clinically when using a holistic approach characterized by *multicomponent* treatment plans. The biochemical and "scientific" reasons for this positive/negative synergism will become more clear during the course of this chapter and textbook.

Single-intervention clinical trials (i.e., clinical trials that utilize only one treatment) are the "gold standard" in allopathic drug-based research because in that setting the goal is to quantify and qualify the nature of positive and negative responses to a single intervention, generally a drug. However, this approach loses much of its luster and relevance in clinical settings where neither patients nor their environments and treatment plans can be standardized due to the unique constitution, lifestyle, history, and other nuances of each patient. Single intervention clinical trials have a place in the researching of all treatments, including natural interventions. However, clinicians—especially recent graduates—must pry themselves away from this research tool when it comes to treating individual patients in clinical practice, where **single interventions are the antithesis of holistic treatment**.

Daily Living: Life occurs on a moment-to-moment and daily basis. Choices that we make in relationships, occupations, exercise, and diet have profound and powerful influence over the course of our lives—particularly our health and happiness. Despite the previous and current obfuscation of health information by allopathic groups[12,13,14,15,16] and the pharmaceutical industry[17,18], enough valid information and common sense is available to doctors and the public such that **ignorance is no longer a viable excuse for deferring responsibility for lifestyle-induced disease and misery**.[19] Eating too much sugar and fat while not eating enough fruits and vegetables is making a choice to have an increased probability of developing diabetes, cancer, heart disease, arthritis, and obesity. Exercising regularly, eating a healthy diet, and supplementing the diet with high-quality nutrients and botanicals is making the choice to greatly reduce one's risk of health problems[20,21] and to nurture one's life and one's body so that one can make the most of one's life experience and enjoy life, hobbies, life purpose(s), travel, creativity, community involvement, and time with friends and family.

When we were children, we looked to other people to provide for us and to "take care of us." **As adults, we have to assume responsibility for the course of our own lives, to make decisions based on long-term considerations rather than instant gratification and selective ignorance.** Of course, this does not mean that we

---

[8] Benton D, Haller J, Fordy J. Vitamin supplementation for 1 year improves mood. *Neuropsychobiology*. 1995;32(2):98-105

[9] Church TS, Earnest CP, Wood KA, Kampert JB. Reduction of C-reactive protein levels through use of a multivitamin. *Am J Med*. 2003;115(9):702-7

[10] Ames BN, Elson-Schwab I, Silver EA. High-dose vitamin therapy stimulates variant enzymes with decreased coenzyme binding affinity (increased K(m)): relevance to genetic disease and polymorphisms. *Am J Clin Nutr*. 2002 Apr;75(4):616-58 http://www.ajcn.org/cgi/content/full/75/4/616

[11] **Vasquez A**. Reducing pain and inflammation naturally - part 4: nutritional and botanical inhibition of NF-kappaB, the major intracellular amplifier of the inflammatory cascade. A practical clinical strategy exemplifying anti-inflammatory nutrigenomics. *Nutritional Perspectives*, July 2005:5-12. www.OptimalHealthResearch.com/part4

[12] Wolinsky H, Brune T. The Serpent on the Staff: The Unhealthy Politics of the American Medical Association. GP Putnam and Sons, New York, 1994

[13] Wilk CA. Medicine, Monopolies, and Malice: How the Medical Establishment Tried to Destroy Chiropractic. Garden City Park: Avery, 1996

[14] Carter JP. Racketeering in Medicine: The Suppression of Alternatives. Norfolk: Hampton Roads Pub; 1993

[15] National Alliance of Professional Psychology Providers. AMA Seeks To Control and Restrict Psychologist's Scope of Practice. http://www.nappp.org/scope.pdf Accessed November 25, 2006

[16] "In an effort to marshal the medical community's resources against the growing threat of expanding scope of practice for allied health professionals, the AMA has formed a national partnership to confront such initiatives nationwide... The committee will use $25,000..." Daly R, American Psychiatric Association. AMA Forms Coalition to Thwart Non-M.D. Practice Expansion. *Psychiatric News* 2006 March; 41: 17 http://pn.psychiatryonline.org/cgi/content/full/41/5/17-a?eaf Accessed November 25, 2006

[17] Angell M. The Truth About the Drug Companies: How They Deceive Us and What to Do About it. Random House; August 2004

[18] "It begins on the first day of medical school... It starts slowly and insidiously, like an addiction, and can end up influencing the very nature of medical decision-making and practice... Attempts to influence the judgment of doctors by commercial interests serving the medical industrial complex are nothing if not thorough." Editorial. Drug-company influence on medical education in USA. *Lancet*. 2000 Sep 2;356(9232):781

[19] "Error is not blindness, error is cowardice. Every acquisition, every step forward in knowledge is the result of courage, of severity towards oneself, of cleanliness with respect to oneself." Nietzsche FW. Ecce Homo: How One Becomes What One Is. [Translator: Hollingdale RJ] Penguin Books:1979,34

[20] Orme-Johnson DW, Herron RE. An innovative approach to reducing medical care utilization and expenditures. *Am J Manag Care*. 1997;3(1):135-44

[21] **Vasquez A**. Five-Part Nutritional Protocol that Produces Consistently Positive Results. *Nutr Wellness* 2005Sept. http://optimalhealthresearch.com/spmd

have to abandon enjoyment; but it does mean that we can make decisions based on priorities, and if health is a priority then we should take steps to attain and maintain it. For people who have chosen to make their health a priority, sugar- and fat-laden food begins to lose its appeal, and exploring new health-building experiences such as healthy cooking, outdoor activities, and community involvement can become an empowering lifestyle that can be transformed into an art—one that is particularly amenable to building relationships and connections with other people. **The improved sense of well-being and improved physical and intellectual performance obtained from consumption of a health-promoting Paleo-Mediterranean diet (described later) supercedes any short-term gratification from the disease-promoting diet commonly referred to as the Standard American Diet (SAD).** When people want to be healthy, exercising and spending enjoyable time outdoors becomes more fun than the inactivity and passivity of watching television. When we consider that the average American watches at least 3-4 hours of television per day then we should not be surprised that, with physical inactivity as such a major component of the day, Americans show progressively higher rates of obesity, cancer, heart disease, and diabetes. Such an inactive lifestyle also affects our children: on average, each American child watches more than 23 hours of television per week[22]—a national habit that unquestionably contributes to the high levels of obesity and (social) illiteracy demonstrated by America's youth. Adults who watch average amounts of television are exposed to—some might say "…indoctrinated by…") more than 30 hours of drug advertisements per year—far exceeding their exposure to other, potentially more authentic, health-promoting health information.[23] Not only does television siphon time and energy that could be used more productively, more socially, or more enjoyably, but at a cost of $50-100 per month ($600 to $1,200 per year) **cable television subtracts from the available resources (i.e., time, money, and attention) that could be directed toward health-promoting choices.** Cable television—because of its financial cost and time commitment—is only one of many examples of how everyday lifestyle choices can have an impact on long-term health/disease outcomes. **Clinicians should encourage patients to become mindful of their choices and the impact these choices have on long-term health and vitality.**

> ### Health living: lifestyle as living art
> "What one should learn from artists: How can we make things beautiful, attractive, and desirable for us when they are not?—and I rather think that in themselves they never are! ... This we should learn from artists, while being wiser than they are in other matters. For with them this subtle power usually comes to an end where art ends and life begins; but we want to be the poets of our lives—first of all in the smallest, most everyday matters."
>
> Nietzsche FW. The Happy Science. 1882. Essay #299.

Lifestyle habits: Without the conscious decision that **health is a priority** and the realization that **optimal health has to be earned rather than taken for granted**, patients and doctors alike can fall into the belief that healthcare and health maintenance are *burdens* and *inconveniences* rather than opportunities for fulfillment and self-care. Taking an **empowered** and **pro-active** role in one's healthcare may include a coordinated program of diet changes (i.e., eating certain foods, avoiding other foods, modulating total intake), regular exercise, nutritional supplementation, stress reduction, and relationship improvement. Unhealthy habits such as eating junk foods, using tobacco, and watching too much television rob people of the time, energy, motivation, and financial resources that could otherwise be used to improve health and prevent unnecessary illness. As described later in this chapter, the choices that are made on a daily basis from this point forward are the most powerful predictors of future health and are generally more powerful than past habits or genetic inheritance. We can all greatly increase our probability of enjoying a future of high-energy health rather than painful illness by consistently choosing health-promoting options instead of foods, behaviors, and emotional states that promote illness.

---

[22] "American children view over 23 hours of television per week. * Teenagers view an average of 21 to 22 hours of television per week. * By the time today's children reach age 70, they will have spent 7 to 10 years of their lives watching television." American Academy of Pediatrics http://www.aapca1.org/aapca1/tv.html accessed September 30, 2003

[23] "…many ads may be targeted specifically at women and older viewers. Our findings suggest that Americans who watch average amounts of television may be exposed to more than 30 hours of direct-to-consumer drug advertisements each year, far surpassing their exposure to other forms of health communication." Brownfield ED, Bernhardt JM, Phan JL, Williams MV, Parker RM. Direct-to-consumer drug advertisements on network television: an exploration of quantity, frequency, and placement. *J Health Commun*. 2004 Nov-Dec;9(6):491-7

One hour of time per day and/or about $2 - $8 per day:

Active self-care lifestyle	Distraction & inactive lifestyle
1. Meditation 2. Yoga, stretching 3. Walking, jogging, biking, no-cost calisthenics 4. Martial arts, Tai Chi 5. Hot bath 6. Cooking new healthy meals 7. Herbal teas (especially green tea) provide anti-inflammatory, anticancer, and antioxidant benefits 8. Basic nutritional supplementation (less than $2 per day): 1) High-potency multivitamin and multimineral supplement, 2) Complete balanced, fatty acid supplementation, 3) 2,000 – 4,000 IU vitamin D per day for adults, 4) probiotics and/or symbiotic.	1. Cable television 2. 1 pack of cigarettes per day 3. Designer coffee such as Grande Café Latte
Benefits 1. Increased flexibility and joint mobility 2. Reduction in blood pressure 3. Reduced risk of cancer 4. Increased strength 5. Improved cognitive function 6. New and enjoyable meals 7. Relaxation 8. New life skills 9. Improved heart health 10. The opportunity to develop social skills and more friends and a better social support network 11. Reduced risk for Alzheimer's and Parkinson's diseases	**Results** 1. Cable television: Cost $2 - $4 per day = average $1,095 per year) 2. 1 pack of cigarettes per day ($3 per day = $1,095 per year) 3. Grande Café Latte ($4 per day = average $1,460 per year)
Cost: At $2 per day for meditation, stretching, calisthenics, (etc.) and basic supplementation, the total comes to $730 per year.	**Cost:** For cable television, cafe coffee, and cigarettes, the total comes to approximately $3,600 per year.

<u>**Motivation**</u>: We all have a combination of reasons, feelings, inclinations, and unconscious influences that support and perpetuate our health behaviors.[24,25,26] Getting in touch with those motivations can help us to better understand the healthy/functional (health-promoting) and unhealthy/dysfunctional (illness-promoting) aspects of our psyches. Uncovering and "upgrading" these motivations can help us and our patients to develop more authentic lives and improved health. Self-defeating behaviors, such as 1) a willingness to remain ignorant of factors which influence health, 2) a willingness to frequently consume disease-promoting processed convenience foods, and 3) submission to confinement within the boundaries of one's insurance coverage (which often confines one to drugs and surgery as the only treatment options), reflect—*at best*—the willingness to settle for mediocrity and—*at worst*—an unconscious movement in the direction of illness and early death—masochism and suicide by lifestyle. Conversely, an unencumbered drive toward health will create the greatest opportunity for wellness. Since **actions originate from beliefs and goals**, we can surmise much about undisclosed beliefs and goals in others and ourselves simply by observing outward behavior. Effectively changing actions (such as diet and lifestyle choices) therefore must include not only behavior modification but also careful examination and reconsideration of largely unconscious goals and beliefs that motivate and underlie those behaviors. **When a fully empowered motivation toward health is matched with accurate informational insight, we have the** *potential* **for health-promoting change—***potential* **which only becomes** *manifest* **after the habitual application of appropriate** *action.* Patients and doctors alike can benefit from considering the factors that incline them *toward* or *away* from behaviors that promote health or disease.

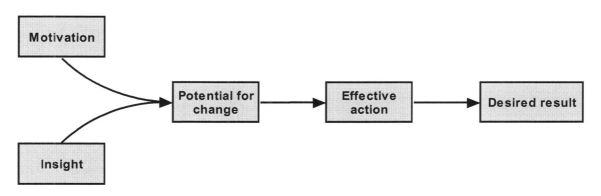

Reasons that I take good care of myself:

_____

_____

_____

_____

Reasons that I don't take good care of myself:

_____

_____

_____

_____

_____

[24] Bradshaw J. <u>Healing the Shame that Binds You</u> [Audio Cassette (April 1990) Health Communications Audio; ISBN: 1558740430]
[25] Miller A. <u>The Drama of the Gifted Child: The Search for the True Self</u>. Basic Books: 1981
[26] Prochaska, JO, Norcross, JC, and DiClemente, CC (1994). <u>Changing for Good: A Revolutionary Six-Stage Program for Overcoming Bad Habits and Moving Your Life Positively Forward</u>. NY, William Morrow and Company; 1994

Motivation: moving from theory to practice: Many recently-graduated doctors start with the erroneous assumption that all patients actually want to become healthier, and furthermore, that all that the doctor has to do is "enlighten" them to the error of their ways and the patient will be dutifully compliant unto the attainment of his or her health-related goals. In reality, many people are surprisingly indifferent about their health. Many people do not care if they are 30 lbs overweight or have hypertension or will die early as a result of their lifestyle; they often have to be encouraged to begin to *consider* making positive changes.

> **Action determines outcome**
> "Knowing is not enough;
> we must apply.
> Willing is not enough;
> we must do."
>
> Johann Wolfgang von Goethe,
> German novelist, poet, and scientist
> (1749 - 1832)

At our 2004 Functional Medicine Symposium, Dr. James Prochaska[27] elucidated the different stages of patient preparedness, and we note that each of these five levels of thought and action produces specific results and requires different types of support from the doctor. I have summarized and modified Dr. Prochaska's lecture in the following table; for additional information and insights, obtain his lecture from the Institute for Functional Medicine (functionalmedicine.org) or obtain his book *Changing for Good*.[28]

Level of preparedness and readiness for change

Stage: representative statement	*Doctor's interventions and social support*
1. **Pre-contemplation**: "I am not seriously thinking about making a change to be healthier."	▪ Outreach ▪ Retainment
2. **Contemplation**: "I am thinking about making a change, but I am not ready for action."	▪ Resolve resistance ▪ Emphasize benefits ▪ Address ambivalence
3. **Preparation**: "I am getting ready to make a change, but I am not taking effective action yet."	▪ Ensure adequate preparation ▪ Prevent relapse following initial action
4. **Action**: "I am beginning to make changes to become healthier."	▪ Support (group support is best) ▪ Encouragement ▪ Reward system
5. **Maintenance**: "I take action every day and on a consistent basis to reach my goals."	▪ Continued provision for continuation of health changes: facilities, supplements, social support, affirmation

Recognizing the different levels of patient preparedness and addressing individual patients with a customized approach not only for their *disease* but also for their *level of preparedness* for action can help doctors deliver more effective healthcare. Also, patients may have different levels of preparedness for different aspects of their treatment plans. He/she may be ready for **action** with regard to exercise, in **preparation** for dietary change, but in **precontemplation** for the use of supplements and botanicals.

---

[27] Prochaska JO. Changing for good: motivating diabetic patients. The Coming Storm: Reversing the Rising Pandemic of Diabetes and Metabolic Syndrome. The Eleventh International Symposium on Functional Medicine. May 13-15, 2004 in Vancouver, British Columbia, Canada. Pages 173-180. Presented by the Institute for Functional Medicine in Gig Harbor, Washington. www.FunctionalMedicine.org
[28] Prochaska, JO, Norcross, JC, and DiClemente, CC (1994). Changing for Good: A Revolutionary Six-Stage Program for Overcoming Bad Habits and Moving Your Life Positively Forward. NY, William Morrow and Company; 1994

<u>The secret to being exceptionally healthy:</u> *One has to live in an exceptional (unique, personalized) way*. We cannot expect to achieve the goal of being vibrantly healthy or exceptionally happy if we live in the same way as everyone else, particularly when our fellow citizens are likely to be overweight, depressed, socially isolated[29], requiring multiple pharmaceutical medications[30], and experiencing a state of progressively declining health.[31] *Healthy lifestyle* not only includes the basics of adequate sleep, healthy whole-foods diet, supportive relationships, and regular exercise, but it also includes preventive medicine and pro-active healthcare. **Despite the fact that we in the United States (US) spend more on medical treatments than does any other country in the world, Americans have the worst health outcomes of all the major industrialized countries.**[32,33,34] This is largely because *American medicine* is centered on a *disease-oriented model of medicine* which means that instead of having a healthcare system and social structure that proactively promotes health and prevents disease before it happens, our systems are *reactive*—treating disease *after* it occurs rather than emphasizing the prevention of disease *before* it occurs. The dominant allopathic model in the US is also reductionistic: focusing on the small problem (micromanagement) rather than the big picture (macromanagement).

Clearly, the most effective method for avoiding expensive and potentially dangerous medical procedures and drug treatments is for us as a nation and as individuals to shift our thinking from a *disease treatment* model of healthcare to a more logical program of aggressive *disease prevention* and *wellness promotion* via the use of safe natural treatments rather than heroic interventions.[35,36] Of course, this means that our concept and view of health and healthcare will have to change. As noted by Shi[37], **"Redesigning the system of health care delivery in the United States may be the only viable option to improve the quality of health care."** In the meantime, while we work for change on a national level, we are wise to change our personal habits and healthcare choices in favor of natural and preventive healthcare.

> **Americans have poor health outcomes compared to citizens of other industrialized nations**
>
> "Basically, you die earlier and spend more time disabled if you're an American rather than a member of most other advanced countries."
>
> Christopher Murray MD PhD, Director of World Health Organization's Global Program on Evidence for Health Policy. Press release on June 4, 2000. http://www.who.int/inf-pr-2000/en/pr2000-life.html

> **Approximately 493 Americans are killed each day by hospital injuries and drug-prescribing errors**
>
> "Recent estimates suggest that each year more than 1 million patients are injured while in the hospital and approximately 180,000 die because of these injuries. Furthermore, drug-related morbidity and mortality are common and are estimated to cost more than $136 billion a year."
>
> Holland EG, Degruy FV. Drug-induced disorders. *Am Fam Physician*. 1997;56:1781-8, 1791-2

> **Medical drug (in)efficacy**
>
> "The vast majority of drugs —more than 90 percent— only work in 30 or 50 percent of the people."
>
> Allen Roses, M.D., worldwide vice-president of genetics at GlaxoSmithKline. Published Dec 8, 2003 http://commondreams.org/headlines03/1208-02.htm

<u>Healthy lifestyle and biochemical individuality credo: Recognize and affirm that you are a unique individual with unique needs</u>: For each of us, our "personality" extends far beyond and far deeper than our sense of humor and our choice of clothing; we are very unique on a physiologic and biochemical level as well. So-called *normal* and *apparently healthy* individuals vary greatly in their biochemical efficiency and nutritional needs. This is the

---

[29] McPherson M, Smith-Lovin L, Brashears ME. Social Isolation in America: Changes in Core Discussion Networks over Two Decades. *American Sociological Review* 2006; 71: 353-75 http://www.asanet.org/galleries/default-file/June06ASRFeature.pdf

[30] "According to the latest available data, total health care costs reached $1.3 trillion in 2000. This represents a per capita health care expenditure of $4,637. The total prescription drug expenditure in 2000 was $121.8 billion, or approximately $430 per person." Presentation to the U.S. Senate Commerce Committee April 23, 2002 "Drug Pricing & Consumer Costs" Kathleen D. Jaeger, R.Ph., J.D. http://commerce.senate.gov/hearings/042302jaegar.pdf

[31] Zack MM, Moriarty DG, Stroup DF, Ford ES, Mokdad AH. Worsening trends in adult health-related quality of life and self-rated health-United States, 1993-2001. *Public Health Rep.* 2004 Sep-Oct;119(5):493-505 http://www.pubmedcentral.nih.gov/articlerender.fcgi?tool=pubmed&pubmedid=15313113

[32] "[America] also has the fewest hospital days per capita, the highest hospital expenditures per day, and substantially higher physician incomes than the other OECD countries. On the available outcome measures, the United States is generally in the bottom half, and its relative ranking has been declining since 1960." Anderson GF, Poullier JP. Health spending, access, and outcomes: trends in industrialized countries. *Health Aff* (Millwood) 1999 May-Jun;18(3):178-92 http://content.healthaffairs.org/cgi/reprint/18/3/178.pdf

[33] "However, on outcomes indicators such as life expectancy and infant mortality, the United States is frequently in the bottom quartile among the twenty-nine industrialized countries, and its relative ranking has been declining since 1960." Anderson GF. In search of value: an international comparison of cost, access, and outcomes. *Health Aff* 1997 Nov-Dec;16(6):163-71

[34] "Basically, you die earlier and spend more time disabled if you're an American rather than a member of most other advanced countries," says Christopher Murray, MD, PhD, Director of WHO's Global Program on Evidence for Health Policy. http://www.who.int/inf-pr-2000/en/pr2000-life.html

[35] "Systematic access to managed chiropractic care not only may prove to be clinically beneficial but also may reduce overall health care costs." Legorreta A, et al N. Comparative Analysis of Individuals With and Without Chiropractic Coverage. *Archives of Internal Medicine* 2004; 164: 1985-1992

[36] Orme-Johnson DW, Herron RE. An innovative approach to reducing medical care utilization and expenditures. *Am J Manag Care*. 1997;3(1):135-44

[37] Shi L. Health care spending, delivery, and outcome in developed countries: a cross-national comparison. *Am J Med Qual* 1997;12(2):83-93

concept of "biochemical individuality" which was first detailed in 1956 by the renowned scientist Roger J Williams from the University of Texas. In his historic work *Biochemical Individuality: The Basis for the Genetotrophic Concept*, Dr. Williams[38] reviews research that conclusively proves that among *apparently healthy* individuals, we can objectively determine great differences in physiology, organ efficiency, enzyme function, and nutritional needs. For example, variables that promote health include increased enzyme efficiency and efficient digestion and assimilation of nutrients, while internal factors that reduce health can include inadequate digestion, inefficient absorption, increased excretion of nutrients, impaired detoxification, poor enzyme function and "partial genetic blocks"—a term now understood to imply single nucleotide polymorphisms[39] and related enzyme defects, which result in **supradietary requirements for specific vitamins and minerals** for the prevention of disease and maintenance of health.[40] What this means for us as doctors and for our patients in practical terms is that in order for us to become as healthy as possible, we will almost certainly have to give attention to each person's unique biochemical abilities/disabilities in order to maximize the function of the various body systems, enzymes, and to optimize genetic expression.[41] This means that what works for one's neighbor, spouse, or best friend in terms of exercise, diet and nutrition may not work for one's unique physiology. We must all muster the courage to affirm that, in order to attain the goal of stable or progressively better health, we will each have to learn about how our unique bodies work—what conditions of health must be created. We will have to learn to make changes in lifestyle and daily routine which reflect and honor our bodies' ways of working. This may mean modifying work, sleep, and exercise schedules, avoiding some foods and eating others, and customizing nutrient intake to meet the body's needs as they are *in the present*—the health program that appears to have worked last year may not be appropriate at the present time. The process of learning how a person's body works requires time, patience, and the process of trial and error—from patient and doctor—but achieving the goal of improved health and increased energy are well worth the effort.

Individuation and the practice of conscious living: Our visions of reality are influenced by religious institutions, large corporations, advertising networks[42], corporate-owned mass media[43], and what Professors Stevens and Glatstein called "the medical-industrial complex."[44] Some of the paradigms that are advocated are both *unhistorical* (having no historical precedent) and *antihistorical* (contrary to the available historical precedent, which includes sustainability). Some of these companies and organizations offer us a view of reality and vision of our individual potentials that is fashioned in such a way as to promote the financial and political interests of the company or organization. Conversely, the actualization of our true physical, emotional, intellectual, and spiritual potentials may require that we separate from or at least attain a conscious appreciation of the (pseudo)reality that we have been advised to follow.[45,46] Critiques of and reasonable alternatives to our current paradigms of school[47], work[48,49], and money[50] have been discussed elsewhere and are worthy of consideration. Becoming mindful of the paradigms and assumptions under which we live is the first step in true individuation, characterized by choosing (*creating* the best option: freedom) rather than deciding

> **The importance of living consciously**
>
> "Consciousness is our basic tool for successful adaptation to reality. The more conscious we are in any situation, the more possibilities we tend to perceive, the more options we have, the more powerful we are — perhaps even the longer we will live.
>
> Living consciously means seeking to be aware of everything that bears on our actions, purposes, values, and goals — and behaving in accordance with that which we see and know."
>
> Branden N. The Art of Living Consciously. http://nathanielbranden.com Accessed Feb 2011

[38] Williams RJ. Biochemical Individuality : The Basis for the Genetotrophic Concept. Austin and London: University of Texas Press, 1956
[39] Ames BN. Cancer prevention and diet: help from single nucleotide polymorphisms. *Proc Natl Acad Sci U S A.* 1999 Oct 26;96(22):12216-8
[40] Ames BN, Elson-Schwab I, Silver EA. High-dose vitamin therapy stimulates variant enzymes with decreased coenzyme binding affinity (increased K(m)): relevance to genetic disease and polymorphisms. *Am J Clin Nutr.* 2002 Apr;75(4):616-58 http://www.ajcn.org/cgi/content/full/75/4/616
[41] "The combination of biochemical individuality and known functional utilities of allelic variants should converge to create a situation in which nutritional optima can be specified as part of comprehensive lifestyle prescriptions tailored to the needs of each person." Eckhardt RB. Genetic research and nutritional individuality. *J Nutr* 2001;131(2):336S-9S
[42] "Patients' requests for medicines are a powerful driver of prescribing decisions. In most cases physicians prescribed requested medicines but were often ambivalent about the choice of treatment. If physicians prescribe requested drugs despite personal reservations, sales may increase but appropriateness of prescribing may suffer." Mintzes B, Barer ML, Kravitz RL, Kazanjian A, Bassett K, Lexchin J, Evans RG, Pan R, Marion SA. Influence of direct to consumer pharmaceutical advertising and patients' requests on prescribing decisions: two site cross sectional survey. *BMJ.* 2002 Feb 2; 324(7332): 278-9
[43] Manufacturing Consent: Noam Chomsky and the Media. Movie directed by Achbar M and Wintonick P. 1992. See also http://zeitgeistmovie.com/
Stevens CW, Glatstein E. Beware the Medical-Industrial Complex. *Oncologist* 1996;1(4):IV-V http://theoncologist.alphamedpress.org/cgi/reprint/1/4/190-iv.pdf on July 4, 2004
[45] Breton D, Largent C. The Paradigm Conspiracy. Center City; Hazelden: 1996
[46] Pearce JC. Exploring the Crack in the Cosmic Egg: Split Minds and Meta-Realities. New York: Washington Square Press; 1974
[47] Gatto JT. Dumbing us down: the hidden curriculum of compulsory education. Gabriola Island, Canada; New Society Publishers: 2005
[48] "No one should ever work. In order to stop suffering, we have to stop working. That doesn't mean we have to stop doing things. It does mean creating a new way of life based on play..." Black B. The abolition of work and other essays. Port Townsend: Loompanics Unlimited; 1985, pages 17-33
[49] Jarow R. Creating the Work You Love: Courage, Commitment and Career; Inner Traditions Intl Ltd; 1995 [ISBN: 0892815426]
[50] Dominguez JR. Transforming Your Relationship With Money. Sounds True; Book and Cassette edition: 2001 Audio tape.

(*selecting* one of the offered options: the illusion of freedom). Various conscious thoughts and unconscious assumptions create our "working reality" which represents the way that we see things and the paradigm by which we *act in* and *interact with* the larger world. These layers come from our own families, schools, teachers, churches, companies, friends, parents, and ourselves—our previous interpretations and misinterpretations of ourselves and events; in sum, our responses to outer events combined with our internal experiences meld into our perception of ourselves (known as "the genesis of personal identity") and how we as individuals relate to our inner ourselves and [our perception of] the outer world. Becoming conscious of these realities and illusions allows us the opportunity to discard those views that are inaccurate, dysfunctional, and harmful and to accept a truer reality based on what we experience, feel, and know to be real—in the present, as adults. Once we are freed from *unreality*, we can live true to ourselves in a way that is authentically responsible to our own needs *and* the needs of our communities so that we can simultaneously sustain our obligations to society[51,52] while being free to be unique individuals.[53,54]

Examples of commonly accepted paradigms and their reasonable alternatives

Commonly advocated/accepted paradigms ↳ *Implication and effect*	*Alternate paradigm* ↳ *Implication and effect*
It is OK to be irresponsible in daily choices and then blame health problems on bad luck, bad genes, or both. ↳ Many people fail to take responsibility for their lives and thereby become victims of circumstances—negative circumstances that they themselves helped to create.	**Lifestyle, especially diet and nutrition, is the most powerful influence on health outcomes. Therefore, an educated patient is empowered to direct his/her health destiny.** ↳ Optimal health *per individual* is attained when people take responsibility for their lives, seek health information, and then incorporate this information into their daily routine in the form of healthy living: health-promoting lifestyle, eating, exercise, supplementation, relationships, and occupational and social activities, including socio-political involvement to protect the environment and resist the privatization of life and the spoliation of the environment in which we live and upon which our lives and health depend.[55,56]
In general, chemical medications are the answer to nearly all health problems. ↳ The belief in medications as the primary treatment of disease creates a patient population that is apathetic, disempowered, and dependent upon the medical-pharmaceutical industry, which grows richer and more powerful despite so-called 'earnest' attempts at cost containment.[57]	**Many acute and chronic problems can be more effectively managed in terms of prevention, safety, efficacy, and cost-effectiveness when phytonutritional interventions are either used as primary therapy or, when necessary, used in conjunction with medications.** ↳ A reduction in disease prevalence via health-promoting diet and lifestyle along with integrative treatments offers the best opportunity for benefit to patients, doctors, and third-party payers.[58]

[51] Bly R. The Sibling Society. Vintage Books USA; Reprint edition (June 1, 1997) ISBN: 0679781285 (Abridged audio edition (May 1, 1996)

[52] Bly R. Where have all the parents gone? A talk on the Sibling Society. New York: Sound Horizons, 1996 Highly recommended.

[53] Bradshaw J. Healing the Shame that Binds You [Audio Cassette (April 1990) Health Communications Audio; ISBN: 1558740430]

[54] Miller A. The truth will set you free: overcoming emotional blindness and finding your true adult self. New York: Basic Books; 2001

[55] "Your lack of interest in the past, your lack of involvement, your unwillingness to develop coherent strategies, your unwillingness to challenge authority - these have created a vacuum in decision-making, that has been filled by professional groups with close relationships with the chemical industries..." Samuel Epstein MD, 1993. Professor of Occupational and Environmental Medicine at the School of Public Health, University of Illinois Medical Center Chicago. http://www.converge.org.nz/pirm/pestican.htm accessed September 11, 2004

[56] Kristin S. Schafer, Margaret Reeves, Skip Spitzer, Susan E. Kegley. Chemical Trespass: Pesticides in Our Bodies and Corporate Accountability. Pesticide Action Network North America. May 2004 Available at http://www.panna.org/campaigns/docsTrespass/chemicalTrespass2004.dv.html on August 1, 2004

[57] "In this paper I offer four hypotheses to help explain why use of pharmaceuticals has continued to grow even as managed care and other cost containment efforts have flourished." Berndt ER. The U.S. pharmaceutical industry: why major growth in times of cost containment? *Health Aff* (Millwood). 2001 Mar-Apr;20(2):100-14

[58] "Hospital admission rates in the control group were 11.4 times higher than those in the MVAH group for cardiovascular disease, 3.3 times higher for cancer, and 6.7 times higher for mental health and substance abuse. ...MVAH patients older than age 45...had 88% fewer total patients days compared with control patients." Orme-Johnson DW, Herron RE. An innovative approach to reducing medical care utilization and expenditures. *Am J Manag Care*. 1997 Jan;3(1):135-44

Examples of commonly accepted paradigms and their reasonable alternatives —*continued*

Commonly accepted paradigms ↳ *Implication and effect*	Alternate paradigm ↳ *Implication and effect*
Work ethic: a belief that "hard work" has moral value and makes a person "better." ↳ Belief in the principle of "work ethic" encourages people to mindlessly engage in work for the sake of engaging in work without considering the implications of their actions or other alternatives that might produce a more beneficial outcome.[59]	**Work is the means rather than an end unto itself (except when the "work" is enjoyable, in which case it is no longer "work").** ↳ Occupations and professions can be designed for the enhancement of life (health, pleasure, relationships, the environment, care of the poor) rather than as an end to themselves at the expense of the individual, society, and the environment.
It is "normal" for adults to give 10.5-12 hours per day 5 days per week to work. ↳ In most corporate environments, employee's work at least 8.5 hours per day, with 1 additional hour spent in commuting[60] and another hour spent in preparation, transportation, and maintenance of work-related clothing, preparing work-related meals, maintaining the auto that is used for work-related tasks. With 10.5 hours given directly to work, 0.5-1 additional hours are needed for recuperation from work-related stress ("daily decompression"); thus the average amount of time given to work-related activities is much larger than commonly believed.[61] Because of the time and energies devoted to "work" the vast majority of people feel that they do not have sufficient time for themselves, their families and friends, their creativity, learning about the world, political involvement, and other more important aspects of life. "Not enough time" is the most common reason given by patients for not exercising.	**A paradigm of a 4-day workweek is just as valid and perhaps more valid than one that advocates a 5-day workweek. A paradigm of a 6-hour workday is at least as valid as one of an 8-10 hour workday.** ↳ Many people in our culture are chronically overworked, undernourished, tired and suffer from an insufficiency of time to simply be in community, to rest, to be creative. Living with such limitations and pressures should be expected to produce a population that is reactively hedonistic, impulsive, and prone to addiction. Behaviors that are addictive (e.g., drugs, alcohol) and destructive (e.g., over-eating, alcohol, sugar, fat) are simply frustrated and maladaptive coping strategies to combat the stress caused by a damaging, unnatural paradigm from which most people cannot escape.[62] Redesigning our societal structures and expectations in ways that conform to our natural humanity and biologic, nutritional, and emotional needs is more rational than forcing *en masse* all of humanity to contort and conform to an artificial posture and cadence of performance, productivity, "professionalism", and other unnatural expectations. Less time dedicated to work and all that it entails leaves more time for 1) healthy cooking, 2) relaxed, conscious, and enjoyable eating, 3) exercise, 4) creativity and hobbies, 5) keeping informed of and involved with political change, and 6) participation in social relationships.[63]

[59] "Conventional wisdom is the habitual, the unexamined life, absorbed into the culture and the fashion of the time, lost in the mad rush of accumulation, lulled to sleep by the easy lies of political hacks and newspaper scribblers, or by priests who wouldn't know a god if they met one." Nisker W. Crazy Wisdom. Berkeley; Ten Speed Press: 1990, page 7

[60] Monday, September 8, 2003 -- The average daily one-way commute to work in the United States takes just over 26 minutes, according to the Bureau of Transportation Statistics' Omnibus Household Survey. Omnibus Household Survey Shows Americans' Average Commuting Time is Just Over 26 Minutes. http://www.bts.gov/press_releases/2003/bts020_03/html/bts020_03.html on August 3, 2004

[61] Dominguez JR. Transforming Your Relationship with Money. Sounds True; Book and Cassette edition: 2001

[62] Breton D, Largent C. The Paradigm Conspiracy: Why Our Social Systems Violate Human Potential-And How We Can Change Them. Hazelden: 1998

Quality and quantity of sleep: A sleep duration of less than 8 hours of deep solid sleep each night is physiologically insufficient for most of people; many people feel best with 9 hours of sleep, yet some people appear to function well on about 6 hours of sleep per night. Not only is it important to get a sufficient *quantity* of sleep, but we need to ensure that the *quality* of the sleep receives appropriate attention, as well. Sleep should be mostly continuous, not "broken" or interrupted. Some experts

> **The Importance of Sleep**
>
> Regulation of sleep-wake cycles and the regular satisfaction of sleep needs are important for preservation of immune function, intellectual performance, emotional stability, and the internal regulation of the body's inflammatory tendency.

believe that people should be able to recall their dreams at night, as this may be a sign of proper neurotransmitter status, especially with regard to serotonin, which is affected by pyridoxine[64] as well as other factors. Going to bed at a regular hour (not later than 10 or 11 at night) helps to synchronize the daily schedule with the body's inherent hormonal rhythms and "physiological clock" which expects one to be in deep sleep by midnight and to be waking at approximately 8 o'clock in the morning. Recent research has shown that **sleep deprivation causes a systemic inflammatory response manifested objectively by increases in high-sensitivity C-reactive protein (hsCRP)**.[65] Correspondingly, sleep apnea, a condition associated with repetitive sleep disturbances, is also associated with an elevation of CRP[66], and effective treatment of sleep apnea results in a normalization of CRP levels.[67] We could therefore conclude that **sleep deprivation creates a proinflammatory condition**. Furthermore, **sleep deprivation has been proven to impair intellectual functioning, emotional state, and immune function**, with abnormalities in immune status already evident the morning after sleep deprivation.[68] Wakefulness and exposure to light at night result in a suppression of melatonin production and may therefore contribute to cancer development since melatonin has anticancer actions that would be abrogated by its reduced endogenous production.[69,70] Limited evidence also suggests that melatonin production is altered in patients with the inflammatory conditions eczema[71] and psoriasis[72] and that this sleep-related hormone has anti-inflammatory/anti-autoimmune benefits that may be relevant for the suppression of diseases such as multiple sclerosis[73] and sarcoidosis.[74]

[63] "Take back your time" is a major U.S./Canadian initiative to challenge the epidemic of overwork, over-scheduling and time famine that now threatens our health, our families and relationships, our communities and our environment. http://www.simpleliving.net/timeday/ on August 3, 2004

[64] " ...a significant difference in dream-salience scores (this is a composite score containing measures on vividness, bizarreness, emotionality, and color) between the 250-mg condition and placebo over the first three days of each treatment... An hypothesis is presented involving the role of B-6 in the conversion of tryptophan to serotonin." Ebben M, Lequerica A, Spielman A. Effects of pyridoxine on dreaming: a preliminary study. *Percept Mot Skills* 2002 Feb;94(1):135-40

[65] "CONCLUSIONS: Both acute total and short-term partial sleep deprivation resulted in elevated high-sensitivity CRP concentrations... We propose that sleep loss may be one of the ways that inflammatory processes are activated and contribute to the association of sleep complaints, short sleep duration, and cardiovascular morbidity observed in epidemiologic surveys." Meier-Ewert HK, Ridker PM, et al. Effect of sleep loss on C-reactive protein, an inflammatory marker of cardiovascular risk. *J Am Coll Cardiol.* 2004 Feb 18;43(4):678-83

[66] "OSA is associated with elevated levels of CRP, a marker of inflammation and of cardiovascular risk. The severity of OSA is proportional to the CRP level." Shamsuzzaman AS, Winnicki M, Lanfranchi P, Wolk R, Kara T, Accurso V, Somers VK. Elevated C-reactive protein in patients with obstructive sleep apnea. *Circulation.* 2002 May 28;105(21):2462-4

[67] "CONCLUSIONS: Levels of CRP and IL-6 and spontaneous production of IL-6 by monocytes are elevated in patients with OSAS but are decreased by nCPAP." Yokoe T, Minoguchi K, Matsuo H, Oda N, Minoguchi H, Yoshino G, Hirano T, Adachi M. Elevated levels of C-reactive protein and interleukin-6 in patients with obstructive sleep apnea syndrome are decreased by nasal continuous positive airway pressure. *Circulation.* 2003 Mar 4;107(8):1129-34 Available on-line at http://circ.ahajournals.org/cgi/reprint/107/8/1129.pdf on August 2, 2004

[68] "Taken together, SD induced a deterioration of both mood and ability to work, which was most prominent in the evening after SD, while the maximal alterations of the host defence system could be found twelve hours earlier, i.e., already in the morning following SD." Heiser P, Dickhaus B, Opper C, Hemmeter U, Remschmidt H, Wesemann W, Krieg JC, Schreiber W. Alterations of host defense system after sleep deprivation are followed by impaired mood and psychosocial functioning. *World J Biol Psychiatry* 2001 Apr;2(2):89-94

[69] "Observational studies support an association between night work and cancer risk. We hypothesise that the potential primary culprit for this observed association is the lack of melatonin, a cancer-protective agent whose production is severely diminished in people exposed to light at night." Schernhammer ES, Schulmeister K. Melatonin and cancer risk: does light at night compromise physiologic cancer protection by lowering serum melatonin levels? *Br J Cancer.* 2004 Mar 8;90(5):941-3

[70] "This is the first biological evidence for a potential link between constant light exposure and increased human breast oncogenesis involving MLT suppression and stimulation of tumor LA metabolism." Blask DE, Dauchy RT, Sauer LA, Krause JA, Brainard GC. Growth and fatty acid metabolism of human breast cancer (MCF-7) xenografts in nude rats: impact of constant light-induced nocturnal melatonin suppression. *Breast Cancer Res Treat.* 2003 Jun;79(3):313-20

[71] "In 6 patients exhibiting low serum levels of melatonin, the circadian melatonin rhythm was found to be abolished. In 8 patients a diminished nocturnal melatonin increase was observed compared with the controls (n = 40)." Schwarz W, Birau N, Hornstein OP, Heubeck B, Schonberger A, Meyer C, Gottschalk J. Alterations of melatonin secretion in atopic eczema. *Acta Derm Venereol.* 1988;68(3):224-9

[72] "Our results show that psoriatic patients had lost the nocturnal peak and usual circadian rhythm of melatonin secretion." Mozzanica N, Tadini G, Radaelli A, et al. Plasma melatonin levels in psoriasis. *Acta Derm Venereol.* 1988;68(4):312-6

[73] "This hypothesis is supported by the observation that administration of melatonin (3 mg, orally) at 2:00 p.m., when the patient experienced severe blurring of vision, resulted within 15 minutes in a dramatic improvement in visual acuity and in normalization of the visual evoked potential latency after stimulation of the left eye." Sandyk R. Diurnal variations in vision and relations to circadian melatonin secretion in multiple sclerosis. *Int J Neurosci.* 1995 Nov;83(1-2):1-6

[74] Cagnoni ML, Lombardi A, Cerinic MC, Dedola GL, Pignone A. Melatonin for treatment of chronic refractory sarcoidosis. *Lancet.* 1995;346:1229-30

Helping patients improve quality and quantity of sleep

- Schedule sufficient time for sleep; generally this is 9 hours to allow time for "winding down" and "daily decompression" so that a full 8 hours of sleep can ensue.
- Reduce intake of stimulants such as caffeine, tobacco, and aspartame. Some patients will need to reduce intake only in the evening, while others will need to reduce intake even in the morning in order to have improved quality and quantity of sleep later at night.
- Exercise early in the day (morning or early afternoon) to promote restful sleep at night.[75]
- Avoid aggressive or arousing physical activity in the evening to avoid increases in norepinephrine, epinephrine, and cortisol, which can discourage sleep.
- Dim lights at night to promote melatonin production. Beginning one to two hours before bedtime, turn off bright lights and use only dim lighting. Bright lights reduce melatonin secretion and stimulate neocortical activity and thereby inhibit sleep.
- Have an evening ritual/pattern that helps the psyche recognize that the time for sleep has arrived. Such practices can include relaxing warm tea, meditation, prayer, and daily reflection.
- For patients with a pattern of falling asleep and then waking approximately 4-6 hours later with feelings of hunger or anxiety (nocturnal hypoglycemia), they should eat a small meal or snack of complex carbohydrates, protein, and fat before going to bed. For example, the combination of nuts (or nut butter) with whole fruit such as apples provides protein, fat, and complex carbohydrate with a low glycemic index to provide sustenance throughout the night. Protein powders and other sources of "predigested" amino acids should generally be avoided late at night because an excess consumption of high protein foods can reduce tryptophan entry into the brain and thus reduce serotonin and melatonin synthesis. Most amino acid-derived neurotransmitters such as dopamine, glutamate, and norepinephrine are excitatory/stimulatory in nature.
- Vitamin and mineral supplementation is commonly beneficial, particularly with thiamine[76], methylcobalamin (weak evidence[77]), and magnesium (particularly sleep disturbance associated with restless leg syndrome[78]). Vitamins should be taken earlier in the day (with breakfast and lunch; not before bed); however calcium and magnesium can be taken before bed.
- Earplugs, window covers, and a quiet, snore-free environment are generally conducive to better sleep.
- For patients with difficulty falling asleep, consider 5-hydroxytryptophan consumed with simple carbohydrate (50-200 mg for adults, up to 2 mg/kg[79] for children), melatonin (0.5-10 mg), valerian-hops tea or capsules[80] 60-90 minutes before bedtime.

[75] "This is the first report to demonstrate that low intensity activity in an elderly population can increase deep sleep and improve memory functioning." Naylor E, Penev PD, Orbeta L, Janssen I, Ortiz R, Colecchia EF, Keng M, Finkel S, Zee PC. Daily social and physical activity increases slow-wave sleep and daytime neuropsychological performance in the elderly. *Sleep*. 2000 Feb 1;23(1):87-95

[76] Wilkinson TJ, Hanger HC, Elmslie J, George PM, Sainsbury R. The response to treatment of subclinical thiamine deficiency in the elderly. *Am J Clin Nutr*. 1997;66(4):925-8

[77] "However, because the percentage of improvement was low and significant improvement was inconsistent, Met-12 might be considered to have a low therapeutic potency and possible use as a booster for other treatment methods of the disorders." Takahashi K, et al. Double-blind test on the efficacy of methylcobalamin on sleep-wake rhythm disorders. *Psychiatry Clin Neurosci*. 1999 Apr;53(2):211-3

[78] "Our study indicates that magnesium treatment may be a useful alternative therapy in patients with mild or moderate RLS-or PLMS-related insomnia." Hornyak M, Voderholzer U, et al. Magnesium therapy for periodic leg movements-related insomnia and restless legs syndrome: an open pilot study. *Sleep*. 1998 Aug 1;21(5):501-5

[79] Bruni O, Ferri R, Miano S, Verrillo E. l -5-Hydroxytryptophan treatment of sleep terrors in children. *Eur J Pediatr*. 2004 May 14

[80] "Sleep improvements with a valerian-hops combination are associated with improved quality of life. Both treatments appear safe and did not produce rebound insomnia upon discontinuation during this study. Overall, these findings indicate that a valerian-hops combination and diphenhydramine might be useful adjuncts in the treatment of mild insomnia." Morin CM, Koetter U, Bastien C, Ware JC, Wooten V. Valerian-hops combination and diphenhydramine for treating insomnia: a randomized placebo-controlled clinical trial. *Sleep*. 2005 Nov 1;28(11):1465-71

Exercise: Human existence has changed radically over the past few millennia, centuries, and decades, and one of the most profound changes has been in our relationship to physical activity. Paleologists and historical scientists agree that physical activity among humans is at its all-time historical low, and that levels of exertion that we now call "vigorous and frequent exercise" would have been *completely normal* in the daily lives of our ancestors, who engaged in at least four times more physical activity than their modern-day progeny.[81] At one time—a time in which vigorous physical activity was a normal part of daily life—probably no word existed for what modern people describe and often resist as "exercise."

Daily exercise is health-promoting and restorative

"The health rewards of exercise extend far beyond its benefits for specific diseases." Exercise reduces blood clotting, lowers blood pressure, lowers cholesterol, improves glucose tolerance and insulin sensitivity, enhances self-image, elevates mood, reduces stress, creates a feeling of well-being, reinforces other positive life-style changes, stimulates creative thinking, increases muscle mass, increases basal metabolic rate, promotes improved sleep, stimulates healthy intestinal function, promotes weight loss, and enhances appearance. "Furthermore, **the ability of exercise to restore function to organs, muscles, joints, and bones is not shared by drugs or surgery.**"

Harold Elrick, MD. Exercise is Medicine. *Physician and Sportsmedicine*. 1996: 24; 2 (February)

Daily exercise is the body's physiological expectation

"Although modern technology has made physical exertion optional, it is still important to exercise as though our survival depended on it, and in a different way it still does. **We are genetically adapted to live an extremely physically active lifestyle.**"

O'Keefe JH Jr, Cordain L. Cardiovascular disease resulting from a diet and lifestyle at odds with our Paleolithic genome: how to become a 21st-century hunter-gatherer. *Mayo Clin Proc.* 2004 Jan;79(1):101-8

Our current mode of compulsory primary and secondary education prioritizes "being still" over physical exertion/expression for the vast majority of students' time. Thus having been separated from their inherent tendency to be physically active and emotionally expressive, many children grow into adults who have to be *retaught to inhabit their bodies* and to engage in physical activity on a daily basis. Basic science has proven that this is true: when animals are restrained, they show less activity when freed and no longer tied down. Conversely, when animals are rigorously exercised, they show higher levels of *spontaneous physical activity* when left to their own discretion. A probable sociological parallel is at work in human cultures where, under the guise of *work* and *entertainment*, people are corralled into lifestyles of physical inactivity in a wide range of apparently divergent activities. Watching television, driving a car, seeing a movie, doing computer/desk work at the office, attending a sports event or educational lecture, seeing the opera—all of these are simply different forms of *sitting*, of physical inactivity. Changing our social structure in a way that prioritizes *life* over *work*, such as moving toward a 4-day work week and/or a 6-hour work day, would allow people more time to live their lives, to pursue healthy diets and relationships, to be creative, and to engage in more physical activity; thus, "escape entertainment" such as fiction books and movies and processed "fast foods"—the latter of which are inherently unhealthy[82]—would become less necessary and less attractive.

Industrialized Westernized societies' disregard for connection with the body

"That I deemed it an imposition to have to make use of my perfectly adequate coordination, or resented—from unexamined principle—the use of time to fill a need, was an arbitrary assignment of values that [this other culture] did not share."

Liedloff J. The Continuum Concept. Cambridge, MA: Da Capo Press; 1977, page 15

---

[81] Eaton SB, Cordain L, Eaton SB. An evolutionary foundation for health promotion. *World Rev Nutr Diet* 2001; 90:5-12
[82] For an additional perspective see movie by Morgan Spurlock (director). Super Size Me. www.supersizeme.com released in 2004

Exploring the spectrum of physical activity from inactivity to athleticism

Inactivity	*Minimally active*	*Active*	*Healthy*	*Athletic*
• Bed-ridden • Chair-ridden • Minimal activity, such as walking to car or bathroom or to buy groceries • Activity in this category is equivalent to or barely above that which is necessary to sustain life	• Periodic performance of more activity than the minimal needed to sustain life, such as walking around the block after dinner, or taking a brief stroll at a park or at the beach	• Regular performance of low/moderate levels of activity at work or leisure, at least 30-60 minutes of physical activity per day	• 60-120 minutes of vigorous activity such as running, swimming, cycling, or other physical training 4-7 days per week	• More than 2 hours devoted to conditioning, strengthening, and skill-building 4-7 days per week

At least 30-45 minutes of exercise four days per week is the *absolute minimum*. Ideally, patients who have been sedentary and are over age 45 years would have a pre-exercise physical exam that might also include electrocardiography before embarking on a program of vigorous exercise. Patients who have been sedentary for many years can start slowly with their new exercise program, gradually increasing the duration and intensity. With the simple addition of regular exercise to their routine, patients will have significantly reduced risk for problems such as depression, chronic pain, cancer, coronary artery disease, stroke, hypertension, diabetes, arthritis, osteoporosis, dyslipidemia, obesity, chronic obstructive pulmonary disease, constipation, and other problems.[83] Furthermore, successful prevention and treatment of health problems with exercise and lifestyle modifications reduces dependency on pharmaceutical drugs, thereby further saving lives. O'Keefe and Cordain[84] report that **during the hunter-gatherer period, humans averaged 5-10 miles of daily running and walking**. Additionally, **other physical activities such as heavy lifting, digging, and climbing would have been considered "normal" aspects of daily life rather than "exercise"—an achievement for which modern/industrialized people seek recognition.** Thus, when sedentary patients achieve the first-step goal of walking around the block after dinner, we can commend them for making a significant stride forward in ultimately attaining better health, but we cannot stop there nor delude them into believing that this is adequate.

Common physical activities: a buffet of options from which to choose
☑ **"Boot camp"-style aerobics classes**: excellent variety and fast-pace maintains oxygen debt for the entire session (generally 60 minutes) even among reasonably well trained "healthy" people
☑ **Aerobic machines such as elliptical runners and stair-climbing machines**: easy on joints; accessible during inclement weather; easy to integrate with weight-lifting which is commonly available at the same facility
☑ **Baseball**: requires some skill in throwing and batting, but otherwise this is a very inactive sport
☑ **Football**: much of the game is spent in inactivity; most of the fitness comes from preparation for the game, not the game itself; high impact activity wherein injuries are expected
☑ **Hiking**: virtually free of expense; allows for conversation, exploration, and time in nature; mountains required
☑ **Indoor aerobics**: excellent for cardiovascular fitness and weight loss, requires and thus promotes coordination and timing
☑ **Indoor cycling**: excellent for cardiovascular fitness and weight loss, easy on the joints; accessible during inclement weather
☑ **Jogging and running**: easy, accessible, virtually free; allows for conversation and exploration; increases endorphin production and promotes a sense of well-being; detoxification via sweating
☑ **Kayaking and canoeing**: excellent combination of relaxation and exertion; develops upper body strength and balance
☑ **Martial arts**: requires more balance, coordination, timing, strategy, endurance; injuries are to be expected, as is enhanced sense of security and confidence
☑ **Outdoor cycling (mountain and trail)**: same as above; requires more balance and coordination
☑ **Outdoor cycling (road)**: same as above with added bonus of being outdoors; promotes independence from automobiles and petroleum products – thereby reducing pollution and sustaining the environment

---

[83] Harold Elrick, MD. Exercise is Medicine. *The Physician and Sportsmedicine* - Volume 24 - No. 2 - February 1996

[84] O'Keefe JH Jr, Cordain L. Cardiovascular disease resulting from a diet and lifestyle at odds with our Paleolithic genome: how to become a 21st-century hunter-gatherer. *Mayo Clin Proc.* 2004 Jan;79(1):101-8. Available on line at http://www.thepaleodiet.com/articles/Hunter-Gatherer%20Mayo.pdf on May 19, 2004

- ☑ **Rock-climbing (indoor and outdoor)**: requires upper body and grip strength; promotes agility, resourcefulness, courage, and trust; good for building stronger relationships assuming that your partner does not drop the rope or get distracted; carries some inherent risk
- ☑ **Skiing, snowboarding, cross-country skiing**: Require balance and coordination, costly equipment, and appropriate season and climate; risk of traumatic injury due to speed in skiing and snowboarding. Cross-country skiing is generally safe from trauma and provides excellent cardiovascular exertion, in addition to exposure to nature
- ☑ **Soccer**: excellent for lower-body conditioning, teamwork, and coordination, the rapid stops and turns can be hard on joints
- ☑ **Surfing**: paddling requires upper body endurance and strength; some leg strength is required but is not strongly developed during the riding portion of surfing, which is mostly technique and "style"; excellent proprioceptive training
- ☑ **Swimming**: requires access to a pool or suitable body of water; excellent for promoting fitness in a way that is generally easy on joints and muscles and is without impact; requires and thus promotes coordination and timing
- ☑ **Tennis and racket sports**: requires more balance, coordination, timing, strategy, endurance; the rapid stops, starts, and turns can be hard on joints; upper body exertion is asymmetric and can promote muscle imbalance
- ☑ **Volleyball**: good team activity; not highly exertional in terms of either aerobic fitness nor strength acquisition
- ☑ **Walking**: easy, accessible, virtually free; allows for conversation and exploration; allows for time outdoors
- ☑ **Weight lifting, bodybuilding, and powerlifting**: excellent for increasing lean body mass – one of the primary determinants of basal metabolic rate; promotes bone strengthening
- ☑ **Yoga, Calisthenics**: inexpensive, can be done alone or in groups; does not require much/any equipment, therefore costs are low and access is near universal

Obesity: Obesity is a major risk factor for cardiovascular disease, cancer, diabetes mellitus, depression, joint degeneration and pain. Obese people also commonly report difficulties with performing daily activities, and they also report higher rates of depression and social isolation than do people of normal weight. Adipose tissue is biologically active, promoting systemic inflammation and estrogen dominance, thereby promoting the development of inflammatory and malignant diseases such as psoriasis and cancers of the breast, prostate, and colon, respectively.

"Body Mass Index" is a clinically valuable measure of height-weight proportionality and therefore adiposity, since an excess of height-proportionate weight is more commonly due to excess adipose than to excess muscle. To calculate BMI simply chart height and weight in the table below. Numbers greater than 25 correlate with being "overweight" while numbers greater than 30 meet the criteria for "obesity." BMI determinations may not be reflective of disease risk for people who are pregnant, highly muscular, or for young children or the frail elderly.

Body mass index (BMI) interpretation
- ❑ Severely underweight: < 16.5
- ❑ Underweight: 16.5 - 18.4
- ❑ **Normal: 18.5 - 24.9**
- ❑ Overweight: 25 - 29.9
- ❑ Obese Class 1: 30 - 34.9
- ❑ Obese Class 2 (severe obesity): 35 - 39.9
- ❑ Obese Class 3 (morbid obesity): 40 - 47.9
- ❑ Obese Class 4 (supermorbid obesity): ≥ 48

WEIGHT in pounds

HEIGHT	100	110	120	130	140	150	160	170	180	190	200	210	220	230	240	250
5'0"	20	21	23	25	27	29	31	33	35	37	39	41	43	45	47	49
5'1"	19	21	23	25	26	28	30	32	34	36	38	40	42	43	45	47
5'2"	18	20	22	24	26	27	29	31	33	35	37	38	40	42	44	46
5'3"	18	19	21	23	25	27	28	30	32	34	35	37	39	41	43	44
5'4"	17	19	21	22	24	26	27	29	31	33	34	36	38	39	41	43
5'5"	17	18	20	22	23	25	27	28	30	32	33	35	37	38	40	42
5'6"	16	18	19	21	23	24	26	27	29	31	32	34	36	37	39	40
5'7"	16	17	19	20	22	23	25	27	28	30	31	33	34	36	38	39
5'8"	15	17	18	20	21	23	24	26	27	29	30	32	33	35	36	38
5'9"	15	16	18	19	21	22	24	25	27	28	30	31	32	34	35	37
5'10"	14	16	17	19	20	22	23	24	26	27	29	30	32	33	34	36
5'11"	14	15	17	18	20	21	22	24	25	26	27	28	30	32	33	35
6'0"	14	15	16	18	19	20	22	23	24	26	27	28	30	31	33	34
6'1"	13	15	16	17	18	20	21	22	24	25	26	28	29	30	32	33
6'2"	13	14	15	17	18	19	21	22	23	24	26	27	28	30	31	32
6'3"	12	14	15	16	17	19	20	21	22	24	25	26	27	29	30	31
6'4"	12	13	15	16	17	18	19	21	22	23	24	26	27	28	29	30

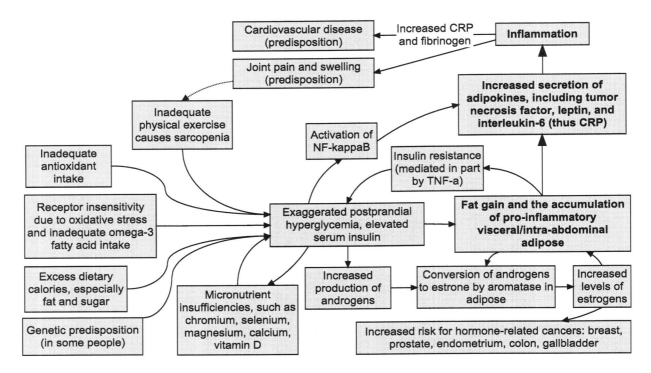

Overview of the proinflammatory and endocrinologic activity of adipose tissue: Adipose tissue is biologically active, promoting systemic inflammation and production of estrogens at the expense of androgens via the enzyme aromatase

The old view that fat (adipose) tissue was merely serving as an inert and inactive depot for lipid/energy storage is now replaced with the view that adipose tissue is biologically-active, influencing overall health via complex mechanisms that are biochemical-inflammatory-endocrinologic and not merely mechanical (i.e., excess weight, excess mass).[85] **Excess fat tissue—especially visceral/abdominal adipose—creates a systemic proinflammatory state** evidenced most readily by the elevations in hsCRP commonly seen in patients with obesity and the metabolic syndrome.[86] Adipokines are cytokines secreted by adipose tissue and include tumor necrosis factor-alpha, interleukin-6, and leptin—a cytokine derived from fat cells that promotes inflammation and immune activation; levels are higher in obese patients and decrease after weight loss. Obese patients also appear to have "leptin resistance" with regard to the suppression of appetite by leptin. **Adipose creates excess estrogens;** concomitant hyperglycemia increases androgen production[87], and these androgens are subsequently converted to estrogens by aromatase in the adipose tissue. For example, the adrenal gland makes androstenedione, which can be converted by aromatase in adipose tissue into estrone.[88] These proinflammatory and hormonal perturbations manifest clinically as an increased risk for breast, prostate, endometrial, colon and gallbladder cancers, and cardiovascular disease. This pattern of inflammation, reduced testosterone, and elevated estrogen is also a predisposition toward the development of autoimmune/inflammatory diseases.

---

[85] "The fat cell is a true endocrine cell that secretes a variety of factors, including metabolites such as lactate, fatty acids, prostaglandin derivatives and a variety of peptides, including cytokines (leptin, tumor necrosis factor, interleukin-1 and -6, adiponectin), angiotensinogen, complement D (adipsin), plasminogen activator inhibitor-1 and undoubtedly many others." Bray GA. The underlying basis for obesity: relationship to cancer. *J Nutr.* 2002 Nov;132(11 Suppl):3451S-3455S

[86] "Our results indicate a strong relationship between adipocytokines and inflammatory markers, and suggest that cytokines secreted by adipose tissue could play a role in increased inflammatory proteins secretion by the liver." Maachi M, Pieroni L, Bruckert E, Jardel C, Fellahi S, Hainque B, Capeau J, Bastard JP. Systemic low-grade inflammation is related to both circulating and adipose tissue TNFalpha, leptin and IL-6 levels in obese women. *Int J Obes Relat Metab Disord.* 2004;28:993-7

[87] Christensen L, Hagen C, Henriksen JE, Haug E. Elevated levels of sex hormones and sex hormone binding globulin in male patients with insulin dependent diabetes mellitus. Effect of improved blood glucose regulation. *Dan Med Bull.* 1997 Nov;44(5):547-50

[88] "The conversion of androstenedione secreted by the adrenal gland into estrone by aromatase in adipose tissue stroma provides an important source of estrogen for the postmenopausal woman. This estrogen may play an important role in the development of endometrial and breast cancer." Bray GA. The underlying basis for obesity: relationship to cancer. *J Nutr.* 2002 Nov;132(11 Suppl):3451S-3455S

The Daily Diet—Powerful Intervention for the Prevention and Treatment of Disease: "Whole foods" should form the foundation and majority of the diet. As doctors and patients, we should emphasize whole fruits, vegetables, nuts, seeds, berries, and lean sources of protein. "Whole foods" are foods that are found in nature, and they should be eaten as closely as possible to their natural state—preferably *unprocessed* and *raw*. Creating a diet based on whole, natural foods by emphasizing the consumption of fruits, vegetables, and lean meats and excluding high-fat factory meats, high-sugar foods like white potatoes, and milled grains like wheat and corn is essential for our efforts of promoting health by matching the human *diet* with the human *genome*.[89] Our genetic make-up was co-created over a period of more than 2.6 million years by interaction with the environment as it exists in its natural state. This environment mandated daily physical activity and a diet that was exclusively composed of 1) fresh fruits, 2) fresh vegetables (mostly uncooked), 3) raw nuts, seeds, berries, roots, and 4) generous portions of lean game meat that was rich in omega-3 fatty acids from free-living animals who were lean because they also ran, fasted, and dealt with limited food supplies. Humans have deviated from this original diet for the sake of ease, conformity, and short-term satisfaction at the expense of health and longevity. Peoples who consume traditional, natural diets have dramatically lower incidences *major* health problems such as cancer, cardiovascular disease, diabetes, obesity and also suffer much less from *milder* problems such as acne, psoriasis, dental cavities, oral

---

The Supplemented Paleo-Mediterranean Diet

My conclusion after reading several hundred articles on epidemiology, nutritional biochemistry, and dietary intervention studies is that the Paleo-Mediterranean diet—particularly its pesco-vegetarian version—is the single most healthy dietary regimen for the broadest range of patients and for the prevention of the widest range of diseases including cancer, hypertension, diabetes, dermatitis, depression, obesity, arthritis and all inflammatory and autoimmune diseases. By definition, this is a diet that helps patients increase their intake of fruits and vegetables (fiber, antioxidants, phytonutrients), increases their intake of fish (for the anti-inflammatory omega-3 fats EPA and DHA) while reducing intake of the pro-cancer and pro-inflammatory omega-6 fats linoleic acid and arachidonic acid), and it is naturally low in sugars and cholesterol (for alleviating hyperglycemia and dyslipidemia). This dietary pattern helps patients avoid grains, particularly wheat (a common allergen), and it reduces the intake of the high-fermentation carbohydrates in breads, pasta, pastries, potatoes, and sucrose which promote overgrowth of bacteria and yeast in the intestines. Supplementing this pesco-vegetarian diet with vitamins, minerals, fatty acids such as fish oil and GLA (from borage oil), and protein from soy and whey makes this diet effective for both the treatment and prevention of many conditions; I have called this "the Supplemented Paleo-Mediterranean Diet."

1. Vasquez A. A Five-Part Nutritional Protocol that Produces Consistently Positive Results. *Nutritional Wellness* 2005 September
2. Vasquez A. Implementing the Five-Part Nutritional Wellness Protocol for the Treatment of Various Health Problems. *Nutritional Wellness* 2005 November
3. Vasquez A. Revisiting the Five-Part Nutritional Wellness Protocol: The Supplemented Paleo-Mediterranean Diet. *Nutritional Perspectives* 2011 January

The complete texts of these articles are included within this book and on-line at http://optimalhealthresearch.com/spmd.html

---

malocclusion, and chronic sinus congestion. Societies that are free of these disorders become overwhelmed with them *within only one or two generations* as soon as they adopt the American/Western style of eating. These facts were conclusively documented by Weston Price in his famous 1945 masterpiece *Nutrition and Physical Degeneration*[90] and have been reiterated recently in an excellent review by O'Keefe and Cordain in *Mayo Clinic Proceedings*.[91]

Most patients (and doctors) need to increase consumption of fruits and vegetables: Encourage consumption of collard greens, broccoli, kale, spinach, chard, lettuce, onions, red peppers, green beans, carrots, apples, oranges, nuts, blueberries and other fruits and vegetables. Patients can find or make a good low-carbohydrate dressing (such as lemon-garlic tahini[92]) to make these vegetables taste great. Fresh fruits and vegetables are best; but frozen fruits and vegetables are acceptable. Patients can buy a package of (organic) frozen vegetables; then when they are ready for a healthy-and-fast meal, simply thaw the vegetables or warm/steam them on the stovetop. In just a few minutes and with only minimal effort, by regularly eating vegetables, they will have significantly reduced their risk for heart disease, diabetes, cancer, hemorrhoids, constipation, and many other chronic health problems. Using frozen vegetables and eating vegetables only twice per day is not *optimal*—it is *minimal*. For many patients,

---

[89] O'Keefe JH Jr, Cordain L. Cardiovascular disease resulting from a diet and lifestyle at odds with our Paleolithic genome: how to become a 21st-century hunter-gatherer. *Mayo Clin Proc.* 2004 Jan;79(1):101-8
[90] Price WA. Nutrition and Physical Degeneration. Santa Monica; Price-Pottinger Nutrition Foundation: 1945
[91] O'Keefe JH Jr,Cordain L.Cardiovascular disease resulting from a diet and lifestyle at odds with our Paleolithic genome. *Mayo Clin Proc.*2004;79:101-8
[92] Mollie Katzen. The New Moosewood Cookbook Ten Speed Press; page 103

consuming two servings of vegetables per day is a major lifestyle change. ***Ultimately, the goal is for fresh fruits and vegetables to form a major portion of the diet, to be the main course rather than simply a side dish.*** A diet based on fruits and vegetables is a powerful nutritional strategy for reducing the risk for cancer, heart disease, and autoimmune and inflammatory disorders.[93]

Proteins, fruits, vegetables—not grains

"Historical and archaeological evidence shows hunter-gatherers generally to be lean, fit, and largely free from signs and symptoms of chronic diseases. When hunter-gatherer societies transitioned to an agricultural grain-based diet, their general health deteriorated. ... When former hunter-gatherers adopt Western lifestyles, obesity, type-2 diabetes, atherosclerosis, and other diseases of civilization become commonplace."

O'Keefe JH Jr, Cordain L. Cardiovascular disease resulting from a diet and lifestyle at odds with our Paleolithic genome. *Mayo Clin Proc.* 2004;79:101-8

<u>**Phytochemicals—important antioxidant and anti-inflammatory nutrients from fruits, vegetables, nuts, seeds, berries, and many herbs and spices**</u>: While we have all commonly thought of the benefits of fruits and vegetables as being derived from the vitamins, minerals, and fiber, we are learning from new research that many if not most of the health-promoting benefits of fruit and vegetable consumption comes from the unique plant-based chemicals—phytochemicals—contained therein. For example, while in the past we might have thought of the benefits of eating apples as being derived from the vitamin C content, we now know that vitamin C only provides 0.4% of the antioxidant action contained within a whole apple—obviously the other components of the apple, namely the phenolic compounds are responsible for most of an apple's antioxidant activity.[94] Recent research has shown that cranberries, apples, red grapes, and strawberries have the most antioxidant power of the fruits[95], while red peppers, broccoli, carrots, and spinach are the best antioxidant vegetables[96]; see the tables that follow. This is a very important concept to appreciate and remember: **the benefits derived from fruits and vegetables are <u>not</u> derived principally from the vitamins and therefore can never be obtained from the use of multivitamin pills as a substitute for whole foods. Multivitamin and multimineral supplements are valuable and worthwhile *supplements* to a whole-foods diet but should not be used as *substitutes* for a whole-foods diet. Fruits and vegetables contain more than 8,000 phytochemicals, most of which have anti-inflammatory, anti-proliferative, and anti-cancer benefits[97]—the best and only way to benefit from these chemicals is to change the diet in favor of relying principally on fruits and vegetables as the major component of the diet**, and the easiest way to do this is to eliminate carbohydrate-rich antioxidant-poor foods such as bread, pasta, rice, sweets, crackers, chips and "junk foods."

Phenolic content and antioxidant capacity of common vegetables and fruits[98,99]

Vegetables		Fruits	
Phenolic content	*Antioxidant capacity*	*Phenolic content*	*Antioxidant capacity*
1. Broccoli	1. Red pepper	1. Cranberry	1. Cranberry
2. Spinach	2. Broccoli	2. Apple	2. Apple
3. Yellow onion	3. Carrot	3. Red grape	3. Red grape
4. Red pepper	4. Spinach	4. Strawberry	4. Strawberry
5. Carrot	5. Cabbage	5. Pineapple	5. Peach
6. Cabbage	6. Yellow onion	6. Banana	6. Lemon
7. Potato	7. Celery	7. Peach	7. Pear
8. Lettuce	8. Potato	8. Lemon	8. Banana
9. Celery	9. Lettuce	9. Orange	9. Orange
10. Cucumber	10. Cucumber	10. Pear	10. Grapefruit
		11. Grapefruit	11. Pineapple

---

[93] "...one of the most consistent research findings is that those who consume higher amounts of fruits and vegetables have lower rates of heart disease and stroke as well as cancer..." Seaman DR. The diet-induced proinflammatory state: a cause of chronic pain and other degenerative diseases? *J Manipulative Physiol Ther.* 2002;25(3):168-79

[94] "We propose that the additive and synergistic effects of phytochemicals in fruit and vegetables are responsible for their potent antioxidant and anticancer activities, and that the benefit of a diet rich in fruit and vegetables is attributed to the complex mixture of phytochemicals present in whole foods." Liu RH. Health benefits of fruit and vegetables are from additive and synergistic combinations of phytochemicals. *Am J Clin Nutr.* 2003 Sep;78(3 Suppl):517S-520S

[95] "Cranberry had the highest total antioxidant activity (177.0 +/- 4.3 micromol of vitamin C equiv/g of fruit), followed by apple, red grape, strawberry, peach, lemon, pear, banana, orange, grapefruit, and pineapple." Sun J, Chu YF, Wu X, Liu RH. Antioxidant and antiproliferative activities of common fruits. *J Agric Food Chem.* 2002 Dec 4;50(25):7449-54

[96] "Red pepper had the highest total antioxidant activity, followed by broccoli, carrot, spinach, cabbage, yellow onion, celery, potato, lettuce, and cucumber." Chu YF, Sun J, Wu X, Liu RH. Antioxidant and antiproliferative activities of common vegetables. *J Agric Food Chem.* 2002;50:6910-6

[97] Liu RH. Health benefits of fruit and vegetables are from additive and synergistic combinations of phytochemicals. *Am J Clin Nutr.* 2003 Sep;78(3 Suppl):517S-520S

[98] Chu YF, Sun J, Wu X, Liu RH. Antioxidant and antiproliferative activities of common vegetables. *J Agric Food Chem.* 2002;50:6910-6

[99] Sun J, Chu YF, Wu X, Liu RH. Antioxidant and antiproliferative activities of common fruits. *J Agric Food Chem.* 2002;50:7449-54

Different fruits and vegetables contain different types, quantities, and ratios of vitamins, minerals, and phytochemicals; therefore, *dietary diversity* **will therefore help patients obtain a broad spectrum of and maximum benefit from these different nutrients**. Taking appropriate action with the data that a fruit/vegetable-based diet has powerful health-promoting benefits means that we as doctors and patients have to change our lifestyles with regard to how we plan our meals, what we buy, what we prepare, and what we eat. Behavior modification is a tremendous challenge for people, especially those who lack sufficient motivation or insight. This text is providing the *insight*—the data, references, and concepts. But without *motivation*—from doctors to help their patients attain the highest levels of health, and from patients to change their lifestyles to become as healthy as possible—the research itself does little to promote health.

<u>**Consuming the right amount of protein**</u>: Dietary protein is eaten to provide the body with amino acids, which are the fundamental components that the body uses to create new tissues (such as skin, mucosal surfaces, hair, and nails), heal wounds (e.g., formation of collagen), fight off infections (e.g., formation of immunoglobulin proteins, antibodies), and to create specific hormones (such as insulin and thyroid hormones) and neurotransmitters, such as dopamine, serotonin, norepinephrine, and gamma-aminobutyric acid (GABA). Amino acid profiles in meats, eggs, and milk is similar to that of the human body and such dietary sources have been described as containing relatively more "complete protein" than most plant-based protein sources. For plant-based diets without concomitant use of animal proteins to provide sufficient quantity and quality of protein, foods must be combined with respect to one another's amino acid profiles.

For most people (without kidney or liver problems) the goal for daily protein intake should be 0.50-0.75 grams of protein per pound of lean body weight, depending on activity level and other health needs (see table).

Recommended <u>Grams of Protein</u> Per <u>Pound of Body Weight</u> Per Day[100]	
Infants and children ages 1-6 years[101]	0.68-0.45
RDA for sedentary adult and children ages 6-18 years[102]	0.4
Adult recreational exerciser	**0.5-0.75**
Adult competitive athlete	0.6-0.9
Adult building muscle mass	0.7-0.9
Dieting athlete	0.7-1.0
Growing teenage athlete	0.9-1.0
Pregnant women need additional protein	Add 15-30 grams/day[103]

Sufficient dietary protein is essential for patients with musculoskeletal injuries because tissue healing relies on the constant availability of amino acids and micronutrients[104], which should be supplied by a healthy, balanced, whole-foods diet that may be supplemented with specific vitamins, minerals, and phytonutrients. Low-protein diets suppress immune function, reduce muscle mass, and impair healing[105,106] whereas intakes of higher amounts of protein safely facilitate healing and the maintenance of muscle mass. Increased protein intake does not adversely affect bone health as long as dietary calcium intake is adequate.[107] According to the 1998 review by Lemon[108], "Those involved in strength training might need to consume as much as …1.7 g protein x kg(-1) x day(-

---

[100] Slightly modified from Nancy Clark, MS, RD. Protein Power. *The Physician and Sportsmedicine* 1996, volume 24, number 4

[101] 1.5-1 g/kg/d (0.68-0.45 grams per pound of body weight. Younger people need proportionately more protein.) Brown ML (ed). Present Knowledge in Nutrition. Sixth Edition. Washington DC: International Life Sciences Institute Nutrition Foundation; 1990 page 68

[102] 0.83 g.kg-1.d-1 (equivalent to 0.37 grams per pound of body weight) Pellet PL. Protein requirements in humans. *Am J Clin Nutr* 1990 May;51:723-37

[103] Weinsier RL, Morgan SL (eds). Fundamentals of Clinical Nutrition. St. Louis: Mosby, 1993 page 50

[104] "Supplementation with protein and vitamins, specifically arginine and vitamins A, B, and C, provides optimum nutrient support of the healing wound." Meyer NA, Muller MJ, Herndon DN. Nutrient support of the healing wound. *New Horiz* 1994 May;2(2):202-14

[105] Castaneda C, Charnley JM, Evans WJ, Crim MC. Elderly women accommodate to a low-protein diet with losses of body cell mass, muscle function, and immune response. *Am J Clin Nutr* 1995 Jul;62(1):30-9 http://www.ajcn.org/cgi/reprint/62/1/30

[106] [No author listed]. Vegetarians and healing. *JAMA* 1995; 273: 910

[107] Heaney RP. Excess dietary protein may not adversely affect bone. *J Nutr* 1998 Jun;128(6):1054-7

[108] Lemon PW. Effects of exercise on dietary protein requirements. *Int J Sport Nutr 1998* Dec;8(4):426-47

1)…while those undergoing endurance training might need about 1.2 to 1.6 g x kg(-1) x day(-1)... **...there is no evidence that protein intakes in the range suggested will have adverse effects in healthy individuals."**

For patients who are completely sedentary, multiply body weight in pounds by 0.4 and this will give the number of grams of protein that should be eaten each day.[109] For patients who are very active (frequent weight lifting, or competitive athlete), multiply body weight in pounds by 0.7-0.9 and this will give the number of grams of protein that should be eaten each day.

Again, compared with sedentary people, *sick people, injured people,* and *athletes* **need more protein** to maintain weight, fight infections, repair injuries, and build and maintain muscle. Not only can insufficient protein intake cause muscle weakness and loss of weight, but recent articles have also suggested that low-protein diets can cause suppression of the immune system[110] and impairment of healing after injury or surgery.[111]

For example, in most instances and according to the data presented in and reviewed for this section, a person weighing 120 pounds should aim for at least 60 grams of protein per day, or 90 grams of protein per day if he/she is more physically active, ill, or injured. A can of tuna has 30 grams of protein; one egg has 6 grams of protein. If she is going to eat eggs as a source of protein for a meal, she might have to eat as many as five eggs to reach a target of 30 grams of protein per meal. When eating meat, visualize the amount of meat in a can of tuna to estimate the amount of protein being eaten—for example, if the portion of meat at a given meal is about the size of a half can of tuna, then we can estimate that the serving contains 15-20 grams of high-quality protein. By knowing the "target intake" for the day, and by estimating the amount of protein eaten with each meal, patients will be able to modify their protein intake to ensure that they reach their protein intake goal.

Protein supplements—most common of which are based on concentrates of or isolated components of egg, soy, or cow's milk— can be used *in conjunction with a healthy diet*. Patients using a protein supplement should eat a healthy diet and then add protein supplements between regular meals. If they substitute a protein supplement for a regular meal, then they may not actually increase protein intake. Whole *real* foods should form the foundation for the diet—patients should not rely too heavily on *protein supplements* when patients can get better results *and improved overall health* with *whole foods*. Whey, casein, and lactalbumin are proteins from milk and dairy products, and may therefore be allergenic in people allergic to cow's milk. Soy protein is safe and a source of high-quality protein for adults[112], and research shows that consumption of soy protein can help reduce the risk of cancer and heart disease[113]; however, I do not recommend the use of large quantities of supplemental soy protein for pregnant women, or for children due to the potential for disrupting endocrine function. Patients may have to experiment with different products until they find one that is suitable in regard to taste, texture, digestibility, hypoallergenicity, nutritional effects, ease of preparation, and affordability.

Recall again that the goal is *improved health*, not simply *adequate protein intake*. If we focus solely on "grams of protein" then we might overlook adverse effects that are associated with certain protein sources. Cow's milk is a high quality protein, but it is commonly allergenic and can exacerbate joint pain in sensitive individuals.[114] Beef, liver, pork and other land animal meats are excellent sources of protein, but they are also generally rich sources of arachidonic acid[115] (if not grass-fed) and iron[116], both of which have been shown to exacerbate joint pain and inflammation. Fish is an excellent source of protein, but fish are often poisoned with mercury and other toxicants, which can be ingested by humans to produce negative health effects.[117,118]

---

[109] Pellet PL. Protein requirements in humans. *Am J Clin Nutr* 1990 May;51(5):723-37

[110] Castaneda C, Charnley JM, Evans WJ, Crim MC. Elderly women accommodate to a low-protein diet with losses of body cell mass, muscle function, and immune response. *Am J Clin Nutr* 1995 Jul;62(1):30-9

[111] Vegetarians and healing. *Journal of the American Medical Association* 1995; 273: 910

[112] "These results indicate that for healthy adults, the isolated soy protein is of high nutritional quality, comparable to that of animal protein sources, and that the methionine content is not limiting for adult protein maintenance." Young VR, Puig M, Queiroz E, Scrimshaw NS, Rand WM. Evaluation of the protein quality of an isolated soy protein in young men: relative nitrogen requirements and effect of methionine supplementation. *Am J Clin Nutr*. 1984 Jan;39(1):16-24

[113] Lissin LW, Cooke JP. Phytoestrogens and cardiovascular health. *J Am Coll Cardiol*. 2000 May;35(6):1403-10

[114] Golding DN. Is there an allergic synovitis? *J R Soc Med* 1990 May;83(5):312-4

[115] Adam O, Beringer C, Kless T, Lemmen C, Adam A, Wiseman M, Adam P, Klimmek R, Forth W. Anti-inflammatory effects of a low arachidonic acid diet and fish oil in patients with rheumatoid arthritis. *Rheumatol Int* 2003 Jan;23(1):27-36

[116] Dabbagh AJ, Trenam CW, Morris CJ, Blake DR. Iron in joint inflammation. *Ann Rheum Dis* 1993; 52:67-73

[117] "These fish often harbor high levels of methylmercury, a potent human neurotoxin." Evans EC. The FDA recommendations on fish intake during pregnancy. *J Obstet Gynecol Neonatal Nurs* 2002 Nov-Dec;31(6):715-20

[118] "Geometric mean mercury levels were almost 4-fold higher among women who ate 3 or more servings of fish in the past 30 days compared with women who ate no fish in that period.." Schober SE, Sinks TH, Jones RL, Bolger PM, McDowell M, Osterloh J, Garrett ES, Canady RA, Dillon CF, Sun Y, Joseph CB, Mahaffey KR. Blood mercury levels in US children and women of childbearing age, 1999-2000. *JAMA* 2003 Apr 2;289(13):1667-74

Eat complex carbohydrates to stabilize blood sugar, mood, and energy: Choose items with a "low glycemic index"[119] to stabilize blood sugar and—for many people—to lower triglycerides and cholesterol levels. Foods with a low Glycemic Index (GI < 55)[120] include yogurt, apple (36), whole orange (43), peach (28), legumes, lentils (28), and soybeans (18), cherries, dried apricots, nuts, most meats, and most vegetables. Healthy foods that have both a low *glycemic index* as well as a low *glycemic load* include: apples, carrots, chick peas, grapes, green peas, kidney beans, oranges, peaches, peanuts, pears, pinto beans, red lentils, and strawberries.[121]

Reduce or eliminate simple sugars from the diet (as necessary): Nearly everyone should minimize intake of table sugar (sucrose), fructose and high-fructose corn syrup, and all artificial sweeteners. Of important and recent note, high-fructose corn syrup has been shown to be contaminated by mercury due to the manufacturing process[122], and fructose has been shown to induce hypertension and the metabolic syndrome in humans.[123] Chronic overconsumption of refined carbohydrates promotes disease by 1) increasing urinary excretion of magnesium and calcium, 2) inducing oxidative stress, 3) promoting fat deposition and obesity, which then generally leads to insulin resistance and hyperinsulinemia with an increase in production of cholesterol, triglycerides, and proinflammatory adipokines[124], and 4) reducing function of leukocytes.[125] Among sweeteners, honey is the best choice since it is the only natural sweetener available with a wide range of health-promoting benefits including anti-inflammatory, antibacterial, antioxidant and anti-allergy effects.[126] Also consider the herb stevia as a non-caloric and nutritive sweetener. Occasional intake of sweets is likely to be of little consequence for people who are generally healthy and who are willing to sustain relatively short-term endothelial dysfunction[127], oxidative stress[128], increased LDL oxidation[129], and activation of NF-kappaB[130] as a result of their self-induced hyperglycemia. Postexertional hyperglycemia can be used to enhance athletic performance by sustaining and inducing glycogen storage following and during exercise (i.e., carbohydrate loading for glycogen "supercompensation"[131,132]). Similarly, consumption of "simple" carbohydrate without protein can be used to

---

[119] For more information on glycemic index, consult a nutrition book or website such as http://www.stanford.edu/~dep/gilists.htm last accessed August 16, 2003

[120] Janette Brand-Miller, Kaye Foster-Powell. Diets with a low glycemic index: from theory to practice. *Nutrition Today* 1999 March. Accessed on-line at: http://www.findarticles.com/cf_dls/m0841/2_34/54654508/p1/article.jhtml on August 16, 2003.

[121] Mendosa D. Glycemic Values of Common American Foods http://www.mendosa.com/common_foods.htm Accessed on August 4, 2004

[122] "Average daily consumption of high fructose corn syrup is about 50 grams per person in the United States. With respect to total mercury exposure, it may be necessary to account for this source of mercury in the diet of children and sensitive populations." Dufault R, LeBlanc B, Schnoll R, Cornett C, Schweitzer L, Wallinga D, Hightower J, Patrick L, Lukiw WJ. Mercury from chlor-alkali plants: measured concentrations in food product sugar. *Environ Health*. 2009 Jan 26;8:2. See also: "High fructose corn syrup has been shown to contain trace amounts of mercury as a result of some manufacturing processes, and its consumption can also lead to zinc loss." Dufault R, Schnoll R, Lukiw WJ, Leblanc B, Cornett C, Patrick L, Wallinga D, Gilbert SG, Crider R. Mercury exposure, nutritional deficiencies and metabolic disruptions may affect learning in children. *Behav Brain Funct*. 2009 Oct 27;5:44.

[123] News release from American Heart Association's 63rd High Blood Pressure Research Conference. High-sugar diet increases men's blood pressure; gout drug protective. Abstract P127. Sept. 23, 2009. http://americanheart.mediaroom.com/index.php?s=43&item=829 Accessed December 19, 2009

[124] "Because visceral and subcutaneous adipose tissues are the major sources of cytokines (adipokines), increased adipose tissue mass is associated with alteration in adipokine production (eg, overexpression of tumor necrosis factor-a, interleukin-6, plasminogen activator inhibitor-1, and underexpression of adiponectin in adipose tissue)." Aldhahi W, Hamdy O. Adipokines, inflammation, and the endothelium in diabetes. *Curr Diab Rep*. 2003 Aug;3(4):293-8

[125] Sanchez A, Reeser JL, Lau HS, Yahiku PY, Willard RE, McMillan PJ, Cho SY, Magie AR, Register UD. Role of sugars in human neutrophilic phagocytosis. *Am J Clin Nutr*. 1973 Nov;26(11):1180-4

[126] Al-Waili NS. Effects of daily consumption of honey solution on hematological indices and blood levels of minerals and enzymes in normal individuals. *J Med Food*. 2003 Summer;6(2):135-4

[127] "Modest hyperinsulinemia, mimicking fasting hyperinsulinemia of insulin-resistant states, abrogates endothelium-dependent vasodilation in large conduit arteries, probably by increasing oxidant stress. These data may provide a novel pathophysiological basis to the epidemiological link between hyperinsulinemia/insulin-resistance and atherosclerosis in humans." Arcaro G, Cretti A, Balzano S, Lechi A, Muggeo M, Bonora E, Bonadonna RC. Insulin causes endothelial dysfunction in humans: sites and mechanisms. *Circulation*. 2002 Feb 5;105(5):576-82

[128] "Hyperglycemia increased plasma MDA concentrations, but the activities of GSH-Px and SOD were significantly higher after a larger dose of glucose only. Plasma catecholamines were unchanged. These results indicate that the transient increase of plasma catecholamine and insulin concentrations did not induce oxidative damage, while glucose already in the low dose was an important triggering factor for oxidative stress." Koska J, Blazicek P, Marko M, Grna JD, Kvetnansky R, Vigas M. Insulin, catecholamines, glucose and antioxidant enzymes in oxidative damage during different loads in healthy humans. *Physiol Res*. 2000;49 Suppl 1:S95-100

[129] "In conclusion, insulin at physiological doses is associated with increased LDL peroxidation independent of the presence of hyperglycemia." Quinones-Galvan A, Sironi AM, Baldi S, Galetta F, Garbin U, Fratta-Pasini A, Cominacini L, Ferrannini E. Evidence that acute insulin administration enhances LDL cholesterol susceptibility to oxidation in healthy humans. *Arterioscler Thromb Vasc Biol*. 1999 Dec;19(12):2928-32

[130] "These data show that the intake of a mixed meal results in significant inflammatory changes characterized by a decrease in IkappaBalpha and an increase in NF-kappaB binding, plasma CRP, and the expression of IKKalpha, IKKbeta, and p47(phox) subunit." Aljada A, Mohanty P, Ghanim H, Abdo T, Tripathy D, Chaudhuri A, Dandona P. Increase in intranuclear nuclear factor kappaB and decrease in inhibitor kappaB in mononuclear cells after a mixed meal: evidence for a proinflammatory effect. *Am J Clin Nutr*. 2004 Apr;79(4):682-90

[131] "A significant glycogen sparing, as well as supercompensation within 24 h of recovery, was observed after [carbohydrate] supplementation." Brouns F, Saris WH, Beckers E, Adlercreutz H, van der Vusse GJ, Keizer HA, Kuipers H, Menheere P, Wagenmakers AJ, ten Hoor F. Metabolic changes induced by sustained exhaustive cycling and diet manipulation. *Int J Sports Med*. 1989 May;10 Suppl 1:S49-62

[132] "The accepted method of increasing muscle glycogen stores is by "glycogen loading," which classically involves depletion of muscle glycogen, usually by exercise, followed by consumption of a high-CHO diet for several days (e.g., 3, 39). ...increase muscle glycogen concentrations ([glycogen]) to between 150 and 200% of normal resting levels." Robinson TM, Sewell DA, Hultman E, Greenhaff PL. Role of submaximal exercise in promoting creatine and glycogen accumulation in human skeletal muscle. *J Appl Physiol*. 1999 Aug;87(2):598-604

promote entry of tryptophan across the blood-brain barrier and into the brain to promote serotonin synthesis.[133] In summary, *habitual overconsumption* of simple carbohydrates promotes disease by oxidative and proinflammatory mechanisms, while conversely *periodic consumption* of simple carbohydrates can be used to promote athletic performance and to increase intracerebral serotonin synthesis for the promotion of enhanced mood and cognitive performance and for the regulation of food intake.

Avoid artificial sweeteners, colors and other additives: Absolutely never use **aspartame**—this is a synthetic chemical that is easily converted to the toxin formaldehyde.[134] Aspartame causes cancer in animals and is strongly linked to brain tumors in humans.[135,136] **Sodium benzoate** is a food preservative that can cause asthma[137] and skin rashes[138] in sensitive individuals. **Tartrazine (yellow dye #5)** is a food/drug coloring agent that can cause asthma and skin rashes in sensitive individuals.[139] **Carrageenan** is a naturally-occurring carbohydrate extracted from red seaweed. Common sources of carrageenan are certain brands of "rice milk" and "soy milk." In addition to suppressing immune function[140], carrageenan causes intestinal ulcers and inflammatory bowel disease in animals[141] and some research indicates that carrageenan consumption is associated with an increased risk for cancer in humans.[142,143]

Consume sufficient daily water in the form of water and health-promoting teas and juices: Daily "water" intake should be approximately 30 ml/kg; thus, for a 150-lb (70-kg) person, fluid intake should be at least 2.1 liters, and for a person who weighs 220 lbs (100 kg) the daily intake should be approximately 3 liters. More fluids may be used during times of exercise, heat exposure, illness, or detoxification, while fluid restriction can be indicated in patients with heart failure, renal failure, anasarca (generalized edema), and hyponatremia.

Consider reducing or eliminating caffeine: This is especially important for people with reactive hypoglycemia, insomnia, anxiety, hypertension, low-back pain, and for women with fibrocystic breast disease. Caffeine ingestion also leads to the activation of brain noradrenergic receptors, which can cause inhibition of dopaminergic pathways.[144] For people who are in good health, 1-3 servings of caffeine per day are not harmful. Herbal teas and green tea appear to have significant health-promoting effects due to their phytonutrient components and antioxidant, anti-inflammatory, and anticancer properties.

To the extent possible, eat "organic" foods rather than industrially-produced foods: Organic foods (i.e., foods which are *naturally grown* rather than being treated with insect poisons, synthetic fertilizers, and chemicals to enhance shelf-life) tend to cost more than chemically-produced foods; but the increased phytonutrient content justifies the cost. Organic foods contain more nutrients than do chemically-produced foods.[145] More importantly,

[133] "Our results suggest that high-carbohydrate meals have an influence on serotonin synthesis. We predict that carbohydrates with a high glycemic index would have a greater serotoninergic effect than carbohydrates with a low glycemic index." Lyons PM, Truswell AS. Serotonin precursor influenced by type of carbohydrate meal in healthy adults. *Am J Clin Nutr*. 1988 Mar;47(3):433-9
[134] Trocho C, Pardo R, Rafecas I, Virgili J, Remesar X, Fernandez-Lopez JA, Alemany M. Formaldehyde derived from dietary aspartame binds to tissue components in vivo. *Life Sci*. 1998;63(5):337-4949
[135] Compared to other environmental factors putatively linked to brain tumors, the artificial sweetener aspartame is a promising candidate to explain the recent increase in incidence and degree of malignancy of brain tumors. ...exceedingly high incidence of brain tumors in aspartame-fed rats compared to no brain tumors in concurrent controls..." Olney JW, Farber NB, Spitznagel E, Robins LN. Increasing brain tumor rates: is there a link to aspartame? *J Neuropathol Exp Neurol* 1996;55(11):1115-23
[136] Russell Blaylock MD. Excitotoxins. Health Press; December 1996 [ISBN: 0929173252] Pages 211-214
[137] "Adverse reactions to benzoate in this patient required avoidance of some drugs, some of those classically prescribed under the form of syrups in asthma." Petrus M, Bonaz S, Causse E, Rhabbour M, Moulie N, Netter JC, Bildstein G. [Asthma and intolerance to benzoates] [Article in French] *Arch Pediatr*. 1996;3(10):984-7
[138] Munoz FJ, et al. Perioral contact urticaria from sodium benzoate in a toothpaste. *Contact Dermatitis*. 1996 Jul;35(1):51
[139] "Tartrazine sensitivity is most frequently manifested by urticaria and asthma... Vasculitis, purpura and contact dermatitis infrequently occur as manifestations of tartrazine sensitivity." Dipalma JR. Tartrazine sensitivity. *Am Fam Physician*. 1990 Nov;42(5):1347-50
[140] "Impairment of complement activity and humoral responses to T-dependent antigens, depression of cell-mediated immunity, prolongation of graft survival and potentiation of tumour growth by carrageenans have been reported." Thomson AW, Fowler EF. Carrageenan: a review of its effects on the immune system. *Agents Actions*. 1981;11(3):265-73
[141] Watt J, Marcus R. Experimental ulcerative disease of the colon. *Methods Achiev Exp Pathol*. 1975;7:56-71
[142] Tobacman JK. Review of harmful gastrointestinal effects of carrageenan in animal experiments. *Environ Health Perspect*. 2001 Oct;109(10):983-94
[143] "However, the gum carrageenan which is comprised of linked, sulfated galactose residues has potent biological activity and undergoes acid hydrolysis to poligeenan, an acknowledged carcinogen." Tobacman JK, Wallace RB, Zimmerman MB. Consumption of carrageenan and other water-soluble polymers used as food additives and incidence of mammary carcinoma. *Med Hypotheses*. 2001 May;56(5):589-98
[144] "The results suggest that noradrenergic innervation of dopamine cells can directly inhibit the activity of dopamine cells." Paladini CA, Williams JT. Noradrenergic inhibition of midbrain dopamine neurons. *J Neurosci*. 2004 May 12;24(19):4568-75
[145] Smith B. Organic Foods versus Supermarket Foods: element levels. *Journal of Applied Nutrition* 1993; 45(1), p35-9

recent research has also indicated that organic foods are better able to prevent the genetic damage that can lead to cancer than are foods that have been grown in an environment of artificial fertilizers and pesticides.[146]

Recognize the importance of avoiding food allergens: Biomedical research has established that adverse food reactions, regardless of the underlying mechanisms or classification of allergy, intolerance, or sensitivity, can exacerbate a wide range of human illnesses, including thyroid disease[147], mental depression[148,149], asthma, rhinitis,[150] recurrent otitis media[151], migraine[152,153,154], attention deficit and hyperactivity disorders[155], epilepsy[156,157,158], gastrointestinal inflammation[159], hypertension[160], joint pain and inflammation[161,162,163,164,165,166,167,168] and a wide range of other health problems. Any program of health promotion and health maintenance must include consideration of food allergies, food intolerances, and food sensitivities. The elimination-and-challenge technique is the most cost-effective and it also teaches patients how to identify their own food allergies and intolerances, which may change for the better or worse over time; when the patient is empowered with this technique, he/she can take an active and on-going role in his/her own healthcare. Patients may be allergic to foods that are generally considered healthy, including whole organic foods. The more common food allergens—exemplified here by a list of offending foods identified in a study of patients with migraine[169]—are wheat (78%), orange (65%), eggs (45%), tea and coffee (40% each), chocolate and milk (37% each), beef (35%), and corn, cane sugar, and yeast (33% each).

Supplement the health-promoting whole-foods diet with specific vitamins, minerals, fatty acids, and probiotics: Despite the fact that America is one of the richest nations on earth, and that we produce more than enough food to feed ourselves and many other nations with a healthy diet, Americans tend to have poor dietary habits and inadequate levels of nutritional intake that do not meet the minimal standards, such as the Recommended Daily Allowance (RDA, now Daily Reference Intake (DRI)).[170] Many people are under the misperception that if they appear healthy or are even overweight then they could not possibly have nutritional deficiencies. The truths of this matter are that 1) gross/obvious nutritional deficiencies are common among "apparently healthy" individuals, 2) common situations like stress, poor diets, and use of medications predispose people to nutritional deficiencies, 3) hereditary/genetic disorders affect a large portion of the population and lead

---

[146] "Against BaP, three species of OC vegetables showed 30-57% antimutagenecity, while GC ones did only 5-30%." Ren H, Endo H, Hayashi T. The superiority of organically cultivated vegetables to general ones regarding antimutagenic activities. *Mutat Res*. 2001 Sep 20;496(1-2):83-8

[147] Sategna-Guidetti C, Volta U, Ciacci C, Usai P, Carlino A, De Franceschi L, Camera A, Pelli A, Brossa C. Prevalence of thyroid disorders in untreated adult celiac disease patients and effect of gluten withdrawal: an Italian multicenter study. *Am J Gastroenterol*. 2001 Mar;96(3):751-7

[148] "The detection and treatment of psychological dysfunction related to food intolerance with particular reference to the problem of objective evaluation is discussed… Long-term follow-up revealed maintenance of marked improvements in psychological and physical functioning." Mills N. Depression and food intolerance: a single case study. *Hum Nutr Appl Nutr*. 1986 Apr;40(2):141-5

[149] "OBJECTIVE: To describe a patient with food intolerance probably contributing to depressive symptoms, intolerance to psychotropic medication and treatment resistance… RESULTS: The patient's course improved considerably with an elimination diet." Parker G, Watkins T. Treatment-resistant depression: when antidepressant drug intolerance may indicate food intolerance. *Aust N Z J Psychiatry*. 2002 Apr;36(2):263-5

[150] Speer F. The allergic child. *Am Fam Physician*. 1975 Feb;11(2):88-94

[151] Juntti H, Tikkanen S, Kokkonen J, Alho OP, Niinimaki A. Cow's milk allergy is associated with recurrent otitis media during childhood. *Acta Otolaryngol*. 1999;119(8):867-73

[152] "Foods which provoked migraine in 9 patients with severe migraine refractory to drug therapy were identified… These observations confirm that a food-allergic reaction is the cause of migraine in this group of patients." Monro J, Carini C, Brostoff J. Migraine is a food-allergic disease. *Lancet*. 1984 Sep 29;2(8405):719-21

[153] Egger J, Carter CM, Wilson J, et al. Is migraine food allergy? A double-blind controlled trial of oligoantigenic diet treatment. *Lancet*. 1983 Oct 15;2(8355):865-9

[154] Monro J, Brostoff J, Carini C, Zilkha K. Food allergy in migraine. Study of dietary exclusion and RAST. *Lancet*. 1980 Jul 5;2(8184):1-4

[155] Boris M, Mandel FS. Foods and additives are common causes of the attention deficit hyperactive disorder in children. *Ann Allergy*. 1994 May;72(5):462-8

[156] Egger J, Carter CM, Soothill JF, Wilson J. Oligoantigenic diet treatment of children with epilepsy and migraine. *J Pediatr*. 1989;114(1):51-8

[157] Pelliccia A, Lucarelli S, Frediani T, D'Ambrini G, Cerminara C, Barbato M, Vagnucci B, Cardi E. Partial cryptogenetic epilepsy and food allergy/intolerance. A causal or a chance relationship? Reflections on three clinical cases. *Minerva Pediatr*. 1999 May;51(5):153-7

[158] Frediani T, Lucarelli S, Pelliccia A, Vagnucci B, et al. Allergy and childhood epilepsy: a close relationship? *Acta Neurol Scand*. 2001;104(6):349-52

[159] Marr HY, Chen WC, Lin LH. Food protein-induced enterocolitis syndrome: report of one case. *Acta Paediatr Taiwan*. 2001;42(1):49-52

[160] Grant EC. Food allergies and migraine. *Lancet*. 1979 May 5;1(8123):966-9

[161] "Food allergy appeared to be responsible for the joint symptoms in three patients and in one it was possible to precipitate swelling of a knee due to synovitis with effusion by drinking milk a few hours beforehand, the synovial fluid having mildly inflammatory features and a relatively high eosinophil count." Golding DN. Is there an allergic synovitis? *J R Soc Med*. 1990 May;83(5):312-4

[162] Panush RS. Food induced ("allergic") arthritis: clinical and serologic studies. *J Rheumatol*. 1990 Mar;17(3):291-4

[163] Pacor ML, Lunardi C, Di Lorenzo G, Biasi D, Corrocher R. Food allergy and seronegative arthritis: report of two cases. *Clin Rheumatol*. 2001;20(4):279-81

[164] Schrander JJ, Marcelis C, de Vries MP, van Santen-Hoeufft HM. Does food intolerance play a role in juvenile chronic arthritis? *Br J Rheumatol*. 1997 Aug;36(8):905-8

[165] van de Laar MA, van der Korst JK. Food intolerance in rheumatoid arthritis. I. A double blind, controlled trial of the clinical effects of elimination of milk allergens and azo dyes. *Ann Rheum Dis*. 1992 Mar;51(3):298-302

[166] Haugen MA, Kjeldsen-Kragh J, Forre O. A pilot study of the effect of an elemental diet in the management of rheumatoid arthritis. *Clin Exp Rheumatol*. 1994;12(3):275-9

[167] van de Laar MA, Aalbers M, Bruins FG, et al. Food intolerance in rheumatoid arthritis. II. Clinical and histological aspects. *Ann Rheum Dis*. 1992;51(3):303-6

[168] Panush RS, Stroud RM, Webster EM. Food-induced (allergic) arthritis. Inflammatory arthritis exacerbated by milk. *Arthritis Rheum* 1986; 29(2): 220-6

[169] Grant EC. Food allergies and migraine. *Lancet*. 1979 May 5;1(8123):966-9

[170] "Most people do not consume an optimal amount of all vitamins by diet alone. Pending strong evidence of effectiveness from randomized trials, it appears prudent for all adults to take vitamin supplements." Fletcher RH, Fairfield KM. Vitamins for chronic disease prevention in adults: clinical applications. *JAMA* 2002 Jun 19;287(23):3127-9

to an increased need for nutritional intake which can generally only be met with supplementation in addition to a healthy whole-foods diet. Taking a "one-a-day" multivitamin is insufficient for people who truly desire significant benefit from supplementation. These one-a-day preparations generally only provide the minimum daily allowance—this dose is not large enough to provide truly preventive medicine results; also, such one-a-day products tend to contain low-quality nutrients, such as ergocalciferol rather than cholecalciferol[171], cyanocobalamin rather than the hydroxyl-, methyl-, or adenosyl- forms[172], and DL-tocopherol or exclusively L-alpha-tocopherol rather than a mix of tocopherols with a high concentration (generally approximately 40%) of gamma tocopherol.[173]

For people still not convinced of the importance of a multi-vitamin/mineral supplement as part of the basic foundation of the health plan, please consider the following data from the medical research:

- Many people think that eating a "healthy diet" will supply them with the nutrients that they need and that they do not need to take a vitamin supplement. This may have been true 2000 years ago, but today's industrially produced "foods" are generally stripped of much of their nutritional value long before they leave the factory. Industrially-produced fruits and vegetables contain lower quantities of nutrients than does naturally raised "organic" produce. [174]

- The reason that people can be of normal weight or can even be overweight and obese and still have nutrient deficiencies is that the body lowers the metabolic rate when the intake of vitamins and minerals is low. This is referred to as the "physiologic adaptation to marginal malnutrition." Even though people may eat enough calories and protein, they can still suffer from growth retardation and behavioral problems as a result of micronutrient malnutrition, even though they *appear* nourished.[175]

- Most nutrition-oriented doctors will agree that magnesium is one of the most important nutrients, especially for helping prevent heart attack and stroke. **Magnesium deficiency is an epidemic in so-called "developed" nations, with 20-40% of different populations showing objective laboratory evidence of magnesium deficiency.**[176,177,178,179]

- Add to the above that every day we are confronted with more chronic emotional stress and toxic chemicals than has ever before existed on the planet, and it becomes easy to see that basic nutritional support and an organic whole foods diet is just the start of attaining improved health.

<u>General Guidelines for the Safe Use of Nutritional Supplements</u>: Supplementation with vitamins and minerals is generally safe, especially if the following guidelines are followed:

- <u>Vitamins and minerals should generally be taken with food in order to eliminate the possibility of nausea and to increase absorption</u>: Most vitamins and other supplements should be taken with food so that nausea is avoided.

- <u>Iron is potentially harmful</u>: Iron promotes the formation of reactive oxygen species ("free radicals") and is thus implicated in several diseases, such as infections, cancer, liver disease, diabetes, and cardiovascular disease. Iron supplements should not be consumed except by people who have been definitively

---

[171] "Vitamin D(2) potency is less than one third that of vitamin D(3). Physicians resorting to use of vitamin D(2) should be aware of its markedly lower potency and shorter duration of action relative to vitamin D(3)." Armas LA, Hollis BW, Heaney RP. Vitamin D2 is much less effective than vitamin D3 in humans. *J Clin Endocrinol Metab*. 2004 Nov;89(11):5387-91

[172] Freeman AG. Cyanocobalamin--a case for withdrawal: discussion paper. *J R Soc Med*. 1992 Nov;85(11):686–687 http://www.ncbi.nlm.nih.gov/pmc/articles/PMC1293728/pdf/jrsocmed00105-0046.pdf

[173] "gamma-tocopherol is the major form of vitamin E in many plant seeds and in the US diet, but has drawn little attention compared with alpha-tocopherol, the predominant form of vitamin E in tissues and the primary form in supplements. However, recent studies indicate that gamma-tocopherol may be important to human health and that it possesses unique features that distinguish it from alpha-tocopherol." Jiang Q, Christen S, Shigenaga MK, Ames BN. gamma-tocopherol, the major form of vitamin E in the US diet, deserves more attention. *Am J Clin Nutr*. 2001 Dec;74(6):714-22 http://www.ajcn.org/content/74/6/714.full.pdf

[174] Smith B. Organic Foods versus Supermarket Foods: element levels. *Journal of Applied Nutrition* 1993; 45(1), p35-9. I recently found that this article is also available on-line at http://journeytoforever.org/farm_library/bobsmith.html as of June 19, 2004

[175] Allen LH. The nutrition CRSP: what is marginal malnutrition, and does it affect human function? *Nutr Rev* 1993 Sep;51(9):255-67

[176] "The American diet is low in magnesium, and with modern water systems, very little is ingested in the drinking water." Innerarity S. Hypomagnesemia in acute and chronic illness. *Crit Care Nurs Q*. 2000 Aug;23(2):1-19

[177] "Altogether 43% of 113 trauma patients had low magnesium levels compared to 30% of noninjured cohorts." Frankel H, Haskell R, Lee SY, Miller D, Rotondo M, Schwab CW. Hypomagnesemia in trauma patients. *World J Surg*. 1999 Sep;23(9):966-9

[178] "There was a 20% overall prevalence of hypomagnesemia among this predominantly female, African American population." Fox CH, Ramsoomair D, Mahoney MC, Carter C, Young B, Graham R. An investigation of hypomagnesemia among ambulatory urban African Americans. *J Fam Pract*. 1999 Aug;48(8):636-9

[179] "Suboptimal levels were detected in 33.7 per cent of the population under study. These data clearly demonstrate that the Mg supply of the German population needs increased attention." Schimatschek HF, Rempis R. Prevalence of hypomagnesemia in an unselected German population of 16,000 individuals. *Magnes Res*. 2001 Dec;14(4):283-90

diagnosed with iron deficiency by measurement of serum ferritin. Iron supplementation without documentation of iron deficiency by measurement of serum ferritin is inappropriate. [180]

- <u>Vitamin A is one of the only vitamins with the potential for serious toxicity even at low doses</u>: Attention should be given to vitamin A intake so that toxicity is avoided. Total intake of vitamin A must account for all sources—foods, fish oils, and vitamin supplements. Manifestations of vitamin A toxicity include: skin problems (dry skin, flaking skin, chapped or split lips, red skin rash, hair loss), joint pain, bone pain, headaches, anorexia (loss of appetite), edema (water retention, weight gain, swollen ankles, difficulty breathing), fatigue, and/or liver damage. Whenever vitamin A is used in high doses, it must be used for a defined period of time in order to avoid the toxicity that will result from high-dose long-term vitamin A supplementation.

  - <u>Adults</u>: Women who are pregnant or might become pregnant and who are planning to carry the baby to full term delivery should not ingest more than 10,000 IU of vitamin A per day. Vitamin A toxicity is seen with chronic ingestion of therapeutic doses (for example: 25,000 IU per day for 6 years, or 100,000 IU per day for 2.5 years[181]). Most patients should not consume more than 25,000 IU of vitamin A per day for more than 2 months without express supervision by a healthcare provider. Vitamin A is present in some multivitamins, in animal liver and products such as fish liver oil, and in other supplements—read labels to ensure that the total daily intake is not greater than 25,000 IU per day.

  - <u>Infants and Children</u>: Different studies have used either daily or monthly schedules of vitamin A supplementation. In a study with extremely low-birth weight infants, 5,000 IU of vitamin A per day for 28 days was safely used.[182] In another study conducted in sick children, those aged less than 12 months received 100,000 IU on two consecutive days, while children between ages 12-60 months received a larger dose of 200,000 IU on two consecutive days.[183]

- <u>Preexisting kidney problems (such as renal insufficiency) increase the risks associated with nutritional supplementation</u>: Supplementation with vitamins and minerals does not cause kidney damage. However, if a patient already has kidney problems, then nutritional supplementation may become hazardous; this is particularly true with magnesium and potassium and perhaps also with vitamin C. Assessment of renal function with serum or urine tests is encouraged before beginning an aggressive plan of supplementation. Conditions which cause kidney damage include use of specific drugs (e.g., acetaminophen, aspirin, contrast and chemotherapy agents, cocaine), acute or chronic high blood pressure, diabetes mellitus and other diseases such as lupus (SLE), polycystic kidney disease, and scleroderma.

- <u>Pre-existing medical conditions may make supplementation unsafe</u>: A few rare medical conditions may cause nutritional supplementation to be unsafe, including severe liver disease, renal failure, electrolyte imbalances, hyperparathyroidism and other vitamin D hypersensitivity syndromes.

- <u>Several drugs/medications may adversely interact with vitamin/mineral supplements and with botanical medicines</u>: Vitamins/minerals may reduce the effectiveness of some prescription medications. For example, taking certain antibiotics such as ciprofloxacin or tetracycline with calcium reduces absorption of the drugs, therefore rendering the drugs much less effective. Taking botanical medicines with medications may make the drugs dangerously less effective (such as when St. John's Wort is combined with protease inhibitor drugs[184]) or may make the drug dangerously more effective (such when Kava is

---

[180] Hollán S, Johansen KS. Adequate iron stores and the 'Nil nocere' principle.*Haematologia* (Budap). 1993;25(2):69-84

[181] "The smallest continuous daily consumption leading to cirrhosis was 25,000 IU during 6 years, whereas higher daily doses (greater than or equal to 100,000 IU) taken during 2 1/2 years resulted in similar histological lesions. ... The data also indicate that prolonged and continuous consumption of doses in the low "therapeutic" range can result in life-threatening liver damage." Geubel AP, De Galocsy C, Alves N, Rahier J, Dive C. Liver damage caused by therapeutic vitamin A administration: estimate of dose-related toxicity in 41 cases. *Gastroenterology*. 1991 Jun;100(6):1701-9

[182] "Infants with birth weight < 1000 g were randomised at birth to receive oral vitamin A supplementation (5000 IU/day) or placebo for 28 days." Wardle SP, Hughes A, Chen S, Shaw NJ. Randomised controlled trial of oral vitamin A supplementation in preterm infants to prevent chronic lung disease. *Arch Dis Child Fetal Neonatal Ed*. 2001 Jan;84(1):F9-F13 Available on-line at http://adc.bmjjournals.com/cgi/content/full/fetalneonatal%3b84/1/F9

[183] "Children were assigned to oral doses of 200 000 IU vitamin A (half that dose if <12 months) or placebo on the day of admission, a second dose on the following day, and third and fourth doses at 4 and 8 months after discharge from the hospital, respectively." Villamor E, Mbise R, Spiegelman D, Hertzmark E, Fataki M, Peterson KE, Ndossi G, Fawzi WW. Vitamin A supplements ameliorate the adverse effect of HIV-1, malaria, and diarrheal infections on child growth. *Pediatrics*. 2002 Jan;109(1):E6

[184] Piscitelli SC, Burstein AH, Chaitt D, Alfaro RM, Falloon J. Indinavir concentrations and St John's wort. *Lancet*. 2000 Feb 12;355(9203):547-8

combined with the anti-anxiety drug alprazolam[185]). If vitamin D is used in doses greater than 1,000 IU/d in patients taking hydrochlorothiazide or other calcium-retaining drugs, serum calcium should be monitored at least monthly until safety (i.e., lack of hypercalcemia) has been established per patient.[186] Patients should not combine nutritional or botanical medicines with chemical/synthetic drugs without specific advice from a knowledgeable doctor. Do not increase vitamin K consumption from supplements or dietary improvements in patients taking coumadin/warfarin. A reasonable recommendation is that nutritional supplements be taken 2 hours away from pharmaceutical medications to avoid complications such as intraintestinal drug-nutrient binding.

[185] Almeida JC, Grimsley EW. Coma from the health food store: interaction between kava and alprazolam. *Ann Intern Med.* 1996 Dec 1;125(11):940-1

[186] **Vasquez A**, Manso G, Cannell J. The clinical importance of vitamin D (cholecalciferol): a paradigm shift with implications for all healthcare providers. *Altern Ther Health Med.* 2004 Sep-Oct;10(5):28-36 http://optimalhealthresearch.com/monograph04.html

Advanced concepts in nutrition—an introduction

Biochemical Individuality and Orthomolecular Medicine:

"Biochemical individuality" was the term coined by biochemist Dr. Roger Williams of the University of Texas[187] to describe the genetic and physiologic variations in human beings that produced different nutritional needs among individuals. Because we all have different genes, each of our bodies therefore creates different protein enzymes, and many of these enzymes—which are essential for proper cellular function—are adversely affected by defects in their construction (i.e., amino acid sequence) that reduce their efficiency. Dr. Linus Pauling[188] noted that single amino acid substitutions could produce dramatic alterations in protein function. Pauling discovered that sickle cell disease was caused by a single amino acid substitution in the hemoglobin molecule, and for this discovery he won the Nobel Prize in Chemistry in 1954.[189] With recognition of the importance of individual molecules in determining health or disease, Pauling coined the phrase "orthomolecular medicine" based on his thesis that many diseases could be effectively prevented and treated if we used the "right molecules" to correct abnormal physiologic function. Pauling contrasted the clinical use of nutrients for the improvement of physiologic function (orthomolecular medicine) with the use of chemical drugs, which generally work by interfering with normal physiology (toximolecular medicine). Since nutrients are the fundamental elements of the human body from which all enzymes, chemicals, and cellular structures are formed, Pauling advocated that the use of customized nutrition and nutritional supplements could promote optimal health by optimizing cellular function and efficiency. More recently, Dr. Bruce Ames has thoroughly documented the science of the orthomolecular precepts[190] and has advocated optimal diets along with nutritional supplementation as a highly efficient and cost-effective method for preventing disease and optimizing health.[191,192] In sum, we see that 1) the foundational diet must be formed from whole foods such as fruits, nuts, seeds, vegetables, and lean meats, 2) processed and artificial foods should be avoided, and 3) the use of nutritional supplements is necessary to provide sufficiently high levels of nutrition to overcome defects in enzymatic activity.

Orthomolecular precepts
▪ The functions of the body are dependent upon thousands of enzymes. Because of genetic defects that are common in the general population, some of these enzymes are commonly defective – even if only slightly – in large portions of the human population.
▪ Enzyme defects reduce the function and efficiency of important chemical reactions. Because enzymes are so important for normal function and the prevention of disease, defects in enzyme function can result in disruptions in physiology and the creation of what later manifests as "disease."
▪ Rather than treating these diseases with synthetic chemical drugs, it is commonly possible to prevent and treat disease with high-doses of vitamins, minerals, and other nutrients to compensate for or bypass metabolic dysfunctions, thus allowing for the promotion of optimal health by promoting optimal physiologic function.
Recent independent review: Ames BN, Elson-Schwab I, Silver EA. High-dose vitamin therapy stimulates variant enzymes with decreased coenzyme binding affinity (increased K(m)): relevance to genetic disease and polymorphisms. *Am J Clin Nutr*. 2002 Apr;75(4):616-58

---

[187] "Every individual organism that has a distinctive genetic background has distinctive nutritional needs which must be met for optimal well-being. ...[N]utrition applied with due concern for individual genetic variations...offers the solution to many baffling health problems." Williams RJ. Biochemical Individuality : The Basis for the Genetotrophic Concept. Austin and London: University of Texas Press, 1956. Page x

[188] "...the concentration of coenzyme [vitamins and minerals] needed to produce the amount of active enzyme required for optimum health may well be somewhat different for different individuals. ...many individuals may require a considerably higher concentration of one or more coenzymes than other people do for optimum health..." Pauling L. On the Orthomolecular Environment of the Mind: Orthomolecular Theory. In: Williams RJ, Kalita DK. A Physician's Handbook on Orthomolecular Medicine. New Cannan; Keats Publishing: 1977. Page 76

[189] http://www.nobel.se/chemistry/laureates/1954/pauling-bio.html on April 4, 2004

[190] "About 50 human genetic dis-eases due to defective enzymes can be remedied or ameliorated by the administration of high doses of the vitamin component of the corresponding coenzyme, which at least partially restores enzymatic activity." Ames BN, Elson-Schwab I, Silver EA. High-dose vitamin therapy stimulates variant enzymes with decreased coenzyme binding affinity (increased K(m)): relevance to genetic disease and polymorphisms. *Am J Clin Nutr*. 2002 Apr;75(4):616-58

[191] "An optimum intake of micronutrients and metabolites, which varies with age and genetic constitution, would tune up metabolism and give a marked increase in health, particularly for the poor and elderly, at little cost." Ames BN. The metabolic tune-up: metabolic harmony and disease prevention. *J Nutr*. 2003 May;133(5 Suppl 1):1544S-8S

[192] "Optimizing micronutrient intake [through better diets, fortification of foods, or multivitamin-mineral pills] can have a major impact on public health at low cost." Ames BN. Cancer prevention and diet: help from single nucleotide polymorphisms. *Proc Natl Acad Sci* U S A. 1999 Oct 26;96(22):12216-8

Nutrigenomics—Nutritional Genomics:

"Genome" refers to all of the genetic material in an organism, and "genomics" is the field of study of this information. The field of nutritional genomics—nutrigenomics—refers to the clinical synthesis of 1) research on the human genome (e.g., the Human Genome Project[193]), and 2) the advancing science of clinical nutrition, including research on nutraceuticals (nutritional medicines) and phytomedicinals (botanical medicines). Nutrigenomics represents a major advance in our understanding of the underlying biochemical and physiologic mechanisms of the effects of nutrition.

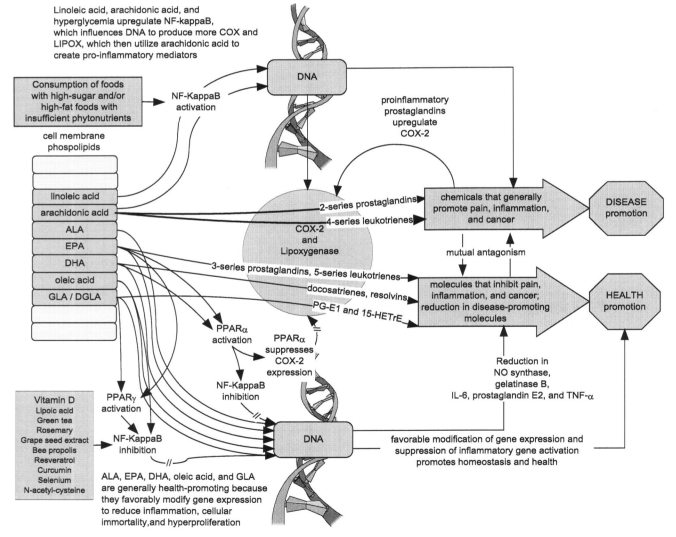

Nutrigenomics—a conceptual diagram: Nutrients influence gene transcription as well as post-translational metabolism.

---

[193] "Begun formally in 1990, the U.S. Human Genome Project is a 13-year effort coordinated by the U.S. Department of Energy and the National Institutes of Health. The project originally was planned to last 15 years, but rapid technological advances have accelerated the expected completion date to 2003. Project goals are to identify all the approximate 30,000 genes in human DNA..." See the official Human Genome website at http://www.ornl.gov/sci/techresources/Human_Genome/home.shtml

Nutrition is far more than "fuel" for our biophysiologic machine; we know now that nutrition—the consumption of specific proteins, amino acids, vitamins, minerals, fatty acids, and phytochemicals—can alter genetic expression and can thus either promote health or disease at the very fundamental level of genetic expression. The commonly employed excuse that many patients use—"I just have bad genes"—now takes on a whole new meaning; it may be that these patients suffer from the expression of "bad genes" *because of the food that they eat*.

The concept and phenomenon of nutrigenomics can be described by saying that each of us has the genes for health, as well as the genes for disease; what largely determines our level of health is how we treat our genes with environmental inputs, especially nutrition. We appear able, to a large extent, to "turn on" disease-promoting genes with poor nutrition and a pro-inflammatory lifestyle[194,195], while, to a lesser extent, we are able to activate or "turn on" health-promoting genes with a healthy diet[196] and with proper nutritional supplementation.[197] For additional details, see the literature cited in this section and the review article by Vasquez available on-line.[198]

Putting it all together with "the supplemented Paleo-Mediterranean diet": The health-promoting diet of choice for the majority of people is a diet based on abundant consumption of fruits, vegetables, seeds, nuts, omega-3 and monounsaturated fatty acids, and lean sources of protein such as lean meats, fatty cold-water fish, soy and whey proteins. This diet prohibits and obviates overconsumption of chemical preservatives, artificial sweeteners, and carbohydrate-dominant foods such as candies, pastries, breads, potatoes, grains, and other foods with a high glycemic load and high glycemic index. This "Paleo-Mediterranean Diet" is a combination of the "Paleolithic" or "Paleo diet" and the well-known "Mediterranean diet", both of which are well described in peer-reviewed journals and the lay press. The Mediterranean diet is characterized by increased proportions of legumes, nuts, seeds, whole grain products, fruits, vegetables (including potatoes), fish and lean meats, and monounsaturated and n-3 fatty acids.[199] Consumption of the Mediterranean diet is associated with improvements in insulin sensitivity and reductions in cardiovascular disease, diabetes, cancer, and all-cause mortality when contrasted to the effects of *ad libitum* eating, particularly in the standard American diet (SAD) eating pattern.[200] The Paleolithic diet detailed by collaborators Eaton[201], O'Keefe[202], and Cordain[203] is similar to the Mediterranean diet except for stronger emphasis on fruits and vegetables (preferably raw or minimally cooked), omega-3-rich lean meats, and reduced consumption of starchy foods such as potatoes and grains, the latter of which were not staples in the human diet until the last few thousand years. Emphasizing the olive oil and red wine of the Mediterranean diet and the absence of grains and potatoes per the Paleo diet appears to be the way to get the best of both dietary worlds; the remaining diet is characterized by fresh whole fruits, vegetables, nuts (especially almonds), seeds, berries, olive oil, lean meats rich in n-3 fatty acids, and red wine in moderation. In sum, this dietary plan along with the inclusion of garlic and dark chocolate (a rich source of cardioprotective, antioxidative, antihypertensive, and anti-inflammatory polyphenolic flavonoids[204,205]) is expected to reduce adverse cardiovascular events by more than 76%.[206] Biochemical justification for this type of diet is ample and is well supported by numerous long-term studies in humans wherein both Mediterranean and Paleolithic diets result in statistically significant and

[194] Rusyn I, Bradham CA, Cohn L, Schoonhoven R, Swenberg JA, Brenner DA, Thurman RG. Corn oil rapidly activates nuclear factor-kappaB in hepatic Kupffer cells by oxidant-dependent mechanisms. *Carcinogenesis*. 1999 Nov;20(11):2095-100 http://carcin.oxfordjournals.org/cgi/content/full/20/11/2095

[195] Aljada A, Mohanty P, Ghanim H, Abdo T, Tripathy D, Chaudhuri A, Dandona P. Increase in intranuclear nuclear factor kappaB and decrease in inhibitor kappaB in mononuclear cells after a mixed meal: evidence for a proinflammatory effect. *Am J Clin Nutr*. 2004 Apr;79(4):682-90

[196] OKeefe JH Jr, Cordain L. Cardiovascular disease resulting from a diet and lifestyle at odds with our Paleolithic genome. *Mayo Clin Proc*.2004;79:101-8

[197] Kaput J, Rodriguez LR. Nutritional genomics: the next frontier in the postgenomic era. *Physiol Genomics* 16: 166–177 http://physiolgenomics.physiology.org/cgi/content/full/16/2/166

[198] **Vasquez A.**Reducing pain and inflammation naturally - Part 4: Nutritional and Botanical Inhibition of NF-kappaB, the Major Intracellular Amplifier of the Inflammatory Cascade.A Clinical Strategy Exemplifying Anti-Inflammatory Nutrigenomics.*Nutr Persp* 2005;Jul:5-12 http://optimalhealthresearch.com/part4

[199] Curtis BM, O'Keefe JH Jr. Understanding the Mediterranean diet. Could this be the new "gold standard" for heart disease prevention? *Postgrad Med*. 2002 Aug;112(2):35-8, 41-5 http://www.postgradmed.com/issues/2002/08_02/curtis.htm

[200] Knoops KT, de Groot LC, Kromhout D, Perrin AE, Moreiras-Varela O, Menotti A, van Staveren WA. Mediterranean diet, lifestyle factors, and 10-year mortality in elderly European men and women: the HALE project. *JAMA*. 2004 Sep 22;292(12):1433-9

[201] Eaton SB, Shostak M, Konner M. The Paleolithic Prescription: A program of diet & exercise and a design for living, New York: Harper & Row, 1988

[202] O'Keefe JH Jr, Cordain L. Cardiovascular disease resulting from a diet and lifestyle at odds with our Paleolithic genome: how to become a 21st-century hunter-gatherer. *Mayo Clin Proc*. 2004 Jan;79(1):101-8

[203] Cordain L. The Paleo Diet: Lose Weight and Get Healthy by Eating the Food You Were Designed to Eat. Indianapolis; John Wiley and Sons, 2002

[204] Schramm DD, Wang JF, Holt RR, Ensunsa JL, Gonsalves JL, Lazarus SA, Schmitz HH, German JB, Keen CL. Chocolate procyanidins decrease the leukotriene-prostacyclin ratio in humans and human aortic endothelial cells. *Am J Clin Nutr*. 2001;73(1):36-40

[205] Engler MB, Engler MM, Chen CY, et al. Flavonoid-rich dark chocolate improves endothelial function and increases plasma epicatechin concentrations in healthy adults. *J Am Coll Nutr*. 2004;23(3):197-204

[206] Franco OH, Bonneux L, de Laet C, Peeters A, Steyerberg EW, Mackenbach JP. The Polymeal: a more natural, safer, and probably tastier (than the Polypill) strategy to reduce cardiovascular disease by more than 75%. *BMJ*. 2004;329(7480):1447-50

clinically meaningful reductions in disease-specific and all-cause mortality.[207,208,209,210] Diets rich in fruits and vegetables are sources of more than 8,000 phytochemicals, many of which have antioxidant, anti-inflammatory, and anti-cancer properties.[211] Oleic acid, squalene, and phenolics in olive oil and phenolics and resveratrol in red wine have antioxidant, anti-inflammatory, and anti-cancer properties and also protect against cardiovascular disease.[212] N-3 fatty acids have numerous health benefits via multiple mechanisms as described in the sections that follow. Increased intake of dietary fiber from fruits and vegetable favorably modifies gut flora, promotes xenobiotic elimination (via flora modification, laxation, and overall reductions in enterohepatic recirculation), and is associated with reductions in morbidity and mortality. Such a "Paleolithic diet" can also lead to urinary alkalinization (average urine pH of ≥ 7.5 according to Sebastian et al[213]) which increases renal *retention of minerals* for improved musculoskeletal health[214,215,216] and which increases *urinary elimination of many toxicants and xenobiotics* for a tremendous reduction in serum levels and thus adverse effects from chemical exposure or drug overdose.[217] Furthermore, therapeutic alkalinization was recently shown in an open trial with 82 patients to reduce symptoms and disability associated with low-back pain and to increase intracellular magnesium concentrations by 11%.[218] **Ample intake of amino acids via dietary proteins supports phase-2 detoxification** (amino acid and sulfate conjugation) for proper xenobiotic elimination[219,220], **provides amino acid precursors for neurotransmitter synthesis** and maintenance of mood, memory, and cognitive performance[221,222,223,224], **and prevents the immunosuppression and decrements in musculoskeletal status caused by low-protein diets.**[225] Described originally by the current author[226], the "supplemented Paleo-Mediterranean diet" provides patients the best of current knowledge in nutrition by relying on a foundational diet plan of fresh fruits, vegetables, nuts, seeds, berries, fish, and lean meats which is adorned with olive oil for its squalene, phenolic antioxidant/anti-inflammatory and monounsaturated fatty acid content. Inclusive of medical foods such as red wine, garlic, and dark chocolate which may synergize to effect at least a 76% reduction in cardiovascular disease[227], this diet also reduces the risk for cancer[228] and can be an integral component of a health-promoting lifestyle.[229] Competitive athletes are allowed increased carbohydrate consumption before and after training and competition to promote glycogen storage supercompensation.[230,231,232]

[207] de Lorgeril M, Salen P, Martin JL, Monjaud I, Boucher P, Mamelle N. Mediterranean dietary pattern in a randomized trial: prolonged survival and possible reduced cancer rate. *Arch Intern Med.* 1998 Jun 8;158(11):1181-7

[208] Knoops KT, de Groot LC, Kromhout D, Perrin AE, Moreiras-Varela O, Menotti A, van Staveren WA. Mediterranean diet, lifestyle factors, and 10-year mortality in elderly European men and women: the HALE project. *JAMA.* 2004 Sep 22;292(12):1433-9

[209] Lindeberg S, Cordain L, and Eaton SB. Biological and clinical potential of a Paleolithic diet. *J Nutri Environ Med* 2003; 13:149-160

[210] O'Keefe JH Jr, Cordain L, Harris WH, Moe RM, Vogel R. Optimal low-density lipoprotein is 50 to 70 mg/dl: lower is better and physiologically normal. *J Am Coll Cardiol.* 2004 Jun 2;43(11):2142-6

[211] Liu RH. Health benefits of fruit and vegetables are from additive and synergistic combinations of phytochemicals. *Am J Clin Nutr.* 2003;78(3 Sup):517S-520S

[212] Alarcon de la Lastra C, Barranco MD, Motilva V, Herrerias JM. Mediterranean diet and health: biological importance of olive oil. *Curr Pharm Des.* 2001;7:933-50

[213] Sebastian A, Frassetto LA, Sellmeyer DE, Merriam RL, Morris RC Jr. Estimation of the net acid load of the diet of ancestral preagricultural Homo sapiens and their hominid ancestors. *Am J Clin Nutr* 2002;76:1308-16

[214] Sebastian A, Harris ST, Ottaway JH, Todd KM, Morris RC Jr. Improved mineral balance and skeletal metabolism in postmenopausal women treated with potassium bicarbonate. *N Engl J Med.* 1994;330(25):1776-81

[215] Tucker KL, Hannan MT, Chen H, Cupples LA, Wilson PW, Kiel DP. Potassium, magnesium, and fruit and vegetable intakes are associated with greater bone mineral density in elderly men and women. *Am J Clin Nutr.* 1999;69(4):727-36

[216] Whiting SJ, Boyle JL, Thompson A, Mirwald RL, Faulkner RA. Dietary protein, phosphorus and potassium are beneficial to bone mineral density in adult men consuming adequate dietary calcium. *J Am Coll Nutr.* 2002;21(5):402-9

[217] Proudfoot AT, Krenzelok EP, Vale JA. Position Paper on urine alkalinization. *J Toxicol Clin Toxicol.* 2004;42(1):1-26

[218] "The results show that a disturbed acid-base balance may contribute to the symptoms of low back pain. The simple and safe addition of an alkaline multimineral preparate was able to reduce the pain symptoms in these patients with chronic low back pain." Vormann J,Worlitschek M,Goedecke T,Silver B. Supplementation with alkaline minerals reduces symptoms in patients with chronic low back pain. J Trace Elem Med Biol. 2001;15:179-83

[219] Liska DJ. The detoxification enzyme systems. *Altern Med Rev.* 1998;3:187-9

[220] Anderson KE, Kappas A. Dietary regulation of cytochrome P450. *Annu Rev Nutr.* 1991;11:141-67

[221] Rogers RD, Tunbridge EM, Bhagwagar Z, Drevets WC, Sahakian BJ, Carter CS. Tryptophan depletion alters the decision-making of healthy volunteers through altered processing of reward cues. *Neuropsychopharmacology.* 2003;28:153-62 Accessed at http://www.acnp.org/sciweb/journal/Npp062402336/default.htm on November 10, 2004

[222] Arnulf I, Quintin P, Alvarez JC, Vigil L, Touitou Y, Lebre AS, Bellenger A, Varoquaux O, Derenne JP, Allilaire JF, Benkelfat C, Leboyer M. Mid-morning tryptophan depletion delays REM sleep onset in healthy subjects. *Neuropsychopharmacology.* 2002;27(5):843-51 http://www.nature.com/npp/journal/v27/n5/pdf/1395948a.pdf

[223] Thomas JR,Lockwood PA,Singh A, Deuster PA.Tyrosine improves working memory in a multitasking environment.*Pharmacol Biochem Behav.*1999;64:495-500

[224] Markus CR, Olivier B, Panhuysen GE, Van Der Gugten J, Alles MS, Tuiten A, Westenberg HG, Fekkes D, Koppeschaar HF, de Haan EE. The bovine protein alpha-lactalbumin increases the plasma ratio of tryptophan to the other large neutral amino acids, and in vulnerable subjects raises brain serotonin activity, reduces cortisol concentration, and improves mood under stress. *Am J Clin Nutr.* 2000;71:1536-44

[225] Castaneda C, Charnley JM, Evans WJ, Crim MC. Elderly women accommodate to a low-protein diet with losses of body cell mass, muscle function, and immune response. *Am J Clin Nutr.* 1995;62:30-9

[226] **Vasquez A.** Five-Part Nutritional Protocol that Produces Consistently Positive Results. *Nutritional Wellness* 2005 Sept. http://optimalhealthresearch.com/protocol

[227] Franco OH, Bonneux L, de Laet C, Peeters A, Steyerberg EW, Mackenbach JP. The Polymeal: a more natural, safer, and probably tastier (than the Polypill) strategy to reduce cardiovascular disease by more than 75%. *BMJ.* 2004;329(7480):1447-50

[228] "The combination of 4 low risk factors lowered the all-cause mortality rate to 0.35 (95% CI, 0.28-0.44). In total, lack of adherence to this low-risk pattern was associated with a population attributable risk of 60% of all deaths, 64% of deaths from coronary heart disease, 61% of deaths from cardiovascular diseases, and 60% from cancer." Knoops KT, de Groot LC, Kromhout D, et al. Mediterranean diet, lifestyle factors, and 10-year mortality in elderly European men and women: the HALE project. *JAMA.* 2004 Sep 22;292(12):1433-9

[229] Orme-Johnson DW, Herron RE. An innovative approach to reducing medical care utilization and expenditures. *Am J Manag Care.* 1997;3(1):135-44

[230] Cordain L, Friel J. The Paleo Diet for Athletes : A Nutritional Formula for Peak Athletic Performance: Rodale Books (September 23, 2005)

Profile of the Supplemented Paleo-Mediterranean Diet[233]

Foods to consume: whole, natural, minimally processed foods include:	Foods to avoid: factory products, high-sugar foods, and chemicals
☺ **Lean sources of protein** • Fish (avoiding tuna which is commonly loaded with mercury) • Chicken and turkey • Lean cuts of free-range grass-fed meats: beef, buffalo, lamb are occasionally acceptable • Soy protein[234] and whey protein[235,236] ☺ **Fruits and fruit juices** ☺ **Vegetables and vegetable juices** ☺ **Nuts, seeds, berries** ☺ **Generous use of olive oil**: On sautéed vegetables and fresh salads ☺ **Daily vitamin/mineral supplementation**: With a high-potency broad-spectrum multivitamin and multimineral supplement[237] ☺ **Sun exposure or vitamin D3 supplementation**: To ensure provision of 2,000-5,000 IU of vitamin D3 per day for adults[238] ☺ **Balanced broad-spectrum fatty acid supplementation**: With ALA, GLA, EPA, and DHA[239] ☺ **Water, tea, home-made fruit/vegetable juices**: Commercial vegetable juices are commonly loaded with sodium chloride; choose appropriately. Fruit juices can be loaded with natural and superfluous sugars. Herbal teas can be selected based on the medicinal properties of the plant that is used.	☒ **Avoid as much as possible fat-laden arachidonate-rich meats like beef, liver, pork, and lamb, as well as high-fat cream and other dairy products with emulsified, readily absorbed saturated fats and arachidonic acid** ☒ **High-sugar pseudofoods**: • Corn syrup • Cola and soda • Donuts, candy, etc…."junk food" ☒ **Grains such as wheat, rye, barley**: These have only existed in the human diet for less than 10,000 years and are consistently associated with increased prevalence of degenerative diseases due to the allergic response they invoke and because of their high glycemic load and high glycemic index. ☒ **Potatoes and rice**: High in sugar, low in phytonutrients ☒ **Avoid allergens**: Determined per individual ☒ **Chemicals to avoid**: • Pesticides, Herbicides, Fungicides • Carcinogenic sweeteners: aspartame[240] • Artificial flavors • Artificial colors: tartrazine • Preservatives: benzoate • Flavor enhancers: carrageenan and monosodium glutamate

[231] "A significant glycogen sparing, as well as supercompensation within 24 h of recovery, was observed after [carbohydrate] supplementation." Brouns F, Saris WH, Beckers E, Adlercreutz H, van der Vusse GJ, Keizer HA, Kuipers H, Menheere P, Wagenmakers AJ, ten Hoor F. Metabolic changes induced by sustained exhaustive cycling and diet manipulation. *Int J Sports Med.* 1989 May;10 Suppl 1:S49-62

[232] "The accepted method of increasing muscle glycogen stores is by "glycogen loading," which classically involves depletion of muscle glycogen, usually by exercise, followed by consumption of a high-CHO diet for several days (e.g., 3, 39). …increase muscle glycogen concentrations ([glycogen]) to between 150 and 200% of normal resting levels." Robinson TM, Sewell DA, Hultman E, Greenhaff PL. Role of submaximal exercise in promoting creatine and glycogen accumulation in human skeletal muscle. *J Appl Physiol.* 1999 Aug;87(2):598-604

[233] **Vasquez A**. Five-Part Nutritional Protocol that Produces Consistently Positive Results. *Nutritional Wellness* 2005 Sept. and Vasquez A. Revisiting the Five-Part Nutritional Wellness Protocol: The Supplemented Paleo-Mediterranean Diet. *Nutritional Perspectives* 2011 January. Both of these articles are included in this textbook and/or on-line at http://optimalhealthresearch.com/spmd.html

[234] "These results indicate that for healthy adults, the isolated soy protein is of high nutritional quality, comparable to that of animal protein sources, and that the methionine content is not limiting for adult protein maintenance." Young VR, Puig M, Queiroz E, Scrimshaw NS, Rand WM. Evaluation of the protein quality of an isolated soy protein in young men: relative nitrogen requirements and effect of methionine supplementation. *Am J Clin Nutr.* 1984 Jan;39(1):16-24

[235] Bounous G. Whey protein concentrate (WPC) and glutathione modulation in cancer treatment. *Anticancer Res.* 2000 Nov-Dec;20(6C):4785-92

[236] Markus CR, Olivier B, Panhuysen GE, Van Der Gugten J, Alles MS, Tuiten A, Westenberg HG, Fekkes D, Koppeschaar HF, de Haan EE. The bovine protein alpha-lactalbumin increases the plasma ratio of tryptophan to the other large neutral amino acids, and in vulnerable subjects raises brain serotonin activity, reduces cortisol concentration, and improves mood under stress. *Am J Clin Nutr.* 2000 Jun;71(6):1536-44 http://www.ajcn.org/cgi/content/full/71/6/1536

[237] "Most people do not consume an optimal amount of all vitamins by diet alone. …it appears prudent for all adults to take vitamin supplements." Fletcher RH, Fairfield KM. Vitamins for chronic disease prevention in adults: clinical applications. *JAMA.* 2002;287:3127-9

[238] **Vasquez A**, MansoG, CannellJ. The clinical importance of vitamin D (cholecalciferol). *Altern Ther Health Med.* 2004 Sep 10:28-36 www.optimalhealthresearch.com

[239] **Vasquez A**. New Insights into Fatty Acid Supplementation and Its Effect on Eicosanoid Production and Genetic Expression. *Nutr Perspectives* 2005; Jan: 5-16

[240] "In the past two decades brain tumor rates have risen in several industrialized countries, including the United States... Compared to other environmental factors putatively linked to brain tumors, the artificial sweetener aspartame is a promising candidate to explain the recent increase in incidence and degree of malignancy of brain tumors." Olney JW, Farber NB, Spitznagel E, Robins LN. Increasing brain tumor rates: is there a link to aspartame? *J Neuropathol Exp Neurol* 1996 Nov;55(11):1115-23

Emotional, Mental, and Social Health

Stress management and authentic living: Mental, emotional, and physical "stress" describes any unpleasant living condition which can lead to negative effects on health, such as increased blood pressure, depression, apathy, increased muscle tension, and, according to some research, increased risk of serious health problems such as early death from cardiovascular disease and cancer. Many people find that their modern lives are characterized by excess amounts of multitasking, job responsibilities, family responsibilities, commuter traffic, financial pressures in combination with an insufficient amount of relaxation, sleep, community support, exercise, time in nature, healthy nutrition, and time to simply *be* rather than *do*. Stress comes in many different forms and includes malnutrition, trauma, insufficient exercise (epidemic), excess exercise (rare), sleep deprivation, emotional turmoil, and exposure to chemicals and radiation. When most people talk about "stress" they are referring to either chronic anxiety (such as with high-pressure work situations or dysfunctional interpersonal relationships) or the acute stress reaction that is typical of unpredictable rapid-onset events such as an injury, accident, or other physically threatening situation. **These "different types of stress" are not separate from each other; rather, they are interconnected:**

- Emotional stress causes nutritional depletion[241],
- Sleep deprivation alters immune response[242],
- Chemical exposure can disrupt endocrine function.[243]

Therefore, **any type of stress can cause other types of stress**. Avoiding stressful situations is, of course, an effective way to avoid being bothered or harmed by them. If work-related stress is the problem, then finding a new position or occupation is certainly an option worth considering and implementing. High-stress jobs are often high-paying jobs; but if in the process of making money, a person ruins her health and loses years from her life, then no one would ever say, "It was worth it." **Money, success, and freedom only have value for the person alive and healthy to enjoy them.**

Toxic relationships, whether at home or work, are relationships that cause more harm than good by re-injuring old emotional wounds and by creating new emotional injuries. We can all benefit from affirming our right to a happy and healthy life by minimizing/eliminating contact with people who cause emotional harm to us—this requires conscious effort.[244] Engel[245] provides a clear articulation and description of abusive relationships, along with checklists for their recognition and exercises for their remediation. Healthy relationships are difficult to create and maintain these days, and probably a few basic components contribute to this phenomenon. ❶ With the society-wide disintegration of the extended family, most people in our society have never even seen a healthy family unit and therefore have no model and no available mentors to help them recreate a lasting family structure. ❷ Due specifically to the structure of our educational systems and (pseudo)culture of entertainment, most people have very short attention spans and are accustomed to inattention, distraction, and externally derived entertainment and gratification. ❸ Modern schools and fragmented families both fail to teach conflict resolution and relationship skills. ❹ Poor nutritional status—very common in the general population—promotes impulsivity, irritability, depression, and mood instability.

> **"Good relationships make you feel loved, wanted, and cared for."**
> Malcolm LL. Health Style. Thorsons: 2001, p 133

---

[241] Ingenbleek Y, Bernstein L. The stressful condition as a nutritionally dependent adaptive dichotomy. *Nutrition* 1999 Apr;15(4):305-20

[242] Heiser P, e. Alterations of host defense system after sleep deprivation are followed by impaired mood and psychosocial functioning. *World J Biol Psychiatry* 2001 Apr;2(2):89-94

[243] "Evidence suggests that environmental exposure to some anthropogenic chemicals may result in disruption of endocrine systems in human and wildlife populations." http://www.epa.gov/endocrine on March 7, 2004

[244] Bryn C. Collins. *How to Recognize Emotional Unavailability and Make Healthier Relationship Choices*. [Mjf Books; ISBN: 1567313442] Recently reprinted as: Emotional Unavailability: Recognizing It, Understanding It, and Avoiding Its Trap [McGraw Hill - NTC (April 1998); ISBN: 0809229145]

[245] Engel B. *The Emotionally Abusive Relationship: How to Stop Being Abused and How to Stop Abusing*. Wiley Publishers: 2003

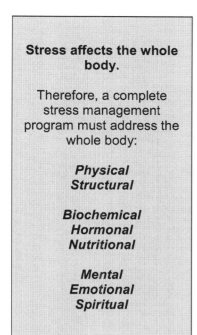

Stress affects the whole body.

Therefore, a complete stress management program must address the whole body:

Physical Structural

Biochemical Hormonal Nutritional

Mental Emotional Spiritual

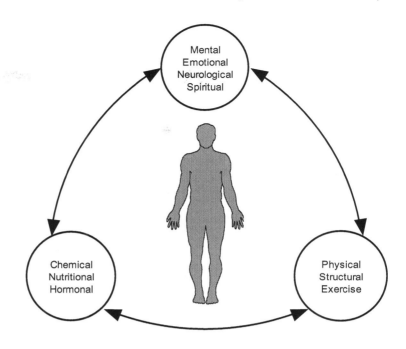

An important concept is that **stress is a "whole body" phenomenon**: affecting the mind, the brain, emotional state, the physical body (including musculoskeletal, immune, and cardiovascular systems), as well as the nutritional status of the individual. The adverse effects of stress can be reduced with an integrated combination of therapeutics that addresses each of the major body systems affected by stress, which are 1) mental/emotional, 2) physical, and 3) nutritional/biochemical.

Approaching stress management from a tripartite perspective

	Mental/emotional	**Physical**	**Nutritional/biochemical**
<u>**Therapeutic considerations**</u>	• Social support • Re-parenting • Conversational style[246] • Meditation, prayer • Healthy boundaries • Books, tapes, groups • Expressive writing[247] • Time to simply rest and relax	• Yoga • Massage • Exercise • Stretching • Swimming • Resting • Biking • Hiking • Affection	• Vitamins, including vitamin C[248] • Fish oil[249] • Hormones, cytokines, neurotransmitters, and eicosanoids • Tryptophan, pyridoxine • Botanical medicines such as *kava*[250], *Ashwaganda,* and *Eleutherococcus*

[246] Rick Brinkman ND and Rick Kirschner ND. *How to Deal With Difficult People* [Audio Cassette. Career Track, 1995]

[247] Smyth JM, Stone AA, Hurewitz A, Kaell A. Effects of writing about stressful experiences on symptom reduction in patients with asthma or rheumatoid arthritis: a randomized trial. *JAMA.* 1999 Apr 14;281(14):1304-9

[248] Brody S, Preut R, Schommer K, Schurmeyer TH. A randomized controlled trial of high dose ascorbic acid for reduction of blood pressure, cortisol, and subjective responses to psychological stress. *Psychopharmacology* (Berl). 2002 Jan;159(3):319-24

[249] Hamazaki T, Itomura M, Sawazaki S, Nagao Y. Anti-stress effects of DHA. *Biofactors.* 2000;13(1-4):41-5

[250] Cagnacci A, et al. Kava-Kava administration reduces anxiety in perimenopausal women. *Maturitas.* 2003 Feb 25;44(2):103-9

Sometimes a stressful situation can be modified into one that is less stressful or dysfunctional, so that the benefits are retained, yet the negative aspects are reduced. Of course, the best example of this is interpersonal relationships, which easily lend themselves to improvement with the application of conscious effort. Many audiotapes, books, and seminars are available for people interested in having improved interpersonal relationships. Selected resources are listed here:

- Men and Women: Talking Together by Deborah Tannen and Robert Bly [Sound Horizons, 1992. ISBN: 1879323095] A lively discussion of the different communication and relationship styles of men and women by two respected experts in their fields.
- How to Deal with Difficult People by Drs. Rick Brinkman and Rick Kirschner. [Audio Cassette. Career Track, 1995] An entertaining format with solutions to common workplace and situational difficulties. Authored and performed by two naturopathic physicians.
- Men are From Mars, Women are From Venus by John Gray. [Audio Cassette and Books]. Phenomenally popular concepts in understanding, accepting, and effectively integrating the differences between men and women.
- The ManKind Project (www.mkp.org). An international organization hosting events for men and women. The men's events, formats, and groups are authentic, clear, and healthy. The ManKind Project has an organization for women called The WomanWithin (www.womanwithin.org). No book or tape can substitute for the dynamics and personal attention that can be experienced by a conscious, empowered, and well-intended group.

When "the problem" cannot be avoided, and the interaction/relationship with the problem cannot be improved, a remaining option is to supplement the internal environment so that it is somewhat "strengthened" to deal with the stress of the bothersome event or situation. For example, when dealing with emotional stress, we can use counseling, support groups, or various relaxation techniques.[251] If we determine that the emotional stress has a biochemical component, then we can use specific botanical and nutritional supplementation to safely and naturally support and restore normal function. Moving deeper into the issue of "stress management" requires that we ask why a person is in a stressful situation to begin with. Of course, with *random acts of chaos* like car accidents, we cannot always ascribe the problem to the person, unless the accident resulted from their own negligence. But **when people are chronically stressed and unhappy about their jobs and/or relationships, then we need to employ more than stress reduction techniques,** and as clinicians we need to offer more than the latest adaptogen. **We have to ask why a person would subject himself/herself to such a situation, and what fears or limitations (self-imposed and/or externally applied) keep him/her from breaking free into a life that works.**[252,253,254,255,256,257]

[251] Martha Davis PhD, Matthew McKay MSW, Elizabeth Robbins Eshelman PhD. The Relaxation & Stress Reduction Workbook 5th edition. New Harbinger Publishers; 2000. [ISBN: 1572242140]
[252] Rick Jarow. Creating the Work You Love: Courage, Commitment and Career; Inner Traditions Intl Ltd; 1995 [ISBN: 0892815426]
[253] Breton D, Largent C. The Paradigm Conspiracy: Why Our Social Systems Violate Human Potential-And How We Can Change Them. Hazelden: 1998
[254] Dominguez JR. Transforming Your Relationship With Money. Sounds True; Book and Cassette edition: 2001 Audio tape.
[255] Miller A. The truth will set you free: overcoming emotional blindness and finding your true adult self. New York: Basic Books; 2001
[256] Bradshaw J. Healing the Shame that Binds You [Audio Cassette (April 1990) Health Communications Audio; ISBN: 1558740430]
[257] Miller A. The Drama of the Gifted Child: The Search for the True Self. Basic Books: 1981

Stress always has a biochemical/physiologic component: Regardless of its origins, stress always takes a toll on the body—*the whole body*. Well-documented effects of stress include:

1. Increased levels of cortisol—higher levels are associated with osteoporosis, memory loss, slow healing, and insulin resistance.
2. Reduced function of thyroid hormones[258] (i.e., induction of peripheral/metabolic hypothyroidism)
3. Reduced levels of testosterone (in men)
4. Increased intestinal permeability and "leaky gut"[259]
5. Increased excretion of minerals in the urine
6. Increased need for vitamins, minerals, and amino acids
7. Suppression of immune function and of natural killer cells that fight viral infections and tumors
8. Decreased production of sIgA—the main defense of the lungs, gastrointestinal tract, and genitourinary tract
9. Increased populations of harmful bacteria in the intestines and an associated increased rate of lung and upper respiratory tract infections
10. Increased incidence of food allergies[260]
11. Sleep disturbance

The body functions as a whole—not as independent, autonomous organ systems: Problems with one aspect of health create problems in other aspects of health. Treatment of disease and promotion of wellness must therefore improve overall health and functioning while simultaneously addressing the disease or presenting complaint.

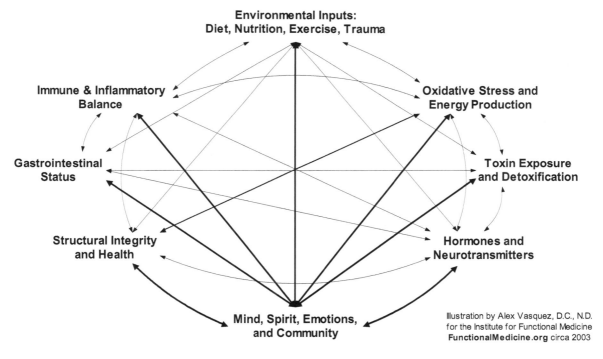

An earlier rendering of the Functional Medicine Matrix, circa 2003: The "Matrix" provides a graphic illustration of the interconnectedness and interdependency of physiologic factors and organ systems; this version was published in *Textbook of Functional Medicine* and published separately as Vasquez A. Web-like Interconnections of Physiological Factors. *Integrative Medicine* 2006, April, 32-37

---

[258] Ingenbleek Y, Bernstein L. The stressful condition as a nutritionally dependent adaptive dichotomy. *Nutrition* 1999 Apr;15(4):305-20

[259] Hart A, Kamm MA. Review article: mechanisms of initiation and perpetuation of gut inflammation by stress. *Aliment Pharmacol Ther* 2002;16(12):2017-28

[260] Anderzen I, Arnetz BB, Soderstrom T, Soderman E. Stress and sensitization in children: a controlled prospective psychophysiological study of children exposed to international relocation. *Journal of Psychosomatic Research* 1997; 43: 259-69

Autonomization, intradependence, emotional literacy, corrective experience:

> "None of us are completely developed people when we reach adulthood.
> We are each incomplete in our own way." *Merle Fossum*[261]

Consciousness-raising is a keystone gift that holistic physicians can impart to their patients and one which may be necessary for true healing to be manifested and maintained. Healthcare providers are quick to enlighten their patients to the details of diet, exercise, nutrition, medications, surgeries, and other *biomechanical* and *biochemical* aspects of health, but are routinely negligent when it comes to sharing with patients the emotional tools that may be necessary to repair or construct the "self" which is supposed to implement the treatment plan that the doctor has designed. Passivity and ignorance are not hindrances to the success of the *medical paradigm*, which requires that patients are "compliant" rather than self-directed; however, for *authentic, holistic healthcare* to be successful, it must empower the patient sufficiently such that he/she attains/regains appropriate *autonomy*—an "internal locus of control"—sufficient for lifelong internally-driven health maintenance. Health implications of autonomy (or its absence) are obvious and intuitive. Patients with an underdeveloped internal locus of control appear to experience greater degrees of social stress which can lead to hypercortisolemia and hippocampal atrophy.[262] A developed internal locus of control correlates strongly with the success of weight-loss programs, and for nonautonomous patients it is necessary to encourage the development of autonomous self-care behavior in addition to the provision of information about diet and exercise.[263]

Six fundamental components of self-esteem
1. Living consciously
2. Self-acceptance
3. Self-responsibility
4. Self-assertiveness
5. Living purposefully
6. Personal integrity
Branden N. <u>The Six Pillars of Self-Esteem</u>. Bantam: 1995

Completely formed internal identities are the natural result of the *continuum* of positive childhood experiences (inclusive of stability, "unconditional love", healthy parenting, and active, conscious intergenerational social contact) which are ideally merged into adolescent and adulthood experiences of success, acceptance, inclusion, independence, interdependence, and intradependence with the end result being a socially-conscious adult with an internal locus of control. Where the patient has experienced a relative absence of these natural and expected prerequisites, a truncated—wounded, reactive, shame-based, dissatisfied—self is likely to result. The failure to develop self-esteem and an internal locus of control largely explains why so many adult patients feign that they are incapable of action, "can't exercise", and "can't leave" their abusive jobs and relationships, and "can't resist" the dietary habits which daily contribute to their physical and psychoemotional decline. Thus, for more than a few patients, a therapeutic path must be explored which helps to re-create the foundation from which an autonomous adult and authentic self can grow—it is a *process* (not an event) of **emotional recovery**.[264] To this extent, interventional or therapeutic *autonomization* resembles a *recovery program* that can include various forms of conscious action, including goal-setting, positive reinforcement, developing emotional literacy[265] and emotional intelligence[266], and consciousness-raising experiences such as therapy and group work—all of which serve to intentionally (re)create and maintain the necessary climate for authentic selfhood. Therewith, the patient can accept challenges to further develop an *empowered self* by participating in exercises in which the ability to decide, choose, and act responsibly and appropriately are reinforced to eventually become second nature, replacing passivity, inaction, and ineffectiveness.[267]

"Empowerment" can only be authentic if it is built on the foundation of a developed self. While *emotional recovery* and *personal empowerment* are separate spheres of activity and attention, they are not mutually exclusive and indeed are synergistic. However, emotional recovery—that process of recounting one's own history, delving

[261] Fossum M. <u>Catching Fire: Men Coming Alive in Recovery</u>. New York; Harper/Hazelden: 1989, 4-7

[262] "Cumulative exposure to high levels of cortisol over the lifetime is known to be related to hippocampal atrophy... Self-esteem and internal locus of control were significantly correlated with hippocampal volume in both young and elderly subjects." Pruessner JC, Baldwin MW, Dedovic K, Renwick R, Mahani NK, Lord C, Meaney M, Lupien S. Self-esteem, locus of control, hippocampal volume, and cortisol regulation in young and old adulthood. *Neuroimage*. 2005 Dec;28(4):815-26

[263] "Their weight loss was significant and associated with an internal locus of control orientation (P < 0.05)... Participants with an internal orientation could be offered a standard weight reduction programme. Others, with a more external locus of control orientation, could be offered an adapted programme, which also focused on and encouraged the participants' internal orientation." Adolfsson B, Andersson I, Elofsson S, Rossner S, Unden AL. Locus of control and weight reduction. *Patient Educ Couns*. 2005 Jan;56(1):55-61

[264] Bradshaw J. <u>Healing the Shame that Binds You</u> [Audio Cassette (April 1990) Health Communications Audio; ISBN: 1558740430]

[265] Dayton T. <u>Trauma and Addiction: Ending the Cycle of Pain through Emotional Literacy</u>. Deerfield Beach; Health Communications, 2000

[266] Goleman D. <u>Emotional Intelligence</u>. New York; Bantam Books: 1995. Although the book as a whole was considered pioneering for its time, and the book continues to make a valuable contribution, a few of the concepts and author's personal stories are embarrassingly simplistic.

[267] Gatto JT. <u>A Schooling Is Not An Education: interview by Barbara Dunlop</u>. http://www.johntaylorgatto.com/bookstore/index.htm

into the depths of one's own psyche, and integrating what is found into a cohesive, functional and healthy whole—must occur before the program of personal development emphasizes empowerment. *Empowerment* cannot succeed without *recovery* because otherwise the so-called "empowerment" is likely to add to the defense mechanisms that protect against pain and thereby block the development of an authentic self. Stated concisely by Janov[268], **"Anything that builds a stronger defense system deepens the neurosis."**

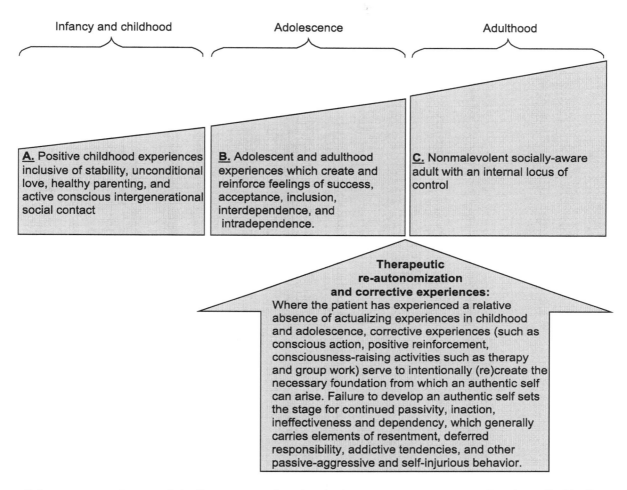

Primary, secondary, and tertiary means for developing an autonomous, authentic self: Ideally, positive childhood experiences (A) merge into adolescent and adult experiences of confidence and maturity (B) for the development of a true adult (C). If A or B is lacking or insufficient, the result is an incomplete self often incapable of *effective* and *appropriate* action. Corrective experiences must then be pursued to re-establish the foundation from which an authentic self can arise.

Patients lacking an internal locus of control are much more likely to succumb to the tantalizing barrage of direct-to-consumer drug advertising[269] which infantilizes patients by 1) oversimplifying diseases, their causes, and treatments, 2) exonerating patients from responsibility and reinforcing the illusion of victimization and helplessness, and 3) encouraging a dependent, passively receptive role by telling patients that they have no proactive role other than to "ask your doctor if a prescription is right for you." Americans consume more prescription and OTC medications per capita than people in any other country.[270,271] With the combined and

---

[268] Janov A. The Primal Scream. New York; GP Putnam's Sons: 1970, page 20

[269] Aronson E. The Social Animal. San Fransisco; WH Freeman and company: 1972: 21-22, 53

[270] America the medicated. http://www.cbsnews.com/stories/2005/04/21/health/printable689997.shtml and http://www.msnbc.msn.com/id/7503122/ . See also http://usgovinfo.about.com/od/healthcare/a/usmedicated.htm Accessed September 17, 2005.

[271] Kivel P. You Call This a Democracy? Apex Press (August, 2004). ISBN: 1891843265 http://www.paulkivel.com/

synergistic effects of 1) the dissolution of first the extended family and now the nuclear family[272], 2) a society-wide famine of mentors, elders, and community[273,274,275], 3) a dearth of autonomous, genuine exploration from childhood to adulthood, and 4) primary and secondary "educational" institutions designed to squelch independence and autonomy in favor of the more efficient,

predictable, and controllable conformity and "standardization"[276,277], **industrialized societies have raised generations of people who lack completely formed internal identities**. Lacking an internal locus of control and identity from which to think independently and critically, these "adults" are easy prey for slick and flashy drug advertisements that promise the illusion of perfect health in exchange for passivity, abdication, and lifelong medicalization. That the typical American watches four hours of television per day[278] is bad enough, what makes this worse is that "Americans who watch average amounts of television may be exposed to more than 30 hours of direct-to-consumer drug advertisements each year, far surpassing their exposure to other forms of health communication."[279] If we are to wean our suckling culture from undue dependence on the pharmaceutical industry, we have to address our patient population directly and transform them from *passive, nonautonomous, and ignorant about health and disease* to pro-active, autonomous, and well-informed about health and the means required to obtain and sustain it.

Insight into a patient's internal dynamic can provide the clinician with an understanding that explains the phenomena of *non-compliance* and *disease identification*. Rather than seeing non-compliance as "weakness of will", non-compliance as a form of "disobedience" may be a reflection of the patient's unconscious need to wrestle with and resolve parental introjects. For example, if a patient had a rejecting, nonaffirming parent, he/she may need to find another rejecting authority figure in order to continue playing the role of the child; by assuming this role and "setting the stage", the patient is unconsciously attempting to create a situation wherein the primary relationship can be healed.[280] Complicating this is *disease identification*—in which patients use their disease as a source of identity and secondary gain for martyrdom, social support, group participation, acceptance, admiration, purpose, excitement, and drama.

---

[272] Bly R. <u>Iron John</u>. Reading, Mass.: Addison Wesley, 1990

[273] Bly R. <u>The Sibling Society</u>. Vintage Books USA; Reprint edition (June 1, 1997) ISBN: 0679781285 (Abridged audio edition (May 1, 1996), ASIN: 0679451609)

[274] Bly R. <u>Where have all the parents gone? A talk on the Sibling Society</u>. New York: Sound Horizons, 1996 Highly recommended.

[275] Bly R, Hillman J, Meade M. <u>Men and the Life of Desire</u>. Oral Tradition Archives. ISBN: 1880155001. Audio Cassette

[276] Gatto JT. <u>Dumbing Us Down: the Hidden Curriculum of Compulsory Education</u>. Gabriola Island, Canada; New Society Publishers: 2005

[277] Gatto JT. <u>The Paradox of Extended Childhood</u>. [From a presentation in Cambridge, Mass. October 2000] http://www.johntaylorgatto.com/bookstore/index.htm

[278] "American children view over 23 hours of television per week. Teenagers view an average of 21 to 22 hours of television per week. By the time today's children reach age 70, they will have spent 7 to 10 years of their lives watching television." American Academy of Pediatrics http://www.aapca1.org/aapca1/tv.html See also TV-Turnoff Network. Facts and Figures About our TV Habit http://www.tvturnoff.org/factsheets.htm Accessed September 17, 2005

[279] Brownfield ED, et al. Direct-to-consumer drug advertisements on network television. *J Health Commun*. 2004 Nov-Dec;9(6):491-7

[280] Miller A. <u>The Drama of the Gifted Child: The Search for the True Self</u>. Basic Books: 1981, page 88

Helping patients create and maintain authentic selves

An absent or underdeveloped locus of control is the key problem that underlies many anxiety disorders, addictive behavioral traits such as overeating, overworking, codependency, as well as chronic ineffectiveness in the pursuit of one's goals. The solutions to this problem are logical, practical, and accessible to everyone; the major costs associated with each are open-mindedness, attentiveness, discipline and persistence. There is scant mention of this concept and its intervention in the biomedical literature; however, it is well described in the psychological literature, particularly that which focuses on various types of "recovery" such as that from addiction, co-dependence, and low self-esteem, the latter two of which are virtually synonymous with an insufficient internal locus of control.

There is no single path here. There are many paths. The goal is not to choose the right path; rather the goal is to travel several paths to the degree necessary, implement what has been learned, travel other paths, and return to the same path again to retrace one's steps in new ways. The process is similar to that of *ceremonial initiation*, the purpose of which is to formally mark the *beginning* of a process that is *ongoing* and *infinite*.[281] Each path and each process has its gifts, significance, and limitations. However, the ultimate goal of each must be a tangible and positive change in the ways which the patient feels and/or behaves in and interacts with the world on a day-to-day basis.

In no particular order (since the proper sequence will have to be customized to the situation and willingness of the patient), the following are some of the more commonly cited exercises, processes, and sources of additional information:

Apprenticeship and Mentoring: books, tapes, and lectures: Children and non-autonomous adults are pulled into authentic adulthood by mentors, elders, and true adults. The therapeutic encounters thus provided—whether interpersonal or vicarious in the form of lectures, books, or audiotapes— serve as sources of information from which new possibilities can be gleaned, and these therefore serve as infinitely valuable resources for expanding the narrow horizons that characterize an underdeveloped internal locus of control. In essence, books, tapes, and lectures allow the patient to become a student and to choose a vicarious mentor. *Advantages*: Books and tapes allow access to many of the best minds in psychology; books and tapes are inexpensive; allow patients to explore and benefit from many different perspectives; books and tapes are always available and are therefore amenable to various schedules of work and responsibility. *Disadvantages*: Books and tapes do not re-create the interpersonal bridge which is essential for authentic recovery; do not provide a direct and objective means of accountably, thus potentially allowing patients to delude themselves about the effectiveness (or lack thereof) of their recovery process. Examples of better-known books, tapes and recorded lectures on the *process* of emotional recovery:

- ***The Six Pillars of Self-Esteem*** by Nathaniel Branden PhD. This is a very accessible yet very structured work in which Dr Branden brilliantly elucidates key concepts in psychology relevant to self-efficacy and self-esteem; also available as an audiobook excellently narrated by Dr Branden.
- ***Healing the Shame that Binds You*** by John Bradshaw [Audio Cassette (April 1990) Health Communications Audio; ISBN: 1558740430] Available as book and cassette with identical titles and different content.
- ***A Little Book on the Human Shadow*** by Robert Bly. Certainly among the most concise, accessible, and complete books ever written on the processes involved in losing and recovering the self; also available as an audio presentation.
- ***The Drama of the Gifted Child*** by Alice Miller. This internationally acclaimed book is considered a true classic among therapists and patients alike. Available as book and a brilliantly performed audio cassette.
- ***You Can Heal Your Life*** by Louise Hay. Another standard for recovery; very "new age."
- ***Codependent No More: How to Stop Controlling Others and Start Caring for Yourself*** by Melody Beattie. Pioneering for its time.
- ***The Artist's Date Book*** by Julia Cameron. Each page has a new creative idea for creative expression and "creative recovery."
- ***The Psychology of Self-Esteem*** by Nathaniel Branden PhD. More advanced and perhaps less widely relevant than his "six pillars" work, this is also an excellent encapsulation of important concepts in personal psychology.

---

[281] Hillman J, Meade M, Some M. Images of initiation. Oral Tradition Archives; 1992

Therapy: *"Therapy is a conversation that matters."* Therapy in this context specifically means face-to-face, active interaction, either one-on-one or in a group setting, with the specific intention to give and/or provide support for personal growth. Whether 12-step groups such as Codependents Anonymous qualify as a form of therapy depends entirely upon the level of engagement of the participant; sitting in a room while *other people* do *their* work provides slow or no benefit for the passive observer. **Recovery is an *active* process, which is why it is antithetical to depression, which is a *passive* state of being.** Patients should go in knowing that this is a *process* and to not expect to be "fixed" after the first hour or even the first month. ***Advantages***: Therapists can provide crucial support and insight while the client wrestles with undecipherable and convoluted emotional and psychic data. Therapists can help the client set goals ("stretches" and "homework") by which the client reaches beyond his/her comfort zone to attain the next expansion in being and experience. Therapists must create a safe space or "container" in which ideas and feelings can be brought forth to intermingle and be consciously appreciated. ***Disadvantages***: Requires a flexible and disciplined schedule; costs money; bad therapists can do more harm than good if they misdirect their clients away from volatile and core issues and authentic expression.[282,283,284,285] Therapy can be disempowering if the patient continues to project his/her locus of control onto the therapist.

Some of the more commonly used tools of the psychotherapeutic trade include:
- **Active listening**
- **Insight, explanation of events**: their origins, reasons, and significance
- **Reminders** of previous conclusions and stories
- **Challenge old ideas and habits**: Therapy that generally or completely lacks confrontation and accountability is ineffective.
- **Encourage exploration and new modes of being and interacting**
- **Creating a safe container wherein the client can review the details, significance, and feelings associated with past events**
- **Modeling the expression of feeling**
- **Defining goals and helping the client focus on what is significant**
- **Correcting distortions of reality**
- **Asking patients to get in touch with and then express their feelings**
- **Support and encourage clients to take calculated risks for the sake of self-expansion**
- **Pointing out errors in logic**
- **Coaching patients in the proper and responsible use of emotional language**
- **Discouraging evasiveness; requiring accountability**[286]

Creativity: All types of self-expression reinforce and validate the patient's sense of self. Creative self-expression, such as writing about thoughts and feelings about significant experiences, can reduce symptomatology in patients with rheumatoid arthritis and asthma.[287]

Experiential: Corrective experiences can be obtained in therapy, with friends and family, in integration groups, and during "experiential" retreats. ***Advantages***: Experiential events orchestrated by therapists and various groups such as ManKind Project (mkp.org) and WomanWithin.org can rapidly facilitate personal growth while also providing an ongoing container and support system that encourages self-development rather than the ego-inflation that accompanies short-term events. ***Disadvantages***: "Adventures" like driving across the nation or climbing a mountain are unconscious and largely impotent attempts at self-initiation; authentic initiation has always been supervised by community elders. However, once a well-founded initiation has taken place, preferably with an on-going community that facilitates continued refinement and self-exploration, then "adventures" can be undertaken consciously to maintain and reinforce the experience of autonomy and competent selfhood. Eventually, transformative and sustentative experiences can be integrated and created in the daily life experience so that dramatic adventures become unnecessary for the continued renewal and "recharging" of the self.

[282] Lee J. Expressing Your Anger Appropriately (Audio Cassette). Sounds True (June 1, 1990); ISBN: 1564550338
[283] Bradshaw J. Healing the Shame that Binds You [Audio Cassette (April 1990) Health Communications Audio; ISBN: 1558740430]
[284] Miller A. The Drama of the Gifted Child: The Search for the True Self. Basic Books: 1981
[285] Miller A. The truth will set you free: overcoming emotional blindness and finding your true adult self. New York: Basic Books; 2001
[286] Kottler JA. The Compleat Therapist. San Francisco; Jossey-Bass publishers; 1991, pages 134-174
[287] Smyth JM, Stone AA, Hurewitz A, Kaell A. Effects of writing about stressful experiences on symptom reduction in patients with asthma or rheumatoid arthritis: a randomized trial. *JAMA*. 1999 Apr 14;281(14):1304-9

Creating and Re-creating the Self:
An on-going process that involves various types of "therapy" such as healthy formal/informal interpersonal and group relationships, creative expression and exploration, the periodic infusion of new ideas from teachers and mentors, attendance in workshops and seminars (or other forms of on-going consciousness-raising), reflection, and the integration of transformative and sustentative significance into everyday life, in such a way that daily life itself becomes *therapeutic* and *affirmative*.

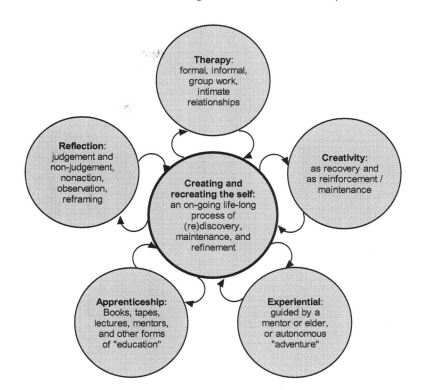

One possible sequence of events for effective, lasting, and authentic autonomization: The caterpillar does not blossom into a butterfly without spending time in its cocoon. The airborne seed descends into the earth for its nourishment before it sprouts and searches for the sun. Similarly, gratification of our ascentionist and impatient ego must be deferred for the sake of allowing the time and descent that provide "grounding" and developing of a solid foundation from which authentic growth can arise. The Western view of "personal development" idealizes a life course of constant ascension that is generally inconsistent with living in a real world fraught with imperfections; two of the major complications arising from such a perfectionistic paradigm are 1) that it causes people to feel anxious and ashamed when confronted with otherwise normal delays and failures, and 2) that it biases people into believing that improvement comes only from advancement rather than also from the return and short-term regression that are characteristic of most historically-proven societal traditions. With modification of the stepwise model proposed by Bradshaw[288], here I propose the following sequence:

1. *Short-term behavior modification*: For people whose behavior is acutely dysfunctional or harmful to themselves or others, they must stop the "acting out" that is the symptom of the underlying emotional injury or schism. Accepting abuse—at work or home—is a form of **acting out** that perpetuates old wounds and saps the strength required for recovery. Enacting addictive behavior is injurious to the psyche because self-injurious behavior reinforces the image of oneself as an object of contempt while also reinforcing the image of psychological dependency and emotional helplessness.

2. *Emotional recovery*: Complete healing is only possible when consciously pursued, and conscious healing can only be pursued after one has become conscious of the wounds, injuries, absences, dynamics, and events that lead to the current state. This process of recovery is referred to mythologically as the "descent" or the time of "eating ashes" that is a recurrent theme in various fairy tales ("Cinderella" literally means "ash girl") and cultural-religious histories (such as Jesus' *descent* into the tomb).[289] The biggest blockades to this process are 1) the ego, which prefers to ascend and to deny intrapersonal "negativity"[290], and 2) the challenge in finding elders and mentors in a society that constantly perpetuates and encourages immaturity, materialism, and superficiality.[291] In the words of famed psychologist Carl Jung, "One does not become enlightened by

---

[288] Bradshaw J. Healing the Shame that Binds You [Audio Cassette (April 1990) Health Communications Audio; ISBN: 1558740430]
[289] Bly R, Hillman J, Meade M. Men and the Life of Desire. Oral Tradition Archives. ISBN: 1880155001
[290] Robert Bly. The Human Shadow. Sound Horizons, New York 1991 [ISBN: 1879323001] and Bly R. A Little Book on the Human Shadow.[ISBN: 0062548476]
[291] Bly R. Where have all the parents gone? A talk on the Sibling Society. New York: Sound Horizons, 1996

imagining figures of light, but by making the darkness *conscious*. The latter procedure, however, is disagreeable, and therefore unpopular." People often have tremendous resistances to the process of self-exploration and internal learning; as Jeffrey Kottler[292] wrote of his own experience in *The Compleat Therapist,* "...like most prospective consumers of therapy, I made up a bunch of excuses for why I could handle this on my own… I was smiling like an idiot…"

3. *Long-term behavior modification and integration*: Insight allows for an illumination of the internal mental-emotional landscape, and effective insight must then be manifested externally by changes/modifications in behavior, habits, and interaction in the world. **Externalized behaviors simultaneously reflect and reinforce thoughts and feelings.** According to Grieneeks[293], patients (and their healthcare providers) can "*think* their way into new ways of *acting*" and "*act* their way into new ways of *thinking*." Eventually, a consciously designed life can be created so that actions, interactions, thoughts, and feelings are melded together in such ways that everyday life itself becomes simultaneously *therapeutic, affirmative, sustentative,* and *empowering*. In this way, the person and his/her life are unified in such ways as to become self-perpetuating and self-sustaining cycles of ascents and descents, thought-feeling and action, reflection and courage, independence and interdependence—in sum: "a wheel rolling from its own center."[294] At this point the self is established, though it must be maintained and developed with the continuous application of consciousness, reflection, and action.

4. *Metapersonal involvement in community, religion, spirituality, and the world*: Many people are tempted to move from a state of woundedness, relative incompleteness and the feelings of shame and disempowerment to a state of illusory *perfection, enlightenment* and *omnipotence* without doing the requisite hard work that makes authentic personal growth possible. People with unhealed emotional wounds often seek to camouflage those deficiencies by becoming pious and projecting an image of completeness and of "having it all figured out" and "having it all together"; religion and the acquisition of power are often misused for this purpose. Many people are successful in wearing this mask for many years; but its crumbling—often manifested as the "midlife crisis"—heralds an opportunity for personal growth if not medicated with anti-depressants, vacations, affairs, gambling, or other distractions.[295] The temptation to bypass Stages 2 [emotional recovery] and 3 [integration] and leapfrog from Stage 1 [woundedness] to Stage 4 [spirituality] should be resisted because the religion or spirituality is then used as a shield *against authenticity* and as a tool for illusory control. Religion can be misused in this way by providing an "identity" and sense of redemption for people with incompletely formed identities and for those with incompletely reconciled shadows and unresolved childhood-parental introjects.[296,297,298] Nietzsche's[299] response to this problem was to encourage self-knowledge and self-reconciliation as prerequisites to religious devotion, hence his admonition, "By all means love your neighbor as yourself – but *first* be such that you love yourself." Historical and recent events remind us of how religion can be misused for misanthropic ends.[300] What is commonly referred to as "spiritual development"— a level of resolution, reconciliation, and autonomy that allows for compassionate interdependence with people, the planet and the larger "world"—is synergistic with and can be supported by religion; but the latter is not a substitute for the former.[301,302] Religion and other forms of metapersonal involvement (e.g., community participation and social generosity) are *important* and *necessary* extensions of self-development. In order for personal development to blossom from the germ of necessary narcissism into its flower of functional completeness, it must eventually manifest in the larger community and the world.

---

[292] Kottler JA. The Compleat Therapist. San Francisco; Jossey-Bass publishers; 1991, pages 2-3
[293] Keith Grieneeks PhD. "Psychological Assessment" taught in 1998 at Bastyr University.
[294] Friedrich Wilhelm Nietzsche, Walter Kaufmann (Translator). Thus Spoke Zarathustra. Penguin USA; 1978, page 27
[295] Robinson JC. Death of a Hero, Birth of a Soul: Answering the Call of Midlife. Council Oak Books, March 1997 ISBN: 1571780432
[296] Bradshaw J. Healing the Shame that Binds You [Audio Cassette (April 1990) Health Communications Audio; ISBN: 1558740430]
[297] Miller A. The Drama of the Gifted Child: The Search for the True Self. Basic Books: 1981
[298] Miller A. The truth will set you free: overcoming emotional blindness and finding your true adult self. New York: Basic Books; 2001
[299] Nietzsche N. Thus spoke Zarathustra. Read by Jon Cartwright and Alex Jennings and published by Naxos AudioBooks. I think this is among the more brilliant achievements in human history. http://naxosaudiobooks.com/nabusa/pages/432512.htm
[300] Bonhoeffer. (movie documentary by director/writer Martin Doblmeier) http://www.bonhoeffer.com/
[301] Lozoff B. It's a Meaningful Life : It Just Takes Practice. March 1, 2001. ISBN: 0140196242
[302] Bradshaw J. Healing the Shame that Binds You [Audio Cassette (April 1990) Health Communications Audio; ISBN: 1558740430]

5. _Acceptance of mortality and death_: No individual person or any system of thought, whether scientific or religious, can feign completeness without accounting for the end of life and incorporating this account into its overarching paradigm. The event is too significant, and the fear and concerns it provokes are too weighty to not be addressed directly and held in consciousness on a periodic—if not frequent—basis. This topic is of practical importance, too, not only in our own lives and those of our friends and family, but also to the national healthcare system, which currently spends the bulk of its money and resources vainly attempting to preserve life in the last few years and months after which disease or age call unrelentingly for the end of life.

Perhaps if we as individuals and as participants in the healthcare system could accept and deal with our own deaths, then we would not have to panic and participate in such superfluous expenditures of time, energy, emotion, and money when death seeks to arrive, either for our patients, our friends and family, or ourselves. Proximal to the panic and aversion that characterizes the West's relationship to death is the "subclinical" panic and aversion that infiltrate the lives, practices, and policies that we experience every day. Surely, many

> "**The event of death is not a tragedy**—to rabbit, fox or man. But **the *concept* of death *is* a tragedy**, for man, and *indirectly* for poor fox, rabbit, bush, bird, just anything and everything in man's path."
>
> Pearce JC, Exploring the Crack in the Cosmic Egg. Washington Square Press; 1974, page 59

unconscious events and subconscious influences contribute to the "lives of quiet desperation"[303] and "universal anxiety"[304] that subtly yet powerfully afflict most people; surely, lack of reconciliation with death is a major contributor. Especially in western cultures, death is commonly seen as some type of failure or shortcoming, either on behalf of the patient or his/her doctors, and the most common questions asked on the topic of death are *"how can this be avoided?"* before the event and *"who is to blame?"* after the event. Other cultures accept death as a natural part of life, and indeed, people are seen to have an obligation to die so that the next generations can have their turn in the cycle of life. Alternatives to western hysteria are founded on acceptance of death, and the prerequisites for the acceptance of death are 1) the dedication of sufficient time for its consideration (most people would rather watch a bad movie or attend spectator sports), 2) reframing the event in terms of its being a natural part of our lives, certainly nothing to be ashamed of (discussed below), 3) making necessary logistical preparations (e.g., writing of wills, providing for dependents, and other obvious technicalities), and 4) living as completely, consciously, compassionately, effectively, and authentically as possible so that remorse can be minimized, perhaps completely mitigated. Reframing the event of death begins with its description in general terms so that its enigma, from which its power over the hearts and minds of humanity is derived, can be deciphered and thus deflated. The main characteristics of death which precipitate its fear are 1) the unpredictability of its arrival, 2) the duration of the dying process, and 3) the quality of that process, for example whether it is painful or associated with or precipitated by severe illness or injury. The first characteristic of *timeliness*—the unpredictability of its arrival—stresses people because of their inadequate preparation and the feeling that they have only recently begun to live or have not quite yet begun to live their authentic lives. These concerns are allayed by preparation, both logistical and intrapersonal. Each of us has the responsibility to "become authentically whole" so that we do not inflict our incompleteness onto others, either directly through various forms of transference or deprivation or indirectly though the more subtle means of politics and cultural mores.[305,306] If a person can live with vitality, authenticity, compassion and effectiveness then little is left to want, and fears of death and its

untimely arrival are diminished. The remaining variables are both controllable and uncontrollable; they are uncontrollable to the extent that we are all subject to chaos and accidents, whether in cars, planes, or bathtubs. *Duration* and *quality* are both controllable on an inpatient setting to the extent that palliative care and autonomous decision-making is made available.[307,308]

> "Once accepted, death is an integral component of every event, as the left hand to the right. The cultural death concept could only be instilled in a mind split from its own life flow."
>
> Pearce JC, Exploring the Crack in the Cosmic Egg. Washington Square Press; 1974, page 59

[303] Throeau HD, (Thomas O, ed). Walden and Civil Disobedience. New York: WW Norton and Company; 1966, page 5
[304] Becker E. The Denial of Death. New York: Free Press; 1973, pages 11 and 21
[305] Miller A. The Drama of the Gifted Child: The Search for the True Self. Basic Books: 1981
[306] Robert Bly. The Human Shadow. Sound Horizons, New York 1991 [ISBN: 1879323001] and Bly R. A Little Book on the Human Shadow.[ISBN: 0062548476
[307] Steinbrook R. Medical marijuana, physician-assisted suicide, and the Controlled Substances Act. *N Engl J Med*. 2004 Sep 30;351(14):1380-3
[308] "Failure to give an effective therapy to seriously ill patients, either adults or children, violates the core principles of both medicine and ethics... Therefore, in the patient's best interest, patients and parents/surrogates, have the right to request medical marijuana under certain circumstances and physicians have the duty to disclose medical marijuana as an

Life can only be authentically and completely experienced after one has created an authentic self and has thereafter accepted life *as it is*. Since death is part of life, the full engagement of life requires *acceptance of* and *reconciliation with* death. Acceptance of death does not necessarily entail that life becomes permeated with nihilistic resignation; on the contrary, it infuses daily events with significance and makes all experiences unique and worthy of appreciation.

Growth, integration, and acceptance: Starting at the top, the progression of personal growth, emotional recovery, integration and daily practice is followed by the more advanced integration of one's chosen purpose, mission, and life work with one's chosen spiritual/religious practice, family and community involvement, and acceptance of and preparation for the end of life and the continuity of society and the environment.

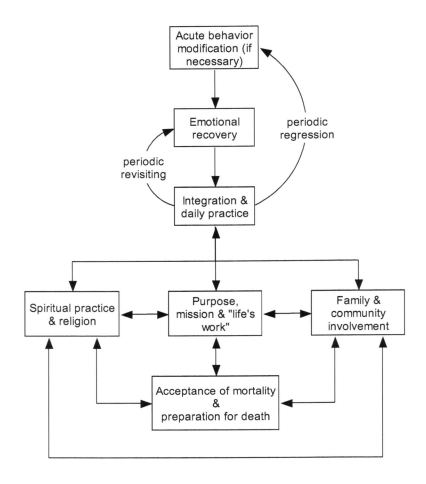

"They say there's no future for us.
They're right,
which is fine with us." *Rumi*[309]

option and prescribe it when appropriate." Clark PA. Medical marijuana: should minors have the same rights as adults? *Med Sci Monit.*2003;9:ET1-9
www.medscimonit.com/pub/vol_9/no_6/3640.pdf
[309] Rumi in Barks C (translator). The Essential Rumi. HarperSanFransisco: 1995, page 2

Environmental Health, Toxicity, and Detoxification

"Man's attitude toward nature is today critically important simply because we have now acquired a fateful power to alter and destroy nature. But man is a part of nature, and his war against nature is inevitably a war against himself." *Rachel Carson*[310]

Environmental exposures to chemicals and toxic substances: Studies using blood tests and tissue samples from Americans across the nation have consistently shown that all Americans have toxic chemical accumulation whether or not they work in chemical factories or are obviously exposed at home or work.[311,312] **The recent report from the CDC found toxic chemicals such as pesticides in all Americans, especially minorities, women, and children.**[313] Nearly all of these chemicals are known to contribute to health problems in humans—problems such as cancer, fatigue, poor memory, endocrinopathy, subfertility/infertility, Parkinson's disease, autoimmune diseases like lupus, and many other serious conditions. Therefore, *detoxification programs are a necessity—not a luxury*.

Examples of toxicants commonly found in Americans

Environmental pollutant (population frequency)	Biologic effects as quoted from HSDB: Hazardous Substances Data Bank. National Library of Medicine, NIH[314] or other reference as noted
DDE (found in 99% of Americans): DDE is the main metabolite of DDT, a pesticide that was presumably banned in the US in 1972	• DDT is known to be immunosuppressive in animals. • A study published in 2004 showed that increasing levels of DDE in African-American male farmers in North Carolina correlated with a higher prevalence of antinuclear antibodies and up to 50% reductions in serum IgG.[315] • Other studies in humans have suggested an estrogenic or anti-androgenic effect.[316] • Virtually all US women have evidence of DDT/DDE accumulation. Women with higher levels of DDT and/or its metabolites show pregnancy and childbirth complications and have higher rates of infant mortality.[317]

[310] Rachel Carson. *Silent Spring*. Boston, Houghton Mifflin Company (2002). ISBN: 0395683297. See also Rachel Carson Dies of Cancer; 'Silent Spring' Author Was 56. New York Times 1956. http://www.rachelcarson.org/ on August 1, 2004

[311] "The average concentration of 2,3,7,8-tetrachlorodibenzo-p-dioxin in the adipose tissue of the US population was 5.38 pg/g, increasing from 1.98 pg/g in children under 14 years of age to 9.40 pg/g in adults over 45." Orban JE, Stanley JS, Schwemberger JG, Remmers JC. Dioxins and dibenzofurans in adipose tissue of the general US population and selected subpopulations. *Am J Public Health* 1994 Mar;84(3):439-45

[312] "Although the use of HCB as a fungicide has virtually been eliminated, detectable levels of HCB are still found in nearly all people in the USA." Robinson PE, Leczynski BA, Kutz FW, Remmers JC. An evaluation of hexachlorobenzene body-burden levels in the general population of the USA. *IARC Sci Publ* 1986;77:183-92

[313] "Many of the pesticides found in the test subjects have been linked to serious short- and long-term health effects including infertility, birth defects and childhood and adult cancers." http://www.panna.org/campaigns/docsTrespass/chemicalTrespass2004.dv.html July 25, 2004

[314] Primary source for this data is the Hazardous Substances Data Bank. National Library of Medicine, National Institutes of Health: http://toxnet.nlm.nih.gov/cgi-bin/sis/htmlgen?HSDB accessed on August 1, 2004

[315] Cooper GS, Martin SA, Longnecker MP, Sandler DP, Germolec DR. Associations between plasma DDE levels and immunologic measures in African-American farmers in North Carolina. *Environ Health Perspect*. 2004 Jul;112(10):1080-4

[316] Dalvie MA, Myers JE, Lou Thompson M, Dyer S, Robins TG, Omar S, Riebow J, Molekwa J, Kruger P, Millar R. The hormonal effects of long-term DDT exposure on malaria vector-control workers in Limpopo Province, South Africa. *Environ Res*. 2004 Sep;96(1):9-19

[317] "The findings strongly suggest that DDT use increases preterm births, which is a major contributor to infant mortality. If this association is causal, it should be included in any assessment of the costs and benefits of vector control with DDT." Longnecker MP, Klebanoff MA, Zhou H, Brock JW. Association between maternal serum concentration of the DDT metabolite DDE and preterm and small-for-gestational-age babies at birth. *Lancet*. 2001 Jul 14;358(9276):110-4

Examples of toxicants commonly found in Americans—*continued*

Environmental pollutant (population frequency)	*Biologic effects as quoted from HSDB: Hazardous Substances Data Bank. National Library of Medicine, NIH[318] or other reference*
2,5-dichlorophenol (88% nationally and up to 96% in select children populations): Dichlorophenols can occur in tap water as a result of standard chlorination treatment. General population may be exposed to 2,5-dichlorophenol through oral consumption or dermal contact with chlorinated tap water. 2,5-Dichlorophenol was identified in 96% of the urine samples of children residing in Arkansas near an herbicide plant at concentrations of 4-1,200 ppb. The sole manufacturer for herbicide use is Sandoz (Clariant Corporation).	▪ Human Toxicity Excerpts: 1. Burning pain in mouth and throat. White necrotic lesions in mouth, esophagus, and stomach. Abdominal pain, vomiting ... and bloody diarrhea. 2. Pallor, sweating, weakness, headache, dizziness, tinnitus. 3. Shock: Weak irregular pulse, hypotension, shallow respirations, cyanosis, pallor, and a profound fall in body temperature. 4. Possibly fleeting excitement and confusion, followed by unconsciousness. ... 5. Stentorous breathing, mucous rales, rhonchi, frothing at nose and mouth and other signs of pulmonary edema are sometimes seen. Characteristic odor of phenol on the breath. 6. Scanty, dark-colored ... urine ... moderately severe renal insufficiency may appear. 7. Methemoglobinemia, Heinz body hemolytic anemia and hyperbilirubinemia have been reported. ... 8. Death from respiratory, circulatory or cardiac failure. 9. If spilled on skin, pain is followed promptly by numbness. The skin becomes blanched, and a dry opaque eschar forms over the burn. When the eschar sloughs off, a brown stain remains.
Chlorpyrifos (found in 93% of Americans): Insecticide used on corn and cotton and for termite control. Conservative estimates hold that 80% of the chlorpyrifos in the US was produced directly or indirectly by Dow Chemical Corporation.[319] **This pesticide is routinely used in schools and is thus found in blood and tissue samples of nearly all American children.**	▪ Toxic if inhaled, in contact with skin, and if swallowed. ▪ All the organophosphorus insecticides have a cumulative effect by progressive inhibition of cholinesterase. ▪ The symptoms of chronic poisoning due to organophosphorus pesticides include headache, weakness, feeling of heaviness in head, decline of memory, quick onset of **fatigue, disturbed sleep,** loss of appetite, and loss of orientation. Other manifestations of accumulation include **tension, anxiety, restlessness, insomnia, headache, emotional instability, fatigue**... ▪ Chlorpyrifos is a suspected endocrine disruptor.[320] ▪ **Higher chlorpyrifos levels in children correlate with higher incidences attention problems, attention-deficit/hyperactivity disorder, and pervasive developmental disorder.**[321]

---

[318] Primary source for this data is the Hazardous Substances Data Bank, National Institutes of Health: http://toxnet.nlm.nih.gov/cgi-bin/sis/htmlgen?HSDB accessed on August 1, 2004

[319] Kristin S. Schafer, Margaret Reeves, Skip Spitzer, Susan E. Kegley. Chemical Trespass: Pesticides in Our Bodies and Corporate Accountability. Pesticide Action Network North America. May 2004 Available at http://www.panna.org/campaigns/docsTrespass/chemicalTrespass2004.dv.html on August 1, 2004

[320] http://www.panna.org/resources/documents/factsChlorpyrifos.dv.html accessed August 1, 2004

[321] "Highly exposed children (chlorpyrifos levels of >6.17 pg/g plasma) scored, on average, 6.5 points lower on the Bayley Psychomotor Development Index and 3.3 points lower on the Bayley Mental Development Index at 3 years of age compared with those with lower levels of exposure. Children exposed to higher, compared with lower, chlorpyrifos levels were also significantly more likely to experience Psychomotor Development Index and Mental Development Index delays, attention problems, attention-deficit/hyperactivity disorder problems, and pervasive developmental disorder problems at 3 years of age." Rauh VA, Garfinkel R, Perera FP, Andrews HF, Hoepner L, Barr DB, Whitehead R, Tang D, Whyatt RW. Impact of prenatal chlorpyrifos exposure on neurodevelopment in the first 3 years of life among inner-city children. *Pediatrics.* 2006 Dec;118(6):e1845-59

Examples of toxicants commonly found in Americans—*continued*

Environmental pollutant (population frequency)	Biologic effects as quoted from HSDB: *Hazardous Substances Data Bank. National Library of Medicine, NIH*[322] *or other reference as noted*
Mercury (8% of American women of reproductive age have mercury levels high enough to cause adverse health effects)	▪ Mercury is a well-known neurotoxin, immunotoxin, and nephrotoxin. Mercury toxicity is also a known cause of hypertension in humans. ▪ A recent study published in *JAMA—Journal of the American Medical Association*[323] noted that "Humans are exposed to methylmercury, a well-established neurotoxin, through fish consumption. The fetus is most sensitive to the adverse effects of exposure. … **approximately 8% of women had concentrations higher than the US EPA's recommended reference dose (5.8 microg/L),** below which exposures are considered to be without adverse effects." **The most obvious interpretation of this data published in *JAMA* is that 8% of American women have chronic mercury poisoning—poisoning in this case refers specifically to elevated blood levels of a known toxicant that consistently demonstrates adverse effects on human health.** Logical deduction holds that such a high prevalence of human poisoning should be unacceptable and should lead directly to legislative restrictions on corporate emissions to protect and salvage the health of the public.
2,4-dichlorophenol (found in 87% of Americans): Pesticide	▪ Human Toxicity Excerpts: same as for 2,5-dichlorophenol ▪ In males, significant increases in relative risk ratios for lung cancer, rectal cancer, and soft tissue sarcomas were reported; in females, there were increases in the relative risk of cervical cancer.

> **"The only thing necessary for the triumph of evil is for good men to do nothing."**
> **Edmond Burke (1729 – 1797)**
>
> "Your lack of interest in the past, your lack of involvement, your unwillingness to develop coherent strategies, your unwillingness to challenge authority - these have created a vacuum in decision-making, that has been filled by professional groups with close relationships with the chemical industries…"   Samuel Epstein, M.D.[324]

---

[322] Primary source for this data is the Hazardous Substances Data Bank, National Institutes of Health: http://toxnet.nlm.nih.gov/cgi-bin/sis/htmlgen?HSDB Accessed Aug 1, 2004
[323] Schober SE, Sinks TH, Jones RL, Bolger PM, McDowell M, Osterloh J, Garrett ES, Canady RA, Dillon CF, Sun Y, Joseph CB, Mahaffey KR. Blood mercury levels in US children and women of childbearing age, 1999-2000. *JAMA*. 2003 Apr 2;289(13):1667-74
[324] Samuel Epstein MD, 1993. Professor of Occupational and Environmental Medicine at the School of Public Health, University of Illinois Medical Center Chicago. http://www.converge.org.nz/pirm/pestican.htm accessed September 11, 2004

<u>Toxicity and detoxification—basics</u>: The physiologic processes by which toxins—whether chemicals or metals—are referred to generally as "detoxification." Clinically, doctors can implement treatment interventions to promote and facilitate the removal of chemical and metal toxins; this, too, is generally referred to as detoxification or clinical/therapeutic detoxification programs. Detoxification programs are popular with patients and some doctors and are most often misused and misapplied.

The recent findings that mercury poisoning can result from once-weekly consumption of tuna[325] and that the average American has 13 pesticides in his/her body[326] should be seen as an indication of how dangerously toxic our environment has become, largely due to irresponsible corporate and government policies that value profitability over sustainability.

<u>Detoxification procedures</u>: Though a detailed clinical explanation of detoxification procedures will not be included here (see Chapter 4 of *Integrative Rheumatology*[327]), the general concepts for detoxification are as follows:
1. *Avoidance*: reduced exposure = reduced problem
   a. If there were less chemical pollution, then our environment would be less toxic and therefore we would not have such problems with environmental poisoning.
   b. Limit or eliminate exposure to paint fumes, car exhaust, new carpet, solvents, adhesives, artificial foods, synthetic chemical drugs, copier fumes, pesticides, herbicides, chemical fertilizers, etc.
2. *Depuration*: "The act or process of freeing from foreign or impure matter"[328]
   a. Exercise and sauna
   b. Bowel cleansing, fiber, probiotics, antibiotics, laxatives
   c. Liver and bile stimulators
   d. Cofactors for phase 1 oxidation and phase 2 conjugation
   e. Chelation for heavy metals
   f. Urine alkalinization
3. *Damage control*: managing the consequences of chemical and heavy metal toxicity
   a. Hormone replacement
   b. Antioxidant therapy
   c. Occupational and rehabilitative training
   d. Management of resultant diseases, particularly autoimmune diseases
4. *Political and social action*: Due in large part to corporate influence and government deregulation, environmental contamination with pesticides from American corporations has increased to such an extent over the past few decades that now all Americans show evidence of pesticide accumulation in their bodies. Failure to hold corporations to tight regulatory standards has jeopardized the future of humanity. Voter passivity combined with collusion between multinational corporations and government officials is the underlying problem. Political action is the solution. The past and recent history on this topic is clear and well documented for those who wish to access the facts.[329,330,331,332,333,334,335, 336,337]

---

[325] "The neurobehavioral performance of subjects who consumed tuna fish regularly was significantly worse on color word reaction time, digit symbol reaction time and finger tapping speed (FT)." Carta P, Flore C, Alinovi R, Ibba A, Tocco MG, Aru G, Carta R, Girei E, Mutti A, Lucchini R, Randaccio FS. Sub-clinical neurobehavioral abnormalities associated with low level of mercury exposure through fish consumption. *Neurotoxicology*. 2003 Aug;24(4-5):617-23

[326] "A comprehensive survey of more than 1,300 Americans has found traces of weed- and bug-killers in the bodies of everyone tested, …. The survey, conducted by the U.S. Centers for Disease Control and Prevention, found that the body of the average American contained 13 of these chemicals." Martin Millelstaedt. 13 pesticides in body of average American. *The Globe and Mail*. Friday, May 21, 2004 - Page A17 Available on-line at http://www.theglobeandmail.com/servlet/ArticleNews/TPStory/LAC/20040521/HPEST21/TPEnvironment/ on August 6, 2004

[327] **Vasquez A**. Integrative Rheumatology. IBMRC. http://optimalhealthresearch.com/textbooks/rheumatology.html

[328] Webster's 1913 Dictionary

[329] Robert Van den Bosch. The pesticide conspiracy. Garden City, NY: Doubleday, 1978. ISBN: 0385133847

[330] "Monsanto Corporation is widely known for its production of the herbicide Roundup and genetically engineered Roundup-ready crops… altered to survive a dousing of the toxic herbicide. …glyphosate, is known to cause eye soreness, headaches, diarrhea, and other flu-like symptoms, and has been linked to non-Hodgkin's lymphoma." Bush Names Former Monsanto Executive as EPA Deputy Administrator. Daily News Archive From March 29, 2001 http://www.beyondpesticides.org/NEWS/daily_news_archive/2001/03_29_01.htm accessed on August 1, 2004

[331] "They pointed to budgets cuts for research and enforcement, to steep declines in the number of cases filed against polluters, to efforts to relax portions of the Clean Air Act, to an acceleration of federal approvals for the spraying of restricted pesticides and more." Patricia Sullivan. Anne Gorsuch Burford, 62, Dies; Reagan EPA Director. *Washington Post*. Thursday, July 22, 2004; Page B06 http://www.washingtonpost.com/wp-dyn/articles/A3418-2004Jul21.html on August 2, 2004

[332] "In fact, amongst the crimes of Reagan and Bush which will go down in history are their emasculation of Federal regulatory apparatus... But in 1988, under the Bush administration, the EPA - illegally, in our view - revoked the Dellaney Law..." Samuel Epstein MD, 1993. Professor of Occupational and Environmental Medicine at the School of Public Health, University of Illinois Medical Center Chicago. http://www.converge.org.nz/pirm/pestican.htm on August 1, 2004

[333] "The Environmental Protection Agency will be free to approve pesticides without consulting wildlife agencies to determine if the chemical might harm plants and animals protected by the Endangered Species Act, according to new Bush administration rules…. It also is intended to head off future lawsuits, the officials said." Associated Press. Bush Eases Pesticide Laws http://www.cbsnews.com/stories/2004/07/29/tech/main633009.shtml accessed August 1, 2004

Personal plans for taking responsible action and avoiding political/social passivity that has created the opportunity for regulatory failure and corporate exploitation of the environment that threatens the sustainability of the human species:

_____
_____
_____
_____
_____
_____
_____
_____
_____
_____
_____
_____
_____
_____
_____
_____
_____
_____
_____
_____
_____
_____
_____
_____
_____
_____
_____
_____
_____
_____
_____
_____

[334] "The new policy also could bolster pesticide makers' contention that federal labeling insulates them from suits alleging that their products cause illness or environmental damage, Olson says. 'It . . . could really be disastrous for public health.'" Bush Exempts Pesticide Companies from Lawsuits. Law on Pesticides Reinterpreted: Government Alters Policy in Effort to Protect Manufacturers. Peter Eisler. *USA TODAY*. October 6, 2003 http://www.organicconsumers.org/foodsafety/bushpesticides100703.cfm Accessed Aug 2004
[335] WASHINGTON (AP) — "The Environmental Protection Agency will be free to approve pesticides without consulting wildlife agencies to determine if the chemical might harm plants and animals protected by the Endangered Species Act, according to new Bush administration rules." Bush eases pesticide reviews for endangered species. http://www.usatoday.com/news/washington/2004-07-29-epa-pesticides_x.htm?csp=34 Accessed August 2004
[336] "It is simply intolerable that the EPA, instead of providing an example for open scientific discussion, has continuously violated key environmental legislation, stifling legitimate dissent. The failure of EPA to properly encourage and protect whistleblowing has undermined the ability of the EPA and state environmental agencies to enforce environmental laws." Letter to Carol Browner, Administrator U.S. Environmental Protection Agency from Stephen Kohn, Chair National Whistleblower Center Board of Directors dated March 23, 1999. Availble at http://www.whistleblowers.org/statements.htm on October 10, 2004
[337] "The Bush administration has imposed a gag order on the U.S. Environmental Protection Agency from publicly discussing perchlorate pollution, even as two new studies reveal high levels of the rocket-fuel component may be contaminating the nation's lettuce supply." Peter Waldman. Rocket Fuel Residues Found in Lettuce: Bush administration issues gag order on EPA discussions of possible rocket fuel tainted lettuce. *THE WALL STREET JOURNAL*. See http://www.organicconsumers.org/toxic/lettuce042903.cfm http://www.rhinoed.com/epa's_gag_order.htm http://www.peer.org/press/508.html http://yubanet.com/artman/publish/article_13637.shtml

Toxicant Exposure: solvents, pesticides, herbicides, plastics, fire-proofing, dioxins, exhaust, PCB, mercury, lead, cadmium, and thousands of others; the ultimate causes and therefore solutions are found primarily in addressing corporate environmental policies and influence on government regulations, societal structure/expectations regarding materialism/independence/convenience/passivity

Biological Persistence: lipolysis/redistribution; detoxification/reabsorption

Promote lipolysis with diet, exercise, sauna

lipophilic chemicals are deposited in cell membranes/adipose

metals circulate and are deposited in tissues where they impair function and thereby contribute to 'disease'

some heavy metals may alter detoxification

treatment

DMSA chelation

Phase One: activation / oxidation
Rapidly inducible by toxicant exposure and some drugs; the main clinical problems here are
1) **inhibition** by SNiPs, nutrient deficiencies, drugs, LPS, heavy metals
2) **relative excess activity**: rapid phase one in relation to slow conjugation: the body is not making a mistake here; it is simply responding to exposure; the solutions are to reduce exposure and support conjugation

Clinical Solutions:
1) nutritional supplementation and diet improvement,
2) reduce exposure to drugs and other 'inducers' including enterohepatic recirculation (check increased permeability and fecal b-glucuronidase)
3) clean the gut to restore mucosal integrity and reduce LPS and b-glucuronidase

hydration/urination, bile formation/expulsion, maintenance of conjugation, botanical adsorbents, daily defecation

failure

excretion in urine, excretion via bile flow and defecation

enterohepatic recirculation

insufficient oxidation

sufficient oxidation

chemical toxicant accumulation: increased disease risk: autoimmunity, Parkinson's disease, cancer, multiple chemical sensitivity, adverse drug reactions

a few chemicals are excreted following Phase 1 (without Conjugation)

sufficient oxidation

Phase Two: conjugation
Insufficiently induced by toxicant exposure; failure of conjugation following oxidation is highly problematic; the main clinical problems here are
1) **slow action**: phase 2 is commonly slower than phase 1; slow action can be caused by nutritional deficiencies, insufficient intake of vegetables/crucifers, and SNiPs, which are surprisingly common and are consistently associated with increased risk for disease;
2) **insufficient nutrient intake for conjugation**: recall that most conjugation factors are, of course, derived from foods: amino acids and sulphur

Clinical Solutions:
1) general nutritional supplementation and diet improvement,
2) reduce exposure to all endogenous and exogenous toxicants: drugs, chemicals, enterohepatic recirculation, hyperabsorption due to increased permeability and fecal b-glucuronidase
3) induce conjugation with cruciferous vegetables and specific botanicals
4) stimulate bile flow and bowel cleansing

insufficient conjugation

successful conjugation

hydration, healthy renal function (and alkalosis)

excretion in urine

Toxicant is solublized for excretion in bile or urine

failure of bile formation, blockage in bile flow, dehydration, dysbiosis causing deconjugation constipation promoting reabsorption, insufficient fiber

bile formation, bile expulsion, maintenance of conjugation, daily defecation

excretion via bile flow and defecation

enterohepatic recirculation

Overview of toxicant exposure and detoxification/depuration: Details are discussed in *Integrative Rheumatology*.[338]

[338] **Vasquez A**. Integrative Rheumatology. IBMRC: 2006, 2009. http://optimalhealthresearch.com/rheumatology.html

Integrative/functional healthcare empowers patients with the ability to understand and effectively participate in the course of their life and health

Drug/surgery-based medicine	Paradigm	Holistic natural healthcare
• Doctor as "savior" and indifferent "objective" observer	Role of the doctor	• Doctor as "teacher" and active caring partner and co-participant in the process
• Helpless victim, disempowered, dependent	Role of the patient	• Active participant, empowered, responsible
• Illness is impossibly complex, and treating this with natural means is generally impossible • Treatment is simple: you have this disease, and you need to take one or more drugs for every problem • Diet and lifestyle modifications are generally viewed as secondary to drugs • The disease is more important than the patient	Nature of illness	• Multifactorial: involving many different aspects of lifestyle, diet, exercise, genetic inheritance, psychology, and environment • Many causes allows for many different treatment approaches and different ways of attaining health • Illness can be modified via selective dietary and lifestyle changes and a custom-tailored treatment plan • The patient is more important than the disease
• Disease-centered, drug-centered	Viewpoint	• Patient-centered, wellness-centered
• Drugs, including chemotherapy • Surgery • Radiation • Electroconvulsive treatment • Vaccinations	Treatment and options	• Diet and lifestyle improvement • Relationship/emotional work • Botanical and nutritional medicines • Physical medicine, chiropractic, exercise • Acupuncture • *Selective* rather than *first-line* use of pharmaceuticals and medical procedures
• Symptom suppression • Drug side-effects are a significant cause of death in the US • Only *treats disease*, does not *promote health*; cannot reach optimal health by only reactively treating established health problems • Enormous expense, often subsidized by private or public "insurance"	Long-term outcome	• Improved health • Potential for successful prevention, treatment or eradication of chronic disease • Potential to become optimally healthy • Proven cost-reduction
• Heightened risk, since drugs are foreign chemicals that have action in the body by interfering with the way that the body normally works • Every drug has side-effects, some of which can be life-threatening • Surgery causes irreparable changes to the body, often for the worse. • Radiation and chemotherapy can cause a secondary cancer to develop	Risks	• Reduced risk, since most of the botanical treatments and all of the nutritional medicines have been a major part of the human diet for centuries/millennia and have proven safety • Delayed onset of action: most treatments are not fast-acting enough to be of value in traumatic or acutely life-threatening situations • Patients must be willing to adopt healthier lifestyles
• Allows a doctor to see many patients within a short amount of time, thus increasing profitability • Since drugs do not cure problems, patients must return for lifelong prescription renewals • Therapeutic passivity: minimal action or effort required by patient and doctor • The doctor holds all the power, and the patient is completely dependent on the doctor for treatment	Benefits	• Improved short-term and long-term health • Empowerment • Understanding of body processes as well as healthcare directions and goals • Options

Health-promoting:

- Frequent exercise and physical activity
- Plenty of sleep
- Maintaining ideal body weight
- Avoiding exposure to chemicals, drugs, pollution, exhaust, tobacco smoke
- Daily consumption of fruits and vegetables
- Ideal protein intake for body size, physical activity, and health status
- Diet high in fiber and complex carbohydrates
- Use of health-promoting beverages such as green tea, fruit/vegetable juices, water, and light consumption of beer or red wine
- Increased intake of ALA, EPA, DHA, GLA, and oleic acid
- Multi-vitamin and multi-mineral supplementation
- Optimal vitamin D and iron status
- Beneficial gastrointestinal flora
- Natural and phytonutraceutical interventions to promote optimal health
- Pro-active healthcare
- Healthy and supportive relationships that foster responsibility, independence, interdependence, health and feelings of being wanted and cared for
- Work environments that promote collaboration and creativity and which appreciate personal time and allow for schedule flexibility

Disease-promoting:

- Physical inactivity and sedentary lifestyle
- Insufficient sleep
- Obesity
- Frequent exposure to chemicals, drugs, pollution, exhaust, tobacco smoke
- Daily consumption of processed and artificial foods
- Insufficient (common) or excessive (rare) protein
- Diet high in simple carbohydrates and sugars
- Use of disease-promoting beverages such as cola, artificially colored/flavored/sweetened drinks, and hard liquor
- Increased intake of linoleic acid (vegetable oils) and arachidonic acid (beef, liver, pork, lamb and most farm-raised land animals)
- Low intake of vitamins and minerals
- Excess iron and insufficient vitamin D
- Dysbiosis: intestinal overgrowth of yeast, parasites, and harmful bacteria
- Use of synthetic chemical drugs to suppress symptoms of poor health
- Reactive healthcare that only responds to problems after they have developed
- Dysfunctional relationships that enable and foster illness, dependency and isolation
- Work environments that promote isolation, pressure, perfectionism and which disapprove of creativity, personal time, and flexibility

Maximize factors that promote health ◆ Minimize factors that promote disease

Opposite influences of health promotion vs. disease promotion: Lifestyle concept: Improved clinical outcomes will be attained when doctors and patients attend to both **prescription of health-promoting activities** and **proscription of disease-promoting activities**. Indeed, attention needs to be given to the **ratio** of these disparate and opposing forces, which ultimately influence genetic expression and physiologic function of many organ systems.

Previously published essays

A Five-Part Nutritional Wellness Protocol That Produces Consistently Positive Results: Brief Review of Scientific Rationale

Alex Vasquez, DC, ND

This article was originally published in *Nutritional Wellness*
http://www.nutritionalwellness.com/archives/2005/sep/09_vasquez.php

When I am lecturing here in the U.S., as well as in Europe, doctors often ask if I will share the details of my protocols with them. Thus, in 2004, I published a 486-page textbook for doctors that includes several protocols and important concepts for the promotion of wellness and treatment of musculoskeletal disorders.[339] In this article, I will share with you what I consider a basic protocol for wellness promotion. I've implemented this protocol as part of the treatment plan for a wide range of clinical problems. In my next column, I will provide several case reports of patients from my office to exemplify the effectiveness of this program and show how it can be the foundation upon which additional treatments can be added as necessary.

Nutrients are required in the proper amounts, forms, and approximate ratios for essential physiologic function; if nutrients are lacking, the body cannot function normally, let alone optimally. Impaired function results in subjective and objective manifestations of what is commonly labeled as "disease." Thus, a powerful and effective alternative to treating diseases with drugs is to re-establish normal/optimal physiologic function by replenishing the body with essential nutrients.

Of course, many diseases are multifactorial and therefore require multicomponent treatment plans, and some diseases actually require the use of drugs. However, while only a relatively small portion of patients actually need drugs for their problems, I am sure we all agree that everyone needs a foundational nutrition plan, as outlined and substantiated below.

1. Health-promoting diet: Following an extensive review of the research literature, I developed what I call the "supplemented Paleo-Mediterranean diet," which I have described in greater detail elsewhere.[340] In essence, this diet plan combines the best of the Mediterranean diet with the best of the Paleolithic diet, the latter of which has been detailed most recently by Dr. Loren Cordain in his book, The Paleo Diet, and his numerous scientific articles.[341] This diet places emphasis on fruits, vegetables, nuts, seeds, and berries that meet the body's needs for fiber, carbohydrates, and most importantly, the 8,000+ phytonutrients that have additive and synergistic health benefits.[342] Preferred protein sources are lean meats such as fish and poultry. In contrast to Cordain's Paleo diet, I also advocate soy and whey for their high-quality protein and anticancer, cardioprotective, and mood-enhancing benefits. Rice and potatoes are discouraged due to their relatively high glycemic indexes and high glycemic loads, and their lack of fiber and phytonutrients (compared to other fruits and vegetables). Generally speaking, grains such as wheat and rye are discouraged due to the high glycemic loads/indexes of most breads and pastries, as well as the allergenicity of gluten, a protein that appears to help trigger disorders such as migraine, celiac disease, psoriasis, epilepsy, and autoimmunity. Sources of simple sugars such as high-fructose corn syrup (e.g., cola, soda) and processed foods (e.g., "TV dinners" and other manufactured snacks and convenience foods) are strictly forbidden. Chemical preservatives, colorants, sweeteners and carrageenan are likewise prohibited. In summary, this diet plan provides plenty of variety, as most dishes comprised of poultry, fish, soy, fruits, vegetables, nuts, berries, and seeds are allowed. The diet also provides plenty of fiber, phytonutrients, carbohydrates, potassium, and protein, while simultaneously being low in fat, sodium, arachidonic acid, and "simple sugars." The diet must be customized with regard to total protein and calorie intake, as determined by the size, status, and activity level of the patient, and individual food allergens should be avoided. Regular consumption of this diet has shown the ability to reduce hypertension, alleviate diabetes, ameliorate migraine headaches, and result in improvement of overall health and a lessening of the severity of many common "diseases." This diet is supplemented with vitamins, minerals, and fatty acids as described below.

2. Multivitamin and multimineral supplementation: Vitamin and mineral supplementation finally received endorsement from "mainstream" medicine when researchers from Harvard Medical School published a review article in Journal of the American Medical Association that concluded, "Most people do not consume an optimal amount of all vitamins by diet alone. ...It appears prudent for all adults to take vitamin supplements."[343] Long-term nutritional insufficiencies experienced by "most people" promote the development of "long-latency deficiency diseases" such as cancer, neuroemotional deterioration, and cardiovascular disease.[344] Impressively, the benefits of multivitamin/multimineral supplementation have been demonstrated in numerous clinical trials. Multivitamin/multimineral supplementation has been shown to improve nutritional status and reduce the risk for chronic diseases[345]. improve mood[346], potentiate antidepressant drug treatment[347], alleviate migraine headaches (when used with diet improvement and fatty acids[348]), improve immune

[339] **Vasquez A.** *Integrative Orthopedics: The Art of Creating Wellness While Managing Acute and Chronic Musculoskeletal Disorders.* 2004, 2007

[340] **Vasquez A.** The Importance of Integrative Chiropractic Health Care in Treating Musculoskeletal Pain and Reducing the Nationwide Burden of Medical Expenses and Iatrogenic Injury and Death: A Concise Review of Current Research and Implications for Clinical Practice and Healthcare Policy. *The Original Internist* 2005; 12(4): 159-182

[341] Cordain L. *The Paleo Diet.* (John Wiley and Sons, 2002). Also: Cordain L. Cereal grains: humanity's double edged sword. *World Rev Nutr Diet* 1999;84:19-73 Access to most of Dr Cordain's articles is available at http://thepaleodiet.com/

[342] Liu RH. Health benefits of fruit and vegetables are from additive and synergistic combinations of phytochemicals. *Am J Clin Nutr* 2003;78(3 Suppl):517S-520S

[343] Fletcher RH, Fairfield KM. Vitamins for chronic disease prevention in adults: clinical applications. *JAMA* 2002;287:3127-9

[344] Heaney RP. Long-latency deficiency disease: insights from calcium and vitamin D. *Am J Clin Nutr* 2003;78:912-9

[345] McKay DL, Perrone G, Rasmussen H, Dallal G, Hartman W, Cao G, Prior RL, Roubenoff R, Blumberg JB. The effects of a multivitamin/mineral supplement on micronutrient status, antioxidant capacity and cytokine production in healthy older adults consuming a fortified diet. *J Am Coll Nutr* 2000;19(5):613-21

[346] Benton D, Haller J, Fordy J. Vitamin supplementation for 1 year improves mood. *Neuropsychobiology* 1995;32(2):98-105

[347] Coppen A, Bailey J. Enhancement of the antidepressant action of fluoxetine by folic acid: a randomised, placebo controlled trial. *J Affect Disord* 2000;60:121-30

function and infectious disease outcomes in the elderly[349] (especially diabetics[350]), reduce morbidity and mortality in patients with HIV infection[351,352] alleviate premenstrual syndrome[353,354] and bipolar disorder[355], reduce violence and antisocial behavior in children[356] and incarcerated young adults (when used with essential fatty acids[357]), and improve scores of intelligence in children.[358] Vitamin supplementation has anti-inflammatory benefits, as evidenced by significant reduction in C-reactive protein, (CRP) in a double-blind, placebo-controlled trial.[359] The ability to safely and affordably deliver these benefits makes multimineral-multivitamin supplementation and essential component of any and all health-promoting and disease-prevention strategies. Vitamin A can result in liver damage with chronic consumption of 25,000 IU or more, and intake should generally not exceed 10,000 IU per day in women of childbearing age. Iron should not be supplemented except in patients diagnosed with iron deficiency by a blood test (serum ferritin). Additional vitamin D should be used, as described in the next section.

3. Physiologic doses of vitamin D3: The prevalence of vitamin D deficiency varies from 40 percent (general population) to almost 100 percent (patients with musculoskeletal pain) in the American population. I described the many benefits of vitamin D3 supplementation in the previous issue of *Nutritional Wellness* and in the major monograph published last year.[360] In summary, vitamin D deficiency causes or contributes to depression, hypertension, seizures, migraine, polycystic ovary syndrome, inflammation, autoimmunity, and musculoskeletal pain such as low-back pain. Clinical trials using vitamin D supplementation have proven the cause-and-effect relationship between vitamin D deficiency and these conditions by showing that each of these could be cured or alleviated with vitamin D supplementation. In our review of the literature, we concluded that daily vitamin D doses should be 1,000 IU for infants, 2,000 IU for children, and 4,000 IU for adults. Cautions and contraindications include the use of thiazide diuretics (e.g., hydrochlorothiazide) or any other medications that can promote hypercalcemia, as well as granulomatous diseases such as sarcoidosis, tuberculosis, and certain types of cancer, especially lymphoma. Effectiveness is monitored by measuring serum 25-OH-vitamin D, and safety is monitored by measuring serum calcium.

4. Balanced and complete fatty acid supplementation: A detailed survey of the literature shows there are at least five health-promoting fatty acids commonly found in the human diet.[361] These are alpha-linolenic acid (ALA; omega-3, from flaxseed oil), eicosapentaenoic acid (EPA; omega-3, from fish oil), docosahexaenoic acid (DHA; omega-3, from fish oil and algae), gamma-linolenic acid (GLA; omega-6, most concentrated in borage oil), and oleic acid (omega-9, from olive oil, also flaxseed and borage oils). Each of these fatty acids has health benefits that cannot be fully attained from supplementing a different fatty acid. The benefits of GLA (borage oil) are not attained by consumption of EPA and DHA (fish oil); in fact, consumption of fish oil can actually promote a deficiency of GLA.[362] Likewise, consumption of GLA alone can reduce EPA levels while increasing levels of proinflammatory arachidonic acid; both of these problems are avoided with co-administration of fish oil any time borage oil is used. Using ALA (flaxseed oil) alone only slightly increases EPA but generally leads to no improvement in DHA status and can lead to a reduction of oleic acid; thus, fish oil, olive oil (and borage oil) should be supplemented when flaxseed oil is used.[363] Obviously, the goal here is a balanced intake of all of the health-promoting fatty acids; using only one or two sources of fatty acids is not balanced and results in suboptimal improvement, at best. In clinical practice, I routinely use combination fatty acid therapy comprised of ALA, EPA, DHA, and GLA for essentially all patients. The product also contains a modest amount of oleic acid, and I encourage use of olive oil for salads and cooking. This approach results in complete and balanced fatty acid intake, and the clinical benefits are impressive.

5. Probiotics /gut flora modification: Proper levels of good bacteria promote intestinal health, proper immune function, and support overall health. Excess bacteria or yeast, or the presence of harmful bacteria, yeast, or "parasites" such as amoebas and protozoas, can cause "leaky gut," systemic inflammation, and a wide range of clinical problems. Intestinal flora can become imbalanced by poor diets, excess stress, immunosuppressive drugs, antibiotics, or exposure to contaminated food or water, all of which are common among American patients. Thus, as a rule, I reinstate the good bacteria by the use of probiotics (good bacteria and yeast), prebiotics (fiber, arabinogalactan, and inulin), and the use of fermented foods such as kefir (in patients not allergic to milk). Harmful yeast, bacteria, and other "parasites" can be eradicated with the combination of dietary change, drugs, and/or herbal extracts. For example, oregano oil in an

[348] Wagner W, Nootbaar-Wagner U. Prophylactic treatment of migraine with gamma-linolenic and alpha-linolenic acids. *Cephalalgia* 1997;17:127-30

[349] Langkamp-Henken B, Bender BS, Gardner EM, Herrlinger-Garcia KA, Kelley MJ, Murasko DM, Schaller JP, Stechmiller JK, Thomas DJ, Wood SM. Nutritional formula enhanced immune function and reduced days of symptoms of upper respiratory tract infection in seniors. *J Am Geriatr Soc* 2004;52:3-12

[350] Barringer TA, Kirk JK, Santaniello AC, Foley KL, Michielutte R. Effect of a multivitamin and mineral supplement on infection and quality of life. A randomized, double-blind, placebo-controlled trial. *Ann Intern Med* 2003;138:365-71

[351] Fawzi WW, Msamanga GI, Spiegelman D, et al. A randomized trial of multivitamin supplements and HIV disease progression and mortality. *N Engl J Med* 2004;351:23-32

[352] Burbano X, Miguez-Burbano MJ, McCollister K, Zhang G, Rodriguez A, Ruiz P, Lecusay R, Shor-Posner G. Impact of a selenium chemoprevention clinical trial on hospital admissions of HIV-infected participants. *HIV Clin Trials* 2002;3:483-91

[353] Abraham GE. Nutritional factors in the etiology of the premenstrual tension syndromes. *J Reprod Med* 1983;28(7):446-64

[354] Stewart A. Clinical and biochemical effects of nutritional supplementation on the premenstrual syndrome. *J Reprod Med* 1987;32:435-41

[355] Kaplan BJ, Simpson JS, Ferre RC, Gorman CP, McMullen DM, Crawford SG. Effective mood stabilization with a chelated mineral supplement: an open-label trial in bipolar disorder. *J Clin Psychiatry* 2001;62:936-44

[356] Kaplan BJ, Crawford SG, Gardner B, Farrelly G. Treatment of mood lability and explosive rage with minerals and vitamins: two case studies in children. *J Child Adolesc Psychopharmacol* 2002;12(3):205-19

[357] Gesch CB, Hammond SM, Hampson SE, Eves A, Crowder MJ. Influence of supplementary vitamins, minerals and essential fatty acids on the antisocial behaviour of young adult prisoners. Randomised, placebo-controlled trial. *Br J Psychiatry* 2002;181:22-8

[358] Benton D. Micro-nutrient supplementation and the intelligence of children. *Neurosci Biobehav Rev* 2001;25:297-309

[359] Church TS, Earnest CP, Wood KA, Kampert JB. Reduction of C-reactive protein levels through use of a multivitamin. *Am J Med* 2003;115:702-7

[360] **Vasquez A**, Manso G, Cannell J. The clinical importance of vitamin D (cholecalciferol): a paradigm shift with implications for all healthcare providers. *Alternative Therapies in Health and Medicine* 2004;10:28-37 http://optimalhealthresearch.com/cholecalciferol.html

[361] **Vasquez A**. Reducing Pain and Inflammation Naturally. Part 2: New Insights into Fatty Acid Supplementation and Its Effect on Eicosanoid Production and Genetic Expression. *Nutritional Perspectives* 2005; January: 5-16 http://optimalhealthresearch.com/part2

[362] Cleland LG, Gibson RA, Neumann M, French JK. The effect of dietary fish oil supplement upon the content of dihomo-gammalinolenic acid in human plasma phospholipids. *Prostaglandins Leukot Essent Fatty Acids* 1990 May;40(1):9-12

[363] Jantti J, Nikkari T, Solakivi T, Vapaatalo H, Isomaki H. Evening primrose oil in rheumatoid arthritis: changes in serum lipids and fatty acids. *Ann Rheum Dis* 1989;48(2):124-7

emulsified, time-released form has proven safe and effective for the elimination of various parasites encountered in clinical practice.[364] Likewise, the herb *Artemisia annua* (sweet wormwood) commonly is used to eradicate specific bacteria and has been used for thousands of years in Asia for the treatment and prevention of infectious diseases, including malaria.[365]

Conclusion:

In this brief review, I have outlined and scientifically substantiated a fundamental protocol that can serve as effective therapy for patients with a wide range of "diseases." Customizing the Paleo-Mediterranean diet to avoid food allergens, using vitamin-mineral supplements along with physiologic doses of vitamin D and broad-spectrum balanced fatty acid supplementation, and ensuring gastrointestinal health with the skillful use of probiotics, prebiotics, and antimicrobial treatments provides an excellent health-promoting and disease-eliminating foundation and lifestyle for many patients. Often, this simple protocol is all that is needed for the effective treatment of a wide range of clinical problems. For other patients with more complex illnesses, of course, additional interventions and laboratory assessments can be used to customize the treatment plan. However, we must always remember that the attainment and preservation of health requires that we meet the body's basic nutritional needs. This five-step protocol begins the process of meeting those needs. In my next article, I'll give you some examples from my clinical practice and additional references to show how safe and effective this protocol can be.

Implementing the Five-Part Nutritional Wellness Protocol for the Treatment of Various Health Problems

Alex Vasquez, DC, ND

This article was originally published in *Nutritional Wellness*
http://www.nutritionalwellness.com/archives/2005/nov/11_vasquez.php

In my last article in *Nutritional Wellness* I described a 5-part nutritional protocol that can be used in the vast majority of patients without adverse effects and with major benefits. For many patients, the basic protocol consisting of 1) the Paleo-Mediterranean diet, 2) multivitamin/multimineral supplementation, 3) additional vitamin D3, 4) combination fatty acid therapy with an optimal balance of ALA, GLA, EPA, DHA, and oleic acid, and 5) probiotics (including the identification and eradication of harmful yeast, bacteria, and other "parasites") is all the treatment that they need. For patients who need additional treatment, this foundational plan still serves as the core of the biochemical aspect of their intervention. Of course, in some cases, we have to use other lifestyle modifications (such as exercise), additional supplements (such as policosanol or antimicrobial herbs), manual treatments (including spinal manipulation) and occasionally select medications (such has hormone modulators) to obtain our goal of maximum improvement.

The following examples show how the 5-part protocol serves to benefit patients with a wide range of conditions. For the sake of saving space, I will use only highly specific citations to the research literature, since I have provided the other references in the previous issue of *Nutritional Wellness* and elsewhere.[366]

- **A Man with High Cholesterol**: This patient is a 41-year-old slightly overweight man with very high cholesterol. His total cholesterol was 290 (normal < 200), LDL cholesterol was 212 (normal <130), and his triglycerides were 148 (optimal <100). I am quite certain that nearly every medical doctor would have put this man on cholesterol-lowering statin drugs for life. ***Treatment***: In contrast, I advised a low-carb Paleo-Mediterranean diet because such diets have been shown to reduce cardiovascular mortality more powerfully that "statin" cholesterol-lowing drugs in older patients.[367] Likewise, fatty acid supplementation is more effective than statin drugs for reducing cardiac and all-cause mortality.[368] We added probiotics, because supplementation with *Lactobacillus* and *Bifidobacterium* has been shown to lower cholesterol levels in humans with high cholesterol.[369] Finally, I also prescribed 20 mg of policosanol for its well-known ability to favorably modify cholesterol levels.[370] ***Results***: Within ***one month*** the patient had lost weight, felt better, and his total cholesterol had dropped to normal at 196 (from 290!), LDL was reduced to 141, and triglycerides were reduced to 80. Basically, this treatment plan was "the protocol + policosanol." Drug treatment of this patient would have been more expensive, more risky, and would not have resulted in global health improvements.
- **A Child with Intractable Seizures**: This is a 4-year-old nonverbal boy with 3-5 seizures per day despite being on two anti-seizure medications and having previously had several other "last resort" medical and surgical procedures. He also had a history of food allergies. ***Treatment***: Obviously, there was no room for error in this case. We implemented a moderately low-carb hypoallergenic diet since both carbohydrate restriction[371] and allergy avoidance[372] can reduce the frequency and

---

[364] Force M, Sparks WS, Ronzio RA. Inhibition of enteric parasites by emulsified oil of oregano in vivo. *Phytother Res* 2000;14:213-4
[365] Schuster BG. Demonstrating the validity of natural products as anti-infective drugs. *J Altern Complement Med* 2001;7 Suppl 1:S73-82
[366] **Vasquez A.** Integrative Orthopedics. www.OptimalHealthResearch.com and Chiropractic and Naturopathic Medicine for the Promotion of Optimal Health and Alleviation of Pain and Inflammation. http://optimalhealthresearch.com/monograph05
[367] Knoops KT, et al. Mediterranean diet, lifestyle factors, and 10-year mortality in elderly European men and women: the HALE project. *JAMA.* 2004 Sep 22;292(12):1433-9
[368] Studer M, et al. Effect of different antilipidemic agents and diets on mortality: a systematic review. *Arch Intern Med.* 2005;165:725-30
[369] Xiao JZ, et al. Effects of milk products fermented by Bifidobacterium longum on blood lipids in rats and healthy adult male volunteers.*J Dairy Sci.* 2003;86:2452-61
[370] Cholesterol-lowering action of policosanol compares well to that of pravastatin and lovastatin. *Cardiovasc J S Afr.* 2003;14(3):161
[371] Freeman JM, et al. The efficacy of the ketogenic diet-1998: a prospective evaluation of intervention in 150 children. *Pediatrics.* 1998;102:1358-63
[372] Egger J, Carter CM, Soothill JF, Wilson J. Oligoantigenic diet treatment of children with epilepsy and migraine. *J Pediatr.* 1989;114:51-8

severity of seizures. Since many "anti-seizure" medications actually cause seizures by causing vitamin D deficiency[373], I added 800 IU per day of emulsified vitamin D3 for its antiseizure benefit.[374] We used 1 tsp per day of a combination fatty acid supplement that provides balanced amounts of ALA, GLA, EPA, and DHA, since fatty acids appear to have potential antiseizure benefits.[375] Vitamin B-6 (250 mg of P5P) and magnesium (bowel tolerance) were also added to reduce brain hyperexcitability.[376] Stool testing showed an absence of *Bifidobacteria* and *Lactobacillus*; probiotics were added for their anti-allergy benefits.[377] *Results*: Within about 2 months seizure frequency reduced from 3-5 per day to one seizure every other day: *an 87% reduction in seizure frequency*. Patient was able to discontinue one of the anti-seizure medications. His parents also noted several global improvements: the boy started making eye contact with people, he was learning again, and intellectually he was "making gains every day." His parents considered this an "amazing difference." Going from 30 seizures per week to 4 seizures per week while reducing medication use by 50% is a major achievement. Notice that we simply used the basic wellness protocol with some additional B6 and magnesium. It is highly unlikely that B6 and magnesium alone would have produced such a favorable response.

- **A Young Woman with Full-Body Psoriasis Unresponsive to Drug Treatment**: This is a 17-year-old woman with head-to-toe psoriasis since childhood. She wears long pants and long-sleeved shirts year-round, and the psoriasis is a major interference to her social life. Medications have ceased to help. *Treatment*: The Paleo-Mediterranean diet was implemented with an emphasis on food allergy identification.[1] We used a multivitamin-mineral supplement with 200 mcg selenium to compensate for the nutritional insufficiencies and selenium deficiency that are common in patients with psoriasis; likewise 10 mg of folic acid was added to address the relative vitamin deficiencies and elevated homocysteine that are common in these patients.[378] Combination fatty acid therapy with EPA and DHA from fish oil and GLA from borage oil was used for the anti-inflammatory and skin-healing benefits.[379] Vitamin E (1200 IU of mixed tocopherols) and lipoic acid (1,000 mg per day) were added for their anti-inflammatory benefits and to combat the oxidative stress that is characteristic of psoriasis.[380] Of course, probiotics were used to modify gut flora, which is commonly deranged in patients with psoriasis.[381] *Results*: Within a few weeks, this patient's "lifelong psoriasis" was essentially gone. Food allergy identification and avoidance played a major role in the success of this case. When I saw the patient again 9 months later for her second visit, she had no visible evidence of psoriasis. Her "medically untreatable" condition was essentially cured by the use of my basic protocol, with the addition of a few extra nutrients.

- **A Man with Fatigue and Recurrent Numbness in Hands and Feet**. This 40-year-old man had seen numerous neurologists and had spent tens of thousands of dollars on MRIs, CT scans, lumbar punctures, and other diagnostic procedures. No diagnosis had been found, and no effective treatment had been rendered by medical specialists. *Assessments*: We performed a modest battery of lab tests which revealed elevations of fibrinogen and C-reactive protein (CRP), two markers of acute inflammation. Assessment of intestinal permeability with the lactulose-mannitol assay showed major intestinal damage ("leaky gut"). Follow-up parasite testing on different occasions showed dysbiosis caused by *Proteus, Enterobacter, Klebsiella, Citrobacter,* and *Pseudomonas aeruginosa*—of course, these are gram-negative bacteria that can induce immune dysfunction and autoimmunity, as described elsewhere.[1] Specifically, *Pseudomonas aeruginosa* has been linked to the development of nervous system autoimmunity, such as multiple sclerosis.[382] *Treatment*: We implemented a plan of diet modification, vitamins, minerals, fatty acids, and probiotics. The dysbiosis was further addressed with specific antimicrobial herbs (including caprylic acid and emulsified oregano oil[383]) and drugs (such as tetracycline, Bactrim, and augmentin). The antibiotic drugs proved to be ineffective based on repeat stool testing. *Results*: Within one month we witnessed impressive improvements, both subjectively and objectively. Subjectively, the patient reported that the numbness and tingling almost completely resolved. Fatigue was reduced, and energy was improved. Objectively, the patient's elevated CRP plummeted from abnormally high at 11 down to completely normal at 1. Eighteen months later, the patient's CRP had dropped to less than 1 and fatigue and numbness were no longer problematic. Notice that this treatment plan was basically "the protocol" with additional attention to eradicating the dysbiosis we found with specialized stool testing.

- **A 50-year-old Man with Rheumatoid Arthritis**. This patient presented with a 3-year history of rheumatoid arthritis that had been treated unsuccessfully with drugs (methotrexate and intravenous Remicade). The first time I tested his hsCRP level, it was astronomically high at 124 (normal is <3). Because of the severe inflammation and other risk factors for sudden cardiac death, I referred this patient to an osteopathic internist for immune-suppressing drugs; the patient refused, stating that he was no longer willing to rely on immune-suppressing chemical medications. His treatment was entirely up to me. *Assessments and Treatments*: We implemented the Paleo-Mediterranean diet and a program of vitamins, minerals, optimal combination fatty acid therapy (providing ALA, GLA, EPA, DHA, and oleic acid), and 4000 IU of vitamin D in emulsified form to overcome defects in absorption that are seen in older patients and those with gastrointestinal problems.[384] Hormone testing showed abnormally low DHEA, low testosterone, and slightly elevated estrogen; these problems were corrected with DHEA supplementation and the use of a hormone-modulating drug (Arimidex) that lowers

[373] Ali FE, Al-Bustan MA, Al-Busairi WA, Al-Mulla FA. Loss of seizure control due to anticonvulsant-induced hypocalcemia. *Ann Pharmacother*. 2004;38:1002-5

[374] Christiansen C, Rodbro P, Sjo O."Anticonvulsant action" of vitamin D in epileptic patients? A controlled pilot study. *Br Med J*. 1974 May 4;2(913):258-9

[375] Yuen AW, et al. Omega-3 fatty acid supplementation in patients with chronic epilepsy: A randomized trial. *Epilepsy Behav*. 2005 Sep;7(2):253-8

[376] Mousain-Bosc M, et al. Magnesium VitB6 intake reduces central nervous system hyperexcitability in children. *J Am Coll Nutr*. 2004;23(5):545S-548S

[377] Majamaa H, Isolauri E.Probiotics: a novel approach in the management of food allergy. *J Allergy Clin Immunol*. 1997 Feb;99(2):179-85

[378] Vanizor Kural B, et al. Plasma homocysteine and its relationships with atherothrombotic markers in psoriatic patients. *Clin Chim Acta*. 2003 Jun;332(1-2):23-3

[379] **Vasquez A**. Reducing Pain and Inflammation Naturally. Part 2: New Insights into Fatty Acid Supplementation and Its Effect on Eicosanoid Production and Genetic Expression. *Nutritional Perspectives* 2005; January: 5-16 www.OptimalHealthResearch.com/part2

[380] Kokcam I, Naziroglu M. Antioxidants and lipid peroxidation status in the blood of patients with psoriasis. *Clin Chim Acta*. 1999 Nov;289(1-2):23-31

[381] Waldman A, et al. Incidence of Candida in psoriasis--a study on the fungal flora of psoriatic patients. *Mycoses*. 2001 May;44(3-4):77-81

[382] Hughes LE, et al. Antibody responses to Acinetobacter spp. and Pseudomonas aeruginosa in multiple sclerosis: prospects for diagnosis using the myelin-acinetobacter-neurofilament antibody index. *Clin Diagn Lab Immunol*. 2001;8(6):1181-8

[383] Force M, Sparks WS, Ronzio RA. Inhibition of enteric parasites by emulsified oil of oregano in vivo. *Phytother Res*. 2000 May;14(3):213-4

[384] **Vasquez A**. Subphysiologic Doses of Vitamin D are Subtherapeutic: Comment on the Study by The Record Trial Group. TheLancet.com Accessed June 16, 2005

estrogen and raises testosterone. Specialized stool testing showed absence of *Lactobacillus* and *Bifidobacteria* and intestinal overgrowth of *Citrobacter* and *Enterobacter* which was corrected with probiotics and antimicrobial treatments including undecylenic acid and emulsified oregano oil. Importantly, I also decided to inhibit NF-kappaB (the primary transcription factor that upregulates the pro-inflammatory response[385]) by using a combination botanical formula that contains curcumin, piperine, lipoic acid, green tea extract, propolis, rosemary, resveratrol, ginger, and phytolens (an antioxidant extract from lentils that may inhibit autoimmunity[386])—all of these herbs and nutrients have been shown to inhibit NF-kappaB and to thus downregulate inflammatory responses.[387] **Results**: Within 6 weeks, this patient had happily lost 10 lbs of excess weight and was able to work without pain for the first time in years. Follow-up testing showed that his previously astronomical hsCRP had dropped from 124 to 7—a drop of 114 points in less than one month: better than had ever been achieved even with the use of intravenous immune-suppressing drugs! This patient continues to make significant progress. Obviously this case was complex, and we needed to do more than the basic protocol. Nonetheless, the basic protocol still served as the foundation for the treatment plan. Note that vitamin D has significant anti-inflammatory benefits and can cause major reductions in inflammation measured by CRP.[388] The correction of the hormonal abnormalities and the dysbiosis, and downregulating NF-kappaB with several botanical extracts were also critical components of this successful treatment plan.[1]

Summary and Conclusions

These examples show how the nutritional wellness protocol that I described in the September issue of *Nutritional Wellness* can be used as the foundational treatment for a wide range of health problems. In many cases, implementation of the basic protocol is all that is needed. In more complex situations, we use the basic protocol and then add more specific treatments to address dysbiosis and hormonal problems, and we can add additional nutrients as needed. However, there will never be a substitute for a healthy diet, sufficiencies of vitamin D and all five of the health-promoting fatty acids (i.e., ALA, GLA, EPA, DHA, and oleic acid), and normalization of gastrointestinal flora. Without these basics, survival and the appearance of health are possible, but true health and recovery from "untreatable" illnesses is not possible. In order to attain optimal health, we have to create the conditions that allow for health to be attained[1,] and we start this process by supplying the body with the nutrients that it needs to function optimally. In the words of naturopathic physician Jared Zeff from the *Journal of Naturopathic Medicine*, "*The work of the naturopathic physician is to elicit healing by helping patients to create or recreate the conditions for health to exist within them. Health will occur where the conditions for health exist. Disease is the product of the conditions which allow for it.*"[389] Although the chiropractic profession has emphasized spinal manipulation as its primary therapeutic tool, the profession has always appreciated holistic, integrative models of therapeutic intervention, health and disease.

Chiropractic was the first healthcare profession in America to specifically claim that the optimization of health requires attention to the spiritual (emotional, psychological), mechanical (physical, structural), and chemical (nutritional, hormonal) aspects of our lives.[1] Chiropractic's founder DD Palmer[390] wrote, "The human body represents the actions of three laws—spiritual, mechanical, and chemical—united as one triune. As long as there is perfect union of these three, there is health." Accordingly, these cornerstones are fundamental to the modern definition of the chiropractic profession recently articulated by the American Chiropractic Association[391]: "*Doctors of Chiropractic are physicians who consider man as an integrated being and give special attention to the physiological and biochemical aspects including structural, spinal, musculoskeletal, neurological, vascular, nutritional, emotional and environmental relationships.*" The cases that I have described in this article demonstrate the importance of attending to the nutritional, hormonal, environmental and gastrointestinal aspects of human physiology for helping our patients attain optimal health.

Common Oversights and Shortcomings in the Study and Implementation of Nutritional Supplementation

Alex Vasquez, D.C., N.D.

This article was originally published in *Naturopathy Digest*
http://www.naturopathydigest.com/archives/2007/jun/vasquez.php

Introduction

An impressive discrepancy often exists between the low efficacy of nutritional interventions reported in the research literature and the higher efficacy achieved in the clinical practices of clinicians trained in the use of interventional nutrition (i.e., chiropractic and naturopathic physicians). This discrepancy is dangerous for at least two reasons. First, it results in an undervaluation of the efficacy of nutritional supplementation, which ultimately leaves otherwise treatable patients untreated. Second, such untreated and undertreated patients are often then forced to use dangerous and expensive pharmaceutical drugs and surgical interventions to treat conditions that could have otherwise been easily and safely treated with nutritional

[385] Tak PP, Firestein GS. NF-kappaB: a key role in inflammatory diseases. *J Clin Invest*. 2001 Jan;107(1):7-11

[386] Sandoval M, et al. Peroxynitrite-induced apoptosis in epithelial (T84) and macrophage (RAW 264.7) cell lines: effect of legume-derived polyphenols (phytolens). *Nitric Oxide*. 1997;1(6):476-83

[387] **Vasquez A**. Reducing pain and inflammation naturally - Part 4: Nutritional and Botanical Inhibition of NF-kappaB, the Major Intracellular Amplifier of the Inflammatory Cascade. A Practical Clinical Strategy Exemplifying Anti-Inflammatory Nutrigenomics. *Nutritional Perspectives* 2005;July: 5-12 www.OptimalHealthResearch.com/part4

[388] Timms PM, et al. Circulating MMP9, vitamin D and variation in the TIMP-1 response with VDR genotype. *QJM*. 2002 Dec;95(12):787-96

[389] Zeff JL. The process of healing: a unifying theory of naturopathic medicine. *Journal of Naturopathic Medicine* 1997; 7: 122-5

[390] Palmer DD. *The Science, Art, and Phiosophy, of Chiropractic*. Portland, OR; Portland Printing House Company, 1910: 107

[391] American Chiropractic Association. What is Chiropractic? http://amerchiro.org/media/whatis/ Accessed January 9, 2005

supplementation and diet modification. Consequently, the burden of suffering, disease, and healthcare expense in the US is higher than it would be if nutritionally-trained clinicians were more fully integrated into the healthcare system.

Obstacles to Efficacy in the Use of Nutritional Supplementation

Below are listed some of the most common causes for the underachievement of nutritional supplementation in practice and in published research. While this list is not all-inclusive, it will serve as a review for clinicians and an introduction for chiropractic/naturopathic students. In both practice and research, the problems listed below often overlap and function synergistically to reduce the efficacy of nutritional supplementation.

1. **Inadequate dosing (quantity)**: Many clinical trials published in major journals and many doctors in clinical practice have used inadequate doses of vitamins (and other natural therapeutics) and have thus failed to achieve the results that would have easily been obtained had they implemented their protocol with the proper physiologic or supraphysiologic dose of intervention. The best example in my experience centers on vitamin D, where so many of the studies are performed with doses of 400-800 IU per day only to conclude that vitamin supplementation is ineffective for the condition being treated. The problem here is that the researchers failed to appreciate that the physiologic requirement for vitamin D3 in adults is approximately 3,000-5,000 IU per day[392] and that therefore their supplemental dose of 400-800 IU is only 10-20% of what is required. Subphysiologic doses are generally subtherapeutic. In this regard, I have had to correct journals such as *The Lancet*[393], *JAMA*[394], and *British Medical Journal*[395] from misleading their readers (many of whom are major policymakers) from concluding that nutritional supplementation is impotent; rather, their researchers and editors were not sufficiently educated in the design and review of studies using nutritional interventions. These journals should hire chiropractic and naturopathic physicians so that they have staff trained in natural treatments and who can thus provide an educated review of studies on these topics.[396]

2. **Inadequate dosing (duration)**: Often the effects of long-term nutritional deficiency are not fully reversible and/or may require a treatment period of months or years to achieve maximal clinical response. For example, full replacement of fatty acids in human brain phospholipids is an ongoing process that occurs over a period of several years; thus studies using fatty acid supplements for a period of weeks or 2-3 months generally underestimate the enhanced effectiveness that can be obtained with administration over many months or several years of treatment. Relatedly, recovery from vitamin D deficiency takes several weeks of high-dose supplementation in order to achieve tissue saturation and subsequent cellular replenishment; studies of short duration are destined to underestimate the results that could have been achieved with supplementation carried out over several months.[397]

3. **Failure to use proper forms of nutrients**: Nutrients are often available in different forms, not the least of which are "active" versus "inactive" and "natural" versus "unnatural." Most vitamin supplements, particularly high-potency B vitamins, are manufactured synthetically and are not from "natural sources" despite the marketing hype promulgated by companies that, for example, mix their synthetic vitamins with a vegetable powder and then call their vitamin supplements "natural." The simple fact is that production of high-potency supplements from purely natural sources would be prohibitively wasteful, inefficient, and expensive. Thus, while it is not necessary for vitamins to be "natural" in order to be useful, it is necessary that the vitamins are useable and preferably not "unnatural." The best example of the use of unnatural supplements is the use of synthetic DL-tocopherol in the so-called "vitamin E" studies; DL-tocopherol is by definition 50% comprised of the L-isomer of tocopherol which is not only unusable by the human body but is actually harmful in that it interferes with normal metabolism and can exacerbate hypertension and cause symptomatic complications (e.g., headaches). Further, tocopherols exist within the body in relationship with the individual forms of the vitamin, such that supplementation with one form (e.g., alpha-tocopherol) can result in a relative deficiency of another form (e.g., gamma-tocopherol). One final example of the failure to use proper forms of nutrients is in the use of pyridoxine HCl as a form of vitamin B6; while this practice itself is not harmful, clinicians need to remember that pyridoxine HCl is ineffective until converted to the more active forms of the vitamin including pyridoxal-5-phosphate. Since this conversion requires co-nutrients such as magnesium and zinc, we can easily see that the reputed failure of B6 supplementation when administered in the form of pyridoxine HCl might actually be due to untreated insufficiencies of required co-nutrients, as discussed in the following section.

4. **Failure to ensure adequacy of co-nutrients**: Vitamins, minerals, amino acids, and fatty acids work together in an intricately choreographed and delicately orchestrated dance that culminates in the successful completion of interconnected physiologic functions. If any of the performers in this event are missing (i.e., nutritional deficiency) or if successive interconversions are impaired due to lack of enzyme function, then the show cannot go on, or—if it does go on—impaired metabolism and defective function will result. So, if we take a patient with "vitamin B6 deficiency" and give him vitamin B6 in the absence of other co-nutrients needed for the proper activation and metabolic utilization of vitamin B6, we cannot honestly expect the "nutritional supplementation" to work in this case; rather, we might see a marginal benefit or perhaps even a negative outcome as an imbalanced system is pushed into a different state of imbalance despite supplementation with the "correct" vitamin. In the case of vitamin B6, necessary co-nutrients include zinc, magnesium, and riboflavin; deficiency of any of these will result in a relative "failure" of B6 supplementation even if a

[392] Heaney RP, Davies KM, Chen TC, Holick MF, Barger-Lux MJ. Human serum 25-hydroxycholecalciferol response to extended oral dosing with cholecalciferol. *Am J Clin Nutr.* 2003 Jan;77(1):204-10 http://www.ajcn.org/cgi/content/full/77/1/204

[393] **Vasquez A**. Subphysiologic Doses of Vitamin D are Subtherapeutic: Comment on the Study by The Record Trial Group. *The Lancet* 2005 Published on-line May 6 http://OptimalHealthResearch.com/lancet

[394] Muanza DN, **Vasquez A**, Cannell J, Grant WB. Isoflavones and Postmenopausal Women. [letter] *JAMA* 2004; 292: 2337

[395] **Vasquez A**, Cannell J. Calcium and vitamin D in preventing fractures: data are not sufficient to show inefficacy. [letter] *BMJ: British Medical Journal* 2005;331:108-9 http://www.optimalhealthresearch.com/reprints/vasquez-cannell-bmj-reprint.pdf

[396] **Vasquez A**. Allopathic Usurpation of Natural Medicine: The Blind Leading the Sighted. *Naturopathy Digest* 2006 February http://www.naturopathydigest.com/archives/2006/feb/vasquez.php

[397] **Vasquez A**, Manso G, Cannell J. The clinical importance of vitamin D (cholecalciferol): a paradigm shift with implications for all healthcare providers. *Altern Ther Health Med.* 2004 Sep-Oct;10(5):28-36 http://optimalhealthresearch.com/monograph04

patient has a B6-responsive condition. Notably, overt magnesium deficiency is alarmingly common among patients and citizens in industrialized nations[398,399,400], and this epidemic of magnesium deficiency is due not only to insufficient intake but also to excessive excretion caused by consumption of high-glycemic foods, caffeine, and a diet that promotes chronic metabolic acidosis with resultant urinary acidification.

5. **Failure to achieve urinary alkalinization**: Western/American-style diets typified by overconsumption of grains, dairy, sugar, and salt result in a state of subclinical chronic metabolic acidosis which results in urinary acidification, relative hypercortisolemia, and consequent hyperexcretion of minerals such as calcium and magnesium.[401 402] Thus, the common conundrum of magnesium replenishment requires not only magnesium supplementation but also dietary interventions to change the internal climate to one that is conducive to bodily retention and cellular uptake of magnesium.[403]

6. **Use of mislabeled supplements**: Even in the professional arena of nutritional supplement manufacturers, some companies habitually underdose their products either in an attempt to spend less in the manufacture of their products or as a consequence of poor quality control. If a product is labeled to contain 1,000 IU of vitamin D but only contains 836 IU of the nutrient, then obviously full clinical efficacy will not be achieved; this was a problem in a recent clinical trial involving vitamin D.[404] The problem for clinicians is in trusting the companies that supply nutritional supplements; some companies do "in house" testing which lacks independent review, while other companies use questionable "independent testing" which is not infrequently performed by a laboratory that is a wholly owned subsidiary of the parent nutritional company. Manufacturing regulations that are sweeping through the industry will cleanse the nutritional supplement world of poorly made products, and these same regulations will sweep some unprepared companies right out the door when they are unable to meet the regulatory requirements.

7. **Assurance of bioavailability and optimal serum/cellular levels**: Clinical trials with nutritional therapies need to monitor serum or cellular levels to ensure absorption, product bioavailability, and the attainment of optimal serum levels. This is particularly relevant in the treatment of chronic disorders such as the autoimmune diseases, wherein so many of these patients have gastrointestinal dysbiosis and often have concomitant nutrient malabsorption.[405] Simply dosing these patients with supplements is not always efficacious; often the gut must be cleared of dysbiosis so that the mucosal lining can be repaired and optimal nutrient absorption can be reestablished.

8. **Coadministration of food with nutritional supplements (sometimes right, sometimes wrong)**: Food can help or hinder the absorption of nutritional supplements. Some supplements, like coenzyme Q10, should be administered with fatty food to enhance absorption. Other supplements, like amino acids, should be administered away from protein-rich foods and are often better administered with simple carbohydrate to enhance cellular uptake; this is especially true with tryptophan.

9. **Correction of gross dietary imbalances enhances supplement effectiveness**: If the diet is grossly imbalanced, then nutritional supplementation is less likely to be effective. The best example of this is in the use of fatty acid supplements, particularly in the treatment of inflammatory disorders. If the diet is laden with dairy, beef, and other sources of arachidonate, then fatty acid supplementation with EPA, DHA, and GLA is much less likely to be effective, or much higher doses of the supplements will need to be used in order to help restore fatty acid balance. Generally speaking, the diet needs to be optimized to enhance the efficacy of nutritional supplementation.

Conclusion

In this brief review, I have listed and discussed some of the most common impediments to the success of nutritional supplementation. I hope that chiropractic and naturopathic students, clinicians, and researchers will find these points helpful in their design of clinical treatment protocols.

---

[398] "Altogether 43% of 113 trauma patients had low magnesium levels compared to 30% of noninjured cohorts." Frankel H, Haskell R, Lee SY, Miller D, Rotondo M, Schwab CW. Hypomagnesemia in trauma patients. *World J Surg*. 1999 Sep;23(9):966-9

[399] "There was a 20% overall prevalence of hypomagnesemia among this predominantly female, African American population." Fox CH, Ramsoomair D, Mahoney MC, Carter C, Young B, Graham R. An investigation of hypomagnesemia among ambulatory urban African Americans. *J Fam Pract*. 1999 Aug;48(8):636-9

[400] "Suboptimal levels were detected in 33.7 per cent of the population under study. These data clearly demonstrate that the Mg supply of the German population needs increased attention." Schimatschek HF, Rempis R. Prevalence of hypomagnesemia in an unselected German population of 16,000 individuals. *Magnes Res*. 2001 Dec;14(4):283-90

[401] Cordain L, Eaton SB, Sebastian A, Mann N, Lindeberg S, Watkins BA, O'Keefe JH, Brand-Miller J. Origins and evolution of the Western diet: health implications for the 21st century. *Am J Clin Nutr*. 2005 Feb;81(2):341-54

[402] Maurer M, Riesen W, Muser J, Hulter HN, Krapf R. Neutralization of Western diet inhibits bone resorption independently of K intake and reduces cortisol secretion in humans. *Am J Physiol Renal Physiol*. 2003 Jan;284(1):F32-40

[403] Vormann J, Worlitschek M, Goedecke T, Silver B. Supplementation with alkaline minerals reduces symptoms in patients with chronic low back pain. *J Trace Elem Med Biol*. 2001;15(2-3):179-83

[404] Heaney RP, Davies KM, Chen TC, Holick MF, Barger-Lux MJ. Human serum 25-hydroxycholecalciferol response to extended oral dosing with cholecalciferol. *Am J Clin Nutr*. 2003 Jan;77(1):204-10 http://www.ajcn.org/cgi/content/full/77/1/204

[405] **Vasquez A**. Reducing Pain and Inflammation Naturally. Part 6: Nutritional and Botanical Treatments Against "Silent Infections" and Gastrointestinal Dysbiosis, Commonly Overlooked Causes of Neuromusculoskeletal Inflammation and Chronic Health Problems. *Nutritional Perspectives* 2006; January http://www.optimalhealthresearch.com/part6

Revisiting the Five-Part Nutritional Wellness Protocol: The Supplemented Paleo-Mediterranean Diet

Alex Vasquez, DC, ND, DO

This article was originally published in the January 2011 issue of the American Chiropractic Association's Council on Nutrition's journal *Nutritional Perspectives*

Abstract: This article reviews the five-part nutritional protocol that incorporates a health-promoting nutrient-dense diet and essential supplementation with vitamins/minerals, specific fatty acids, probiotics, and physiologic doses of vitamin D3. This foundational nutritional protocol has proven benefits for disease treatment, disease prevention, and health maintenance and restoration. Additional treatments such as botanical medicines, additional nutritional supplements, and pharmaceutical drugs can be used atop this foundational protocol to further optimize clinical effectiveness. The rationale for this five-part protocol is presented, and consideration is given to adding iodine-iodide as the sixth component of the protocol.

<u>Introduction</u>: In 2004 and 2005 I first published a "five-part nutrition protocol"[406,407] that provides the foundational treatment plan for a wide range of health disorders. This protocol served and continues to serve as the foundation upon which other treatments are commonly added, and without which those other treatments are likely to fail, or attain suboptimal results at best.[408] Now as then, I will share with you what I consider a basic foundational protocol for wellness promotion and disease treatment. I have used this protocol in my own self-care for many years and have used it in the treatment of a wide range of health-disease conditions in clinical practice.

<u>Review</u>: This nutritional protocol is validated by biochemistry, physiology, experimental research, peer-reviewed human trials, and the clinical application of common sense. It is the most nutrient-dense diet available, satisfying nutritional needs and thereby optimizing metabolic processes while promoting satiety and weight loss/optimization. Nutrients are required in the proper amounts, forms, and approximate ratios for critical and innumerable physiologic functions; if nutrients are lacking, the body cannot function *normally*, let alone *optimally*. Impaired function results in subjective and objective manifestations of what is eventually labeled as "disease." Thus, a powerful and effective alternative to treating diseases with drugs is to re-establish normal/optimal physiologic function by replenishing the body with essential nutrients, reestablishing hormonal balance ("orthoendocrinology"), promoting detoxification of environmental toxins, and by reestablishing the optimal microbial milieu, especially the eradication of (multifocal) dysbiosis; this multifaceted approach can be applied to several diseases, especially those of the inflammatory and autoimmune varieties.[409]

Of course, most diseases are multifactorial and therefore require multicomponent treatment plans, and some diseases actually require the use of drugs in conjunction with assertive interventional nutrition. However, while only a smaller portion of patients actually need drugs for the long-term management of their problems, all clinicians should agree that everyone needs a foundational nutrition plan because nutrients—not drugs—are universally required for life and health. This five-part nutrition protocol is briefly outlined below; a much more detailed substantiation of the underlying science and clinical application of this protocol was recently published in a review of more than 650 pages and approximately 3,500 citations.[410]

1. <u>Health-promoting Paleo-Mediterranean diet</u>: Following an extensive review of the research literature, I developed what I call the "supplemented Paleo-Mediterranean diet." In essence, this diet plan combines the best of the Mediterranean diet with the best of the Paleolithic diet, the latter of which has been best distilled by Dr. Loren Cordain in his book "The Paleo Diet"[411] and his numerous scientific articles.[412,413,414] The Paleolithic diet is superior to the Mediterranean diet in nutrient density for promoting satiety, weight loss, and improvements/normalization in overall metabolic function.[415,416] This diet places emphasis on fruits, vegetables, nuts, seeds, and berries that meet the body's needs for fiber, carbohydrates, and

---

[406] **Vasquez A**. *Integrative Orthopedics: The Art of Creating Wellness While Managing Acute and Chronic Musculoskeletal Disorders*. 2004, 2007

[407] Vasquez A. A Five-Part Nutritional Protocol that Produces Consistently Positive Results. *Nutritional Wellness* 2005 September Available in the printed version and on-line at http://www.nutritionalwellness.com/archives/2005/sep/09_vasquez.php

[408] **Vasquez A**. Common Oversights and Shortcomings in the Study and Implementation of Nutritional Supplementation. *Naturopathy Digest* 2007 June. http://www.naturopathydigest.com/archives/2007/jun/vasquez.php

[409] **Vasquez A**. Integrative Rheumatology. IBMRC: 2006, 2009. http://optimalhealthresearch.com/rheumatology.html

[410] **Vasquez A**. Chiropractic and Naturopathic Mastery of Common Clinical Disorders. IBMRC: 2009. http://optimalhealthresearch.com/clinical_mastery.html

[411] Cordain L. *The Paleo Diet*. John Wiley and Sons, 2002

[412] O'Keefe JH Jr, Cordain L. Cardiovascular disease resulting from a diet and lifestyle at odds with our Paleolithic genome: how to become a 21st-century hunter-gatherer. *Mayo Clin Proc*. 2004 Jan;79(1):101-8

[413] Cordain L. Cereal grains: humanity's double edged sword. *World Rev Nutr Diet* 1999;84:19-73

[414] Cordain L, Eaton SB, Sebastian A, Mann N, Lindeberg S, Watkins BA, O'Keefe JH, Brand-Miller J. Origins and evolution of the Western diet: health implications for the 21st century. *Am J Clin Nutr*. 2005 Feb;81(2):341-54

[415] "A high micronutrient density diet mitigates the unpleasant aspects of the experience of hunger even though it is lower in calories. Hunger is one of the major impediments to successful weight loss. Our findings suggest that it is not simply the caloric content, but more importantly, the micronutrient density of a diet that influences the experience of hunger. It appears that a high nutrient density diet, after an initial phase of adjustment during which a person experiences "toxic hunger" due to withdrawal from pro-inflammatory foods, can result in a sustainable eating pattern that leads to weight loss and improved health." Fuhrman J, Sarter B, Glaser D, Acocella S. Changing perceptions of hunger on a high nutrient density diet. *Nutr J*. 2010 Nov 7;9:51 http://www.nutritionj.com/content/9/1/51

[416] "The Paleolithic group were as satiated as the Mediterranean group but consumed less energy per day (5.8 MJ/day vs. 7.6 MJ/day, Paleolithic vs. Mediterranean, p=0.04). Consequently, the quotients of mean change in satiety during meal and mean consumed energy from food and drink were higher in the Paleolithic group (p=0.03). Also, there was a strong trend for greater Satiety Quotient for energy in the Paleolithic group (p=0.057). Leptin decreased by 31% in the Paleolithic group and by 18% in the Mediterranean group with a trend for greater relative decrease of leptin in the Paleolithic group." Jonsson T, Granfeldt Y, Erlanson-Albertsson C, Ahren B, Lindeberg S. A Paleolithic diet is more satiating per calorie than a Mediterranean-like diet in individuals with ischemic heart disease. *Nutr Metab* (Lond). 2010 Nov 30;7(1):85.

most importantly, the 8,000+ phytonutrients that have additive and synergistic health effects[417]—including immunomodulating, antioxidant, anti-inflammatory, and anti-cancer benefits. High-quality protein sources such as fish, poultry, eggs, and grass-fed meats are emphasized. Slightly modifying Cordain's paleo diet, I also advocate soy and whey protein isolates for their high-quality protein and their anticancer, cardioprotective, and mood-enhancing (due to the high tryptophan content) benefits. Potatoes and other starchy vegetables, wheat and other grains including rice are discouraged due to their high glycemic indexes and high glycemic loads, and their relative insufficiency of fiber and phytonutrients compared to fruits and vegetables. Grains such as wheat, barley, and rye are discouraged due to the high glycemic loads/indexes of most breads, pastries, and other grain-derived products, as well as due to the immunogenicity of constituents such as gluten, a protein composite (consisting of a prolamin and a glutelin) that can contribute to disorders such as migraine, epilepsy, eczema, arthritis, celiac disease, psoriasis and other types of autoimmunity. Sources of simple sugars and foreign chemicals such as colas/sodas (which contain artificial colors, flavors, and high-fructose corn syrup, which contains mercury[418] and which can cause the hypertensive-diabetic metabolic syndrome[419]) and processed foods (e.g., "TV dinners" and other manufactured snacks and convenience foods) are strictly forbidden. Chemical preservatives, colorants, sweeteners, flavor-enhancers such as monosodium glutamate and carrageenan are likewise avoided. In summary, this diet plan provides plenty of variety, as most dishes comprised of poultry, fish, lean meats, soy, eggs, fruits, vegetables, nuts, berries, and seeds are allowed. The diet provides an abundance of fiber, phytonutrients, carbohydrates, potassium, and protein, while simultaneously being low in fat, sodium, arachidonic acid, and "simple sugars." The diet must be customized with regard to total protein and calorie intake, as determined by the size, status, and activity level of the patient; individual per-patient food allergens should be avoided. Regular consumption of this diet has shown the ability to reduce hypertension, alleviate diabetes, ameliorate migraine headaches, and result in improvement of overall health and a lessening of the severity of many common "diseases", particularly those with an autoimmune or inflammatory component. This Paleo-Mediterranean diet is supplemented with vitamins, minerals, fatty acids, and probiotics—making it the "supplemented Paleo-Mediterranean diet" as described below.

2. <u>Multivitamin and multimineral supplementation</u>: Vitamin and mineral supplementation has been advocated for decades by the chiropractic/naturopathic professions while being scorned by so-called "mainstream medicine." Vitamin and mineral supplementation finally received bipartisan endorsement when researchers from Harvard Medical School published a review article in *Journal of the American Medical Association* that concluded, "Most people do not consume an optimal amount of all vitamins by diet alone. ...it appears prudent for all adults to take vitamin supplements."[420] Long-term nutritional insufficiencies experienced by "most people" promote the development of "long-latency deficiency diseases"[421] such as cancer, neuroemotional deterioration, and cardiovascular disease. Impressively, the benefits of multivitamin/multimineral supplementation have been demonstrated in numerous clinical trials. Multivitamin/multimineral supplementation has been shown to improve nutritional status and reduce the risk for chronic diseases[422], improve mood[423], potentiate antidepressant drug treatment[424], alleviate migraine headaches (when used with diet improvement and fatty acids[425]), improve immune function and infectious disease outcomes in the elderly[426] (especially diabetics[427]), reduce morbidity and mortality in patients with HIV infection[428,429], alleviate premenstrual syndrome[430,431] and bipolar disorder[432], reduce violence and antisocial behavior in children[433] and incarcerated young adults (when used with essential fatty acids[434]), and improve scores of intelligence in children.[435] Multivitamin and multimineral supplementation provides anti-inflammatory benefits, as evidenced by significant reduction in C-reactive protein (CRP) in a double-blind,

[417] Liu RH. Health benefits of fruit and vegetables are from additive and synergistic combinations of phytochemicals. *Am J Clin Nutr* 2003;78(3 Suppl):517S-520S

[418] "With daily per capita consumption of HFCS in the US averaging about 50 grams and daily mercury intakes from HFCS ranging up to 28 μg, this potential source of mercury may exceed other major sources of mercury especially in high-end consumers of beverages sweetened with HFCS." Dufault R, LeBlanc B, Schnoll R, Cornett C, Schweitzer L, Wallinga D, Hightower J, Patrick L, Lukiw WJ. Mercury from chlor-alkali plants: measured concentrations in food product sugar. *Environ Health.* 2009 Jan 26;8:2 http://www.ehjournal.net/content/8/1/2

[419] **Vasquez A**. Integrative Medicine and Functional Medicine for Chronic Hypertension: An Evidence-based Patient-Centered Monograph for Advanced Clinicians. IBMRC; 2011. http://optimalhealthresearch.com/hypertension_functional_integrative_medicine.html See also: Reungjui S, Roncal CA, Mu W, Srinivas TR, Sirivongs D, Johnson RJ, Nakagawa T. Thiazide diuretics exacerbate fructose-induced metabolic syndrome. *J Am Soc Nephrol.* 2007 Oct;18(10):2724-31 http://jasn.asnjournals.org/content/18/10/2724.full.pdf

[420] Fletcher RH, Fairfield KM. Vitamins for chronic disease prevention in adults: clinical applications. *JAMA* 2002;287:3127-9

[421] Heaney RP. Long-latency deficiency disease: insights from calcium and vitamin D. *Am J Clin Nutr* 2003;78:912-9

[422] McKay DL, Perrone G, Rasmussen H, Dallal G, Hartman W, Cao G, Prior RL, Roubenoff R, Blumberg JB. The effects of a multivitamin/mineral supplement on micronutrient status, antioxidant capacity and cytokine production in healthy older adults consuming a fortified diet. *J Am Coll Nutr* 2000;19(5):613-21

[423] Benton D, Haller J, Fordy J. Vitamin supplementation for 1 year improves mood. *Neuropsychobiology* 1995;32(2):98-105

[424] Coppen A, Bailey J. Enhancement of the antidepressant action of fluoxetine by folic acid: a randomised, placebo controlled trial. *J Affect Disord* 2000;60:121-30

[425] Wagner W, Nootbaar-Wagner U. Prophylactic treatment of migraine with gamma-linolenic and alpha-linolenic acids. *Cephalalgia* 1997;17:127-30

[426] Langkamp-Henken B, Bender BS, Gardner EM, Herrlinger-Garcia KA, Kelley MJ, Murasko DM, Schaller JP, Stechmiller JK, Thomas DJ, Wood SM. Nutritional formula enhanced immune function and reduced days of symptoms of upper respiratory tract infection in seniors. *J Am Geriatr Soc* 2004;52:3-12

[427] Barringer TA, Kirk JK, Santaniello AC, Foley KL, Michielutte R. Effect of a multivitamin and mineral supplement on infection and quality of life. A randomized, double-blind, placebo-controlled trial. *Ann Intern Med* 2003;138:365-71

[428] Fawzi WW, Msamanga GI, Spiegelman D, et al. A randomized trial of multivitamin supplements and HIV disease progression and mortality. *N Engl J Med* 2004;351:23-32

[429] Burbano X, Miguez-Burbano MJ, McCollister K, Zhang G, Rodriguez A, Ruiz P, Lecusay R, Shor-Posner G. Impact of a selenium chemoprevention clinical trial on hospital admissions of HIV-infected participants. *HIV Clin Trials* 2002;3:483-91

[430] Abraham GE. Nutritional factors in the etiology of the premenstrual tension syndromes. *J Reprod Med* 1983;28(7):446-64

[431] Stewart A. Clinical and biochemical effects of nutritional supplementation on the premenstrual syndrome. *J Reprod Med* 1987;32:435-41

[432] Kaplan BJ, Simpson JS, Ferre RC, Gorman CP, McMullen DM, Crawford SG. Effective mood stabilization with a chelated mineral supplement: an open-label trial in bipolar disorder. *J Clin Psychiatry* 2001;62:936-44

[433] Kaplan BJ, Crawford SG, Gardner B, Farrelly G. Treatment of mood lability and explosive rage with minerals and vitamins: two case studies in children. *J Child Adolesc Psychopharmacol* 2002;12(3):205-19

[434] Gesch CB, Hammond SM, Hampson SE, Eves A, Crowder MJ. Influence of supplementary vitamins, minerals and essential fatty acids on the antisocial behaviour of young adult prisoners. Randomised, placebo-controlled trial. *Br J Psychiatry* 2002;181:22-8

[435] Benton D. Micro-nutrient supplementation and the intelligence of children. *Neurosci Biobehav Rev* 2001;25:297-309

placebo-controlled trial.[436] The ability to safely and affordably deliver these benefits makes multimineral-multivitamin supplementation an essential component of any and all health-promoting and disease-prevention strategies. A few cautions need to be observed; for example, vitamin A can (rarely) result in liver damage with chronic consumption of 25,000 IU or more, and intake should generally not exceed 10,000 IU per day in women of childbearing age. Also, iron should not be supplemented except in patients diagnosed with iron deficiency by a blood test (serum ferritin).

3. <u>Physiologic doses of vitamin D3</u>: The prevalence of vitamin D deficiency varies from 40-80 percent (general population) to almost 100 percent (patients with musculoskeletal pain) among Americans and Europeans. Vasquez, Manso, and Cannell described the many benefits of vitamin D3 supplementation in an assertive review published in 2004.[437] Our publication showed that vitamin D deficiency causes or contributes to depression, hypertension, seizures, migraine, polycystic ovary syndrome, inflammation, autoimmunity, and musculoskeletal pain, particularly low-back pain. Clinical trials using vitamin D supplementation have proven the cause-and-effect relationship between vitamin D deficiency and most of these conditions by showing that each could be cured or alleviated with vitamin D supplementation. In our review of the literature, we concluded that daily vitamin D doses should be 1,000 IU for infants, 2,000 IU for children, and 4,000 IU for adults, although some adults respond better to higher doses of 10,000 IU per day. Cautions and contraindications include the use of thiazide diuretics (e.g., hydrochlorothiazide) or any other medications that promote hypercalcemia, as well as granulomatous diseases such as sarcoidosis, tuberculosis, and certain types of cancer, especially lymphoma. Effectiveness is monitored by measuring serum 25-OH-vitamin D, and safety is monitored by measuring serum calcium. Dosing should be tailored for the attainment of optimal serum levels of 25-hydroxy-vitamin D3, generally 50-100 ng/ml (125-250 nmol/l) as illustrated.

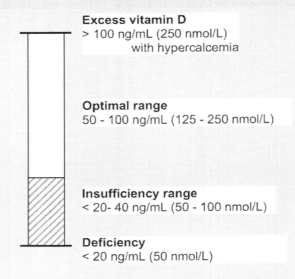

Excess vitamin D
> 100 ng/mL (250 nmol/L)
    with hypercalcemia

Optimal range
50 - 100 ng/mL (125 - 250 nmol/L)

Insufficiency range
< 20- 40 ng/mL (50 - 100 nmol/L)

Deficiency
< 20 ng/mL (50 nmol/L)

Interpretation of serum 25(OH) vitamin D levels.
Modified from Vasquez et al, *Alternative Therapies in Health and Medicine* 2004 and Vasquez A. *Musculoskeletal Pain: Expanded Clinical Strategies* (Institute for Functional Medicine) 2008.

4. <u>Balanced and complete fatty acid supplementation</u>: A detailed survey of the literature shows that five fatty acids have major health-promoting disease-preventing benefits and should therefore be incorporated into the daily diet and/or regularly consumed as dietary supplements.[438] These are alpha-linolenic acid (ALA; omega-3, from flaxseed oil), eicosapentaenoic acid (EPA; omega-3, from fish oil), docosahexaenoic acid (DHA; omega-3, from fish oil and algae), gamma-linolenic acid (GLA; omega-6, most concentrated in borage oil but also present in evening primrose oil, hemp seed oil, black currant seed oil), and oleic acid (omega-9, most concentrated in olive oil, which contains in addition to oleic acid many anti-inflammatory, antioxidant, and anticancer phytonutrients). Supplementing with one fatty acid can exacerbate an insufficiency of other fatty acids; hence the importance of balanced combination supplementation. Each of these fatty acids has health benefits that cannot be fully attained from supplementing a different fatty acid; hence, again, the importance of balanced combination supplementation. The benefits of GLA are not attained by consumption of EPA and DHA; in fact, consumption of fish oil can actually promote a deficiency of GLA.[439] Likewise, consumption of GLA alone can reduce EPA levels while increasing levels of proinflammatory arachidonic acid; both of these problems are

[436] Church TS, Earnest CP, Wood KA, Kampert JB. Reduction of C-reactive protein levels through use of a multivitamin. *Am J Med* 2003;115:702-7
[437] **Vasquez A**, Manso G, Cannell J. The clinical importance of vitamin D (cholecalciferol): a paradigm shift with implications for all healthcare providers. *Alternative Therapies in Health and Medicine* 2004;10:28-37 http://optimalhealthresearch.com/cholecalciferol.html
[438] **Vasquez A**. Reducing Pain and Inflammation Naturally - Part 1: New Insights into Fatty Acid Biochemistry and the Influence of Diet. *Nutritional Perspectives* 2004; October: 5, 7-10, 12, 14 http://optimalhealthresearch.com/reprints/series/
[439] Cleland LG, Gibson RA, Neumann M, French JK. The effect of dietary fish oil supplement upon the content of dihomo-gammalinolenic acid in human plasma phospholipids. *Prostaglandins Leukot Essent Fatty Acids* 1990 May;40(1):9-12

avoided with co-administration of EPA any time GLA is used because EPA inhibits delta-5-desaturase, which converts dihomo-GLA into arachidonic acid. Using ALA alone only slightly increases EPA but generally leads to no improvement in DHA status and can lead to a reduction of oleic acid; thus, DHA and oleic acid should be supplemented when flaxseed oil is used.[440] Obviously, the goal here is physiologically-optimal (i.e., "balanced") intake of all of the health-promoting fatty acids; using only one or two sources of fatty acids is not balanced and results in suboptimal improvement. In clinical practice, I routinely use combination fatty acid therapy comprised of ALA, EPA, DHA, and GLA for essentially all patients; when one appreciates that the average daily Paleolithic intake of n-3 fatty acids was 7 grams per day contrasted to the average daily American intake of 1 gram per day, we can see that—by using combination fatty acid therapy emphasizing n-3 fatty acids—we are simply meeting physiologic expectations via supplementation, rather than performing an act of recklessness or heroism. The product I use also contains a modest amount of oleic acid that occurs naturally in flax and borage seed oils, and I encourage use of olive oil for salads and cooking. This approach results in complete and balanced fatty acid intake, and the clinical benefits are impressive. Benefits are to be expected in the treatment of premenstrual syndrome, diabetic neuropathy, respiratory distress syndrome, Crohn's disease, lupus, rheumatoid arthritis, cardiovascular disease, hypertension, psoriasis, eczema, migraine headaches, bipolar disorder, borderline personality disorder, mental depression, schizophrenia, osteoporosis, polycystic ovary syndrome, multiple sclerosis, and musculoskeletal pain. The discovery in September 2010 that the G protein-coupled receptor 120 (GPR120) functions as an n-3 fatty acid receptor that, when stimulated with EPA or DHA, exerts broad anti-inflammatory effects (in cell experiments) and enhances systemic insulin sensitivity (in animal study) confirms a new mechanism of action of fatty acid supplementation and shows that we as clinician-researchers are still learning the details of the beneficial effects of commonly used treatments.[441]

5. <u>Probiotics /gut flora modification</u>: Proper levels of good bacteria promote intestinal health, support proper immune function, and encourage overall health. Excess bacteria or yeast, or the presence of harmful bacteria, yeast, or "parasites" such as amoebas and protozoas, can cause "leaky gut," systemic inflammation, and a wide range of clinical problems, especially autoimmunity. Intestinal flora can become imbalanced by poor diets, excess stress, immunosuppressive drugs, and antibiotics, and all of these factors are common among American patients. Thus, as a rule, I reinstate the good bacteria by the use of probiotics (good bacteria and yeast), prebiotics (fiber, arabinogalactan, and inulin), and the use of fermented foods such as kefir and yogurt for patients not allergic to milk. Harmful yeast, bacteria, and other "parasites" can be eradicated with the combination of dietary change, antimicrobial drugs, and/or herbal extracts. For example, oregano oil in an emulsified, time-released form has proven safe and effective for the elimination of various parasites encountered in clinical practice.[442] Likewise, the herb *Artemisia annua* (sweet wormwood) commonly is used to eradicate specific bacteria and has been used for thousands of years in Asia for the treatment and prevention of infectious diseases, including drug-resistant malaria.[443] Restoring microbial balance by providing probiotics, restoring immune function (immunorestoration) and eliminating sources of dysbiosis, especially in the gastrointestinal tract, genitourinary tract, and oropharynx, is a very important component in the treatment plan of autoimmunity and systemic inflammation.[444]

<u>Should combinations of iodine and iodide be the sixth component of the Protocol?</u>: Both iodine and iodide have biological activity in humans. An increasing number of clinicians are using combination iodine-iodide products to provide approximately 12 mg/d; this is consistent with the average daily intake of iodine-iodide in countries such as Japan with a high intake of seafood, including fish, shellfish, and seaweed. Collectively, iodine and iodide provide antioxidant, antimicrobial, mucolytic, immunosupportive, antiestrogen, and anticancer benefits that extend far beyond the mere incorporation of iodine into thyroid hormones.[5] Benefits of iodine/iodide in the treatment of asthma[445,446] and systemic fungal infections[447,448] have been documented, and many clinicians use combination iodine/iodide supplementation for the treatment of estrogen-driven conditions such as fibrocystic breast disease.[449] While additional research is needed and already underway to further establish the role of iodine-iodide as a routine component of clinical care, clinicians should begin incorporating this nutrient into their protocols based on the above-mentioned physiologic roles and clinical benefits.

<u>Summary and Conclusions</u>: In this brief review, I have described and substantiated a fundamental protocol that can serve as effective therapy for patients with a wide range of diseases and health disorders. Customizing the Paleo-Mediterranean diet to avoid patient-specific food allergens, using vitamin-mineral supplements along with physiologic doses of vitamin D and broad-spectrum balanced fatty acid supplementation, and ensuring "immunomicrobial" health with the skillful use of probiotics, prebiotics, immunorestoration, and antimicrobial treatments provides an excellent health-promoting and disease-eliminating foundation and lifestyle for many patients. Often, this simple protocol is all that is needed for the effective treatment of a wide range of clinical problems, even those that have been "medical failures" for many years. For other patients with more complex illnesses, of course, additional interventions and laboratory assessments can be used to optimize and further customize the

[440] Jantti J, Nikkari T, Solakivi T, Vapaatalo H, Isomaki H. Evening primrose oil in rheumatoid arthritis: changes in serum lipids and fatty acids. *Ann Rheum Dis* 1989;48(2):124-7
[441] Oh da Y, Talukdar S, Bae EJ, Imamura T, Morinaga H, Fan W, Li P, Lu WJ, Watkins SM, Olefsky JM. GPR120 is an omega-3 fatty acid receptor mediating potent anti-inflammatory and insulin-sensitizing effects. Cell. 2010 Sep 3;142(5):687-98 http://www.cell.com/abstract/S0092-8674%2810%2900888-3?switch=standard
[442] Force M, Sparks WS, Ronzio RA. Inhibition of enteric parasites by emulsified oil of oregano in vivo. *Phytother Res* 2000;14:213-4
[443] Schuster BG. Demonstrating the validity of natural products as anti-infective drugs. *J Altern Complement Med* 2001;7 Suppl 1:S73-82
[444] **Vasquez A.** Integrative Rheumatology. IBMRC: 2006, 2009. http://optimalhealthresearch.com/rheumatology.html
[445] Tuft L. Iodides in bronchial asthma. *J Allergy Clin Immunol*. 1981 Jun;67(6):497
[446] Falliers CJ, McCann WP, Chai H, Ellis EF, Yazdi N. Controlled study of iodotherapy for childhood asthma. *J Allergy*. 1966 Sep;38(3):183-92
[447] Tripathy S, Vijayashree J, Mishra M, Jena DK, Behera B, Mohapatra A. Rhinofacial zygomycosis successfully treated with oral saturated solution of potassium iodide: a case report. *J Eur Acad Dermatol Venereol*. 2007 Jan;21(1):117-9
[448] Bonifaz A, Saúl A, Paredes-Solis V, Fierro L, Rosales A, Palacios C, Araiza J. Sporotrichosis in childhood: clinical and therapeutic experience in 25 patients. *Pediatr Dermatol*. 2007 Jul-Aug;24(4):369-72
[449] Ghent WR, Eskin BA, Low DA, Hill LP. Iodine replacement in fibrocystic disease of the breast. *Can J Surg*. 1993 Oct;36(5):453-60

treatment plan. Clinicians should avoid seeking "silver bullet" treatments that ignore overall metabolism, immune function, and inflammatory balance, and we must always remember that the attainment and preservation of health requires that we first meet the body's basic nutritional and physiologic needs. This five-step protocol begins the process of meeting those needs. With it, health can be restored and the need for disease-specific treatment is obviated or reduced; without it, fundamental physiologic needs are not met, and health cannot be obtained and maintained. Addressing core physiologic needs empowers doctors to deliver the most effective healthcare possible, and it allows patients to benefit from such treatment.

Chapter 3:
Comprehensive Musculoskeletal Care

Introduction
Nonpharmacologic management of musculoskeletal problem should be seen as the treatment of choice because of the collateral benefits, safety, and cost-effectiveness associated with manual, dietary, botanical, and physiologic/physiotherapeutic treatments.

Topics:
- **Comprehensive Musculoskeletal Care**
  - Protect, prevent re-injury
  - Relative rest
  - Ice/heat, individualize treatment
  - Compression
  - Elevation, establish treatment program
  - Anti-inflammatory & analgesic treatments
  - Treat with physical/manual medicine
  - Uncover the underlying problem
  - Re-educate, rehabilitate, resourcefulness, return to active life, refer to specialist
  - Nutrition, diet, and supplements
- **Myofascial trigger points (MFTP): diagnosis and treatment**
- **Musculoskeletal Manipulative Manual Medicine**
- **Proprioceptive retraining/rehabilitation**
- **Reasons to avoid the use of nonsteroidal anti-inflammatory drugs (NSAIDs) and COX-2 inhibitors (coxibs)**

Core Competencies:
- Provide one example from each letter of the "p.r.i.c.e. a. t.u.r.n." and/or "b.e.n.d. s.t.e.m.s." mnemonic acronyms for holistic and comprehensive acute care for musculoskeletal injuries.
- List at least 6 of the 10 mechanisms of action of spinal manipulative therapy.
- List the two most common clinical findings associated with myofascial trigger points and describe appropriate physical/manual and nutritional treatments.
- Describe plans for low-back and ankle proprioceptive retraining/rehabilitation for a patient who has no exercise equipment.
- Describe the effects of stereotypic NSAIDs on chrondrocyte metabolism and the long-term effects on joint structure.
- Name four biochemical/physiologic mechanisms by which COX-2 inhibiting drugs predispose to cardiovascular death.
- By the time you finish reading this chapter (if necessary, see additional information in the chapter on *Therapeutics*), you should be able to describe 1) indications, 2) contraindications, 3) drug interactions, 4) adult doses and administration, and 5) molecular/physiologic mechanisms of action for each of the following commonly employed therapeutics:
  - Flaxseed oil: Alpha-linolenic acid (ALA)
  - Fish oil: Eicosapentaenoic acid (EPA), Docosahexaenoic acid (DHA)
  - Gamma-linolenic acid (GLA)
  - Vitamin D3: Cholecalciferol
  - Vitamin E: Alpha-tocopherol, beta-tocopherol, delta-tocopherol, gamma-tocopherol
  - Niacinamide
  - Glucosamine sulfate and Chondroitin Sulfate
  - Pancreatin, bromelain, papain, trypsin and alpha-chymotrypsin: "proteolytic enzymes" and "pancreatic enzymes"
  - *Zingiber officinale*, Ginger
  - *Uncaria tomentosa, Uncaria guianensis*, "Cat's claw", "una de gato"
  - *Salix alba*, Willow Bark
  - *Capsicum annuum, Capsicum frutescens*, Cayenne pepper, hot chili pepper
  - *Boswellia serrata*, Frankincense, Salai guggal
  - *Harpagophytum procumbens*, Devil's claw

Introduction: Whether dealing with a *recent and acutely painful injury* or an *exacerbation of a chronic injury or musculoskeletal disease*, all integrative clinicians are wise to have at their disposal a comprehensive protocol for the management of acute and subacute pain and exacerbations of joint inflammation. Incompetence in musculoskeletal medicine, which is common among allopathic physicians[1,2,3,4,5], forces doctors to overuse simplistic and dangerous treatments (i.e., pharmaceutical drugs) because they are unaware of better options.[6] Failure to understand how to arrive at an accurate diagnosis and subsequent failure to know how to manage musculoskeletal pain leaves doctors *and thus their patients* with no other option than the overuse of so-called anti-inflammatory drugs such as non-steroidal anti-inflammatory drugs (NSAIDs, such as aspirin), which kill at least 17,000 patients per year[7], and the cyclooxygenase-2 inhibiting drugs (COX-2 inhibitors, coxibs, such as Vioxx and Celebrex) which have killed tens of thousands of patients.[8,9,10,11]

Previously, any medical treatment that was non-surgical was commonly described as "conservative" simply because it was *non-invasive/non-surgical*. However, many so-called "conservative" drug treatments are dangerously lethal and expensive, as the coxibs, with their lethality and high costs, have demonstrated. Further, "conservative" has become such a confusing term in modern politics that even people who identify themselves as such are often at a loss for an accurate definition of the term. Thus, I have replaced the previous "holistic conservative care" with the current "comprehensive acute care" to indicate the consideration and selective implementation of the treatments described in this chapter.

Throughout the other chapters this text, when the phrase "**comprehensive musculoskeletal care**" is included in the list of therapeutic considerations, readers should understand that this implies these treatments for musculoskeletal problems *in addition to reestablishing the foundation for health*, which was detailed in Chapter 2. While all of us are familiar with the components of basic care for injuries—"*rice*": r̲est, i̲ce, c̲ompression, e̲levation—I have expanded this list to include p̲rotect, p̲revent re-injury, r̲elative rest, i̲ce, individualize treatment, c̲ompression, e̲levation, establish treatment program, a̲nti-inflammatory and analgesic treatments, t̲reat with physical/manual medicine, u̲ncover the underlying problem, r̲e-educate, rehabilitate, retrain, resourcefulness, return to active life, and n̲utrition including diet and nutritional and botanical supplements. The mnemonic acronym spells "*price a turn*" which is cumbersome but perhaps easy to remember and therefore useful. The major point is to think outside of the "rice" box; as integrative clinicians, we have much more to offer our patients than rest, ice, compression, and elevation.

Understanding the shorthand that is conveyed by *comprehensive musculoskeletal care* is important for grasping the important differences between our medicine and the myopic and pharmacocentric allopathic approach. Whereas the allopathic approach stops with minimal disease treatment and provides essentially nothing in terms of prevention or comprehensive patient management—let alone promotion of optimal health—the holistic and integrative approach is centered on the *patient* and seeks to help him/her attain optimal health while being treated for the musculoskeletal disorder. We can and must help our patients attain optimal health while effectively managing their acute and chronic musculoskeletal problems.[12,13,14] **Indeed, since for many patients their only interaction with the healthcare system is when they are injured, we must seize upon this opportunity to enroll patients in preventive and pro-active healthcare.**

[1] Joy EA, Hala SV. Musculoskeletal Curricula in Medical Education: Filling In the Missing Pieces. *The Physician and Sportsmedicine*. 2004; 32: 42-45
[2] Freedman KB, Bernstein J. The adequacy of medical school education in musculoskeletal medicine. *J Bone Joint Surg Am*. 1998;80(10):1421-7
[3] Freedman KB, Bernstein J. Educational deficiencies in musculoskeletal medicine. *J Bone Joint Surg Am*. 2002;84-A(4):604-8
[4] Matzkin E, Smith ME, Freccero CD, Richardson AB. Adequacy of education in musculoskeletal medicine. *J Bone Joint Surg Am*. 2005 Feb;87-A(2):310-4
[5] Schmale GA. More evidence of educational inadequacies in musculoskeletal medicine. *Clin Orthop Relat Res*. 2005 Aug;(437):251-9
[6] Vasquez A. The Importance of Integrative Chiropractic Health Care in Treating Musculoskeletal Pain and Reducing the Nationwide Burden of Medical Expenses and Iatrogenic Injury and Death: Concise Review of Current Research and Implications for Clinical Practice and Healthcare Policy. *The Original Internist* 2005;12:159-182 www.optimalhealthresearch.com/monograph06
[7] Singh G. Recent considerations in nonsteroidal anti-inflammatory drug gastropathy. *Am J Med*. 1998;105(1B):31S-38S
[8] "The results from VIGOR showed that the relative risk of developing a confirmed adjudicated thrombotic cardiovascular event (myocardial infarction, unstable angina, cardiac thrombus, resuscitated cardiac arrest, sudden or unexplained death, ischemic stroke, and transient ischemic attacks) with rofecoxib treatment compared with naproxen was 2.38." Mukherjee D, Nissen SE, Topol EJ. Risk of cardiovascular events associated with selective COX-2 inhibitors. *JAMA*. 2001 Aug 22-29;286(8):954-9
[9] Topol EJ. Failing the public health--rofecoxib, Merck, and the FDA. *N Engl J Med*. 2004 Oct 21;351(17):1707-9
[10] Ray WA, Griffin MR, Stein CM. Cardiovascular toxicity of valdecoxib. *N Engl J Med*. 2004;351(26):2767
[11] "Patients in the clinical trial taking 400 mg. of Celebrex twice daily had a 3.4 times greater risk of CV events compared to placebo. For patients in the trial taking 200 mg. of Celebrex twice daily, the risk was 2.5 times greater. The average duration of treatment in the trial was 33 months." FDA Statement on the Halting of a Clinical Trial of the cox-2 Inhibitor Celebrex. http://www.fda.gov/bbs/topics/news/2004/NEW01144.html Available on January 4, 2005
[12] Vasquez A. Reducing Pain and Inflammation Naturally. Part 2: New Insights into Fatty Acid Supplementation and Its Effect on Eicosanoid Production and Genetic Expression. *Nutritional Perspectives* 2005; January: 5-16 www.optimalhealthresearch.com/part2
[13] Vasquez A. Reducing pain and inflammation naturally - Part 3: Improving overall health while safely and effectively treating musculoskeletal pain. *Nutritional Perspectives* 2005; 28: 34-38, 40-42 http://optimalhealthresearch.com/part3
[14] Vasquez A. The Importance of Integrative Chiropractic Health Care in Treating Musculoskeletal Pain and Reducing the Nationwide Burden of Medical Expenses and Iatrogenic Injury and Death: A Concise Review of Current Research and Implications for Clinical Practice and Healthcare Policy. *The Original Internist* 2005; 12(4): 159-182

Basic Treatment Concepts and Commonly Employed Therapeutics

The following pages summarize the basic therapeutics most commonly employed by integrative physicians in the treatment of acute and chronic musculoskeletal conditions. Knowledge of some of the clinical skills relied upon in orthopedics[15] is necessary when treating rheumatic musculoskeletal problems[16] because an acutely inflamed joint associated with a *chronic* and *systemic* disorder may need to be treated as if it were a *recent* and *focal* injury.

Orthopedics generally centers on the clinical management of 1) **acute injuries** (e.g., whiplash), 2) **chronic injuries** (tendonitis and myofasciitis/myofascitis), and 3) **congenital/developmental anomalies**, (odontoid hypoplasia and scoliosis). For most clinicians, management of congenital anomalies centers on accurate diagnosis and then either observation or appropriate referral. For the treatment of common acute and chronic injuries encountered in general practice, **comprehensive acute care** can include the facets described in the following section, modified for the clinical situation and individual patient. Although *rheumatology* is generally concerned with the treatment of *non-traumatic* disorders of an inflammatory or autoimmune nature, knowledge of orthopedics is necessary during the course of evaluating and treating patients with autoimmunity because differential diagnosis, qualification/quantification, and comanagement of joint disorders *within the same patient* are commonly necessary. For example, a patient with rheumatoid arthritis (chronic autoimmune disease) affecting the knees and hips may also develop carpal tunnel syndrome (orthopedic problem) and later present with neck pain and leg spasticity secondary to atlantoaxial instability (neuro-orthopedic emergency).

Generally, different types and locations of injuries can be treated from a common framework of interventions that are then customized for the three following primary considerations:

1) Location: The specific location and associated functional considerations, e.g., lower extremity injuries may require crutches while upper extremity injuries may benefit from a brace or sling,
2) Tissue: The type of tissue that is injured—i.e., muscle, cartilage, tendons, or ligaments—may respond to a particular nutritional and rehabilitative protocol,
3) Patient: The specific goals, needs, comorbidities, medications, occupation, recreational activities, age, and other characteristics of the individual patient.

Protect & prevent re-injury:

- **Avoid motions and activities that cause significant pain, as pain indicates that damaged/inflamed tissues are being stressed.** The goals are 1) to allow healing of injured tissues, and 2) to promote maximal physical restoration and functional ability. An excess of rest promotes functional disability, muscle atrophy, and psychological dysfunction (e.g., iatrogenic neurosis, inaccurate perception of patient being permanently damaged or defective, loss of confidence, loss of social contact [especially for children, and adults for whom physical activity is important]). Returning to activities and work too quickly may not allow time for sufficient healing and may thus promote re-injury, temporary exacerbation, progression from mild to severe injury, and/or progression to repetitive strain injury.
- **Use bracing, taping, bandages, wrapping, canes, crutches, and walkers as needed.**[17,18]

Relative rest:

- **"Relative rest" simply means to take time away from the activities that either promote additional injury or that unnecessarily drain energies which could otherwise be used for healing and recuperation.** For some patients, this means avoiding certain exercises during a workout, while for other patients this may mean using a crutch or taking days off from work.
- "Bed rest" is generally to be avoided since it promotes muscle atrophy, intraarticular adhesions, loss of neuromuscular coordination, constipation, and patients' assumption of the sick role.[19]

---

[15] Vasquez A. Integrative Orthopedics. http://optimalhealthresearch.com/orthopedics.html
[16] Vasquez A. Integrative Rheumatology. http://www.optimalhealthresearch.com/rheumatology.html
[17] Van Hook FW, Demonbreun D, Weiss BD. Ambulatory devices for chronic gait disorders in the elderly. *Am Fam Physician.* 2003 Apr 15;67(8):1717-24 http://www.aafp.org/afp/20030415/1717.html and http://www.aafp.org/afp/20030415/1717.pdf Accessed July 23, 2006
[18] Joyce BM, Kirby RL. Canes, crutches and walkers. *Am Fam Physician.* 1991 Feb;43(2):535-42
[19] "Glucose intolerance, anorexia, constipation, and pressure sores might develop. Central nervous system changes could affect balance and coordination and lead to increasing dependence on caregivers." Teasell R, Dittmer DK. Complications of immobilization and bed rest. Part 2: Other complications. *Can Fam Physician.* 1993 Jun;39:1440-2, 1445-6

Ice/heat:

- **First 48-72 hours after injury**: Apply ice or cold pack for 10 minutes each 30-60 minutes for reduction in pain and inflammation. The best protocol appears to be interrupted application of ice to maximize deep cooling of tissues while minimizing cold-induced damage to the skin.[20] Ice massage is more effective than stationary application of ice or an ice bag.[21] Intraarticular temperatures can be lowered with topical application of ice[22], and immersion into ice water appears to be the best method for reducing intraarticular temperature according to an animal study.[23] Greater skin thickness due to subcutaneous adipose increases the amount of time needed to achieve clinically significant cooling of deep tissues.[24] Avoid frostbite and cold injuries to skin and superficial nerves. Use caution in patients with decreased skin sensitivity, circulatory insufficiency, and/or suboptimal ability to follow directions and employ good judgment.

- **After 48-72 hours post-injury**: Apply gentle heat as needed for the relief of pain and reduction in muscle spasm and to promote healing by increasing circulation. Avoid heat injuries to skin. Use caution in patients with decreased skin sensitivity (e.g., diabetics and the elderly) or suboptimal ability to follow directions and employ good judgment.

Individualize treatment:

- The cornerstone of effective holistic and integrative treatment is to design treatment plans that simultaneously 1) address "the problem" while also 2) improving the patient's overall health. Often, serious and so-called "untreatable" diseases can be ameliorated or eradicated simply with general, non-specific, overall health improvement even when these conditions repeatedly fail to respond to specific "disease-targeting" medical treatments.

Compression:

- Snug bandages/wraps may help to reduce swelling and can provide support for injured tissues and weakened joints. Care must be utilized to avoid arterial, venous, or lymphatic obstruction.

Educate, establish treatment program, elevation:

- Educate patient about the injury.
- Educate patient about the need for appropriate follow-up office visits for reexamination, reassessment, and treatment.
- Estimate the amount of time during which most recovery will take place.
- Estimate the extent of return to previous status.
- Elevate the injured part to minimize swelling and edema.

Anti-inflammatory & analgesic treatments:

- Anti-inflammation versus hemostasis: Anti-inflammatory/analgesic medications that impair coagulation (e.g., aspirin) are contraindicated in patients with possible internal bleeding such as severe hematoma, hemarthrosis, spleen injury, intracranial hemorrhage (i.e., subdural hematoma following a whiplash injury) and in patients about to undergo surgery. Caution should also be used with nutritional/botanical supplements that have anti-coagulant effects, such as ginkgo biloba[25] and garlic.[26]
- Avoidance of pro-inflammatory foods: **Arachidonic acid** (high in cow's milk, beef, liver, pork, and lamb) is the direct precursor to pro-inflammatory prostaglandins and leukotrienes[27] and pain-

---

[20] "The evidence from this systematic review suggests that melting iced water applied through a wet towel for repeated periods of 10 minutes is most effective." MacAuley DC. Ice therapy: how good is the evidence? *Int J Sports Med*. 2001 Jul;22(5):379-84

[21] Zemke JE, Andersen JC, Guion WK, McMillan J, Joyner AB. Intramuscular temperature responses in the human leg to two forms of cryotherapy: ice massage and ice bag. *J Orthop Sports Phys Ther*. 1998 Apr;27(4):301-7

[22] Martin SS, Spindler KP, Tarter JW, Detwiler K, Petersen HA. Cryotherapy: an effective modality for decreasing intraarticular temperature after knee arthroscopy. *Am J Sports Med*. 2001 May-Jun;29(3):288-91

[23] Bocobo C, Fast A, Kingery W, Kaplan M. The effect of ice on intra-articular temperature in the knee of the dog. *Am J Phys Med Rehabil*. 1991 Aug;70(4):181-5

[24] Otte JW, Merrick MA, Ingersoll CD, Cordova ML. Subcutaneous adipose tissue thickness alters cooling time during cryotherapy. *Arch Phys Med Rehabil*. 2002 Nov;83(11):1501-5

[25] "A structured assessment of published case reports suggests a possible causal association between using ginkgo and bleeding events... Patients using ginkgo, particularly those with known bleeding risks, should be counseled about a possible increase in bleeding risk." Bent S, Goldberg H, Padula A, Avins AL. Spontaneous bleeding associated with ginkgo biloba: a case report and systematic review of the literature: a case report and systematic review of the literature. *J Gen Intern Med*. 2005 Jul;20(7):657-61 http://www.pubmedcentral.gov/picrender.fcgi?artid=1490168&blobtype=pdf

[26] "The authors report a case of spontaneous spinal epidural hematoma causing paraplegia secondary to a qualitative platelet disorder from excessive garlic ingestion." Rose KD, Croissant PD, Parliament CF, Levin MB. Spontaneous spinal epidural hematoma with associated platelet dysfunction from excessive garlic ingestion: a case report. *Neurosurgery*. 1990 May;26(5):880-2

[27] Vasquez A. Reducing Pain and Inflammation Naturally. Part 2: New Insights into Fatty Acid Supplementation and Its Effect on Eicosanoid Production and Genetic Expression. *Nutritional Perspectives* 2005; January: 5-16 www.optimalhealthresearch.com/part2

promoting isoprostanes.[28] **Saturated fats** promote inflammation by activating/enabling pro-inflammatory Toll-like receptors, which are otherwise "specific" for inducing pro-inflammatory responses to microorganisms.[29] Consumption of saturated fat in the form of **cream** creates marked oxidative stress and lipid peroxidation that lasts for at least 3 hours postprandially.[30] **Corn oil** rapidly activates NF-kappaB (in hepatic Kupffer cells) for a pro-inflammatory effect[31]; similarly, consumption of PUFA and linoleic acid promotes intracellular antioxidant depletion and may thus promote oxidation-mediated inflammation via activation of NF-kappaB. **Linoleic acid** causes intracellular oxidative stress and calcium influx and results in increased NF-kappaB-stimulated transcription of pro-inflammatory genes.[32] **High glycemic foods** cause oxidative stress[33,34] and inflammation via activation of NF-kappaB and other mechanisms—e.g., *white bread causes inflammation*[35] as does *a high-fat high-carbohydrate fast-food breakfast.*[36] **High glycemic foods** suppress immune function[37,38] and thus promote the development of infection/dysbiosis.[39] Delivery of a **high carbohydrate load** to the gastrointestinal lumen promotes bacterial overgrowth[40,41], which is inherently pro-inflammatory[42,43] and which appears to be myalgenic in humans[44] at least in part due to the ability of endotoxin to impair muscle function.[45] Overconsumption of high-carbohydrate low-phytonutrient **grains, potatoes, and manufactured foods** displaces phytonutrient-dense foods such as fruits, vegetables, nuts, seeds, and berries which contain more than 8,000 phytonutrients, many of which have antioxidant and thus anti-inflammatory actions.[46,47]

- Anti-inflammatory diet, the "supplemented Paleo-Mediterranean diet": The health-promoting diet of choice for the majority of people is a diet based on **abundant consumption of fruits, vegetables, seeds, nuts, berries, omega-3 and monounsaturated fatty acids, and lean sources of protein such as lean meats, fatty cold-water fish, soy and whey proteins.** This diet obviates overconsumption of chemical preservatives, artificial sweeteners, and carbohydrate-dominant foods such as candies, pastries, breads, potatoes, grains, and other foods with a high glycemic load and high glycemic index. This "Paleo-Mediterranean Diet" is a combination of the "Paleolithic" or "Paleo diet" and the well-known "Mediterranean diet", both of which are well described in peer-reviewed journals and the lay press, particularly by Eaton[48], O'Keefe[49], and Cordain.[50] See Chapter 2 and my other reviews[51,52] for

[28] Evans AR, Junger H, Southall MD, Nicol GD, Sorkin LS, Broome JT, Bailey TW, Vasko MR. Isoprostanes, novel eicosanoids that produce nociception and sensitize rat sensory neurons. *J Pharmacol Exp Ther.* 2000 Jun;293(3):912-20

[29] Lee JY, Sohn KH, Rhee SH, Hwang D. Saturated fatty acids, but not unsaturated fatty acids, induce the expression of cyclooxygenase-2 mediated through Toll-like receptor 4. *J Biol Chem.* 2001 May 18;276(20):16683-9. Epub 2001 Mar 2 http://www.jbc.org/cgi/content/full/276/20/16683

[30] "CONCLUSIONS: Both fat and protein intakes stimulate ROS generation. The increase in ROS generation lasted 3 h after cream intake and 1 h after protein intake. Cream intake also caused a significant and prolonged increase in lipid peroxidation." Mohanty P, Ghanim H, Hamouda W, Aljada A, Garg R, Dandona P. Both lipid and protein intakes stimulate increased generation of reactive oxygen species by polymorphonuclear leukocytes and mononuclear cells. *Am J Clin Nutr.* 2002 Apr;75(4):767-72 http://www.ajcn.org/cgi/content/full/75/4/767

[31] Rusyn I, Bradham CA, Cohn L, Schoonhoven R, Swenberg JA, Brenner DA, Thurman RG. Corn oil rapidly activates nuclear factor-kappaB in hepatic Kupffer cells by oxidant-dependent mechanisms. *Carcinogenesis.* 1999 Nov;20(11):2095-100 http://carcin.oxfordjournals.org/cgi/content/full/20/11/2095

[32] "Exposing endothelial cells to 90 micromol linoleic acid/L for 6 h resulted in a significant increase in lipid hydroperoxides that coincided with an increase in intracellular calcium concentrations." Hennig B, Toborek M, Joshi-Barve S, Barger SW, Barve S, Mattson MP, McClain CJ. Linoleic acid activates nuclear transcription factor-kappa B (NF-kappa B) and induces NF-kappa B-dependent transcription in cultured endothelial cells. *Am J Clin Nutr.* 1996 Mar;63(3):322-8 http://www.ajcn.org/cgi/reprint/63/3/322

[33] Mohanty P, Hamouda W, Garg R, Aljada A, Ghanim H, Dandona P. Glucose challenge stimulates reactive oxygen species (ROS) generation by leucocytes. *J Clin Endocrinol Metab.* 2000 Aug;85(8):2970-3 http://jcem.endojournals.org/cgi/content/full/85/8/2970 Glucose/carbohydrate and saturated fat consumption appear to be the two biggest offenders in the food-stimulated production of oxidative stress. The effect by protein is much less. "CONCLUSIONS: Both fat and protein intakes stimulate ROS generation. The increase in ROS generation lasted 3 h after cream intake and 1 h after protein intake. Cream intake also caused a significant and prolonged increase in lipid peroxidation." Mohanty P, Ghanim H, Hamouda W, Aljada A, Garg R, Dandona P. Both lipid and protein intakes stimulate increased generation of reactive oxygen species by polymorphonuclear leukocytes and mononuclear cells. *Am J Clin Nutr.* 2002 Apr;75(4):767-72 http://www.ajcn.org/cgi/content/full/75/4/767

[34] Koska J, Blazicek P, Marko M, Grna JD, Kvetnansky R, Vigas M. Insulin, catecholamines, glucose and antioxidant enzymes in oxidative damage during different loads in healthy humans. *Physiol Res.* 2000;49 Suppl 1:S95-100 http://www.biomed.cas.cz/physiolres/pdf/2000/49_S95.pdf

[35] "Conclusion - The present study shows that high GI carbohydrate, but not low GI carbohydrate, mediates an acute proinflammatory process as measured by NF-kappaB activity." Dickinson S, Hancock DP, Petocz P, Brand-Miller JC..High glycemic index carbohydrate mediates an acute proinflammatory process as measured by NF-kappaB activation. *Asia Pac J Clin Nutr.* 2005;14 Suppl:S120

[36] Aljada A, Mohanty P, Ghanim H, Abdo T, Tripathy D, Chaudhuri A, Dandona P. Increase in intranuclear nuclear factor kappaB and decrease in inhibitor kappaB in mononuclear cells after a mixed meal: evidence for a proinflammatory effect. *Am J Clin Nutr.* 2004 Apr;79(4):682-90 http://www.ajcn.org/cgi/content/full/79/4/682

[37] Sanchez A, Reeser JL, Lau HS, et al. Role of sugars in human neutrophilic phagocytosis. *Am J Clin Nutr.* 1973 Nov;26(11):1180-4

[38] "Postoperative infusion of carbohydrate solution leads to moderate fall in the serum concentration of inorganic phosphate. ... The hypophosphatemia was associated with significant reduction of neutrophil phagocytosis, intracellular killing, consumption of oxygen and generation of superoxide during phagocytosis." Rasmussen A, Segel E, Hessov I, Borregaard N. Reduced function of neutrophils during routine postoperative glucose infusion. *Acta Chir Scand.* 1988 Jul-Aug;154(7-8):429-33

[39] Vasquez A. Reducing Pain and Inflammation Naturally. Part 6: Nutritional and Botanical Treatments Against "Silent Infections" and Gastrointestinal Dysbiosis, Commonly Overlooked Causes of Neuromusculoskeletal Inflammation and Chronic Health Problems. *Nutritional Perspectives* 2006; January http://optimalhealthresearch.com/part6

[40] Ramakrishnan T, Stokes P. Beneficial effects of fasting and low carbohydrate diet in D-lactic acidosis associated with short-bowel syndrome. *JPEN J Parenter Enteral Nutr.* 1985 May-Jun;9(3):361-3

[41] Gottschall E. Breaking the Vicious Cycle: Intestinal Health Through Diet. Kirkton Press; Rev edition (August 1, 1994)

[42] Lin HC. Small intestinal bacterial overgrowth: a framework for understanding irritable bowel syndrome. *JAMA.* 2004 Aug 18;292(7):852-8

[43] Lichtman SN, Wang J, Sartor RB, Zhang C, Bender D, Dalldorf FG, Schwab JH. Reactivation of arthritis induced by small bowel bacterial overgrowth in rats: role of cytokines, bacteria, and bacterial polymers. *Infect Immun.* 1995 Jun;63(6):2295-301

[44] Pimentel M, et al. A link between irritable bowel syndrome and fibromyalgia may be related to findings on lactulose breath testing. *Ann Rheum Dis.* 2004 Apr;63(4):450-2

[45] Bundgaard H, Kjeldsen K, Suarez Krabbe K, van Hall G, Simonsen L, Qvist J, Hansen CM, Moller K, Fonsmark L, Lav Madsen P, Klarlund Pedersen B. Endotoxemia stimulates skeletal muscle Na+-K+-ATPase and raises blood lactate under aerobic conditions in humans. *Am J Physiol Heart Circ Physiol.* 2003 Mar;284(3):H1028-34. Epub 2002 Nov 21 http://ajpheart.physiology.org/cgi/reprint/284/3/H1028

[46] "We propose that the additive and synergistic effects of phytochemicals in fruit and vegetables are responsible for their potent antioxidant and anticancer activities, and that the benefit of a diet rich in fruit and vegetables is attributed to the complex mixture of phytochemicals present in whole foods." Liu RH. Health benefits of fruit and vegetables are from additive and synergistic combinations of phytochemicals. *Am J Clin Nutr.* 2003 Sep;78(3 Suppl):517S-520S

[47] **Seaman DR. The diet-induced proinflammatory state: a cause of chronic pain and other degenerative diseases?** *J Manipulative Physiol Ther.* 2002;25(3):168-79

[48] Eaton SB, Shostak M, Konner M. The Paleolithic Prescription: A program of diet & exercise and a design for living. New York: Harper & Row, 1988

[49] O'Keefe JH Jr, Cordain L. Cardiovascular disease resulting from a diet and lifestyle at odds with our Paleolithic genome: how to become a 21st-century hunter-gatherer. *Mayo Clin Proc.* 2004 Jan;79(1):101-8

details. This diet is the most nutrient-dense diet available, and its benefits are further enhanced by supplementation with vitamins, minerals, probiotics, and the health-promoting polyunsaturated fatty acids: ALA, GLA, EPA, DHA.

- Anti-inflammatory nutrients and botanicals: Nutritional and botanical therapeutics are prescribed *per patient* and *per condition*. Select botanicals and therapeutics are detailed later in this book. Doses listed are for adults and can be reduced when numerous interventions are simultaneously applied.

  - Fish oil, EPA with DHA: Three grams per day (3,000 mg/d) of combined EPA and DHA is a reasonable therapeutic dose[53] and is generally supplied in one tablespoon of liquid fish oil. Encapsulated fish oil supplements vary tremendously in their concentration of EPA and DHA and may require consumption of as few as five and as many as 21 capsules per day to achieve the same dosage and of EPA+DHA found in one tablespoon of liquid fish oil; encapsulated fish oil supplements also generally cost significantly more than do liquid fish oil supplements. The routine use of eicosapentaenoic acid (EPA) and docosahexaenoic acid (DHA) supplements is justified based on the following data:

    1. Most modern diets are profoundly deficient in omega-3 fatty acids.[54]
    2. Dietary/supplemental intake of omega-3 fatty acids is a necessary prerequisite to reducing the pro-inflammatory effects of omega-6 fatty acids.[55]
    3. Supplementation with EPA+DHA is safe and reduces all-cause mortality.[56]
    4. Supplementation with EPA+DHA consistently provides clinically significant benefits in the treatment of a wide range of inflammatory conditions.[57,58]

  - GLA, Gamma-linolenic acid: Approximately 500 mg per day is the common anti-inflammatory dose[59] although higher doses of 2.8 grams per day have been safely used in patients with rheumatoid arthritis.[60] Except in the rarest circumstances (perhaps including temporal lobe epilepsy[61]), **GLA (most concentrated in borage oil) should always be co-administered with EPA and DHA (from fish oil) in order to obtain maximal benefit and avoid the increased formation of arachidonic acid that occurs when GLA is administered alone and the reduction in GLA/DGLA that occurs when fish oil is administered alone.** For more details on fatty acid metabolism, see the final chapter in this text on *Therapeutics* and the 2005 fatty acid review published by Vasquez available on-line.[62]

  - *Uncaria guianensis* and *Uncaria tomentosa* ("cat's claw", "una de gato")*: A double-blind placebo-controlled study using 100 mg daily of highly-concentrated freeze-dried aqueous extract of *Uncaria tomentosa* found significant pain relief (reduction by 36%) and minimal adverse effects after 4 weeks of treatment in 30 male patients with osteoarthritis of the knees, a benefit mediated via antioxidant activities and inhibition of NF-kappaB, TNFα, COX-2, and PGE-2 production.[63] Inhibition of NF-kappaB and iNOS are of primary importance in the treatment of inflammatory conditions.[64] A year-long study of patients with active rheumatoid

[50] Cordain L. The Paleo Diet: Lose Weight and Get Healthy by Eating the Food You Were Designed to Eat. Indianapolis; John Wiley and Sons, 2002

[51] **Vasquez A. A Five-Part Nutritional Protocol that Produces Consistently Positive Results. *Nutritional Wellness* 2005 September Available in the printed version and on-line at** http://www.nutritionalwellness.com/archives/2005/sep/09_vasquez.php **and** http://optimalhealthresearch.com/protocol

[52] **Vasquez A. Implementing the Five-Part Nutritional Wellness Protocol for the Treatment of Various Health Problems. *Nutritional Wellness* 2005 November. Available on-line at** http://www.nutritionalwellness.com/archives/2005/nov/11_vasquez.php **and** http://optimalhealthresearch.com/protocol

[53] "...clinical benefits of the n-3 fatty acids were not apparent until they were consumed for > or =12 wk. It appears that a minimum daily dose of 3 g eicosapentaenoic and docosahexaenoic acids is necessary to derive the expected benefits [in patients with rheumatoid arthritis]." Kremer JM. n-3 fatty acid supplements in rheumatoid arthritis. *AmJ Clin Nutr*. 2000;71(1Suppl):349S-51S

[54] Simopoulos AP. Essential fatty acids in health and chronic disease. *Am J Clin Nutr*. 1999 Sep;70(3 Suppl):560S-569S

[55] Rubin D, Laposata M. Cellular interactions between n-6 and n-3 fatty acids: a mass analysis of fatty acid elongation/desaturation, distribution among complex lipids, and conversion to eicosanoids. *J Lipid Res*. 1992 Oct;33(10):1431-40.

[56] "The recent GISSI (Gruppo Italiano per lo Studio della Sopravvivenza nell'Infarto miocardico)-Prevention study of 11,324 patients showed a 45% decrease in risk of sudden cardiac death and a 20% reduction in all-cause mortality in the group taking 850 mg/d of omega-3 fatty acids. These fatty acids have potent anti-inflammatory effects and may also be antiatherogenic." O'Keefe JH Jr, Harris WS. From Inuit to implementation: omega-3 fatty acids come of age. *Mayo Clin Proc*. 2000 Jun;75(6):607-14

[57] "Many of the placebo-controlled trials of fish oil in chronic inflammatory diseases reveal significant benefit, including decreased disease activity and a lowered use of anti-inflammatory drugs." Simopoulos AP. Omega-3 fatty acids in inflammation and autoimmune diseases. *J Am Coll Nutr*. 2002 Dec;21(6):495-505

[58] **Vasquez A. Reducing Pain and Inflammation Naturally. Part 2: New Insights into Fatty Acid Supplementation and Its Effect on Eicosanoid Production and Genetic Expression. *Nutritional Perspectives* 2005; January: 5-16** www.optimalhealthresearch.com/part2

[59] "Forty patients with rheumatoid arthritis and upper gastrointestinal lesions due to non-steroidal anti-inflammatory drugs entered a prospective 6-month double-blind placebo controlled study of dietary supplementation with gamma-linolenic acid 540 mg/day..." Brzeski M, Madhok R, Capell HA. Evening primrose oil in patients with rheumatoid arthritis and side-effects of non-steroidal anti-inflammatory drugs. *Br J Rheumatol*. 1991 Oct;30(5):370-2

[60] Zurier RB, Rossetti RG, Jacobson EW, DeMarco DM, Liu NY, Temming JE, White BM, Laposata M. gamma-Linolenic acid treatment of rheumatoid arthritis. A randomized, placebo-controlled trial. *Arthritis Rheum*. 1996 Nov;39(11):1808-17

[61] "Three long-stay, hospitalised schizophrenics who had failed to respond adequately to conventional drug therapy were treated with gamma-linolenic acid and linoleic acid in the form of evening primrose oil. They became substantially worse and electroencephalographic features of temporal lobe epilepsy became apparent." Vaddadi KS. The use of gamma-linolenic acid and linoleic acid to differentiate between temporal lobe epilepsy and schizophrenia. *Prostaglandins Med*. 1981 Apr;6(4):375-9

[62] Vasquez A. Reducing Pain and Inflammation Naturally. Part 2: New Insights into Fatty Acid Supplementation and Its Effect on Eicosanoid Production and Genetic Expression. *Nutritional Perspectives* 2005; January: 5-16 www.optimalhealthresearch.com/part2

[63] Piscoya J, Rodriguez Z, Bustamante SA, Okuhama NN, Miller MJ, Sandoval M. Efficacy and safety of freeze-dried cat's claw in osteoarthritis of the knee: mechanisms of action of the species Uncaria guianensis. *Inflamm Res*. 2001 Sep;50(9):442-8

[64] Sandoval-Chacon M, Thompson JH, Zhang XJ, Liu X, Mannick EE, Sadowska-Krowicka H, Charbonnet RM, Clark DA, Miller MJ. Antiinflammatory actions of cat's claw: the role of NF-kappaB. *Aliment Pharmacol Ther*. 1998 Dec;12(12):1279-89

arthritis (RA) treated with sulfasalazine or hydroxychloroquine showed "relative safety and modest benefit" of coadministration of *Uncaria tomentosa*.[65] Other studies with *Uncaria tomentosa* have shown enhancement of post-vaccination immunity[66] and enhancement of DNA repair in humans.[67] Traditional uses have included the use of the herb as a contraceptive and as treatment for gastrointestinal ulcers.

o   <u>Topical application of *Capsicum annuum*, *Capsicum frutescens* (Cayenne pepper, hot chili pepper)</u>: Controlled clinical trials have conclusively demonstrated capsaicin's ability to deplete sensory fibers of substance P to thus reduce pain. Capsaicin also blocks transport and de-novo synthesis of substance P. Topical capsaicin alleviates diabetic neuropathy[68], chronic low back pain[69], chronic neck pain[70], osteoarthritis[71], rheumatoid arthritis[72], notalgia paresthetica[73], reflex sympathetic dystrophy[74], and cluster headache (intranasal application).[75,76,77] Doctors should experiment on themselves with this treatment before administering to patients in order to gain understanding by experience.

o   *Boswellia serrata*: *Boswellia* inhibits 5-lipoxygenase[78] with no apparent effect on cyclooxygenase[79] and has been shown effective in the treatment of osteoarthritis of the knees[80] as well as asthma[81] and ulcerative colitis.[82] When used as monotherapy, the target dose is approximately 150 mg of boswellic acids TID.

o   *Zingiber officinale* (Ginger): Ginger is a well known spice and food with a long history of use as an anti-inflammatory, anti-nausea, and gastroprotective agent[83], and components of ginger have been shown to reduce production of the leukotriene LTB4 by inhibiting 5-lipoxygenase and to reduce production of the prostaglandin PGE2 by inhibiting cyclooxygenase.[84,85] With its dual reduction in the formation of pro-inflammatory prostaglandins and leukotrienes, ginger has been shown to safely reduce nonspecific musculoskeletal pain[86,87] and to provide relief from osteoarthritis of the knees[88] and migraine headaches.[89] Ginger can be consumed somewhat liberally as a supplement or as whole food, and it is safe for use in pregnancy up to one gram per day.[90]

o   *Harpagophytum procumbens* (Devil's claw): The safety and effectiveness of *Harpagophytum* has been established in patients with hip pain, low-back pain, and knee pain.[91,92,93] The mechanisms of action include weak anti-inflammatory effects and a stronger analgesic

[65] "This small preliminary study demonstrates relative safety and modest benefit to the tender joint count of a highly purified extract from the pentacyclic chemotype of UT in patients with active RA taking sulfasalazine or hydroxychloroquine." Mur E, Hartig F, Eibl G, Schirmer M. Randomized double blind trial of an extract from the pentacyclic alkaloid-chemotype of uncaria tomentosa for the treatment of rheumatoid arthritis. *J Rheumatol.* 2002 Apr;29(4):678-81

[66] "...Uncaria tomentosa or Cat's Claw which is known to possess immune enhancing and antiinflammatory properties in animals. There were no toxic side effects observed as judged by medical examination, clinical chemistry and blood cell analysis. However, statistically significant immune enhancement for the individuals on C-Med-100 supplement was observed..." Lamm S, Sheng Y, Pero RW. Persistent response to pneumococcal vaccine in individuals supplemented with a novel water soluble extract of Uncaria tomentosa, C-Med-100. *Phytomedicine.* 2001;8(4):267-74

[67] Sheng Y, Li L, Holmgren K, Pero RW. DNA repair enhancement of aqueous extracts of Uncaria tomentosa in a human volunteer study. *Phytomedicine.* 2001 Jul;8(4):275-82

[68] "Study results suggest that topical capsaicin cream is safe and effective in treating painful diabetic neuropathy. "[No authors listed] Treatment of painful diabetic neuropathy with topical capsaicin. A multicenter, double-blind, vehicle-controlled study. The Capsaicin Study Group. *Arch Intern Med.* 1991 Nov;151(11):2225-9

[69] Keitel W, Frerick H, Kuhn U, Schmidt U, Kuhlmann M, Bredehorst A. Capsicum pain plaster in chronic non-specific low back pain. *Arzneimittelforschung.* 2001 Nov;51(11):896-903

[70] Mathias BJ, Dillingham TR, Zeigler DN, Chang AS, Belandres PV. Topical capsaicin for chronic neck pain. A pilot study. *Am J Phys Med Rehabil* 1995 Jan-Feb;74(1):39-44

[71] McCarthy GM, McCarty DJ. Effect of topical capsaicin in the therapy of painful osteoarthritis of the hands. *J Rheumatol.* 1992;19(4):604-7

[72] Deal CL, Schnitzer TJ, Lipstein E, Seibold JR, Stevens RM, Levy MD, Albert D, Renold F. Treatment of arthritis with topical capsaicin: a double-blind trial. *Clin Ther.* 1991 May-Jun;13(3):383-95

[73] Leibsohn E. Treatment of notalgia paresthetica with capsaicin. *Cutis* 1992 May;49(5):335-6

[74] "Capsaicin is effective for psoriasis, pruritus, and cluster headache; it is often helpful for the itching and pain of postmastectomy pain syndrome, oral mucositis, cutaneous allergy, loin pain/hematuria syndrome, neck pain, amputation stump pain, and skin tumor; and it may be beneficial for neural dysfunction (detrusor hyperreflexia, reflex sympathetic dystrophy, and rhinopathy)." Hautkappe M, Roizen MF, Toledano A, Roth S, Jeffries JA, Ostermeier AM. Review of the effectiveness of capsaicin for painful cutaneous disorders and neural dysfunction. *Clin J Pain* 1998 Jun;14(2):97-106

[75] "Capsaicin application to human nasal mucosa was found to induce painful sensation, sneezing, and nasal secretion. All of these factors exhibit desensitization upon repeated applications." Sicuteri F, Fusco BM, Marabini S, Campagnolo V, Maggi CA, Geppetti P, Fanciullacci M. Beneficial effect of capsaicin application to the nasal mucosa in cluster headache. *Clin J Pain.* 1989;5(1):49-53

[76] "The efficacy of repeated nasal applications of capsaicin in cluster headache is congruent with previous reports on the therapeutic effect of capsaicin in other pain syndromes (post-herpetic neuralgia, diabetic neuropathy, trigeminal neuralgia) and supports the use of the drug to produce a selective analgesia." Fusco BM, Marabini S, Maggi CA, Fiore G, Geppetti P. Preventative effect of repeated nasal applications of capsaicin in cluster headache. *Pain.* 1994 Dec;59(3):321-5

[77] "These results indicate that intranasal capsaicin may provide a new therapeutic option for the treatment of this disease." Marks DR, Rapoport A, Padla D, Weeks R, Rosum R, Sheftell F, Arrowsmith F. A double-blind placebo-controlled trial of intranasal capsaicin for cluster headache. *Cephalalgia.* 1993 Apr;13(2):114-6

[78] Wildfeuer A, Neu IS, Safayhi H, Metzger G, Wehrmann M, Vogel U, Ammon HP. Effects of boswellic acids extracted from a herbal medicine on the biosynthesis of leukotrienes and the course of experimental autoimmune encephalomyelitis. *Arzneimittelforschung* 1998 Jun;48(6):668-74

[79] Safayhi H, Mack T, Sabieraj J, Anazodo MI, Subramanian LR, Ammon HP. Boswellic acids: novel, specific, nonredox inhibitors of 5-lipoxygenase. *J Pharmacol Exp Ther* 1992 Jun;261(3):1143-6

[80] Kimmatkar N, Thawani V, Hingorani L, Khiyani R. Efficacy and tolerability of Boswellia serrata extract in treatment of osteoarthritis of knee--a randomized double blind placebo controlled trial. *Phytomedicine.* 2003 Jan;10(1):3-7

[81] Gupta I, Gupta V, Parihar A, Gupta S, Ludtke R, Safayhi H, Ammon HP. Effects of Boswellia serrata gum resin in patients with bronchial asthma: results of a double-blind, placebo-controlled, 6-week clinical study. *Eur J Med Res.* 1998 Nov 17;3(11):511-4

[82] Gupta I, Parihar A, Malhotra P, Singh GB, Ludtke R, Safayhi H, Ammon HP. Effects of Boswellia serrata gum resin in patients with ulcerative colitis. *Eur J Med Res.* 1997 Jan;2(1):37-43

[83] Langner E, Greifenberg S, Gruenwald J. Ginger: history and use. *Adv Ther* 1998 Jan-Feb;15(1):25-44

[84] Kiuchi F, Iwakami S, Shibuya M, Hanaoka T, Sankawa U. Inhibition of prostaglandin and leukotriene biosynthesis by gingerols and diarylheptanoids. *Chem Pharm Bull* (Tokyo) 1992 Feb;40(2):387-91

[85] Tjendraputra E, Tran VH, Liu-Brennan D, Roufogalis BD, Duke CC. Effect of ginger constituents and synthetic analogues on cyclooxygenase-2 enzyme in intact cells. *Bioorg Chem* 2001 Jun;29(3):156-63

[86] Srivastava KC, Mustafa T. Ginger (Zingiber officinale) in rheumatism and musculoskeletal disorders. *Med Hypotheses.* 1992 Dec;39(4):342-8

[87] Srivastava KC, Mustafa T. Ginger (Zingiber officinale) and rheumatic disorders. *Med Hypotheses.* 1989 May;29(1):25-8

[88] Altman RD, Marcussen KC. Effects of a ginger extract on knee pain in patients with osteoarthritis. *Arthritis Rheum.* 2001 Nov;44(11):2531-8

[89] Mustafa T, Srivastava KC. Ginger (Zingiber officinale) in migraine headache. *J Ethnopharmacol.* 1990 Jul;29(3):267-73

[90] "...oral ginger 1 g per day... No adverse effect of ginger on pregnancy outcome was detected." Vutyavanich T, Kraisarin T, Ruangsri R. Ginger for nausea and vomiting in pregnancy: randomized, double-masked, placebo-controlled trial. *Obstet Gynecol* 2001 Apr;97(4):577-82.

[91] Chrubasik S, Thanner J, Kunzel O, Conradt C, Black A, Pollak S. Comparison of outcome measures during treatment with the proprietary Harpagophytum extract doloteffin in patients with pain in the lower back, knee or hip. *Phytomedicine* 2002 Apr;9(3):181-94

[92] Chantre P, Cappelaere A, Leblan D, Guedon D, Vandermander J, Fournie B. Efficacy and tolerance of Harpagophytum procumbens versus diacerhein in treatment of osteoarthritis. *Phytomedicine* 2000 Jun;7(3):177-83

[93] Leblan D, Chantre P, Fournie B. Harpagophytum procumbens in the treatment of knee and hip osteoarthritis. Four-month results of a prospective, multicenter, double-blind trial versus diacerhein. *Joint Bone Spine* 2000;67(5):462-7

effect.[94,95] Research suggests that *Harpagophytum* is an effective analgesic for low back pain[96], including low back pain with radiculitis and radiculopathy.[97] The common dose is 60 mg harpagoside per day.[98]

o   *Willow bark (Salix spp)*: In a double-blind placebo-controlled clinical trial in 210 patients with moderate/severe low-back pain (20% of patients had positive straight-leg raising test), willow bark extract showed a dose-dependent analgesic effect with benefits beginning in the first week of treatment.[99] In a head-to-head study of 228 patients comparing willow bark (standardized for 240 mg salicin) with Vioxx (rofecoxib), treatments were equally effective yet willow bark was safer and 40% less expensive.[100] Because willow bark's salicylates were the original source for the chemical manufacture of acetylsalicylic acid (aspirin), researchers and clinicians have erroneously mistaken willow bark to be synonymous with aspirin; this is certainly inaccurate and therefore clarification of willow's mechanism of action will be provided here. Aspirin has two primary effects via three primary mechanisms of action: 1) anticoagulant effects mediated by the acetylation and permanent inactivation of thromboxane-A synthase, which is the enzyme that makes the powerfully proaggregatory thromboxane-A2; 2) antiprostaglandin action via acetylation of both isoforms of cyclooxygenase (COX-1 inhibition 25-166x more than COX-2) with widespread inhibition of prostaglandin formation, and 3) antiprostaglandin formation via retroconversion of acetylsalicylate into salicylic acid which then inhibits cyclooxygenase-2 gene transcription.[101] Notice that the acetylation reactions are specific to aspirin and thus actions #1 and #2 are not seen with willow bark; whereas #3 — inhibition of COX-2 transcription by salicylates — appears to be the major mechanism of action of willow bark extract. Proof of this principle is supported by the lack of adverse effects associated with willow bark in the research literature. If willow bark were pharmacodynamically synonymous with aspirin, then we would expect case reports of gastric ulceration, hemorrhage, and Reye's syndrome to permeate the research literature; this is not the case and therefore — **with the exception of possible allergic reactions in patients previously allergic/anaphylactic to aspirin and salicylates — extensive "warnings" on willow bark products[102] are unnecessary.**[103] Salicylates are widely present in fruits, vegetables, herbs and spices and are partly responsible for the anti-cancer, anti-inflammatory, and health-promoting benefits of fruit and vegetable consumption.[104,105] With willow bark products, the daily dose should not exceed 240 mg of salicin, and products should include other components of the whole plant. **Except for rare allergy in patients previously sensitized to aspirin or salicylates, no adverse effects are known**; to be on the medicolegal safe side, use is discouraged during pregnancy, before surgery, or when anti-coagulant medications are being used.

Treat with physical/manual medicine:

- Massage: Gentle massage provides comfort, increases circulation, reduces edema, and promotes healing. After the acute phase, deeper massage may help restore range of motion by breaking adhesions and reducing the feeling of vulnerability that may occur after injury. Research indicates that massage can reduce adolescent aggression[106], improve outcome in preterm infants[107], alleviate

[94] Whitehouse LW, Znamirowska M, Paul CJ. Devil's Claw (Harpagophytum procumbens): no evidence for anti-inflammatory activity in the treatment of arthritic disease. *Can Med Assoc J* 1983 Aug 1;129(3):249-51

[95] Moussard C, Alber D, Toubin MM, Thevenon N, Henry JC. A drug used in traditional medicine, harpagophytum procumbens: no evidence for NSAID-like effect on whole blood eicosanoid production in human. *Prostaglandins Leukot Essent Fatty Acids* 1992 Aug;46(4):283-6

[96] Chrubasik S, Model A, Black A, Pollak S. A randomized double-blind pilot study comparing Doloteffin and Vioxx in the treatment of low back pain. *Rheumatology* (Oxford). 2003 Jan;42(1):141-8

[97] "The majority of responders' were patients who had suffered less than 42 days of pain, and subgroup analyses suggested that the effect was confined to patients with more severe and radiating pain accompanied by neurological deficit... There was no evidence for Harpagophytum-related side-effects, except possibly for mild and infrequent gastrointestinal symptoms." Chrubasik S, Junck H, Breitschwerdt H, Conradt C, Zappe H. Effectiveness of Harpagophytum extract WS 1531 in the treatment of exacerbation of low pain: a randomized, placebo-controlled, double-blind study. *Eur J Anaesthesiol* 1999 Feb;16(2):118-29

[98] "They took an 8-week course of Doloteffin at a dose providing 60 mg harpagoside per day... Doloteffin is well worth considering for osteoarthritic knee and hip pain and nonspecific low back pain." Chrubasik S, Thanner J, Kunzel O, Conradt C, Black A, Pollak S. Comparison of outcome measures during treatment with the proprietary Harpagophytum extract doloteffin in patients with pain in the lower back, knee or hip. *Phytomedicine* 2002 Apr;9(3):181-94

[99] Chrubasik S, Eisenberg E, Balan E, Weinberger T, Luzzati R, Conradt C. Treatment of low-back pain exacerbations with willow bark extract: a randomized double-blind study. *Am J Med*. 2000;109:9-14

[100] Chrubasik S, Kunzel O, Model A, Conradt C, Black A. Treatment of low-back pain with a herbal or synthetic anti-rheumatic: a randomized controlled study. Willow bark extract for low-back pain. *Rheumatology* (Oxford). 2001;40:1388-93

[101] Hare LG, Woodside JV, Young IS. Dietary salicylates. *J Clin Pathol* 2003 Sep;56(9):649-50 http://jcp.bmj.com/cgi/content/full/56/9/649

[102] Clauson KA, Santamarina ML, Buettner CM, Cauffield JS. Evaluation of Presence of Aspirin-Related Warnings with Willow Bark (July/August). *Ann Pharmacother*. 2005 May 31; [Epub ahead of print]

[103] **Vasquez A, Muanza DN. Evaluation of Presence of Aspirin-Related Warnings with Willow Bark: Comment on the Article by Clauson et al. *Ann Pharmacotherapy* 2005 Oct;39(10):1763**

[104] Lawrence JR, Peter R, Baxter GJ, Robson J, Graham AB, Paterson JR. Urinary excretion of salicyluric and salicylic acids by non-vegetarians, vegetarians, and patients taking low dose aspirin. *J Clin Pathol*. 2003 Sep;56(9):651-3

[105] Paterson JR, Lawrence JR. Salicylic acid: a link between aspirin, diet and the prevention of colorectal cancer. *QJM*. 2001 Aug;94(8):445-8 http://qjmed.oxfordjournals.org/cgi/content/full/94/8/445

[106] Diego MA, Field T, Hernandez-Reif M, Shaw JA, Rothe EM, Castellanos D, Mesner L. Aggressive adolescents benefit from massage therapy. *Adolescence* 2002 Fall;37(147):597-607

premenstrual syndrome[108], improve flexibility, reduce pain, increase serotonin and dopamine in patients with low back pain[109], and improve function and alleviate depression in patients with Parkinson's disease (Alexander technique).[110]

- <u>Joint mobilization and manipulation</u> as appropriate (after contraindications have been excluded) and to the level of patient comfort. Mechanisms of action are listed later in this section.
- <u>Treatment of associated muscle spasm and myofascial trigger points (MFTP)</u>: Such treatment can increase range of motion and decrease pain. See notes on the diagnosis and treatment of MFTP in the following section in this chapter.
- <u>Consider physiotherapy</u>: As appropriate.[111]

Uncover the underlying problem:

- In the case of most acute injuries, the underlying problem is often the injury itself. However, the physician must not be overly naïve and must conduct a thorough history and examination to assess for possible underlying pathologies that cause or contribute to the problem that "appears" to be injury related. Congenital anomalies, underlying pathology, previous injury, and psychoemotional disorders may have been present before the "injury."
    o **In children and young adults, 5% of "sports-related" injuries are associated with preexisting infection, anomalies, or other conditions.**
    o In adult women: "In three cases of carcinoma, the breast mass was not noticed until after the [auto accident] and was initially thought by the patient to have been caused by the trauma. **Indeed between 9% and 20% of women with breast cancer attribute their symptoms to previous trauma to the breast**."[112]
- Look for leg length inequalities and biomechanical faults such as hyperpronation and pelvic torque.
- Assess and correct poor posture, poor ergonomics, lack of flexibility, muscle strength imbalances, and proprioceptive/coordination deficits.
- Patients may experience a reduction in pain—particularly low-back pain and osteoarthritis pain—when they eliminate coffee/caffeine, food allergens, and/or specific foods to which they are sensitive, most notably the *Solanaceae*/nightshade family—eggplant, tobacco, tomatoes, potatoes, and bell peppers. Foods in the *Solanaceae* family contain anti-acetylcholinesterases[113] that may effect increased synaptic transmission of afferent pain sensations, particularly via NMDA receptors.
- Correction of **diet-induced chronic metabolic acidosis** with the use of alkalinizing diets/supplements[114] can alleviate musculoskeletal pain[115], at least in part by raising/normalizing intracellular magnesium levels and by reducing intracellular calcium levels. Additional benefits of alkalinization include increased mineral retention, reduced bone resorption[116] and enhanced clearance of toxic xenobiotics[117], especially many pesticides and pharmacologic agents.

[107] Mainous RO. Infant massage as a component of developmental care: past, present, and future. *Holist Nurs Pract* 2002 Oct;16(5):1-7
[108] Hernandez-Reif M, Martinez A, Field T, Quintero O, Hart S, Burman I. Premenstrual symptoms are relieved by massage therapy. *J Psychosom Obstet Gynaecol* 2000 Mar;21(1):9-15
[109] "RESULTS: By the end of the study, the massage therapy group, as compared to the relaxation group, reported experiencing less pain, depression, anxiety and improved sleep. They also showed improved trunk and pain flexion performance, and their serotonin and dopamine levels were higher." Hernandez-Reif M, Field T, Krasnegor J, Theakston H. Lower back pain is reduced and range of motion increased after massage therapy. *Int J Neurosci* 2001;106(3-4):131-45
[110] Stallibrass C, Sissons P, Chalmers C. Randomized controlled trial of the Alexander technique for idiopathic Parkinson's disease. *Clin Rehabil* 2002 Nov;16(7):695-708
[111] Download the free notes at http://www.OptimalHealthResearch.com/physiotherapy
[112] Seifert S. Medical Illness Simulating Trauma (MIST) syndrome: case reports and discussion of syndrome. *Fam Med* 1993 Apr;25(4):273-6
[113] Krasowski MD, McGehee DS, Moss J. Natural inhibitors of cholinesterases: implications for adverse drug reactions. *Can J Anaesth*. 1997 May;44(5 Pt 1):525-34 www.cja-jca.org/cgi/reprint/44/5/525.pdf
[114] For long-term out-patient treatment of patients who do not achieve alkalinization with diet alone, oral administration of potassium citrate and/or sodium bicarbonate can be implemented. See the following article for concepts: "Urine alkalinization is a treatment regimen that increases poison elimination by the administration of intravenous sodium bicarbonate to produce urine with a pH > or = 7.5." Proudfoot AT, Krenzelok EP, Vale JA. Position Paper on urine alkalinization. *J Toxicol Clin Toxicol*. 2004;42:1-26
http://www.eapcct.org/publicfile.php?folder=congress&file=PS_UrineAlkalinization.pdf Also see: Vormann J, Worlitschek M, Goedecke T, Silver B. Supplementation with alkaline minerals reduces symptoms in patients with chronic low back pain. *J Trace Elem Med Biol*. 2001;15(2-3):179-83 Also see: Maurer M, Riesen W, Muser J, Hulter HN, Krapf R. Neutralization of Western diet inhibits bone resorption independently of K intake and reduces cortisol secretion in humans. *Am J Physiol Renal Physiol*. 2003 Jan;284(1):F32-40. Epub 2002 Sep 24.
http://ajprenal.physiology.org/cgi/content/full/284/1/F32
[115] "The results show that a disturbed acid-base balance may contribute to the symptoms of low back pain. The simple and safe addition of an alkaline multimineral preparate was able to reduce the pain symptoms in these patients with chronic low back pain." Vormann J, Worlitschek M, Goedecke T, Silver B. Supplementation with alkaline minerals reduces symptoms in patients with chronic low back pain. *J Trace Elem Med Biol*. 2001;15(2-3):179-83
[116] "In postmenopausal women, the oral administration of potassium bicarbonate at a dose sufficient to neutralize endogenous acid improves calcium and phosphorus balance, reduces bone resorption, and increases the rate of bone formation." Sebastian A, Harris ST, Ottaway JH, Todd KM, Morris RC Jr. Improved mineral balance and skeletal metabolism in postmenopausal women treated with potassium bicarbonate. *N Engl J Med*. 1994 Jun 23;330(25):1776-81 http://content.nejm.org/cgi/content/abstract/330/25/1776
[117] "Urine alkalinization is a treatment regimen that increases poison elimination by the administration of intravenous sodium bicarbonate to produce urine with a pH > or = 7.5." Proudfoot AT, Krenzelok EP, Vale JA. Position Paper on urine alkalinization. *J Toxicol Clin Toxicol*. 2004;42:1-26 http://www.eapcct.org/publicfile.php?folder=congress&file=PS_UrineAlkalinization.pdf

Re-educate, rehabilitate, resourcefulness, return to active life, reassure, referral:
- Educate patient on ways to avoid re-injury and to decrease likelihood of recurrence.
- Pre-rehabilitation assessment has three main goals: 1) identification of the type of injury, 2) quantification of the severity of the injury, and 3) determining the appropriate interventions.[118] Rehabilitative exercises **emphasizing strength, coordination, proprioception, range of motion, and functional utility** (appropriate per occupation and hobbies) should be employed.
- **Isometric exercises** can be used to maintain/increase muscle strength in patients for whom range-of-motion exercises are painful or contraindicated.
- **Work hardening** has been defined by the American Physical Therapy Association as "a highly structured goal-oriented, individualized treatment program designed to return a person to work. Work Hardening programs...use real or simulated work activities designed to restore physical, behavioral, and vocational functions."[119] Teperman[120] defined the specific goals of work hardening as:
    1. Improved lifting strength (loading and unloading) to/from different heights, including overhead,
    2. Improved carrying capacity (various objects, different distances, unilateral and bilateral),
    3. Improved functional tolerance (coordination and manipulation) at different levels,
    4. Improved cardiovascular endurance,
    5. Improved dexterity tasks (counting, weighing, sorting, packaging/unpacking)
    6. Improved biomechanics in any setting (work/leisure).
- **Work conditioning** has been defined as "a work-related, intensive, and goal-oriented treatment program specifically designed to restore an individual's systemic, neuromuscular (strength, endurance, flexibility, etc.) and cardiopulmonary function."[121] While overlaps exist between work hardening and work conditioning, and both are generally designed to "return the patient to work", work hardening is focused more on the performance of work-related tasks (task-oriented) while work conditioning tends to focus more on the cardiopulmonary and neuromuscular fitness of the patient (fitness-oriented).
- **Rehabilitation can become more than *restorative*; if the plan is comprehensive and it effects long-term improvements in overall health, then such a program can become *transformative*.** For example, while the oversimplified medical model as commonly practiced in HMO and PPO systems might describe a patient's problem as "low-back pain, refer for physiotherapy and begin Vioxx 25 mg b.i.d.", a more comprehensive assessment and treatment of the same patient's problem might be described as "low-back pain secondary to sedentary lifestyle, obesity, mild systemic inflammation, hypovitaminosis D, and proprioceptive deficits. Begin program of daily general exercise along with specific exercises for low-back region, low-carbohydrate diet to promote weight loss, balance training twice daily, begin supplementation with cholecalciferol 4,000 IU/d and fish oil 3 g/d." Notice that the typical allopathic plan *requires* and *thus ensures* patient passivity and does nothing to promote overall health, whereas the comprehensive natural/integrative plan is more in accord with current biomedical literature, requires active patient participation, offers the probability of improved overall health, and will reduce the severity and risk of present and future diseases, respectively.
- Patients should be supported in the tolerance of minor discomfort to avoid overuse of analgesics, to avoid an excessive reduction in activities, and to avoid playing the "sick role." While validating the patient's concerns, physicians should not encourage dysfunctional behavior or contribute to "iatrogenic neurosis."
- **Symptomatic treatment that provides no lasting benefit can foster therapeutic dependency and therapeutic passivity.** "Therapeutic dependency" describes the situation wherein the patient becomes dependent on treatment sessions for secondary gain of attention, physical contact, and time off from work (etc.) rather than focusing on the goal of getting as healthy as possible as quickly as possible. Therapeutic dependency is fostered by doctors who fail to educate patients to take an active role in

---

[118] Geffen SJ. 3: Rehabilitation principles for treating chronic musculoskeletal injuries. *Med J Aust.* 2003 Mar 3;178(5):238-42

[119] American Physical Therapy Association, "Guidelines for Programs for Injured Workers" 1995. Quoted by Washington State Department of Labor and Industries. http://www.lni.wa.gov/Main/MostAskedQuestions/ClaimsIns/WorkHardFaq.asp. Accessed July 23, 2006

[120] Teperman LJ. Active functional restoration and work hardening program returns patient with 2½-year-old elbow fracture-dislocation to work after 6 months: a case report. *J Can Chiropr Assoc* 2002; 46(1): 22-30 http://www.jcca-online.org/client/cca/JCCA.nsf/objects/Active+functional+restoration+elbow+fracture-dislocation/$file/5-Teperman.pdf

[121] Howar JM. Keys to Effective Work Hardening and Limited Duty Programs. http://www.eh.doe.gov/feosh/contacts/LimitedDutyPrograms.pdf Accessed July 23, 2006. Ironically, even though the third page of this presentation clearly shows the use of spinal manipulation, chiropractic doctors are notably absent from the list of "Industrial Rehab Specialists" having been usurped even by Occupational Nurses.

their own care and by doctors who take on the role of "savior" rather than empowering patients to take effective action in improving their health. **Therapeutic passivity** is related to **therapeutic dependency** since patients who fail to take responsible action tend to become dependent on healthcare providers to "cure me" and "rescue me."

- While detailed individual descriptions of therapeutic exercise and rehabilitative programs are not the subject of this book, we can readily appreciate the many options that are available to us for the rehabilitation of injuries:

  o Therapeutic exercise: Includes strength training, stretching, improving endurance, and functional training specific to the patient's occupational or athletic activities. These can be tailored to great detail to the patient's condition and goals.[122]

  o Proprioceptive retraining/rehabilitation: As discussed later in this chapter, restoration and optimization of proprioceptive function and balance control is especially important for the long-term functional improvement of patients with proprioceptive deficits, commonly seen in patients with chronic low-back pain[123], neck pain[124], knee arthritis[125], and ankle instability.[126]

  o Weight optimization: For the majority of patients living in our society where obesity is pandemic, weight reduction is important not only to improve overall health and to reduce mechanical stresses on joints, but perhaps even more importantly to reduce the production of proinflammatory chemicals made in adipose tissue (adipokines) which promote an overall internal climate of pain and inflammation. Some patients may need to gain muscle strength to promote healing and avoid re-injury; this can generally be achieved with resistance training and increased protein consumption.

  o Eicosanoid modulation: Historically, the balance of omega-3 to omega-6 fatty acids in the human diet has been approximately 1:1 or 1:2.[127] Since omega-3 fatty acids are generally *anti-inflammatory* while omega-6 fatty acids are generally proinflammatory (with the exception of GLA/DGLA), the former *quantitative* dietary balance translated to a *qualitative* balance with regard to the body's inherent inflammatory tendency. Modern diets today, however, provide a ratio of 1:30, with anti-inflammatory omega-3 fatty acids greatly outnumbered by the proinflammatory omega-6 fatty acids. Thus, human physiology has been altered by the widespread consumption of a *pro-inflammatory diet*.[128] Correction of this problem at the level of dietary intake rather than by the use of anti-inflammatory medications is essential for the attainment of health and the long-term relief of pain and inflammation.[129,130]

  o Alkalinization: The American/Western style of eating results in subclinical diet-induced pathogenic chronic metabolic acidosis[131] which can be corrected with a Paleo-Mediterranean diet[132] or alkalinizing supplements[133] for the alleviation of musculoskeletal pain in general and low-back pain in particular.[134]

  o Analgesia: Safe and effective natural means for achieving a timely reduction in pain include topical capsaicin, *Harpagophytum*, *Uncaria*, acupuncture, willow, and spinal manipulation.

  o Anti-inflammatory botanicals and nutraceuticals: Fish oil, GLA, vitamin E, *Boswellia*, willow bark, *Harpagophytum*, and *Zingiber* are just a few of the effective natural anti-inflammatory treatments available.

[122] Basmajian JV (ed). Therapeutic Exercise. Fourth Edition. Baltimore: Williams and Wilkins. 1984
[123] Newcomer KL, Jacobson TD, Gabriel DA, Larson DR, Brey RH, An KN. Muscle activation patterns in subjects with and without low back pain. Arch Phys Med Rehabil. 2002;83(6):816-21
[124] McPartland JM, Brodeur RR, Hallgren RC. Chronic neck pain, standing balance, and suboccipital muscle atrophy--a pilot study. J Manipulative Physiol Ther. 1997 Jan;20(1):24-9
[125] Callaghan MJ, Selfe J, Bagley PJ, Oldham JA. The Effects of Patellar Taping on Knee Joint Proprioception. J Athl Train. 2002 Mar;37(1):19-24
[126] Olmsted LC, Carcia CR, Hertel J, Shultz SJ. Efficacy of the Star Excursion Balance Tests in Detecting Reach Deficits in Subjects With Chronic Ankle Instability. J Athl Train. 2002 Dec;37(4):501-506
[127] Simopoulos AP. Essential fatty acids in health and chronic disease. Am J Clin Nutr. 1999 Sep;70(3 Suppl):560S-569S
[128] Seaman DR. The diet-induced proinflammatory state: a cause of chronic pain and other degenerative diseases? J Manipulative Physiol Ther. 2002;25(3):168-79
[129] Vasquez A. A Five-Part Nutritional Protocol that Produces Consistently Positive Results. Nutritional Wellness 2005 September Available in the printed version and on-line at http://www.nutritionalwellness.com/archives/2005/sep/09_vasquez.php and http://optimalhealthresearch.com/protocol
[130] Vasquez A. Dietary, Nutritional and Botanical Interventions to Reduce Pain and Inflammation. Naturopathy Digest 2006, March Nutritional Wellness 2006, March http://optimalhealthresearch.com/archives/anti-inflammation-nutrition
[131] "As a result, healthy adults consuming the standard US diet sustain a chronic, low-grade pathogenic metabolic acidosis that worsens with age as kidney function declines." Cordain L, Eaton SB, Sebastian A, Mann N, Lindeberg S, Watkins BA, O'Keefe JH, Brand-Miller J. Origins and evolution of the Western diet: health implications for the 21st century. Am J Clin Nutr. 2005 Feb;81(2):341-54 http://www.ajcn.org/cgi/content/full/81/2/341
[132] Cordain L. The Paleo Diet: Lose Weight and Get Healthy by Eating the Food You Were Designed to Eat. Indianapolis; John Wiley and Sons, 2002
[133] "An acidogenic Western diet results in mild metabolic acidosis in association with a state of cortisol excess, altered divalent ion metabolism, and increased bone resorptive indices." Maurer M, Riesen W, Muser J, Hulter HN, Krapf R. Neutralization of Western diet inhibits bone resorption independently of K intake and reduces cortisol secretion in humans. Am J Physiol Renal Physiol. 2003 Jan;284(1):F32-40. Epub 2002 Sep 24. http://ajprenal.physiology.org/cgi/content/full/284/1/F32
[134] "The results show that a disturbed acid-base balance may contribute to the symptoms of low back pain. The simple and safe addition of an alkaline multimineral preparate was able to reduce the pain symptoms in these patients with chronic low back pain." Vormann J, Worlitschek M, Goedecke T, Silver B. Supplementation with alkaline minerals reduces symptoms in patients with chronic low back pain. J Trace Elem Med Biol. 2001;15(2-3):179-83

- o <u>Treatment of myofascial trigger points</u>: Since joint injuries and chronic pain—*especially in the neck, back and shoulder*—are commonly associated with trigger points[135], addressing this secondary and occult cause of pain is important to maximize pain relief and functional restoration.
- o <u>Manipulation, mobilization, and massage</u>: Joint manipulation has numerous physiologic and anatomic effects, most of which are relevant for the alleviation of pain and improvement of joint function. These mechanisms include:
    1. Releasing entrapped intraarticular menisci and synovial folds,
    2. Acutely reducing intradiscal pressure, thus promoting replacement of decentralized disc material,
    3. Stretching of deep periarticular muscles to break the cycle of chronic autonomous muscle contraction by lengthening the muscles and thereby releasing excessive actin-myosin binding,
    4. Promoting restoration of proper kinesthesia and proprioception,
    5. Promoting relaxation of paraspinal muscles by stretching facet joint capsules,
    6. Promoting relaxation of paraspinal muscles via "postactivation depression", which is the temporary depletion of contractile neurotransmitters,
    7. Temporarily elevating plasma beta-endorphin,
    8. Temporarily enhancing phagocytic ability of neutrophils and monocytes,
    9. Activating the diffuse descending pain inhibitory system located in the periaqueductal gray matter—this is an important aspect of nociceptive inhibition by intense sensory/mechanoreceptor stimulation, and
    10. Improving neurotransmitter balance and reducing pain (soft-tissue manipulation).[136]
    Additional details are provided in numerous published reviews and primary research[137,138,139,140,141,142,143] and by Leach[144], whose extensive description of the mechanisms of action of spinal manipulative therapy is unsurpassed. Given such a wide base of experimental and clinical support published in peer-reviewed journals and widely-available textbooks, denigrations directed toward spinal manipulation on the grounds that it is "unscientific" or "unsupported by research" are unfounded and are indicative of selective ignorance.[145]
- o <u>Reassurance</u>: Education, explanation, reassurance, and support help to address the mental and emotional aspects of injury.
- o <u>Referral</u>: **Patients with severe pain, serious conditions/complications, or documented noncompliance are excellent candidates for co-management or unidirectional referral**.
- Modify home and occupational workstations to minimize strain and stress on injured tissues. Educate patients to use tools, machines, props, and stepstools to work efficiently and to reduce unnecessary lifting and straining motions.
- Physical activities can be fully resumed when symptoms have decreased and when physical examination findings (e.g., reflexes, strength, range of motion, spinal segmental function, and trigger points) are within normal limits. Note that in many situations returning the patient to their previous duration, frequency, and intensity of activity may predispose to re-injury since the patient is re-entering the situation wherein the original injury occurred; therefore at least one of these lifestyle/occupational/recreational variables must change in order to reduce the likeliness of re-injury.
- Books, websites, and national/local support groups and organizations may be available for emotional, physical, psychological-emotional, and legal assistance.

[135] "The mean number of TrPs present on each neck pain patient was 4.3, of which 2.5 were latent and 1.8 were active TrPs. Control subjects also exhibited TrPs (mean: 2; SD: 0.8). All were latent TrPs." Fernandez-de-Las-Penas C, Alonso-Blanco C, Miangolarra JC. Myofascial trigger points in subjects presenting with mechanical neck pain: A blinded, controlled study. *Man Ther*. 2006 Jun 10
[136] "RESULTS: By the end of the study, the massage therapy group, as compared to the relaxation group, reported experiencing less pain, depression, anxiety and improved sleep. They also showed improved trunk and pain flexion performance, and their serotonin and dopamine levels were higher." Hernandez-Reif M, Field T, Krasnegor J, Theakston H. Lower back pain is reduced and range of motion increased after massage therapy. *Int J Neurosci* 2001;106(3-4):131-45
[137] Maigne JY, Vautravers P. Mechanism of action of spinal manipulative therapy. *Joint Bone Spine*. 2003;70(5):336-41
[138] Brennan PC, Triano JJ, McGregor M, Kokjohn K, Hondras MA, Brennan DC. Enhanced neutrophil respiratory burst as a biological marker for manipulation forces: duration of the effect and association with substance P and tumor necrosis factor. *J Manipulative Physiol Ther*. 1992 Feb;15(2):83-9
[139] Brennan PC, Kokjohn K, Kaltinger CJ, Lohr GE, Glendening C, Hondras MA, McGregor M, Triano JJ. Enhanced phagocytic cell respiratory burst induced by spinal manipulation: potential role of substance P. *J Manipulative Physiol Ther*. 1991 Sep;14(7):399-408
[140] Heikkila H, Johansson M, Wenngren BI. Effects of acupuncture, cervical manipulation and NSAID therapy on dizziness and impaired head repositioning of suspected cervical origin: a pilot study. *Man Ther*. 2000 Aug;5(3):151-7
[141] Rogers RG. The effects of spinal manipulation on cervical kinesthesia in patients with chronic neck pain: a pilot study. *J Manipulative Physiol Ther*. 1997;20(2):80-5
[142] Bergman, Peterson, Lawrence. <u>Chiropractic Technique</u>. New York: Churchill Livingstone 1993. An updated edition is now availabe published by Mosby.
[143] Herzog WH. Mechanical and physiological responses to spinal manipulative treatments. *JNMS: J Neuromusculoskeletal System* 1995; 3: 1-9
[144] Leach RA. (ed). <u>The Chiropractic Theories: A Textbook of Scientific Research, Fourth Edition</u>. Baltimore: Lippincott, Williams & Wilkins, 2004
[145] Vasquez A. The Science of Chiropractic and Spinal Manipulation, Part 2. http://www.mercola.com/2005/mar/12/chiropractic_spine.htm

Nutrition:

- Protein: In otherwise healthy patients with no liver, renal, or other metabolic disorders, ensure adequate intake of 0.5-0.9 gram of protein per pound of body weight.[146] Vegetarians may heal more slowly after injury than do omnivores; vegetarians and lacto-vegetarians undergoing cosmetic surgery reportedly have more complications and slower healing than do people eating a diet containing meat.[147] Additionally, low-protein diets have shown to reduce muscle mass and suppress immune function.[148] See the table below for protein intake recommendations:

Recommended Grams of Protein Per Pound of Body Weight Per Day[149]	
Infants and children ages 1-6 years[150]	0.68-0.45
RDA for sedentary adult and children ages 6-18 years[151]	0.4
Adult recreational exerciser	**0.5-0.75**
Adult competitive athlete	0.6-0.9
Adult building muscle mass	0.7-0.9
Dieting athlete	0.7-1.0
Growing teenage athlete	0.9-1.0
Pregnant women need additional protein	Add 15-30 grams/day[152]

- Water: Adequate intake of water is important to flush out wastes, toxins, and to prevent constipation. Eight glasses per day is the classic recommendation; however increased fluid intake is appropriate during exercise, heat exposure, stress, and to promote clearance of nitrogenous wastes and xenobiotics. Fluid restriction may be appropriate for persons with adrenal insufficiency to avoid hyponatremia and those with cardiovascular failure, fluid overload, or edema.

- Vegetables, fruit, and fiber: Whole foods provide micronutrients, natural anti-inflammatory components, and immune modulators; the fiber/phytonutrient content provides positive effects on gut flora while maintaining proper waste elimination and reducing straining (e.g., reduced need for the Valsalva maneuver).

- Carbohydrates: Carbohydrate intake should be adequate to supply energy-expenditure needs and to support healing but should not be excessive such as to unfavorably increase body weight during times of decreased physical activity. Preferred sources of carbohydrates are fruits and vegetables.

- Identification and elimination of adverse food reactions: Adverse food reactions—regardless of the underlying mechanism(s) or classification of allergy, intolerance, or sensitivity—can precipitate joint pain and inflammation[153,154,155,156,157,158,159] and a wide range of other health problems.

- Supplementation with a high-potency broad-spectrum multivitamin and multimineral product: This will help correct common nutritional deficiencies and support optimal healing. Certain nutrients such as vitamin C, zinc, and copper are commonly considered "specific" for promoting optimal repair of connective tissue.

- Specific supplements/botanicals: Supplementation is tailored to the type of tissue that has been injured, such as calcium, magnesium, and vitamins D and K for bone fractures, glucosamine sulfate and niacinamide for cartilage injuries, and proteolytic enzymes for muscle strains.
    - Niacinamide: The niacinamide form of vitamin B3 was proven effective against osteoarthritis by Kaufman more than 50 years ago.[160] Furthermore, Kaufman's documentation of an "anti-aging" effect of vitamin supplementation in general and niacinamide therapy in particular[161]

[146] Nancy Clark, MS, RD. The Power of Protein. *The Physician and Sportsmedicine* 1996, volume 24, number 4. http://www.physsportsmed.com/issues/1996/04_96/protein.htm
[147] Vegetarians and healing. *JAMA* 1995; 273: 910
[148] Castaneda C, Charnley JM, Evans WJ, Crim MC. Elderly women accommodate to a low-protein diet with losses of body cell mass, muscle function, and immune response. *Am J Clin Nutr* 1995 Jul;62(1):30-9
[149] Slightly modified from Nancy Clark, MS, RD. The Power of Protein. *The Physician and Sportsmedicine* 1996, volume 24, number 4
[150] 1.5-1 g/kg/d (0.68-0.45 grams per pound of body weight. Younger people need proportionately more protein.) Brown ML (ed). Present Knowledge in Nutrition. Sixth Edition. Washington DC: International Life Sciences Institute Nutrition Foundation; 1990 page 68
[151] 0.83 g.kg-1.d-1 (equivalent to 0.37 grams per pound of body weight) "By use of an age-specific scoring system and the mean amino acid composition and digestibility of the US diet, this allowance became 0.83 g.kg-1.d-1 of mixed US dietary protein--a value similar to the previous RDA but derived in a different manner." Pellet PL. Protein requirements in humans. *Am J Clin Nutr*. 1990 May;51(5):723-37
[152] Weinsier RL, Morgan SL (eds). Fundamentals of Clinical Nutrition. St. Louis: Mosby, 1993 page 50
[153] Golding DN. Is there an allergic synovitis? *J R Soc Med*. 1990 May;83(5):312-4
[154] Panush RS. Food induced ("allergic") arthritis: clinical and serologic studies. *J Rheumatol*. 1990 Mar;17(3):291-4
[155] Pacor ML, Lunardi C, Di Lorenzo G, Biasi D, Corrocher R. Food allergy and seronegative arthritis: report of two cases. *Clin Rheumatol*. 2001;20(4):279-81
[156] Schrander JJ, Marcelis C, de Vries MP, van Santen-Hoeufft HM. Does food intolerance play a role in juvenile chronic arthritis? *Br J Rheumatol*. 1997 Aug;36(8):905-8
[157] van de Laar MA, van der Korst JK. Food intolerance in rheumatoid arthritis. I. A double blind, controlled trial of the clinical effects of elimination of milk allergens and azo dyes. *Ann Rheum Dis*. 1992 Mar;51(3):298-302
[158] Haugen MA, Kjeldsen-Kragh J, Forre O. A pilot study of the effect of an elemental diet in the management of rheumatoid arthritis. *Clin Exp Rheumatol*. 1994 May-Jun;12(3):275-9
[159] van de Laar MA, Aalbers M, Bruins FG, van Dinther-Janssen AC, van der Korst JK, Meijer CJ. Food intolerance in rheumatoid arthritis. II. *Ann Rheum Dis*. 1992 Mar;51(3):303-6
[160] Kaufman W. Niacinamide therapy for joint mobility. Therapeutic reversal of a common clinical manifestation of the "normal" aging process. *Conn State Med J* 1953;17:584-591
[161] Kaufman W. The use of vitamin therapy to reverse certain concomitants of aging. *J Am Geriatr Soc* 1955;3:927-936

is consistent with recent experimental data demonstrating rapid reversion of aging phenotypes by niacinamide through modulation of histone acetylation.[162] A recent double-blind placebo-controlled repeat study found that niacinamide therapy improved joint mobility, reduced objective inflammation as assessed by ESR, reduced the impact of the arthritis on the activities of daily living, and allowed a reduction in analgesic/anti-inflammatory medication use.[163] While the mechanism of action is probably multifaceted, inhibition of joint-destroying nitric oxide appears to be an important benefit.[164] The standard dose of 500 mg given orally 6 times per day is more effective than 1,000 mg 3 times per day. Hepatic dysfunction is rare when daily doses are kept below 3,000 mg per day, yet Gaby[165] suggests measurement of liver enzymes after 3 months of treatment and yearly thereafter. Antirheumatic benefit is generally significant following 2-6 weeks of treatment, and patients may also notice an anxiolytic benefit, possibly mediated by the binding of niacinamide to GABA/benzodiazepine receptors.[166]

- o Glucosamine sulfate and chondroitin sulfate: Glucosamine and chondroitin are the "building blocks" from which cartilage is built and oral supplementation is intended to enhance cartilage anabolism and to thus counteract the enhanced cartilage catabolism seen in destructive arthritic processes.[167] Clinical trials with glucosamine and chondroitin sulfates have shown consistently positive results in clinical trials involving patients with osteoarthritis of the hands, hips, knees, temporomandibular joint, and low-back.[168,169,170,171,172,173,174] For example, glucosamine sulfate was superior to placebo for pain reduction and preservation of joint space in a 3-year clinical trial in patients with knee osteoarthritis.[175] Arguments against the use of glucosamine due to inflated concern about inefficacy or exacerbation of diabetes[176] are without scientific merit[177,178] as evidenced by a 90-day trial of diabetic patients consuming 1500 mg of glucosamine hydrochloride with 1200 mg of chondroitin sulfate which showed no significant alterations in serum glucose or hemoglobin A1c[179] and by the previously cited 3-year study which found significant clinical benefit and no adverse effects on glucose homeostasis.[180] The adult dose of glucosamine sulfate is generally 1500-2000 mg per day in divided doses, and the dose of chondroitin sulfate is approximately 1000 mg daily; these treatments can be used singly, in combination, and with other treatments. Both treatments are safe for multiyear use, and rare adverse effects include allergy and nonpathologic gastrointestinal upset. Clinical benefit is generally significant following 4-6 weeks of treatment and is maintained for the duration of treatment. In contrast to coxib and other mislabeled "anti-inflammatory" drugs that consistently elevate the incidence of cardiovascular disease, death, and other adverse effects[181,182,183,184,185], supplementation with

[162] Matuoka K, Chen KY, Takenawa T. Rapid reversion of aging phenotypes by nicotinamide through possible modulation of histone acetylation. *Cell Mol Life Sci.* 2001;58(14):2108-16
[163] Jonas WB, Rapoza CP, Blair WF. The effect of niacinamide on osteoarthritis: a pilot study. *Inflamm Res* 1996 Jul;45(7):330-4
[164] McCarty MF, Russell AL. Niacinamide therapy for osteoarthritis--does it inhibit nitric oxide synthase induction by interleukin 1 in chondrocytes? *Med Hypotheses.* 1999;53(4):350-60
[165] Gaby AR. Literature review and commentary: Niacinamide for osteoarthritis. *Townsend Letter for Doctors and Patients.* 2002: May; 32
[166] Mohler H, Polc P, Cumin R, Pieri L, Kettler R. Nicotinamide is a brain constituent with benzodiazepine-like actions. *Nature.* 1979; 278(5704): 563-5
[167] Vidal y Plana RR, Bizzarri D, Rovati AL. Articular cartilage pharmacology: I. In vitro studies on glucosamine and non steroidal antiinflammatory drugs. *Pharmacol Res Commun.* 1978 Jun;10(6):557-69
[168] "...patients taking GS had a significantly greater decrease in TMJ pain with function, effects of pain, and acetaminophen used between Day 90 and 120 compared with patients taking ibuprofen." Thie NM, Prasad NG, Major PW. Evaluation of glucosamine sulfate compared to ibuprofen for the treatment of temporomandibular joint osteoarthritis: a randomized double blind controlled 3 month clinical trial. *J Rheumatol.* 2001;28(6):1347-55
[169] Braham R, Dawson B, Goodman C. The effect of glucosamine supplementation on people experiencing regular knee pain. *Br J Sports Med.* 2003;37(1):45-9
[170] "...oral glucosamine therapy achieved a significantly greater improvement in articular pain score than ibuprofen, and the investigators rated treatment efficacy as 'good' in a significantly greater proportion of glucosamine than ibuprofen recipients. In comparison with piroxicam, glucosamine significantly improved arthritic symptoms after 12 weeks of therapy..." Matheson AJ, Perry CM. Glucosamine: a review of its use in the management of osteoarthritis. *Drugs Aging.* 2003; 20(14): 1041-60
[171] Uebelhart D, Malaise M, Marcolongo R, DeVathaire F, Piperno M, Mailleux E, Fioravanti A, Matoso L, Vignon E. Intermittent treatment of knee osteoarthritis with oral chondroitin sulfate: a one-year, randomized, double-blind, multicenter study versus placebo. *Osteoarthritis Cartilage.* 2004;12:269-76
[172] van Blitterswijk WJ, van de Nes JC, Wuisman PI. Glucosamine and chondroitin sulfate supplementation to treat symptomatic disc degeneration: biochemical rationale and case report. *BMC Complement Altern Med.* 2003;3(1):2
[173] Morreale P, Manopulo R, Galati M, Boccanera L, Saponati G, Bocchi L. Comparison of the antiinflammatory efficacy of chondroitin sulfate and diclofenac sodium in patients with knee osteoarthritis. *J Rheumatol.* 1996;23(8):1385-91
[174] Mazieres B, Combe B, Phan Van A, Tondut J, Grynfeltt M. Chondroitin sulfate in osteoarthritis of the knee: a prospective, double blind, placebo controlled multicenter clinical study. *J Rheumatol.* 2001;28(1):173-81
[175] Reginster JY, Deroisy R, Rovati LC, Lee RL, Lejeune E, Bruyere O, Giacovelli G, Henrotin Y, Dacre JE, Gossett C. Long-term effects of glucosamine sulphate on osteoarthritis progression: a randomised, placebo-controlled clinical trial. *Lancet.* 2001;357(9252):251-6
[176] Adams ME. Hype about glucosamine. *Lancet.* 1999;354(9176):353-4
[177] Cumming A. Glucosamine in osteoarthritis. *Lancet.* 1999;354(9190):1640-1
[178] Rovati LC, Annefeld M, Giacovelli G, Schmid K, Setnikar I. *Glucosamine in osteoarthritis.* Lancet. 1999;354(9190):1640
[179] Scroggie DA, Albright A, Harris MD. The effect of glucosamine-chondroitin supplementation on glycosylated hemoglobin levels in patients with type 2 diabetes mellitus: a placebo-controlled, double-blinded, randomized clinical trial. *Arch Intern Med.* 2003;163(13):1587-90
[180] Reginster JY, Deroisy R, Rovati LC, Lee RL, Lejeune E, Bruyere O, Giacovelli G, Henrotin Y, Dacre JE, Gossett C. Long-term effects of glucosamine sulphate on osteoarthritis progression: a randomised, placebo-controlled clinical trial. *Lancet.* 2001;357(9252):251-6
[181] Topol EJ. Failing the public health--rofecoxib, Merck, and the FDA. *N Engl J Med.* 2004 Oct 21;351(17):1707-9
[182] Mukherjee D, Nissen SE, Topol EJ. Risk of cardiovascular events associated with selective cox-2 inhibitors. *JAMA* 2001; 286(8):954-9
[183] Ray WA, Griffin MR, Stein CM. Cardiovascular toxicity of valdecoxib. *N Engl J Med.* 2004;351(26):2767

chondroitin sulfate appears to safely reduce the pain and disability associated with osteoarthritis while simultaneously reducing incidence of cardiovascular morbidity and mortality.[186,187] In a study with animals that spontaneously develop atherosclerosis[188], administration of chondroitin sulfate induced regression of existing atherosclerosis. In a six-year study with 120 patients with established cardiovascular disease, 60 chondroitin-treated patients suffered 6 coronary events and 4 deaths compared to 42 events and 14 deaths in a comparable group of 60 patients receiving "conventional" therapy; chondroitin-treated patients reported enhancement of well-being while no adverse clinical or laboratory effects were noted during the 6 years of treatment.[189]

o Pancreatic/proteolytic enzymes: Orally-administered pancreatic and proteolytic enzymes are absorbed from the gastrointestinal tract into the systemic circulation[190,191] to exert analgesic, anti-inflammatory, anti-edematous benefits with therapeutic relevance for acute and chronic musculoskeletal disorders.[192,193,194,195]

o Vitamin C: Doses of 1-2 grams per day have been suggested to reduce pain and the need for surgery in patients with low-back pain by improving disc integrity.[196] Vitamin C reduces production of isoprostanes, which promote inflammation and pain. Ascorbate is also necessary for the production of the anti-inflammatory prostaglandin E-1. Supplemental vitamin C may also reduce the severity and progression of osteoarthritis.[197]

o Vitamin E, with an emphasis on gamma-tocopherol: The *gamma* form of vitamin E inhibits cyclooxygenase and thus has anti-inflammatory activity.[198] Clinical trials and case reports have suggested benefit of vitamin E supplementation in patients with rheumatoid arthritis[199,200], spondylosis and back pain[201], osteoarthritis[202,203,204], and autoimmune diseases including scleroderma, discoid lupus erythematosus, porphyria cutanea tarda, vasculitis, and polymyositis.[205,206,207]

[184] "Patients in the clinical trial taking 400 mg. of Celebrex twice daily had a 3.4 times greater risk of CV events compared to placebo. For patients in the trial taking 200 mg. of Celebrex twice daily, the risk was 2.5 times greater. The average duration of treatment in the trial was 33 months." FDA Statement on the Halting of a Clinical Trial of the cox-2 Inhibitor Celebrex. http://www.fda.gov/bbs/topics/news/2004/NEW01144.html Available on January 4, 2005

[185] "Preliminary information from the study showed some evidence of increased risk of cardiovascular events, when compared to placebo, to patients taking naproxen." FDA Statement on Naproxen. http://www.fda.gov/bbs/topics/news/2004/NEW01148.html Available on January 4, 2005

[186] Morrison LM. Treatment of coronary arteriosclerotic heart disease with chondroitin sulfate-A: preliminary report. *J Am Geriatr Soc.* 1968;16(7):779-85

[187] Morrison LM, Branwood AW, Ershoff BH, Murata K, Quilligan JJ Jr, Schjeide OA, Patek P, Bernick S, Freeman L, Dunn OJ, Rucker P. The prevention of coronary arteriosclerotic heart disease with chondroitin sulfate A: preliminary report. *Exp Med Surg.* 1969;27(3):278-89

[188] Morrison LM, Bajwa GS. Absence of naturally occurring coronary atherosclerosis in squirrel monkeys (Saimiri sciurea) treated with chondroitin sulfate A. *Experientia.* 1972 Dec 15;28(12):1410-1

[189] Morrison LM, Enrick N. Coronary heart disease: reduction of death rate by chondroitin sulfate A. *Angiology.* 1973 May;24(5):269-87

[190] Gotze H, Rothman SS. Enteropancreatic circulation of digestive enzymes as a conservative mechanism. *Nature* 1975; 257(5527): 607-609

[191] Liebow C, Rothman SS. Enteropancreatic Circulation of Digestive Enzymes. *Science* 1975; 189(4201): 472-474

[192] Trickett P. Proteolytic enzymes in treatment of athletic injuries. *Appl Ther.* 1964;30:647-52

[193] Walker JA, Cerny FJ, Cotter JR, Burton HW. Attenuation of contraction-induced skeletal muscle injury by bromelain. *Med Sci Sports Exerc.* 1992 Jan;24(1):20-5

[194] Walker AF, Bundy R, Hicks SM, Middleton RW. Bromelain reduces mild acute knee pain and improves well-being in a dose-dependent fashion in an open study of otherwise healthy adults. *Phytomedicine.* 2002; 9: 681-6

[195] Brien S, Lewith G, Walker A, Hicks SM, Middleton D. Bromelain as a Treatment for Osteoarthritis: a Review of Clinical Studies. *Evidence-based Complementary and Alternative Medicine.* 2004;1(3)251–257

[196] Greenwood J. Optimum vitamin C intake as a factor in the preservation of disc integrity. *Med Ann Dist Columbia.* 1964 Jun;33:274-6

[197] "A 3-fold reduction in risk of OA progression was found for both the middle tertile and highest tertile of vitamin C intake. This related predominantly to a reduced risk of cartilage loss. Those with high vitamin C intake also had a reduced risk of developing knee pain." McAlindon TE, Jacques P, Zhang Y, Hannan MT, Aliabadi P, Weissman B, Rush D, Levy D, Felson DT. Do antioxidant micronutrients protect against the development and progression of knee osteoarthritis? *Arthritis Rheum.* 1996 Apr;39(4):648-56

[198] Jiang Q, Christen S, Shigenaga MK, Ames BN. gamma-tocopherol, the major form of vitamin E in the US diet, deserves more attention. *Am J Clin Nutr* 2001 Dec;74(6):714-22

[199] Helmy M, Shohayeb M, Helmy MH, el-Bassiouni EA. Antioxidants as adjuvant therapy in rheumatoid disease. A preliminary study. *Arzneimittelforschung.* 2001;51(4):293-8

[200] Edmonds SE, Winyard PG, Guo R, Kidd B, Merry P, Langrish-Smith A, Hansen C, Ramm S, Blake DR. Putative analgesic activity of repeated oral doses of vitamin E in the treatment of rheumatoid arthritis. Results of a prospective placebo controlled double blind trial. *Ann Rheum Dis.* 1997 Nov;56(11):649-55

[201] "Vitamin E administration at a dose of 100 mg daily for three weeks resulted in a significant increase in serum vitamin E level accompanied by complete relief of pain... The results therefore strongly indicate that vitamin E is effective in curing spondylosis and most probably due to its antioxidant activity." Mahmud Z, Ali SM. Role of vitamin A and E in spondylosis. *Bangladesh Med Res Counc Bull.* 1992 Apr;18(1):47-59

[202] "The results of this double-blind controlled clinical trial showed that vitamin E was superior to placebo with respect to the relief of pain (pain at rest, pain during movement, pressure-induced pain) and the necessity of additional analgetic treatment. Improvement of mobility was better in the group treated with vitamin E." Blankenhorn G. [Clinical effectiveness of Spondyvit (vitamin E) in activated arthroses. A multicenter placebo-controlled double-blind study] [Article in German] *Z Orthop Ihre Grenzgeb.* 1986 May-Jun;124(3):340-3

[203] This is a very interesting study because the clinical response to vitamin E was proportional to the increase in plasma levels of vitamin E, thus confirming the dose-response relationship that implies causality as well as indicating that the failure of such treatment in some patients may be due to malabsorption or unquenchable systemic oxidative stress rather than the inefficacy of vitamin E supplementation, per se. "There were no significant differences in the efficacy of the two drugs, although one patient of the V-group refused further treatment after 8 days because of inefficacy. V reduced or abolished the pain at rest in 77% (D in 85%), the pain on pressure in 67% (D in 50%), and the pain on movement in 62% (D in 63%). Both treatments appeared to be equally effective in reducing the circumference of the knee joints (p = 0.001) and the walking time (p less than 0.001) and in increasing the joint mobility (p less than 0.002)." Scherak O, Kolarz G, Schodl C, Blankenhorn G. [High dosage vitamin E therapy in patients with activated arthrosis] [Article in German] *Z Rheumatol.* 1990 Nov-Dec;49(6):369-73

[204] Machtey I, Ouaknine L. Tocopherol in Osteoarthritis: a controlled pilot study. *J Am Geriatr Soc.* 1978 Jul;26(7):328-30

[205] Killeen RN, Ayres S Jr, Mihan R. Polymyositis: response to vitamin E. *South Med J.* 1976 Oct;69(10):1372-4

[206] Ayres S Jr, Mihan R. Lupus erythematosus and vitamin E: an effective and nontoxic therapy. *Cutis.* 1979 Jan;23(1):49-52, 54

[207] Ayres S Jr, Mihan R. Is vitamin E involved in the autoimmune mechanism? *Cutis.* 1978 Mar;21(3):321-5

Myofascial trigger points (MFTP)

<u>Description/pathophysiology</u>:

- Many patients suffer from chronic pain that originates from myofascial trigger points—localized areas within muscle tissue that produce chronic pain, promote muscle contraction and tightness, and which mediate autonomous autonomic responses. Physicians who take the time to locate and treat MFTP and educate patients about effective home care can often rapidly and permanently reduce their patients' pain in a safe and highly cost-effective manner.
- MFTP have been defined as "a highly localized and hyperirritable spot in a palpable taut band of skeletal muscle fibers"[208] characterized by the following:
  1. <u>Referred pain with compression</u>: Digital compression of the MFTP causes local pain and most often causes referred pain in a distribution similar or identical to the patient's presenting complaint. The distribution of pain may appear radicular and may thus be described as "pseudoradicular."
  2. <u>Twitch response</u>: When digital pressure is applied perpendicularly to the direction of muscle fibers at the location of the MFTP and the muscle is "plucked" or allowed to "snap" as if one were plucking a taut rubber band or the string of a guitar, the muscle being assessed undergoes a rapid contraction.
  3. <u>Muscle tightness</u>: The muscle involved is tighter than usual, and it is resistant to stretch.
  4. <u>Associated autonomic phenomena</u>: Regions of the body near a localized MFTP may display associated autonomic dysregulation such as vasoconstriction, sweating, pilomotor response, and the patient may experience nausea, dizziness, light-headedness[209] or atrial fibrillation.[210]
  5. <u>MFTP may be "active" or "latent"</u>: Active MFTP are those which cause spontaneous pain with joint motion or muscle contraction, whereas latent MFTP cause pain only when provoked by an examiner's deep palpation and physical compression. [211]
  6. <u>Normal muscle strength</u>: Muscle weakness and atrophy are not associated with MFTP unless the weakness or atrophy is secondary to pain.
- The initiation and perpetuation of MFTP is complex and commonly associated with previous injury or chronic static posturing (such as sitting in front of a computer for 8-14 hours per day) and also with emotional stress. Since **intrafusal fibers of muscle spindles receive direct sympathetic innervation**, and since adrenaline/epinephrine directly increases the contractile tone and tension of muscles, it is reasonable to conclude that attention to emotional stress and stress management techniques should be part of the comprehensive treatment plan for MFTP. A significant reduction in emotional tension and work-related repetitive strain injuries may follow a comprehensive and "body-based" approach to healthy living and appropriate career choices.[212]
- The pathogenesis and physiology-based treatment of MFTP follow this route are as follows:
  <u>Pathogenesis</u>[213]
  1. Excess calcium is released from the sarcoplasmic reticulum, leading to local muscle fiber contraction.
  2. Intense and chronic muscle contractions cause relative local ischemia.
  3. The reduction in local blood supply limits energy replacement and leads to the depletion of adenosine triphosphate (ATP).
  4. The muscle cell now has insufficient ATP for the active return of calcium from the contractile elements to the sarcoplasmic reticulum, thus maintaining the muscle fibers in a contracted state.

[208] Hong CZ, Simons DG. Pathophysiologic and electrophysiologic mechanisms of myofascial trigger points. *Arch Phys Med Rehabil*. 1998;79(7):863-72
[209] Hubbard DR, Berkoff GM. Myofascial trigger points show spontaneous needle EMG activity. *Spine*. 1993 Oct 1;18(13):1803-7
[210] Simons DG. Cardiology and myofascial trigger points: Janet G. Travell's contribution. *Tex Heart Inst J*. 2003;30(1):3-7
[211] Hubbard DR, Berkoff GM. Myofascial trigger points show spontaneous needle EMG activity. *Spine*. 1993 Oct 1;18(13):1803-7
[212] Jarrow R. <u>Creating the Work You Love: Courage, Commitment and Career</u>. Inner Traditions Intl Ltd; December 1995) [ISBN: 0892815426]
[213] Simons DG. Cardiology and myofascial trigger points: Janet G. Travell's contribution. *Tex Heart Inst J*. 2003;30(1):3-7

Physiology-based treatment:

5. Stretching the muscle fibers reduces the overlap between actin and myosin, which then leads to a reduction in energy demand of the cell and thus helps to "break the cycle" of **contraction** *leading to* **energy depletion** *leading to* **contraction** *leading to* **energy depletion...**

6. Application of ice (or other benign, intense afferent stimuli such as capsaicin or spinal manipulation) floods the dorsal horn and thus blocks transmission of nociceptive stimuli via the hypothesized "gate control" mechanism of pain reception.

7. Magnesium supplementation is appropriate for many patients with MFTP since many patients do not consume sufficient dietary magnesium and since magnesium inhibits calcium release from the sarcoplasmic reticulum[214] and thereby has a muscle relaxing effect. **Magnesium deficiency is an epidemic** in so-called "developed" nations, with 20-40% of different populations showing objective serologic/cytologic evidence of magnesium deficiency.[215,216,217,218]

Clinical presentations:

- The pain pattern from MFTP is varied and is dependent on the muscle(s) involved. Each muscle has a unique pattern of pain referral; e.g., a MFTP in the deltoid or supraspinatus may cause shoulder pain and arm pain that can mimic cervical radiculitis. MFTP in the sternocleidomastoid commonly causes "headache" and pain over the side of the face and TMJ; MFTP in the psoas can cause low back and leg pain. Patients may also subjectively notice numbness or tingling in addition to pain.[219] Differentiation of MFTP pain from radiculitis and radiculopathy should be pursued clinically and documented in the patient chart.

Major differential diagnoses:

- Arthropathy and arthritis: Passive joint provocation tests are negative with MFTP; no laboratory abnormalities (such as elevated CRP) are seen with MFTP.
- Acute muscle injury, strain: History of *recent* injury is often negative; history of *chronic* strain and *previous* injury are common with MFTP
- Radiculitis: The pain associated with MFTP is not dermatomal and is reproduced with local muscle compression, whereas the pain of radiculitis is dermatomal and reproduced with nerve tension tests.
- Radiculopathy: Radiculopathy is associated with muscle weakness, which is not a characteristic of MFTP.

Clinical assessments:

- History/subjective: Pain is always present (although it may be mild or latent).
- Physical examination/objective: The most reliable physical signs of MFTP are **1) spot tenderness within a taut band of muscle, 2) reproduction of pain and referred pain with palpation and provocation**, and 3) local twitch response with palpation and provocation.
- Imaging & laboratory assessments: Lab tests and imaging assessments are normal. Myofascial trigger points show spontaneous electromyographic activity.[220]

[214] "Mg2+ inhibits Ca2+ release from the sarcoplasmic reticulum." Mathew R, Altura BM. The role of magnesium in lung diseases: asthma, allergy and pulmonary hypertension. *Magnes Trace Elem*. 1991-92;10(2-4):220-8

[215] "The American diet is low in magnesium, and with modern water systems, very little is ingested in the drinking water." Innerarity S. Hypomagnesemia in acute and chronic illness. *Crit Care Nurs Q*. 2000 Aug;23(2):1-19

[216] "Altogether 43% of 113 trauma patients had low magnesium levels compared to 30% of noninjured cohorts." Frankel H, Haskell R, Lee SY, Miller D, Rotondo M, Schwab CW. Hypomagnesemia in trauma patients. *World J Surg*. 1999 Sep;23(9):966-9

[217] "There was a 20% overall prevalence of hypomagnesemia among this predominantly female, African American population." Fox CH, Ramsoomair D, Mahoney MC, Carter C, Young B, Graham R. An investigation of hypomagnesemia among ambulatory urban African Americans. *J Fam Pract*. 1999 Aug;48(8):636-9

[218] "Suboptimal levels were detected in 33.7 per cent of the population under study. These data clearly demonstrate that the Mg supply of the German population needs increased attention." Schimatschek HF, Rempis R. Prevalence of hypomagnesemia in an unselected German population of 16,000 individuals. *Magnes Res*. 2001 Dec;14(4):283-90

[219] Hubbard DR, Berkoff GM. Myofascial trigger points show spontaneous needle EMG activity. *Spine*. 1993 Oct 1;18(13):1803-7

[220] Hubbard DR, Berkoff GM. Myofascial trigger points show spontaneous needle EMG activity. *Spine*. 1993 Oct 1;18(13):1803-7

Establishing the diagnosis:
- Reasonable clinical exclusion of acute strain, radiculopathy and radiculitis combined with characteristic clinical findings mentioned above, including at least **1) spot tenderness within a taut band of muscle, 2) reproduction of pain and referred pain with palpation/provocation**.

Complications:
- Many patients with MFTP suffer from pain for years before being properly diagnosed. Many patients are prescribed hazardous and inappropriate medications to treat the pain and symptoms of MFTP, and surgical interventions are periodically used inappropriately in patents who have not been accurately diagnosed. For example when a patient with low back pain due to MFTP is found to have an incidental disc herniation, the patient may undergo surgery on the intervertebral disc only to have pain continue postoperatively until it is treated with simple techniques directed at the MFTP.[221]

Clinical management:
- Simple nutritional and physical treatments as described below.
- Patients should be advised that deep massage of the area is often necessary and that pain may be temporarily exacerbated.
- A sample of notes for educating patients about natural treatment for cervical MFTP and neck pain is available at http://OptimalHealthResearch.com/neck

Treatments:
- Post-isometric stretching: Lewit and Simons described this simple and highly effective treatment succinctly in a highly recommended article[222], "The post-isometric relaxation technique begins by placing the muscle in a stretched position. Then an isometric contraction is exerted against minimal resistance. Relaxation and then gentle stretch follow as the muscle releases." In a large study involving 244 patients, post-isometric stretching "produced **immediate pain relief in 94%, lasting pain relief in 63%**, as well as lasting relief of point tenderness in 23% of the sites treated. Patients who practiced autotherapy on a home program were more likely to realize lasting relief." Clinically the technique is simultaneously performed, explained, and taught by the clinician: 1) stretch the target muscle, 2) weakly contract the target muscle against resistance for 10 seconds, 3) stretch the target muscle to a greater length than before for at least 20 seconds, 4) repeat this procedure 2-3 times. Pretreatment heating or exercising of the target muscles along with post-treatment application of ice helps to increase treatment efficacy and minimize post-treatment soreness, respectively.
- Cold and stretch: The application of cold and the simultaneous stretching of the muscle is an effective treatment for MFTP.[223] Cold can be applied with ice. The previously popular "spray and stretch" technique that used a vapocoolant spray such as Fluori-Methane is unnecessary and is environmentally irresponsible.
- Topical application: Capsaicin helps to relieve neuromuscular pain, too, and may help break the cycle of pain and spasm by 1) providing afferent stimuli to block nociceptive stimuli, and 2) by depleting local tissues of substance P, which not only serves as a transmitter of pain sensations, but may also perpetuate muscle contraction and spasm. Another mechanism by which capsaicin can alleviate trigger points is by desensitizing the vanilloid receptor (VR-1) to ultimately decrease local neurotransmitter release.[224]
- Dry needling or injection of local anesthetic or saline: While local injection of anesthetic or saline may appear more complex and therefore more effective, dry needling (rapid insertion and withdrawal of a needle) directly into the MFTP is just as effective, safer, and is less complicated than using anesthetic or saline solution. Increased efficacy of this technique is associated with the elicitation of a local twitch response immediately upon insertion and withdrawal of the needle. The accuracy of the needle

---

[221] Rubin D. Myofascial trigger point syndromes: an approach to management. *Arch Phys Med Rehabil*. 1981 Mar;62(3):107-10
[222] Lewit K, Simons DG. Myofascial pain: relief by post-isometric relaxation. *Arch Phys Med Rehabil*. 1984 Aug;65(8):452-6
[223] Rubin D. Myofascial trigger point syndromes: an approach to management. *Arch Phys Med Rehabil*. 1981 Mar;62(3):107-10
[224] "Massage with capsaicin cream (0.075%, available over the counter) is useful for treating TrPs located in surgical scars,36 which are particularly refractory to treatment." McPartland JM. Travell trigger points--molecular and osteopathic perspectives. *J Am Osteopath Assoc*. 2004 Jun;104(6):244-9 http://www.jaoa.org/cgi/content/full/104/6/244

insertion directly into the "sensitive locus" of the MFTP is essential for the effectiveness of this approach. Common locations for MFTP correlate with commonly used acupuncture points, and the technique of acupuncture is analogous to the dry needling technique except that dry needling is performed more quickly and with highly localized precision into the MFTP sensitive locus. [225]

- <u>Adjunctive nutritional support</u>: Supplementation with **magnesium** (600 mg per day or to bowel tolerance[226]) and **calcium** are often helpful, particularly when used with an **alkalinizing Paleo-Mediterranean diet** (as discussed in Chapter 2), which—at the very least—promotes renal retention of calcium and magnesium to thus facilitate mineral retention. Other treatments to reduce intracellular calcium levels (intracellular hypercalcinosis[227]) include supplementation with **physiologic doses of vitamin D3**[228] and **fish oil for EPA**[229] along with avoidance/reduction of factors which promote renal loss of calcium and magnesium such as caffeine, sugar, alcohol/ethanol, and psychoemotional stress.

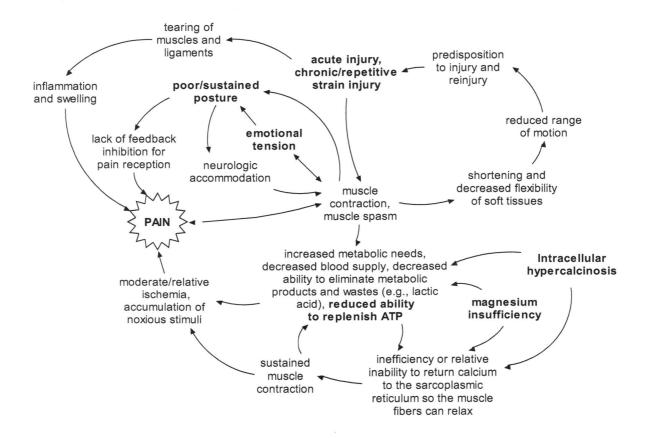

Hypothesized model for the initiation and promotion of myofascial trigger points with self-perpetuating cycles

[225] Hong CZ, Simons DG. Pathophysiologic and electrophysiologic mechanisms of myofascial trigger points. *Arch Phys Med Rehabil.* 1998 Jul;79(7):863-72
[226] "When the practitioner has been convinced to start Mg on the basis of his diagnosis or through insistence of the patient, the often recommended dose of 300 mg per day is insufficient. Experience of successful therapy indicates that no less than 600 mg per day is required." Liebscher DH, Liebscher DE. About the misdiagnosis of magnesium deficiency. *J Am Coll Nutr.* 2004 Dec;23(6):730S-1S http://www.coldcure.com/html/misdiagnosis-magnesium-deficiency.pdf
[227] See http://optimalhealthresearch.com/archives/intracellular-hypercalcinosis and www.naturopathydigest.com/archives/2006/sep/vasquez.php for additional discussion
[228] Vasquez A, Manso G, Cannell J. The clinical importance of vitamin D (cholecalciferol): a paradigm shift with implications for all healthcare providers. *Altern Ther Health Med.* 2004 Sep-Oct;10(5):28-36 http://optimalhealthresearch.com/monograph04
[229] "This is a consequence of the ability of EPA to release Ca2+ from intracellular stores while inhibiting their refilling via capacitative Ca2+ influx that results in partial emptying of intracellular Ca2+ stores and thereby activation of protein kinase R." Palakurthi SS, Fluckiger R, Aktas H, Changolkar AK, Shahsafaei A, Harneit S, Kilic E, Halperin JA. Inhibition of translation initiation mediates the anticancer effect of the n-3 polyunsaturated fatty acid eicosapentaenoic acid. *Cancer Res.* 2000 Jun 1;60(11):2919-25

Musculoskeletal Manipulation and Manual Medicine: Selection of Commonly Used Chiropractic and Osteopathic Techniques

Manual medicine in general and spinal manipulation in particular are mentioned in nearly every section of **Integrative Orthopedics**, and select techniques are described with accompanying text and photographs. Manipulative techniques are included in this textbook to remind practitioners of a few of the more useful and commonly applied maneuvers and to provide descriptions and citations for refinement of their application. However, the level of detail provided here is insufficient unless the reader has received hands-on professionally-supervised training in an accredited institution wherein other important concepts have been taught and implemented under experienced guidance. Competence and proficiency in the art and skill of manipulation cannot be learned from a textbook; these can only be approached with personal mentoring and in-person coursework amply provided in colleges and post-graduate trainings specializing in manipulative technique. **Manipulative medicine** is a *time-space* objective-subjective-intuitive **kinesthetic phenomenon** which might be described as occurring in four dimensions—*anteroposterior, transverse/horizontal, vertical,* and *chronological* due to variations in speed and power; all the while, the doctor is monitoring subjective and objective responses of the what might be considered the fifth dimension—the doctor's dynamic *perception of, influence upon,* and *interaction with* the patient's affect, posture, muscle tension, dynamic joint positioning, tissue response, and compressive tension. As the doctor assesses and provides force, the patient's response changes the target, and so the doctor must adapt to a constantly moving target—the lesion being treated.

These sections presume professional training by the reader has already been begun or completed and that the reader is familiar with manipulative concepts, technique, terminology, and commonly used abbreviations. Again, the intention here is to remind clinicians of manipulation in general and these specific techniques in particular; only a few *subjectively chosen* techniques are included from the several hundred vertebral, myofascial, visceral, and extravertebral/extremity maneuvers that are available.

General Layout and Description of Manipulative Techniques	
Patient position:	• Patient position may be prone, supine, lateral recumbent or "side-posture", standing, or seated
Doctor position:	• Usually standing, either *upright, forward flexed,* or using an oblique *fencer's stance*; knees are almost always bent in order to bring doctor's torso near treatment area to increase mechanical force from the upper limbs
Assessment:	• <u>Subjective</u>: Patient's experience, sensations, and effect on daily living • <u>Motion palpation</u>: Intersegmental motion analysis generally used for assessing the presence of vertebral motion restrictions or aberrant motion. The patient is relaxed and passive while the doctor takes the joint that is being assessed through its normal range of motion in various directions while palpating near adjacent joint surfaces for nuance of pattern and end-feel. Motion lesions are generally described as **restrictions** and/or **hypermobility** • <u>Static palpation</u>: Boney and other landmarks are compared symmetrically and to the practitioner's experience for the detection of abnormality consistent with subjective, motion, and soft tissue findings; static palpations are usually described in terms of prominence or relative superiority/inferiority when compared symmetrically • <u>Soft tissue palpation</u>: Subcutaneous tissues, tendons, ligaments, muscles, and joint spaces can be palpated to assess myofascial status and function. Soft tissue findings commonly include edema, joint swelling, bogginess, "ropiness" of muscles, tenderness, restricted motion of soft tissues, hypertonicity, spasm, and adhesions
Treatment contact, directive hand:	• Generally the doctor provides therapeutic contact with one of the contact surfaces of the hands—digital, hypothenar, pisiform, index, thumb, thenar, or "calcaneal" when using the heel of the hand[230]; other contacts such as the elbow or chest might be used for deep myofascial or compressive manipulative procedures, respectively. The *treatment contact* is

[230] Kirk CR, Lawrence DJ, Valvo NL. <u>States Manual of Spinal, Pelvic, and Extravertebral Technics, Second Edition</u>. Lombard, Illinois: National College of Chiropractic; 1985, page 20

	provided by the *directive hand*—the hand that is delivering the therapeutic *thrust* or *direction*; the treatment contact of the directive hand works in cooperation with the *supporting contact* of the *supporting hand*
Supporting contact:	This generally refers to the supportive hand, the one that is either holding or stabilizing the patient in contrast to the hand that is delivering the manipulative force. The indirect hand can provide at least three different types of support • Neutral/stabilizing support: The supportive hand plays a relatively neutral role with regard to the manipulative force • Synergistic/cooperative/assistive support: In this situation, the supportive hand moves with the therapeutic force in the same direction. An example of this would be the head-holding hand moving in the same direction as the directive/treatment hand when performing manipulation of the upper cervical spine • Counterthrust/resistive support: In this situation, the supportive hand moves counter/against the direction of the directive force. A common example is the force applied to the upper torso when performing a side-posture manipulation of the lumbar spine or pelvis. Another important example is the counterthrust by the supportive hand when performing a more forceful manipulation of the cervical spine; in this case the supportive hand is serving to limit the motion that would otherwise be imposed by forceful motion by the directive hand; more forceful manipulations such as used to increase afferent input to joint proprioceptors should *not* result in more motion; rather the increased speed and force of the directive hand is countered rather than assisted by the supportive hand
Pretreatment positioning:	• Joints are generally—but not always—taken to the end range of motion before the manipulative thrust is applied because the general purpose of high-velocity low-amplitude manipulation is to break myofascial restrictions and/or forcefully activate joint proprioceptors. In chiropractic terms, this is described as taking the joint into the **paraphysiologic space** because the physiologic range of motion is temporarily though safely exceeded[231]; in osteopathic terms, this part of the range of motion is described as being within the range of **passive motion** but still within the **anatomic barrier**[232]
Therapeutic action:	• For joint manipulation, this is usually the **chiropractic adjustment** or the **osteopathic HVLA** (high-velocity low-amplitude thrust); <u>**thrust vectors**</u> can be *straight, curvilinear,* or *rotary* into **segmental directions** of *rotation, extension, flexion, side-bending, traction,* and combinations of those directions • Other common manual techniques include stretching, post-isometric stretching, massage, compression, percussion, joint springing, mobilization, articulation, traction
Image:	• Photographs will be provided when relevant and available
Resources:	Textbook and article citations for additional information will be provided in this last row when relevant and available; the most commonly cited works include: • States Manual, Second Edition[233] by Constance Kirk DC, Dana Lawrence DC, Nila Valvo DC • Kimberly Manual, 2006 Edition[234] by Paul Kimberly DO • Chiropractic Technique[235] by Thomas Bergmann DC, David Peterson DC, Dana Lawrence DC • Chiropractic Management of Spine-Related Disorders[236] edited by Meridel Gatterman DC

> The following samples are an obvious underrepresentation of the diversity of manipulative techniques available, which easily numbers into the hundreds. Various techniques are—of course—described with greater range and depth in textbooks wholly dedicated to the topic of manipulation, which by itself is not the subject of this text. Rather, **use these samples as reminders to include or at least consider manipulative therapy** when composing your treatment plan; oftentimes, the manipulative therapy is the fastest and shortest route between *pain* and *relief from pain*.

[231] Leach RA. (ed). The Chiropractic Theories: A Textbook of Scientific Research, Fourth Edition. Baltimore: Lippincott, Williams & Wilkins, 2004, page 32-33
[232] Kimberly PE. Outline of Osteopathic Manipulative Procedures. The Kimberly Manual 2006. Kirksville College of Osteopathic Medicine. Walsworth Publishing , Marceline, Mo, page 7
[233] Kirk CR, Lawrence DJ, Valvo NL. States Manual of Spinal, Pelvic, and Extravertebral Technics. Second Edition. Lombard, Illinois: National College of Chiropractic; 1985
[234] Kimberly PE. Outline of Osteopathic Manipulative Procedures. The Kimberly Manual 2006. Kirksville College of Osteopathic Medicine. Walsworth Publishing , Marceline, Mo
[235] Bergmann TF, Peterson DH, Lawrence DJ. Chiropractic Technique. New York; Churchill Livingstone: 1993
[236] Gatterman MI. Chiropractic Management of Spine Related Disorders. Baltimore; Williams and Wilkins: 1990

Cervical Spine: Rotation Emphasis	
Patient position:	• Supine, neck slightly flexed
Doctor position:	• At 45° angle from head of table; may also be in a more lateral position aside the patient's head and neck; while it is acceptable to assess and set-up with straight legs, at the time of impulse, doctor's legs should be bent to provide the doctor with greater power, stability, and biomechanical safety
Assessment:	• <u>Subjective</u>: neck pain, headaches
	• <u>Motion palpation</u>: rotation restriction; primary or compensatory hypermobile segments may be detected above or below the restricted segment
	• <u>Static palpation</u>: vertebra may feel relatively posterior on the side opposite the rotational restriction, e.g., a right rotational restriction may present with a relative left rotational malposition that brings the vertebral lamina and articular pillars posterior on the left
	• <u>Soft tissue</u>: tenderness, may also have muscle spasm
Treatment contact:	• Doctor uses either an index or proximal phalange contact on the posterior aspect of the transverse process and/or articular pillar
	• The doctor's vector and hence the positioning of the forearm of the contact hand must change depending on the level of the cervical spine that is being treated
	• Notice in this photograph that the thumb of the doctor's contact hand is placed on the angle of the mandible, this is more to help anchor the contact and stabilize the doctor's wrist than to assist with the manipulation; very little pressure and zero thrust are applied to the mandible
Supporting contact:	• Head is held into rotation and slight flexion; as with all techniques, nuanced adjustments in flexion-extension, rotation, and side-bending are made until the premanipulative tension is localized to the specific direction/tissue of restriction
Pretreatment positioning:	• Slight flexion and extension may be used below and above the treatment contact to create motion restriction at the adjacent motion segments; this helps to focus the motion and therapeutic force at the specific; importantly the support hand is largely responsible for proper positioning with the correct amount of nuanced flexion-extension and side-bending so that the rotational force is accurately delivered
Therapeutic action:	• Rotational thrust with contact hand; support hand keeps head off table so that rotational motion can occur
Image:	

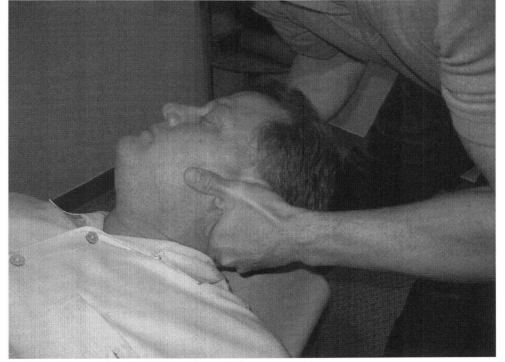

Resources:	• <u>States Manual, Second Edition</u>[237] page 47

---

[237] Kirk CR, Lawrence DJ, Valvo NL. <u>States Manual of Spinal, Pelvic, and Extravertebral Technics, Second Edition</u>. Lombard, Illinois: National College of Chiropractic; 1985

Cervical Spine: Lateral Flexion (Side-Bending) Emphasis; Treatment of Lateral Malposition

Patient position:	• Supine, head is neutrally placed—neither flexed nor extended; slight flexion is allowed; this technique can also be adapted for use in a seated position
Doctor position:	• At 45° angle from head of table; may also be in a more lateral position aside the patient's head and neck
Assessment:	• <u>Subjective</u>: neck pain, headaches • <u>Motion palpation</u>: lateral flexion restriction • <u>Static palpation</u>: vertebra may feel laterally displaced • <u>Soft tissue</u>: tenderness, may also have muscle spasm
Treatment contact:	• Using an index (metacarpal-phalangeal) contact at the tip of the transverse process or slightly posterior to the transverse process; an index phalangeal contact can also be used on the articular pillars as long as doctor is careful not to thrust in a rotational direction; notice in this picture how Dr Harris has the forearm of his contact hand perfectly aligned in the treatment vector, which is almost purely in the patient's transverse/horizontal plane; notice also that Dr Harris has his knees bent and is forward flexed to bring his torso closer to his contact and thereby minimize stress and strain on his own shoulders; with slight modifications in vector direction, this technique can be applied throughout the cervical spine from C0-C7
Supporting contact:	• Lateral aspect of head, opposite contact; generally the supporting hand is neutral, however it can supply some traction and can help induce lateral flexion at impulse; with more aggressive adjustments, the supporting hand can supply a counterforce to minimize motion following the application of a faster and more powerful thrust
Pretreatment positioning:	• Lateral flexion at the targeted segment; the slightest amount of contralateral rotation is applied
Therapeutic action:	• Establish minimal premanipulative tension once the end range of motion has been reached, then use quick and very shallow trust to induce lateral flexion
Image:	

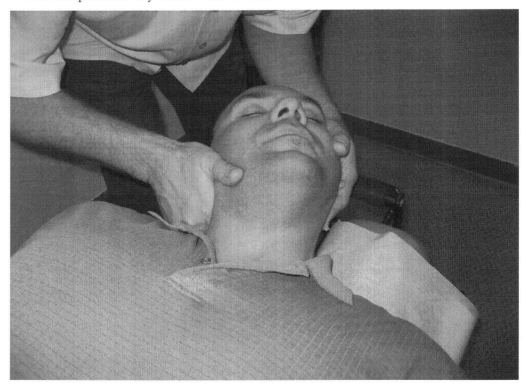

Resources:	• <u>States Manual, Second Edition</u>[238] page 39 • <u>Kimberly Manual, 2006 Edition</u>[239] page 79 • <u>Chiropractic Technique</u>[240] pages 268, 271, 285

[238] Kirk CR, Lawrence DJ, Valvo NL. <u>States Manual of Spinal, Pelvic, and Extravertebral Technics. Second Edition</u>. Lombard, Illinois: National College of Chiropractic; 1985
[239] Kimberly PE. <u>Outline of Osteopathic Manipulative Procedures. The Kimberly Manual 2006</u>. Kirksville College of Osteopathic Medicine. Walsworth Publishing , Marceline, Mo
[240] Bergmann TF, Peterson DH, Lawrence DJ. <u>Chiropractic Technique</u>. New York; Churchill Livingstone: 1993

Thoracic Spine: Supine Thoracic Flexion, "Anterior Thoracic"

Patient position:	• Supine on table; to facilitate positioning, patient's leg opposite doctor may be flexed at hip and knee with foot flat on table • Patient is instructed to place right hand on right trapezius and left hand on left trapezius; the patient is instructed, "Do not place your hands behind your neck and do not interlace your fingers."
Doctor position:	• Facing table at 45° angle in fencer stance with feet apart and knees bent • Doctor must be midline and balanced at time of impulse in order to provide symmetric force
Assessment:	• <u>Subjective</u>: mechanical midback pain • <u>Motion palpation</u>: flexion restriction • <u>Static palpation</u>: extension malposition; focal loss of thoracic kyphosis; focal approximation of spinous processes consistent with extension malposition; vertebra may feel anteriorly displaced • <u>Soft tissue</u>: local paravertebral myohypertonicity is common; local paresthesia is very common, and patients are often exquisitely sensitive to the lightest touch
Treatment contact:	• Closed fist contact with spinous processes between doctor's distal interphalangeal joints and thenar eminence; the trust is delivered from the doctor's chest through the patient's arms which compress the patient's chest; Dr Harris (pictured as patient) prefers to use a forearm contact to reduce wear-and-tear on his hands and wrists
Supporting contact:	• The supporting contact is the hand-arm that supports the patient's upper torso; the supporting contact pulls toward the doctor and superiorly at time of impulse
Pretreatment positioning:	• Patient lifts head from table; doctor uses supporting hand and arm to lift patient off table to allow placement of contact hand and to facilitate spinal flexion
Therapeutic action:	• Doctor uses **body drop thrust** technique at 45° toward ground and toward the head of the table; the trust should simultaneously generate compression and long-axis traction; the contact hand remains tense to provide solid leverage *inferior* to the targeted motion segment; the supporting hand and arm pull toward doctor at time of impulse to accentuate traction and spinal flexion; patient is instructed to breath deeply then relax and exhale; upon exhalation, the doctor establishes and maintains premanipulative tension to achieve joint flexion, then applies HVLA thrust; the thrust must be fast and shallow; slow and deep impulses can sprain the interspinous ligaments
Image:	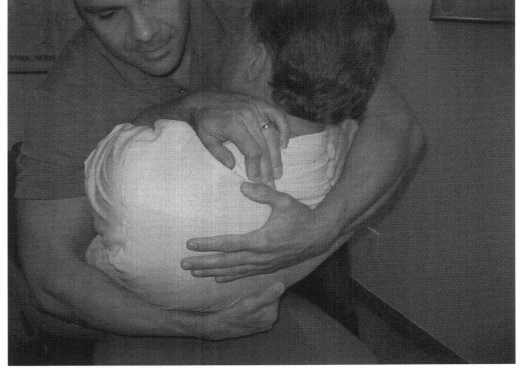
Resources:	• <u>States Manual, Second Edition</u>[241] page 67 • <u>Kimberly Manual, 2006 Edition</u>[242] page 93-94 • <u>Chiropractic Technique</u>[243] page 349

[241] Kirk CR, Lawrence DJ, Valvo NL. <u>States Manual of Spinal, Pelvic, and Extravertebral Technics. Second Edition</u>. Lombard, Illinois: National College of Chiropractic; 1985
[242] Kimberly PE. <u>Outline of Osteopathic Manipulative Procedures. The Kimberly Manual 2006</u>. Kirksville College of Osteopathic Medicine. Walsworth Publishing , Marceline, Mo

Lumbar Side-Posture Rotational Manipulation/Mobilization, "Lumbar Roll"

Patient position:	• Side-posture, lateral recumbent; lower leg is straight; upper leg is flexed at hip and knee with foot behind calf of the leg that is straight on the table
Doctor position:	• Facing table at 45° angle in fencer stance with feet apart and knees bent
	• Notice in the photograph how Dr Harris approximates his center of gravity and biomechanical leverage directly over his therapeutic contact
Assessment:	• <u>Subjective</u>: asymptomatic or with lumbar pain; lumbar disc herniation[244], use a cautious and gentle technique if the patient has radicular symptoms, and as a rule of thumb the patient should be positioned with the symptomatic leg down on the table (e.g., "good leg *up*, bad leg *down*")
	• <u>Motion palpation</u>: focal restrictions with focal pain are perhaps better treated with a lesion-specific technique such as the "push-pull" maneuver; this is an excellent technique if the patient has general discomfort without localization, or has pain and will benefit from rotational manipulation for its muscle stretching and afferent-stimulating analgesic benefits
	• <u>Static palpation</u>: minor displacements and malpositions may be noted; if specific biomechanical lesions are found, use a more specific technique such as the "push-pull" maneuver
	• <u>Soft tissue</u>: palpate for hypertonicity/spasm with or without relative muscle atrophy; patients with chronic low-back pain tend to have weaker extensor muscles than the general population; however, during an acutely painful episode, their otherwise weakened muscles will be hypertonic thus leading to a paradoxical **atrophic hypertonicity**
Treatment contact:	• Doctor uses a palmar/calcaneal ("heel of the hand") contact over the lumbar facet joints
	• Rotation and traction are provided at the time of impulse with the doctor's thigh which is compressed and providing long-axis traction against the patient's upper leg, which is flexed at the hip and knee
Support:	• Doctor's cephalad hand applies rotational resistance to patient's shoulder as shown
Pretreatment positioning:	• Premanipulative tension is attained and maintained prior to **body drop impulse**
	• The premanipulative tension and the therapeutic impulse are established and delivered through the contact hand and the doctor's caudad leg which has compressive contact with the patient's flexed leg
Therapeutic action:	• Body drop thrust impulse with rotational emphasis
	• Notice how Dr Harris has the forearm of his contact hand perpendicular to the patient's coronal plane to direct his impulse in a posterior-to-anterior direction
Image:	

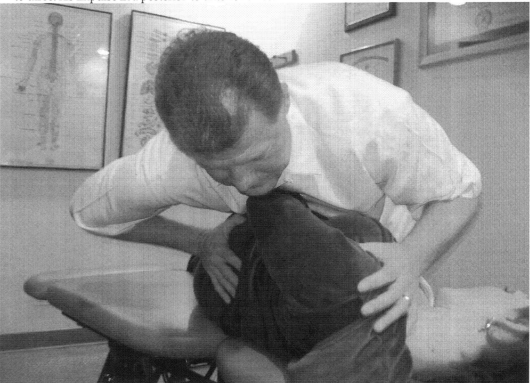

Resources:	• <u>States Manual, Second Edition</u>[245] pages 95, 105, 106

---

[243] Bergmann TF, Peterson DH, Lawrence DJ. <u>Chiropractic Technique</u>. New York; Churchill Livingstone: 1993

[244] Quon JA, Cassidy JD, O'Connor SM, Kirkaldy-Willis WH. Lumbar intervertebral disc herniation: treatment by rotational manipulation. *J Manipulative Physiol Ther*. 1989 Jun;12(3):220-7

[245] Kirk CR, Lawrence DJ, Valvo NL. <u>States Manual of Spinal, Pelvic, and Extravertebral Technics. Second Edition</u>. Lombard, Illinois: National College of Chiropractic; 1985

Lumbar Spine: Side-Posture Segmental Rotation (Lumbar "Push-Pull")

Patient position:	• Lateral recumbent (side-posture) with no/minimal lateral flexion and minimal thoracic rotation; upper leg is flexed at hip and knee, with foot placed/locked behind the calf that is on the table; the patient grasps his/her own forearms and maintains modest tension to provide anchoring for the doctor's caudad arm, which is placed under the patient's superior arm; the patient's lower leg is straight
Doctor position:	• Doctor is facing the table standing on the cephalad leg while the caudad leg is flexed at the hip and knee and placed atop the patient's flexed upper leg to provide additional leverage at the time of manipulative thrust
	• Regarding the doctor's cephalad arm, the humerus is directed toward the patient's shoulder, and the elbow is bent allowing the forearm to push into the sulcus formed by the pectoralis major and deltoid; doctors forearm emerges under patient's elbow, so that fingertips are on the superior/lateral aspect of the lumbar spinous process of the superior vertebra of the targeted motion segment
	• Regarding the doctor's caudad arm, the elbow is flexed and the forearm is placed along the posterior aspect of the patient's superior ilium; fingers hook the inferior/lateral aspect of the lumbar spinous process of the inferior vertebra of the targeted motion segment
Assessment:	• <u>Subjective</u>: asymptomatic or lumbar pain, which may not be at the affected segment
	• <u>Motion palpation</u>: rotational restriction
	• <u>Static palpation</u>: may have rotational malposition
	• <u>Soft tissue</u>: may have muscle spasm at nearby area of hypermobility
Treatment contact:	• The doctor's cephalad contacts are at the patient's deltopectoral sulcus and directly on the superior/lateral aspect of the lumbar spinous process of the superior vertebra of the targeted motion segment
	• This maneuver has three caudad contacts: 1) doctor's fingertips pull directly on the inferior/lateral aspect of the lumbar spinous process of the inferior vertebra of the targeted motion segment; 2) doctor's forearm on patient's ilium; 3) doctors caudad lower leg is atop patient's flexed leg
Support:	• All contacts are active
Pretreatment positioning:	• Rotational tension is applied and focused at the lumbar spinal segment being treated
	• Thoracic rotation and lateral flexion are minimized to the extent possible
	• Modest lumbar lateral flexion toward the table helps to gap the inferior articular process of the superior segment from the superior articular process of the inferior segment
Therapeutic action:	• 1) Doctor's cephalad elbow thrusts toward patient's shoulder to create simultaneous rotation and long-axis traction; 2) cephalad fingertips push toward the ground while atop the superior/lateral aspect of the lumbar spinous process of the superior vertebra of the targeted motion segment; 3) doctor's caudad fingertips hook and pull the inferior vertebra; 4) forearm pushes patient's ilium into rotation; 5) extension "kick" of doctor's knee quickly creates rotational force. All five actions must occur simultaneously
Image:	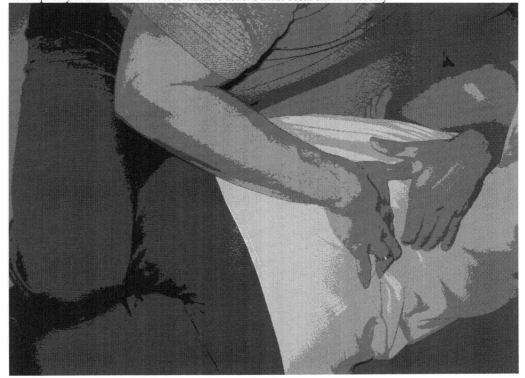
Resources:	• <u>Chiropractic Technique</u>[246] page 428

[246] Bergmann TF, Peterson DH, Lawrence DJ. <u>Chiropractic Technique</u>. New York; Churchill Livingstone: 1993

Proprioceptive Rehabilitation and Retraining: An Essential Component in the Comprehensive Management of Chronic Neck and Back Pain as Well as Recurrent Knee and Ankle Injuries

The central nervous system plays a silent and often underappreciated role in the maintenance of joint integrity and the prevention of joint injuries. Finely coordinated, minute alterations in muscle tension and joint position are essential for proper musculoskeletal biomechanics. Impaired coordination of this delicate neuromuscular system—either by injury or more commonly by disuse—predisposes to subtle and gross injuries and the perpetuation of chronic pain. **Muscle spasm, myofascial trigger points, and neuromuscular uncoupling must be viewed within a context that appreciates how the Western diet and lifestyle contribute to the genesis and perpetuation of painful musculoskeletal problems.**

Proprioceptive deficits are common in patients with chronic low-back pain[247], neck pain[248], knee pain and arthritis[249], and ankle instability.[250] Not only does poor proprioception leave joints vulnerable to recurrent microtrauma, but also lack of proprioceptive inhibition of nociceptors negates the proposed "gate-control" mechanism of pain inhibition and thus opens the door to the perception of chronic pain.[251] Thus, **proprioceptive deficits both increase joint injury and increase pain perception.** Chronic pain may lead to functional reorganization in the central nervous system and self-perpetuate pain as "pain memories."[252]

An important component to injury rehabilitation and prevention is proprioceptive retraining.[253] Proprioceptive retraining programs have been shown to reduce the severity of pain and the occurrence and recurrence of injuries. With the simple investment of a few minutes per day, patients and athletes

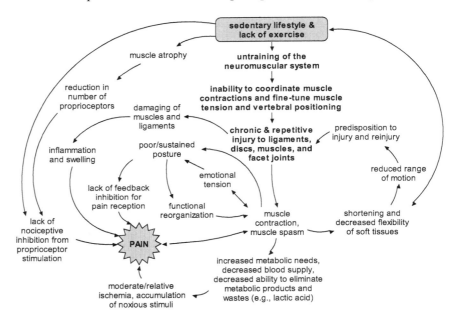

can retrain their nervous systems to respond more quickly and to increase the accuracy of proprioception. Muscle-strengthening rehabilitative programs that fail to address proprioceptive retraining do not result in improved neuromuscular coordination as evaluated by electromyography.[254] Furthermore, muscle-strengthening programs may actually lead to a reduction in postural stability when compared to balance training.[255]

[247] Newcomer KL, Jacobson TD, Gabriel DA, Larson DR, Brey RH, An KN. Muscle activation patterns in subjects with and without low back pain. *Arch Phys Med Rehabil.* 2002;83(6):816-21
[248] McPartland JM, Brodeur RR, Hallgren RC. Chronic neck pain, standing balance, and suboccipital muscle atrophy--a pilot study. *J Manipulative Physiol Ther.* 1997 Jan;20(1):24-9
[249] Callaghan MJ, Selfe J, Bagley PJ, Oldham JA. The Effects of Patellar Taping on Knee Joint Proprioception. *J Athl Train.* 2002 Mar;37(1):19-24
[250] Olmsted LC, Carcia CR, Hertel J, Shultz SJ. Efficacy of the Star Excursion Balance Tests in Detecting Reach Deficits in Subjects With Chronic Ankle Instability. *J Athl Train.* 2002 Dec;37(4):501-506 http://www.pubmedcentral.gov/articlerender.fcgi?tool=pubmed&pubmedid=12937574
[251] "The lack of proprioceptive inhibition of nociceptors at the dorsal horn of the spinal cord would result in chronic pain and a loss of standing balance." McPartland JM, Brodeur RR, Hallgren RC. Chronic neck pain, standing balance, and suboccipital muscle atrophy--a pilot study. *J Manipulative Physiol Ther.* 1997 Jan;20(1):24-9
[252] "Functional reorganisation in both the somatosensory and motor system... In patients with chronic low back pain and fibromyalgia... reorganisational change increases with chronicity; ...cortical reorganisation is correlated with the amount of pain... central alterations may be viewed as pain memories ... influence the processing of both painful and nonpainful input..." Flor H. Cortical reorganisation and chronic pain: implications for rehabilitation. *J Rehabil Med.* 2003 May;(41 Suppl):66-72
[253] Murphy DR. Chiropractic rehabilitation of the cervical spine. *J Manipulative Physiol Ther.* 2000 Jul-Aug; 23(6): 404-8
[254] "Unbalanced electromyographic patterns found in patients with LBP given symmetrical tasks were not affected by rehabilitation treatment." Lu WW, Luk KD, Cheung KM, Wong YW, Leong JC. Back muscle contraction patterns of patients with low back pain before and after rehabilitation treatment: an electromyographic evaluation. *J Spinal Disord.* 2001 Aug;14(4):277-82
[255] "RESULTS: After 1 month, back extensor strengthening led to decreased postural stability on hard surface... Balance skill training, however, increased postural stability as indicated by a decreased low-frequency component." Kollmitzer J, Ebenbichler GR, Sabo A, Kerschan K, Bochdansky T. Effects of back extensor strength training versus balance training on postural control. *Med Sci Sports Exerc.* 2000 Oct;32(10):1770-6

The **physical medicine portion** of musculoskeletal rehabilitative programs should generally include:

- <u>Correction of faulty movement patterns</u>: Addressing each of the three major components: 1) initial posture, 2) quality of somatosensory input, and 3) CNS motor programs,
- <u>Promotion of spinal stability</u>: Addressing both the *active* and the *passive* components,
- <u>Proprioceptive/sensorimotor training</u>: Target the neck, torso, lumbar spine, pelvis, and lower extremity,
- <u>Strengthening exercises</u>: Strengthen the neck, shoulders, back, legs, and abdominal and oblique muscles,
- <u>Myofascial and spinal manipulative therapy</u>: Use manual medicine to alleviate pain, facilitate and effect proprioceptive/sensorimotor restoration, and promote optimal joint biomechanics.

A very comprehensive and dense review of this topic was published by Murphy[256] in 2000, and this article is highly recommended for practitioners specializing in rehabilitation.

Clinical techniques for proprioceptive/sensorimotor retraining and rehabilitation:

- <u>Wobble board, balance shoes, foam, exercise ball, or other labile support surface</u>: At the very least, patients should be advised to use a wobble board, balance board, balance shoes or exercise sandals for *at least* 5 minutes 2 times per day every day of the week. Exercise sandals appear to be highly efficient for increasing muscular activity in the lower leg and ankle.[257] Sedentary patients can easily integrate proprioceptive training into their lives — they can use the wobble board or balance shoes while they are watching television. This easy treatment has been shown to facilitate rapid subconscious neuromuscular coordination of the gluteal muscles, thus enhancing pelvic and low-back stability.[258] Other techniques include standing on thick foam or walking in thick sand, which are labile surfaces that require increased neuromuscular control. Standing on one leg and performing gentle motions while blindfolded or with closed eyes further challenges *and therefore improves* the coordination of proprioceptive input with neuromuscular responsiveness.[259,260,261]
- <u>Spinal manipulation</u>: Spinal manipulation appears to improve proprioceptive function.[262]
- <u>Skin taping to increase afferent stimuli</u>: Applying tape to the skin can increase sensory input from cutaneous mechanoreceptors and can improve sensorimotor coordination.[263,264,265,266]
- <u>Vigorous full-body exercise of any and all types</u>, especially those that are relatively fast and require high-frequency complex neuromuscular responses, such as:
  - <u>Swimming</u>: Excellent for promoting fitness in a way that is generally easy on joints and muscles and is without impact; requires and thus promotes coordination and timing
  - <u>Indoor aerobics</u>: Excellent for cardiovascular fitness and weight loss, requires and thus promotes coordination and timing
  - <u>Outdoor cycling (road)</u>: Excellent for cardiovascular fitness and weight loss, easy on the joints; requires and promotes coordination and balance
  - <u>Outdoor cycling (mountain and trail)</u>: Same as above; requires more balance and coordination than road cycling due to unpredictability of surface; rough surfaces provide flood of afferent stimuli through feet and hands
  - <u>Yoga, Pilates, Calisthenics</u>: Inexpensive, can be done alone or in groups; does not require expensive equipment, can be tailored for low-back rehabilitation[267,268,269]
  - <u>Hiking</u>: Excellent combination of lower extremity strengthening and aerobics; random and uneven trails provide proprioceptive challenge; helps people get in touch with nature.

---

[256] **Murphy DR. Chiropractic rehabilitation of the cervical spine.** *J Manipulative Physiol Ther*. 2000 Jul-Aug;23(6):404-8

[257] Troy Blackburn J, Hirth CJ, Guskiewicz KM. Exercise Sandals Increase Lower Extremity Electromyographic Activity During Functional Activities. *J Athl Train*. 2003 Sep;38(3):198-203

[258] Bullock-Saxton JE, **Janda V**, Bullock MI.Reflex activation of gluteal muscles in walking. An approach to restoration of muscle function for patients with low-back pain. *Spine* 1993 May;18(6):704-8

[259] Olmsted LC, Carcia CR, Hertel J, Shultz SJ. Efficacy of the Star Excursion Balance Tests in Detecting Reach Deficits in Subjects with Chronic Ankle Instability. *J Athl Train*. 2002 Dec;37(4):501-506

[260] Troy Blackburn J, Hirth CJ, Guskiewicz KM. Exercise Sandals Increase Lower Extremity Electromyographic Activity During Functional Activities. *J Athl Train*. 2003 Sep;38(3):198-203

[261] Willems T, Witvrouw E, Verstuyft J, Vaes P, De Clercq D. Proprioception and Muscle Strength in Subjects With a History of Ankle Sprains and Chronic Instability. *J Athl Train*. 2002 Dec;37(4):487-493

[262] "RESULTS: Subjects receiving manipulation demonstrated a mean reduction in visual analogue scores of 44%, along with a 41% improvement in mean scores for the head repositioning skill." Rogers RG. The effects of spinal manipulation on cervical kinesthesia in patients with chronic neck pain: a pilot study. *J Manipulative Physiol Ther* 1997 Feb;20(2):80-5

[263] "This suggests that ankle taping partly corrects impaired proprioception caused by modern athletic footwear and exercise." Robbins S, Waked E, Rappel R. Ankle taping improves proprioception before and after exercise in young men. *Br J Sports Med*. 1995 Dec;29(4):242-7

[264] "We concluded that increased cutaneous sensory feedback provided by strips of athletic tape applied across the ankle joint of healthy individuals can help improve ankle joint position perception in nonweightbearing, especially for a midrange plantar-flexed ankle position." Simoneau GG, Degner RM, Kramper CA, Kittleson KH. Changes in Ankle Joint Proprioception Resulting From Strips of Athletic Tape Applied Over the Skin. *J Athl Train*. 1997 Apr;32(2):141-147 http://www.pubmedcentral.nih.gov/picrender.fcgi?artid=1319817&blobtype=pdf

[265] Callaghan MJ, Selfe J, Bagley PJ, Oldham JA. The Effects of Patellar Taping on Knee Joint Proprioception. *J Athl Train*. 2002 Mar;37(1):19-24 http://www.pubmedcentral.nih.gov/articlerender.fcgi?tool=pubmed&pubmedid=12937439

[266] "Application of stretch to the skin over VMO via the tape can increase VMO activity, suggesting that cutaneous stimulation may be one mechanism by which patella taping produces a clinical effect." Macgregor K, Gerlach S, Mellor R, Hodges PW. Cutaneous stimulation from patella tape causes a differential increase in vasti muscle activity in people with patellofemoral pain. *J Orthop Res*. 2005 Mar;23(2):351-8

[267] Shiple B. Relieving Low-Back Pain With Exercise. *Physician and Sportsmedicine* 1997; 25: http://www.physsportsmed.com/issues/1997/08aug/shiplepa.htm

[268] Drezner JA. Exercises in the Treatment of Low- Back Pain. *Physician and Sportsmedicine* 2001; 29: http://www.physsportsmed.com/issues/2001/08_01/pa_drezner.htm

[269] Kuritzky L, White J. Extend Yourself for Low-Back Pain Relief. *Physician and Sportsmedicine* 1997; 25: http://www.physsportsmed.com/issues/1997/01jan/back_pa.htm

Reasons to Avoid the Use of Pharmaceutical Nonsteroidal Anti-inflammatory Drugs (NSAIDs) and Selective Cyclooxygenase-2 Inhibitors (coxibs)

<u>Introduction</u>: Nonsteroidal anti-inflammatory drugs (NSAIDs) have many common and serious adverse effects, including the promotion of joint destruction. Paradoxically, these drugs *cause* or *exacerbate* the very symptoms and disease they are supposed to treat: joint pain and destruction. In a tragic exemplification of Orwellian newspeak[270], the habitual utilization and long-term prescription of NSAIDs for joint pain and inflammation as advocated by the pharmaceutical industry[271] and medical textbooks[272] is not described as *malpractice*; rather it is described as the *"standard of care"* and *"first-line therapy."* Adverse effects include:

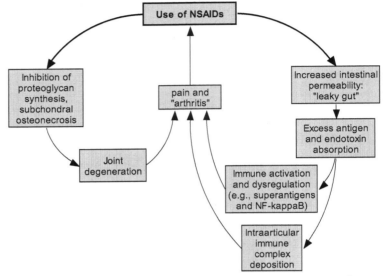

The Vicious Cycle of NSAID Use: Pain prompts doctors and patients to use NSAIDS, which then promote joint destruction and increased intestinal permeability that promotes systemic inflammation which then contribute to the perpetuation of joint pain.

- <u>Gastric ulceration and gastrointestinal bleeding</u>: Nearly all NSAIDs promote gastric ulceration and gastrointestinal bleeding. Among patients who chronically use NSAIDs 65% will develop intestinal inflammation[273] and up to 30% will develop gastroduodenal ulceration.[274] Drugs differ greatly in their propensity to damage the gastrointestinal mucosa and cause bleeding, and aspirin appears to be the most problematic.[275] NSAIDs can also promote and exacerbate colitis and inflammation of the large intestine.[276]

- <u>Increased intestinal permeability</u>: NSAIDs damage the mucosa of the small intestine and promote macromolecular absorption and paracellular permeability—"leaky gut." As described in greater detail later in this text, increased intestinal permeability most certainly contributes to the exacerbation and perpetuation of many rheumatic and musculoskeletal disorders by inducing inflammation via immune activation and by promoting the formation of immune complexes that are then deposited into synovial tissues for the induction of a local inflammatory response inside the joint.[277]

- <u>Promotion of bone necrosis and cartilage destruction</u>: Several NSAIDs cause osteonecrosis[278] and many of these drugs interfere with chondrocyte function and cartilage formation and thus promote the destruction of joints.[279] As noted by Newman and Ling[280], **"...femoral head collapse and acceleration of osteoarthritis have been well documented in association with the NSAIDs..."** The subchondral osteonecrosis induced by many NSAIDs may both necessitate and complicate arthroplasty (joint

[270] Orwell G. <u>1984</u>. New York; Harcourt Brace Jovanovich: 1949. The term "newspeak" is defined by the Merriam-Webster Dictionary (http://www.m-w.com) as "propagandistic language marked by euphemism, circumlocution, and the inversion of customary meanings" and as "a language designed to diminish the range of thought," in the novel *1984* (1949) by George Orwell.
[271] "Congratulations—you've joined the 20 million people who have taken CELEBREX, the #1 doctor-prescribed brand of arthritis medication." http://www.celebrex.com January 24, 2004
[272] "The first drug to treat rheumatoid arthritis is an NSAID." Tierney ML. McPhee SJ, Papadakis MA (eds). <u>Current Medical Diagnosis and Treatment 2002, 41ˢᵗ Edition</u>. New York: Lange Medical Books; 2002. Page 856
[273] "NSAIDs cause small intestinal inflammation in 65% of patients receiving the drugs long-term." Bjarnason I, Macpherson AJ. Intestinal toxicity of non-steroidal anti-inflammatory drugs. *Pharmacol Ther*. 1994 Apr-May;62(1-2):145-57
[274] "Endoscopic studies indicate that up to 30% of chronic NSAID users will develop gastroduodenal ulceration." Blower AL. Considerations for nonsteroidal anti-inflammatory drug therapy: safety. *Scand J Rheumatol Suppl*. 1996;105:13-24
[275] "ASA (1,500 mg/day for 5 days) caused about a 6-fold increase in blood loss. Four days after withdrawal of ASA, faecal blood was still about twice as high as in faeces of subjects given ibuprofen and indoprofen." Porro GB, Corvi G, Fuccella LM, Goldaniga GC, Valzelli G. Gastro-intestinal blood loss during administration of indoprofen, aspirin and ibuprofen. *J Int Med Res* 1977;5(3):155-60
[276] "Non-steroidal anti-inflammatory drugs (NSAIDs) may adversely affect the colon, either by causing a non-specific colitis or by exacerbating a preexisting colonic disease. ... Local and/or systemic effects of NSAIDs on mucosal cells might lead to an increased intestinal permeability, which is a prerequisite for colitis." Faucheron JL, Parc R. Non-steroidal anti-inflammatory drug-induced colitis. *Int J Colorectal Dis*. 1996;11(2):99-101
[277] Inman RD. Antigens, the gastrointestinal tract, and arthritis. *Rheum Dis Clin North Am*. 1991 May; 17(2): 309-21
[278] "The case of a young healthy man, who developed avascular necrosis of head of femur after prolonged administration of indomethacin, is reported here." Prathapkumar KR, Smith I, Attara GA. Indomethacin induced avascular necrosis of head of femur. *Postgrad Med J*. 2000 Sep; 76(899): 574-5
[279] "At...concentrations comparable to those... in the synovial fluid of patients treated with the drug, several NSAIDs suppress proteoglycan synthesis... These NSAID-related effects on chondrocyte metabolism ... are much more profound in osteoarthritic cartilage than in normal cartilage, due to enhanced uptake of NSAIDs by the osteoarthritic cartilage." Brandt KD. Effects of nonsteroidal anti-inflammatory drugs on chondrocyte metabolism in vitro and in vivo. *Am J Med*. 1987 Nov 20; 83(5A): 29-34
[280] Newman NM, Ling RS. Acetabular bone destruction related to non-steroidal anti-inflammatory drugs. *Lancet*. 1985 Jul 6; 2(8445): 11-4

replacement with prosthesis) because of extensive joint damage and because the underlying bone that must hold the new implant is too weak to provide a stable foundation.[281] *In vivo* studies have shown that salicylate, acetylsalicylic acid, fenoprofen, isoxicam, tolmetin, and ibuprofen reduce glycosaminoglycan synthesis.[282] COX-2 inhibition impairs anabolic bone activity that is necessary for the preservation of bone strength.[283,284]

- Promotion of hepatic and renal injury and failure: Chronic use of NSAIDs is an important risk factor for the development of renal failure.[285] Hepatic injury is less common than NSAID-induced renal failure but can be achieved with higher drug doses (especially with the non-NSAID analgesic acetaminophen), coadministration of drugs, and concomitant consumption of alcohol.

- Death: NSAIDs are an impressively significant cause of death in America. According to the review by Singh[286], "**Conservative calculations estimate that approximately 107,000 patients are hospitalized annually for nonsteroidal anti-inflammatory drug (NSAID)-related gastrointestinal (GI) complications and at least 16,500 NSAID-related deaths occur each year among arthritis patients alone. The figures for all NSAID users would be overwhelming, yet the scope of this problem is generally under-appreciated.**"

- Adverse effects specific to Coxibs: Drugs specifically designed to inhibit the isoform of cyclooxygenase known as cyclooxygenase-2 (coxibs) carry their own list of adverse effects, namely membranous glomerulopathy and acute interstitial nephritis[287], acute cholestatic hepatitis[288], toxic epidermal necrolysis[289,290], and—perhaps most importantly—increased risk for cardiovascular disease (e.g., stroke, hypertension, myocardial infarction) and cardiovascular death. Immediately following the withdrawal of the arthritis drug rofecoxib (Vioxx) in late September 2004, Topol[291] extrapolated that as many as 160,000 adverse cardiovascular events (including stroke, myocardial infarction, and death) may have resulted from the overuse of Vioxx/rofecoxib due to the collusion of Merck's intentional failure to withdraw what was known for years to be a dangerous drug, the FDA's failure to enforce regulatory standards to protect the public, and the overutilization of Vioxx by the medical profession, which was well informed of the lethality of Vioxx for several years[292] before Merck's confessionary and belated withdrawal of the drug. Soon thereafter, several other so-called "anti-inflammatory drugs" such as valdecoxib (Bextra)[293], celecoxib (Celebrex)[294], and naproxen (Aleve)[295] were likewise associated with excess cardiovascular injury and death. Although the advertising-induced feeding frenzy on Celebrex made it the most "successful" drug launch in US history with more than 7.4 million prescriptions written within its first 6 months[296], major adverse effects due to the drug were noted within 2 years of its release onto the medical market[297]; current guidelines hold that patients must be informed of the excess cardiovascular risk associated with this drug and that its use should be limited to the lowest dose for the shortest time possible (weeks).[298] When compared with placebo in cardiac surgery patients, Bextra/valdecoxib is associated with a 3-fold to 4-fold increased risk of heart attack,

[281] "This highly significant association between NSAID use and acetabular destruction gives cause for concern, not least because of the difficulty in achieving satisfactory hip replacements in patients with severely damaged acetabula." Newman NM, Ling RS. Acetabular bone destruction related to non-steroidal anti-inflammatory drugs. *Lancet*. 1985 Jul 6; 2(8445): 11-4

[282] Brandt KD. Effects of nonsteroidal anti-inflammatory drugs on chondrocyte metabolism in vitro and in vivo. *Am J Med*. 1987 Nov 20; 83(5A): 29-34

[283] "Histological observations suggest that cox-2 is required for normal endochondral ossification during fracture healing. Because mice lacking Cox2 form normal skeletons, our observations indicate that fetal bone development and fracture healing are different and that cox-2 function is specifically essential for fracture healing." Simon AM, Manigrasso MB, O'Connor JP. Cyclo-oxygenase 2 function is essential for bone fracture healing. *J Bone Miner Res*. 2002 Jun;17(6):963-76

[284] "The results indicate that cox-2 and constitutive NOS are important signaling molecules in the anabolic responses of neonatal tibial bone to the micromechanical load in vitro." Kunnel JG, Igarashi K, Gilbert JL, Stern PH. Bone anabolic responses to mechanical load in vitro involve cox-2 and constitutive NOS. *Connect Tissue Res*. 2004;45(1):40-9

[285] "Patients with chronic arthritis who consume excessive amount of NSAIDs are at risk of developing renal papillary necrosis and chronic renal impairment." Segasothy M, Chin GL, Sia KK, Zulfiqar A, Samad SA. Chronic nephrotoxicity of anti-inflammatory drugs used in the treatment of arthritis. *Br J Rheumatol*. 1995 Feb; 34(2): 162-5

[286] Singh G. Recent considerations in nonsteroidal anti-inflammatory drug gastropathy. *Am J Med*. 1998 Jul 27; 105(1B): 31S-38S

[287] Markowitz GS, Falkowitz DC, Isom R, Zaki M, Imaizumi S, Appel GB, D'Agati VD. Membranous glomerulopathy and acute interstitial nephritis following treatment with celecoxib. *Clin Nephrol*. 2003;59(2):137-42

[288] Grieco A, Miele L, Giorgi A, Civello IM, Gasbarrini G. Acute cholestatic hepatitis associated with celecoxib. *Ann Pharmacother*. 2002;36(12):1887-9

[289] Berger P, Dwyer D, Corallo CE. Toxic epidermal necrolysis after celecoxib therapy. *Pharmacotherapy*. 2002 Sep;22(9):1193-5.

[290] Friedman B, Orlet HK, Still JM, Law E. Toxic epidermal necrolysis due to administration of celecoxib (Celebrex). *South Med J*. 2002;95(10):1213-4

[291] Topol EJ. Failing the public health--rofecoxib, Merck, and the FDA. *N Engl J Med*. 2004 Oct 21;351(17):1707-9

[292] Mukherjee D, Nissen SE, Topol EJ. Risk of cardiovascular events associated with selective cox-2 inhibitors. *JAMA* 2001; 286(8):954-9

[293] Ray WA, Griffin MR, Stein CM. Cardiovascular toxicity of valdecoxib. *N Engl J Med*. 2004;351(26):2767

[294] "Patients in the clinical trial taking 400 mg. of Celebrex twice daily had a 3.4 times greater risk of CV events compared to placebo. For patients in the trial taking 200 mg. of Celebrex twice daily, the risk was 2.5 times greater. The average duration of treatment in the trial was 33 months." FDA Statement on the Halting of a Clinical Trial of the cox-2 Inhibitor Celebrex. http://www.fda.gov/bbs/topics/news/2004/NEW01144.html Available on January 4, 2005

[295] "Preliminary information from the study showed some evidence of increased risk of cardiovascular events, when compared to placebo, to patients taking naproxen." FDA Statement on Naproxen. http://www.fda.gov/bbs/topics/news/2004/NEW01148.html Available on January 4, 2005

[296] Monsanto, Pfizer celebrate Celebrex. *St. Louis Business Journal*. July 20, 1999 http://www.bizjournals.com/stlouis/stories/1999/07/19/daily5.html Accessed on January 5, 2005

[297] Mukherjee D, Nissen SE, Topol EJ. Risk of cardiovascular events associated with selective cox-2 inhibitors. *JAMA*. 2001 Aug 22-29;286(8):954-9

[298] "Celecoxib should be used in the lowest effective doses for short periods (weeks) only. A risk-benefit discussion is necessary for those requiring the drug for a longer period." Cotter J, Wooltorton E. New restrictions on celecoxib (Celebrex) use and the withdrawal of valdecoxib (Bextra). *CMAJ*. 2005 May 10;172(10):1299. Epub 2005 Apr 15 http://www.cmaj.ca/cgi/content/full/172/10/1299 Accessed September 28, 2005

stroke, and death[299], and recently 7 million arthritis patients, many of whom were already at high risk for cardiovascular disease, were being treated with this drug.[300] Use of Bextra was also strongly associated with toxic epidermal necrolysis, a potentially fatal condition.[301] Due primarily to the adverse cardiovascular effects[302], in the interest of protecting the public from additional adverse effects and unnecessary deaths, in April 2005 the FDA ordered that Bextra/valdecoxib be taken off the market in the US[303], and Health Canada followed suit by removing the drug from Canadian markets.[304] **It is inexcusable that these drugs were so highly utilized despite evidence of relative analgesic inefficacy (not better than earlier NSAIDs like aspirin), exorbitant costs (US $90-180 per month[305]) and clear evidence of danger (e.g., cardiovascular death) by two well-identified biochemical/physiologic mechanisms, namely: 1) inhibiting the formation of vasodilating and anti-aggregatory prostacyclin, which is formed by COX-2, and 2) shunting arachidonate toward formation of pro-atherosclerotic leukotrienes[306] by blocking cyclooxygenase.** Inhibition of prostacyclin formation promotes thrombosis and hypertension.

Perspective: If we summarize that at least 17,000 people die each year from NSAIDs, that other "medication errors" kill over 7,000 people in America[307] and that an additional 180,000 Americans die due to hospital errors[308], then we have a situation where at least 200,000 Americans die each year due to drug effects and hospital/physician errors. Furthermore, according to estimates by David Graham, MD, MPH, (Associate Director for Science, Office of Drug Safety, US FDA), more than 139,000 Americans who took Vioxx suffered serious side effects and between 26,000 and 55,000 people died from using the drug.[309] This aggregate is significantly more than the annual deaths due to diabetes (71,000), suicide (30,000), homicide (20,000) [310], and the September 11, 2001 terrorist attack (up to 3,000) *combined*.[311] Preliminary data indicates that natural treatments such as spinal manipulation[312], glucosamine sulfate[313], and *Harpagophytum*[314] are safer and/or more effective than NSAIDs for the relief of many types of pain. The increased utilization of these nonpharmacologic treatments will result in reductions in morbidity, mortality, and overall healthcare expenses when compared to our current overutilization of NSAIDs and other medical/allopathic pharmacosurgical treatments.[315]

> **"Only that day dawns to which we are awake."**
>
> *Henry David Thoreau*[316]

---

[299] Lenzer J. Pfizer criticised over delay in admitting drug's problems. *BMJ*. 2004;329(7472):935

[300] Ray WA, Griffin MR, Stein CM. Cardiovascular toxicity of valdecoxib. *N Engl J Med*. 2004;351(26):2767

[301] "There is a strong association between Stevens-Johnson syndrome/toxic epidermal necrolysis and the use of the sulfonamide cox-2 inhibitors, particularly valdecoxib." La Grenade L, Lee L, Weaver J, Bonnel R, Karwoski C, Governale L, Brinker A. Comparison of Reporting of Stevens-Johnson Syndrome and Toxic Epidermal Necrolysis in Association with Selective cox-2 Inhibitors. *Drug Saf*. 2005;28(10):917-24

[302] Nussmeier NA, Whelton AA, Brown MT, Langford RM, Hoeft A, Parlow JL, Boyce SW, Verburg KM. Complications of the cox-2 inhibitors parecoxib and valdecoxib after cardiac surgery. *N Engl J Med*. 2005 Mar 17;352(11):1081-91. Epub 2005 Feb 15

[303] "On April 7, the Food and Drug Administration requested that Pfizer suspend sales of BEXTRA in the United States. As a result, BEXTRA will no longer be available to patients in the United States... In light of the FDA's position that there is an increased cardiovascular risk for all prescription non-steroidal anti-inflammatory arthritis medicines, as well as the increased rate of rare, serious skin reactions with BEXTRA, the FDA has requested that sales of BEXTRA be suspended." http://www.bextra.com/ Accessed September 28, 2005

[304] Sibbald B. Pfizer withdraw valdecoxib (Bextra) at Health Canada's request. *CMAJ*. 2005 May 10;172(10):e1298. Epub 2005 Apr 7 http://www.cmaj.ca/cgi/reprint/172/10/e1298 Accessed September 28, 2005

[305] http://www.walgreens.com/library/finddrug/druginfo1.jsp?particularDrug=Celebrex&id=15102 Accessed September 29, 2005

[306] "CONCLUSIONS: Variant 5-lipoxygenase genotypes identify a subpopulation with increased atherosclerosis. The observed diet-gene interactions further suggest that dietary n-6 polyunsaturated fatty acids promote, whereas marine n-3 fatty acids inhibit, leukotriene-mediated inflammation that leads to atherosclerosis in this subpopulation." Dwyer JH, Allayee H, Dwyer KM, Fan J, Wu H, Mar R, Lusis AJ, Mehrabian M. Arachidonate 5-lipoxygenase promoter genotype, dietary arachidonic acid, and atherosclerosis. *N Engl J Med*. 2004 Jan 1;350(1):29-37

[307] "In 1983, 2876 people died from medication errors. ... By 1993, this number had risen to 7,391 - a 2.57-fold increase." Phillips DP, Christenfeld N, Glynn LM. Increase in US medication-error deaths between 1983 and 1993. *Lancet*. 1998 Feb 28;351(9103):643-4

[308] "Recent estimates suggest that each year more than 1 million patients are injured while in the hospital and approximately 180,000 die because of these injuries. Furthermore, drug-related morbidity and mortality are common and are estimated to cost more than $136 billion a year." Holland EG, Degruy FV. Drug-induced disorders. *Am Fam Physician*. 1997;56(7):1781-8, 1791-2

[309] http://www.commondreams.org/views05/0223-35.htm and http://www.fda.gov/cder/drug/infopage/vioxx/vioxxgraham.pdf Accessed July 26, 2006

[310] Centers for Disease Control and Prevention (CDC), National Center for Health Statistics. Deaths: Final Data for 2001. 116 pp. (PHS) 2003-1120. Available at http://www.cdc.gov/nchs/releases/03facts/mortalitytrends.htm on January 18, 2004

[311] "On September 11, 2001, four U.S. planes hijacked by terrorists crashed into the World Trade Center, the Pentagon and a field in Pennsylvania killing nearly 3,000 people in a matter of hours." From http://www.cnn.com/SPECIALS/2001/memorial/ on January 26, 2004

[312] "CONCLUSION: The best evidence indicates that cervical manipulation for neck pain is much safer than the use of NSAIDs, by as much as a factor of several hundred times. There is no evidence that indicates NSAID use is any more effective than cervical manipulation for neck pain." Dabbs V, Lauretti WJ. A risk assessment of cervical manipulation vs. NSAIDs for the treatment of neck pain. *J Manipulative Physiol Ther*. 1995 Oct;18(8):530-6

[313] Muller-Fassbender H, Bach GL, Haase W, Rovati LC, Setnikar I. Glucosamine sulfate compared to ibuprofen in osteoarthritis of the knee. *Osteoarthritis Cartilage*. 1994 Mar;2(1):61-9

[314] Chrubasik S, Model A, Black A, Pollak S. A randomized double-blind pilot study comparing Doloteffin and Vioxx in the treatment of low back pain. *Rheumatology* (Oxford). 2003 Jan;42(1):141-8

[315] Orme-Johnson DW, Herron RE. An innovative approach to reducing medical care utilization and expenditures. *Am J Manag Care*. 1997 Jan;3:135-44 http://www.ajmc.com/Article.cfm?Menu=1&ID=2154

[316] Thoreau HD. (Owen Thomas, Ed). Walden and Civil Disobedience. New York; WW Norton and Company: 1966, page 221

Another Clinically Useful Mnemonic Acronym: "B.e.n.d. S.t.e.m.s."

As an alternative to the "p.r.i.c.e. a. t.u.r.n." acronym previously described, clinicians may use the following alternate, either additively or substitutionally. "B.e.n.d. s.t.e.m.s." is aesthetically more appealing, though it is less complete than *price a turn*. The goal, of course, is to have a useful memory key available when the clinician is formulating the treatment plan. Just as all doctors are familiar with the *s.o.a.p.* format for writing chart notes to ensure their inclusion of *subjective, objective, assessment,* and *plan* for each visit, when arriving to the "p" portion of the note, integrative clinicians can use *price a turn* and/or *bend stems* to help remember key components to integrative and holistic care.

B   **Botanical**: Numerous botanical medicines are available for a wide range of indications. Among the botanical medicines with the best research support for the treatment of musculoskeletal pain and inflammation are willow bark, *Boswellia, Harpagophytum, Uncaria,* ginger, and *Capsicum*.

E   **Ergonomics/posture and Exercise**: Patients can improve their ergonomics at home, at work, and (occasionally) in the car. Likewise, attention to posture—the "style" with which one holds one's body—is important in the prevention of repetitive strain injuries, particularly to the shoulders and neck region. Most patients are overweight, out of shape, weak, and neuromuscularly uncoordinated; problems correctible with exercise.

N   **Nutrition**: Nutritional supplements are extremely valuable in the treatment and prevention of a wide range of mild and serious health problems. Use of high-dose "supranutritional" levels of vitamins can be used to help patients overcome their enzyme and receptor defects to facilitate improved physiological function and improved overall health.[317]

D   **Diet**: In order to remain consistent with the time-proven wisdom of the *Hierarchy of Therapeutics* (discussed in Chapter 2) and to avoid becoming an aimless horde of drug-pushing symptom-suppressors, holistic integrative clinicians must always attend to the basics—the foundational influences which powerfully affect metabolism and thus overall health. Clearly, diet is one of those basics, along with emotions and lifestyle—exercise, work, stress management, outlook, and relationships.

S   **Stretching, strengthening, and stabilization**: Tight muscles can be stretched in the office, where the doctor is able to teach the patient proper methods and is able to refine the diagnosis and specificity of the stretch to ensure that targeted muscles are effectively addressed. Thereafter, the patient *must* continue these stretches at home—both physically and mentally. *Physical stretching* involves the therapeutic lengthening of muscles and fascia to maintain or restore ease of myofascial motion and to alleviate adhesions or restrictions that impair function. *Mental stretching* involves the patient's active use of reframing and discipline in order to attain a higher level of functioning and effectiveness in his/her relationships, lifestyle, work situation, mental outlook, habits and other phenomena in order to overcome the external or internal *adhesions* or *restrictions* that are impairing and preventing optimal function *of the patient as a whole*. Exercise and proproceptive rehabilitation for spinal and peripheral joint stabilization are essential requirements for neuromusculoskeletal health.

T   **Trigger points**: Always remember to address the trigger point component (discussed previously in this chapter) when working with musculoskeletal pain. Seek and ye shall find; treat and the patient will improve. Think outside the region. A trigger point in the low-back or gluteal region may cause the patient to assume an antalgic posture that results in altered biomechanics and leads to a clinical presentation of shoulder or neck pain with chronic tension headaches; direct treatment of the painful shoulders or neck will provide improvement, but cure will not be effected until the cause—often distant from the region of complaint—is effectively addressed.[318]

E   **Educate and Ensure return**: Educate the patient about the condition, its cause and solutions. Educate about PAR-B—procedures, risks, alternatives, and benefits of treatment. Also, educate the patient *in writing* about the importance of follow-up visits and time limitations on treatments; failure to ensure that the patient was educated to return for follow-up visits is grounds for malpractice if the patient's condition changes or deteriorates due to complications associated with the presenting complaint at the last office visit.

M   **Manual medicine—mobilization, manipulation, massage**: Treat the problem effectively and directly with the skilled use of your hands. Practice produces proficiency.

S   **Spirituality (emotions, psychology)**: Perceptions create our emotional and mental realities, and from these subjective realities do we engage the world. Inaccurate perceptions skew and misshape one's interactions with the world. Creating more accurate perceptions—a process that requires intentionality and hard work—enhances *effectiveness* and ultimately *enjoyment* of one's life experience.

---

[317] Ames BN, Elson-Schwab I, Silver EA. High-dose vitamin therapy stimulates variant enzymes with decreased coenzyme binding affinity (increased K(m)): relevance to genetic disease and polymorphisms. *Am J Clin Nutr*. 2002 Apr;75(4):616-58 http://www.ajcn.org/cgi/content/full/75/4/616
[318] "This patient seemed to respond favorably to conservative care that included regions of spine not traditionally associated with headache pain." Stude DE, Sweere JJ. A holistic approach to severe headache symptoms in a patient unresponsive to regional manual therapy. *J Manipulative Physiol Ther*. 1996 Mar-Apr;19(3):202-7

Reducing Pain and Inflammation Naturally – Part 3: Improving Overall Health While Safely and Effectively Treating Musculoskeletal Pain

Alex Vasquez, D.C., N.D.

Abstract: Following the optimization of diet and fatty acid balance, the next therapeutic steps in the treatment of pain and inflammation can include the use of vitamin D, chondroitin sulfate, niacinamide, and botanical medicines such as Boswellia. In direct contrast to so-called "anti-inflammatory drugs" which always have significant toxicity, each of these natural treatments has been proven in controlled clinical trials to significantly reduce pain and inflammation without major adverse effects. Chondroitin sulfate has actually been shown to reduce cardiovascular mortality in humans while it safely and effectively ameliorates the pain and inflammation of osteoarthritis. Similarly, vitamin D supplementation has been proven effective in the treatment of hypertension, depression, migraine headaches, polycystic ovary syndrome and in the prevention of type-1 diabetes. By failing to fully cover chiropractic and naturopathic healthcare services, insurance companies which comprise and contribute to the American healthcare system are losing profitability and forcing patients to use drug and surgical treatments that are commonly less effective, more dangerous, and more expensive than the natural treatments described in this paper. Services provided by chiropractic and naturopathic physicians are supported by peer-reviewed research and deserve equitable coverage and status in America's healthcare system.

INTRODUCTION

As primary care providers with specialized training in musculoskeletal medicine, chiropractic physicians typically play a dual role in clinical practice on a daily basis, generally striving to simultaneously accomplish two related goals in each patient: 1) promoting overall wellness and professionally-supervised patient-implemented preventive healthcare, and 2) alleviating acute and chronic musculoskeletal pain. Both of these goals are important given the tremendous financial and social impact of musculoskeletal pain and the progressive deterioration of Americans' health. At any given time, nearly thirty percent of the American population suffers from musculoskeletal pain, joint swelling, or limitation of movement, and approximately 1 of every 7 (14% of total) visits to a primary healthcare provider is for the treatment of musculoskeletal pain or dysfunction. Resulting in more than $100 billion in US healthcare costs each year, back pain is the most prevalent medical problem in the US, is the leading cause of long-term disability, and is the second leading cause of restricted activity and the use of prescription and non-prescription drugs.[1] The preventive healthcare and wellness promotion advocated and implemented by chiropractic and naturopathic physicians is now more important than ever since the health of the American population is consistently and progressively declining: obesity and diabetes are "ever-growing" epidemics among children and adults,[2] infant mortality has recently increased for the first time in 40 years,[3] and self-reported health status and health-related quality of life among adults are declining.[4] In the 25 years between 1975 and 2000, the incidence of cancer increased significantly, and the number of people diagnosed with cancer is expected to double in the next several decades.[5] Despite these negative health trends, America spends more on healthcare than does any other nation—an unprecedented $1.55 trillion, which is roughly 15% of the US gross domestic product.[6] From the perspective of cost-effectiveness, the medically-dominated American healthcare system delivers a very poor return on investment, and it appears that assertive wellness promotion and increased utilization of chiropractic and naturopathic healthcare may provide improved outcomes and decreased overall healthcare costs.[7,8]

Numerous adverse effects are produced as a direct result of medical/pharmaceutical management of benign musculoskeletal pain. According to a 1998 review by Singh,[9] "Conservative calculations estimate that approximately 107,000 patients are hospitalized annually for nonsteroidal anti-inflammatory drug (NSAID)-related gastrointestinal (GI) complications and at least 16,500 NSAID-related deaths occur each year among arthritis patients alone. The figures for all NSAID users would be overwhelming, yet the scope of this problem is generally under-appreciated." More recently following the withdrawal of the arthritis drug rofecoxib (Vioxx) in late September 2004, Topol[10] extrapolated that as many as 160,000 adverse cardiovascular events (including stroke, myocardial infarction, and death) may have resulted from the collusion of Merck's intentional failure to withdraw what was known for years to be a dangerous drug, the FDA's failure to enforce regulatory standards to protect the public, and the overutilization of Vioxx by the medical profession, which was well informed of the lethality of Vioxx for several years[11] before Merck's confessionary and belated withdrawal of the drug. Soon thereafter, several other so-called "anti-inflammatory drugs" such as valdecoxib (Bextra),[12] celecoxib (Celebrex),[13] and naproxen (Aleve)[14] were likewise associated with excess cardiovascular injury and death. Although the advertising-induced feeding frenzy on Celebrex made it the most successful drug launch in US history with more than 7.4 million prescriptions written within its first 6 months,[15] within 2 years of its release, evidence linking the drug to increased cardiovascular events (including death) was accumulating,[11] and the drug has since been linked to a wide range of adverse effects such as membranous glomerulopathy and acute interstitial nephritis,[16] acute cholestatic hepatitis,[17] and toxic epidermal necrolysis.[18] When compared with placebo in cardiac surgery patients, Bextra/valdecoxib is associated with a 3-fold to 4-fold increased risk of heart attack, stroke, and death,[19] and currently 7 million arthritis patients, many of whom are already at high risk for cardiovascular disease, are being treated with this drug.[12]

Increasingly aware of the negative effects of pharmaceutical management of musculoskeletal pain, patients and healthcare providers alike are looking to natural treatments and chiropractic healthcare[20,21] with the hopes of avoiding the risks of iatrogenic disease, such as drug-induced renal failure,[22] hepatotoxicity,[23] gastrointestinal ulceration and hemorrhage,[24] osteonecrosis,[25,26] joint degeneration,[27,28] hypertension,[28] myocardial infarction,[11] and premature death[11,12] that are associated with the non-steroidal anti-inflammatory drugs ("NSAIDs"), non-NSAID analgesics such as acetaminophen, and the relatively new selective cyclooxygenase-2 inhibitors (cox-2 inhibitors, or "coxibs"). It is tragically paradoxical that many of the pharmaceutical drugs used for the suppression of arthritis symptoms and advertised as "arthritis relief" actually exacerbate joint destruction and chronic inflammation by interfering with the biosynthesis of the glycosaminoglycans that are essential components of joint cartilage while also promoting destruction of subchondral bone.[25,26,27,28] This places chiropractic physicians in an ethical dilemma when helping patients who have been prescribed potentially dangerous medications by their medical doctors. On the one hand, chiropractic physicians are aware of the research showing that, for example, coxibs provide little clinical benefit while promoting increased cardiovascular mortality and other potentially lethal adverse effects. On the other hand, if a chiropractic physician advises discontinuation of the medication, he or she may be reprimanded for "practicing medicine." It appears that chiropractic physicians will need to obtain limited prescription rights for the sake of helping protect their patients from iatrogenic and drug-induced disease. Given that chiropractic physicians are already duly trained in basic and clinical sciences sufficient for primary care, post-graduate certification courses in pharmacology would be sufficient if additional training is deemed necessary to obtain these prescription rights.

The first two articles in this series reviewed the importance of diet and fatty acids in the alleviation of pain and inflammation. This article reviews the most commonly used and well-researched nutritional and botanical interventions for the treatment of pain and inflammation, namely vitamin D, glucosamine and chondroitin sulfate, niacinamide, vitamin D, proteolytic enzymes, Devil's Claw (*Harpagophytum procumbens*), Willow bark (*Salix* spp), and Boswellia *(Boswellia serrata)*. This review will provide chiropractic and naturopathic physicians with clinically useful information to help their patients attain improved health and well-being. Osteoarthritis and chronic low-back pain, the two most prevalent musculoskeletal afflictions, will serve as prototypes for this discussion.

SELECTED NUTRITIONAL AND BOTANICAL THERAPEUTICS FOR THE ALLEVIATION OF JOINT PAIN AND INFLAMMATION

Subsequent to the overall health improvement and anti-inflammatory benefits provided by the supplemented Paleo-Mediterranean diet described previously, many patients who require additional anti-inflammatory interventions can be safely and effectively treated with the following phytonutraceuticals, each of which is supported by experimental and clinical data in humans. Mechanism(s) of action, indications, contraindications, dosage, and common drug interactions (if any) are listed for each.

Glucosamine and chondroitin sulfate: Glucosamine and chondroitin are the "building blocks" from which cartilage is built and oral supplementation is intended to enhance cartilage anabolism and to thus counteract the enhanced cartilage catabolism seen in destructive arthritic processes. Clinical trials with glucosamine and chondroitin sulfates have shown consistently positive results in clinical trials involving patients with osteoarthritis of the hands, hips, knees, temporomandibular joint, and low-back.[29,30,31,32,33,34] For example, glucosamine sulfate was superior to placebo for pain reduction and preservation of joint space in a 3-year clinical trial in patients with knee osteoarthritis.[36] Arguments against the use of glucosamine due to inflated concern about inefficacy or exacerbation of diabetes[37] are without scientific merit[38,39] as evidenced by a 90-day trial[40] of diabetic patients consuming 1500 mg of glucosamine hydrochloride with 1200 mg of chondroitin sulfate which showed no significant alterations in serum glucose or hemoglobin A1c and by the previously cited 3-year study which found significant clinical benefit and no adverse effects on glucose homeostasis. The adult dose of glucosamine sulfate is generally 1500-2000 mg per day in divided doses, and the dose of chondroitin sulfate is approximately 1000 mg daily. Both treatments are safe for multiyear use, and rare adverse effects include allergy and nonpathologic gastrointestinal upset. Clinical benefit is generally significant following 4-6 weeks of treatment and is maintained for the duration of treatment. In contrast to coxib and other mislabeled "anti-inflammatory " drugs that consistently elevate the incidence of cardiovascular disease, death, and other adverse effects, supplementation with chondroitin sulfate appears to safely reduce the pain and disability associated with osteoarthritis while simultaneously reducing incidence of cardiovascular morbidity and mortality.[41,42] In a study with animals that spontaneously develop atherosclerosis,[43] administration of chondroitin sulfate appears to have induced regression of existing atherosclerosis. In a six-year study with 120 patients with established cardiovascular disease, 60 chondroitin-treated patients suffered 6 coronary events and 4 deaths compared to 42 events and 14 deaths in a comparable group of 60 patients receiving "conventional" therapy; chondroitin-treated patients reported enhancement of well-being while no adverse clinical or laboratory effects were noted during the 6 years of treatment.[44]

Vitamin D (cholecalciferol): Vitamin D insufficiency is epidemic in the United States and is extremely prevalent (>90%) among patients with chronic musculoskeletal pain[45] limb pain,[46] and low-back pain.[47] The mechanism by which this pain is produced has been clearly elucidated: 1) vitamin D deficiency causes a reduction in calcium absorption, 2) production of parathyroid hormone (PTH) is increased to maintain blood calcium levels, 3) PTH results in increased urinary excretion of phosphorus, which leads to hypophosphatemia, 4) insufficient calcium phosphate results in deposition of unmineralized collagen matrix on the endosteal (inside) and periosteal (outside) of bones, 5) when the collagen matrix hydrates and swells, it causes pressure on the sensory-innervated periosteum resulting in pain.[48] In patients with vitamin D deficiency, oral supplementation with vitamin D clearly produces anti-inflammatory benefits,[49,50] and treatment with vitamin D can safely lead to dramatic reductions in musculoskeletal pain in a large percentage of patients.[46,47] Routine annual measurement of vitamin D status should be the standard of care[51] since failure to diagnose vitamin D deficiency and to provide adequate replacement doses are both ethically questionable and scientifically unjustifiable in light of the low cost, manifold benefits, rare adverse effects, and high prevalence of vitamin D deficiency.[52,53] Physiologic requirements are approximately 4,000 IU per day in men[54] and can only be achieved with high-dose oral supplementation or full-body sun exposure on a frequent or preferably daily basis. As reviewed in the recent monograph by Vasquez et al,[55] relative contraindications include the use of thiazide diuretics or presence of a vitamin D hypersensitivity syndrome such as primary hyperparathyroidism, adrenal insufficiency, hyperthyroidism, hypothyroidism, or granulomatous disease such as sarcoidosis, Crohn's disease, or tuberculosis). Serum calcium is periodically monitored in patients receiving moderate doses of vitamin D (adult range 4,000 – 10,000 IU per day), since hypercalcemia is the best laboratory indicator of vitamin D excess.

High doses of vitamin D (up to 100,000 IU per day) have been safely used during pregnancy[56,57] periodic testing of serum calcium is required to monitor and for hypercalcemia. Vitamin D supplementation has been proven effective in the treatment of hypertension, depression, migraine headaches, polycystic ovary syndrome and in the prevention of cancer and type-1 diabetes. [55]

Figure 2. Normal and optimal ranges for serum 25(OH) vitamin D levels based on current research. Used with permission from Vasquez A. Integrative Orthopedics. (OptimalHealthResearch.com): 2004

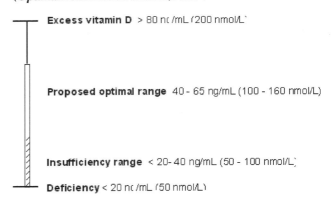

Proteolytic enzymes: Oral administration of proteolytic enzymes (such as pancreatin, bromelain, papain, trypsin and alpha-chymotrypsin) for therapeutic purposes is well established on physiologic, biochemical, and clinical grounds, and a brief review of their historical use is warranted. One of the first experimental studies was published by Beard in 1906 in the *British Medical Journal* wherein he showed that proteolytic enzymes significantly inhibited tumor growth in mice with implanted tumors,[58] and a year later in that same journal, Cutfield[59] reported tumor regression and other objective improvements in a patient treated with proteolytic enzymes. In the American research literature, anti-cancer effects of proteolytic enzymes were reported during this same time in the *Journal of the American Medical Association* in anecdotal case reports of patients with fibrosarcoma,[60] breast cancer,[61] and head and neck malignancy[62]—all of whom responded positively to the administration of proteolytic enzymes; no adverse effects were seen. Although nearly a century would pass before Beard's study and results were replicated with modern techniques,[63,64] by now it is well established that orally administered proteolytic enzymes are well absorbed from the gastrointestinal tract into the systemic circulation[65,66] and that the anti-tumor, anti-metastatic, anti-infectious, anti-inflammatory , analgesic, and anti-edematous actions result from synergism between a variety of mechanisms of action, including the dose-dependent stimulation of reactive oxygen species production and anti-cancer cytotoxicity in human neutrophils,[67] a pro-differentiative effect,[68]

reduction in PG-E2 production,[69] reduction in substance P production,[70] modulation of adhesion molecules and cytokine levels,[71] fibrinolytic effects and a anti-thrombotic effect mediated at least in part by a reduction in 2-series thromboxanes.[72] Unfortunately, enthusiasm for the enzyme treatment of cancer waned prematurely when trypsin was judged to not be a "miracle cure", when the mechanism of action could not be determined, and as enthusiasm surrounding drug and radiation treatments grabbed the attention of allopaths.[73] However, modern controlled clinical trials in cancer patients have established the value of enzyme therapy, which produces important clinical benefit (e.g., symptom reduction and prolonged survival) for little cost and with negligible adverse effects.[74,75,76] Research in other clinical applications for proteolytic enzymes has consistently shown benefit when properly formulated and manufactured preparations are administered appropriately in the treatment of cellulitis, diabetic ulcers, sinusitis, and bronchitis.[77] For example, in a double-blind placebo-controlled trial with 59 patients, Taub[78] documented that oral administration of bromelain significantly promoted the resolution of congestion, inflammation, and edema in patients with acute and chronic refractory sinusitis; no adverse effects were seen in any patient.

When not treating patients with cancer or infectious disease, chiropractic and naturopathic physicians today use these enzymes mostly for the treatment of inflammatory and injury-related disorders. Reporting from the Tulane University Health Service Center, Trickett[79] reported that a papain-containing preparation benefited 40 patients with various injuries (e.g., contusions, sprains, lacerations, strains, fracture, surgical repair, and muscle tears); no adverse effects were seen. In a recent open trial of patients with knee pain, Walker et al[80] found a dose-dependent reduction in pain and disability as well as a significant improvement in psychological well-being in patients consuming bromelain orally. Most of the studies reviewed by Brien et al[69] were suggestive of a positive benefit in patients with knee osteoarthritis, but inadequate dosing clearly prohibited the attainment of optimal results. Bromelain also attenuates experimental contraction-induced skeletal muscle injury,[81] reduces production of hyperalgesic PG-E2 and substance P, is generally effective in the amelioration of trauma-induced injury, edema, and inflammation, and is practically non-toxic.[70] Although bromelain may be used in isolation, enzyme therapy is generally delivered in the form of polyenzyme preparations containing pancreatin, bromelain, papain, trypsin and alpha-chymotrypsin.

Niacinamide: Niacinamide is a form of vitamin B3 that was first shown to be highly effective in the treatment of

osteoarthritis by Kaufman more than 50 years ago.[82] Furthermore, Kaufman's documentation of an "anti-aging" effect of vitamin supplementation in general and niacinamide therapy in particular[83] is consistent with recent experimental data demonstrating rapid reversion of aging phenotypes by niacinamide through possible modulation of histone acetylation.[84] A recent double-blind placebo-controlled repeat study found that niacinamide therapy improved joint mobility, reduced objective inflammation as assessed by ESR, reduced the impact of the arthritis on the activities of daily living, and allowed a reduction in medication use.[85] While the mechanism of action is probably multifaceted, inhibition of joint-destroying nitric oxide appears to be an important benefit.[86] The standard dose of 500 mg given orally 6 times per day is more effective than 1,000 mg 3 times per day. Hepatic dysfunction is rare when daily doses are kept below 3,000 mg per day, yet Gaby[87] suggests measurement of liver enzymes after 3 months of treatment and yearly thereafter. Antirheumatic benefit is generally significant following 2-6 weeks of treatment, and patients may also notice an anxiolytic benefit, which is probably due to the binding of niacinamide to GABA/benzodiazepine receptors.[88]

Boswellia (Boswellia serrata): Boswellia shows anti-inflammatory action via inhibition of 5-lipoxygenase with no apparent effect on cyclooxygenase. A recent clinical study showed that Boswellia was able to reduce pain and swelling while increasing joint flexion and walking distance in patients with osteoarthritis of the knee.[89] While reports from clinical trials published in English are relatively rare, a recent abstract from the German medical research[90] stated, "In clinical trials promising results were observed in patients with rheumatoid arthritis, chronic colitis, ulcerative colitis, Crohn's disease, bronchial asthma and peritumoral brains edemas." Additional recent studies have confirmed the effectiveness of Boswellia in the treatment of asthma[91] and ulcerative colitis.[92] Minor gastrointestinal upset has been reported. Products are generally standardized to contain 37.5–65% boswellic acids, which are currently considered the active constituents with clinical benefit. The target dose is approximately 150 mg of boswellic acids thrice daily; dose and number of capsules/tablets will vary depending upon the concentration found in differing products. Lower doses are effective when used as a part of a comprehensive, multicomponent treatment plan.

Devil's Claw (Harpagophytum procumbens): Harpagophytum has a long history of use in the treatment of musculoskeletal complaints, and recent clinical trials have substantiated its role as a moderately effective analgesic suitable for clinical utilization. At least 12 clinical trials have been published on the use of Harpagophytum in the treatment of musculoskeletal pain, and all trials have found the botanical to be clinically valuable and with adverse effects comparable to placebo.[93] *Harpagophytum's* clinical benefit appears to derive chiefly from its analgesic effect, since administration of the herb does not alter eicosanoid production in humans. In patients with osteoarthritis of the hip and knee, *Harpagophytum* is just as effective yet safer and better tolerated than the drug diacerhein.[94,95] In a study involving 183 patients with low-back pain, *Harpagophytum* was found to be safe and moderately effective in patients with "severe and unbearable pain" and radiating pain with neurologic deficit.[96] Most recently, *Harpagophytum* was studied in a head-to-head clinical trial with the formerly popular but dangerous selective cox-2 inhibitor Vioxx (rofecoxib); the data indicate that *Harpagophytum* was safer and at least as effective.[97] About 8% of patients may experience diarrhea or other mild gastrointestinal effects, and fewer patients may experience dizziness; *Harpagophytum* may potentiate anticoagulants. Treatment should be continued for at least 4 weeks, and many patients will continue to improve after 8 weeks from the initiation of treatment.[98] Products are generally standardized for the content of harpagosides, with a target dose of at least 30 and up to 60 mg harpagoside per day. However, the whole plant is considered to contain effective constituents, not only the iridoid glycosides. Chrubasik[99] noted that while *Harpagophytum* appears to be safe and moderately effective for the treatment musculoskeletal pain, different proprietary products show significant variances in potency and clinical effectiveness. Data suggest that *Harpagophytum* is better than placebo and at least as good as commonly used NSAIDs, suggesting that Harpagophytum should be clinically preferred over NSAIDs due to the lower cost and what appears to be greater safety.

Willow bark (Salix spp): In a double-blind placebo-controlled clinical trial in 210 patients with moderate/severe low-back pain (20% of patients had positive straight-leg raising test), extract of willow bark showed a dose-dependent analgesic effect with benefits beginning in the first week of treatment.[100] In a head-to-head study of 228 patients comparing willow bark (standardized for 240 mg salicin) with Vioxx (rofecoxib), treatments were equally effective yet willow bark was safer and 40% less expensive.[101] Actions of willow bark are manifold including anti-oxidative, anti-cytokine, along with cyclooxygenase- and lipoxygenase-inhibiting effects. A non-purified extract of the phytomedicinal is required for full clinical benefit. The daily dose should not exceed 240 mg of salicin, and products should include other components of the whole plant. Except for rare allergy, no adverse effects are known, yet use during pregnancy and with anti-coagulant medication is discouraged.

SPINAL MANIPULATION: MECHANISMS OF ACTION AND SYNERGISM WITH NUTRITIONAL/BOTANICAL INTERVENTIONS

Select nutritional interventions as surveyed in this paper may have enhanced effects and benefits when combined with spinal manipulative therapy. For example, enhanced respiratory burst clearly carries both antitumor and antimicrobial benefits, and this physiologic effect can be induced by oral consumption of proteolytic enzymes as well as by chiropractic spinal manipulative therapy.[102] Likewise, we would expect synergism between spinal manipulative therapy[103] and nutritional[104] and botanical (e.g., Boswellia) interventions in the treatment of asthma, particularly since these treatments are mediated primarily via different mechanisms—namely the neurophysiologic inhibition of neurogenic inflammation and the biochemical reduction in pro-inflammatory mediators such as leukotrienes, respectively. As a final example, synergism would be expected in the treatment of low-back pain when spinal manipulation, therapeutic exercise, proprioceptive retraining, oral vitamin D supplementation, and botanical medicines such as *Harpagophytum* and Willow Bark are used together in holistic, integrative, multicomponent treatment plans.[105] Taken together, these data form an integrative model that incorporates and mechanistically validates the chiropractic "triad of health" which appreciates the interconnectedness of physical, biochemical, and neurologic aspects of human physiology.[105]

CONCLUSIONS

The chiropractic profession continues to develop and mature over time and with advances in research that further our understanding of health and disease and the value of diet, nutrition, exercise, spinal manipulation and other natural therapeutics. In contrast to our allopathic counterparts, chiropractic and naturopathic physicians are the only healthcare providers trained to consider each patient as an integrated being and to give specific attention to the physiological and biochemical aspects of health and disease, including structural, spinal, musculoskeletal, neurological, vascular, nutritional, emotional and environmental relationships.[106] The anti-inflammatory and analgesic nutritional and botanical medicines described in this review are generally appropriate for the treatment of inflammatory and degenerative musculoskeletal conditions, and they comprise an attractive alternative to the too-often lethal effects of pharmacologic anti-inflammatory and anti-rheumatic drugs.

If we consider that medical/surgical interventions result in an excess of 110,000 – 225,000 iatrogenic American deaths each year,[107,108] we could reasonably conclude that undue restriction of chiropractic and naturopathic physicians to practice preventive healthcare and the discriminatory legal and financial barriers that inhibit patients from accessing alternatives to drugs and surgery ultimately deny patients' access to safe, effective, cost-effective, empowering, affordable healthcare by simultaneously restricting them to interventions that carry greater risk for harm and greater financial expense. With ever-increasing costs and ever-worsening health outcomes, the American healthcare system is destined for collapse unless we change the model upon which our healthcare system is founded—namely the belief that surgery and chemical drugs are the solutions to chronic diseases induced by nutritional deficiencies, oxidative stress, impaired detoxification, defects in fatty acid metabolism, altered gastrointestinal function, and neuromusculoskeletal dysfunction. We have reached an irrevocable impasse in which our current healthcare system dominated by drugs and surgery is no longer consistent with the balance of scientific research.[109] The time has come for patients and practitioners of natural healthcare to demand change and equitable access within the healthcare arena.

ABOUT THE AUTHOR:

Dr. Alex Vasquez is a licensed naturopathic physician in Washington and Oregon, and licensed chiropractor in Texas, where he maintains a private practice and is a member of the Research Team at Biotics Research Corporation. As former Adjunct Professor of Orthopedics and Rheumatology for the Naturopathic Medicine Program at Bastyr University, he is the author of more than 20 published articles and a recently published 486-page textbook for the chiropractic and naturopathic professions, "Integrative Orthopedics: The Art of Creating Wellness While Managing Acute and Chronic Musculoskeletal Disorders" available from OptimalHealthResearch.com.

ACKNOWLEDGEMENTS:

Pepper Grimm BA of Biotics Research Corporation reviewed the draft of this manuscript before submission.

REFERENCES:

1. Legorreta AP, Metz RD, Nelson CF, Ray S, Chernicoff HO, Dinubile NA. Comparative analysis of individuals with and without chiropractic coverage: patient characteristics, utilization, and costs. Arch Intern Med. 2004;164:1985-92
2. Bloomgarden ZT. Type 2 diabetes in the young: the evolving epidemic. Diabetes Care. 2004;27:998-1010
3. Nelson R. US infant mortality shows first rise in 40 years. Lancet. 2004;363(9409):626
4. Zack MM, Moriarty DG, Stroup DF, Ford ES, Mokdad AH. Worsening trends in adult health-related quality of life and self-rated health-United States, 1993-2001. Public Health Rep. 2004;119:493-505
5. Weir HK, Thun MJ, Hankey BF, Ries LA, Howe HL, Wingo PA, Jemal A, Ward E, Anderson RN, Edwards BK. Annual report to the nation on the status of cancer, 1975-2000, featuring the uses of surveillance data for cancer prevention and control. J Natl Cancer Inst. 2003;95(17):1276-99
6. US health care: a state lottery? Lancet. 2004 Nov 20;364(9448):1829-30
7. Legorreta AP, Metz RD, Nelson CF, Ray S, Chernicoff HO, Dinubile NA. Comparative analysis of individuals with and without chiropractic coverage: patient characteristics, utilization, and costs. Arch Intern Med. 2004;164:1985-92
8. Orme-Johnson DW, Herron RE. An innovative approach to reducing medical care utilization and expenditures. Am J Manag Care. 1997 Jan;3(1):135-44
9. Singh G. Recent considerations in nonsteroidal anti-inflammatory drug gastropathy. Am J Med. 1998;105(1B):31S-38S
10. Topol EJ. Failing the public health—rofecoxib, Merck, and the FDA. N Engl J Med. 2004 Oct 21;351(17):1707-9
11. Mukherjee D, Nissen SE, Topol EJ. Risk of cardiovascular events associated with selective COX-2 inhibitors. JAMA 2001; 286(8):954-9
12. Ray WA, Griffin MR, Stein CM. Cardiovascular toxicity of valdecoxib. N Engl J Med. 2004;351(26):2767
13. "Patients in the clinical trial taking 400 mg. of Celebrex twice daily had a 3.4 times greater risk of CV events compared to placebo. For patients in the trial taking 200 mg. of Celebrex twice daily, the risk was 2.5 times greater. The average duration of treatment in the trial was 33 months." FDA Statement on the Halting of a Clinical Trial of the Cox-2 Inhibitor Celebrex.http://www.fda.gov/bbs/topics /news/ 2004/NEW01144.html Available on January 4, 2005
14. "Preliminary information from the study showed some evidence of increased risk of cardiovascular events, when compared to placebo, to patients taking naproxen." FDA Statement on Naproxen. http://www.fda.gov/bbs/topics/news/2004/NEW01148.html Available on January 4, 2005
15. Monsanto, Pfizer celebrate Celebrex. St. Louis Business Journal. July 20, 1999
16. Markowitz GS, Falkowitz DC, Isom R, Zaki M, Imaizumi S, Appel GB, D'Agati VD. Membranous glomerulopathy and acute interstitial nephritis following treatment with celecoxib. Clin Nephrol. 2003;59(2):137-42
17. Grieco A, Miele L, Giorgi A, Civello IM, Gasbarrini G. Acute cholestatic hepatitis associated with celecoxib. Ann Pharmacother. 2002;36(12):1887-9
18. Berger P, Dwyer D, Corallo CE. Toxic epidermal necrolysis after celecoxib therapy. Pharmacotherapy. 2002 Sep;22(9): 1193-5

19. Lenzer J. Pfizer criticised over delay in admitting drug's problems. BMJ. 2004;329(7472):935

20. The Growth of Chiropractic and CAM: More Bad News for Medicine. Dynamic Chiropractic October 8, 2001, Volume 19, Issue 21 http://www.chiroweb.com/archives/19/21 /03.html accessed November 11, 2004

21. Kessler RC, Davis RB, Foster DF, Van Rompay MI, Walters EE, Wilkey SA, Kaptchuk TJ, Eisenberg DM. Long-term trends in the use of complementary and alternative medical therapies in the United States. Ann Intern Med. 2001 Aug 21;135(4):262-8

22. Segasothy M, Chin GL, Sia KK, Zulfiqar A, Samad SA. Chronic nephrotoxicity of anti-inflammatory drugs used in the treatment of arthritis. Br J Rheumatol. 1995 Feb; 34(2): 162-5

23. O'Connor N, Dargan PI, Jones AL. Hepatocellular damage from non-steroidal anti-inflammatory drugs. QJM. 2003 Nov;96(11): 787-91

24. Blower AL. Considerations for nonsteroidal anti-inflammatory drug therapy: safety. Scand J Rheumatol Suppl. 1996;105:13-24

25. Prathapkumar KR, Smith I, Attara GA. Indomethacin induced avascular necrosis of head of femur. Postgrad Med J. 2000 Sep; 76(899): 574-5

26. Newman NM, Ling RS. Acetabular bone destruction related to non-steroidal anti-inflammatory drugs. Lancet. 1985 Jul 6; 2(8445): 11-4

27. Brandt KD. Effects of nonsteroidal anti-inflammatory drugs on chondrocyte metabolism in vitro and in vivo. Am J Med. 1987; 83(5A): 29-34

28. "Systolic blood pressure increased significantly in 17% of rofecoxib- compared with 11% of celecoxib-treated patients (P = 0.032) at any study time point." Whelton A, Fort JG, Puma JA, Normandin D, Bello AE, Verburg KM; SUCCESS VI Study Group.Cyclooxygenase-2—specific inhibitors and cardiorenal function: a randomized, controlled trial of celecoxib and rofecoxib in older hypertensive osteoarthritis patients. Am J Ther 2001 Mar-Apr;8(2):85-95

29. Thie NM, Prasad NG, Major PW. Evaluation of glucosamine sulfate compared to ibuprofen for the treatment of temporomandibular joint osteoarthritis: a randomized double blind controlled 3 month clinical trial. J Rheumatol. 2001;28(6):1347-55

30. Braham R, Dawson B, Goodman C. The effect of glucosamine supplementation on people experiencing regular knee pain. Br J Sports Med. 2003;37(1):45-9

31. Matheson AJ, Perry CM. Glucosamine: a review of its use in the management of osteoarthritis. Drugs Aging. 2003; 20(14): 1041-60

32. Uebelhart D, et al. Intermittent treatment of knee osteoarthritis with oral chondroitin sulfate: a one-year, randomized, double-blind, multicenter study versus placebo. Osteoarthritis Cartilage. 2004;12:269-76

33. van Blitterswijk WJ, van de Nes JC, Wuisman PI. Glucosamine and chondroitin sulfate supplementation to treat symptomatic disc degeneration: biochemical rationale and case report. BMC Complement Altern Med. 2003;3(1):2

34. Morreale P, Manopulo R, Galati M, Boccanera L, Saponati G, Bocchi L. Comparison of the antiinflammatory efficacy of chondroitin sulfate and diclofenac sodium in patients with knee osteoarthritis. J Rheumatol. 1996;23(8):1385-91

35. Mazieres B, Combe B, Phan Van A, Tondut J, Grynfeltt M. Chondroitin sulfate in osteoarthritis of the knee: a prospective, double blind, placebo controlled multicenter clinical study. J Rheumatol. 2001;28(1):173-81

36. Reginster JY, Deroisy R, Rovati LC, Lee RL, Lejeune E, Bruyere O, Giacovelli G, Henrotin Y, Dacre JE, Gossett C. Long-term effects of glucosamine sulphate on osteoarthritis progression: a randomised, placebo-controlled clinical trial. Lancet. 2001;357(9252):251-6

37.Adams ME. Hype about glucosamine. Lancet. 1999;354(9176):353-4

38. Cumming A. Glucosamine in osteoarthritis. Lancet. 1999;354(9190):1640-1

39. Rovati LC, Annefeld M, Giacovelli G, Schmid K, Setnikar I. Glucosamine in osteoarthritis. Lancet. 1999;354(9190):1640

40. Scroggie DA, Albright A, Harris MD. The effect of glucosamine-chondroitin supplementation on glycosylated hemoglobin levels in patients with type 2 diabetes mellitus: a placebo-controlled, double-blinded, randomized clinical trial. Arch Intern Med. 2003;163(13):1587-9

41. Morrison LM. Treatment of coronary arteriosclerotic heart disease with chondroitin sulfate-A: preliminary report. J Am Geriatr Soc. 1968;16(7):779-85

42. Morrison LM, Branwood AW, Ershoff BH, Murata K, Quilligan JJ Jr, Schjeide OA, Patek P, Bernick S, Freeman L, Dunn OJ, Rucker P. The prevention of coronary arteriosclerotic heart disease with chondroitin sulfate A: preliminary report. Exp Med Surg. 1969;27(3):278-89

43. Morrison LM, Bajwa GS. Absence of naturally occurring coronary atherosclerosis in squirrel monkeys (Saimiri sciurea) treated with chondroitin sulfate A. Experientia. 1972 Dec 15;28(12):1410-1

44. Morrison LM, Enrick N. Coronary heart disease: reduction of death rate by chondroitin sulfate A. Angiology. 1973 May;24(5):269-87

45. Plotnikoff GA, Quigley JM. Prevalence of severe hypovitaminosis D in patients with persistent, nonspecific musculoskeletal pain. Mayo Clin Proc. 2003;78(12):1463-70

46. Masood H, Narang AP, Bhat IA, Shah GN. Persistent limb pain and raised serum alkaline phosphatase the earliest markers of subclinical hypovitaminosis D in Kashmir. Indian J Physiol Pharmacol. 1989;33:259-61

47. Al Faraj S, Al Mutairi K. Vitamin D deficiency and chronic low-back pain in Saudi Arabia. Spine. 2003;28:177-9

48. Holick MF. Vitamin D deficiency: what a pain it is. Mayo Clin Proc. 2003 Dec;78(12):1457-9

49. Timms PM, Mannan et al.. Circulating MMP9, vitamin D and variation in the TIMP-1 response with VDR genotype: mechanisms for inflammatory damage in chronic

disorders? QJM. 2002;95:787-96

50. Van den Berghe G, Van Roosbroeck D, Vanhove P, Wouters PJ, De Pourcq L, Bouillon R. Bone turnover in prolonged critical illness: effect of vitamin D. J Clin Endocrinol Metab. 2003;88(10):4623-32

51. Holick MF. Vitamin D: importance in the prevention of cancers, type 1 diabetes, heart disease, and osteoporosis. Am J Clin Nutr. 2004;79(3):362-71

52. Heaney RP. Vitamin D, nutritional deficiency, and the medical paradigm. J Clin Endocrinol Metab. 2003;88(11):5107-8

53. Hollis BW, Wagner CL. Assessment of dietary vitamin D requirements during pregnancy and lactation. Am J Clin Nutr. 2004;79(5):717-26

54. Heaney RP, Davies KM, Chen TC, Holick MF, Barger-Lux MJ. Human serum 25-hydroxycholecalciferol response to extended oral dosing with cholecalciferol. Am J Clin Nutr. 2003;77(1):204-10

55. Vasquez A, Manso G, Cannell J. The Clinical Importance of Vitamin D (Cholecalciferol): A Paradigm Shift with Implications for All Healthcare Providers. Alternative Therapies in Health and Medicine 2004; 10: 28-37

56. O'Leary JA, Klainer LM, Neuwirth RS. The management of hypoparathyroidism in pregnancy. Am J Obstet Gynecol. 1966;94(8):1103-7

57. Goodenday LS, Gordon GS. No risk from vitamin D in pregnancy. Ann Intern Med. 1971;75(5):807-8

58. Beard J. The action of trypsin upon the living cells of Jensen's mouse-tumour. Br Med J 1906; 4 (Jan 20): 140-1

59. Cutfield A. Trypsin Treatment in Malignant Disease. Br Med J. 1907; 5: 525

60. Wiggin FH. Case of Multiple Fibrosarcoma of the Tongue, With Remarks on the Use of Trypsin and Amylopsin in the Treatment of Malignant Disease." Journal of the American Medical Association 1906; 47: 2003-8

61. Goeth RA. Pancreatic treatment of cancer, with report of a cure. Journal of the American Medical Association 1907; (March 23) 48: 1030

62. Campbell JT. Trypsin Treatment of a Case of Malignant Disease. Journal of the American Medical Association 1907; 48: 225-226

63. Saruc M, Standop S, Standop J, Nozawa F, Itami A, Pandey KK, Batra SK, Gonzalez NJ, Guesry P, Pour PM. Pancreatic enzyme extract improves survival in murine pancreatic cancer. Pancreas. 2004;28(4):401-12

64. Batkin S, Taussig SJ, Szekerezes J. Antimetastatic effect of bromelain with or without its proteolytic and anticoagulant activity. J Cancer Res Clin Oncol. 1988;114(5):507-8

65. Gotze H, Rothman SS. Enteropancreatic circulation of digestive enzymes as a conservative mechanism. Nature 1975; 257(5527): 607-609

66. Liebow C, Rothman SS. Enteropancreatic Circulation of Digestive Enzymes. Science 1975; 189(4201): 472-474

67. Zavadova E, Desser L, Mohr T. Stimulation of reactive oxygen species production and cytotoxicity in human neutrophils in vitro and after oral administration of a polyenzyme preparation. Cancer Biother. 1995;10(2):147-52

68. Maurer HR, Hozumi M, Honma Y, Okabe-Kado J. Bromelain induces the differentiation of leukemic cells in vitro: an explanation for its cytostatic effects? Planta Med. 1988 Oct;54(5):377-81

69. Brien S, Lewith G, Walker A, Hicks SM, Middleton D. Bromelain as a Treatment for Osteoarthritis: a Review of Clinical Studies. Evidence-based Complementary and Alternative Medicine. 2004;1(3)251-257

70. Gaspani L, Limiroli E, Ferrario P, Bianchi M. In vivo and in vitro effects of bromelain on PGE(2) and SP concentrations in the inflammatory exudate in rats. Pharmacology. 2002;65(2):83-6

71. Leipner J, Saller R. Systemic enzyme therapy in oncology: effect and mode of action. Drugs. 2000 Apr;59(4):769-80

72. Vellini M, Desideri D, Milanese A, Omini C, Daffonchio L, Hernandez A, Brunelli G. Possible involvement of eicosanoids in the pharmacological action of bromelain. Arzneimittelforschung. 1986;36(1):110-2

73. The trypsin treatment of cancer. British Medical Journal 1907; March 2: 519-20

74. Gonzalez NJ, Isaacs LL. Evaluation of pancreatic proteolytic enzyme treatment of adenocarcinoma of the pancreas, with nutrition and detoxification support. Nutr Cancer. 1999;33(2):117-24

75. Sakalova A, Bock PR, Dedik L, Hanisch J, Schiess W, Gazova S, Chabronova I, Holomanova D, Mistrik M, Hrubisko M. Retrolective cohort study of an additive therapy with an oral enzyme preparation in patients with multiple myeloma. Cancer Chemother Pharmacol. 2001 Jul;47 Suppl:S38-44

76. Popiela T, Kulig J, Hanisch J, Bock PR. Influence of a complementary treatment with oral enzymes on patients with colorectal cancers—an epidemiological retrolective cohort study. Cancer Chemother Pharmacol. 2001;47 Suppl:S55-63

77. Taussig SJ, Yokoyama MM, Chinen A, Onari K, Yamakido M. Bromelain: a proteolytic enzyme and its clinical application. A review. Hiroshima J Med Sci. 1975;24(2-3):185-93

78. Taub SJ. The use of bromelains in sinusitis: a double-blind clinical evaluation. Eye Ear Nose Throat Mon. 1967 Mar;46(3):361-5

79. Trickett P. Proteolytic enzymes in treatment of athletic injuries. Appl Ther. 1964;30:647-52

80. Walker AF, Bundy R, Hicks SM, Middleton RW. Bromelain reduces mild acute knee pain and improves well-being in a dose-dependent fashion in an open study of otherwise healthy adults.Phytomedicine.2002;9:681-6

81. Walker JA, Cerny FJ, Cotter JR, Burton HW. Attenuation of contraction-induced skeletal muscle injury by bromelain. Med Sci Sports Exerc. 1992 Jan;24(1):20-5

82. Kaufman W. Niacinamide therapy for joint mobility. Therapeutic reversal of a common clinical manifestation of the "normal" aging process. Conn State Med J 1953;17:584-591

83. Kaufman W. The use of vitamin therapy to reverse cer-

tain concomitants of aging. J Am Geriatr Soc 1955;3:927-936

84. Matuoka K, Chen KY, Takenawa T. Rapid reversion of aging phenotypes by nicotinamide through possible modulation of histone acetylation. Cell Mol Life Sci. 2001;58(14):2108-16

85. Jonas WB, Rapoza CP, Blair WF. The effect of niacinamide on osteoarthritis: a pilot study. Inflamm Res 1996 Jul;45(7):330-4

86. McCarty MF, Russell AL. Niacinamide therapy for osteoarthritis—does it inhibit nitric oxide synthase induction by interleukin 1 in chondrocytes? Med Hypotheses. 1999;53(4):350-60

87. Gaby AR. Literature review and commentary: Niacinamide for osteoarthritis. Townsend Letter for Doctors and Patients. 2002: May; 32

88. Mohler H, Polc P, Cumin R, Pieri L, Kettler R. Nicotinamide is a brain constituent with benzodiazepine-like actions. Nature. 1979; 278(5704): 563-5

89. Kimmatkar N, Thawani V, Hingorani L, Khiyani R. Efficacy and tolerability of Boswellia serrata extract in treatment of osteoarthritis of knee—a randomized double blind placebo controlled trial. Phytomedicine. 2003 Jan;10(1):3-7

90. Ammon HP. [Boswellic acids (components of frankincense) as the active principle in treatment of chronic inflammatory diseases] [Article in German] Wien Med Wochenschr. 2002;152(15-16):373-8

91. Gupta I, Gupta V, Parihar A, Gupta S, Ludtke R, Safayhi H, Ammon HP. Effects of Boswellia serrata gum resin in patients with bronchial asthma: results of a double-blind, placebo-controlled, 6-week clinical study. Eur J Med Res. 1998 Nov 17;3(11):511-4

92. Gupta I, Parihar A, Malhotra P, Singh GB, Ludtke R, Safayhi H, Ammon HP. Effects of Boswellia serrata gum resin in patients with ulcerative colitis. Eur J Med Res. 1997 Jan;2(1):37-43

93. Gagnier JJ, Chrubasik S, Manheimer E. Harpgophytum procumbens for osteoarthritis and low-back pain: a systematic review. BMC Complement Altern Med. 2004 Sep 15;4(1):13

94. Chantre P, Cappelaere A, Leblan D, Guedon D, Vandermander J, Fournie B. Efficacy and tolerance of Harpagophytum procumbens versus diacerhein in treatment of osteoarthritis. Phytomedicine 2000;7(3):177-83

95. Leblan D, Chantre P, Fournie B. Harpagophytum procumbens in the treatment of knee and hip osteoarthritis. Four-month results of a prospective, multicenter, double-blind trial versus diacerhein. Joint Bone Spine 2000;67(5):462-7

96. Chrubasik S, Junck H, Breitschwerdt H, Conradt C, Zappe H. Effectiveness of Harpagophytum extract WS 1531 in the treatment of exacerbation of low-back pain: a randomized, placebo-controlled, double-blind study. Eur J Anaesthesiol 1999 Feb;16(2):118-29

97. Chrubasik S, Model A, Black A, Pollak S. A randomized double-blind pilot study comparing Doloteffin and Vioxx in the treatment of low-back pain. Rheumatology (Oxford). 2003 Jan;42(1):141-8 See www.WellBody-Book.com/articles.htm for the full-text of this article.

98. Chrubasik S, Thanner J, Kunzel O, Conradt C, Black A, Pollak S. Comparison of outcome measures during treatment with the proprietary Harpagophytum extract doloteffin in patients with pain in the lower back, knee or hip. Phytomedicine 2002 Apr;9(3):181-94

99. Chrubasik S, Conradt C, Roufogalis BD. Effectiveness of Harpagophytum extracts and clinical efficacy. Phytother Res. 2004 Feb;18(2):187-9

100. Chrubasik S, Eisenberg E, Balan E, Weinberger T, Luzzati R, Conradt C. Treatment of low-back pain exacerbations with willow bark extract: a randomized double-blind study. Am J Med. 2000;109:9-14

101. Chrubasik S, Kunzel O, Model A, Conradt C, Black A. Treatment of low-back pain with a herbal or synthetic anti-rheumatic: a randomized controlled study. Willow bark extract for low-back pain. Rheumatology (Oxford). 2001;40:1388-93

102. Brennan PC, Triano JJ, McGregor M, Kokjohn K, Hondras MA, Brennan DC. Enhanced neutrophil respiratory burst as a biological marker for manipulation forces: duration of the effect and association with substance P and tumor necrosis factor. J Manipulative Physiol Ther. 1992 Feb;15(2):83-9

103. Balon J, Aker PD, Crowther ER, Danielson C, Cox PG, O'Shaughnessy D, Walker C, Goldsmith CH, Duku E, Sears MR. A comparison of active and simulated chiropractic manipulation as adjunctive treatment for childhood asthma. N Engl J Med. 1998 Oct 8;339(15):1013-20

104. Vasquez A. Reducing Pain and Inflammation Naturally. Part 2: New Insights into Fatty Acid Supplementation and Its Effect on Eicosanoid Production and Genetic Expression. Nutr Perspect 2005; January: 5-16

105. Vasquez A. Integrative Orthopedics: The Art of Creating Wellness While Managing Acute and Chronic Musculoskeletal Disorders. Houston; Natural Health Consulting Corporation. (OptimalHealthResearch.com): 2004

106. American Chiropractic Association. What is Chiropractic? http://amerchiro.org/media/whatis/ Accessed January 9, 2005

107. Starfield B. Is US health really the best in the world? JAMA. 2000 Jul 26;284(4):483-5

108. Holland EG, Degruy FV. Drug-induced disorders. Am Fam Physician. 1997 Nov 1;56(7):1781-8, 1791-2

109. Hyman M. Paradigm shift: the end of "normal science" in medicine understanding function in nutrition, health, and disease. Altern Ther Health Med. 2004;10(5):10-5, 90-4

Chapter 4:
Skull Dysfunction,
Temporomandibular Joint Disorders,
Headaches, and Migraine

Introduction:

Painful conditions of the head and jaw—TMJ, migraine and other headache disorders—are discussed here. In particular, the section on migraine headaches is very clinically useful.

Topics:
- Skull dysfunction
- Headache, head pain, and migraine headaches
- Temporomandibular joint dysfunction and bruxism

Core Competencies:
- Differentiate the characteristics of a benign headache from one that is potentially life-threatening.
- Name two natural treatments for cluster headaches.
- List the characteristics of migraine headaches and the migraine-specific mechanisms and proper administration—including contraindications—of the following treatments:
   - Riboflavin, vitamin D, CoQ-10, niacin, magnesium, hypoallergenic diet
- Review concepts of neurologic diagnosis and localization described in your neurology courses/text and Chapter 1.

Skull Dysfunction and Cranial Manipulation:

- Anatomical and clinical evidence supports the hypothesis that, in some patients, dysfunction of the joints of the skull may lead to clinical manifestations and that skillful correction of this dysfunction with manual, intranasal, and intraoral techniques can lead to clinical improvement, such as in patients with chronic sinusitis.[1] For clinicians interested in learning more about this concept and technique, I defer to the treatise by Berman[2] which details the anatomic basis and clinical treatment of "skull dysfunction." A more recent article by Blum[3] provides a case report of a woman with severe scoliosis who benefited from the combination of spinal manipulation, Pilates exercises, sacro-occipital technique, and cranial manipulation. The number of studies on cranial manipulation appears to have increased in the past few years, perhaps owing to the converging effects of 1) generalized increased interest and utilization of natural medicine, 2) improved technology for evaluating minute physiologic parameters, and specifically 3) the osteopathic profession's resurging interest in scientifically documenting the effects of osteopathic manipulative medicine. Although studies showing objective effects of cranial manipulation (e.g., cranial manipulation alters specific parameters of cranial blood flow[4]) validate the fundamental concepts that 1) cranial bones can be manually manipulated and that 2) manipulation of cranial bones has physiologic effects, the clinical significance of some studies is not immediately clear. Recent articles with clinically relevance include the findings by Cutler et al[5] that the CV4 technique reduces both sympathetic nervous activity and sleep latency, and the case report by Elliot et al[6] documenting subjective and objective improvement after cranial manipulation in a patient with post-traumatic facial palsy. Balloon insufflation of the sinuses for the purpose of cranial manipulation is a controversial treatment that should be considered only by highly qualified clinicians; it has resulted in at least one death (due to inhalation of the inflating balloon and subsequent suffocation). Manual intraoral and extracranial techniques are generally safe when applied with dexterity and common sense.

---

[1] "When additional interventions (nasal specific technique and light force cranial adjusting) were added to the treatment regimen, significant relief of symptoms was achieved after the nasal specific technique was performed." Folweiler DS, Lynch OT. Nasal specific technique as part of a chiropractic approach to chronic sinusitis and sinus headaches. *J Manipulative Physiol Ther*. 1995 Jan;18(1):38-41

[2] Berman S. Skull dysfunction. *Cranio*. 1991 Jul;9(3):268-79. This highly detailed article is strongly recommended for those with an interest in cranial manipulation.

[3] Blum CL. Chiropractic and pilates therapy for the treatment of adult scoliosis. *J Manipulative Physiol Ther*. 2002 May;25(4):E3
http://www.journals.elsevierhealth.com/periodicals/ymmt/article/PIIS0161475402932549/fulltext

[4] "Compression of the fourth ventricle (CV-4) is a manual, noninvasive procedure that reportedly affects the cranial rhythmic impulse, a phenomenon recognized by practitioners of cranial manipulation… CONCLUSIONS: This study showed that CV-4 has an effect on the TH frequency component of blood flow velocity." Nelson KE, Sergueef N, Glonek T. The effect of an alternative medical procedure upon low-frequency oscillations in cutaneous blood flow velocity. *J Manipulative Physiol Ther*. 2006 Oct;29(8):626-36

[5] "The current study is the first to demonstrate that cranial manipulation, specifically the CV4 technique, can alter sleep latency and directly measured MSNA [muscle sympathetic nerve activity] in healthy humans." Cutler MJ, Holland BS, Stupski BA, Gamber RG, Smith ML. Cranial manipulation can alter sleep latency and sympathetic nerve activity in humans: a pilot study. *J Altern Complement Med*. 2005 Feb;11(1):103-8

[6] Elliott JM, Jacobson EJ, Centeno CJ, Emerson PL. Cranial manipulation with possible neurovascular contact injury at the cerebello-pontine angle: a case report. *Altern Ther Health Med*. 2003 Jul-Aug;9(4):112, 108-9

Headache and head pain
Migraine headaches

<u>Description/pathophysiology</u>:
- <u>Introduction</u>: Headaches are a common symptom-based diagnosis with a wide variety of underlying causes ranging from commonplace and benign (e.g., muscle tension headache) to catastrophic (e.g., meningitis or stroke). This section deals only with the pathophysiology and amelioration of routine benign headaches (migraine, cluster, allergic, tension, and cervicogenic); emphasis is placed on migraine headaches as the prototype for thesedisorders. The differential diagnosis of headache by history, examination, and laboratory and imaging assessments should be familiar to clinicians. In particular, the neurological examination should include psychoemotional assessment, as well as cranial nerve and fundoscopic examination, and any new headache symptoms, even in a patient with a history of headaches, must receive due diligence on the part of the clinician. Once serious pathological causes of headache have been excluded, the headache can be treated with symptom-suppressing drugs or by biological interventions that address the underlying causative mechanisms.

- <u>Significance</u>: Headaches, head pain, and dysfunction of the temporomandibular joint (TMJ)—while seemingly insignificant compared to life-threatening diseases such as cancer and autoimmune diseases—account for huge losses in quality of life and productivity. Headache is a diagnosis based on the patient's subjective report of pain in (deep) or on (superficial) the head. The potential causes are numerous, ranging from benign muscle tension to life-threatening intracranial hemorrhage or meningitis. Relief of headache with analgesic medications does not exclude serious underlying disease.

- <u>Mechanism of pain sensation in headache</u>: The final common pathway for headaches is currently reported to be neurogenic inflammation—in this case, release of neuropeptides from trigeminal nerve (cranial nerve V) neurons to local blood vessels, dura mater, and pia mater.[7] Since this sensory pathway is operative regardless of underlying cause, relief of headache with analgesic medications does not exclude serious underlying disease such as hemorrhage or meningitis.

- <u>Pathophysiology</u>: The sensation of headache pain results from activation and sensitization of sensory trigeminal pain neurons that service intracranial blood vessels and meninges. The debate continues as to whether *vasculogenic* or *neurogenic* influences predominate, and most if not all headaches appear to involve both of these main components, thus allowing for the consensus that headaches are *neurovascular* in origin. That said, the weight of evidence increasingly supports the neurological origin of headaches in general and migraines in particular. "Brain-initiated events" such as cortical spreading depression culminate in the release of nociceptive substances including hydrogen ions and arachidonate metabolites, which irritate trigeminovascular sensory neurons surrounding pial vessels.[8,9] Neurogenic inflammation (e.g., the release of neuropeptides from trigeminal nerve [cranial nerve V] neurons to local blood vessels and meninges) is also important and contributes to a vicious cycle of pain and inflammation.[10] Elevated intracellular calcium levels that trigger inflammatory pathways can be promoted by arachidonate, secondary hyperparathyroidism due to vitamin D deficiency, a relative insufficiency of magnesium, and mitochondrial impairment. Mast cell degranulation releases inflammatory mediators such as serotonin, prostaglandin I-2, and histamine, which induce local inflammation and activation of meningeal nociceptors[11,12] and might serve as a pathophysiological link between emotional stress or allergen exposure and headache (i.e., the link between environmental stressors and headache pain). Mast cells can also be activated by neuropeptides that originate from neurons in the brain parenchyma. Further substantiating the role of local inflammation in migraine is the finding of increased activity of nuclear

[7] Tierney ML. McPhee SJ, Papadakis MA (eds). <u>Current Medical Diagnosis and Treatment 2006, 45th Edition</u>. New York: Lange Medical Books; 2006, pages 31-33
[8] Moskowitz MA. Pathophysiology of headache--past and present. *Headache*. 2007 Apr;47 Suppl 1:S58-63
[9] Moskowitz MA. Genes, proteases, cortical spreading depression and migraine: impact on pathophysiology and treatment. *Funct Neurol*. 2007 Jul-Sep;22(3):133-6
[10] Tierney ML. McPhee SJ, Papadakis MA (eds). <u>Current Medical Diagnosis and Treatment 2006, 45th Edition</u>. New York: Lange Medical Books; 2006, pages 31-33
[11] Levy D, Burstein R, Kainz V, Jakubowski M, Strassman AM. Mast cell degranulation activates a pain pathway underlying migraine headache. *Pain*. 2007 Jul;130(1-2):166-76
[12] Zhang XC, Strassman AM, Burstein R, Levy D. Sensitization and activation of intracranial meningeal nociceptors by mast cell mediators. *J Pharmacol Exp Ther*. 2007 Aug;322(2):806-12

transcription factor-kappa B (NF-κB) in jugular blood of migraine patients during migraine episode[13]; NF-κB is an important mediator of inflammation through its ability to enhance transcription of genes that encode for inflammatory mediators.[14] This model provides for the often observed continuum between external and biopsychosocial factors such as exposure to bright lights, hypoglycemia, stress, anxiety, allergen exposure, and hormonal fluctuations with the triggering of new or recurrent headaches. An appreciation for the intraneuronal genesis of headaches such as migraines sharpens our focus on events occurring within the neuronal cell, in particular mitochondrial bioenergetics, intraneuronal calcium homeostasis, and the elaboration of inflammatory mediators derived from polyunsaturated fatty acids. With the realization of mitochondrial and eicosanoid contributions to headache, clinicians can intervene with nutritional intervention and fatty acid supplementation to enhance mitochondrial function and modulate eicosanoid production, respectively. Failure to appreciate these underlying pathophysiological mechanisms forces clinicians and patients to rely on pharmacological symptom suppression while the underlying processes remain unaddressed.

Clinical presentations:
- Head pain
- Additional symptoms of aura, photophobia, periodic recurrence, chronicity, family history, and nausea suggest the specific headache subtype of migraine.
- Concomitant subjective complaints (e.g., lethargy, sleepiness, mood/cognitive changes, changed vision) and/or objective presentations (e.g., fever, skin rash, galactorrhea, or neurologic deficits) indicate the need for additional evaluation to exclude important intracranial lesions such as pituitary adenoma, meningitis, tumor, subdural hematoma, etc.

Major differential diagnoses:
- Cervical spondylosis: Cervical spine dysfunction and arthropathy can cause and contribute to head pain and headaches; confer with history and examination.
- Cluster headache: Presents with intense unilateral periorbital pain often associated with ipsilateral nasal congestion, rhinorrhea, lacrimation, eye redness, and transient/chronic Horner's syndrome; more common in men, especially in smokers; exacerbated by alcohol; tend to recur at the same time every day, most often at night.
- Cough headache: Severe transient headache triggered by coughing, straining, sneezing, or laughing; patients with recurrent complaints need to be evaluated with a complete neurologic examination and are candidates for CT/MRI since 10% of patients with persistent cough headache have an intracranial lesion.[15]
- Dental or occlusive disorders: Mouth examination, history, oral/dental exam.
- Depression: Check for history consistent with depression: apathy, recent stressful life events.
- Drug side-effect: Check each drug that the patient is taking to see if side-effects correlate with clinical complaints.
- Food allergy: Evaluate with elimination/challenge, history; consider blood tests for recalcitrant cases.
- Head injury: Evaluate with history and examination.
- Hyperparathyroidism: Begin by assessing serum calcium.
- Hypertension: Assess blood pressure; although most patients with hypertension do not have headaches, and most patients with headaches do not have hypertension, acute exacerbations of hypertension commonly precipitate headache. Assess for papilledema and hyperreflexia.
- Hyperthyroidism: Assess TSH (generally low) and free T4 (always high); additional testing and treatment as indicated.
- Hypothyroidism: Assess TSH (may be high or low, depending on pituitary or thyroid lesion), free T4 (generally low), free T3 (may be low or normal), anti-TPO antibodies (seen with autoimmune

[13] Sarchielli P, Floridi A, Mancini ML, Rossi C, Coppola F, Baldi A, Pini LA, Calabresi P. NF-kappaB activity and iNOS expression in monocytes from internal jugular blood of migraine without aura patients during attacks. *Cephalalgia*. 2006 Sep;26(9):1071-9
[14] Tak PP, Firestein GS. NF-kappaB: a key role in inflammatory diseases. *J Clin Invest*. 2001 Jan;107(1):7-11
[15] Tierney ML. McPhee SJ, Papadakis MA (eds). Current Medical Diagnosis and Treatment 2002, 41st Edition. New York: Lange; 2002. Page 999-1005

hypothyroidism: Hashimoto's disease); effective treatment with thyroid hormone alleviates most headaches in hypothyroid-headache patients.[16]

- <u>HIV infection</u>: Patients with HIV are at increased risk for infections, including intracranial infections, particularly toxoplasmosis; intracranial lymphoma is also more common in HIV-positive patients.

- <u>Intracranial aneurysm</u>: May present with throbbing pain; assessed with contrast angiography. In one large international study with 1449 patients[17], the risk of rupture was less than 1% per year, whereas complications from surgery were seen in approximately 14%. A Japanese study[18] found that 95% of patients had a favorable outcome with surgery, implying that 5% had an unfavorable outcome, which is still greater than the risk of rupture, being less than 1% per year for untreated aneurysms reported previously.[19] A more recent study also suggested that the risks of treatment might exceed the risk of spontaneous rupture.[20] Thus the clinical management of intracranial aneurysms must be determined per patient, neurologic location, available and techniques and research, and experience of the neurosurgeon.

- <u>Iron overload</u>: For reasons reviewed in Chapter 1 in the section on serum ferritin, all patients must be tested for iron overload. Iron overload is positively associated with headaches.[21,22]

- <u>Magnesium deficiency</u>: Magnesium deficiency is common in industrialized nations[23,24,25,26] and can be assessed clinically (e.g., response to supplementation) or with laboratory tests (e.g., intracellular magnesium). Associated findings common with magnesium deficiency are muscle cramps, bruxism, constipation, and cravings of sweets/candies and especially chocolate.

- <u>Meningitis</u>: Evaluate fundoscopic examination, skin rash, fever, CBC, CRP; immediate transport to emergency department if meningitis is suspected.

- <u>Migraine</u>: Classic presentation includes periodicity, unilaterality, with prodrome, photophobia, nausea, vomiting, visual changes, and positive family history and onset in early teens or adulthood; a large percentage of migraine patients do not have the classic presentation. Migraine can be associated with transient neurologic deficits: numbness, aphasia, clumsiness, and weakness.

- <u>Muscle tension and tension headaches</u>: Assessed with palpation/provocation of cervical/cranial musculature; worse with stress and generally worse at the end of the workday; generally responsive to manual therapies, stress reduction, stretching of affected musculature, and magnesium supplementation.

- <u>Myofascial trigger points</u>: Palpation/provocation of cervical/cranial musculature; treat with post-isometric stretching, ergonomic improvements, and the supplemented Paleo-Mediterranean diet[27] with an emphasis on supplementation with vitamin D, calcium, and magnesium.

[16] "Thirty-one patients with hypothyroidism of 102 (30%) presented with headache 1 to 2 months after the first symptoms of hypothyroidism. The headache was slight, nonpulsatile, continuous, bilateral, and salicylate responsive and disappeared with thyroid hormone therapy. " Moreau T, Manceau E, Giroud-Baleydier F, Dumas R, Giroud M. Headache in hypothyroidism. Prevalence and outcome under thyroid hormone therapy. *Cephalalgia* 1998 Dec;18(10):687-9

[17] International Study of Unruptured Intracranial Aneurysms Investigators. Unruptured intracranial aneurysms--risk of rupture and risks of surgical intervention. *N Engl J Med* 1998 Dec 10;339(24):1725-33

[18] Orz YI, Hongo K, Tanaka Y, Nagashima H, Osawa M, Kyoshima K, Kobayashi S. Risks of surgery for patients with unruptured intracranial aneurysms. *Surg Neurol* 2000 Jan;53(1):21-7; discussion 27-9

[19] International Study of Unruptured Intracranial Aneurysms Investigators. Unruptured intracranial aneurysms--risk of rupture and risks of surgical intervention. *N Engl J Med* 1998 Dec 10;339(24):1725-33

[20] Risks associated with spontaneous rupture "were often equaled or exceeded by the risks associated with surgical or endovascular repair of comparable lesions." Wiebers DO, Whisnant JP, Huston J 3rd, Meissner I, Brown RD Jr, Piepgras DG, Forbes GS, Thielen K, Nichols D, O'Fallon WM, Peacock J, Jaeger L, Kassell NF, Kongable-Beckman GL, Torner JC; International Study of Unruptured Intracranial Aneurysms Investigators. Unruptured intracranial aneurysms: natural history, clinical outcome, and risks of surgical and endovascular treatment. *Lancet*. 2003 Jul 12; 362(9378): 103-10

[21] In a study involving more than 51,000 patients: "Phenotypic hemochromatosis and the C282Y/C282Y genotype were both associated with an 80% increase in headache prevalence evident only among women. The reason for this association is unclear, but one may speculate that iron overload alters the threshold for triggering a headache by disturbing neuronal function." Hagen K, Stovner LJ, Asberg A, Thorstensen K, Bjerve KS, Hveem K. High headache prevalence among women with hemochromatosis: the Nord-Trondelag health study. *Ann Neurol* 2002;51(6):786-9

[22] "The coexistence of the two disorders may be a mere coincidence, but the temporary improvement of headache from depletion of iron stores may indicate a causal relation, possibly mediated by iron deposits in pain-modulating centres in the brainstem." Stovner LJ, Hagen K, Waage A, Bjerve KS. Hereditary haemochromatosis in two cousins with cluster headache. *Cephalalgia* 2002 May;22(4):317-9

[23] "The American diet is low in magnesium, and with modern water systems, very little is ingested in the drinking water." Innerarity S. Hypomagnesemia in acute and chronic illness. *Crit Care Nurs Q*. 2000 Aug;23(2):1-19

[24] "Altogether 43% of 113 trauma patients had low magnesium levels compared to 30% of noninjured cohorts." Frankel H, Haskell R, Lee SY, Miller D, Rotondo M, Schwab CW. Hypomagnesemia in trauma patients. *World J Surg*. 1999 Sep;23(9):966-9

[25] "There was a 20% overall prevalence of hypomagnesemia among this predominantly female, African American population." Fox CH, Ramsoomair D, Mahoney MC, Carter C, Young B, Graham R. An investigation of hypomagnesemia among ambulatory urban African Americans. *J Fam Pract*. 1999 Aug;48(8):636-9

[26] "Suboptimal levels were detected in 33.7 per cent of the population under study. These data clearly demonstrate that the Mg supply of the German population needs increased attention." Schimatschek HF, Rempis R. Prevalence of hypomagnesemia in an unselected German population of 16,000 individuals. *Magnes Res*. 2001 Dec;14(4):283-90

[27] Vasquez A. A Five-Part Nutritional Protocol that Produces Consistently Positive Results. *Nutritional Wellness* 2005Sept. http://optimalhealthresearch.com/protocol.html

- **Ocular disorders**: Assess with history (e.g., recent change in prescription, new glasses or contacts), and neurologic, eye, and fundoscopic examination; consider diabetes mellitus, multiple sclerosis, and glaucoma and test or refer appropriately.
- **Preeclampsia**: Headache in a pregnant woman may indicate preeclampsia; assess for hypertension, edema, and proteinuria; emergency or urgent obstetrical referral will be indicated in most cases.
- **Pheochromocytoma**: Common presentation is periodic headache concurrent with exacerbations of hypertension, sweats, and tachycardia/palpitations.
- **Sinusitis or sinus infection**: History, fever, pain with palpation of sinuses, nasal discharge; test CBC and CRP; consider radiographic or CT imaging.
- **Temporal arteritis (TA) and polymyalgia rheumatica (PMR)**: History of diffuse head/shoulder pain and jaw claudication generally with systemic complaints of myalgia and fatigue in a patient over 50 years of age; if suspected, must assess CRP/ESR and palpation of artery. **Remember that temporal arteritis can result in blindness; any visual change in a patient with TA/PMR should be considered a medical emergency.** "Loss of vision is the most feared manifestation and occurs quite commonly."[28]
- **TMJ dysfunction**: Assess with examination, history, oral/dental exam, pain worse with chewing (DDX temporal arteritis).
- **Tumor or other intracranial mass lesion**: One-third of brain tumor patients present with an initial complaint of headache[29]; symptoms are typically worse upon waking and worse with exertion. Assess with neurologic exam, CT, and MRI as indicated.

Clinical assessment:
- **History/subjective**:
  - **Subacute or chronic/periodic head pain**: Most likely benign if course is not progressive and if no neurologic deficits and other findings are present.
  - **Acute headache**: Recent onset of severe headache in a previously healthy patient suggests intracranial lesion or meningitis.[30] Approximately 1% of patients with acute headache who present to emergency departments will have a life-threatening disorder.[31]
- **Physical examination/objective**:
  - Neurologic examination should be performed on all patients with a recent onset of new headaches or a change from their previous headache. **The finding of any mental abnormality or neurologic deficit indicates immediate need for further evaluation: brain CT/MRI and/or emergency department referral.**[32]
  - Muscle strength
  - Reflexes
  - Fundoscopic examination for papilledema
  - Cranial nerve examination
  - Blood pressure
  - Signs for meningeal irritation:
    - **Nuchal rigidity (previously referred to as Soto-Hall maneuver)**: patient supine on examining table; doctor gently-yet-assertively forces patient's neck into flexion: positive sign for meningeal irritation is undue pain or resistance. **This test must not be performed in patients who may have atlantoaxial instability or cervical spine fracture.**
    - **Kernig sign**: patient supine with hip flexed, slowly extend knee; positive sign: pain in posterior thigh with or without flexion of opposite knee
    - **Brudzinski sign**: bilateral hip flexion following forced cervical flexion when the patient is supine

[28] Tierney ML. McPhee SJ, Papadakis MA (eds). Current Medical Diagnosis and Treatment 2002, 41st Edition. New York: Lange; 2002, page 999-1005
[29] Tierney ML. McPhee SJ, Papadakis MA (eds). Current Medical Diagnosis and Treatment 2002, 41st Edition. New York: Lange; 2002, page 999-1005
[30] "The onset of severe headache in a previously well patient is more likely than chronic headache to relate to an intracranial disorder such as subarachnoid hemorrhage or meningitis." Tierney ML. McPhee SJ, Papadakis MA (eds). Current Medical Diagnosis and Treatment 2002, 41st Edition. New York: Lange Medical Books; 2002, page 999
[31] Tierney ML. McPhee SJ, Papadakis MA (eds). Current Medical Diagnosis and Treatment 2006, 45th Edition. New York: Lange Medical Books; 2006, pages 31-33
[32] Tierney ML. McPhee SJ, Papadakis MA (eds). Current Medical Diagnosis and Treatment 2006, 45th Edition. New York: Lange Medical Books; 2006, pages 31-33

- **Imaging & laboratory assessments**:
  - <u>Imaging</u>: Rarely required except to assess for or exclude intracranial pathology or cervical spondylosis. Importantly, **new onset of headache in an elderly patient or a patient with HIV warrants neuroimaging** *even if the neurologic examination is normal.*[33]
  - <u>Lumbar puncture for CSF analysis</u>: This procedure assesses for infection and subarachnoid hemorrhage and must not be performed unwittingly in patients with increased intracranial hypertension/papilledema.
  - <u>Laboratory evaluation</u> is generally routine and includes the following:
    - <u>CBC</u>: Assess for anemia and evidence of infection.
    - <u>Chemistry panel</u>: Screening evaluation for diabetes, hypercalcemia/electrolytes, liver and kidney function.
    - <u>CRP</u>: Helps to exclude an infectious or inflammatory etiology
    - <u>Ferritin</u>: Assessment for iron overload is indicated in African Americans[34,35], white men over age 30 years[36], patients with peripheral arthropathy[37], diabetics[38] and is advisable in children[39], women[40], young adults[41] and the general population.[42] Iron overload causes headaches.[43,44]
    - <u>Thyroid assessment</u>: Especially in patients with classic manifestations of hypothyroidism: fatigue, depression, cold hands and feet, dry skin, constipation, and delayed Achilles return.[45] See Chapter 1 for interpretive guide.
    - <u>Food allergy testing</u>: May be helpful when elimination-and-challenge procedures are nonproductive and when other therapeutic measures have failed.
- **Establishing the diagnosis**:
  - Headache is considered a diagnosis based on the patient's subjective report of head pain. However, the headache is always secondary to some other cause of pain, which is the true diagnosis. A clinical or empirical process of elimination must consider common and dangerous causes of head pain, including meningitis, temporal arteritis, sinus infections, cervicogenic pain, intracranial lesions such as brain tumors, hypertension, drug side-effects, and food intolerances.
  - **Serious causes of head pain must be considered with each recurrence, as a patient with a long-term history of benign headaches may contract meningitis or develop hypertension as a new or additive cause of his/her headaches.**

<u>Complications</u>:
- Pain and secondary inability to engage in work, play, and other daily activities.
- Nausea, vomiting, diarrhea are common with migraine.
- Complications may arise if the underlying cause (e.g., tumor, meningitis, hemorrhage) is undiagnosed and unsuccessfully managed.

[33] Tierney ML. McPhee SJ, Papadakis MA (eds). <u>Current Medical Diagnosis and Treatment 2006, 45th Edition</u>. New York: Lange Medical Books; 2006, pages 31-33

[34] Barton JC, Edwards CQ, Bertoli LF, Shroyer TW, Hudson SL. Iron overload in African Americans. *Am J Med*. 1995 Dec;99(6):616-23

[35] Wurapa RK, Gordeuk VR, Brittenham GM, Khiyami A, Schechter GP, Edwards CQ. Primary iron overload in African Americans. *Am J Med*. 1996;101(1):9-18

[36] Baer DM, Simons JL, Staples RL, Rumore GJ, Morton CJ. Hemochromatosis screening in asymptomatic ambulatory men 30 years of age and older. *Am J Med*. 1995 May;98(5):464-8

[37] Olynyk J, Hall P, Ahern M, KwiatekR, MackinnonM. Screening for hemochromatosis in a rheumatology clinic. *Aust NZ J Med* 1994; 24: 22-5

[38] Phelps G, Chapman I, Hall P, Braund W, Mackinnon M. Prevalence of genetic haemochromatosis among diabetic patients. *Lancet* 1989; 2: 233-4

[39] Kaikov Y, Wadsworth LD, Hassall E, Dimmick JE, Rogers PCJ. Primary hemochromatosis in children: report of three newly diagnosed cases and review of the pediatric literature. *Pediatrics* 1992; 90: 37-42

[40] Edwards CQ, Kushner JP. Screening for hemochromatosis. *N Engl J Med* 1993; 328: 1616-20

[41] Gushusrt TP, Triest WE. Diagnosis and management of precirrhotic hemochromatosis. *W Virginia Med J* 1990; 86: 91-5

[42] Balan V, Baldus W, Fairbanks V, Michels V, Burritt M, Klee G. Screening for hemochromatosis: a cost-effectiveness study based on 12, 258 patients. *Gastroenterology* 1994; 107: 453-9

[43] Hagen K, Stovner LJ, Asberg A, Thorstensen K, Bjerve KS, Hveem K. High headache prevalence among women with hemochromatosis: the Nord-Trondelag health study. *Ann Neurol* 2002 Jun;51(6):786-9

[44] Stovner LJ, Hagen K, Waage A, Bjerve KS. Hereditary haemochromatosis in two cousins with cluster headache. *Cephalalgia* 2002 May;22(4):317-9

[45] DeQowin RL. <u>DeQowin and DeQowin's Diagnostic Examination. Sixth Edition</u>. New York, McGraw-Hill; 1994, page 900

Clinical management:

- *Medical standard for migraine*: "Management of migraine consists of avoidance of any precipitating factors, together with prophylactic or symptomatic pharmacologic treatment if necessary."[46]

- For benign headaches including migraine, standard medical treatment is targeted at the alleviation of symptoms. To this end, analgesics and anti-inflammatory drugs such as acetaminophen, aspirin, ibuprofen, naproxen, and ketoprofen are the medical mainstays. Antidepressant drugs ranging from amitriptyline to fluoxetine also might be used for both migraine and tension headaches. Other drugs used for migraine include beta-adrenergic blockers such as propanolol, calcium-channel antagonists such as verapamil, anticonvulsants such as gabapentin and topirmate, and serotonin-modulating drugs such as methysergide and sumatriptan, as well as monoamine oxidase inhibitors and angiotensin-2 receptor blockers. Treatments unique to cluster headaches include inhaled oxygen, lithium carbonate, and prednisone. Migraine patients may become dependent on prescription narcotic drugs, which carry inherent risks of dependence and abuse. Topiramate (Topomax®) is one of the most commonly used pharmaceutical drugs for the treatment of migraine, and a brief description of its efficacy and expense is warranted in order to provide clinical perspective. A recent clinical trial in a leading headache journal concluded that topiramate "resulted in statistically significant improvements" and that the drug is "safe and generally well tolerated"[47]; these statements would appear to support clinical use of the drug. However, more than 10% of patients stopped using the drug due to adverse effects, and the statistically significant benefit largely consisted of a reduction in headache days by 1.5 days per 91 days of treatment compared to placebo. The out-of-pocket cost for 3 months of this drug treatment (not including physician fees, recommended laboratory monitoring, and management of adverse effects) is in the range of $400 to $600. Thus, for a yearly cost of approximately $2000, the total reduction in headache days over placebo would be approximately 6 days per year. This study was funded by the company that makes the drug, and 11 of the 13 authors received funding, employment, or direct payment from Ortho-McNeil Neurologics, Inc.

- A complete patient history and the above-mentioned lab tests and a physical examination with neurologic assessment will exclude most of the lethal differential diagnoses, allowing the provisional assessment of "benign headache" or "migraine headache" to be established.

- Therapeutic trials are implemented to address the underlying problem(s); natural treatments may be superior to drug treatments especially when used in combination.[48]

- New onset of headaches or a progressive headache disorder always requires investigation. Refer to neurologist if clinical outcome is unsatisfactory or if complications become evident.

Treatments (all benign headaches): Standard medical treatment for headaches is expensive and fraught with adverse effects, drug dependence, and suboptimal efficacy. Further, such symptom-suppressive treatment fails to address the causative food intolerances, nutritional deficiencies, and mitochondrial defects that are common in headache patients and migraineurs. Following the exclusion of serious underlying disease, headache patients should be counseled on allergen identification (free and highly efficacious) and should receive nutritional supplementation with combination fatty acids (e.g., ALA, GLA, EPA, DHA) and therapeutic doses of vitamins and minerals, particularly riboflavin, vitamin D3, and magnesium. CoQ10, 5-HTP, melatonin, spinal manipulation, post-isometric stretching, and the other treatments listed above can be used in combination as appropriate per patient to optimize the therapeutic response.

- Lifestyle optimization: Patients with cluster headaches show a greater percentage of increased work-related stress, self-employment, tobacco smoking, and alcohol use or abuse. These concerns should be addressed per patient as indicated. Lifestyle factors such the standard American diet, overconsumption of caffeine and alcohol, and use of tobacco can result in mitochondrial impairment through various

---

[46] Tierney ML. McPhee SJ, Papadakis MA (eds). Current Medical Diagnosis and Treatment 2002, 41st Edition. New York: Lange; 2002. Page 999-1005
[47] Silberstein SD, Lipton RB, Dodick DW, Freitag FG, Ramadan N, Mathew N, Brandes JL, Bigal M, Saper J, Ascher S, Jordan DM, Greenberg SJ, Hulihan J; Topiramate Chronic Migraine Study Group. Efficacy and safety of topiramate for the treatment of chronic migraine: a randomized, double-blind, placebo-controlled trial. *Headache*. 2007 Feb;47(2):170-80
[48] Vasquez A. Interventions need to be consistent with osteopathic philosophy. *J Am Osteopath Assoc*. 2006 Sep;106(9):528-9 http://www.jaoa.org/cgi/content/full/106/9/528

mechanisms, not the least of which are nutrient (especially magnesium) deficiency and accumulation of cyanide, a known mitochondrial poison and constituent of tobacco smoke.

- <u>Food allergy elimination</u>: Food allergy is among the most common causes of headaches[49,50], particularly migraine headaches, particularly those that do not respond to drug treatments.[51,52] In the important study by Grant[53], the following foods were identified as the most common headache triggers: wheat (78%), orange (65%), eggs (45%), tea and coffee (40% each), chocolate and milk (37% each), beef (35%), corn, cane sugar, and yeast (33% each); when an average of 10 triggering foods were avoided, patients experienced a "dramatic fall in the number of headaches per month, 85% of patients becoming headache-free." Food allergen identification via the elimination and challenge technique is accurate and inexpensive, and problem-causing foods are then eliminated from the daily diet. In addition to food allergen avoidance, immunomodulatory and anti-inflammatory techniques can be used (including hormonal correction, eradication of gastrointestinal dysbiosis, and supplementation with vitamin C, mixed tocopherols, balanced combination fatty acids, probiotics, vitamin B-12, bioflavonoids, pancreatic/proteolytic enzymes, honey, calcium and magnesium butyrate, and cromolyn and other prescription agents) as has been reviewed elsewhere.[54]

- <u>Avoidance of food additives</u>: Red wine, aged cheeses, sardines, sausage, bacon, and monosodium glutamate (MSG)-containing foods are common triggers for headache and migraine in susceptible patients and should therefore be avoided. Most of these foods contain tyramine, nitrites, or other neuroexcitatory or vasoactive substances, in addition to components (allergens) to which migraine patients tend to be immunologically sensitized. Sulfites in red wine are also noted to trigger migraine and headache in some patients; many wines are available on the market now which contain no detectable sulfites.

- <u>Magnesium supplementation to bowel tolerance (generally with additional pyridoxine)</u>: Magnesium deficiency is common, affecting approximately 30% of different populations in various industrialized nations.[55,56,57,58] Regardless of headache etiology or classification, magnesium deficiency is more common in headache patients than in headache-free controls. Magnesium deficiency directly contributes to headache by at least 4 mechanisms: (1) facilitating brain cortex hyperexcitability and hypesthesia due to a reduction in the partial blockade of N-methyl-D-aspartate (NMDA) neurotransmitter receptor sites by magnesium[59], (2) impairing cellular energy production, (3) promoting vasoconstriction, and (4) promoting increased muscle tension, with the latter 2 mechanisms caused in part by impaired energy production, as well as altered intracellular calcium-to-magnesium ratios. Conversely, adequate magnesium nutriture and use of magnesium supplementation help prevent headaches by modulation of NMDA receptor sensitivity and support of energy production, vasorelaxation, and myorelaxation. Not only is magnesium deficiency common in female patients with menstrual migraine[60] and in patients with post-traumatic headaches[61], but magnesium supplementation is justified in headache patients based on the findings of "disturbances in magnesium ion homeostasis" which appear to contribute to brain cortex

[49] Egger J, Carter CM, Wilson J, Turner MW, Soothill JF. Is migraine food allergy? A double-blind controlled trial of oligoantigenic diet treatment. *Lancet* 1983 Oct ;2:865-9

[50] Monro J, Brostoff J, Carini C, Zilkha K. Food allergy in migraine. Study of dietary exclusion and RAST. *Lancet* 1980 Jul 5;2(8184):1-4

[51] Monro J, Carini C, Brostoff J. Migraine is a food-allergic disease. *Lancet* 1984 Sep 29;2(8405):719-21

[52] Finn R, Cohen HN. "Food allergy": Fact or Fiction? *Lancet* 1978 Feb 25;1(8061):426-8

[53] Grant EC. Food allergies and migraine. *Lancet* 1979 May 5;1(8123):966-9

[54] Vasquez A. Improving neuromusculoskeletal health by optimizing immune function and reducing allergic reactions: a review of 16 treatments and a 3-step clinical approach. Nutritional Perspectives 2005; October: 27-35, 40 http://optimalhealthresearch.com/part5.html

[55] Innerarity S. Hypomagnesemia in acute and chronic illness. *Crit Care Nurs Q.* 2000 Aug;23(2):1-19

[56] Frankel H, Haskell R, Lee SY, Miller D, Rotondo M, Schwab CW. Hypomagnesemia in trauma patients. *World J Surg.* 1999 Sep;23(9):966-9

[57] Fox CH, Ramsoomair D, Mahoney MC, Carter C, Young B, Graham R. An investigation of hypomagnesemia among ambulatory urban African Americans. *J Fam Pract.* 1999 Aug;48(8):636-9

[58] Schimatschek HF, Rempis R. Prevalence of hypomagnesemia in an unselected German population of 16,000 individuals. *Magnes Res.* 2001 Dec;14(4):283-90

[59] Boska MD, Welch KM, Barker PB, Nelson JA, Schultz L. Contrasts in cortical magnesium, phospholipid and energy metabolism between migraine syndromes. *Neurology* 2002 Apr 23;58(8):1227-33

[60] "CONCLUSIONS: The high incidence of IMg2+ deficiency and the elevated ICa2+/IMg2+ ratio during menstrual migraine confirm previous suggestions of a possible role for magnesium deficiency in the development of menstrual migraine." Mauskop A, Altura BT, Altura BM. Serum ionized magnesium levels and serum ionized calcium/ionized magnesium ratios in women with menstrual migraine. *Headache* 2002 Apr;42(4):242-8

[61] "Abnormalities in serum IMg(2+) concentrations and ICa(2+)/IMg(2+) ratios were found in children with post-traumatic headaches, but total magnesium levels were normal." Marcus JC, Altura BT, Altura BM. Serum ionized magnesium in post-traumatic headaches. *J Pediatr* 2001 Sep;139(3):459-62

hyperexcitability.[62] **Except when contraindicated due to renal failure or drug interaction, magnesium supplementation is safe, effective, and reasonable for essentially all patients with headache.**[63,64,65,66,67] A reasonable clinical approach is to 1) evaluate patient with history, physical examination, and screening laboratory tests to exclude contraindications such as renal insufficiency (assess with BUN, creatinine, and urinalysis), 2) assess for possible drug interactions, and then 3) begin the patient with 200 mg elemental magnesium (citrate or malate) with the dose increased by 200 mg every 1-2 days until bowel tolerance is

<table>
<tr><td>Clinical Pearl: Urinary Alkalinization</td></tr>
<tr><td>The importance of alkalinization for the renal retention and intracellular uptake of magnesium can hardly be overemphasized; so-called failure of magnesium therapy is generally due to failure to attain systemic alkalinization, without which magnesium is both hyperexcreted in the urine and underabsorbed into the intracellular space. As discussed in this context, systemic pH can be assessed by measuring urine pH, which should range from 7.5 up to approximately 8.5.</td></tr>
</table>

reached. Reduce dose if excessively loose stools or diarrhea occur. When high-dose magnesium supplementation is used in patients with renal insufficiency or drugs that predispose to hypermagnesemia, cautious professional supervision is warranted, with periodic measurement of serum or ionized magnesium. Efficacy of magnesium supplementation is enhanced with concomitant pyridoxine supplementation (e.g., 100-250 mg per day with food) and with an alkalinizing Paleo-Mediterranean Diet as described in Chapter 2. The Paleo-Mediterranean Diet can promotes alkalinization[68] which facilitates systemic mineral and magnesium retention[69,70] and increases intracellular magnesium levels.[71] Alkalinization and increased intracellular magnesium levels are associated with reductions in low-back pain according to a clinical trial.[72]

- o **Caution must be employed when using magnesium with the medications mentioned here: Magnesium may decrease the absorption or effectiveness of several drugs,** including: Azithromycin (Zithromax), Cimetidine (Tagamet), Ciprofloxacin (Ciloxan, Cipro), Doxycycline (Atridox, Doryx, Doxy, Monodox, Periostat, Vibramycin), Famotidine (Mylanta-AR, Pepcid, Pepcid AC), Hydroxychloroquine (Plaquenil), Levofloxacin (Levaquin), Nitrofurantoin (Furadantin, Macrobid, Macrodantin), Nizatidine (Axid, Axid AR), Ofloxacin (Floxin, Ocuflox), Tetracycline (Achromycin, Sumycin, Helidac), and Warfarin (Coumadin). Misoprostol (Cytotec, Arthrotec) with magnesium may result in diarrhea. **Spironolactone (Aldactone, Aldactazide) or Amiloride (Midamor, Moduretic) may cause hypermagnesemia.**
- Vitamin D3 (cholecalciferol): Several case reports have documented the effectiveness of vitamin D supplementation in the treatment and prevention of migraine.[73,74] Vitamin D is anti-inflammatory and

[62] "...disturbances in magnesium ion homeostasis may contribute to brain cortex hyperexcitability and the pathogenesis of migraine syndromes associated with neurologic symptoms." Boska MD, Welch KM, Barker PB, Nelson JA, Schultz L. Contrasts in cortical magnesium, phospholipid and energy metabolism between migraine syndromes. *Neurology* 2002 Apr 23;58(8):1227-33

[63] Mazzotta G, Sarchielli P, Alberti A, Gallai V. Intracellular Mg++ concentration and electromyographical ischemic test in juvenile headache. *Cephalalgia* 1999 Nov;19(9):802-9

[64] Mishima K, Takeshima T, Shimomura T, Okada H, Kitano A, Takahashi K, Nakashima K. Platelet ionized magnesium, cyclic AMP, and cyclic GMP levels in migraine and tension-type headache. *Headache* 1997 Oct;37(9):561-4

[65] " After a prospective baseline period of 4 weeks they received oral 600 mg (24 mmol) magnesium (trimagnesium dicitrate) daily for 12 weeks or placebo... High-dose oral magnesium appears to be effective in migraine prophylaxis." Peikert A, Wilimzig C, Kohne-Volland R. Prophylaxis of migraine with oral magnesium: results from a prospective, multi-center, placebo-controlled and double-blind randomized study. *Cephalalgia* 1996 Jun;16(4):257-63

[66] Mauskop A, Altura BT, Cracco RQ, Altura BM. Intravenous magnesium sulfate rapidly alleviates headaches of various types. *Headache* 1996 Mar;36(3):154-60

[67] Wang F, Van Den Eeden SK, Ackerson LM, Salk SE, Reince RH, Elin RJ. Oral magnesium oxide prophylaxis of frequent migrainous headache in children: a randomized, double-blind, placebo-controlled trial. *Headache*. 2003;43:601 –610

[68] Sebastian A, Frassetto LA, Sellmeyer DE, Merriam RL, Morris RC Jr. Estimation of the net acid load of the diet of ancestral preagricultural Homo sapiens and their hominid ancestors. *Am J Clin Nutr* 2002;76:1308-16

[69] Sebastian A, Harris ST, Ottaway JH, Todd KM, Morris RC Jr. Improved mineral balance and skeletal metabolism in postmenopausal women treated with potassium bicarbonate. *N Engl J Med*. 1994;330(25):1776-81

[70] Tucker KL, Hannan MT, Chen H, Cupples LA, Wilson PW, Kiel DP. Potassium, magnesium, and fruit and vegetable intakes are associated with greater bone mineral density in elderly men and women. *Am J Clin Nutr*. 1999;69(4):727-36

[71] "The results show that a disturbed acid-base balance may contribute to the symptoms of low back pain. The simple and safe addition of an alkaline multimineral preparate was able to reduce the pain symptoms in these patients with chronic low back pain." Vormann J,Worlitschek M,Goedecke T,Silver B. Supplementation with alkaline minerals reduces symptoms in patients with chronic low back pain. *J Trace Elem Med Biol*. 2001;15(2-3):179-83

[72] "The results show that a disturbed acid-base balance may contribute to the symptoms of low back pain. The simple and safe addition of an alkaline multimineral preparate was able to reduce the pain symptoms in these patients with chronic low back pain." Vormann J,Worlitschek M,Goedecke T,Silver B. Supplementation with alkaline minerals reduces symptoms in patients with chronic low back pain. *J Trace Elem Med Biol*. 2001;15(2-3):179-83

[73] "Therapeutic replacement with vitamin D and calcium resulted in a dramatic reduction in the frequency and duration of their migraine headaches." Thys-Jacobs S. Alleviation of migraines with therapeutic vitamin D and calcium. *Headache*. 1994 Nov-Dec;34(10):590-2

[74] "These observations suggest that vitamin D and calcium therapy should be considered in the treatment of migraine headaches." Thys-Jacobs S. Vitamin D and calcium in menstrual migraine. *Headache*. 1994 Oct;34(9):544-6

immunomodulatory[75] and also modulates vascular tone by reducing intracellular hypercalcinosis.[76] Reasonable replacement doses are 2,000 IU per day for children and 4,000 IU per day for adults; monitoring serum calcium ensures safety. Optimal vitamin D status correlates with serum 25(OH)D levels of 50 – 100 ng/mL (125 - 250 nmol/L)—see our review article for more details[77]; levels greater than 100 ng/mL are unnecessary and increase the risk of hypercalcemia.[78]

> **Clinical Pearl: Find and treat MFTP**
>
> If deep palpation of the upper cervical musculature produces referred pain to the head or face, then you know the patient has MFTP, and you can then treat them with at-home and in-office stretching and exercises. Generally their "chronic pain" will be greatly reduced within 3-10 days. Better results will be obtained with alkalinization and concomitant supplementation with magnesium, vitamin D, and fish oil.

- <u>Fish oil supplying 3,000 mg of EPA and DHA per day, with additional 400 IU mixed tocopherols</u>: Fish oil has been shown to reduce the frequency, duration, and intensity of migraine headaches[79] and the effectiveness of fish oil may be mediated via alterations in cytokine production.[80]

- <u>Gamma-linolenic acid and alpha-linolenic acid</u>: Supplementation with GLA and ALA—along with the use of a multivitamin and multimineral supplement and avoidance of dietary arachidonic acid—has been shown to significantly reduce the intensity, frequency, and duration of migraine headaches.[81] The standard minimal dose of GLA for antiinflammatory effect is 500 mg per day.

- <u>Treatment of cervical myofascial trigger points</u>: Check the upper cervical spine musculature (especially suboccipital muscles and sternocleidomastoid) for the characteristic manifestations of myofascial trigger points (MFTP, see Chapter 3): palpable nodule, twitch response, and elicitation of referred pain with deep palpation/provocation. Myofascial trigger points are much more common in patients with migraine[82] than in non-headache controls, and they are an important cervicogenic contribution to chronic headaches.[83,84] If located, the MFTP can be effectively treated with in-office post-isometric stretching and exercises performed at home[85] as outlined on an upcoming page.

- <u>Spinal manipulation</u>: Myofascial, arthrogenic, and dyskinetic contributions to headache are significant, and these cervicogenic problems can

> **Osteopathic treatment should include manual musculoskeletal medicine and nutritional interventions**
>
> "In contrast to the description of the osteopathic medical profession by the American Osteopathic Association, namely, "doctors of osteopathic medicine, or D.O.s, apply the philosophy of treating the whole person to the prevention, diagnosis and treatment of illness, disease and injury," [the authors of the article in question] essentially reviewed only pharmacologic treatment.
>
> …
>
> It is hoped that future reviews in this journal can include a more balanced survey of the literature, inclusive of non-pharmacologic and "holistic" interventions that are consistent with osteopathic philosophy."
>
> **Vasquez A**. Interventions Need to be Consistent With Osteopathic Philosophy. [Letter] *JAOA: Journal of the American Osteopathic Association* 2006 Sep;106(9):528-9
> http://www.jaoa.org/cgi/content/full/106/9/528

[75] Timms PM, Mannan N, Hitman GA, Noonan K, Mills PG, Syndercombe-Court D, Aganna E, Price CP, Boucher BJ. Circulating MMP9, vitamin D and variation in the TIMP-1 response with VDR genotype: mechanisms for inflammatory damage in chronic disorders? *QJM*. 2002 Dec;95(12):787-96

[76] Vasquez A. Intracellular Hypercalcinosis: A Functional Nutritional Disorder With Implications Ranging From Myofascial Trigger Points to Affective Disorders, Hypertension and Cancer. *Naturopathy Digest* 2006 September http://www.naturopathydigest.com/archives/2006/sep/vasquez.php

[77] **Vasquez A, Manso G, Cannell J. The Clinical Importance of Vitamin D (Cholecalciferol): A Paradigm Shift with Implications for All Healthcare Providers.** *Alternative Therapies in Health and Medicine* **2004; 10: 28-37.** www.optimalhealthresearch.com/monograph04.html

[78] Vasquez A, Manso G, Cannell J. The Clinical Importance of Vitamin D (Cholecalciferol): A Paradigm Shift with Implications for All Healthcare Providers. *Alternative Therapies in Health and Medicine* 2004; 10: 28-37. Also published in *Integrative Medicine: A Clinician's Journal* 2004; 3: 44-54. See www.optimalhealthresearch.com/monograph04.html

[79] "In fact, results of this preliminary study suggest that both fish oil and olive oil may be beneficial in the treatment of recurrent migraines in adolescents." Harel Z, Gascon G, Riggs S, Vaz R, Brown W, Exil G. Supplementation with omega-3 polyunsaturated fatty acids in the management of recurrent migraines in adolescents. *J Adolesc Health* 2002 Aug;31(2):154-61

[80] Smith RS.The cytokine theory of headache. *Med Hypotheses* 1992 Oct;39(2):168-74

[81] "In 129 patients available for study, 86% experienced reduction in severity, frequency and duration of migraine attacks, 22% became free of migraine and more than 90% had reduced nausea and vomiting." Wagner W, Nootbaar-Wagner U.Prophylactic treatment of migraine with gamma-linolenic and alpha-linolenic acids. *Cephalalgia*. 1997 Apr;17(2):127-30

[82] "Trigger points were found in 92 (93.9%) migraineurs and in nine (29%) controls (P < 0.0001). The number of individual migraine trigger points varied from zero to 14, and was found to be related to both the frequency of migraine attacks, and the duration of the disease." Calandre EP, Hidalgo J, Garcia-Leiva JM, Rico-Villademoros F. Trigger point evaluation in migraine patients: an indication of peripheral sensitization linked to migraine predisposition? *Eur J Neurol*. 2006 Mar;13(3):244-9

[83] "Myofascial trigger points can refer pain to the head and face in the cervical region, thus contributing to cervicogenic headache." Borg-Stein J. Cervical myofascial pain and headache. *Curr Pain Headache Rep*. 2002 Aug;6(4):324-30

[84] "Because treating myofascial problems may be the only way to offer complete relief from certain types of headache, clinicians must learn to diagnose and manage trigger points in neck, shoulder, and head muscles." Davidoff RA. Trigger points and myofascial pain: toward understanding how they affect headaches. *Cephalalgia*. 1998 Sep;18(7):436-48

[85] Lewit K, Simons DG. Myofascial pain: relief by post-isometric relaxation. *Arch Phys Med Rehabil* 1984 Aug;65(8):452-6

be addressed with manual spinal and myofascial manipulation. Spinal manipulation safely alleviates headaches with efficacy comparable to commonly used first-line prophylactic prescription medications for tension-type headache and migraine headache. [86,87,88,89] Spinal manipulation should be performed only by professionals with graduate and postgraduate training in relevant spinal biomechanics, patient assessment, and manipulative technique.[90,91,92,93]

- Ginger: Components of ginger reduce production of the leukotriene LTB4 by inhibiting 5-lipoxygenase and reduce production of the prostaglandin PG-E2 by inhibiting cyclooxygenase.[94,95] With its dual reduction in the formation of inflammation-promoting prostaglandins and leukotrienes, ginger has been shown to safely reduce musculoskeletal pain in general[96,97] and to provide relief from osteoarthritis of the knees[98] and migraine headaches.[99]

- Intentional relaxation and biofeedback: Biofeedback is proven effective in the prevention of chronic headaches, including pediatric migraine.[100,101] Relaxation and stress management are more effective than drug treatment with metoprolol for pediatric migraine.[102]

- 5-Hydroxytryptophan (5-HTP)—typical dose is 50-300 mg per day in divided doses: 5-Hydroxytryptophan (5-HTP) is a natural constituent of the human body and is also found in some plants and is thus available as a nutritional supplement. Altered serotonin metabolism has been observed in headache patients, and this observation serves to support the use of selective serotonin reuptake inhibitors (SSRIs) in headache patients, while supplementation with 5-HTP increases serotonin levels naturally. Among various types of headache, migraine would be expected to show the best response to 5-HTP because the conversion of serotonin to melatonin would extend the benefits of serotonin-mediated analgesia to include the protection of mitochondrial function, an important benefit of melatonin. Conversion of serotonin to melatonin occurs in non-migraine headaches but is of lesser therapeutic importance since these disorders (cluster headaches excepted) are not associated directly with mitochondrial dysfunction. 5-HTP has a better safety and efficacy profile than does the drug

Tryptophan insufficiency: common in migraine, chronic pain, and fibromyalgia
"The recently shown **high prevalence of migraine in the population of fibromyalgia sufferers,** suggests a common ground shared by fibromyalgia and migraine. Migraine has been demonstrated to be characterized by a defect in the serotonergic and adrenergic systems. A parallel dramatic failure of serotonergic systems and a defect of adrenergic transmission have been evidenced to affect fibromyalgia sufferers, too."
Nicolodi M, Sicuteri F.Fibromyalgia and migraine, two faces of the same mechanism. Serotonin as the common clue for pathogenesis and therapy. *Adv Exp Med Biol.* 1996;398:373-9

[86] Bronfort G, Assendelft WJ, Evans R, Haas M, Bouter L. Efficacy of spinal manipulation for chronic headache: a systematic review. *J Manipulative Physiol Ther* 2001 Sep;24(7):457-66

[87] Tuchin PJ, Pollard H, Bonello R. A randomized controlled trial of chiropractic spinal manipulative therapy for migraine. *J Manipulative Physiol Ther.* 2000 Feb;23(2):91-5

[88] "CONCLUSIONS: SMT appears to have a better effect than massage for cervicogenic headache. It also appears that SMT has an effect comparable to commonly used first-line prophylactic prescription medications for tension-type headache and migraine headache." Bronfort G, Assendelft WJ, Evans R, Haas M, Bouter L. Efficacy of spinal manipulation for chronic headache: a systematic review. *J Manipulative Physiol Ther* 2001 Sep;24(7):457-66

[89] "The average response of the treatment group (n = 83) showed statistically significant improvement in migraine frequency (P < .005), duration (P < .01), disability, and medication use..." Tuchin PJ, Pollard H, Bonello R. A randomized controlled trial of chiropractic spinal manipulative therapy for migraine. *J Manipulative Physiol Ther.* 2000 Feb;23(2):91-5

[90] Kirk CR, Lawrence DJ, Valvo NL. States Manual of Spinal, Pelvic, and Extravertebral Technics. Second Edition. Lombard, Illinois: National College of Chiropractic; 1985

[91] Kimberly PE. Outline of Osteopathic Manipulative Procedures. The Kimberly Manual 2006. Kirksville College of Osteopathic Medicine. Walsworth Publishing , Marceline, Mo

[92] Bergmann TF, Peterson DH, Lawrence DJ. Chiropractic Technique. New York; Churchill Livingstone: 1993

[93] Gatterman MI. Chiropractic Management of Spine Related Disorders. Baltimore; Williams and Wilkins: 1990

[94] Kiuchi F, Iwakami S, Shibuya M, Hanaoka F, Sankawa U. Inhibition of prostaglandin and leukotriene biosynthesis by gingerols and diarylheptanoids. *Chem Pharm Bull* (Tokyo) 1992 Feb;40(2):387-91

[95] Tjendraputra E, Tran VH, Liu-Brennan D, Roufogalis BD, Duke CC. Effect of ginger constituents and synthetic analogues on cyclooxygenase-2 enzyme in intact cells. *Bioorg Chem* 2001 Jun;29(3):156-63

[96] Srivastava KC, Mustafa T. Ginger (Zingiber officinale) in rheumatism and musculoskeletal disorders. *Med Hypotheses.* 1992 Dec;39(4):342-8

[97] Srivastava KC, Mustafa T. Ginger (Zingiber officinale) and rheumatic disorders. *Med Hypotheses.* 1989 May;29(1):25-8

[98] Altman RD, Marcussen KC. Effects of a ginger extract on knee pain in patients with osteoarthritis. *Arthritis Rheum.* 2001 Nov;44(11):2531-8

[99] "It is proposed that administration of ginger may exert abortive and prophylactic effects in migraine headache without any side-effects." Mustafa T, Srivastava KC. Ginger (Zingiber officinale) in migraine headache. *J Ethnopharmacol.* 1990 Jul;29(3):267-73

[100] Scharff L, Marcus DA, Masek BJ. A controlled study of minimal-contact thermal biofeedback treatment in children with migraine. *J Pediatr Psychol.*2002; 27:109 –119 http://jpepsy.oxfordjournals.org/cgi/content/abstract/27/2/109

[101] "Feedback training was accompanied by significant reduction of cortical excitability. This was probably responsible for the clinical efficacy of the training; a significant reduction of days with migraine and other headache parameters was observed." Siniatchkin M, Hierundar A, Kropp P, Kuhnert R, Gerber WD, Stephani U. Self-regulation of slow cortical potentials in children with migraine: an exploratory study. *Appl Psychophysiol Biofeedback.*2000; 25:13 –32

[102] "The overall results of the study showed that relaxation training combined with stress management training was significantly more effective in reducing the headache index than treatment with the betablocker metoprolol." Sartory G, Muller B, Metsch J, Pothmann R.A comparison of psychological and pharmacological treatment of pediatric migraine. *BehavResTher*1998;36:1155-1170

methysergide in the treatment of migraine according to a study of 124 adults and children with migraine.[103]

- <u>Melatonin</u>: Melatonin is a hormone made in the pineal gland from the neurotransmitter serotonin which is derived from the amino acid tryptophan and 5-hydroxytryptophan. Melatonin levels are low in patients with migraine and cluster headache. According to case reports and studies with small numbers of patients, 10 mg of melatonin taken at night relieves cluster headaches in approximately 50% of patients, with results beginning 3 to 5 days after the start of treatment and continuing for the duration of treatment.[104,105] Clinical trials using melatonin in migraine patients have shown consistently positive results, with a significant number of patients becoming completely migraine-free.[106] Melatonin is generally administered at night in doses ranging from 3 to 10 mg, although studies in cancer patients have safely used doses as high as 20 to 40 mg and have shown antitumor and pro-survival benefits. Melatonin has antioxidant and immunomodulatory actions in addition to its ability to preserve mitochondrial function, which is particularly relevant to migraine and cluster headaches (see below).

- <u>Hydroxocobalamin (hydroxo-vitamin-B12, OH-B12)</u>: Hydroxocobalamin is a nitric oxide scavenger and appears to benefit the majority of patients with migraine headaches; this study used OH-B12 1 mg/d via aqueous intranasal administration to obviate the need for parenteral administration.[107] If the route of administration is unimportant, then high-dose oral supplementation with 2,000-6,000 mcg/d may prove to be just as effective, according to comparable research using cyanocobalamin.[108]

- <u>Feverfew (*Tanacetum parthenium*)</u>: Results of numerous studies support the use of feverfew for the safe and cost-effective treatment and prevention of migraine headaches. Feverfew has several mechanisms of action including antithrombosis and inhibition of NF-κB. Feverfew products are generally concentrated to 0.2% to 0.7% parthenolide, and a reasonable starting dose is 250 mcg/d of parthenolide; lower doses can be used within a context of multicomponent treatment. Feverfew can be used alone, with other nutrients, or with other botanical medicines. The combination of ginger and feverfew has shown efficacy for halting incipient migraine attacks when started within 2 hours of pain onset.[109] Similarly, the combination of feverfew and willow extract was shown to be remarkably safe and effective in preventing and reducing migraine.[110]

- <u>Eradication of dysbiosis, particularly gastrointestinal dysbiosis due to *Helicobacter pylori*</u>: Patients with migraine have a higher-than-average prevalence of gastric infection with *H. pylori*, and significant symptomatic improvement is obtained following eradication of *H. pylori* in these patients, according to two studies[111,112] and refuted by two others.[113,114] As usual, gastrointestinal dysbiosis should be assessed and corrected on a *per patient* (rather than *per disease*) basis—see Chapter 4 of *Integrative Rheumatology*[115]

[103] "The most beneficial effect of 5-HTP appears to be felt with regard to the intensity and duration rather than the frequency of the attacks... These results suggest that 5-HTP could be a treatment of choice in the prophylaxis of migraine." Titus F, Davalos A, Alom J, Codina A. 5-Hydroxytryptophan versus methysergide in the prophylaxis of migraine. Randomized clinical trial. *Eur Neurol*.1986; 25:327-329

[104] Leone M, D'Amico D, Moschiano F, Fraschini F, Bussone G. Melatonin versus placebo in the prophylaxis of cluster headache: a double-blind pilot study with parallel groups. *Cephalalgia* 1996 Nov;16(7):494-6

[105] "Melatonin levels have been found to be decreased in cluster headache patients. ... We report two chronic cluster headache patients who had both daytime and nocturnal attacks that were alleviated with melatonin." Peres MF, Rozen TD. Melatonin in the preventive treatment of chronic cluster headache. *Cephalalgia*. 2001 Dec;21(10):993-5

[106] Vogler B, Rapoport AM, Tepper SJ, Sheftell F, Bigal ME. Role of melatonin in the pathophysiology of migraine: implications for treatment. CNS Drugs. 2006;20(5):343-50

[107] van der Kuy PH, Merkus FW, Lohman JJ, ter Berg JW, Hooymans PM. Hydroxocobalamin, a nitric oxide scavenger, in the prophylaxis of migraine: an open, pilot study. *Cephalalgia*.2002; 22:513 –519

[108] "In cobalamin deficiency, 2 mg of cyanocobalamin administered orally on a daily basis was as effective as 1 mg administered intramuscularly on a monthly basis and may be superior." Kuzminski AM, Del Giacco EJ, Allen RH, Stabler SP, Lindenbaum J. Effective treatment of cobalamin deficiency with oral cobalamin. *Blood* 1998 Aug 15;92(4):1191-8 http://www.bloodjournal.org/cgi/content/full/92/4/1191

[109] Cady RK, Schreiber CP, Beach ME, Hart CC. Gelstat Migraine (sublingually administered feverfew and ginger compound) for acute treatment of migraine when administered during the mild pain phase. *Med Sci Monit*. 2005 Sep;11(9):PI65-9

[110] Shrivastava R, Pechadre JC, John GW. Tanacetum parthenium and Salix alba (Mig-RL) combination in migraine prophylaxis: a prospective, open-label study. Clin Drug Investig. 2006;26(5):287-96

[111] "CONCLUSIONS: H. pylori is common in subjects with migraine. Bacterium eradication causes a significant decrease in attacks of migraine. The reduction of vasoactive substances produced during infection may be the pathogenetic mechanism underlying the phenomenon." Gasbarrini A, De Luca A, Fiore G, Gambrielli M, Franceschi F, Ojetti V, Torre ES, Gasbarrini G, Pola P, Giacovazzo M. Beneficial effects of Helicobacter pylori eradication on migraine. *Hepatogastroenterology*. 1998 May-Jun;45(21):765-70

[112] "CONCLUSION: Helicobacter pylori should be examined in migranous patients and eradication of the infection may be helpful for the treatment of the disease." Tunca A, Turkay C, Tekin O, Kargili A, Erbayrak M. Is Helicobacter pylori infection a risk factor for migraine? A case-control study. *Acta Neurol Belg*. 2004 Dec;104(4):161-4

[113] "CONCLUSIONS: Our study suggests that chronic Helicobacter pylori infection is not more frequent in patients with migraine than in controls and that infection does not modify clinical features of the disease." Pinessi L, Savi L, Pellicano R, Rainero I, Valfre W, Gentile S, Cossotto D, Rizzetto M, Ponzetto A. Chronic Helicobacter pylori infection and migraine: a case-control study. *Headache*. 2000 Nov-Dec;40(10):836-9

[114] "In conclusion, our results do not support any specific correlation between Hp infection and migraine." Ciancarelli I, Di Massimo C, Tozzi-Ciancarelli MG, De Matteis G, Marini C, Carolei A. Helicobacter pylori infection and migraine. *Cephalalgia*. 2002 Apr;22(3):222-5

[115] Vasquez A. *Integrative Rheumatology*. Fort Worth, Texas; Integrative and Biological Medicine Research and Consulting, 2006: http://OptimalHealthResearch.com

for details and interventions. For patients with recalcitrant headaches (and for those seeking comprehensive whole-patient health care), assessment of digestion, absorption, and gastrointestinal microecology is a reasonable component of evaluation that can help guide treatment. Although *Helicobacter pylori* is a common inhabitant of the human gastrointestinal tract (found in more than 50% of Americans over age 50), immunologic responses to the organism can range from nonreactive on one end of the spectrum to diverse diseases like chronic gastritis, chronic urticaria, autoimmune thrombocytopenia, or reactive arthritis on the more severe and systemic end of the spectrum. Thus, the host-microbe relationship is of greater significance than the identity and microbiological characteristics of the microbe.

- Surgical closure of patent foramen ovale: While the prevalence of patent foramen ovale in the general adult population is approximately 20% to 30%, patients with migraine—especially migraine with aura— show a higher prevalence (55–65%) of this physiological cardiopulmonary shunt. Surgical closure of a patent foramen ovale can provide relief from headache in many migraine patients.[116,117] If the cardiopulmonary shunt is severe enough to result in reduced blood oxygenation, it can exacerbate the already reduced energy production caused by the aforementioned mitochondrial dysfunction. More likely, bypassing the lungs results in failure of pulmonary degradation of proinflammatory mediators. The lungs inactivate proinflammatory mediators such as prostaglandins E1, E2, and F2-alpha, all of the leukotrienes, and norepinephrine (30% reduction). Thus, surgical closure of the patent foramen ovale stops inflammatory mediators from bypassing the lungs and may provide a systemic anti-inflammatory benefit that reduces migraine severity.

- Psychological exploration of emotional tension: If someone has chronic "tension headaches" then the question becomes *"Why does this person have chronic tension?"* Generally, the answer is a combination of magnesium deficiency along with some underlying emotional issue(s). If someone feels compelled to maintain a static posture all day without taking a necessary and healthful break to stretch and relax, this suggests that they are over-focusing on their work at the expense of taking care of their body and health—this is not a sign of health, and it suggest an underlying compulsion or dissociation.

- Acupuncture: Acupuncture is effective symptomatic treatment for migraine and tension headaches, with cost-effectiveness comparable to standard medical treatment.[118,119,120] Acupuncture is known to affect regional blood flow, and the neurophysiological mechanisms involved include increased release of endogenous analgesics such as endomorphin-1, beta-endorphin, encephalin, and serotonin.[121] In a head-to-head study of acupuncture versus drug treatment with metoprolol, "2 of 59 patients randomized to acupuncture withdrew prematurely from the study compared to 18 of 55 randomized to metoprolol ... The proportion of responders was 61% for acupuncture and 49% for metoprolol. Both physicians and patients reported fewer adverse effects in the acupuncture group."[122] While pain relief is an important benefit, it should not be the primary goal in treatment if an underlying physiological or biochemical disturbance (including nutritional deficiencies or imbalances) can be corrected.

- Mitochondrial resuscitation: We must appreciate that migraine is a multifaceted phenomenon with neuroemotional, structural, allergic-immunologic-inflammatory, and mitochondrial components. With regard to the latter, we can understand migraine from the perspective of defects in the mitochondrial electron transport chain (ETC), namely **NADH-dehydrogenase, citrate synthase** and **cytochrome-c-**

[116] Rigatelli G, Braggion G, Aggio S, Chinaglia M, Cardaioli P. Primary patent foramen ovale closure to relieve severe migraine. *Ann Intern Med.* 2006 Mar 21;144(6):458-60 http://www.annals.org/cgi/reprint/144/6/458-a.pdf

[117] Dubiel M, Bruch L, Schmehl I, Liebner M, Winkelmann A, Stretz A, Grad MO, Kleber FX. Migraine Headache Relief after Percutaneous Transcatheter Closure of Interatrial Communications. J Interv Cardiol. 2007 Dec 18; [Epub ahead of print]

[118] Endres HG, Bowing G, Diener HC, Lange S, Maier C, Molsberger A, Zenz M, Vickers AJ, Tegenthoff M. Acupuncture for tension-type headache: a multicentre, sham-controlled, patient-and observer-blinded, randomised trial. J Headache Pain. 2007 Oct 23; [Epub ahead of print]

[119] Vickers AJ, Rees RW, Zollman CE, McCarney R, Smith CM, Ellis N, Fisher P, Van Haselen R, Wonderling D, Grieve R. Acupuncture of chronic headache disorders in primary care: randomised controlled trial and economic analysis. Health Technol Assess. 2004 Nov;8(48):iii, 1-35

[120] Wonderling D, Vickers AJ, Grieve R, McCarney R. Cost effectiveness analysis of a randomised trial of acupuncture for chronic headache in primary care. BMJ. 2004 Mar 27;328(7442):747

[121] Cabyoglu MT, Ergene N, Tan U. The mechanism of acupuncture and clinical applications. Int J Neurosci. 2006 Feb;116(2):115-25

[122] Streng A, Linde K, Hoppe A, Pfaffenrath V, Hammes M, Wagenpfeil S, Weidenhammer W, Melchart D. Effectiveness and tolerability of acupuncture compared with metoprolol in migraine prophylaxis. Headache. 2006 Nov-Dec;46(10):1492-502

oxidase; defects in **NADH-cytochrome-c-reductase** appear to be specific to migraine with aura.[123] Thus, not surprisingly, nutrients which are intimately involved with these steps of the ETC have shown impressive efficacy in the treatment and prevention of migraine via the Le Chatelier principle which states—from the perspective of orthomolecular nutrition—that metabolic defects can be compensated for by the administration of supraphysiologic quantities of nutrients to push defective pathways toward completion; in the case of migraine, we are bypassing or compensating for defects in mitochondrial function by supplying supraphysiologic doses of the nutrients involved in those pathways with the end result being enhanced function of mitochondrial function. In the world of nutritional medicine, we would probably not be familiar with these concepts were it not for the independent and synergistic works of Roger Williams, Linus Pauling, Jeff Bland, and Bruce Ames; to these men do we owe gratitude for our understanding of this phenomenon and its clinical application. Furthermore however, we must also appreciate that nutrients have numerous functions and *affect* and *effect* numerous (not singular) pathways and processes, such that a "mitochondrial nutrient" may exert its action via a *non-mitochondrial* effect, as mentioned per nutrient in the itemized section that follows:

- o <u>Niacin, including inositol hexaniacinate and niacinamide—dose varies per type used</u>: High-dose niacin alleviates migraine headaches and headaches of various etiologies, whether administered orally, intramuscularly, or intravenously; niacin can also be used to halt acute migraine attacks.[124,125] Niacinamide adenine dinucleotide (NADH) is an essential component of the first stage (Complex 1) of the ETC, a step that is commonly defective in migraine patients. High-dose niacin facilitates this step and thus enhances energy production. Another anti-migraine benefit of high-dose niacin is its sparing effect on tryptophan, allowing its conversion to serotonin. Niacin also has a vasodilating action and may thereby address the vasculogenic component of headache. Efficacious oral doses of niacin can range from 300 to 1500 mg/d; lower doses are used for children. High-dose niacin, particularly in time-released tablets, presents some risk for hepatic damage, and thus safer forms of niacin such as plain niacin, slow-release niacin (e.g., Niaspan®), and inositol hexaniacinate are preferred; niacinamide and NADH might also be efficacious but neither has vasodilating actions provided by the other forms of niacin. Doses of niacin exceeding 500 to 1000 mg/d are probably unnecessary in headache patients if other treatments such as coenzyme Q10 (CoQ10), vitamin D, and fatty acids are being used; before implementing high-dose niacin, patients should be selected, informed, and monitored appropriately.

- o <u>CoQ-10—100-400 mg per day</u>: CoQ-10 supplementation significantly reduces migraine headache frequency, duration, and intensity.[126] As shown in the diagram below, CoQ-10 shuttles electrons from Complex 1 to Complex 2, and from "Complex 2" to Complex 3. Thus, CoQ-10 supplementation helps to bypass defects in Complex 1 and perhaps Complex 2. Furthermore, research by Folkers et al[127] strongly suggests that CoQ-10 has an anti-allergy and immunomodulatory role; thus the anti-migraine benefits of CoQ-10 may be mediated via immunomodulation in addition to enhancement of mitochondrial function.

- o <u>Riboflavin (vitamin B2)—400 mg per day</u>: Flavin adenine dinucleotide is required at Complex 2 of the ETC. High-dose vitamin B2 shows "high efficacy, excellent tolerability, and low cost" in the prevention of migraine headaches.[128]

- o <u>Lipoic acid—600 mg/d</u>: Lipoic (thiotic) acid is an essential component of the pyruvate dehydrogenase complex. A placebo-controlled clinical trial showed benefit of lipoic acid (600

[123] "NADH-dehydrogenase, citrate synthase and cytochrome-c-oxidase activities in both patient groups were significantly lower than in controls (p < 0.01), while NADH-cytochrome-c-reductase activity was reduced only in migraine with aura (p < 0.01)." Sangiorgi S, Mochi M, Riva R, Cortelli P, Monari L, Pierangeli G, Montagna P. Abnormal platelet mitochondrial function in patients affected by migraine with and without aura. *Cephalalgia*. 1994 Feb;14(1):21-3

[124] Velling DA, Dodick DW, Muir JJ. Sustained-release niacin for prevention of migraine headache. *Mayo Clin Proc*. 2003 Jun;78(6):770-1

[125] Prousky J, Seely D. The treatment of migraines and tension-type headaches with intravenous and oral niacin (nicotinic acid): systematic review of the literature. Nutr J. 2005 Jan 26;4:3

[126] Rozen TD, Oshinsky ML, Gebeline CA, Bradley KC, Young WB, Shechter AL, Silberstein SD. Open label trial of coenzyme Q10 as a migraine preventive. *Cephalalgia* 2002;22(2):137-41

[127] Ye CQ, Folkers K, Tamagawa H, Pfeiffer C. A modified determination of coenzyme Q10 in human blood and CoQ10 blood levels in diverse patients with allergies. *Biofactors*. 1988 Dec;1(4):303-6

[128] Schoenen J, Jacquy J, Lenaerts M. Effectiveness of high-dose riboflavin in migraine prophylaxis. A randomized controlled trial. *Neurology* 1998;50(2):466-70

mg/d) supplementation in migraine patients.[129] Lipoic acid also inhibits NF-κB activation and thus may have at least 2 separate anti-headache mechanisms: promotion of ATP production and inhibition of NF-κB-activated inflammation.

- Melatonin—5-20 mg at night: As mentioned previously, melatonin is a potent protector of mitochondrial function, which has been demonstrated in experimental models of mitochondrial inhibition by bacterial endotoxin. As a powerful antioxidant, melatonin scavenges oxygen and nitrogen-based reactants generated in mitochondria and thereby limits the loss of the intramitochondrial glutathione; this prevents mitochondrial protein and DNA damage. Melatonin increases the activity of Complexes 1 and 4 of the ETC, improving mitochondrial respiration and increasing ATP synthesis under various physiological and experimental conditions.[130]

- Carnitine—300-2,000 mg/d taken between meals: The amino acid L-carnitine is necessary for fatty acid transport into the mitochondria for oxidative metabolism and energy production. Deficiency of or metabolic inability to use carnitine can precipitate or perpetuate migraine headaches, which can be alleviated by carnitine supplementation.[131] As a natural component of the human diet, carnitine has a wide safety margin, and supplemental doses ranging from 300 to 2000 mg/d are commonly used.

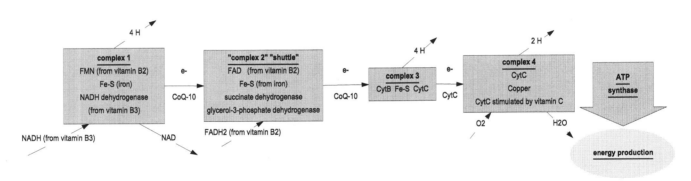

Schematic diagram of the electron transport chain, function of which is wholly dependent upon niacin, riboflavin, CoQ-10, iron, copper, and—to a lesser extent— vitamin C

---

129 Magis D, Ambrosini A, Sandor P, Jacquy J, Laloux P, Schoenen J. A randomized double-blind placebo-controlled trial of thioctic acid in migraine prophylaxis. Headache. 2007 Jan;47(1):52-7

130 León J, Acuña-Castroviejo D, Escames G, Tan DX, Reiter RJ. Melatonin mitigates mitochondrial malfunction. J Pineal Res. 2005 Jan;38(1):1-9

131 Kabbouche MA, Powers SW, Vockell AL, LeCates SL, Hershey AD. Carnitine palmityltransferase II (CPT2) deficiency and migraine headache: two case reports. Headache. 2003 May;43(5):490-5

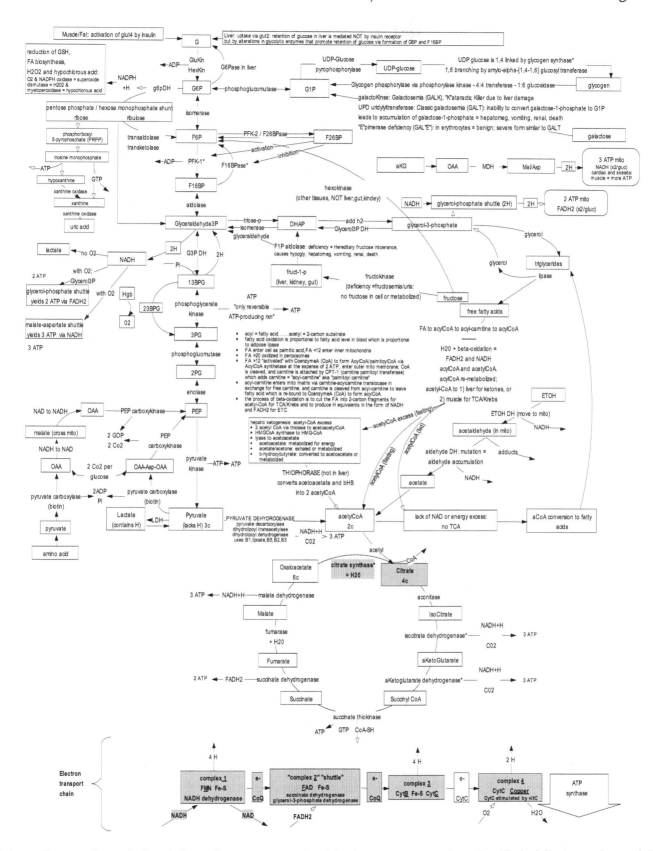

Schematic overview of glycolytic pathways, pyruvate dehydrogenase complex, the Krebs/citrate cycle, and the electron transport chain: items in bold/gray are those which are commonly defective in patients with migraine headaches—consult your biochemistry text for details and definitions

Musculoskeletal Manipulation and Manual Medicine: Samples of Commonly Used Chiropractic and Osteopathic Techniques

Manual medicine in general and spinal manipulation in particular are mentioned in nearly every section of *Integrative Orthopedics*, and select techniques are described with accompanying text and photographs. Manipulative techniques are included in this textbook to remind practitioners of a few of the more useful and commonly applied maneuvers and to provide descriptions and citations for refinement of their application. However, the level of detail provided here is insufficient unless the reader has received hands-on professionally-supervised training in an accredited institution wherein other important concepts have been taught and implemented under experienced guidance. Competence and proficiency in the art and skill of manipulation cannot be learned from a textbook; these can only be approached with personal mentoring and in-person coursework amply provided in colleges and post-graduate trainings specializing in manipulative technique. **Manipulative medicine** is a *time-space* objective-subjective-intuitive **kinesthetic phenomenon** which might be described as occurring in four dimensions—*anteroposterior, transverse/horizontal, vertical,* and *chronological* due to variations in speed and power; all the while, the doctor is monitoring subjective and objective responses of the what might be considered the fifth dimension—the doctor's dynamic *perception of, influence upon,* and *interaction with* the patient's affect, posture, muscle tension, dynamic joint positioning, tissue response, and compressive tension. As the doctor assesses and provides force to the spinal lesion, the patient's response changes the quality of the lesion, and so the doctor must adapt to a moving target—the lesion being treated. These sections presume professional training by the reader has already been begun or completed and that the reader is familiar with manipulative concepts, technique, terminology, and commonly used abbreviations. Again, the intention here is to remind clinicians of manipulation in general and these specific techniques in particular; only a few *subjectively chosen* techniques are included from the several hundred vertebral, myofascial, visceral, and extravertebral/extremity maneuvers that are available.

General Layout and Description of Manipulative Techniques

- **Patient position**: Patient position may be prone, supine, lateral recumbent or "side-posture", standing, or seated.
- **Doctor position**: Usually standing, either upright, forward flexed, or using an oblique fencer's stance; knees are almost always bent in order to bring doctor's torso near treatment area to increase mechanical force from the upper limbs.
- **Assessment**: *Subjective*: Patient's experience, sensations, and effect on daily living. *Motion palpation*: Intersegmental motion analysis generally used for assessing the presence of vertebral (and extravertebral) motion restrictions or aberrant motion. The patient is relaxed and passive while the doctor takes the joint that is being assessed through its normal range of motion in various directions while palpating near adjacent joint surfaces for nuance of pattern and end-feel. Motion lesions are generally described as **restrictions** and/or **hypermobility**. *Static palpation*: Boney and other landmarks are compared symmetrically and to the practitioner's experience for the detection of abnormality consistent with subjective, motion, and soft tissue findings; static palpations are usually described in terms of prominence or relative superiority/inferiority when compared symmetrically. *Soft tissue palpation*: Subcutaneous tissues, tendons, ligaments, muscles, and joint spaces can be palpated to assess myofascial status and function. Soft tissue findings commonly include edema, joint swelling, bogginess, "ropiness" of muscles, tenderness, restricted motion of soft tissues, hypertonicity, spasm, and adhesions.
- **Treatment contact, directive hand**: Generally the doctor provides therapeutic contact with one of the contact surfaces of the hands—digital, hypothenar, pisiform, index, thumb, thenar, or "calcaneal" (when using the "heel" of the hand)[132]; other contacts such as the elbow or chest might be used for deep myofascial or compressive manipulative procedures, respectively. The treatment contact is provided by the directive hand—the hand that is delivering the therapeutic thrust or direction; the treatment contact of the directive hand works in cooperation with the supporting contact of the supporting hand.
- **Supporting contact**: This generally refers to the supportive hand, the one that is either holding or stabilizing the patient in contrast to the hand that is delivering the manipulative force. The indirect hand can provide at least three different types of support.
- **Neutral/stabilizing support**: The supportive hand plays a relatively neutral role with regard to the manipulative force.
- **Synergistic/cooperative/assistive support**: In this situation, the supportive hand moves with the therapeutic force in the same direction. An example of this would be the head-holding hand moving in the same direction as the directive/treatment hand when performing manipulation of the upper cervical spine.
- **Counterthrust/resistive support**: In this situation, the supportive hand moves counter/against the direction of the directive force. A common example is the force applied to the upper torso when performing a side-posture manipulation of the lumbar spine or pelvis.
- **Pretreatment positioning**: Joints are generally—but not always—taken to the end range of motion before the manipulative thrust is applied because the general purpose of high-velocity low-amplitude manipulation is to break myofascial restrictions and/or forcefully activate joint proprioceptors. In chiropractic terms, this is described as taking the joint into the **paraphysiologic space** because the physiologic range of motion is temporarily though safely exceeded[133];

---

[132] Kirk CR, Lawrence DJ, Valvo NL. States Manual of Spinal, Pelvic, and Extravertebral Technics. Second Edition. Lombard, Illinois: National College of Chiropractic; 1985, page 20

[133] Leach RA. (ed). The Chiropractic Theories: A Textbook of Scientific Research, 4th Edition. Baltimore:Lippincott,Williams,Wilkins,2004,page 32-33

in osteopathic terms, this part of the range of motion is described as being within the range of **passive motion** but still within the **anatomic barrier.**[134]

- **Therapeutic action**: For joint manipulation, this is usually the **chiropractic adjustment** or the **osteopathic HVLA** (high-velocity low-amplitude thrust); <u>**thrust vectors**</u> can be straight, curvilinear, or rotary into <u>**segmental directions**</u> of rotation, extension, flexion, side-bending, traction, and combinations of those directions. Other common manual techniques include stretching, post-isometric stretching, massage, compression, percussion, joint springing, mobilization, articulation, traction.

- **Resources**: The most commonly cited works here include: *States Manual, Second Edition* by Constance Kirk DC, Dana Lawrence DC, Nila Valvo DC; *Kimberly Manual, 2006 Edition* by Paul Kimberly DO; *Chiropractic Technique* by Thomas Bergmann DC, David Peterson DC, Dana Lawrence DC; *Chiropractic Management of Spine-Related Disorders* edited by Meridel Gatterman DC.

- **Context**: The following samples are an obvious underrepresentation of the diversity of manipulative techniques available, which easily numbers into the hundreds. Various techniques are—of course—described with greater range and depth in textbooks wholly dedicated to the topic of manipulation, which by itself is not the subject of this text. Rather, **use these samples as reminders to include *or at least consider* manipulative therapy** when composing your treatment plan; oftentimes, the manipulative therapy is the fastest and shortest route between *pain* and *relief from pain* and also from *dysfunction* toward *homeostasis*.

---

[134] Kimberly PE. <u>Outline of Osteopathic Manipulative Procedures. The Kimberly Manual 2006</u>. Kirksville College of Osteopathic Medicine. Walsworth Publishing , Marceline, Mo, page 7

Cervical Spine: Rotation Emphasis for Treatment of Rotational Restriction

- **Patient position**: Supine, neck slightly flexed.
- **Doctor position**: At 45° angle from head of table; may also be in a more lateral position aside the patient's head and neck; while it is acceptable to assess and set-up with straight legs, at the time of impulse, doctor's legs should be bent to provide the doctor with greater power, stability, and biomechanical safety.
- **Assessment**: Subjective: neck pain, headaches. Motion palpation: rotation restriction; primary or compensatory hypermobile segments may be detected above or below the restricted segment. Static palpation: vertebra may feel relatively posterior on the side opposite the rotational restriction, e.g., a right rotational restriction may present with a relative left rotational malposition that brings the vertebral lamina and articular pillars posterior on the left. Soft tissue: tenderness, may also have muscle spasm.
- **Treatment contact**: Doctor uses either an index or proximal phalange contact on the posterior aspect of the transverse process and/or articular pillar. The doctor's vector and hence the positioning of the forearm of the contact hand must change depending on the level of the cervical spine that is being treated. Notice in this photograph that the thumb of the doctor's contact hand is placed on the angle of the mandible, this is more to help anchor the contact and stabilize the doctor's wrist than to assist with the manipulation; very little pressure and zero thrust are applied to the mandible.
- **Supporting contact**: Head is held into rotation and slight flexion; as with all techniques, nuanced adjustments in flexion-extension, rotation, and side-bending are made until the premanipulative tension is localized to the specific direction/tissue of restriction.
- **Pretreatment positioning**: Slight flexion and extension may be used below and above the treatment contact to create motion restriction at the adjacent motion segments; this helps to focus the motion and therapeutic force at the specific; importantly the support hand is largely responsible for proper positioning with the correct amount of nuanced flexion-extension and side-bending so that the rotational force is accurately delivered.
- **Therapeutic action**: Rotational thrust with contact hand; support hand keeps head off table so that rotational motion can occur.
- **Resources**: *States Manual, Second Edition*[135] page 47

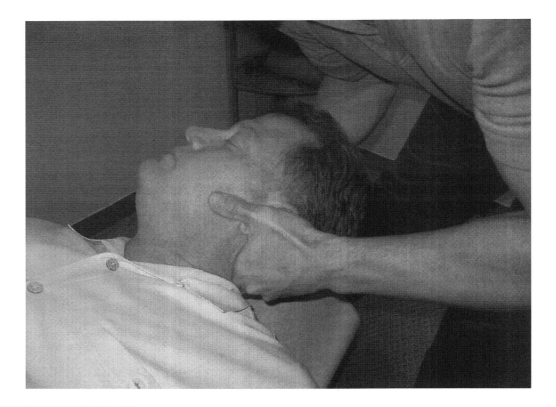

[135] Kirk CR, Lawrence DJ, Valvo NL. States Manual of Spinal, Pelvic, and Extravertebral Technics. Second Edition. Lombard, Illinois: National College of Chiropractic; 1985

> **Cervical Spine: Lateral Flexion (Side-Bending) Emphasis; Treatment of Lateral Malposition or Lateral Flexion Restriction**

- **Patient position**: Supine, head is neutrally placed—neither flexed nor extended; slight flexion is allowed; this technique can also be adapted for use in a seated position.
- **Doctor position**: At 45° angle from head of table; may also be in a more lateral position aside the patient's head and neck.
- **Assessment**: <u>Subjective</u>: neck pain, headaches. <u>Motion palpation</u>: lateral flexion restriction. <u>Static palpation</u>: vertebra may feel laterally displaced. <u>Soft tissue</u>: tenderness, may also have muscle spasm.
- **Treatment contact**: Using an index (metacarpal-phalangeal) contact at the tip of the transverse process or slightly posterior to the transverse process; an index phalangeal contact can also be used on the articular pillars as long as doctor is careful not to thrust in a rotational direction; notice in this picture how Dr Harris has the forearm of his contact hand perfectly aligned in the treatment vector, which is almost purely in the patient's transverse/horizontal plane; notice also that Dr Harris has his knees bent and is forward flexed to bring his torso closer to his contact and thereby minimize stress and strain on his own shoulders; with slight modifications in vector direction, this technique can be applied throughout the cervical spine from C0-C7.
- **Supporting contact**: Lateral aspect of head, opposite contact; generally the supporting hand is neutral, however it can supply some traction and can help induce lateral flexion at impulse; with more aggressive adjustments, the supporting hand can supply a counterforce to minimize motion following the application of a faster and more powerful thrust.
- **Pretreatment positioning**: Lateral flexion at the targeted cervical segment; the slightest amount of contralateral rotation is applied. The doctor establishes an "index" contact on the posterolateral aspect of the cervical vertebrae (i.e., the "paravertebral gutter"[136]).
- **Therapeutic action**: Establish minimal premanipulative tension once the end range of motion has been reached, then use quick and very shallow trust to induce lateral flexion.
- **Resources**:[137, 138, 139]

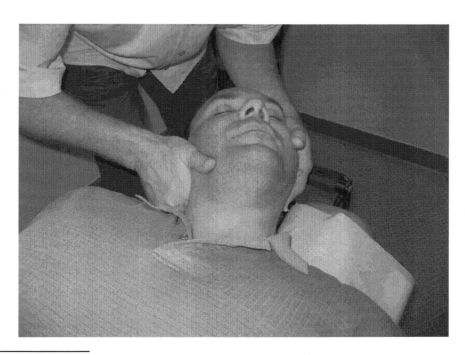

---

[136] "There are eleven pairs of thoracic zygapophysial joints, with one pair located between each vertebral level. These joints contribute to the floor of the 'paravertebral gutter', the region between the spinous and transverse processes. In the cervical and lumbar regions this gutter is shallow, formed mainly by the laminae and articular pillars, whereas in the thoracic region the gutter is deeper and broader, being formed by the laminae, articular pillars and transverse processes." Cornwall J, Mercer s. Thoracic Zygapophysial joint palpation. *New Zealand Journal of Physiotherapy* 2006: 34(2); 56-59

[137] Kirk CR, Lawrence DJ, Valvo NL. <u>States Manual of Spinal, Pelvic, and Extravertebral Technics. Second Edition</u>. Lombard, Illinois: National College of Chiropractic; 1985

[138] Kimberly PE. <u>Outline of Osteopathic Manipulative Procedures. The Kimberly Manual 2006</u>. Kirksville College of Osteopathic Medicine. Walsworth Publishing , Marceline, Mo

[139] Bergmann TF, Peterson DH, Lawrence DJ. <u>Chiropractic Technique</u>. New York; Churchill Livingstone: 1993

Thoracic Spine: Supine Thoracic Flexion, "Anterior Thoracic"

- **Patient position**: Supine on table; to facilitate positioning, patient's leg opposite doctor may be flexed at hip and knee with foot flat on table. Patient is instructed to place right hand on right trapezius and left hand on left trapezius; the patient is instructed, "Place your hands behind your neck and do not interlace your fingers."
- **Doctor position**: Facing table at 45° angle in fencer stance with feet apart and knees bent. Doctor must be midline and balanced at time of impulse in order to provide symmetric force.
- **Assessment**: Subjective: mechanical midback pain. Motion palpation: flexion restriction. Static palpation: extension malposition; focal loss of thoracic kyphosis; focal approximation of spinous processes consistent with extension malposition; vertebra may feel anteriorly displaced. Soft tissue: local paravertebral myohypertonicity is common; local paresthesia is very common, and patients are often exquisitely sensitive to the lightest touch.
- **Treatment contact**: Closed fist contact with spinous processes between doctor's distal interphalangeal joints and thenar eminence; the trust is delivered from the doctor's chest through the patient's arms which compress the patient's chest; Dr Harris (pictured as patient) prefers to use a forearm contact to reduce wear-and-tear on his hands and wrists.
- **Supporting contact**: The supporting contact is the hand-arm that supports the patient's upper torso; the supporting contact pulls toward the doctor and superiorly at time of impulse.
- **Pretreatment positioning**: Patient lifts head from table; doctor uses supporting hand and arm to lift patient off table to allow placement of contact hand and to facilitate spinal flexion.
- **Therapeutic action**: Doctor uses **body drop thrust** technique at 45° toward ground and toward the head of the table; the trust should simultaneously generate compression and long-axis traction; the contact hand remains tense to provide solid leverage inferior to the targeted motion segment; the supporting hand and arm pull toward doctor at time of impulse to accentuate traction and spinal flexion; patient is instructed to breath deeply then relax and exhale; upon exhalation, the doctor establishes and maintains premanipulative tension to achieve joint flexion, then applies HVLA thrust; the thrust must be fast and shallow; slow and deep impulses can sprain the interspinous ligaments.
- **Resources**: *States Manual*[140] page 67, *Kimberly Manual, 2006 Edition*[141] page 93-94, *Chiropractic Technique*[142] page 349

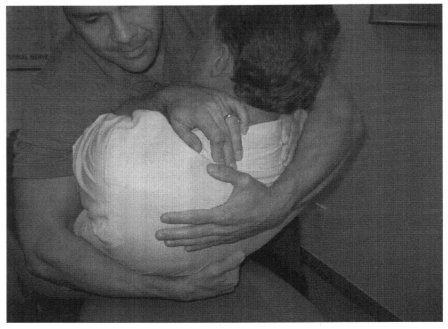

[140] Kirk CR, Lawrence DJ, Valvo NL. States Manual of Spinal, Pelvic, and Extravertebral Technics. Second Edition. Lombard, Illinois: National College of Chiropractic; 1985
[141] Kimberly PE. Outline of Osteopathic Manipulative Procedures. The Kimberly Manual 2006. Kirksville College of Osteopathic Medicine. Walsworth Publishing , Marceline, Mo
[142] Bergmann TF, Peterson DH, Lawrence DJ. Chiropractic Technique. New York; Churchill Livingstone: 1993

Posterior Ribs: Manipulation of the Costovertebral Junction

- **Patient position**: Supine on table; to facilitate positioning, patient's leg opposite doctor may be flexed at hip and knee with foot flat on table. Patient's arms are crossed over the front of their body; my preference is that the arm closest to the doctor (the arm opposite to the side of the thorax being treated) is atop.
- **Doctor position**: Modified fencer's stance facing cephalad.
- **Assessment**: <u>Subjective</u>: mechanical paraspinal pain; often discomfort with inhalation. <u>Motion palpation</u>: stiffness at the affected costo-transverse junction. <u>Static palpation</u>: prominence in the posterior direction of the rib near the costo-transverse junction. <u>Soft tissue</u>: local tenderness to palpation is very common.
- **Treatment contact**: Contact on the specific rib immediately lateral to the costo-transverse junction is made with the doctor's thenar eminence with the doctor's hand in a firm, pursed position. Initial contact is made superior and lateral to the final location of manipulative contact in order to attain proper premanipulative tissue tension.
- **Supporting contact**: The doctor's supporting (noncontact) hand along with the doctor's torso deliver the manipulative thrust through the patient's arm atop the patient's thorax.
- **Pretreatment positioning**: Patient is supine; after positioning the contact hand posteriorly, the doctor grasps the patient's upper arm, then pulls downward and then applies progressively compressive force (body weight, not muscular force) while raising the supporting contact and rolling the patient over atop the contact hand.
- **Therapeutic action**: Body-drop thrust generally superiorly and laterally in the direction of the patient's opposite shoulder; the angle of the thrust changes depending on the spinal-costal level being treated, with more superior segments requiring a more superiorly directed thrust, while lower segments require a progressively laterally-yet-sagittally directed thrust. Notably, the manipulative thrust is applied to the anterior thorax via contact with the patient's upper arm, yet the true manipulative force is from posterior to anterior via the doctor's thenar eminence positioned posteriorly.
- **Resources**: See appropriate sections in previously listed textbooks, particularly *States Manual, Second Edition*[143], and *Chiropractic Technique*.[144]

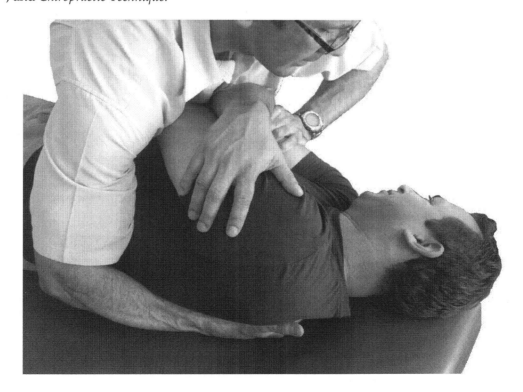

---

[143] Kirk CR, Lawrence DJ, Valvo NL. <u>States Manual of Spinal, Pelvic, and Extravertebral Technics. Second Edition</u>. Lombard, Illinois: National College of Chiropractic; 1985
[144] Bergmann TF, Peterson DH, Lawrence DJ. <u>Chiropractic Technique</u>. New York; Churchill Livingstone: 1993

Additional treatments for cluster headaches (CH):

- <u>Lifestyle modification</u>: Patients with cluster headaches show a greater percentage of increased work-related stress, self-employment, tobacco smoking and alcohol use and abuse.[145] Address as indicated.

- <u>Melatonin 10 mg at night</u>: According to small studies and case reports with small numbers of patients, 10 mg of melatonin taken at night relieves cluster headaches in approximately 50% of patients.[146,147]

- <u>Intranasal capsaicin</u>: capsaicin is the "hot" spicy component of hot chili peppers; when applied to the skin or mucus membranes, it damages pain-sensing nerves and thereby reduces the sensation of pain after an intial exacerbation of pain. Intranasal capsaicin (300 mcg/100 microliters) is remarkably well studied in the treatment and prevention of cluster headaches, beginning with the first report published by Sicuteri et al in 1989.[148] Treatment of active cluster headache with intranasal capsaicin (compared with placebo) reduced severity after 7 days of treatment.[149] In a small controlled clinical trial, patients stated that intranasal capsaicin alleviated chronic migraine suffering by 50% to 80%.[150] Burning pain, sneezing, and increased nasal secretions induced by topical capsaicin application are intense for the first few applications but decrease over time, generally within a week or so; clinical benefits generally begin on the eighth day of consecutive treatment. Episodic cluster headache patients appear to benefit more than do chronic cluster headache patients. Cluster headaches are typically unilateral, and capsaicin should be applied to the nostril on the same side as the head pain.[151]

- <u>Oxygen</u>: One hundred percent oxygen delivered by facial mask at 8 L/min for 10 minutes can help abort an attack of cluster headache. Oxygen is the required terminal component of the mitochondrial electron transport chain (ETC) for ATP production; thus, supraphysiological oxygen, like supraphysiological doses of mitochondria-specific nutrients, generally improves mitochondrial energy (ATP) production.

[145] Manzoni GC. Cluster headache and lifestyle: remarks on a population of 374 male patients. *Cephalalgia* 1999 Mar;19(2):88-94

[146] "Five of the 10 treated patients were responders whose attack frequency declined 3-5 days after treatment, and they experienced no further attacks until melatonin was discontinued." Leone M, D'Amico D, Moschiano F, Fraschini F, Bussone G. Melatonin versus placebo in the prophylaxis of cluster headache: a double-blind pilot study with parallel groups. *Cephalalgia* 1996 Nov;16(7):494-6

[147] "Melatonin levels have been found to be decreased in cluster headache patients. ... We report two chronic cluster headache patients who had both daytime and nocturnal attacks that were alleviated with melatonin." Peres MF, Rozen TD. Melatonin in the preventive treatment of chronic cluster headache. *Cephalalgia*. 2001 Dec;21(10):993-5

[148] Sicuteri F, Fusco BM, Marabini S, Campagnolo V, Maggi CA, Geppetti P, Fanciullacci M. Beneficial effect of capsaicin application to the nasal mucosa in cluster headache. Clin J Pain. 1989;5(1):49-53

[149] Marks DR, Rapoport A, Padla D, Weeks R, Rosum R, Sheftell F, Arrowsmith F. A double-blind placebo-controlled trial of intranasal capsaicin for cluster headache. Cephalalgia. 1993 Apr;13(2):114-6

[150] Fusco BM, Barzoi G, Agrò F. Repeated intranasal capsaicin applications to treat chronic migraine. Br J Anaesth. 2003 Jun;90(6):812

[151] Fusco BM, Marabini S, Maggi CA, Fiore G, Geppetti P. Preventative effect of repeated nasal applications of capsaicin in cluster headache. *Pain*. 1994 Dec;59(3):321-5

Temporomandibular Joint Dysfunction and Bruxism

"The TMJ is one of the most active joints in the body, moving more than 2,000 times per day in its functions of mastication, swallowing, respiration, and speech."[152]

<u>Description/pathophysiology</u>:
- The temporomandibular joint is a complex hinge-sliding joint comprised of the condyle of the mandible with articulates with the mandibular fossa on the inferior aspect of the temporal bone of the skull by means of a bicameral synovial joint with an intra-articular disc. Opening the mouth involves both axial rotation of the joint along with anterior and inferior translational motion; the joint also allows for accessory motions such as lateral translation and combinations of opening/closing along with translational motion in the anterior/posterior, superior/inferior, medial/lateral directions.

<u>Clinical presentations</u>:
- Patient reports pain in the head, face, and/or TMJ regions. Pain is often worse with chewing (DDX temporal arteritis). Patients often have a history of bruxism and muscle cramps, and often anxiety, tension, or depression; constipation and chocolate cravings (associated with depression and magnesium deficiency) may also be seen.
- As the TMJ is a synovial joint, it can be affected by systemic rheumatologic processes such as lupus, rheumatoid arthritis, psoriatic arthritis, etc.

<u>Major differential diagnoses</u>:
- Temporal arteritis—generally seen in older patients, commonly with systemic complaints of fatigue and muscle pain and weakness; assess CRP for elevation and CBC for the anemia of chronic disease.

<u>Clinical assessment</u>:
- **History/subjective**: Patient reports pain in the head, face, and/or TMJ regions. Pain is often worse with chewing and exacerbated by nocturnal bruxism.

<u>Physical examination/objective</u>:
- Physical examination should include the cervical spine as well as the cervical musculature and TMJ. Clinical assessments for TMJ dysfunction have been reviewed elsewhere in considerable detail[153] but generally consist of the following:
  1. <u>Assess alignment</u> of the mandible in relation to the skull both in the static closed position, as well as during the dynamic process of opening and closing. Dynamic and/or static malalignment suggests imbalances within the surrounding musculature, ligaments and/or osseous structures.
  2. <u>Range of motion</u>: the mouth should open to accommodate three "stacked" fingers between the incisors; insufficient motion suggests hypomobility due to disc displacement or musculature or ligamentous restriction is probable, while hypermobilty suggests excess laxity and instability of the joint capsule and surrounding ligaments.
  3. <u>Joint palpation</u>: can be accomplished externally, internally from the ear canal, and intraorally. Motion palpation and assessment of dynamic function of the joint is best performed with the examiner in front of the patient while palpating either externally or from within the ear canal with the tip of the 5th digit. Intraoral palpation of the joint and surrounding structures may be used for the identification of joint tenderness as well as tenderness and swelling of associated muscular and ligamentous structures.
  4. <u>Assessment of general posture and biomechanics</u>

---

[152] Bergmann TF, Peterson DH, Lawrence DJ. <u>Chiropractic Technique: Principles and Procedures</u>. New York, Churchill Livingstone: 1993, pages 523-543
[153] Bergmann TF, Peterson DH, Lawrence DJ. <u>Chiropractic Technique: Principles and Procedures</u>. New York, Churchill Livingstone: 1993, pages 523-543

Imaging & laboratory assessments:

- Laboratory assessments are not generally indicated for the evaluation of TMJ dysfunction unless an underlying disease process such as septic arthritis or rheumatic disease is suspected. However, laboratory assessment may prove beneficial for the evaluation of the patient as a whole and may provide insight into interventions that can assist the overall treatment and management of the patient.
- CT and MRI are used for the evaluation of severe disease, especially when concomitant diseases are present (e.g., rheumatoid arthritis) or when surgical intervention is being considered.

Establishing the diagnosis:

- TMJ dysfunction is a diagnosis established based on the doctor's overall evaluation of the patient's complaint and examination findings.

Complications:

- Pain in the TMJ, head, and face
- Malnutrition due to insufficient eating (pain avoidance) or poor mastication

Clinical management:

- Referral if clinical outcome is unsatisfactory or if serious complications are evident.

Treatments:

- <u>Manipulation of the TMJ, cervical spine, and/or thoracic spine</u>: as indicated[154,155]
- <u>Magnesium</u>: Start at 300 mg per day, and then escalate up to bowel tolerance if necessary. TMJ dysfunction is commonly secondary to bruxism, and bruxism is commonly a form of tetany responsive to magnesium supplementation.[156]
- <u>Food allergy identification and elimination</u>: Bruxism may result from allergy.[157,158]
- <u>Treatment of myofascial trigger points</u>: these are commonly seen as part of the spectrum of problems in patients with TMJ disorder. The underlying food allergy, magnesium deficiency, and postural strain may result in chronic muscle tension that eventually becomes a MFTP—a self-feeding cycle of pain and muscle tension resulting in referred and chronic pain. Treatment of the MFTP with exercises, stretching, warmth, and post-isometric stretching is highly effective.[159] Overall stress reduction is commonly helpful.
- <u>Anti-inflammatory, analgesic, and joint-health promoting botanical and nutritional medicines</u>: **Consider treating the TMJ as you would any chronically inflamed painful joint.**[160] Consider niacinamide, ginger, MSM, glucosamine sulfate[161], fish oil, and *Boswellia*. **Glucosamine sulfate 500 mg TID is superior to ibuprofen 400 mg TID for the treatment of TMJ osteoarthritis.**[162]
- <u>Treatment to stabilize blood sugar levels</u>: Reactive hypoglycemia has been reported in patients with TMJ disorder, and dietary modifications (e.g., small frequent meals, avoidance of sugars and simple carbohydrates, supplementation with chromium and magnesium) can help reduce the "psychic tension" (neuromuscular tension) that contributes to and perpetuates the problem.[163]

---

[154] Bergmann TF, Peterson DH, Lawrence DJ. <u>Chiropractic Technique: Principles and Procedures</u>. New York, Churchill Livingstone: 1993, pages 523-543

[155] Alcantara J, Plaugher G, Klemp DD, Salem C. Chiropractic care of a patient with temporomandibular disorder and atlas subluxation. *J Manipulative Physiol Ther* 2002 Jan;25(1):63-70

[156] "Bruxism and facial tics are most often atypical forms of tetany. Prolonged treatment by magnesium administration nearly always leads to their disappearance and also an improvement in associated functional disorders." Plocieniak C. [Bruxism and magnesium, my clinical experiences since 1980] [Article in French] *Rev Stomatol Chir Maxillofac* 1990;91 Suppl 1:127

[157] "Nocturnal bruxism may be initiated reflexly by increased negative pressures in the tympanic cavities from intermittent allergic edema of the mucosa of the Eustachian tubes. ... Chronic middle ear disturbances may promote reflex action to the jaws by stimulating the trigeminal nuclei in the brain." Marks MB. Bruxism in allergic children. *Am J Orthod* 1980 Jan;77(1):48-59

[158] "Bruxism and malocclusion may also be related to an allergic diathesis." Marks MB. Recognizing the allergic person. *Am Fam Physician* 1977 Jul;16(1):72-9

[159] Lewit K, Simons DG. Myofascial pain: relief by post-isometric relaxation. *Arch Phys Med Rehabil* 1984 Aug;65(8):452-6

[160] Vasquez A. Reducing pain and inflammation naturally - Part 3: Improving overall health while safely and effectively treating musculoskeletal pain. *Nutritional Perspectives* 2005; 28: 34-38, 40-42 http://optimalhealthresearch.com/part3

[161] Modest improvement was seen in TMJ patients consuming a daily dose of 1500 mg of glucosamine hydrochloride and 1200 mg of chondroitin sulfate taken for twelve weeks. "Subjects taking CS-GH had improvements in their pain as measured by one index of the McGill Pain Questionnaire, in TMJ tenderness, in TMJ sounds, and in the number of daily over-the-counter medications needed." Nguyen P, Mohamed SE, Gardiner D, Salinas T. A randomized double-blind clinical trial of the effect of chondroitin sulfate and glucosamine hydrochloride on temporomandibular joint disorders: a pilot study. *Cranio*. 2001 Apr;19(2):130-9

[162] "GS and ibuprofen reduce pain levels in patients with TMJ degenerative joint disease. In the subgroup that met the initial efficacy criteria, GS had a significantly greater influence in reducing pain produced during function and effect of pain with daily activities. GS has a carryover effect." Thie NM, Prasad NG, Major PW. Evaluation of glucosamine sulfate compared to ibuprofen for the treatment of temporomandibular joint osteoarthritis: a randomized double blind controlled 3 month clinical trial. *J Rheumatol.* 2001 Jun;28(6):1347-55

[163] Oles RD. Glucose intolerance associated with temporomandibular joint pain-dysfunction syndrome. *Oral Surg Oral Med Oral Pathol* 1977 Apr;43(4):546-53

Six-part Self-treatment Protocol for the Alleviation of Pain Secondary to Muscle Tension and Myofascial Trigger Points in the Neck

1—APPLICATION OF HEAT: *Gentle heat softens muscles and tissues and allows for safer and more effective stretching and exercising.*
- You may find that applying heat before you begin your home treatment routine allows you to have increased range of motion and decreased pain. Heat softens muscles and tissues and can promote healing by increasing circulation—these positive effects can help you get the most out of your treatment plan. (Of course, use applications of heat that are safe and not damaging to skin.)
  - *Hot shower*—Moist heat seems to be the best for getting the warmth deep into the tissues where it is needed. Directing the hot water onto your neck and shoulders for 10-15 minutes will help to increase circulation and to soften the tissues before you perform the other exercises.
  - *Heating pads*—These are good if you are applying the heat away from home and need maximal convenience with minimal cleanup.

2—RANGE OF MOTION EXERCISES: *Allow enough time so that you can move in each direction for 20-100 repetitions.*
- *Flexion*—Start by brining your chin straight downward to your chest; return to neutral and repeat.
- *Extension*—From the neutral position, gently tilt your head straight backward then return to the neutral position.
- *Rotation*—Gently turn your head to the left, then back to center, then turn to the right and then repeat in the opposite direction.
- *Lateral bending*—From the neutral position, gently lean your head to one side, then return to neutral, then lean again and repeat toward the opposite side.
  - ***How much and how often?*** In a clinical research study with 77 women who suffered from chronic neck and shoulder pain, women who performed their exercises **three times per week for 5 sets of 20 repetitions** had better results than those who performed their exercises three times per week for 1 set of 20 repetitions.[164] ***More exercise gives better results—faster and more complete relief of neck pain.***

3—GENTLE STRETCHING: *"Gentle" is the key to effective stretching.* Apply a bit of end-of-range pressure with your hand (as demonstrated in the office) to stretch the muscles. Stretching needs to be *gentle* and *slow* to maximize benefits and minimize the introduction of new injury.
- *Flexion*—Bringing your chin straight downward to your chest.
- *Extension*—From the neutral position, gently tilt your head straight backward then return to the neutral position.
- *Rotation*—As above. Use care to not overstretch, and you do not need to turn your head past 90° or past your shoulder when you turn.
- *Lateral bending*—From the neutral position, gently lean your head to one side, then return to neutral, then lean again and repeat toward the opposite side.

4—POST-ISOMETRIC STRETCHING: Post-isometric stretching provides immediate relief of pain in 94% of patients, lasting relief of general pain in 63% of patients, and lasting relief of "point tenderness" in 23% of patients.[165] Follow these five steps: stretch, contract, stretch, relax, repeat
1. Position yourself with **target muscle in __stretched__ position** just short of pain or to the place where you begin to feel resistance.
2. While in the stretched position, **__contract__ the target muscle against slight resistance**, such as with your hands, for about 10-30 seconds.
3. Now breathe, relax for a few seconds, and then **gently __stretch__ the muscle** with slight pressure and allow the muscle to continue to lengthen with slight pressure; the duration of the stretch can range from 10-30 seconds followed by 10-30 seconds of relaxation.
4. **Relax** back into the neutral position.
5. **Repeat** steps 1-3 for 3-5 repetitions.

[164] Randlov A, Ostergaard M, Manniche C, Kryger P, Jordan A, Heegaard S, Holm B. Intensive dynamic training for females with chronic neck/shoulder pain. A randomized controlled trial. *Clin Rehabil*. 1998 Jun;12(3):200-10
[165] "The method produced immediate pain relief in 94%, lasting pain relief in 63%, as well as lasting relief of point tenderness in 23% of the sites treated. Patients who practiced autotherapy on a home program were more likely to realize lasting relief." Lewit K, Simons DG. Myofascial pain: relief by post-isometric relaxation. *Arch Phys Med Rehabil*. 1984 Aug;65(8):452-6

- o *How much and how often?* In a research study, the frequency recommendation was 2 times per week up to 2 times per day.
- o *Be specific!* Your efforts for stretching and contracting the muscles must be specific for the fibers of the muscle that are affected—with practice, you will learn to localize and affect the specific muscle fibers for efficient treatment.
- o *Proof of effectiveness from the clinical research*: "*...the increased tension of the affected muscles and the resulting pain and dysfunction are both relieved by restoring the full stretch length of the muscle... Post-isometric stretching-relaxation appears to be a simple, harmless, noninvasive, and effective way of restoring full stretch length to relieve pain originating in tense musculature.*[166]

5—APPLY ICE OR COLD PACK: You can apply a cold pack "generally" to most muscles of the neck, or you can target specific problem areas by applying local cold to muscles that continue to produce pain.
- **Apply cold for 10-20 minutes each 1-2 hours for reduction in pain and inflammation after your exercises.** Use your good judgment to avoid "frostbite" and cold injuries to skin.
- **Ice-and-stretch for the problematic/painful muscles**: A final bit of attention can be directed toward the problematic and painful muscles with trigger points. You can apply ice (or any source of cold) to the area for approximately 30 seconds to 2 minutes *as you continue to gently stretch the muscle.* The application of cold helps to decrease the pain and swelling that might arise from minor injuries incurred during stretching and exercising, and the cold has an important neurologic effect by helping to interrupt the cycle of pain and muscle spasm.

6—COMPLETE YOUR TREATMENT WITH THE APPLICATION OF A *natural* ANALGESIC CREAM: You can finish your routine with the application of a heating neck cream containing capsaicin or menthol to help your neck feel better for the rest of the day.

---

[166] Lewit K, Simons DG. Myofascial pain: relief by post-isometric relaxation. *Arch Phys Med Rehabil*. 1984 Aug;65(8):452-6

Chapter 5:
Cervical Spine and Neck

Introduction

Mechanical disorders—either post-traumatic or secondary to repetitive use—are common in the region of the cervical spine and neck. Unfortunately, many general practitioners are undertrained in the assessment and management of these disorders[1,2,3,4,5,6,7]; in particular, they lack a systematic method for evaluating and treating these conditions. In this chapter, practitioners are introduced to a 5-part system of categorization of the most common causes for patients to present with neck pain, and this is followed by several of the more common miscellaneous regional disorders.

---

[1] Freedman KB, Bernstein J. The adequacy of medical school education in musculoskeletal medicine. *J Bone Joint Surg Am*. 1998;80(10):1421-7

[2] Freedman KB, Bernstein J. Educational deficiencies in musculoskeletal medicine. *J Bone Joint Surg Am*. 2002;84-A(4):604-8

[3] Joy EA, Hala SV. Musculoskeletal curricula in medical education: filling in the missing pieces. The *Physician and Sportsmedicine*. 2004;32:42-45

[4] Matzkin E, Smith ME, Freccero CD, Richardson AB. Adequacy of education in musculoskeletal medicine. *J Bone Joint Surg Am*. 2005 Feb;87-A(2):310-4

[5] Schmale GA. More evidence of educational inadequacies in musculoskeletal medicine. *Clin Orthop Relat Res*. 2005 Aug;(437):251-9

[6] Stockard AR, Allen TW. Competence levels in musculoskeletal medicine: comparison of osteopathic and allopathic medical graduates. *J Am Osteopath Assoc*. 2006 Jun;106(6):350-5

[7] Humphreys BK, Sulkowski A, McIntyre K, Kasiban M, Patrick AN. An examination of musculoskeletal cognitive competency in chiropractic interns. *J Manipulative Physiol Ther*. 2007 Jan;30(1):44-9

Topics:

- **Introduction**: Concepts and Perspectives
- **Common Clinical Disorders of the Cervical Spine:**[*]
  - **Type 1—Nonspecific/Functional:**
    - Non-traumatic, Non-radicular, Non-degenerative Neck Pain
    - Cervical Myofascial Pain Syndrome
    - General Considerations and Management Protocol for Neck Pain
  - **Type 2—Degenerative:**
    - Cervical Osteoarthritis
    - Cervical Arthrosis/spondylosis
    - Foraminal Encroachment
    - Cervical Disc Protrusion/herniation
  - **Type 3—Radicular:**
    - Cervical Radiculitis
    - Cervical Radiculopathy
  - **Type 4—Myelopathic:**
    - Cervical Disc Protrusion/herniation
    - Cervical Myelopathy
    - Cervical Spine Canal Stenosis
  - **Type 5—Post-traumatic:**
    - Cervical Strain/sprain
    - Whiplash: Cervical Acceleration-Deceleration Syndrome
- **Miscellaneous Problems of the Neck:**
  - Torticollis, "wry neck"
  - Vertebral Osteomyelitis
  - Atlantoaxial Instability: Os Odontoidium, Agenesis/hypoplasia of the Dens, Fracture of the Odontoid, Rupture of the Transverse Ligament of the Atlas at the Axis
  - Klippel-Feil Syndrome

Core Competencies:

- Describe the pre-manipulative assessment of the cervical spine. Be able to list the relative and absolute contraindications to cervical spine manipulation.
- Describe the presentation, assessment/diagnosis, and management of the following:
  - Neck pain
  - Radiculitis
  - Radiculopathy
  - Myelopathy
  - Atlantoaxial instability
  - Os odontoidium
  - Vertebral osteomyelitis
  - Klippel-Feil Syndrome

Concepts and Perspectives:

- From an *embryological and developmental perspective*, we see that the atlantoaxial joint is subject to anomalies such as agenesis of the dens and os odontoidium, both of which can leave the cervical spinal cord vulnerable to compression due to the lack of stabilization usually provided by the relationship of the transverse ligament to the dens. Other congenital changes in the cervical region can include congenital fusion of vertebrae and the presence of hemivertebrae, as seen with Klippel-Feil syndrome; often these conditions are not diagnosed during childhood and present clinically in adults who complain of chronic neck pain.
- From a *musculoskeletal-anatomical perspective*, we see that the facet joints and other articular structures of the cervical spine and neck are very richly innervated with proprioceptors and

---

[*] The categorization of "Type 1, Type 2...etc" in this chapter is for organization and ease of apprehension; these are not officially recognized nomenclature for neuromusculoskeletal disorders.

nociceptors; thus the opportunities for aberrant kinesthesis and chronic pain are readily apparent. The great range of motion provided by the neck is afforded by the lack of osseous restriction and a reliance therefore upon joint capsules, ligaments, muscles and tendons for structural stability; these soft tissues are relatively weak compared to the osseous stabilization seen in joints such as the hip, and thus the neck is extremely vulnerable to traumatic injuries, such as the flexion-extension injuries seen with "whiplash" and the compressive and lateral bending injuries seen with many sports injuries. Further, the chronic muscle tension required to maintain the head's upright position sets the stage for the development of myofascial trigger points and resultant local and referred pain.

- From an *orthopedic and rheumatologic perspective*, we see that the neck is vulnerable not only to acute trauma, but also to degenerative changes that can occur gradually or subacutely with inflammatory arthropathies such as rheumatoid arthritis and ankylosing spondylitis, which are known to precipitate atlantoaxial instability due to erosive lysis of the transverse ligament.

- From a *clinical medicine perspective*, we see that the neck is the conduit and location for many delicate structures of vital importance, particularly the spinal cord, cervical nerve roots, brachial plexus, cervical sympathetic chains, phrenic nerves, cranial nerves 9-12, vertebral arteries, carotid arteries, trachea, and esophagus. At the anterior base of the neck are the thyroid and parathyroid glands.

- From a *clinical management perspective*, we can categorize common problems involving the neck into general groups or types distinguished by their prevailing characteristic. The most common problems involving the neck have here been separated into five subtypes; this categorization allows clinicians to quickly focus on the type of problem and its attendant complications and details which need attention for successful management. These are detailed later in this chapter and are summarized here:

Category	*Key Assessments and Considerations*	*Keys to Successful Management*
1. Pain (without serious cause and without serious complications)	• Baseline assessment to quantify status and exclude serious disorders: history, examination, laboratory tests; radiographs are generally not necessary unless history, age, or symptoms are suggestive	• Alleviation of pain • Prevention of recurrence *via health optimization, lifestyle-ergonomic-exercise interventions, preventive treatment*
2. Degeneration	• Baseline assessment to quantify status and exclude serious disorders: history, examination, laboratory tests; radiographs help establish and quantify the degenerative nature of the problem but are not always required	• Alleviation of pain • Slowing or reversal of degenerative process • Promotion of optimal functional status
3. Radiculitis, radiculopathy	• Baseline assessment to quantify status and exclude serious disorders: history, examination, laboratory tests • *Slow onset* is characteristic of degenerative compression • *Rapid onset* is characteristic of recent disc herniation • *Sensory-only* changes suggests nerve root irritation, commonly due to local inflammation from acute disc herniation • *Sensory and motor* lesions suggests nerve root compression due to combination of degenerative changes in disc, joints of Luschka, and facet joints	• Comprehensive-holistic management as reviewed in Chapter 3 *as long as no serious underlying problems are present and as long as pain is reasonably controlled and motor deficits are not severe or progressing* • Alleviation of pain • Constant monitoring of muscle strength to determine and re-confirm the appropriateness of nonsurgical treatment
4. Myelopathy	• Identification	• Surgical referral
5. Post-traumatic	• Exclusion of serious complications: vascular, neurologic, and orthopedic (i.e., fractures) • Patients with pain immediately following trauma should be evaluated with comprehensive neurologic examination and radiographs, including flexion/extension views	• Comprehensive-holistic management (Chapter 3) • Whole-body treatment • Alleviation of pain • Promote optimal functionality

Premanipulative cervical spine assessment:

For many years, premanipulative assessment was considered the *standard of care* for practitioners of manual medicine prior to their first utilization of cervical spine manipulation in a new patient. The purpose of this battery of assessments was specifically to identify those patients at increased risk for neurovascular complications (vertebral artery dissection, brainstem stroke (e.g., lateral medullary syndrome), or cerebrovascular accident [CVA]) from manipulation of the cervical spine. While such screening was performed for what was then thought to be in the best interest of the patient, **the specific procedure for provoking vertebrobasilar insufficiency (VBI)—holding the patient's head in a rotated and extended position for 30-60 seconds in an attempt to identify those patients with insufficient vertebrobasilar circulation—has not been proven effective in identifying those patients for whom cervical manipulation confers an important risk.** A clinical trial by Licht et al[8] found that **VBI testing correlated poorly with alterations in posterior cerebral blood flow and that—more importantly—patients who "failed" VBI testing could still be safely treated with manual manipulation of the cervical spine.** A follow-up study by Licht et al[9] further proved this point by showing that a "positive" (symptom-inducing) test was not associated with diminutions of peak or average blood flow velocity in the carotid or the vertebral arteries; the authors concluded, **"If premanipulative testing is used solely for the detection of vascular insufficiency as a potential substrate for CVAs after cervical manipulation, we believe that premanipulative testing is of little clinical value."** These conclusions are in accord with an earlier publication by Cote et al[10] who analyzed the clinical use of VBI testing; their conclusion reads, **"From an ethical point of view, the consequences of unnecessarily alarming patients about the risk of a potential stroke are unsupported and unacceptable."**

While the specific maneuver for testing for VBI as a surrogate indicator for post-manipulative CVA risk appears to have no clinical merit, other components of the "premanipulative assessment" are worthwhile parts of basic patient assessment and physical examination for the purpose of quantifying the patient's overall health, identifying occult and concomitant disorders (i.e., hypertension), and identifying other possible contraindications to manipulation (i.e., osteomyelitis or fracture).

Premanipulative assessment of the cervical spine:

1) History: as extensive and complete as possible and reasonable, specifically for the following:
- Trauma, injury, fracture, strain
- Transient ischemic attacks (TIA), fainting, neurologic symptoms, stroke, CVD
- Cancer
- Medication, especially OCA/BCP and anticoagulants
- Inflammatory arthropathy: increased risk for atlantoaxial instability
- Down's syndrome (increased risk of os odontoidium and dens agenesis)
- Infection
- Radiculopathy, myelopathy
- Overall physical, mental, and emotional health

2) Regional examination of the neck:
- Passive *before* active neck flexion: use caution with all passive (doctor-forced) maneuvers until you are quite sure that the patient has no fracture or instability
- Orthopedic tests, motion and static palpation

3) Cardiovascular and circulatory assessment:
- Bilateral carotid auscultation
- Bilateral blood pressure: finding a 10 mm Hg systolic difference suggests the possibility of arterial occlusion such as due to atherosclerosis or congenital anomaly. If positive, consider Doppler or imaging study to evaluate circulation
- Auscultate: (use the *bell* for *bruits*): carotid arteries in anterolateral neck; Subclavian arteries: instruct patient to "inhale and hold" as you auscultate the supraclavicular fossa
- Testing for vertebrobasilar insufficiency (VBI): expert council that was consulted during the preparation of this section advised against the inclusion of VBI testing due to its consistently reported lack of value in identifying patients at increased risk for manipulation-induced VBI and CVA. That said, a technical description of this procedure has been included here for the sake of completeness and licensure examinations; clinicians may exclude this test, or include it more for *orthopedic* rather than *neurovascular* reasons, *per se*: patient is positioned into cervical rotation and extension 30-60 seconds per side (head is rotated to the same side as the vertebral artery being tested); patient keeps eyes open and answers questions for the assessment of subtle cerebral ischemia

4) Test peripheral nerves and circulation: assess upper and lower extremities for strength, coordination, reflexes, sensory, circulation, and trophic changes

5) Clinical assessment for infection: temperature, clinical assessment, may include WBC and CRP

6) Radiographs and imaging as necessary: Radiographic assessment before spinal manipulation is generally unnecessary except when specifically indicated by the patient's history or physical examination findings

7) Laboratory tests: as indicated

8) Informed consent (PAR-B): Procedures, alternatives, risks, and benefits

9) Monitor response to treatment:

10) Chart all procedures, findings, referrals, treatment

---

[8] "It appears that a positive premanipulative test is not an absolute contraindication to manipulation of the cervical spine. If the test is able to identify patients at risk for cerebrovascular accidents, we suggest patients with a reproducible positive test should be referred for a duplex examination of the vertebral artery flow." Licht PB, Christensen HW, Hoilund-Carlsen PF. Is there a role for premanipulative testing before cervical manipulation? *J Manipulative Physiol Ther*. 2000 Mar-Apr;23(3):175-9

[9] Licht PB, Christensen HW, Hoilund-Carlsen PF. Carotid artery blood flow during premanipulative testing. *J Manipulative Physiol Ther*. 2002 Nov-Dec;25:568-72

[10] Cote P, Kreitz BG, Cassidy JD, Thiel H. The validity of the extension-rotation test as a clinical screening procedure before neck manipulation: a secondary analysis. *J Manipulative Physiol Ther*. 1996 Mar-Apr; 19(3): 159-64

Clinical assessments of the cervical spine

Clinical assessments	*Positive finding and Implications*
1. **History**: *see Chapter 1 for more details.*	• **Systemic symptoms and signs** (such as fever, weight loss, lymphadenopathy) • **Complications** (such as loss of function) • **Indicators from the history** (trauma, risk factors, positive medical history, systemic inflammatory/autoimmune disorder) • **Mechanical/non-mechanical pain** (non mechanical pain suggests pathologic etiology rather than simple joint dysfunction) **Abnormal findings indicate that the patient is at increased risk for serious pathology and potential complications. Proceed with caution. Obtain laboratory and imaging studies as indicated. Defer or modify physical examination. Refer as indicated.**
2. **Shoulder abduction test, Bakody sign**[11]: Patient places the forearm or palm on top of head	• **Relief of radicular pain** with placing the forearm or palm on top of the head (maximal abduction with elbow flexion) suggests nerve root irritation, commonly of C4 or C5. This procedure relieves tension on irritated nerve roots.
3. **Swallowing test**[12]	• **Difficulty swallowing solid food** suggests physical lesion: space-occupying lesion (SOL) near the pharynx or esophagus such as osteophytes, hematoma, infection/abscess, or tumor. • **Difficulty swallowing liquids** suggests neurologic problem in the neck such as paralysis of nerve, neurologic disease, lesion of CN-9 (glossopharyngeal nerve).
4. **Dejerine's triad, Valsalva test**: patient takes a deep breath and bears down	• Increased neurogenic/dermatomal pain with coughing, sneezing, straining, laughing suggests a space-occupying lesion in the spinal canal (e.g., tumor, disc herniation, hematoma, abscess) compressing the spinal cord or nerve root; locate the site of pain and use imaging as necessary
5. **Auscultation of the carotid arteries**	• An audible bruit suggests atherosclerosis or arterial occlusion; refer for ultrasound evaluation; defer cervical spine manipulation until cause of bruit is determined
6. **Active motion of the cervical spine**: patient moves head and neck into full flexion, extension, rotation and lateral bending to both sides	Inability to move the head and neck though a **complete and painless range of motion (ROM)** in all directions may suggest any of the following: • Joint restriction • Muscle spasm, myofascial trigger points (MFTP) • Tight muscles • **Fracture** • **Dislocation** • **Disc herniation/injury** • Facet syndrome, capsular adhesions

[11] Magee DJ. Orthopedic Physical Assessment. Third edition. Philadelphia: WB Saunders, 1997 page 107, 126
[12] Hoppenfeld S. Physical examination of the spine and extremities. Norwalk: Appleton and Lange, 1976, p.127

Clinical assessment of the cervical spine—*continued*

Assessments	Positive finding and Implications
7. **O'Donoghue maneuver**, active resisted motion of the cervical spine: Doctor resists patient's active cervical ROM in all directions, then the doctor passively moves patient's cervical spine in ROM of all directions[13]	▪ Exacerbation of pain with **resisted** ROM suggests **strain** of affected **muscles** ▪ Exacerbation of pain with **passive** ROM suggests **sprain** of affected **ligaments**
8. **Rust's sign**[14]	▪ **Patient needs to support head/neck with hands during normal motions/positions to prevent pain: this suggests severe cervical injury: ligamentous instability or fracture—strongly consider immediate immobilization and imaging**
9. **Cervical distraction**: doctor applies traction to cervical spine, often by standing behind patient and lifting up by applying traction from patient's occiput, temporal bone and mandible	Decrease in pain suggests: ▪ Joint irritation, facet syndrome ▪ Disc herniation ▪ Cervicogenic radiculopathy due to disc herniation or foraminal encroachment Increase in pain suggests: ▪ Muscle spasm or tightness ▪ Stretching of injured ligaments
10. **Cervical compression**: doctor applies downward compressive force with patient's head and neck in neutral, lateral flexion, extension, and extension with lateral flexion with ipsilateral rotation	**Pain may indicate any of the following:** ▪ **Disc injury** ▪ **Facet injury** ▪ Radiculopathy or radiculitis (dermatomal symptoms) ▪ Muscle strain ▪ Other lesion to disc or bone
11. **Cervical compression with rotation**, Jackson's compression test[15]	▪ Radicular pain suggests radiculitis or radiculopathy
12. **Spurling's test, foramina compression test**: doctor applies percussive or compressive force to top of patient's head in neutral, lateral bending, and lateral bending with extension)[16]	▪ Exacerbation of local or radicular pain with this maneuver may indicate radiculopathy due to compression from foraminal encroachment or disc herniation, or possibly facet irritation, especially if the pain is worse on same side as the lateral bending. Exacerbation of pain on the contralateral side may suggest the stretching of injured or tight muscles, or nerve root irritation due to traction

[13] Irene Gold Associates. National Board Review Book 2000. PO Box 306 Gladwyne, PA 19035 Phone (610) 649-8300; Page O-3
[14] Brier S. Primary Care Orthopedics. St. Louis: Mosby, 1999 page 143
[15] Magee DJ. Orthopedic Physical Assessment. Third edition. Philadelphia: WB Saunders, 1997 page 126
[16] Gatterman MI (Ed.). Chiropractic Management of Spine-Related Disorders. Baltimore; Williams and Wilkins, 1990. Page 78, 312

Clinical assessment of the cervical spine — *continued*

Assessments	Positive finding and Implications
13. <u>**Shoulder depression test**</u>: Patient laterally flexes neck while doctor is behind the patient applying pressure downward on contralateral shoulder and gently assisting patient's head in lateral bending	<ul><li>**Pain on the convex/stretched side of the neck is likely due to provocation of injured/tight muscles. Radicular pain on this side is likely due to traction of injured or inflamed nerves.**</li><li>Pain on the concave side of the neck is likely due to compression of facets or closure of foramina. Radicular pain on this side is likely due to foraminal encroachment.</li></ul>
14. <u>**Supine active and passive neck flexion**</u>, Soto-Hall test: patient is supine on the table; patient actively raises head from table into cervical flexion and then relaxes head back to table; doctor then lifts patient's head while stabilizing sternum with other hand.[17,18] *This test must <u>never</u> be performed in patients with a possibility of cervical spine fracture or atlantoaxial instability until imaging and clinical assessments have excluded fracture or instability.*	Neck pain or referred pain to head or arm suggests:<ul><li>**Ligament sprain or instability**</li><li>Fracture</li><li>Meningitis: especially with cognitive changes and fever, may have skin rash[19]</li><li>Disc herniation</li><li>Dislocation</li><li>Muscle spasm, contracture, or strain</li></ul>Also look for:<ul><li>Atlantoaxial instability: myelopathic signs and symptoms</li><li>Lhermitte's sign</li><li>Brudzinski's sign</li></ul>
15. <u>**Lhermitte's sign**</u>: elicited from performing forced neck flexion (Soto-Hall maneuver); variation may be performed by performing straight leg raising concomitantly with cervical flexion[20]	Sharp pain or "electric shock" into upper or lower limbs with neck flexion is associated with:<ul><li>Dural irritation/adhesion; consider meningitis as a possible diagnosis if clinical presentation is suggestive</li><li>Possible cervical myelopathy or spinal cord injury</li><li>Multiple sclerosis</li><li>**New onset of positive Lhermitte's sign strongly suggests need for neurological referral[21]**</li></ul>
16. <u>**Brudzinski's sign**</u>: patient is supine on the table, doctor forces neck into flexion[22,23]	<ul><li>Involuntary flexion of the hip/knees with passive cervical flexion suggests meningeal irritation, such as with meningitis[24], subarachnoid hemorrhage, or dural adhesions</li></ul>

---

[17] Gatterman MI (Ed.). <u>Chiropractic Management of Spine-Related Disorders</u>. Baltimore; Williams and Wilkins, 1990. Page 186
[18] Brier S. <u>Primary Care Orthopedics</u>. St. Louis: Mosby, 1999 page 431
[19] No orthopedic tests have sufficient sensitivity or specificity for meningitis. Clinical findings of neck stiffness, fever, and altered mental status (with or without skin rash) mandate the need for lumbar puncture even if provocative orthopedic tests are negative. Attia J, Hatala R, Cook DJ, Wong JG. The rational clinical examination. Does this adult patient have acute meningitis? *JAMA* 1999 Jul 14;282(2):175-81
[20] Magee DJ. <u>Orthopedic Physical Assessment. Third edition</u>. Philadelphia: WB Saunders, 1997 page 126
[21] Gatterman MI (Ed.). <u>Chiropractic Management of Spine-Related Disorders</u>. Baltimore; Williams and Wilkins, 1990. Page 186
[22] Goldberg S. <u>The Four-Minute Neurologic Exam</u>. Miami, Medimaster, Inc, 1992 page 39
[23] Gatterman MI (Ed.). <u>Chiropractic Management of Spine-Related Disorders</u>. Baltimore; Williams and Wilkins, 1990. Page 186
[24] Unreliable as a screening test for meningitis. See: Thomas KE, Hasbun R, Jekel J, Quagliarello VJ. The diagnostic accuracy of Kernig's sign, Brudzinski's sign, and nuchal rigidity in adults with suspected meningitis. *Clin Infect Dis* 2002 Jul 1;35(1):46-52

Assessments	Positive finding and Implications
17. **Kernig sign**: patient is supine and lying flat; hip and knee are then bent to 90° of flexion, and then the knee is straightened[25]	Pain in the low back with passive extension of the knee: ▪ **Meningeal irritation**, such as with meningitis or subarachnoid hemorrhage ▪ Nerve tension and radicular signs suggest nerve root compression, possibly due to disc herniation
18. **VBI testing, assessing for vertebrobasilar insufficiency: cervical extension and rotation for 30-60 seconds** (Houle's test, de Kleyn's test)	**Any of the following: nystagmus, dizziness, nausea, diplopia, confusion, difficulty speaking, loss of memory suggests vertebral artery occlusion or unilateral agenesis** ▪ **Generally considered a contraindication to cervical manipulation, *especially manipulations that involve rotation and/or and extension*** ▪ **Consider Doppler studies or other follow-up to assess vertebrobasilar circulation** ▪ **This test was previously considered the standard of care prior to use of cervical spine manipulation even though its value in preventing manipulation-induced CVA/VBI was never proven; its use in clinical practice has been discouraged.[26]**
19. **Hautant's test**: This test is a variation of VBI testing: patient is seated, eyes closed, cervical extension and rotation held for 30 seconds with arms outstretched and palms facing upward	Any of the following: nystagmus, dizziness, nausea, diplopia, confusion, difficulty speaking, loss of memory **with deviation or falling of the hands:** ▪ Possible vertebral artery occlusion or unilateral agenesis ▪ Consider Doppler studies or other follow-up to assess vertebrobasilar circulation ▪ Possible contraindication to manipulation *especially that involves rotation and extension*; educate patient, PAR, and informed consent
20. **Maigne's maneuver**: This test is a variation of VBI testing: doctor holds the patient in the premanipulative position. In this procedure, the doctor is prepared to manipulate the cervical spine but holds the patient in the premanipulative position for 15-30 seconds before delivering the manipulative thrust	A positive result is noted with any of the following: nystagmus, dizziness, nausea, diplopia, confusion, difficulty speaking, or loss of memory. Implications include: ▪ Possible vertebral artery occlusion or unilateral agenesis ▪ Consider Doppler studies or other follow-up to assess vertebrobasilar circulation ▪ Possible contraindication to manipulation *especially that involves rotation and extension*; educate patient, PAR, and informed consent

[25] Goldberg S. The Four-Minute Neurologic Exam. Miami, Medimaster, Inc, 1992 page 39

[26] "CONCLUSION: We were unable to demonstrate that the extension-rotation test is a valid clinical screening procedure to detect decreased blood flow in the vertebral artery. The value of this test for screening patients at risk of stroke after cervical manipulation is questionable..." Cote P, Kreitz BG, Cassidy JD, Thiel H. The validity of the extension-rotation test as a clinical screening procedure before neck manipulation: a secondary analysis. *J Manipulative Physiol Ther*. 1996 Mar-Apr; 19(3): 159-64.

Clinical assessment of the cervical spine—*continued*

Assessments	Positive finding and Implications
21. <u>**Underberg's test**</u>: This test is a variation of VBI testing: patient marches-in-place, eyes closed, cervical extension and rotation for 30 seconds with arms outstretched and palms up; doctor stands next to patient to ensure patient safety if balance is lost	A positive result is noted with any of the following: nystagmus, dizziness, nausea, diplopia, confusion, difficulty speaking, or loss of memory. Implications include: ▪ Possible vertebral artery occlusion or unilateral agenesis ▪ Consider Doppler studies or other follow-up to assess vertebrobasilar circulation ▪ Possible contraindication to manipulation *especially that involves rotation and extension*; educate patient, PAR, and informed consent ▪ *Considered the most sensitive of all tests for evaluating vertebrobasilar insufficiency*[27]
22. <u>**Muscle testing**</u>: doctor provides resistance in rotation, extension, lateral flexion, forward flexion against patient's muscle contraction	Weakness or pain may indicate: ▪ Muscle lesion: injury, myopathy ▪ MFTP ▪ Nerve injury: cerebrum, brainstem, spinal cord, peripheral nerve, neuromuscular junction ▪ Electrolyte imbalance
23. <u>**Spinal percussion**</u>[28]: Doctor uses a reflex hammer to percuss the spinous processes of the thoracic and lumbar spine; cervical spine percussion requires the doctor to compress the ligamentum nuchae and apply the percussive force to the doctor's fingers	▪ **Spinal pain with percussion of the spine with a reflex hammer or with the fingertips: strongly consider obtaining radiographs or other imaging in any patient with exacerbation of pain following spinal percussion, as this indicates the possibility of a bone lesion: spinal fracture, spinal tumor, or vertebral osteomyelitis. Other considerations are acute herniated disc and joint or ligament injury**
24. <u>**Adson test**</u>: assess for thoracic outlet syndrome (TOS): patient stands with arms in neutral position, doctor assesses radial pulse of patient, then extends and externally rotates patient's arm; patient takes a deep breath, with head turned to opposite side, then same side	Diminution of pulse accompanied by shoulder/arm pain or paresthesia suggests: ▪ **Thoracic outlet syndrome**: underlying causes include cervical rib, scalene hypertrophy, poor posture, and hypertonic cervical musculature. A positive Adson test has been suggested to indicate **compression of the subclavian artery by a cervical rib and/or hypertonic scalene muscles.**[29] Also consider pathology in the region of the supraclavicular fossa
25. <u>**Eden's test**</u>, costoclavicular maneuver: patient places chin on chest; from behind the patient, doctor pulls patient's arms into slight extension while palpating radial pulse[30]	▪ Diminution of pulse accompanied by shoulder/arm pain or paresthesia suggests **thoracic outlet syndrome**: underlying causes include costoclavicular compression of the subclavicular neurovascular bundle

[27] Carey PF. A suggested protocol for the examination and treatment of the cervical spine: managing the risk. *Journal of the Canadian Chiropractic Association* 1995: 39: 35-40
[28] Gatterman MI (Ed.). <u>Chiropractic Management of Spine-Related Disorders</u>. Baltimore; Williams and Wilkins, 1990. Page 187
[29] Hoppenfeld S. <u>Physical examination of the spine and extremities</u>. Norwalk: Appleton and Lange, 1976, p. 127
[30] Gatterman MI (Ed.). <u>Chiropractic Management of Spine-Related Disorders</u>. Baltimore; Williams and Wilkins, 1990. Page 222

Assessments	*Positive finding and Implications*
26. <u>Wright test</u>: patient is seated with arms down; from behind patient, the doctor holds the patient's wrist and assess the radial pulse while the arm is straight and brought into full abduction; repeat bilaterally[31]	▪ Diminution of pulse accompanied by shoulder/arm pain or paresthesia suggests **thoracic outlet syndrome**: underlying causes include cervical rib, scalene hypertrophy, poor posture, and hypertonic cervical musculature. This test is thought to indicate neurovascular compression due to tight pectoralis minor
27. <u>Roos test</u>: patient abducts both shoulders to 90°, externally rotates arm and flexes elbow to 90°; patient then opens and closes hands for 2 minutes while the doctor simply observes.[32] Some experts consider this to be the best test for thoracic outlet syndrome.	▪ This test attempts to provoke ischemia that manifests as shoulder/arm pain or paresthesia and suggests **thoracic outlet syndrome**: underlying causes include cervical rib, scalene hypertrophy, poor posture, and hypertonic cervical musculature. ▪ Some *normal* people cannot perform this test without significant discomfort
28. <u>Halstead maneuver, (modified Adson)</u>: downward traction on the arm as the doctor palpates the radial pulse[33]	▪ Pain, pallor, reduced pulse, paresthesia in the upper limb suggests thoracic outlet syndrome
29. <u>Motion palpation</u>: a chiropractic technique for assessing subtleties of joint motion to determine the appropriateness and type of spinal manipulation to be applied[34]	▪ Hypermobility and/or hypomobility indicates segmental dysfunction which may indicate simple joint restriction or degenerative changes, or congenital anomalies ▪ Point tenderness may indicate spinal fracture or instability
30. <u>Neurologic assessment</u>: reflexes, muscle strength, sensory perception, coordination 31. <u>Cranial nerve examination</u>: must be performed in patients with neurologic lesions or recent trauma	▪ **Weakness, loss of function, loss of sensation, hyporeflexia, hyperreflexia suggest neurologic compromise at the cord, nerve root, or peripheral nerve** ▪ Also consider double crush syndromes, vitamin B-12 deficiency, diabetes mellitus, and other peripheral nerve lesions
32. <u>Palpation</u>: manual and digital assessment of bones, ligaments, muscles, fascia and general tone and feel of the patient's body	▪ Pain, mass, or enlargement may suggest any of several problems: abscess, thyroid enlargement, muscle spasm, fracture, tumor, etc.
33. <u>Imaging</u>: Radiographs, CT, MRI	▪ Radiographs are fast, inexpensive, and excellent for detecting degenerative changes, obvious fractures and dislocations ▪ CT is faster and less expensive than MRI, and is preferred over MRI when searching for fractures ▪ MRI is best for visualizing soft tissue lesions such as disc herniation causing spinal cord or nerve root compression.

---

[31] Gatterman MI (Ed.). <u>Chiropractic Management of Spine-Related Disorders</u>. Baltimore; Williams and Wilkins, 1990. Page 222-223

[32] Howard TM, O'Connor FG. The injured shoulder. Primary care assessment. *Arch Fam Med*. 1997 Jul-Aug;6(4):376-84

[33] Gatterman MI (Ed.). <u>Chiropractic Management of Spine-Related Disorders</u>. Baltimore; Williams and Wilkins, 1990. Page 221

[34] Motion Palpation Institute information is available at www.motionpalpation.com as of December 20, 2006

Suggested examination flow for the cervical spine and neck

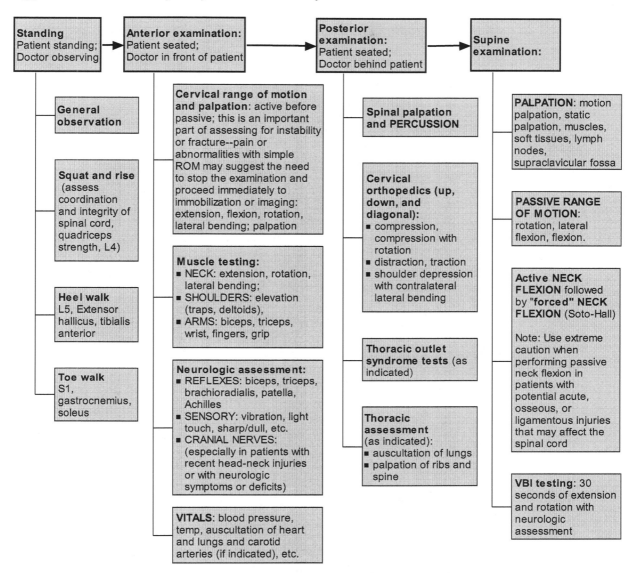

Standing	Anterior	Posterior	Supine
1. Observation 2. Squat and rise 3. Toe walk 4. Heel walk	1. ROM (active) 2. Muscle testing 3. Nerve tests (reflex and sensory, consider cranial nerves) 4. Vital signs	1. Orthopedics tests for the neck can be though of as occurring in 3 directions: <u>up</u>—traction, <u>down</u>—compression, <u>diagonal</u>—lateral bending with contralateral shoulder depression. 2. Percussion and palpation 3. TOS tests 4. Thoracic spine and cardiopulmonary examination	1. Palpation 2. ROM (passive) 3. Neck flexion 4. VBI testing (practitioner's option)

Type 1—Nonspecific Neck Pain:
- ## Non-traumatic, Non-radicular, Non-degenerative Neck Pain
- ## Cervical Myofascial Pain Syndrome
- ## General Considerations and Management Protocol

<u>Description/pathophysiology</u>:
- This section deals with basic concepts in the assessment and treatment of benign neck pain—that which is acute, subacute, or chronic. "Simple neck pain" for this discussion is defined by the *absence* of serious associated or underlying problems, specifically:
  - No evidence of neurologic complications:
    - Sensory, strength, and reflexes are intact in the upper and lower extremities
    - No radiculitis (dermatomal sensory changes), radiculopathy, myelopathy, or Horner's syndrome
    - No bowel/bladder changes, and no anogenital numbness (characteristics of cervical myelopathy and cauda equina syndrome)
  - No evidence or suspicion of underlying pathology or metabolic disorder:
    - No systemic manifestations or changes: weight loss, weight gain, fever, chills, fatigue
    - No past history of severe head-neck-shoulder trauma
    - No history of cancer or skeletal deformity/anomaly
    - No recent or current infections, which may have infiltrated bones or discs
    - No clinical or laboratory evidence of rheumatic diseases that commonly affect the neck and shoulder region: dermatomyositis, polymyositis, polymyalgia rheumatica[35]
    - No metabolic disorder such as fibromyalgia, which typically presents with neck and shoulder pain along with widespread tender points, sleep disturbance, gastrointestinal symptoms, and fatigue
    - Imaging studies (if performed) are essentially normal with the possible exception of *very mild* degenerative changes in the cervical spine
    - Screening laboratory tests—specifically: chemistry/metabolic panel, CBC, CRP, TSH, free T4, 25-OH-vitamin D, and ferritin—are within normal limits. **Diagnoses of exclusion can only be made after alternate diagnoses are excluded, and this unequivocally requires the performance of laboratory tests.**
- Common terms and phenomena associated with neck pain (particularly *chronic* neck and shoulder pain) include **fibrositis** (an archaic and erroneous term implying inflammation (generally absent) of muscle fibers, **myofascial trigger points** (MFTP, generally present; see Chapter 3 for description and treatment), **fibromyalgia** (a complex systemic phenomenon with a major contribution from bacterial overgrowth of the small bowel[36]; see Chapter 4 of *Integrative Rheumatology*[37] for discussion and treatment of gastrointestinal dysbiosis, including bacterial overgrowth); **cervical myofascial pain syndrome** may be a regional form of the more widely distributed **myofascial pain syndrome** and can be addressed with the protocol outlined in this section. To what extent these latter syndromic phenomena are truly valid and distinct clinical entities rather different names for each other and fibromyalgia, and to what extent these conditions are simply a misdiagnosis of the much more common problems of **hypothyroidism** (a common disorder which can cause neck-shoulder regional pain or widespread pain with **inflammatory arthropathy and myopathy**) and **vitamin D deficiency** (a pandemic problem that causes musculoskeletal pain[38] and inflammation[39], particularly of the spine[40]) has not been determined. In the real world, we can be quite certain that most clinicians and

[35] For diagnostic and treatment details, see: Vasquez A. *Integrative Rheumatology*. Fort Worth, Texas; Integrative and Biological Medicine LLC, 2006: http://OptimalHealthResearch.com
[36] Pimentel M, et al. A link between irritable bowel syndrome and fibromyalgia may be related to findings on lactulose breath testing. *Ann Rheum Dis*. 2004 Apr;63(4):450-2
[37] Vasquez A. *Integrative Rheumatology*. Fort Worth, Texas; Integrative and Biological Medicine Research and Consulting, 2006: http://OptimalHealthResearch.com
[38] Masood H, Narang AP, Bhat IA, Shah GN. Persistent limb pain and raised serum alkaline phosphatase the earliest markers of subclinical hypovitaminosis D in Kashmir. *Indian J Physiol Pharmacol*. 1989 Oct-Dec;33(4):259-61
[39] Timms PM, Mannan N, Hitman GA, et al. Circulating MMP9, vitamin D and variation in the TIMP-1 response with VDR genotype: mechanisms for inflammatory damage in chronic disorders? *QJM*. 2002 Dec;95(12):787-96 http://qjmed.oxfordjournals.org/cgi/content/full/95/12/787
[40] Al Faraj S, Al Mutairi K. Vitamin D deficiency and chronic low back pain in Saudi Arabia. *Spine*. 2003 Jan 15;28(2):177-9

researchers do not differentiate between these conditions with a high degree of accuracy and therefore these terms when used clinically carry some inherent inaccuracy and misapplication; newer generations of clinicians have more knowledge and better tools with which to distinguish these conditions and so these terms, if not discarded, will be refined and re-defined in the upcoming years.

Complications:
- Pain, discomfort, reduction in quality of life, reduction in productivity.
- Chronic pain in any part of the body but particularly the neck and shoulder region can literally "take on a life of its own" and become progressive and debilitating. **Myofascial pain syndrome** or **cervical myofascial pain syndrome** can be treated with many of the concepts and interventions discussed in this section and reviewed previously in Chapters 2 and 3. Myofascial pain syndrome is different from the more complex and serious **complex regional pain syndrome**, also named **reflex sympathetic dystrophy**.
- May coexist and/or synergize with migraine headaches and TMJ dysfunction.

Clinical presentations:
- Onset may be acute, subacute, chronic.
- Onset may occur weeks, months, or years after a traumatic event.
- Neck pain may radiate (without neurologic deficit or dermatomal pattern) into the shoulders and upper arms.
- Cervical and upper thoracic paraspinal muscles tend to be hypertonic, tender, and tight/shortened with one or more latent or active MFTP.
- Fibromyalgia and myofascial pain syndromes are more common in women although both genders are affected; the age incidences are highest from the 20s-40s; thereafter the incidences decline sharply while the incidence of inflammatory rheumatic diseases increases.
- The radiation of pain from MFTP can mimic radiculitis/radiculopathy, and the autonomic features rarely seen with MFTP can include ptosis and disequilibrium, thus mimicking Horner's syndrome and vestibulocochlear nerve and/or brainstem lesion.

Major differential diagnoses:
- <u>Facet syndrome</u>: can cause referred neck and arm pain; generally exacerbated with ipsilateral lateral flexion with compression; no change in radial pulse.
- <u>Fracture</u>: Especially after trauma; fracture can occur in osteoporotic (e.g., steroid-treated) patients with minimal force.
- <u>Infections that affect neurologic structures</u>: Herpes zoster and Lyme disease may present with sensory and/or motor disturbances, respectively.
- <u>Intra-abdominal pathology</u>: Gall bladder disease can cause shoulder pain which could mimic the shoulder-neck-arm pain of cervical nerve root dysfunctions.
- <u>Ligamentous instability</u>: Instability may occur following acute trauma due to tearing of ligaments, or ligaments such as the transverse ligament at the dens may be lesioned by chronic inflammatory diseases such as rheumatoid arthritis and ankylosing spondylitis. Atlantoaxial instability can be the presenting complaint of inflammatory arthropathies.[41]
- <u>Myocardial infarction</u>: Can cause pain in the neck, face, and arm and may thus mimic cervical spine disease or cervical radiculopathy.
- <u>Occult pathology</u>: Particularly bone tumor or Pancoast tumor of the lung apex.
- <u>Osteomyelitis</u>: Assess for fever, lymphadenopathy, and elevations in WBC and CRP.
- <u>Pathologies and metabolic diseases</u>: Such as ALS (concomitant upper and lower motor neuron lesions) or syringomyelia (presents with bilateral sensory and motor changes in the upper extremity with "shawl" distribution of shoulder and upper extremity numbness.[42]

---

[41] "Atlantoaxial instability has been recognized as a late complication in only one patient and has not been reported as an early manifestation. This paper presents a case in which atlantoaxial instability and neck pain without neurologic involvement was a presenting manifestation." Thompson GH, Khan MA, Bilenker RM. Spontaneous atlantoaxial subluxation as a presenting manifestation of juvenile ankylosing spondylitis. A case report. *Spine*. 1982 Jan-Feb;7(1):78-9
[42] Beers MH, Berkow R (eds). The Merck Manual. Seventeenth Edition. Whitehouse Station; Merck Research Laboratories 1999 page 1481-2

- Thoracic outlet syndrome (TOS): TOS can cause neck and arm pain; exacerbated with tests for TOS and generally associated with unilateral/provoked decrease in radial pulse with provocative testing.

Clinical assessments:
- History: History is often unremarkable or may include a past history of neck injury and/or a more recent history of chronic posturing or poor ergonomics. Pain of neck tension may be better in the morning and worse in the afternoon and evening as stresses of the day accumulate. Neurologic or systemic manifestations indicate the need for more comprehensive evaluation.
- Physical examination:
  - Routine assessments: Testing of muscle strength, reflexes, and sensory function in the upper and lower extremity; perform screening orthopedic examination.
  - Range of motion: Assess cervical, scapulothoracic, glenohumeral, and thoracolumbar range of motion and posture.
  - Categorization, focus, and triage: Categorize patient into "low risk" or "high risk" and modify the level of detail in your examination and management appropriately.
  - Analyze posture and home/work ergonomics: Poor posture and static posturing are common in patients with chronic neck pain
  - Assess painful areas for active and latent trigger points: Apply digital pressure to taut muscle fibers to determine local and/or radiating pain patterns.

Imaging & laboratory assessments:
- Radiographs should be normal with the possible exception of mild degenerative changes (common in the asymptomatic general population).
- Lab tests are performed to exclude metabolic, nutritional, hormonal, and pathologic causes of musculoskeletal pain. Recommended tests include:
  - Chemistry/metabolic panel: Screen for diabetes, renal and hepatic disease, and electrolyte/mineral disturbances.
  - CBC: Exclude infection and anemia.
  - CRP or ESR: Exclude inflammatory disorders; the finding of an elevated CRP or ESR requires clinical correlation and exclusion of underlying disease.
  - 25-OH-vitamin D: Vitamin D deficiency is extremely common and is a direct cause of musculoskeletal pain. Measurement of serum 25(OH) vitamin D (or empiric treatment with 2,000 – 4,000 IU vitamin D3 per day for adults[43]) is indicated in patients with chronic musculoskeletal pain, particularly low-back pain.[44]
  - TSH and free T4: Hypothyroidism is a common cause of chronic recalcitrant musculoskeletal pain. Screen with TSH, T4, and perhaps anti-thyroid peroxidase antibodies (anti-TPO). Implement treatment for overt and so-called "subclinical" hypothyroidism as appropriate. See Chapter 4 of *Integrative Rheumatology*[45] for discussion and treatments for hypothyroidism.

Clinical management:
- Symptom management with active home care.
- Re-evaluate symptoms and neurologic exam at each visit.
- Referral to specialist with evidence of neurologic deficits, severe pain, or underlying disease.

Treatment for non-specific neck pain
"In the absence of trauma or evidence of infection, malignancy, neurologic findings, or systemic inflammation, the patient can be treated conservatively. Conservative therapy can include rest, analgesics, or physical therapy."
Tierney ML. McPhee SJ, Papadakis MA (eds). Current Medical Diagnosis and Treatment 2006, 45th Edition. Lange Medical; page 815

[43] Vasquez A, Manso G, Cannell J. The Clinical Importance of Vitamin D (Cholecalciferol): A Paradigm Shift with Implications for All Healthcare Providers. *Alternative Therapies in Health and Medicine* 2004; 10: 28-37. Also published in *Integrative Medicine: A Clinician's Journal* 2004; 3: 44-54. See www.optimalhealthresearch.com/monograph04.html

[44] Al Faraj S, Al Mutairi K. Vitamin D deficiency and chronic low back pain in Saudi Arabia. *Spine*. 2003 Jan 15;28(2):177-9

[45] Vasquez A. *Integrative Rheumatology*. Fort Worth, Texas; Integrative and Biological Medicine Research and Consulting, 2006: http://OptimalHealthResearch.com

Therapeutic considerations: *also review Chapter 3 for additional details and citations*

- Medical treatments include trigger point injection, stretching, physical therapy, massage, ergonomic and postural modifications, stress reduction, and drugs such as NSAIDs, tricyclic antidepressants, muscle relaxants, non-narcotic analgesics such as Tramodol/Ultram (weak opioid and reuptake inhibitor of serotonin and norepinephrine in the dorsal horn), and anticonvulsants.[46]

- Active care with in-office and at-home exercises, relaxation, and behavioral, psychological, and ergonomic modification.[47,48,49,50] See the website at OptimalHealthResearch.com/neck for a four-page handout of these instructions for patients.

> **"Bend Stems" mnemonic acronym: a useful reminder of components of holistic musculoskeletal care:**
> - **Botanicals**: analgesic and anti-inflammatory
> - **Exercise, ergonomics** and posture
> - **Nutritional** supplementation
> - **Diet**: anti-inflammatory, hypoallergenic, Paleo-Mediterranean
> - **Stretching, strengthening, stabilizing**: physically, emotionally, and mentally
> - **Trigger points**: doctor treats and coaches in office, patient treats daily at home
> - **Educate, Ensure return visit**: Educate about the condition and its treatments; ensure that patient is informed about duration of treatment, limitations, and importance of follow-up visits with specific time limits
> - **Manual medicine**: mobilization, manipulation, massage
> - **Spirituality**: promote emotional and mental wellness

- **Protect, and prevent re-injury: Avoid motions and activities that cause significant pain, as pain indicates that damaged/inflamed tissues are being stressed. Use bracing, taping, bandages, wrapping, canes, crutches, and walkers as needed.[51,52]**

- Relative rest: Take time away from the activities that either promote additional injury or that unnecessarily drain energies which could otherwise be used for healing and recuperation.

- Ice/heat: During the acute phase, apply ice or cold pack for 10 minutes each 30-60 minutes for reduction in pain and inflammation. During the subacute and chronic phase, apply gentle heat as needed for the relief of pain and reduction in muscle spasm and to promote healing by increasing circulation.

- Individualize treatment: The cornerstone of effective holistic and integrative treatment is to design treatment plans that simultaneously 1) address "the problem" while also 2) improving the patient's overall health.

- Compression: Snug bandages/wraps may help to reduce swelling and can provide support for injured tissues and weakened joints. Care must be utilized to avoid arterial, venous, or lymphatic obstruction.

- Educate, establish treatment program, elevation of injured limb (as applicable), exercise, ergonomic improvements: Educate patient about the need for appropriate follow-up office visits for reexamination, reassessment, and treatment. Educate patient on ways to avoid re-injury and to decrease likelihood of recurrence. Therapeutic exercise can include strength training, stretching, improving endurance, and functional training specific to the patient's occupational or athletic activities; these can be tailored to great detail to the patient's condition and goals.[53] Proprioceptive retraining/rehabilitation is especially important for the long-term functional improvement of patients with proprioceptive deficits, commonly seen in patients with chronic low-back pain[54], neck pain[55],

[46] Froese BB. Childers MK et al (eds). Cervical Myofascial Pain. Updated: January 23, 2006. *eMedicine* http://www.emedicine.com/pmr/topic26.htm Accessed December 18, 2006
[47] Taimela S, Takala EP, Asklof T, Seppala K, Parviainen S. Active treatment of chronic neck pain: a prospective randomized intervention. *Spine* 2000 Apr 15;25(8):1021-7
[48] Graff-Radford SB, Reeves JL, Jaeger B. Management of chronic head and neck pain: effectiveness of altering factors perpetuating myofascial pain. *Headache* 1987 Apr;27(4):186-90
[49] Randlov A, Ostergaard M, Manniche C, Kryger P, Jordan A, Heegaard S, Holm B. Intensive dynamic training for females with chronic neck/shoulder pain. A randomized controlled trial. *Clin Rehabil* 1998 Jun;12(3):200-10
[50] Jordan A, Bendix T, Nielsen H, Hansen FR, Host D, Winkel A. Intensive training, physiotherapy, or manipulation for patients with chronic neck pain. A prospective, single-blinded, randomized clinical trial. *Spine* 1998 Feb 1;23(3):311-8
[51] Van Hook FW, Demonbreun D, Weiss BD. Ambulatory devices for chronic gait disorders in the elderly. *Am Fam Physician*. 2003 Apr 15;67(8):1717-24 http://www.aafp.org/afp/20030415/1717.html and http://www.aafp.org/afp/20030415/1717.pdf Accessed July 23, 2006
[52] Joyce BM, Kirby RL. Canes, crutches and walkers. *Am Fam Physician*. 1991 Feb;43(2):535-42
[53] Basmajian JV (ed). Therapeutic Exercise. Fourth Edition. Baltimore: Williams and Wilkins. 1984
[54] Newcomer KL, Jacobson TD, Gabriel DA, Larson DR, Brey RH, An KN. Muscle activation patterns in subjects with and without low back pain. *Arch Phys Med Rehabil*. 2002;83(6):816-21
[55] McPartland JM, Brodeur RR, Hallgren RC. Chronic neck pain, standing balance, and suboccipital muscle atrophy--a pilot study. *J Manipulative Physiol Ther*. 1997 Jan;20(1):24-9

knee arthritis[56], and ankle instability.[57] Exercise promotes loss of superfluous body fat; thus the short-term myokine-mediated anti-inflammatory benefits of exercise[58] are extended by adipose reduction and the associated reduction in pro-inflammatory adipokines.[59,60.61] Modify home and occupational workstations to minimize strain and stress on injured tissues; educate patients to use tools, machines, props, and stepstools to work efficiently and to reduce unnecessary lifting and straining motions.

- Active patient participation is required for optimal results: Active patient participation is therapeutic and empowering and obviates the **sick role** and prevents **iatrogenic neurosis** and **therapeutic dependency**. Patients who actively participate in rehabilitative/transformative home exercises heal faster, more completely, and with greater duration of pain relief and functional restoration; this action-dependent benefit has been particularly well researched in women with chronic pain in the upper back, shoulders, and neck.[62,63,64]

- Anti-inflammatory & analgesic diet, nutrients, and botanicals:
  o Anti-inflammatory healing-supportive diet: **Pro-inflammatory foods** and food components such as arachidonic acid (high in cow's milk, beef, liver, pork, and lamb)[65,66], saturated fats[67,68], corn oil[69,70], high glycemic foods[71,72], white bread[73], high-fat high-carbohydrate fast-food breakfast[74] should be avoided generally and especially during times of musculoskeletal inflammation. The **Paleo-Mediterranean diet** is based on abundant consumption of fruits, vegetables, seeds, nuts, berries, omega-3 and monounsaturated fatty acids, and lean sources of protein such as lean meats, fatty cold-water fish, soy and whey proteins.[75,76,77,78,79] The

[56] Callaghan MJ, Selfe J, Bagley PJ, Oldham JA. The Effects of Patellar Taping on Knee Joint Proprioception. *J Athl Train*. 2002 Mar;37(1):19-24

[57] Olmsted LC, Carcia CR, Hertel J, Shultz SJ. Efficacy of the Star Excursion Balance Tests in Detecting Reach Deficits in Subjects With Chronic Ankle Instability. *J Athl Train*. 2002 Dec;37(4):501-506

[58] Petersen AM, Pedersen BK. The anti-inflammatory effect of exercise. *J Appl Physiol*. 2005 Apr;98(4):1154-62 http://jap.physiology.org/cgi/content/full/98/4/1154

[59] Monzillo LU, Hamdy O, Horton ES, Ledbury S, Mullooly C, Jarema C, Porter S, Ovalle K, Moussa A, Mantzoros CS. Effect of lifestyle modification on adipokine levels in obese subjects with insulin resistance. *Obes Res*. 2003 Sep;11(9):1048-54 http://www.obesityresearch.org/cgi/content/full/11/9/1048

[60] "Serum TNF-alpha also decreased with weight loss..." Xenachis C, Samojlik E, Raghuwanshi MP, Kirschner MA. Leptin, insulin and TNF-alpha in weight loss. *J Endocrinol Invest*. 2001 Dec;24(11):865-70

[61] "Body mass index decreased more in the intervention group than in controls (-4.2), as did serum concentrations of IL-6 (-1.1 pg/mL), IL-18 (-57 pg/mL), and CRP (-1.6), while adiponectin levels increased significantly (2.2 microg/mL)." Esposito K, Pontillo A, Di Palo C, Giugliano G, Masella M, Marfella R, Giugliano D. Effect of weight loss and lifestyle changes on vascular inflammatory markers in obese women: a randomized trial. *JAMA*. 2003 Apr 9;289(14):1799-804

[62] "Patients in both groups that completed the trial demonstrated statistically significant improvements in nearly all of the outcome measurements at completion. ... pain scores were only significantly improved in the intensive group at 12 mths follow-up." Randlov A, Ostergaard M, Manniche C, Kryger P, Jordan A, Heegaard S, Holm B. Intensive dynamic training for females with chronic neck/shoulder pain. A randomized controlled trial. *Clin Rehabil*. 1998 Jun;12(3):200-10

[63] "Stretching and fitness training are commonly advised for patients with chronic neck pain, but stretching and aerobic exercising alone proved to be a much less effective form of training than strength training. Ylinen J, Takala EP, Nykanen M, Hakkinen A, Malkia E, Pohjolainen T, Karppi SL, Kautiainen H, Airaksinen O. Active neck muscle training in the treatment of chronic neck pain in women: a randomized controlled trial. *JAMA*. 2003 May 21;289(19):2509-16

[64] "Treatment of repetitive stress injuries that combines maintenance of daily active exercises prescribed and modeled by a professional therapist, which emphasize postural awareness to correct poor posture and provide a basic physiological understanding of the disorder, is as crucial to reducing upper back and neck pain and stiffness as hands-on therapy with active exercise provided in a clinical setting." Pesco MS, Chosa E, Tajima N. Comparative study of hands-on therapy with active exercises vs education with active exercises for the management of upper back pain. *J Manipulative Physiol Ther*. 2006 Mar-Apr;29(3):228-35

[65] Vasquez A. Reducing Pain and Inflammation Naturally. Part 2: New Insights into Fatty Acid Supplementation and Its Effect on Eicosanoid Production and Genetic Expression. *Nutritional Perspectives* 2005; January: 5-16 www.optimalhealthresearch.com/part2

[66] Evans AR, Junger H, Southall MD, Nicol GD, Sorkin LS, Broome JT, Bailey TW, Vasko MR. Isoprostanes, novel eicosanoids that produce nociception and sensitize rat sensory neurons. *J Pharmacol Exp Ther*. 2000 Jun;293(3):912-20

[67] Lee JY, Sohn KH, Rhee SH, Hwang D. Saturated fatty acids, but not unsaturated fatty acids, induce the expression of cyclooxygenase-2 mediated through Toll-like receptor 4. *J Biol Chem*. 2001 May 18;276(20):16683-9. Epub 2001 Mar 2 http://www.jbc.org/cgi/content/full/276/20/16683

[68] "CONCLUSIONS: Both fat and protein intakes stimulate ROS generation. The increase in ROS generation lasted 3 h after cream intake and 1 h after protein intake. Cream intake also caused a significant and prolonged increase in lipid peroxidation." Mohanty P, Ghanim H, Hamouda W, Aljada A, Garg R, Dandona P. Both lipid and protein intakes stimulate increased generation of reactive oxygen species by polymorphonuclear leukocytes and mononuclear cells. *Am J Clin Nutr*. 2002 Apr;75(4):767-72 http://www.ajcn.org/cgi/content/full/75/4/767

[69] Rusyn I, Bradham CA, Cohn L, Schoonhoven R, Swenberg JA, Brenner DA, Thurman RG. Corn oil rapidly activates nuclear factor-kappaB in hepatic Kupffer cells by oxidant-dependent mechanisms. *Carcinogenesis*. 1999 Nov;20(11):2095-100 http://carcin.oxfordjournals.org/cgi/content/full/20/11/2095

[70] "Exposing endothelial cells to 90 micromol linoleic acid/L for 6 h resulted in a significant increase in lipid hydroperoxides that coincided wih an increase in intracellular calcium concentrations." Hennig B, Toborek M, Joshi-Barve S, Barger SW, Barve S, Mattson MP, McClain CJ. Linoleic acid activates nuclear transcription factor-kappa B (NF-kappa B) and induces NF-kappa B-dependent transcription in cultured endothelial cells. *Am J Clin Nutr*. 1996 Mar;63(3):322-8 http://www.ajcn.org/cgi/reprint/63/3/322

[71] Mohanty P, Hamouda W, Garg R, Aljada A, Ghanim H, Dandona P. Glucose challenge stimulates reactive oxygen species (ROS) generation by leucocytes. *J Clin Endocrinol Metab*. 2000 Aug;85(8):2970-3 http://jcem.endojournals.org/cgi/content/full/85/8/2970 Glucose/carbohydrate and saturated fat consumption appear to be the two biggest offenders in the food-stimulated production of oxidative stress. The effect by protein is much less. "CONCLUSIONS: Both fat and protein intakes stimulate ROS generation. The increase in ROS generation lasted 3 h after cream intake and 1 h after protein intake. Cream intake also caused a significant and prolonged increase in lipid peroxidation." Mohanty P, Ghanim H, Hamouda W, Aljada A, Garg R, Dandona P. Both lipid and protein intakes stimulate increased generation of reactive oxygen species by polymorphonuclear leukocytes and mononuclear cells. *Am J Clin Nutr*. 2002 Apr;75(4):767-72 http://www.ajcn.org/cgi/content/full/75/4/767

[72] Koska J, Blazicek P, Marko M, Grna JD, Kvetnansky R, Vigas M. Insulin, catecholamines, glucose and antioxidant enzymes in oxidative damage during different loads in healthy humans. *Physiol Res*. 2000;49 Suppl 1:S95-100 http://www.biomed.cas.cz/physiolres/pdf/2000/49_S95.pdf

[73] "Conclusion - The present study shows that high GI carbohydrate, but not low GI carbohydrate, mediates an acute proinflammatory process as measured by NF-kappaB activity." Dickinson S, Hancock DP, Petocz P, Brand-Miller JC..High glycemic index carbohydrate mediates an acute proinflammatory process as measured by NF-kappaB activation. *Asia Pac J Clin Nutr*. 2005;14 Suppl:S120

[74] Aljada A, Mohanty P, Ghanim H, Abdo T, Tripathy D, Chaudhuri A, Dandona P. Increase in intranuclear nuclear factor kappaB and decrease in inhibitor kappaB in mononuclear cells after a mixed meal: evidence for a proinflammatory effect. *Am J Clin Nutr*. 2004 Apr;79(4):682-90 http://www.ajcn.org/cgi/content/full/79/4/682

[75] Eaton SB, Shostak M, Konner M. The Paleolithic Prescription: A program of diet & exercise and a design for living, New York: Harper & Row, 1988

American/Western style of eating results in subclinical pathogenic chronic diet-induced metabolic acidosis[80,81] which can be corrected with a Paleo-Mediterranean diet[82,] or alkalinizing supplements[83] for the alleviation of musculoskeletal pain in general and low-back pain in particular.[84] Ensure adequate fluid intake; teas—especially green teas—provide anti-inflammatory and antioxidant benefits that are clinically significant. Adequate/increased protein intake expedites recovery following injury and shows numerous other benefits[85,86]; in otherwise healthy patients with no liver, renal, or other metabolic disorders, ensure adequate intake of 0.5-0.9 gram of protein per pound of body weight.[87] Physiologically, the body's limit for handling nitrogenous groups from dietary protein is reached when protein intake is greater than 200-300 grams/d; as long as protein intake is kept below this level or below 30-40% of daily calories and/or combined with a *whole foods* fruit- and vegetable-rich diet, patients and doctors need not worry about the familiar myth of "too much protein."[88]

Recommended <u>Grams of Protein</u> Per <u>Pound of Body Weight</u> Per Day[89]	
Infants and children ages 1-6 years[90]	0.68-0.45
RDA for sedentary adult and children ages 6-18 years[91]	0.4
Adult recreational exerciser	0.5-0.75
Adult competitive athlete	0.6-0.9
Adult building muscle mass	0.7-0.9
Dieting athlete	0.7-1.0
Growing teenage athlete	0.9-1.0
Pregnant women need additional protein	Add 15-30 grams/day[92]

    o <u>Fatty acid supplementation for eicosanoid and genomic modulation</u>: Combination therapy with EPA-DHA (fish oil) and GLA (borage oil) is preferred for optimal results.[93]

---

[76] O'Keefe JH Jr, Cordain L. Cardiovascular disease resulting from a diet and lifestyle at odds with our Paleolithic genome: how to become a 21st-century hunter-gatherer. *Mayo Clin Proc*. 2004 Jan;79(1):101-8

[77] Cordain L. <u>The Paleo Diet: Lose Weight and Get Healthy by Eating the Food You Were Designed to Eat</u>. Indianapolis; John Wiley and Sons, 2002

[78] Vasquez A. A Five-Part Nutritional Protocol that Produces Consistently Positive Results. *Nutritional Wellness* 2005 September Available in the printed version and on-line at http://www.nutritionalwellness.com/archives/2005/sep/09_vasquez.php and http://optimalhealthresearch.com/protocol

[79] Vasquez A. Implementing the Five-Part Nutritional Wellness Protocol for the Treatment of Various Health Problems. *Nutritional Wellness* 2005 November. Available on-line at http://www.nutritionalwellness.com/archives/2005/nov/11_vasquez.php and http://optimalhealthresearch.com/protocol

[80] "As a result, healthy adults consuming the standard US diet sustain a chronic, low-grade pathogenic metabolic acidosis that worsens with age as kidney function declines." Cordain L, Eaton SB, Sebastian A, Mann N, Lindeberg S, Watkins BA, O'Keefe JH, Brand-Miller J. Origins and evolution of the Western diet: health implications for the 21st century. *Am J Clin Nutr*. 2005 Feb;81(2):341-54 http://www.ajcn.org/cgi/content/full/81/2/341

[81] "An acidogenic Western diet results in mild metabolic acidosis in association with a state of cortisol excess, altered divalent ion metabolism, and increased bone resorptive indices." Maurer M, Riesen W, Muser J, Hulter HN, Krapf R. Neutralization of Western diet inhibits bone resorption independently of K intake and reduces cortisol secretion in humans. *Am J Physiol Renal Physiol*. 2003 Jan;284(1):F32-40. Epub 2002 Sep 24. http://ajprenal.physiology.org/cgi/content/full/284/1/F32

[82] Cordain L. <u>The Paleo Diet: Lose Weight and Get Healthy by Eating the Food You Were Designed to Eat</u>. Indianapolis; John Wiley and Sons, 2002

[83] For long-term out-patient treatment of patients who do not achieve alkalinization with diet alone, oral administration of potassium citrate and/or sodium bicarbonate can be implemented. See the following article for concepts: "Urine alkalinization is a treatment regimen that increases poison elimination by the administration of intravenous sodium bicarbonate to produce urine with a pH > or = 7.5." Proudfoot AT, Krenzelok EP, Vale JA. Position Paper on urine alkalinization. *J Toxicol Clin Toxicol*. 2004;42:1-26 http://www.eapcct.org/publicfile.php?folder=congress&file=PS_UrineAlkalinization.pdf Also see: Vormann J, Worlitschek M, Goedecke T, Silver B. Supplementation with alkaline minerals reduces symptoms in patients with chronic low back pain. *J Trace Elem Med Biol*. 2001;15(2-3):179-83 Also see: Maurer M, Riesen W, Muser J, Hulter HN, Krapf R. Neutralization of Western diet inhibits bone resorption independently of K intake and reduces cortisol secretion in humans. *Am J Physiol Renal Physiol*. 2003 Jan;284(1):F32-40. Epub 2002 Sep 24. http://ajprenal.physiology.org/cgi/content/full/284/1/F32

[84] "The results show that a disturbed acid-base balance may contribute to the symptoms of low back pain. The simple and safe addition of an alkaline multimineral preparate was able to reduce the pain symptoms in these patients with chronic low back pain." Vormann J, Worlitschek M, Goedecke T, Silver B. Supplementation with alkaline minerals reduces symptoms in patients with chronic low back pain. *J Trace Elem Med Biol*. 2001;15(2-3):179-83

[85] Vegetarians and healing. *JAMA* 1995; 273: 910

[86] Castaneda C, Charnley JM, Evans WJ, Crim MC. Elderly women accommodate to a low-protein diet with losses of body cell mass, muscle function, and immune response. *Am J Clin Nutr* 1995 Jul;62(1):30-9

[87] Nancy Clark, MS, RD. The Power of Protein. *The Physician and Sportsmedicine* 1996, volume 24, number 4. http://www.physsportsmed.com/issues/1996/04_96/protein.htm

[88] "I can assure you that as long as you eat plenty of fresh fruits and vegetables, there is no such thing as too much protein." (page 41). Cordain L. <u>The Paleo Diet: Lose Weight and Get Healthy by Eating the Food You Were Designed to Eat</u>. Indianapolis; John Wiley and Sons: 2002, pages 41, 67, 101

[89] Slightly modified from Nancy Clark, MS, RD. The Power of Protein. *The Physician and Sportsmedicine* 1996, volume 24, number 4

[90] 1.5-1 g/kg/d (0.68-0.45 grams per pound of body weight. Younger people need proportionately more protein.) Brown ML (ed). <u>Present Knowledge in Nutrition. Sixth Edition</u>. Washington DC: International Life Sciences Institute Nutrition Foundation; 1990 page 68

[91] 0.83 g.kg-1.d-1 (equivalent to 0.37 grams per pound of body weight) "By use of an age-specific scoring system and the mean amino acid composition and digestibility of the US diet, this allowance became 0.83 g.kg-1.d-1 of mixed US dietary protein--a value similar to the previous RDA but derived in a different manner." Pellet PL. Protein requirements in humans. *Am J Clin Nutr*. 1990 May;51(5):723-37

[92] Weinsier RL, Morgan SL (eds). <u>Fundamentals of Clinical Nutrition</u>. St. Louis: Mosby, 1993 page 50

[93] Vasquez A. Reducing Pain and Inflammation Naturally. Part 2: New Insights into Fatty Acid Supplementation and Its Effect on Eicosanoid Production and Genetic Expression. *Nutritional Perspectives* 2005; January: 5-16 www.optimalhealthresearch.com/part2

- **Fish oil, EPA with DHA**: Up to three grams per day (3,000 mg/d) of combined EPA and DHA is a reasonable therapeutic dose.[94,95,96,97]
- **GLA, Gamma-linolenic acid**: Approximately 500 mg per day is the common anti-inflammatory dose[98] although higher doses of 2.8 grams per day have been safely used in patients with rheumatoid arthritis.[99]

o Botanical medicines: Tailor the selection, dose, and combinations to the patient's size, age, and other clinical characteristics.

- *Uncaria guianensis* and *Uncaria tomentosa* ("cat's claw", "una de gato")**: Analgesic and anti-inflammatory benefits have been shown in osteoarthritis[100] and rheumatoid arthritis.[101]
- *Boswellia serrata*: Boswellia inhibits 5-lipoxygenase[102] with no apparent effect on cyclooxygenase[103] and has been shown effective in the treatment of osteoarthritis of the knees[104] as well as asthma[105] and ulcerative colitis.[106] When used as monotherapy, the target dose is approximately 150 mg of boswellic acids TID (thrice daily).
- *Zingiber officinale* (Ginger)**: Ginger is a well known spice and food with a long history of use as an anti-inflammatory, anti-nausea, and gastroprotective agent[107], and components of ginger have been shown to reduce production of the leukotriene LTB4 by inhibiting 5-lipoxygenase and to reduce production of the prostaglandin PGE2 by inhibiting cyclooxygenase.[108,109] Ginger has been shown to safely reduce nonspecific musculoskeletal pain[110,111] and to provide relief from osteoarthritis of the knees[112], migraine headaches,[113] and nausea/vomiting of pregnancy.[114]
- *Harpagophytum procumbens* (Devil's claw)**: The safety and analgesic effectiveness of Harpagophytum has been established in patients with hip pain, low-back pain, and knee pain.[115,116,117,118,119,120,121]

[94] "…clinical benefits of the n-3 fatty acids were not apparent until they were consumed for > or =12 wk. It appears that a minimum daily dose of 3 g eicosapentaenoic and docosahexaenoic acids is necessary to derive the expected benefits [in patients with rheumatoid arthritis]." Kremer JM. n-3 fatty acid supplements in rheumatoid arthritis. *Am J Clin Nutr*.2000;71(1Suppl):349S-51S

[95] Rubin D, Laposata M. Cellular interactions between n-6 and n-3 fatty acids: a mass analysis of fatty acid elongation/desaturation, distribution among complex lipids, and conversion to eicosanoids. *J Lipid Res*. 1992 Oct;33(10):1431-40.

[96] "The recent GISSI (Gruppo Italiano per lo Studio della Sopravvivenza nell'Infarto miocardico)-Prevention study of 11,324 patients showed a 45% decrease in risk of sudden cardiac death and a 20% reduction in all-cause mortality in the group taking 850 mg/d of omega-3 fatty acids. These fatty acids have potent anti-inflammatory effects and may also be antiatherogenic." O'Keefe JH Jr, Harris WS. From Inuit to implementation: omega-3 fatty acids come of age. *Mayo Clin Proc*. 2000 Jun;75(6):607-14

[97] "Many of the placebo-controlled trials of fish oil in chronic inflammatory diseases reveal significant benefit, including decreased disease activity and a lowered use of anti-inflammatory drugs." Simopoulos AP. Omega-3 fatty acids in inflammation and autoimmune diseases. *J Am Coll Nutr*. 2002 Dec;21(6):495-505

[98] "Forty patients with rheumatoid arthritis and upper gastrointestinal lesions due to non-steroidal anti-inflammatory drugs entered a prospective 6-month double-blind placebo controlled study of dietary supplementation with gamma-linolenic acid 540 mg/day…" Brzeski M, Madhok R, Capell HA. Evening primrose oil in patients with rheumatoid arthritis and side-effects of non-steroidal anti-inflammatory drugs. *Br J Rheumatol*. 1991 Oct;30(5):370-2

[99] Zurier RB, Rossetti RG, Jacobson EW, DeMarco DM, Liu NY, Temming JE, White BM, Laposata M. gamma-Linolenic acid treatment of rheumatoid arthritis. A randomized, placebo-controlled trial. *Arthritis Rheum*. 1996 Nov;39(11):1808-17

[100] Piscoya J, Rodriguez Z, Bustamante SA, Okuhama NN, Miller MJ, Sandoval M. Efficacy and safety of freeze-dried cat's claw in osteoarthritis of the knee: mechanisms of action of the species Uncaria guianensis. *Inflamm Res*. 2001 Sep;50(9):442-8

[101] "This small preliminary study demonstrates relative safety and modest benefit to the tender joint count of a highly purified extract from the pentacyclic chemotype of UT in patients with active RA taking sulfasalazine or hydroxychloroquine." Mur E, Hartig F, Eibl G, Schirmer M. Randomized double blind trial of an extract from the pentacyclic alkaloid-chemotype of uncaria tomentosa for the treatment of rheumatoid arthritis. *J Rheumatol*. 2002 Apr;29(4):678-81

[102] Wildfeuer A, Neu IS, Safayhi H, Metzger G, Wehrmann M, Vogel U, Ammon HP. Effects of boswellic acids extracted from a herbal medicine on the biosynthesis of leukotrienes and the course of experimental autoimmune encephalomyelitis. *Arzneimittelforschung* 1998 Jun;48(6):668-74

[103] Safayhi H, Mack T, Sabieraj J, Anazodo MI, Subramanian LR, Ammon HP. Boswellic acids: novel, specific, nonredox inhibitors of 5-lipoxygenase. *J Pharmacol Exp Ther* 1992 Jun;261(3):1143-6

[104] Kimmatkar N, Thawani V, Hingorani L, Khiyani R. Efficacy and tolerability of Boswellia serrata extract in treatment of osteoarthritis of knee--a randomized double blind placebo controlled trial. *Phytomedicine*. 2003 Jan;10(1):3-7

[105] Gupta I, Gupta V, Parihar A, Gupta S, Ludtke R, Safayhi H, Ammon HP. Effects of Boswellia serrata gum resin in patients with bronchial asthma: results of a double-blind, placebo-controlled, 6-week clinical study. *Eur J Med Res*. 1998 Nov 17;3(11):511-4

[106] Gupta I, Parihar A, Malhotra P, Singh GB, Ludtke R, Safayhi H, Ammon HP. Effects of Boswellia serrata gum resin in patients with ulcerative colitis. *Eur J Med Res*. 1997 Jan;2(1):37-43

[107] Langner E, Greifenberg S, Gruenwald J. Ginger: history and use. *Adv Ther* 1998 Jan-Feb;15(1):25-44

[108] Kiuchi F, Iwakami S, Shibuya M, Hanaoka F, Sankawa U. Inhibition of prostaglandin and leukotriene biosynthesis by gingerols and diarylheptanoids. *Chem Pharm Bull* (Tokyo) 1992 Feb;40(2):387-91

[109] Tjendraputra E, Tran VH, Liu-Brennan D, Roufogalis BD, Duke CC. Effect of ginger constituents and synthetic analogues on cyclooxygenase-2 enzyme in intact cells. *Bioorg Chem* 2001 Jun;29(3):156-63

[110] Srivastava KC, Mustafa T. Ginger (Zingiber officinale) in rheumatism and musculoskeletal disorders. *Med Hypotheses*. 1992 Dec;39(4):342-8

[111] Srivastava KC, Mustafa T. Ginger (Zingiber officinale) and rheumatic disorders. *Med Hypotheses*. 1989 May;29(1):25-8

[112] Altman RD, Marcussen KC. Effects of a ginger extract on knee pain in patients with osteoarthritis. *Arthritis Rheum*. 2001 Nov;44(11):2531-8

[113] Mustafa T, Srivastava KC. Ginger (Zingiber officinale) in migraine headache. *J Ethnopharmacol*. 1990 Jul;29(3):267-73

[114] "…oral ginger 1 g per day… No adverse effect of ginger on pregnancy outcome was detected." Vutyavanich T, Kraisarin T, Ruangsri R. Ginger for nausea and vomiting in pregnancy: randomized, double-masked, placebo-controlled trial. *Obstet Gynecol* 2001 Apr;97(4):577-82.

[115] Chantre P, Cappelaere A, Leblan D, Guedon D, Vandermander J, Fournie B. Efficacy and tolerance of Harpagophytum procumbens versus diacerhein in treatment of osteoarthritis. *Phytomedicine* 2000 Jun;7(3):177-83

[116] Leblan D, Chantre P, Fournie B. Harpagophytum procumbens in the treatment of knee and hip osteoarthritis. Four-month results of a prospective, multicenter, double-blind trial versus diacerhein. *Joint Bone Spine* 2000;67(5):462-7

[117] Whitehouse LW, Znamirowska M, Paul CJ. Devil's Claw (Harpagophytum procumbens): no evidence for anti-inflammatory activity in the treatment of arthritic disease. *Can Med Assoc J* 1983 Aug 1;129(3):249-51

[118] Moussard C, Alber D, Toubin MM, Thevenon N, Henry JC. A drug used in traditional medicine, harpagophytum procumbens: no evidence for NSAID-like effect on whole blood eicosanoid production in human. *Prostaglandins Leukot Essent Fatty Acids* 1992 Aug;46(4):283-6

- Willow bark (*Salix* spp): Numerous studies—especially among patients with low-back pain—have validated the analgesic and anti-inflammatory benefits of willow bark extract.[122,123,124] Contraindications to the use of willow include aspirin/salicylate allergy and perhaps pregnancy, use of anticoagulant medication, or impending surgery.[125,126] The daily dose is generally kept below 240 mg of salicin, and products should include other components of the whole plant.

- Topical application of *Capsicum annuum, Capsicum frutescens* (Cayenne pepper, hot chili pepper): Controlled clinical trials have conclusively demonstrated capsaicin's ability to deplete sensory fibers of substance P to thus reduce pain in diabetic neuropathy[127], chronic low back pain[128], **chronic neck pain**[129], osteoarthritis[130], rheumatoid arthritis[131], notalgia paresthetica[132], reflex sympathetic dystrophy[133], and cluster headache (intranasal application).[134,135,136]

  o Anti-inflammation versus hemostasis: Anti-inflammatory/analgesic medications that impair coagulation (e.g., aspirin) are contraindicated in patients with possible internal bleeding such as severe hematoma, hemarthrosis, spleen injury, intracranial hemorrhage (i.e., subdural hematoma following a whiplash injury) and in patients about to undergo surgery. Caution should be used with nutritional/botanical supplements that have anti-coagulant effects, such as ginkgo biloba[137] and garlic.[138]

- Treat with physical/manual medicine, massage, mobilization, and manipulation: Gentle massage provides comfort, increases circulation, reduces edema, and promotes healing. After the acute phase, deeper massage may help restore range of motion by breaking adhesions and reducing the feeling of vulnerability that may occur after injury. Joint mobilization and manipulation can be used as appropriate (after contraindications have been excluded) and to the level of patient comfort; mechanisms are listed below and citations were provided previously in Chapter 3. Treat MFTP with

---

[119] Chrubasik S, Model A, Black A, Pollak S. A randomized double-blind pilot study comparing Doloteffin and Vioxx in the treatment of low back pain. *Rheumatology* (Oxford). 2003 Jan;42(1):141-8

[120] "The majority of responders' were patients who had suffered less than 42 days of pain, and subgroup analyses suggested that the effect was confined to patients with more severe and radiating pain accompanied by neurological deficit… There was no evidence for Harpagophytum-related side-effects, except possibly for mild and infrequent gastrointestinal symptoms." Chrubasik S, Junck H, Breitschwerdt H, Conradt C, Zappe H. Effectiveness of Harpagophytum extract WS 1531 in the treatment of exacerbation of low back pain: a randomized, placebo-controlled, double-blind study. *Eur J Anaesthesiol* 1999 Feb;16(2):118-29

[121] "They took an 8-week course of Doloteffin at a dose providing 60 mg harpagoside per day… Doloteffin is well worth considering for osteoarthritic knee and hip pain and nonspecific low back pain." Chrubasik S, Thanner J, Kunzel O, Conradt C, Black A, Pollak S. Comparison of outcome measures during treatment with the proprietary Harpagophytum extract doloteffin in patients with pain in the lower back, knee or hip. *Phytomedicine* 2002 Apr;9(3):181-94

[122] Chrubasik S, Eisenberg E, Balan E, Weinberger T, Luzzati R, Conradt C. Treatment of low-back pain exacerbations with willow bark extract: a randomized double-blind study. *Am J Med*. 2000;109:9-14

[123] Chrubasik S, Kunzel O, Model A, Conradt C, Black A. Treatment of low-back pain with a herbal or synthetic anti-rheumatic: a randomized controlled study. Willow bark extract for low-back pain. *Rheumatology* (Oxford). 2001;40:1388-93

[124] Hare LG, Woodside JV, Young IS. Dietary salicylates. *J Clin Pathol* 2003 Sep;56(9):649-50 http://jcp.bmj.com/cgi/content/full/56/9/649

[125] **Vasquez A, Muanza DN. Evaluation of Presence of Aspirin-Related Warnings with Willow Bark: Comment on the Article by Clauson et al. *Ann Pharmacotherapy* 2005 Oct;39:1763**

[126] Clauson KA, Santamarina ML, Buettner CM, Cauffield JS. Evaluation of Presence of Aspirin-Related Warnings with Willow Bark (July/August). *Ann Pharmacother* 2005;39(7-8):1234-7

[127] "Study results suggest that topical capsaicin cream is safe and effective in treating painful diabetic neuropathy. "[No authors listed] Treatment of painful diabetic neuropathy with topical capsaicin. A multicenter, double-blind, vehicle-controlled study. The Capsaicin Study Group. *Arch Intern Med*. 1991 Nov;151(11):2225-9

[128] Keitel W, Frerick H, Kuhn U, Schmidt U, Kuhlmann M, Bredehorst A. Capsicum pain plaster in chronic non-specific low back pain. *Arzneimittelforschung*. 2001 Nov;51(11):896-903

[129] Mathias BJ, Dillingham TR, Zeigler DN, Chang AS, Belandres PV. Topical capsaicin for chronic neck pain. A pilot study. *Am J Phys Med Rehabil* 1995 Jan-Feb;74(1):39-44

[130] McCarthy GM, McCarty DJ. Effect of topical capsaicin in the therapy of painful osteoarthritis of the hands. *J Rheumatol*. 1992;19(4):604-7

[131] Deal CL, Schnitzer TJ, Lipstein E, et al. Treatment of arthritis with topical capsaicin: a double-blind trial. *Clin Ther*. 1991 May-Jun;13(3):383-95

[132] Leibsohn E. Treatment of notalgia paresthetica with capsaicin. *Cutis* 1992 May;49(5):335-6

[133] "Capsaicin is effective for psoriasis, pruritus, and cluster headache; it is often helpful for the itching and pain of postmastectomy pain syndrome, oral mucositis, cutaneous allergy, loin pain/hematuria syndrome, neck pain, amputation stump pain, and skin tumor; and it may be beneficial for neural dysfunction (detrusor hyperreflexia, reflex sympathetic dystrophy, and rhinopathy)." Hautkappe M, Roizen MF, Toledano A, Roth S, Jeffries JA, Ostermeier AM. Review of the effectiveness of capsaicin for painful cutaneous disorders and neural dysfunction. *Clin J Pain* 1998 Jun;14(2):97-106

[134] "Capsaicin application to human nasal mucosa was found to induce painful sensation, sneezing, and nasal secretion. All of these factors exhibit desensitization upon repeated applications." Sicuteri F, Fusco BM, Marabini S, Campagnolo V, Maggi CA, Geppetti P, Fanciullacci M. Beneficial effect of capsaicin application to the nasal mucosa in cluster headache. *Clin J Pain*. 1989;5(1):49-53

[135] "The efficacy of repeated nasal applications of capsaicin in cluster headache is congruent with previous reports on the therapeutic effect of capsaicin in other pain syndromes (post-herpetic neuralgia, diabetic neuropathy, trigeminal neuralgia) and supports the use of the drug to produce a selective analgesia." Fusco BM, Marabini S, Maggi CA, Fiore G, Geppetti P. Preventative effect of repeated nasal applications of capsaicin in cluster headache. *Pain*. 1994 Dec;59(3):321-5

[136] "These results indicate that intranasal capsaicin may provide a new therapeutic option for the treatment of this disease." Marks DR, Rapoport A, Padla D, Weeks R, Rosum R, Sheftell F, Arrowsmith F. A double-blind placebo-controlled trial of intranasal capsaicin for cluster headache. *Cephalalgia*. 1993 Apr;13(2):114-6

[137] "A structured assessment of published case reports suggests a possible causal association between using ginkgo and bleeding events… Patients using ginkgo, particularly those with known bleeding risks, should be counseled about a possible increase in bleeding risk." Bent S, Goldberg H, Padula A, Avins AL. Spontaneous bleeding associated with ginkgo biloba: a case report and systematic review of the literature: a case report and systematic review of the literature. *J Gen Intern Med*. 2005 Jul;20(7):657-61 http://www.pubmedcentral.gov/picrender.fcgi?artid=1490168&blobtype=pdf

[138] "The authors report a case of spontaneous spinal epidural hematoma causing paraplegia secondary to a qualitative platelet disorder from excessive garlic ingestion." Rose KD, Croissant PD, Parliament CF, Levin MB. Spontaneous spinal epidural hematoma with associated platelet dysfunction from excessive garlic ingestion: a case report. *Neurosurgery*. 1990 May;26(5):880-2

post-isometric stretching and nutrition as reviewed in Chapter 3. Consider physiotherapy, as appropriate.[139] Mechanisms of manipulative therapy:

- o Releasing entrapped intraarticular menisci and synovial folds,
- o Acutely reducing intradiscal pressure, thus promoting replacement of decentralized disc material,
- o Stretching of deep periarticular muscles to break the cycle of chronic autonomous muscle contraction by lengthening the muscles and thereby releasing excessive actin-myosin binding,
- o Promoting restoration of proper kinesthesia and proprioception,
- o Promoting relaxation of paraspinal muscles by stretching facet joint capsules,
- o Promoting relaxation of paraspinal muscles via "postactivation depression", which is the temporary depletion of contractile neurotransmitters,
- o Temporarily elevating plasma beta-endorphin,
- o Temporarily enhancing phagocytic ability of neutrophils and monocytes,
- o Activating the diffuse descending pain inhibitory system located in the periaqueductal gray matter—this is an important aspect of nociceptive inhibition by intense sensory/mechanoreceptor stimulation, and
- o Improving neurotransmitter balance and reducing pain (soft-tissue manipulation).
- o <u>Manual/in-office therapy for myofascial trigger points (MFTP)</u>:
    - ▪ <u>Post-isometric stretching</u>: 1) stretch the target muscle, 2) weakly contract the target muscle against resistance for 10 seconds, 3) stretch the target muscle to a greater length than before for at least 20 seconds, 4) repeat this procedure 2-3 times.[140] Prewarm muscles with exercise, heating pad, or hot shower; follow treatment with cold to reduce stretch-induced inflammation (if any).
    - ▪ <u>Cold and stretch</u>: The application of cold and the simultaneous stretching of the muscle is an effective treatment for MFTP.[141] Cold can be applied with ice. The previously popular "spray and stretch" technique that used a vapocoolant spray such as Fluori-Methane is unnecessary and is environmentally irresponsible.
    - ▪ <u>Topical application</u>: Topical capsaicin alleviates neuromuscular pain, too, and may aid in the treatment of MFTP.
    - ▪ <u>Dry needling or injection of local anesthetic or saline</u>: Dry needling (rapid insertion and withdrawal of a needle) directly into the MFTP is an effective treatment for MFTP. [142]

- <u>Uncover the underlying problem and contributing factors</u>: Congenital anomalies, underlying pathology, previous injury, and psychoemotional disorders may have been present before the "injury."[143] Look for leg length inequalities and biomechanical faults such as hyperpronation and pelvic torque. Assess and correct poor posture, poor ergonomics, lack of flexibility, muscle strength imbalances, and proprioceptive/coordination deficits. Patients may experience a reduction in pain—particularly low-back pain and osteoarthritis pain—when they eliminate coffee/caffeine, food allergens, and/or specific foods to which they are sensitive, most notably the Solanaceae/nightshade family—eggplant, tobacco, tomatoes, potatoes, and bell peppers. Correction of diet-induced chronic metabolic acidosis with the use of alkalinizing diets/supplements can alleviate musculoskeletal pain.[144]
- <u>Rehabilitate, resourcefulness, return to active life, reassure, referral</u>:
    - o <u>Rehabilitation</u>: Pre-rehabilitation assessment has three main goals: 1) identification of the type of injury, 2) quantification of the severity of the injury, and 3) determining the appropriate interventions.[145] **Rehabilitative exercises** emphasizing strength, coordination, proprioception, range of motion, and functional utility (appropriate per occupation and hobbies) should be

[139] Download the free notes at http://www.OptimalHealthResearch.com/physiotherapy
[140] Lewit K, Simons DG. Myofascial pain: relief by post-isometric relaxation. *Arch Phys Med Rehabil.* 1984 Aug;65(8):452-6
[141] Rubin D. Myofascial trigger point syndromes: an approach to management. *Arch Phys Med Rehabil.* 1981 Mar;62(3):107-10
[142] Hong CZ, Simons DG. Pathophysiologic and electrophysiologic mechanisms of myofascial trigger points. *Arch Phys Med Rehabil.* 1998 Jul;79(7):863-72
[143] Seifert S. Medical Illness Simulating Trauma (MIST) syndrome: case reports and discussion of syndrome. *Fam Med* 1993 Apr;25(4):273-6
[144] "The results show that a disturbed acid-base balance may contribute to the symptoms of low back pain. The simple and safe addition of an alkaline multimineral preparate was able to reduce the pain symptoms in these patients with chronic low back pain." Vormann J, Worlitschek M, Goedecke T, Silver B. Supplementation with alkaline minerals reduces symptoms in patients with chronic low back pain. *J Trace Elem Med Biol.* 2001;15(2-3):179-83
[145] Geffen SJ. 3: Rehabilitation principles for treating chronic musculoskeletal injuries. *Med J Aust.* 2003 Mar 3;178(5):238-42

employed. Isometric exercises can be used to maintain/increase muscle strength in patients for whom range-of-motion exercises are painful or contraindicated.

o <u>Rehabilitation for alleviation of pain and promotion of optimal function</u>: Local rehabilitation of the cervical spine should generally include ❶ **correction of faulty movement patterns** by addressing each of the three major components: 1) initial posture, 2) quality of somatosensory input, and 3) CNS motor programs, ❷ **promotion of spinal stability** by addressing both the *active* and the *passive* components, ❸ **proprioceptive/sensorimotor training** targeting the neck, torso, lumbar spine, pelvis, and lower extremity, ❹ **strengthening exercises** for the neck, shoulders, back, and legs, and ❺ **myofascial and spinal manipulative therapy** to alleviate pain, facilitate and effect proprioceptive/sensorimotor restoration, and promote optimal joint biomechanics. A very comprehensive and dense review of this topic was published by Murphy in 2000, and this article is highly recommended for all practitioners.[146]

o <u>Rehabilitation for lifestyle transformation</u>: Rehabilitation can become more than restorative; if the plan is comprehensive and it effects long-term improvements in overall health, then such a program can become transformative. The plan must be comprehensive and require active participation of the patient in order to attain optimal *short-term effectiveness* and *long-term sustainable success*.

o <u>Reassurance and resourcefulness</u>: Education, explanation, reassurance, and support help to address the mental and emotional aspects of injury. Books, websites, and national/local support groups and organizations may be available for emotional, physical, psychological-emotional, and legal assistance.

o **<u>Referral</u>: Patients with severe pain, serious complications, or documented noncompliance are excellent candidates for medical co-management or unidirectional referral.**

o <u>Proprioceptive Rehabilitation</u>: Proprioceptive deficits are common in patients with chronic low-back pain[147], neck pain[148], knee pain and arthritis[149], and ankle instability.[150] Means of challenging and thus developing neuromuscular coordination include use of vigorous full-body exercise, wobble board, balance shoes, foam, exercise ball, or other labile support surface.[151,152,153,154,155] Spinal manipulation appears to improve proprioceptive function.[156]

- <u>Nutritional supplementation</u>: Upon the foundation of a health-promoting healing-supportive anti-inflammatory diet such as the Paleo-Mediterranean diet, a patient-tailored program of nutritional supplementation can be built to expedite restoration/optimization of tissue structure and function. Since vitamin deficiencies are common and because multivitamin/multimineral supplementation generally has a very high benefit:risk ratio, essentially all adults should take a multivitamin/multimineral supplement[157], upon which additional problem-specific nutritional supplementation can be added. Supplementation can be tailored to the type of tissue that has been injured, such as calcium, magnesium, and vitamins D and K for bone fractures, glucosamine sulfate and niacinamide for cartilage injuries, and proteolytic enzymes for muscle strains.

---

[146] Murphy DR. Chiropractic rehabilitation of the cervical spine. *J Manipulative Physiol Ther.* 2000 Jul-Aug;23(6):404-8

[147] Newcomer KL, Jacobson TD, Gabriel DA, Larson DR, Brey RH, An KN. Muscle activation patterns in subjects with and without low back pain. *Arch Phys Med Rehabil.* 2002;83(6):816-21

[148] McPartland JM, Brodeur RR, Hallgren RC. Chronic neck pain, standing balance, and suboccipital muscle atrophy--a pilot study. *J Manipulative Physiol Ther.* 1997 Jan;20(1):24-9

[149] Callaghan MJ, Selfe J, Bagley PJ, Oldham JA. The Effects of Patellar Taping on Knee Joint Proprioception. *J Athl Train.* 2002 Mar;37(1):19-24

[150] Olmsted LC, Carcia CR, Hertel J, Shultz SJ. Efficacy of the Star Excursion Balance Tests in Detecting Reach Deficits in Subjects With Chronic Ankle Instability. *J Athl Train.* 2002 Dec;37(4):501-506 http://www.pubmedcentral.gov/articlerender.fcgi?tool=pubmed&pubmedid=12937574

[151] Troy Blackburn J, Hirth CJ, Guskiewicz KM. Exercise Sandals Increase Lower Extremity Electromyographic Activity During Functional Activities. *J Athl Train.* 2003 Sep;38(3):198-203

[152] Bullock-Saxton JE, Janda V, Bullock MI.Reflex activation of gluteal muscles in walking. An approach to restoration of muscle function for patients with low-back pain. *Spine* 1993 May;18(6):704-8

[153] Olmsted LC, Carcia CR, Hertel J, Shultz SJ. Efficacy of the Star Excursion Balance Tests in Detecting Reach Deficits in Subjects With Chronic Ankle Instability. *J Athl Train.* 2002 Dec;37(4):501-506

[154] Troy Blackburn J, Hirth CJ, Guskiewicz KM. Exercise Sandals Increase Lower Extremity Electromyographic Activity During Functional Activities. *J Athl Train.* 2003 Sep;38(3):198-203

[155] Willems T, Witvrouw E, Verstuyft J, Vaes P, De Clercq D. Proprioception and Muscle Strength in Subjects With a History of Ankle Sprains and Chronic Instability. *J Athl Train.* 2002 Dec;37(4):487-493

[156] "RESULTS: Subjects receiving manipulation demonstrated a mean reduction in visual analogue scores of 44%, along with a 41% improvement in mean scores for the head repositioning skill." Rogers RG. The effects of spinal manipulation on cervical kinesthesia in patients with chronic neck pain: a pilot study. *J Manipulative Physiol Ther.* 1997 Feb;20(2):80-5

[157] "Most people do not consume an optimal amount of all vitamins by diet alone. Pending strong evidence of effectiveness from randomized trials, it appears prudent for all adults to take vitamin supplements." Fletcher RH, Fairfield KM. Vitamins for chronic disease prevention in adults: clinical applications. *JAMA.* 2002 Jun 19;287(23):3127-9

- o Niacinamide: Niacinamide alleviates osteoarthritis pain and appears to have an anti-aging benefit.[158,159,160,161,162] The standard dose of 500 mg given orally 6 times per day is more effective than 1,000 mg 3 times per day. Hepatic dysfunction is rare when daily doses are kept below 3,000 mg per day; measure liver enzymes after 3 months of treatment and yearly thereafter.[163]
- o Pancreatic/proteolytic enzymes: Orally-administered pancreatic and proteolytic enzymes are absorbed from the gastrointestinal tract into the systemic circulation[164,165] to exert analgesic, anti-inflammatory, anti-edematous benefits with therapeutic relevance for acute and chronic musculoskeletal disorders.[166,167,168,169]
- o Glucosamine sulfate and chondroitin sulfate: Glucosamine and chondroitin are the "building blocks" from which cartilage is built and oral supplementation is intended to enhance cartilage anabolism and to thus counteract the enhanced cartilage catabolism seen in destructive arthritic processes. The adult dose of glucosamine sulfate is generally 1500-2000 mg per day in divided doses, and the dose of chondroitin sulfate is approximately 1000 mg daily; these treatments can be used singly, in combination, and with other treatments.
- o Vitamin C: Doses of 1-2 grams per day have been suggested to reduce pain and the need for surgery in patients with low-back pain by improving disc integrity[170], and increased vitamin C intake is also associated with improved joint health and musculoskeletal function.[171]
- o Vitamin E, with an emphasis on gamma-tocopherol: The gamma form of vitamin E inhibits cyclooxygenase and thus has anti-inflammatory activity[172] that appears clinically significant in conditions such as rheumatoid arthritis[173,174], spondylosis and back pain[175], osteoarthritis[176,177,178], and several autoimmune diseases.[179,180,181]

[158] Kaufman W. Niacinamide therapy for joint mobility. Therapeutic reversal of a common clinical manifestation of the "normal" aging process. *Conn State Med J* 1953;17:584-591

[159] Kaufman W. The use of vitamin therapy to reverse certain concomitants of aging. *J Am Geriatr Soc* 1955;3:927-936

[160] Matuoka K, Chen KY, Takenawa T. Rapid reversion of aging phenotypes by nicotinamide through possible modulation of histone acetylation. *Cell Mol Life Sci.* 2001;58(14):2108-16

[161] Jonas WB, Rapoza CP, Blair WF. The effect of niacinamide on osteoarthritis: a pilot study. *Inflamm Res* 1996 Jul;45(7):330-4

[162] McCarty MF, Russell AL. Niacinamide therapy for osteoarthritis--does it inhibit nitric oxide synthase induction by interleukin 1 in chondrocytes? *Med Hypotheses.* 1999;53(4):350-60

[163] Gaby AR. Literature review and commentary: Niacinamide for osteoarthritis. *Townsend Letter for Doctors and Patients.* 2002: May; 32

[164] Gotze H, Rothman SS. Enteropancreatic circulation of digestive enzymes as a conservative mechanism. *Nature* 1975; 257(5527): 607-609

[165] Liebow C, Rothman SS. Enteropancreatic Circulation of Digestive Enzymes. *Science* 1975; 189(4201): 472-474

[166] Trickett P. Proteolytic enzymes in treatment of athletic injuries. *Appl Ther.* 1964;30:647-52

[167] Walker JA, Cerny FJ, Cotter JR, Burton HW. Attenuation of contraction-induced skeletal muscle injury by bromelain. *Med Sci Sports Exerc.* 1992 Jan;24(1):20-5

[168] Walker AF, Bundy R, Hicks SM, Middleton RW. Bromelain reduces mild acute knee pain and improves well-being in a dose-dependent fashion in an open study of otherwise healthy adults. *Phytomedicine.* 2002; 9: 681-6

[169] Brien S, Lewith G, Walker A, Hicks SM, Middleton D. Bromelain as a Treatment for Osteoarthritis: a Review of Clinical Studies. *Evidence-based Complementary and Alternative Medicine.* 2004;1(3)251-257

[170] Greenwood J. Optimum vitamin C intake as a factor in the preservation of disc integrity. *Med Ann Dist Columbia.* 1964 Jun;33:274-6

[171] "A 3-fold reduction in risk of OA progression was found for both the middle tertile and highest tertile of vitamin C intake. This related predominantly to a reduced risk of cartilage loss. Those with high vitamin C intake also had a reduced risk of developing knee pain." McAlindon TE, Jacques P, Zhang Y, Hannan MT, Aliabadi P, Weissman B, Rush D, Levy D, Felson DT. Do antioxidant micronutrients protect against the development and progression of knee osteoarthritis? *Arthritis Rheum.* 1996 Apr;39(4):648-56

[172] Jiang Q, Christen S, Shigenaga MK, Ames BN. gamma-tocopherol, the major form of vitamin E in the US diet, deserves more attention. *Am J Clin Nutr* 2001 Dec;74(6):714-22

[173] Helmy M, Shohayeb M, Helmy MH, el-Bassiouni EA. Antioxidants as adjuvant therapy in rheumatoid disease. A preliminary study. *Arzneimittelforschung.* 2001;51(4):293-8

[174] Edmonds SE, Winyard PG, Guo R, Kidd B, Merry P, Langrish-Smith A, Hansen C, Ramm S, Blake DR. Putative analgesic activity of repeated oral doses of vitamin E in the treatment of rheumatoid arthritis. Results of a prospective placebo controlled double blind trial. *Ann Rheum Dis.* 1997 Nov;56(11):649-55

[175] "Vitamin E administration at a dose of 100 mg daily for three weeks resulted in a significant increase in serum vitamin E level accompanied by complete relief of pain... The results therefore strongly indicate that vitamin E is effective in curing spondylosis and most probably due to its antioxidant activity." Mahmud Z, Ali SM. Role of vitamin A and E in spondylosis. *Bangladesh Med Res Counc Bull.* 1992 Apr;18(1):47-59

[176] "The results of this double-blind controlled clinical trial showed that vitamin E was superior to placebo with respect to the relief of pain (pain at rest, pain during movement, pressure-induced pain) and the necessity of additional analgetic treatment. Improvement of mobility was better in the group treated with vitamin E." Blankenhorn G. [Clinical effectiveness of Spondyvit (vitamin E) in activated arthroses. A multicenter placebo-controlled double-blind study] [Article in German] *Z Orthop Ihre Grenzgeb.* 1986 May-Jun;124(3):340-3

[177] This is a very interesting study because the clinical response to vitamin E was proportional to the increase in plasma levels of vitamin E, thus confirming the dose-response relationship that implies causality as well as indicating that the failure of such treatment in some patients may be due to malabsorption or unquenchable systemic oxidative stress rather than the inefficacy of vitamin E supplementation, per se. "There were no significant differences in the efficacy of the two drugs, although one patient of the V-group refused further treatment after 8 days because of inefficacy. V reduced or abolished the pain at rest in 77% (D in 85%), the pain on pressure in 67% (D in 50%), and the pain on movement in 62% (D in 63%). Both treatments appeared to be equally effective in reducing the circumference of the knee joints (p = 0.001) and the walking time (p less than 0.001) and in increasing the joint mobility (p less than 0.002)." Scherak O, Kolarz G, Schodl C, Blankenhorn G. [High dosage vitamin E therapy in patients with activated arthrosis] [Article in German] *Z Rheumatol.* 1990 Nov-Dec;49(6):369-73

[178] Machtey I, Ouaknine L. Tocopherol in Osteoarthritis: a controlled pilot study. *J Am Geriatr Soc.* 1978 Jul;26(7):328-30

[179] Killeen RN, Ayres S Jr, Mihan R. Polymyositis: response to vitamin E. *South Med J.* 1976 Oct;69(10):1372-4

[180] Ayres S Jr, Mihan R. Lupus erythematosus and vitamin E: an effective and nontoxic therapy. *Cutis.* 1979 Jan;23(1):49-52, 54

[181] Ayres S Jr, Mihan R. Is vitamin E involved in the autoimmune mechanism? *Cutis.* 1978 Mar;21(3):321-5

Six-part Self-treatment Protocol for the Alleviation of Pain Secondary to Muscle Tension and Myofascial Trigger Points in the Neck

1—APPLICATION OF HEAT: *Gentle heat softens muscles and tissues and allows for safer and more effective stretching.*

- Heat softens muscles and tissues and can promote healing by increasing circulation—these positive effects can maximize the effectiveness of the treatment plan.
  - *Hot shower*—Moist heat seems to be the best for getting the warmth deep into the tissues where it is needed. Directing the hot water onto the neck and shoulders for 10-15 minutes will help to increase circulation and to soften the tissues before the exercises are started.
  - *Heating pads*—These are good when applying the heat away from home and when heat is needed with maximal convenience with minimal cleanup.

2—RANGE OF MOTION EXERCISES: *Allow enough time to move in each direction for 20-100 repetitions.*

- *Flexion*—Start by brining the chin straight downward to the chest; return to neutral and repeat.
- *Extension*—Gently tilt the head straight backward, then return to the neutral position.
- *Rotation*—Gently turn the head to the left, back to center, then to the right and then repeat in the opposite direction.
- *Lateral bending*—From the neutral position, gently lean the head to one side, then return to neutral, then lean again and repeat toward the opposite side.
  - ***How much and how often?*** In a clinical research study with 77 women who suffered from chronic neck and shoulder pain, women who performed their exercises **three times per week for 5 sets of 20 repetitions** had better results than those who performed their exercises three times per week for 1 set of 20 repetitions.[182] *More exercise gives better results—faster and more complete relief of pain.*

3—GENTLE STRETCHING: *"Gentle" is the key to effective stretching.* Apply a bit of end-of-range pressure with a hand (as demonstrated in the office) to stretch the muscles. Stretching needs to be *gentle* and *slow* to maximize benefits and minimize the introduction of new injury.

- *Flexion*—Bring the chin straight downward to the chest.
- *Extension*—Gently tilt the head straight backward, then return to the neutral position.
- *Rotation*—Gently turning the head to the left, then back to center, then turning again and then repeating in the opposite direction. Use care to not overstretch; do not turn the head past 90° or past the shoulder when turning.
- *Lateral bending*—From the neutral position, gently lean the head to one side, then return to neutral, then lean again and toward the opposite side.

4—POST-ISOMETRIC STRETCHING: Post-isometric stretching provides immediate relief of pain in 94% of patients, lasting relief of general pain in 63% of patients, and lasting relief of "point tenderness" in 23% of patients.[183] Follow these five steps: stretch, contract, stretch, relax, repeat

- Position the **target muscle in <u>stretched</u> position** just short of pain or to the place where the first resistance is felt.
- While in the stretched position, <u>**contract**</u> **the target muscle against slight resistance**, such as pressure applied from the opposite hand, for about 10-30 seconds.
- Now breathe, relax for a few seconds, and then **gently <u>stretch</u> the muscle** with slight pressure and allow the muscle to continue to lengthen with slight pressure; the duration of the stretch can range from 10-30 seconds followed by 10-30 seconds of relaxation.
- <u>**Relax**</u>; return back into the neutral position.
- <u>**Repeat**</u>; repeat steps 1-3 for 3-5 repetitions.
  - ***How much and how often?*** In a research study, the frequency recommendation was 2 times per week up to 2 times per day.
  - ***Be specific!*** Efforts for stretching and contracting the muscles must be specific for the fibers of the muscle that are affected—with practice, patients will learn to localize and affect the specific muscle fibers for efficient treatment.
  - ***Proof of effectiveness from the clinical research***: *"…the increased tension of the affected muscles and the resulting pain and dysfunction are both relieved by restoring the full stretch length of the muscle… Post-isometric stretching-relaxation appears to be a simple, harmless, noninvasive, and effective way of restoring full stretch length to relieve pain originating in tense musculature.*[184]

5—APPLY ICE OR COLD PACK: Apply a cold pack "generally" to most muscles of the neck, or target specific problem areas by applying local cold to muscles that continue to produce pain.

- **Apply cold for 10-20 minutes each 1-2 hours for reduction in pain and inflammation after the exercises.** Use good judgment to avoid "frostbite" and cold injuries to skin.
- **Ice-and-stretch for the problematic/painful muscles**: A final bit of attention can be directed toward the problematic and painful muscles with trigger points. Apply ice (or any source of cold) to the area for approximately 30 seconds to 2 minutes *as a gentle stretch is continually applied to the targeted muscle*. The application of cold helps to decrease the pain and swelling that might arise from minor injuries incurred during stretching and exercising, and the cold has an important neurologic effect by helping to interrupt the cycle of pain and muscle spasm.

6—COMPLETE THE TREATMENT WITH THE APPLICATION OF A *natural* ANALGESIC CREAM: Patients can finish the routine with the application of a heating cream containing capsaicin or menthol to help the neck feel better for the rest of the day.

---

[182] "Patients in both groups that completed the trial demonstrated statistically significant improvements in nearly all of the outcome measurements at completion. ... pain scores were only significantly improved in the intensive group at 12 nths follow-up." Randlov A, Ostergaard M, Manniche C, Kryger P, Jordan A, Heegaard S, Holm B. Intensive dynamic training for females with chronic neck/shoulder pain. A randomized controlled trial. *Clin Rehabil*. 1998 Jun;12(3):200-10

[183] "The method produced immediate pain relief in 94%, lasting pain relief in 63%, as well as lasting relief of point tenderness in 23% of the sites treated. Patients who practiced autotherapy on a home program were more likely to realize lasting relief." Lewit K, Simons DG. Myofascial pain: relief by post-isometric relaxation. *Arch Phys Med Rehabil*. 1984 Aug;65(8):452-6

[184] Lewit K, Simons DG. Myofascial pain: relief by post-isometric relaxation. *Arch Phys Med Rehabil*. 1984 Aug;65(8):452-6

Cervical Spine: Rotation Emphasis

Patient position:	• Supine, neck slightly flexed
Doctor position:	• At 45° angle from head of table; may also be in a more lateral position aside the patient's head and neck; while it is acceptable to assess and set-up with straight legs, at the time of impulse, doctor's legs should be bent to provide the doctor with greater power, stability, and biomechanical safety
Assessment:	• <u>Subjective</u>: neck pain, headaches
	• <u>Motion palpation</u>: rotation restriction; primary or compensatory hypermobile segments may be detected above or below the restricted segment
	• <u>Static palpation</u>: vertebra may feel relatively posterior on the side opposite the rotational restriction, e.g., a right rotational restriction may present with a relative left rotational malposition that brings the vertebral lamina and articular pillars posterior on the left
	• <u>Soft tissue</u>: tenderness, may also have muscle spasm
Treatment contact:	• Doctor uses either an index or proximal phalange contact on the posterior aspect of the transverse process and/or articular pillar
	• The doctor's vector and hence the positioning of the forearm of the contact hand must change depending on the level of the cervical spine that is being treated
	• Notice in this photograph that the thumb of the doctor's contact hand is placed on the angle of the mandible, this is more to help anchor the contact and stabilize the doctor's wrist than to assist with the manipulation; very little pressure and zero thrust are applied to the mandible
Supporting contact:	• Head is held into rotation and slight flexion; as with all techniques, nuanced adjustments in flexion-extension, rotation, and side-bending are made until the premanipulative tension is localized to the specific direction/tissue of restriction
Pretreatment positioning:	• Slight flexion and extension may be used below and above the treatment contact to create motion restriction at the adjacent motion segments; this helps to focus the motion and therapeutic force at the specific; importantly the support hand is largely responsible for proper positioning with the correct amount of nuanced flexion-extension and side-bending so that the rotational force is accurately delivered
Therapeutic action:	• Rotational thrust with contact hand; support hand keeps head off table so that rotational motion can occur
Image:	

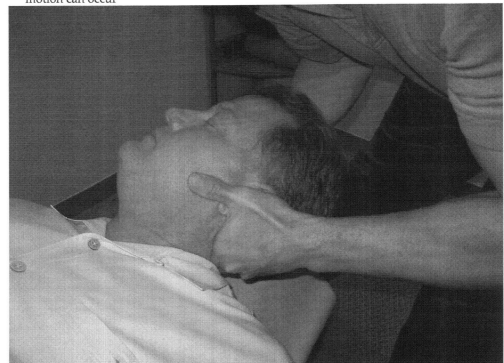

Resources:	• <u>States Manual, Second Edition</u>[185] page 47

---

[185] Kirk CR, Lawrence DJ, Valvo NL. <u>States Manual of Spinal, Pelvic, and Extravertebral Technics. Second Edition</u>. Lombard, Illinois: National College of Chiropractic; 1985

Cervical Spine: Lateral Flexion (Side-Bending) Emphasis; Treatment of Lateral Malposition	
Patient position:	• Supine, head is neutrally placed—neither flexed nor extended; slight flexion is allowed; this technique can also be adapted for use in a seated position
Doctor position:	• At 45° angle from head of table; may also be in a more lateral position aside the patient's head and neck
Assessment:	• <u>Subjective</u>: neck pain, headaches • <u>Motion palpation</u>: lateral flexion restriction • <u>Static palpation</u>: vertebra may feel laterally displaced • <u>Soft tissue</u>: tenderness, may also have muscle spasm
Treatment contact:	• Using an index (metacarpal-phalangeal) contact at the tip of the transverse process or slightly posterior to the transverse process; an index phalangeal contact can also be used on the articular pillars as long as doctor is careful not to thrust in a rotational direction; notice in this picture how Dr Harris has the forearm of his contact hand perfectly aligned in the treatment vector, which is almost purely in the patient's transverse/horizontal plane; notice also that Dr Harris has his knees bent and is forward flexed to bring his torso closer to his contact and thereby minimize stress and strain on his own shoulders; with slight modifications in vector direction, this technique can be applied throughout the cervical spine from C0-C7
Supporting contact:	• Lateral aspect of head, opposite contact; generally the supporting hand is neutral, however it can supply some traction and can help induce lateral flexion at impulse; with more aggressive adjustments, the supporting hand can supply a counterforce to minimize motion following the application of a faster and more powerful thrust
Pretreatment positioning:	• Lateral flexion at the targeted segment; the slightest amount of contralateral rotation is applied
Therapeutic action:	• Establish minimal premanipulative tension once the end range of motion has been reached, then use quick and very shallow trust to induce lateral flexion
Image:	

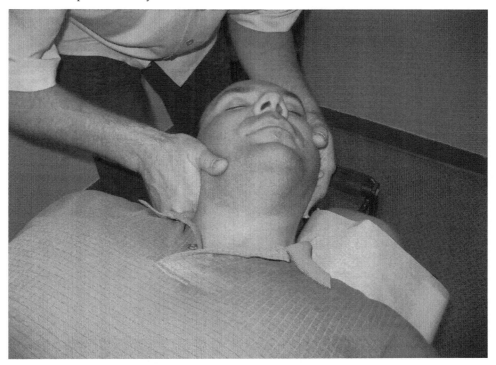

Resources:	• <u>States Manual, Second Edition</u>[186] page 39 • <u>Kimberly Manual, 2006 Edition</u>[187] page 79 • <u>Chiropractic Technique</u>[188] pages 268, 271, 285

[186] Kirk CR, Lawrence DJ, Valvo NL. <u>States Manual of Spinal, Pelvic, and Extravertebral Technics. Second Edition</u>. Lombard, Illinois: National College of Chiropractic; 1985

[187] Kimberly PE. <u>Outline of Osteopathic Manipulative Procedures. The Kimberly Manual 2006</u>. Kirksville College of Osteopathic Medicine. Walsworth Publishing, Marceline, Mo

Type 2—Degenerative Disorders of the Cervical Spine:
- **Cervical Osteoarthritis/arthrosis/spondylosis**
- **Foraminal Encroachment**
- **Cervical Disc Protrusion/herniation**

Description/pathophysiology:
- **Degenerative changes (disc narrowing, facet hypertrophy, osteophytes, joint space narrowing)** in the cervical spine related to normal aging, "wear and tear", and/or previous injury.
- The **intervertebral foramen (IVF)** is bounded anteriorly by the intervertebral disc, **uncinate process**, and **joints of Luschka** and posteriorly by the facet joints; the inferior aspect of the superior pedicle makes the superior border, and the superior aspect of the inferior pedicle makes inferior border. **Degeneration analogous to osteoarthritis** can occur at the joints of Luschka and/or the facet joints; this can result in osteoarthritis-like pain and/or joint hypertrophy and osteophytosis which can alter cervical biomechanics and also result in compression of nearby structures. Narrowing the IVF— **foraminal encroachment**—can easily result in compression of the traversing nerve root. Generally these changes in surrounding bony architecture are degenerative in nature and thus of slow onset; neck pain can be mild or minimal, and motor deficits may appear before or along with sensory changes. This presentation contrasts with that of acute disc herniation, in which the neck and radicular symptoms/deficits present with a more acute or subacute onset. Subclinical degenerative foraminal encroachment may become clinically manifest with a relatively minor disc herniation; i.e., mild/subclinical foraminal encroachment exacerbated by a relatively mild/subclinical disc herniation can additively result in sufficient IVF narrowing to produce clinically important nerve compression.
- The presence of cervical foraminal encroachment can be determined radiographically with oblique cervical views—these are generally performed along with anteroposterior (**AP**) and lateral cervical films, with or without AP open-mouth (**APOM**) and flexion-extension views. Foraminal encroachment does not always result in irritation or compression of the nerve root for **radiculitis (characterized by sensory changes)** or **radiculopathy (characterized by the combination of sensory changes and motor deficits)**; however, the structural boundaries of the IVF leave little space for degenerative changes, and nerve irritation and compression are common sequelae of IVF narrowing.

Complications:
- Pain, similar to that seen in osteoarthritis
- Cervical osteoarthritis/arthrosis/spondylosis can result in foraminal encroachment, which may cause nerve root compression (discussed in the following section, Part 3)[189]
- Loss of disc height and integrity along with cartilage thinning may be accompanied by segmental *hyper*mobility; as degeneration progresses, motion restriction and *hypo*mobility may ensue due to osteophytosis, fibrosis, facet hypertrophy, and joint ankylosis
- Excessive degeneration may contribute to myelopathy, particularly if overlaid atop congenital spinal stenosis

Clinical presentations:
- Pain: the location of pain differs in quality and etiology per region:
  - Head: cervicogenic head pain results from referred pain from active MFTP and facet joints and from direct irritation of the occipital nerves.[190]
  - Neck: cervicogenic neck pain results from joint inflammation and hyperemia/congestion as well as from local pain from muscle spasm, muscle tightness and MFTP.
  - Shoulder: cervicogenic shoulder pain can result from tightness of supporting muscles, compression of the neurovascular bundle exiting between the anterior and middle scalenes

---

[188] Bergmann TF, Peterson DH, Lawrence DJ. Chiropractic Technique. New York; Churchill Livingstone: 1993
[189] Chapter 10 in Gatterman MI (Ed.). Chiropractic Management of Spine-Related Disorders. Baltimore; Williams and Wilkins, 1990.
[190] "The repeated nerve stimulator-guided occipital nerve blockade is a treatment mode that may relieve cervicogenic headache with no recurrence for at least six months in addition to alleviation of associated symptoms." Naja ZM, El-Rajab M, Al-Tannir MA, Ziade FM, Tawfik OM. Repetitive occipital nerve blockade for cervicogenic headache: expanded case report of 47 adults. Pain Pract. 2006 Dec;6(4):278-84

(i.e., thoracic outlet syndrome: discussed later in this text), referred pain from joints, muscles, and MFTP, and possibly from mild nerve root compression.

- o <u>Upper extremity</u>: cervicogenic upper extremity pain can result from referred pain from MFTP and/or facet joints and from cervical nerve root compression.
- o <u>Torso, pelvis, and lower extremity</u>: Symptoms—particularly neurologic sensory/motor deficits—in the torso, pelvis, and/or lower extremity in a patient with neck pain indicates the need to consider cervical spinal cord compression; test lower extremity reflexes, dorsal columns; inquire about anogenital numbness/weakness and changes in bowel/bladder/sexual function.
- Generally in older patients and/or patients with a history of cervical trauma
- Reduced ROM, stiffness
- Myelopathy and radiculopathy, especially with preexisting/congenital spinal stenosis

Major differential diagnoses:
- Myelopathy and radiculopathy
- Instability
- Occult pathology

Clinical assessment:
- History: may be unremarkable or positive for a history of injury
- Physical examination:
  - o Testing of muscle strength, reflexes, and sensory function in the upper and lower extremity.
  - o Regional assessment of neck and shoulders

Imaging & laboratory assessments:
- Lab results should be normal; otherwise suspect and find the pathology.
- Radiographs demonstrate findings characteristic of joint degeneration: disc narrowing, facet hypertrophy, osteophytes, joint space narrowing, and sclerosis. Foraminal encroachment is best seen radiographically on the 55° oblique cervical view.[191]

Clinical management:
- Conservative treatment is appropriate for most cases; see protocol in Part 1.
- <u>Therapeutic and management goals include</u>:
  - o Delay, prevention, and possible reversal of degeneration with integrated use of diet, nutritional and botanical anti-inflammatory supplements, in-office manual treatments, home exercises and stretching, and judicious use of manual or mechanical cervical traction. One single case report suggested that disc degeneration might be reversed with chondroitin/glucosamine supplementation[192]; results would be expected to be more robust with a more comprehensive multicomponent interventional plan as previously outlined in Part 1 of this chapter.
  - o Monitor for signs of progression: onset of severe pain or neurologic deficits strongly suggests the need for additional treatment, referral, and/or decompressive surgery.
  - o Treatments—physician-directed and patient directed—should aim to improve the patient's overall health while also helping alleviate the neck symptoms. For example, systemic inflammation due to nutritional/hormonal imbalances will require a whole-patient approach rather than a "neck only" approach if the patient is to attain maximal improvement.
- Referral if clinical outcome is unsatisfactory or if serious complications (radiculopathy and/or myelopathy) become manifest.

---

[191] "IVF size was substantially increased on the 55 degrees AP oblique projection at all lower cervical levels. The 55 degrees AP oblique view of the cervical spine is optimal for evaluating the lower cervical foramina and can be a routine alternative to the 45 degrees oblique view in the analysis of all cervical foramina." Marcelis S, Seragini FC, Taylor JA, Huang GS, Park YH, Resnick D. Cervical spine: comparison of 45 degrees and 55 degrees anteroposterior oblique radiographic projections. *Radiology*. 1993 Jul;188(1):253-6 http://radiology.rsnajnls.org/cgi/reprint/188/1/253.pdf
[192] "The case suggests that long-term glucosamine and chondroitin sulfate intake may counteract symptomatic spinal disc degeneration, particularly at an early stage." van Blitterswijk WJ, van de Nes JC, Wuisman PI. Glucosamine and chondroitin sulfate supplementation to treat symptomatic disc degeneration: biochemical rationale and case report. *BMC Complement Altern Med*. 2003 Jun 10;3:2 http://www.biomedcentral.com/1472-6882/3/2

Type 3—Nerve Root Compression:

- **Cervical Radiculitis**: nerve root irritation leading to dermatomal sensory changes but no motor deficits
- **Cervical Radiculopathy**: nerve root compression resulting in dermatomal sensory deficits and motor weakness

Description/pathophysiology:

- Cervical radiculitis: inflammation of or near the nerve root that results in *dermatomal* **sensory changes** *without* **motor deficits.**[193] Causes include local inflammation due to injury to the cervical intervertebral disc, infections (herpes, zoster) and others. Pain can be managed conservatively unless it becomes severe, in which case appropriate analgesic management is indicated.
- Cervical radiculopathy: inflammation of or near the nerve root that results in *dermatomal* **sensory changes** *as well as* **deficits in muscle strength.** Causes include 1) protrusion or extrusion of the nucleus pulposus and/or extension of the annulus fibrosis in the posterolateral direction toward the nerve root, 2) foraminal encroachment, and 3) pathology such as infection, tumor, or fracture. Loss of muscle strength is serious and can become permanent and therefore must be managed appropriately: either conservatively or with appropriate referral.
- Cervical disc protrusion/herniation: acute injuries and/or degenerative changes affecting the cervical intervertebral disc predisposes to protrusion or extrusion of the nucleus pulposus and/or diametric enlargement of the annulus fibrosis, thus resulting in inflammatory and/or compressive effects on nearby structures, such as nerve roots and/or the spinal cord. Most common level of herniation is C5-6. Disc protrusion/herniation can result in radiculitis, radiculopathy, or myelopathy, each of which must be managed appropriately.
- Foraminal encroachment: due to degenerative changes, described previously in Part 2

Complications:

- Nerve root irritation with resultant sensory changes, particularly dermatomal paresthesias/tingling and/or pain
- Nerve root compression with resultant loss of neuromuscular function: numbness and weakness
- Altered cervical spine biomechanics

Simplified Conceptual Schema of Interconnected Problems, Presentations, Complications, and Management Strategies

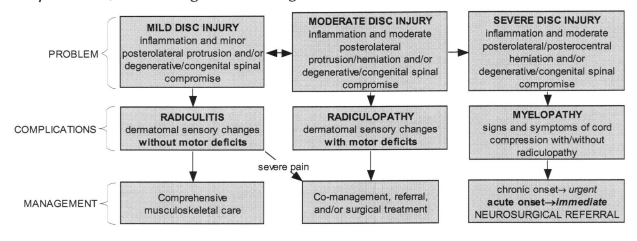

---

[193] Here I use the term "radiculitis" to indicate inflammatory pathologies that result in sensory changes without motor disturbances. I use the term "radiculopathy" to denote primarily compressive mechanisms of injury that result in both sensory and motor changes. Although this outline covers primarily discogenic causes of nerve compromise, other infectious, metabolic, and pathologic causes of radiculitis and radiculopathy should be considered and treated per patient. Many articles and texts do not distinguish radiculitis from radiculopathy; however, I find the differentiation both conceptually and clinically valuable.

Clinical presentations:
- Acute or subacute onset
- Sensory changes may include numbness, tingling, paresthesias, and diminution of reflex
- Motor deficits can include weakness and diminution of reflex
- Pain in the neck, arms, shoulders; often exacerbated with neck motion, coughing, straining, or sneezing
- Paraspinal muscle spasm
- Risk factors: lifting heavy objects, cigarette smokers, divers, workers who operate vibrating equipment, drivers

Major differential diagnoses:
- <u>Myocardial infarction</u>: can cause neck and arm pain
- <u>Occult pathology</u>: such as bone tumor, Pancoast/apical lung tumor, ALS, or syringomyelia[194]
- <u>Osteomyelitis</u>: assess for fever, lymphadenopathy, and elevations in WBC and CRP
- <u>Intra-abdominal pathology</u>: such as <u>gall bladder disease</u> can cause shoulder pain which could mimic the shoulder-neck-arm pain of cervical nerve root dysfunctions
- <u>Myofascial trigger point</u>: causing neck and arm pain
- <u>Facet syndrome</u>: causing neck and arm pain
- <u>Thoracic outlet syndrome</u>: causing neck and arm pain
- <u>Infections that affect nerves</u>: herpes zoster and Lyme disease[195] may present with sensory and/or motor disturbances.

Clinical assessments:
- When neurologic symptoms—sensory changes or motor deficits—are present, the clinician's history and physical examination must become more detailed because **the stakes are higher** and because differentiation of severity, etiology, and concomitant problems becomes more important and complex compared to the evaluation and differential diagnosis of patients with simple non-traumatic non-radicular/neurologic neck pain.
- **History**: OPP-QRST-A
  - Onset
  - Provocation: *"What makes it worse?"*
  - Palliation: *"What makes it better?"*
  - Quality: *"What does it feel like? Can you describe what sensation you are feeling?"*
  - Radiation: *"Does the pain stay localized or does it extend down your arm or into your legs?"*
  - Severity: *"On a scale of 1 to 10, with 1 being almost no pain and 10 being the worst pain you could imagine, how would you rate the pain?"*
  - Timing: *"Do you notice that it is worse at certain times of the day or during certain times of the week? When is it more/less bothersome?"*
  - Associated symptoms: For example, *"Do you notice any other problems that might be associated with your neck injury/pain, such as muscle weakness, lack of sensation, alterations in bowel, bladder, or sexual functioning?"*
- **Physical examination**: Testing of muscle strength, reflexes, and sensory function in the upper and lower extremity. Only perform physical examination tests on patients who are neurologically stable and who are unlikely to have spinal fracture, dislocation, instability, etc.
  - Neurologic exam: upper and lower extremities: "Sensory and motor deficits with asymmetric reflexes should be referred for a neurological evaluation."[196]
  - Cervical regional assessment:
    - Local tenderness and spasm with resultant decreased motion
    - Interspinous tenderness

---

[194] Beers MH, Berkow R (eds). <u>The Merck Manual. Seventeenth Edition</u>. Whitehouse Station; Merck Research Laboratories 1999 page 1481-2

[195] [Persistent leg pain]. [Article in German] *Schweiz Rundsch Med Prax* 1990 Jul 3;79(27-28):866-8

[196] Chapter 10 in Gatterman MI (Ed.). <u>Chiropractic Management of Spine-Related Disorders</u>. Baltimore; Williams and Wilkins, 1990.

- Cervical distraction/traction
- Lateral bending and extension with compression
- Lateral bending with shoulder depression
- Shoulder abduction with elbow flexion (shoulder abduction test)

Imaging & laboratory assessments:
- Lab tests should be completely normal (with the possible exception of high sensitivity CRP).
- Radiographs may demonstrate decreased disc height, foraminal encroachment (oblique view), and signs of degeneration. CT may show osteophytes and osseous hypertrophy. MRI shows disc herniation and nerve root and/or spinal cord compression.

Clinical management: Re-evaluate symptoms and neurologic function before and after each treatment.
- **Cervical disc protrusion/herniation**: Monitor for complications such as radiculopathy and myelopathy. Provide good nutrition, massage (to relieve muscle spasm and relax tightness), manipulation (as appropriate), and good posture as indicated. Cervical disc injury is not per se a serious concern in itself; the major problems/complications arise from neurologic compromise secondary to nerve root or spinal cord compression; many asymptomatic people have MRI and radiographic evidence of disc protrusion and spinal degeneration.[197] For cervical disc herniation with or without nerve root compression, chiropractic management including bracing, physiotherapy, cervical manipulative procedures, traction and exercises can be highly effective.[198] In the treatment of cervical/lumbar disc herniation, interventions including traction, flexion distraction, spinal manipulative therapy, physiotherapy and rehabilitative exercises can benefit the majority of patients, some of whom will have MRI-documented resolution (i.e., "disappearance") of their disc herniation.[199] Modified flexion-distraction manipulation may also be successful.[200] Results from a clinical series of 8 patients with disc herniation and radicular signs/symptoms treated with chiropractic spinal manipulation suggest that cervical manipulation is more likely to be successful if applied with 1) the patient in the supine position, 2) lateral flexion *toward* the radicular side, 3) rotation *away from* the radicular side, 4) arm abducted during manipulation to lessen nerve tension if this is associated with pain relief.[201]
- **Cervical radiculitis:** Conservative care is generally appropriate and can include combinations of anti-inflammatory and analgesic therapies, ergonomic improvements, temporary limitations in activity, use of a soft cervical collar, manual medicine treatments, including manipulation, traction, massage and other myofascial techniques as appropriate *per patient*. Simple "over the door" type cervical traction devices can be successfully used in the treatment of cervical disc herniation with radiculitis.[202]
- **Cervical radiculopathy:** Conservative management—consisting of traction, specific exercises, oral anti-inflammatory treatments, and ergonomic education—can be successful in the vast majority of cases.[203] Referral if clinical outcome is unsatisfactory or if serious complications such as intractable pain or motor deficits are persistent or progressive.

---

[197] Cervical and lumbar MRI in asymptomatic older male lifelong athletes: frequency of degenerative findings. *J Comput Assist Tomogr* 1996 Jan-Feb;20(1):107-12

[198] "Patients with and without nerve root compression secondary to cervical disk herniation can and do respond well to chiropractic care. Chiropractic management of this condition can and should be employed prior to more invasive treatment." Beneliyahu DJ. Chiropractic management and manipulative therapy for MRI documented cervical disk herniation. *J Manipulative Physiol Ther.* 1994 Mar-Apr;17(3):177-85

[199] "Clinically, 80% of the patients studied had a good clinical outcome with postcare visual analog scores under 2 and resolution of abnormal clinical examination findings. Anatomically, after repeat MRI scans, 63% of the patients studied revealed a reduced size or completely resorbed disc herniation." BenEliyahu DJ. Magnetic resonance imaging and clinical follow-up: study of 27 patients receiving chiropractic care for cervical and lumbar disc herniations. *J Manipulative Physiol Ther.* 1996 Nov-Dec;19(9):597-606

[200] "Given the research supporting the effectiveness of flexion distraction on the lumbar spine and the success of this clinical trial, flexion distraction might be an asset in the management of cervical spine nerve root irritation. Kruse RA, Imbarlina F, De Bono VF. Treatment of cervical radiculopathy with flexion distraction. *J Manipulative Physiol Ther.* 2001 Mar-Apr;24(3):206-9

[201] "Six of eight patients had a good outcome associated with receiving manipulation performed by contacting the cervical spine at the level of the radiculopathy, laterally flexing toward the side of radiculopathy, rotating the neck away from the side of the radiculopathy and applying a gentle high-velocity, low-amplitude thrust." Hubka MJ, Phelan SP, Delaney PM, Robertson VL. Rotary manipulation for cervical radiculopathy: observations on the importance of the direction of the thrust. *J Manipulative Physiol Ther.* 1997 Nov-Dec;20(9):622-7

[202] "Cervical spine traction could be considered as a therapy of choice for radiculopathy caused by herniated disks, even in cases of large-volume herniated disks or recurrent episodes." Constantoyannis C, Konstantinou D, Kourtopoulos H, Papadakis N. Intermittent cervical traction for cervical radiculopathy caused by large-volume herniated disks. *J Manipulative Physiol Ther.* 2002 Mar-Apr;25(3):188-92

[203] "Many cervical disc herniations can be successfully managed with aggressive nonsurgical treatment (24 of 26 in the present study). Progressive neurologic loss did not occur in any patient, and most patients were able to continue with their preinjury activities with little limitation. High patient satisfaction with nonoperative care was achieved on outcome analysis." Saal JS, Saal JA, Yurth EF. Nonoperative management of herniated cervical intervertebral disc with radiculopathy. Spine. 1996 Aug 15;21(16):1877-83

o Moderate sensory disturbances and/or mild motor deficits indicate the need for patient education, PAR discussion[204], **informed consent** for patients who *choose* conservative/non-surgical management. An aggressive course of conservative therapy may be undertaken if *both* **doctor** *and* **patient** are willing; however the physician must realize the great significance of motor deficits and must refer the patient for neurosurgical evaluation if the deficits do not improve quickly and/or if they worsen. Conservative management for radiculopathy with motor deficits may be seen as controversial, especially if the patient is not satisfied with treatment. Some experts have recommended "Sensory and motor deficits with asymmetric reflexes should be referred for a neurological evaluation."[205]

o Moderate-severe motor deficits indicate the need for neurosurgical/orthopedic referral.

o Re-evaluate symptoms and neurologic function before and after each treatment.

- <u>Cervical myelopathy</u>: **referral to orthopedist/neurosurgeon.**

  o Chronic, mild, and slow-onset myelopathy should be referred for neurosurgical consultation, although mild cases may ultimately be managed conservatively. Decompressive surgery is indicated for patients with moderate to severe neurologic symptoms.[206]

  o Acute and progressing neurologic deterioration must be treated as a medical emergency: **"Compression of the spinal cord from a central disc herniation with lower extremity symptoms requires immediate referral for surgical evaluation."**[207]

<u>Therapeutic considerations:</u>

- *See overview in Chapter 3, and Therapeutics for Non-specific Neck Pain in this chapter*

- <u>High-dose vitamin supplementation, with emphasis on thiamine, pyridoxine, and cobalamin</u>: In patients with radicular signs and symptoms, consider testing/treating for possible B-12 deficiency neuropathy by measuring serum methylmalonic acid (elevated with B-12 deficiency) or treating empirically with oral hydroxocobalamin/methylcobalamin 2,000-4,000 mcg/d or intramuscular injection of hydroxocobalamin/methylcobalamin at 1,000 mcg/d a few days per week. Clinical experience and an abstract from the German literature[208] reporting positive benefits among "1,149 patients with polyneuropathy, neuralgia, radiculopathy and neuritis associated with pain and paresthesias" has shown that—when they are supplemented with vitamins in general and B1, B6, and B12 in particular—the majority of patients gain symptomatic improvement and appear to heal faster than would otherwise be expected. Similarly, given the role of fatty acids in modulating inflammation as well as promoting maintenance/healing of peripheral nerves, combined supplementation with GLA and EPA-DHA should be considered for its therapeutic and preventive benefits.

- *Harpagophytum procumbens* (Devil's claw): Numerous studies have proven the safety and effectiveness of Harpagophytum in the treatment of neuromusculoskeletal pain[209,210,211,212,213,214], and Harpagophytum has specifically been used in patients with radiculitis and radiculopathy secondary to acute lumbar

---

[204] "P.A.R." should always be charted to indicate that the patient was fully educated about the Procedures, Alternatives, and Risks associated with treatment. Only when patients have been properly educated can they give informed consent to treatment.

[205] Chapter 10 in Gatterman MI (Ed.). <u>Chiropractic Management of Spine-Related Disorders</u>. Baltimore; Williams and Wilkins, 1990.

[206] Tierney ML. McPhee SJ, Papadakis MA (eds). <u>Current Medical Diagnosis and Treatment 2006, 45th Edition</u>. Lange Medical; page 816

[207] Chapter 10 in Gatterman MI (Ed.). <u>Chiropractic Management of Spine-Related Disorders</u>. Baltimore; Williams and Wilkins, 1990.

[208] Abstract: "Under treatment, there was a clear improvement in these symptoms. At a second examination approximately three weeks after initiation of treatment, a positive effect on pain in particular was observed in 69% of the cases." Eckert M, Schejbal P. [Therapy of neuropathies with a vitamin B combination. Symptomatic treatment of painful diseases of the peripheral nervous system with a combination preparation of thiamine, pyridoxine and cyanocobalamin] *Fortschr Med.* 1992 Oct 20;110(29):544-8. German.

[209] Chantre P, Cappelaere A, Leblan D, Guedon D, Vandermander J, Fournie B. Efficacy and tolerance of Harpagophytum procumbens versus diacerhein in treatment of osteoarthritis. *Phytomedicine* 2000 Jun;7(3):177-83

[210] Leblan D, Chantre P, Fournie B. Harpagophytum procumbens in the treatment of knee and hip osteoarthritis. Four-month results of a prospective, multicenter, double-blind trial versus diacerhein. *Joint Bone Spine* 2000;67(5):462-7

[211] Whitehouse LW, Znamirowska M, Paul CJ. Devil's Claw (Harpagophytum procumbens): no evidence for anti-inflammatory activity in the treatment of arthritic disease. *Can Med Assoc J* 1983 Aug 1;129(3):249-51

[212] Moussard C, Alber D, Toubin MM, Thevenon N, Henry JC. A drug used in traditional medicine, harpagophytum procumbens: no evidence for NSAID-like effect on whole blood eicosanoid production in human. *Prostaglandins Leukot Essent Fatty Acids* 1992 Aug;46(4):283-6

[213] Chrubasik S, Model A, Black A, Pollak S. A randomized double-blind pilot study comparing Doloteffin and Vioxx in the treatment of low back pain. *Rheumatology* (Oxford). 2003 Jan;42(1):141-8

[214] "They took an 8-week course of Doloteffin at a dose providing 60 mg harpagoside per day... Doloteffin is well worth considering for osteoarthritic knee and hip pain and nonspecific low back pain." Chrubasik S, Thanner J, Kunzel O, Conradt C, Black A, Pollak S. Comparison of outcome measures during treatment with the proprietary Harpagophytum extract doloteffin in patients with pain in the lower back, knee or hip. *Phytomedicine* 2002 Apr;9(3):181-94

disc herniation.[215] The mechanism appears to be a central neurologic effect rather than a peripheral anti-inflammatory effect.[216] Thus, among the many treatments/interventions listed earlier in this chapter and also in Chapter 3, Harpagophytum may show some prominence among available choices. Clinically, the "right treatment" is whatever works for the patient in terms of safety, effectiveness, tolerability, affordability, and personal preference.

Cervical radiculopathy with 1) moderate-severe pain and/or 2) mild motor deficits: managing the risk/benefit ratio for both doctor and patient:
A wise strategy for both the treating doctor and the patient with significant radiculopathy (dermatomal sensory abnormalities and muscle/reflex weakness) is for the conservative physician to refer the patient to a neurosurgeon/orthopedist for evaluation and consultation. This allows for **1) physician-physician communication**, and **2) complete patient education**, thus allowing for the patient to **3) give informed consent** based on the risks and benefits of conservative treatment versus surgical treatment. This referral also demonstrates that the conservative physician was **4) aware of the potential complications of unsuccessful treatment** and that he/she **5) acted in the best interest of the patient by providing an appropriate and timely referral**. "Conservative management of cervical radiculopathy is effective for the majority of patients in the absence of advancing neurological and motor deficits. ... Prompt referral for decompression is necessary in cases with severe pain, advancing sensory or motor deficits, and lower extremity symptoms."* *Gatterman MI (Ed.). <u>Chiropractic Management of Spine-Related Disorders</u>. Williams & Wilkins, 1990

---

[215] "The majority of responders' were patients who had suffered less than 42 days of pain, and subgroup analyses suggested that the effect was confined to patients with more severe and radiating pain accompanied by neurological deficit... There was no evidence for Harpagophytum-related side-effects, except possibly for mild and infrequent gastrointestinal symptoms." Chrubasik S, Junck H, Breitschwerdt H, Conradt C, Zappe H. Effectiveness of Harpagophytum extract WS 1531 in the treatment of exacerbation of low back pain: a randomized, placebo-controlled, double-blind study. *Eur J Anaesthesiol* 1999 Feb;16(2):118-29

[216] Shin MC, Chang HK, Jang HM, Kim CJ, Kim Y, Kim EH. Modulation of Harpagophytum procumbens on ion channels in acutely dissociated periaquedeuctal gray neurons of rats. *Korean J Meridian Acupoint* 2003; 20: 17-29

Type 4—Cervical Myelopathy:
- **Cervical Disc Protrusion/herniation**
- **Cervical Myelopathy**
- **Cervical Spine Canal Stenosis**

<u>Description/pathophysiology</u>:
- Protrusion/herniation of cervical disc may result in radiculitis or radiculopathy if the disc lesion is posteriorlaterally located; the cervical disc herniation may cause direct compression of the spinal cord if large, located posterocentrally, and/or proceeded by congenital or acquired spinal stenosis.
- Compressive myelopathy—transient or permanent compression of the spinal cord—may be due to any of the following:
  - o Cervical disc herniation
  - o Degenerative changes leading to central canal stenosis
  - o Congenital spinal stenosis, easily exacerbated by mild cervical trauma or degenerative changes
  - o Inflammation, swelling, or hematoma following injury
  - o Tumor
  - o Paget's disease of bone can result in cervical cord compression
- Compression/lesion of the spinal cord can also occur with the following disorders that mandate immediate referral and treatment:
  - o <u>Spinal cord injury</u>: Spinal cord injury can occur with whiplash-type injuries classically seen in **motor vehicle accidents (MVA)** but may also occur in sports injuries. **SCIWORA syndrome** (spinal cord injury without radiographic abnormality) is occasionally seen in children following neck trauma; the laxity of the child's cervical ligaments allow so much movement to occur that the cord can be traumatically bent, twisted, or torn, resulting in internal hemorrhage, neuronal necrosis, or severance of the cord.[217]
  - o <u>Infection: osteomyelitis, infectious discitis</u>: Infection of bone and/or adjacent intervertebral disc; can result in compression due to local inflammatory edema, epidural abscess, or due to collapse of vertebra; patients are generally febrile and have laboratory abnormalities (i.e., leukocytosis, elevated CRP/ESR, and positive blood cultures), *Staphylococcus aureus* is one of the most common infecting agents.
  - o <u>Vertebral tumor, spinal/epidural metastasis</u>: Cancer can lead to cord lesion by direct extension from bone, from epidural metastasis leading to cord compression, or from complications resultant from vertebral collapse.
  - o <u>Inflammatory myelopathy/myelitis</u>: Inflammatory infiltration and subsequent cord destruction leading to motor/sensory deficits may occur from an adverse drug effect or occur as a result of the systemic autoimmune diseases, such as rheumatoid arthritis (RA) or anti-phospholipid antibody syndrome (APLAS); inflammatory myelopathy/myelitis mandates immediate pharmacologic immunosuppression.

<u>Clinical presentations</u>:
- Onset may be acute or subacute; manifestations may be transient or chronic.
- **The classic presentation of cervical myelopathy is upper extremity weakness with lower extremity hyperreflexia, spasticity, and weakness.**
- Characteristics of the neurologic lesion depend upon patient-specific variables such as speed of onset, severity of compression, location of compression (i.e., compression of the anterior cord is likely to present with motor-dominant lesions, whereas compression of the posterior cord is likely to present with sensory-dominant lesions characteristic of lesions of the dorsal columns—fasciculus gracilis and

---

[217] Graber MA, Kathol M. Cervical spine radiographs in the trauma patient. *Am Fam Physician*. 1999 Jan 15;59(2):331-42
http://www.aafp.org/afp/990115ap/331.html

fasciculus cuneatus), size of the lesion, degree of inflammation, and anatomical variation (e.g., collateral circulation, etc).

- Sensory lesions may include pain, numbness, weakness, tingling, paresthesias, and proprioceptive loss
- Loss of bowel/bladder function: fecal/urinary incontinence, urinary retention, sexual dysfunction
- Lower extremity spasticity—strongly suggests myelopathy or other upper motor neuron lesion
- Risk factors: lifting heavy objects, cigarette smokers, workers who operate vibrating equipment, drivers, cervical trauma, inflammatory arthropathy such as rheumatoid arthritis or psoriasis.
- Spinal canal diameter is generally reduced with cervical extension and increased with cervical flexion; therefore patients may report relief of pain with cervical flexion and exacerbation of pain or discomfort with neck extension.

Complications:
- Loss of neuromuscular function
- Sensory deficits
- Loss of bowel/bladder function: fecal/urinary incontinence, urinary retention
- Sexual dysfunction
- Unhappiness, suffering, decreased quality of life, depression: remember that clinical disorders do not occur without impacting the life, feelings, and emotions of the patient.

Major differential diagnoses:
- Compressive pathology such as tumor, osteomyelitis, abscess, hematoma, spine fracture, edema

Clinical assessment:
- History: unremarkable or positive for previous abnormality or injury; assess qualities of signs and symptoms
- Physical examination: Testing of muscle strength, reflexes, and sensory function in the upper and lower extremity. Only perform physical examination tests on patients who are neurologically stable.
    - Take care not to exacerbate or introduce injury. Always begin with history, then if appropriate proceed to active patient motion, then if appropriate proceed to neuro-orthopedic assessments.
    - Never perform aggressive physical examination procedures (such as forced cervical flexion; Soto-Hall) in a patient with possible spinal instability or fracture. Always stabilize and image these patients before proceeding to proceeding to examination and physical treatment.
    - Cervical spine examination and neurologic examination
    - Muscles distal to lesion may be weak, spastic, hyper-reflexive
    - Assess bowel function by history and rectal examination, assessing for sensation and sphincter muscle tone
    - Assess bladder function by history and abdominal examination for suprapubic tenderness or bladder distention
    - Assess genital/bowel/bladder function by history, asking about changes in function or reduction in sensation:
        - *Do you have any numbness, weakness or tingling in your arms, hands, legs, or feet?*
        - *Have you noticed any changes or are you having any problems with bowel or bladder function-fecal incontinence, urinary retention, urinary incontinence?*
        - *Do you notice any numbness or change in sensation near your anus or genitals?*
        - Women: *Have you noticed any loss of vaginal muscle tone or genital numbness?*
        - Men: *Have you noticed any difficulty with obtaining or maintaining erections?*

Imaging & laboratory assessments:
- Lab tests should be normal; otherwise diagnose and treat the pathology.
- Radiographs may demonstrate signs of degeneration and stenosis.
- CT may show osteophytes and osseous hypertrophy.
- MRI shows disc herniation and nerve root and/or spinal cord compression.

Clinical management:

- Referral if clinical outcome is unsatisfactory or if serious complications are evident.
- **Cervical myelopathy**: referral to orthopedist/neurosurgeon.
  - "Compression of the spinal cord from a central disc herniation with lower extremity symptoms requires immediate referral for surgical evaluation."[218]
  - Evidence of *acute* spinal cord injury mandates immediate referral for treatment with methylprednisolone, which should be administered within the first 8 hours after injury: "Once an [acute] injury to the spinal cord is diagnosed, methylprednisolone should be administered as soon as possible in an attempt to limit neurologic injury."[219]
- **Spinal stenosis**: assess neurologic function, initiate protective lifestyle practices, and other ergonomic considerations.
  - Assess other regions of spine in cases of congenital stenosis as other anomalies and areas of stenosis (especially in the lumbar spine) may occur.
  - Refer for neurosurgical or neurologic evaluation with signs of motor deficits.
  - Provide education and proper referral as necessary, since patients with spinal stenosis are at increased risk for spinal cord injury following trauma and may be candidates for surgical decompression.

Therapeutic considerations:

- *See overview in Chapter 3, and Therapeutics for Non-specific Neck Pain in this chapter*
- Orthopedic/neurosurgical referral for patients with severe pain or neurologic deficits.
- Use of a stiff cervical collar may provide pain relief.
- Manual/mechanical traction and gentle manipulative therapy can be successfully used in patients with cervical disc herniation, including those with nerve root compression[220]; traction is not applied to patients with any suspicion or manifestations of spinal cord lesion.
- **Massage:** Massage can help alleviate pain and muscle spasm and can provide comfort.
- **Mobilization:** Mobilization (low-velocity, high amplitude), if applied at all, must be gentle, slow, and within the patient's tolerance.
- **Manipulation:** Due to risk of serious neurologic injury[221], cervical spinal stenosis and myelopathy are both independent absolute contraindications to forceful high-velocity spinal manipulation.
- **Acupuncture:** One author reported a 92% success rate (i.e., either "cured" or "markedly effective") in the treatment of spinal stenosis with a specific acupuncture technique.[222]
- **Martial Art Therapy and Qigong:** In a single case report with minimal neurologic deficits, an exercise and martial art routine including Qigong was self-administered for 20 minutes on a daily and then weekly basis. The patient was followed for one year, and resolution of radicular pain was achieved without change in MRI findings.[223]

Cervical myelopathy/radiculopathy caused or aggravated by spinal manipulation
"In patients with pre-existing stenosis of the canal or those with vertebral instability, these movements [from cervical spine manipulation] may cause (or aggravate) myelopathy... This report describes four patients with cervical myelopathy and/or radiculopathy caused or aggravated by spinal manipulation." Padua L, et al. Radiculomedullary complications of cervical spinal manipulation. *Spinal Cord* 1996 Aug;34(8):488-92

[218] Chapter 10 in Gatterman MI (Ed.). Chiropractic Management of Spine-Related Disorders. Baltimore; Williams and Wilkins, 1990.
[219] "If a cervical fracture or dislocation is found, orthopedic or neurosurgical consultation should be obtained immediately. Any patient with a spinal cord injury should begin therapy with methylprednisolone within the first eight hours after the injury, with continued administration for up to 24 hours." Graber MA, Kathol M. Cervical spine radiographs in the trauma patient. *Am Fam Physician*. 1999 Jan 15;59(2):331-42
[220] "Conservative treatment including chiropractic manipulative therapy seems to be a reasonable alternative to surgery, for cervical radiculopathy caused by a herniated cervical disc." Brouillette DL, Gurske DT. Chiropractic treatment of cervical radiculopathy caused by a herniated cervical disc. *J Manipulative Physiol Ther*. 1994 Feb;17(2):119-23
[221] Padua L, Padua R, LoMonaco M, Tonali PA. Radiculomedullary complications of cervical spinal manipulation. *Spinal Cord* 1996 Aug;34(8):488-92 Manipulative complication of stenosis/myelopathy appears to have been reported here as well: Nijman JJ. [Cervical myelopathy as complication of manual therapy in a patient with a narrow cervical canal]. *Ned Tijdschr Geneeskd* 1993 Aug 7;137(32):1617-8
[222] Yuhua C. Step-by-step needling along Du Channel in Treating Spinal Canal Stenosis. *International J Clin Acupuncture* 1993; 4: 437-9
[223] Massey PB, Kisling GM. A single case report of healing through specific martial art therapy: comparison of MRI to clinical resolution in severe cervical stenosis: a case report. *J Altern Complement Med* 1999 Feb;5(1):75-9

Type 5 — Post-traumatic Neck Pain and Complications:
- **Cervical strain, cervical sprain**
- **Whiplash: Cervical Acceleration-Deceleration Syndrome**

Description/pathophysiology:
- Introduction: Injuries to the neck can occur following occupational repetitive strain, sports injury, falls, assault, or motor vehicle accident (MVA). While post-traumatic pain clearly indicates that tissues have been injured and suggests the need for radiographic evaluation, the absence of pain does not exclude significant injury, since patients may be functionally anesthetized due to shock, confusion, distraction, drugs, medications, or alcohol. Some patients with clinically important injures may have virtually no pain; I recall learning of a patient who "strained his neck" when lifting a heavy object and presented to a chiropractic office where the doctor's insistence upon radiographs led to a diagnosis of a Jefferson's fracture — an open "burst" fracture of the atlas.
- Cervical strain: "Strain" denotes injury to the muscles and tendons rather than discs and ligaments. Strains result from acute or chronic over-stretch or over-contraction injuries. Muscle strain injuries that are mild or due to chronic overuse can be treated as simple neck pain as described in the first section in this chapter on common clinical disorders of the cervical spine.
- Cervical sprain: "Sprain" denotes injury to ligamentous structures (rather than muscles or tendons); acute ligament and disc injuries are typically the result of trauma. Force sufficient to sprain a ligament is generally sufficient to strain a muscle or injure the more delicate neurovascular structures in the neck.
- Whiplash/ cervical acceleration-deceleration syndrome: Signs and symptoms resulting from a mechanism of injury whereby the body and head are exposed to different inertial/external forces at the same time, resulting in motion of the head in a sudden whip-like action.[224] Biomechanical forces commonly include variations and combinations of compression, distraction, as well as flexion, extension, rotation, and shear. Although classically associated with MVAs, these injuries can also occur secondary to falls and sports injuries. Whiplash classically and perhaps exclusively occurs when a stationary or slowly moving vehicle is hit from behind thus forcing the driver's neck into extreme extension and often compression (due to impact with the ceiling of the car) and then flexion (as the car decelerates). The only biomechanical/anatomic limitations to cervical extension are the pain-prone and injury-prone soft tissues of the anterior neck and cervical spine.[225] Other types of injuries (involving predominately flexion or lateral bending) do not generally result in chronic complications because anatomic limitations help reduce excessive tissue injury; cervical flexion is limited anatomically by the chin contacting the sternum, and lateral bending is limited in part by the shoulder. Injuries involving greater speeds and more force are more likely to produce injury, regardless of the direction(s) of force application. Estimates of the prevalence and persistence of symptoms attributable to cervical spine injury vary; some authors[226] report that approximately 95% percent of patients involved in whiplash injuries are relatively healed within one year and that 5% of whiplash patients may continue to have chronic symptoms and impairment, while other authors[227] cite a much higher incidence of morbidity — namely that 55% of whiplash patients are symptomatic at 8-year follow-up, and that the chance of full recovery is only about 60%. In determining the prognosis, although the severity of the accident must be considered, the prognosis is more often influenced by other variables, namely: the patient's attitude, the experience-knowledge-skill of the physician, the diversity and appropriate use of therapeutics (physical, dietary, nutritional, botanical), and lifestyle/ergonomic modifications; importantly, the degree of tissue injury does not always show direct correlation to the severity of the accident or the degree of structural damage to the vehicle(s).
- Limitations of the scope of this section: This section deals with post-traumatic neck pain characteristic of what is typically seen in an out-patient setting; this section does not cover emergency department,

---

[224] Modified from Gatterman MI (Ed.). Chiropractic Management of Spine-Related Disorders. Baltimore: Williams and Wilkins, 1990
[225] Bogduk N. The anatomy and pathophysiology of whiplash. *Clin Biomech* 1986; 1: 92-101
[226] Cisler TA. Whiplash as a total-body injury. *J Am Osteopath Assoc.* 1994 Feb;94(2):145-8
[227] Tarola GA. Whiplash: contemporary considerations in assessment, management, treatment, and prognosis. *JNMS: Journal of the Neuromuscular System* 1993; 1: 156-66

roadside, or "playing field" situations which are typically more severe and more acute. With all conditions described in your texts, articles, and in the course notes, each physician must be sure to consider the balance between what is best for the patient and the physician's own level of knowledge, expertise, and experience. When in doubt, or if the physician is not a specialist in the treatment of a given severe condition, referral is appropriate. These notes are written with the routine "outpatient" in mind and are not tailored to severely injured patients or emergency, "roadside," or "playing field" situations. Consult your First Aid and Emergency Response texts and course materials for additional information; for quick reference, internet sites such as *eMedicine* can provide additional information.[228]

<u>**Complications**</u>:
- Muscle strain (common)
- Ligament sprain (common)
- Intervertebral disc injury, protrusion/herniation with possible resultant radiculopathy or myelopathy
- Brachial plexus injuries, especially with lateral flexion injuries
- Facet joint injury: compression of articular surfaces
- Vertebral fracture (emergency)
- Joint dislocation (emergency)
- Vascular rupture, such as of the vertebral arteries (emergency)
- Nerve injuries, such as of the cervical sympathetic nerves, causing Horner's syndrome
- Segmental dysfunction: commonly reported is the combination of upper and lower cervical hypomobility with mid-cervical hypermobility and distraction injuries[229]
- Concomitant head injury, contusions to brain and spinal cord
- Thoracic outlet syndrome
- Neural and dural adhesions
- Injuries to the low back, hips and feet, and other parts of the body need to be considered and assessed: "**...injury sustained in accidents extends beyond the neck region itself.**"[230]

<u>**Additional considerations**</u>:
- Litigation
- Reinforcement of previous self-perceived victimization
- Secondary gain:
  - The initial onset of symptoms after 72 hours followed by progressive deterioration is unusual and may be viewed with skepticism.[231]
  - Chronicity of symptoms has been reported to be more common in persons with immature or maladaptive coping strategies.[232]
    - Care must also be taken to not disparage the genuine suffering of patients with real injuries.
    - Physicians and patients can both benefit when the physician maintains a demeanor of "compassionate detachment."[Ψ]

<u>**Clinical presentations**</u>:
- Pain: head, neck, shoulder, arm, hands, back...
  - "**If the pain was immediate at the time of a trauma, treat it as a cervical spine fracture until proven otherwise.**"[233]
- Tenderness and swelling of injured tissues

---

[228] Levy D. Neck trauma. Updated June 19, 2006. *eMedicine* http://www.emedicine.com/emerg/topic331.htm Accessed December 23, 2006
[229] Chapter 10 in Gatterman MI (Ed.). <u>Chiropractic Management of Spine-Related Disorders</u>. Baltimore; Williams and Wilkins, 1990.
[230] Cisler TA. Whiplash as a total-body injury. *J Am Osteopath Assoc.* 1994 Feb;94(2):145-8
[231] Tarola GA. Whiplash: contemporary considerations in assessment, management, treatment, and prognosis. *JNMS: Journal of the Neuromusculoskeletal System.* 1993;1:156-66
[232] Tarola GA. Whiplash: contemporary considerations in assessment, management, treatment, and prognosis. *JNMS: Journal of the Neuromusculoskeletal System.* 1993;1:156-66
[Ψ] I coined this phrase to denote the importance of caring for patients without getting "too involved" in their suffering. Excessive pampering and coddling of the patient by the physician is unhealthy for both people involved as it creates dependency and exacerbates symptom amplification by the patient and codependence on the part of the physician.
[233] Pearson JK. A prompt response to acute neck pain. *Patient Care* 1995; February 28: 14-24

- Limited motion
- Segmental dysfunction of the spine and ribs
- Muscle spasm
- Myofascial trigger points
- Thoracic outlet syndrome
- Many other complaints: visual disturbances, disequilibrium, dyscognition
  - Severe/significant disturbances in brain function may require further evaluation for concussion or subdural hematoma. **Following head injury, "Any observed depression of the sensorium should be evaluated with a computed tomographic (CT) scan of the brain..."**[234]

<u>Major differential diagnoses</u>:
- Myelopathy
- Radiculopathy
- Fracture
- Dislocation
- Instability
- Occult pathology or congenital anomalies
- Secondary gain
  - **"The practitioner must readily recognize and deal with those few patients who may not authentically want to recover,** such as the patient who is comfortable with the legal compensation arrangement."[235]

<u>Clinical assessment</u>:
- **Careful history** detailing the mechanisms of injury, positioning, tension, impacts, speeds, restraints/protection, litigation, signs and symptoms, etc.
- **Physical examination** *as appropriate*: muscle testing of the neck and arms and legs and anal sphincter[236], palpation, vibration for sensation and/or as a screen for occult fracture, reflexes, sensory, orthopedic assessments, and assessment of neighboring regions and organs.
- **Assess the degree of** *functional loss* to help assess severity of injury, appropriate interventions, and response to treatment. **Clinical assessment of brain and neurologic function is mandatory** in any patient with whiplash or possible head-cord-nerve injury. Alterations in mental status and/or depression of the sensorium mandate CT/MRI of the brain.[237]
- **Take care not to exacerbate or introduce injury.** Always begin with history, then if appropriate proceed to active patient motion, then if appropriate proceed to neuro-orthopedic assessments. Never perform assertive physical examination procedures in a patient with possible spinal instability or fracture. Always stabilize and image these patients before proceeding to examination or physical treatment.

<u>Imaging & laboratory assessments</u>:
- Laboratory tests are generally not indicated when assessing cervical strain-sprain per se; however, lab evaluation may be used to guide whole-patient care and to exclude comorbid conditions.
- <u>**Strongly consider at least the basic 3-view cervical radiographs**</u>: follow with oblique, flexion-extension views, CT, MRI, bone scan, or other study as indicated.
  - Consider to repeat the original views and/or add new views if pain or immobility persist or if clinical suspicion of fracture is high. Swelling and muscle spasm may initially obscure the detection of clinically significant spinal instability and hypermobility.[238] Fractures that are not visible may become visible after two weeks of callus formation.
  - All spinal fractures, dislocations, or orthopedic subluxations must be visualized with CT and other imaging as indicated.[239]

---

[234] Chiles BW 3rd, Cooper PR. Acute spinal injury. *N Engl J Med* 1996 Feb 22;334(8):514-20
[235] Cisler TA. Whiplash as a total-body injury. *J Am Osteopath Assoc.* 1994 Feb;94(2):145-8
[236] Assessment of the bulbocavernosus reflex and the strength of the anal sphincter are recommended in patients with severe spinal trauma to assess the integrity of the spinal cord and cauda equina. Chiles BW 3rd, Cooper PR. Acute spinal injury. *N Engl J Med* 1996 Feb 22;334(8):514-20
[237] Chiles BW 3rd, Cooper PR. Acute spinal injury. *N Engl J Med* 1996 Feb 22;334(8):514-20
[238] Chiles BW 3rd, Cooper PR. Acute spinal injury. *N Engl J Med* 1996 Feb 22;334(8):514-20
[239] Chiles BW 3rd, Cooper PR. Acute spinal injury. *N Engl J Med* 1996 Feb 22;334(8):514-20

Although criteria for clinically excluding cervical spine fractures have been published,[240] **any patient with neck pain following trauma is a candidate for radiographic evaluation, even when the physical examination is unremarkable.**

- o **The risks and expense associated with radiographic imaging are insignificant compared to the risk and expense associated with failure to diagnose a cervical spine fracture.**
- o Assess for congenital/acquired spinal stenosis.
- o A decrease from the normal cervical lordosis is not necessarily abnormal. However, sharp reversal of cervical lordosis suggests instability and is associated with an unfavorable prognosis.
- o "Dislocations of the cervical spine can be more serious than fractures, because they almost always result in cord compression as well as nerve root compression with loss of motor and sensory function."[241]
- o If a spinal fracture is found, strong consideration should be given to radiographically imaging the entire spine since **up to 17 percent of patients with a spinal fracture in one region will have a spinal fracture in another region.**[242]
- o **High-speed helical CT is more sensitive than plain radiography for detection of fractures and can be used as initial imaging assessment (e.g., prior to plain radiography) in patients with a high probability of spinal injury; patients with multiple injuries and normal plain radiographic and CT studies may still be candidates for MRI to evaluate ligamentous and spinal cord injury.**[243]
- o **Importantly, patients with ligamentous instability following trauma may initially have normal alignment and normal flexion-extension radiographs due to the stabilization provided by muscle spasm; thus a repeat radiographic evaluation for instability should be performed within one week of the initial evaluation in patients suspected of having instability despite an initially normal radiographic series.**[244]

<u>Clinical management</u>:
- Treatment and clinical management must be individualized based on the patient's history and current health, the mechanism of injury, symptoms, examination findings, laboratory, and imaging studies.
- **Treatment must be individualized per patient.**
- Patients with whiplash-type injures must take an active role in their own care with doctor-instructed self-directed home exercises performed at least twice daily. **Active home care**—self-treatment implemented by the patient at home without professional supervision yet under the direction of their healthcare provider—is one of the most important components of an effective treatment plan: "...**minimal practitioner intervention combined with advice on home exercises and to return to usual activities is the best approach for acute whiplash associated disorders.**"[245]
- Patient-implemented exercises performed at home or gym twice or more per day expedite and optimize tissue repair and functional restoration while also empowering the patient to take on the role of active participant rather than helpless victim: "...**the practitioner should aim to make the patient as free of symptoms and as independent of treatment as soon as possible.**"[246]
- Following trauma, early-onset of pain increases the probability of significant tissue injury; immediate-onset pain requires evaluation for fracture, dislocation, and neurovascular injury. Delayed-onset pain is to be expected and is typical of strain-sprain injuries as edema and inflammatory mediators accumulate. Pain typically peaks at 72 hours post-injury.
- Depending on the severity of the injury, the rapidity of healing, and the efficacy of treatment, patients may be biomechanically/physiologically "brittle" for up to 3 months and should be careful to avoid

[240] Graber MA, Kathol M. Cervical spine radiographs in the trauma patient. *Am Fam Physician*. 1999 Jan 15;59(2):331-42
[241] Chapter 10 in Gatterman MI (Ed.). Chiropractic Management of Spine-Related Disorders. Baltimore; Williams and Wilkins, 1990.
[242] Graber MA, Kathol M. Cervical spine radiographs in the trauma patient. *Am Fam Physician*. 1999 Jan 15;59(2):331-42
[243] Shum NT, Magnus W. Cervical strain. Updated June 30, 2006. *eMedicine* http://www.emedicine.com/emerg/topic93.htm Accessed December 23, 2006
[244] Shum NT, Magnus W. Cervical strain. Updated June 30, 2006. *eMedicine* http://www.emedicine.com/emerg/topic93.htm Accessed December 23, 2006
[245] Cassidy JD. Point of view. *Spine* 2000; 25: 1786-7
[246] Cisler TA. Whiplash as a total-body injury. *J Am Osteopath Assoc*. 1994 Feb;94(2):145-8

jarring motions, repetitive strain, and other potentially injurious events until they are pain-free and functionally restored.

- All spinal fractures/dislocations/instability should be immediately co-managed with a specialist: orthopedist or neurosurgeon.
- Evidence of acute spinal cord injury mandates immediate referral for treatment with methylprednisolone, which must be administered within the first 8 hours after injury for optimal outcome. [247]
- Any patient with a recent head-neck injury who demonstrates depressed sensorium must be evaluated with CT/MRI to assess for possible subdural hematoma or other intracranial or brainstem lesion.
- Trauma patients are re-evaluated with orthopedic tests and neurological examination at each visit until they are out of the acute phase and have shown stability over several visits.

<u>Treatment</u>:

- *Medical standard*: According to the 2006 Edition of *Current Medical Diagnosis and Treatment*, medical treatment of whiplash centers on the use of "a cervical collar and administration of analgesics."[248]
- *See overview in Chapter 3, and Therapeutics for Non-specific Neck Pain in this chapter*; additional therapeutic and management considerations are provided below:
- Promote safe driving and proper placement of headrests. **Headrests are only protective against whiplash if they are in contact with the head at the time of impact.**[249]
- Avoid motions and activities that cause significant pain, as pain indicates that damaged/inflamed tissues are being stressed.
- Maintain proper posture and neutral positioning as much as possible.
- The use of soft cervical collars is controversial—generally discouraged—and should be tailored to the patient's needs as appropriate:
  - o <u>Benefits of soft cervical collars</u>:
    - ▪ Support the head and neck thus allowing injured muscle/tendons/ligaments to "rest" and to hurt less;
    - ▪ *Soft* collars allow for some motion and thus allow some *diminished* motion to joints, which are dependent on motion for nutrition and thus healing;
    - ▪ The more rigid cervical collars are indicated for patients with instability/fracture/dislocation until the condition has stabilized and/or is surgically/medically managed.[250]
  - o <u>Disadvantages of cervical collars</u>:
    - ▪ False sense of security, especially with soft collars that do not meet the needs for biomechanical stabilization.
    - ▪ Decreased motion during acute stage may promote motion-limiting adhesions and muscle contracture resulting in limited/abnormal range of motion.
    - ▪ Decreased motion decreases nutrient supply to joints thus inhibiting healing;
    - ▪ Psychologic dependence.
    - ▪ Muscle atrophy and weakness.
  - o <u>Considerations in the use of cervical collars</u>:
    - ▪ The collar should hold the head in an optimal upright position: head straight, neck straight, chin in.
    - ▪ The collar can be used intermittently for 2 weeks following mild-moderate injury: collars are removed to allow motion and are replaced to alleviate pain.

[247] Graber MA, Kathol M. Cervical spine radiographs in the trauma patient. *Am Fam Physician*. 1999 Jan 15;59(2):331-42
[248] Tierney ML. McPhee SJ, Papadakis MA (eds). <u>Current Medical Diagnosis and Treatment 2006, 45th Edition</u>. Lange Medical; page 815
[249] Bogduk N. The anatomy and pathophysiology of whiplash. *Clin Biomech* 1986; 1: 92-101
[250] Clarification/disagreement from Brier (<u>Primary Care Orthopedics</u> page 161) states, "Soft-collar immobilization is appropriate for … clinical instability of the cervical spine." Perhaps Brier means "clinical" (i.e., mild), as opposed to neurologic or orthopedic instability, in which case he might have used the term "hypermobility"; however he does not make this clear. The use of soft-collars can not be considered immobilization such as would be necessary in the case of ligamentous instability, fracture, or dislocation that could result in neurologic compromise—these cases mandate the use of a hard cervical collar. Although a soft collar is better than nothing, it does not provide adequate stabilization for significant post-traumatic "clinical instability of the cervical spine."

- The use of soft collars can not be considered "immobilization" such as would be necessary in the case of ligamentous instability, fracture, or dislocation that could result in neurologic compromise—these cases mandate the use of a hard cervical collar. Although a soft collar is better than nothing, it does not provide adequate stabilization for significant post-traumatic instability of the cervical spine.
  - Selection of the type of collar to use is based on the degree of injury and the goal of the use of the collar:
    - <u>Soft collars</u>: Used for the reduction of pain due to muscular strain and spasm and for mild ligament injuries. These can be used intermittently and are for symptomatic relief only.
    - <u>Rigid/hard collars</u>: Used if with evidence of mild-moderate hypermobility *and no evidence of gross instability or fracture*; patients with this degree of injury should be co-managed with an orthopedist and/or neurologist.
    - <u>Philadelphia collars, shoulder-to-chin collars</u>: Used with instability, dislocations, and fractures; patients with this degree of injury are always co-managed with an orthopedist and/or neurologist.
- Bed rest may be appropriate for 24-72 hours for both physiologic and psychologic reasons. However, prolonged rest and immobility promotes joint degeneration, connective tissue contractures and adhesions, muscle atrophy, and maladaptive proprioceptive responses.
- Prognosis following whiplash is difficult to estimate since objective data such as physical examination findings and radiographic abnormalities do not consistently correlate with long-term outcome[251] and because other factors such as comorbid conditions and secondary gain can influence the long-term outcome.
- Muscle relaxants do not appear to provide benefit in the treatment of "whiplash."
- <u>Acupuncture</u>: Acupuncture may improve proprioceptive/kinesthetic function following whiplash.[252,253]
- **First, do no harm.**
  - <u>Massage</u>: Gentle massage following injury. After the acute phase, deeper massage may help restore range of motion and decrease pain and reduce feeling of vulnerability.
  - <u>Joint mobilization and manipulation</u>: *as appropriate*, only after contraindications have been excluded, and to the level of patient comfort. Manipulation may be contraindicated during the acute phase and when injured and therefore functionally compromised tissues may be stressed or injured further.
  - <u>Gentle manual traction</u>: *use caution not to exacerbate injuries.*
- Treatment of associated muscle spasm and myofascial trigger points can increase range of motion and decrease pain.
- Consider ultrasound and physiotherapy if appropriate.
- Consider using a "neck roll" or rolled towel under neck of supine patient to induce traction and lordosis.
- Modify behavior and home/occupational workstations to minimize strain and stress on injured tissues. Use tools/machines to work efficiently and to reduce unnecessary lifting and straining motions. "Hands off" devices such as speakerphones and telephone headsets will reduce neck strain.

> Double-check to ensure that your patient is safe (no forthcoming complications or predictable emergencies) and that your treatment is safe (appropriate, clearly communicated, and time-limited with return office visit).

- **Supplementation with a high-potency broad-spectrum multivitamin and multimineral product**: will help to treat previous deficiencies and to support optimal healing.
- **Double-check** to ensure that the patient does not have any incipient complications and that the treatment program is generally safe as well as appropriate for the individual patient, his/her concomitant health problems and any medications.

---

[251] Tarola GA. Whiplash: contemporary considerations in assessment, management, treatment, and prognosis. *JNMS: J Neuromusculoskeletal System* 1993;1:156-66

[252] "We observed a significant difference between the two groups regarding the reduction of the CER Length of the statokinesigram just before each session of acupuncture and reduction of the frequency oscillations (FFT) of the patients on the sagittal plane in the study group, in CER..." Fattori B, Borsari C, Vannucci G, Casani A, Cristofani R, Bonuccelli L, Ghilardi PL. Acupuncture treatment for balance disorders following whiplash injury. *Acupunct Electrother Res.* 1996;21:207-17

[253] "The high percentage of positive results in whiplash injury patients leads us to advocate acupuncture for balance disorders due to cervical pathology." Fattori B, Ursino F, Cingolani C, Bruschini L, Dallan I, Nacci A. Acupuncture treatment of whiplash injury. *Int Tinnitus J.* 2004;10(2):156-60

Torticollis, "Wryneck"

Description/pathophysiology: Functional rotational deformity of the head/neck; most commonly unilateral.
1. Congenital: Often due to injury to the sternocleidomastoid (SCM) at birth with resultant shortening and fibrosis of the injured SCM, leading to cervical flexion, cervical rotation, head extension, and limited motion. May also be secondary to osseous vertebral deformity.[254]
2. Acquired: May follow cervical injury, URI, or exposure to cold.
3. Functional: May follow sleeping in awkward position, poor posture, etc.
4. Pathologic: May be secondary to occult pathology, such as parapharyngeal abscess, osteomyelitis or cancer.[255,256]
5. Spasmodic: Spontaneous intermittent or persistent torticollis caused by neuromuscular dysfunction; resistant to conservative treatment; often requires surgical nerve section.

Complications:
- Pain
- Cosmetic deformity
- Reduced range of motion
- Reduced quality of life

Clinical presentations:
- Spasm/contracture of the SCM with resultant cervical flexion, head extension, contralateral rotation, and ipsilateral lateral flexion of the head/neck

Major differential diagnoses:
- Neuromuscular disease
- Abscess, infection
- Fibrous tumor (in congenital torticollis)
- Malignancy

Clinical assessment:
- History: ask about recent injury, illness, weight loss, fever, pharyngitis, and other clues
- Physical examination: identity problems and rule out pathologies per patient

Imaging & laboratory assessments:
- Should be normal—otherwise find and treat the problem

Clinical management:
- Based on the history and physical examination, the doctor will determine the need for laboratory tests and imaging assessments
- If patient does not respond to treatment, perform additional assessments, modify the treatment plan, and consider referral
- Rule out underlying pathology
- Identify and treat the underlying cause; referral if necessary

Treatment for simple muscular torticollis:
- Massage
- Moist heat
- Stretching of contracted muscles/tissues
- Manipulation and mobilization
- Postural correction

---

[254] Brougham DI, Cole WG, Dickens DR, Menelaus MB. Torticollis due to a combination of sternomastoid contracture and congenital vertebral anomalies. *J Bone Joint Surg Br*. 1989 May;71(3):404-7

[255] "The most common causes were upper respiratory infection, sinusitis, otomastoiditis, cervical adenitis, and retropharyngeal abscess or cellulitis. Four patients had subluxation of the atlantoaxial joint... Children with acute torticollis need careful evaluation for either overt or occult otolaryngologic infections. Computed tomography and magnetic resonance imaging are helpful..." Bredenkamp JK, Maceri DR. Inflammatory torticollis in children. *Arch Otolaryngol Head Neck Surg*. 1990 Mar;116(3):310-3

[256] "In children there is often an association between acute torticollis and retropharyngeal cellulitis/abscess." Harries PG. Retropharyngeal abscess and acute torticollis. *J Laryngol Otol*. 1997 Dec;111(12):1183-5

Vertebral Osteomyelitis
Infectious Discitis

"Up to 10-15% of patients with vertebral osteomyelitis will develop neurologic findings or frank spinal-cord compression."

King RW, Johnson D. Osteomyelitis. Updated July 13, 2006. *eMedicine* http://www.emedicine.com/emerg/topic349.htm Accessed December 2006

Description/pathophysiology:
- Bacterial or fungal infection of the spine
- Back pain is common; spinal infection is relatively rare. Spinal infections are "a rare cause of common symptoms."[257]

Clinical presentations:
- Classic presentation: "...the diagnosis is suggested by the clinical findings: a sick patient with severe pain, a rigid back, fever, and a raised WBC and sedimentation rate."[258]
    - Patient generally appears sick with systemic manifestations: fatigue, sweats, anorexia, fever
    - Back/neck/spine pain (90%): Most common region for spinal osteomyelitis is the lumbar spine, followed by the thoracic spine, then the cervical spine. Cervical spine infections are more common in IV drug abusers.
    - Pain may be acute, subacute, or chronic:
        - 30% of patients with vertebral osteomyelitis have had pain for 3 weeks to 3 months at time of diagnosis.
        - 50% of patients with vertebral osteomyelitis have had pain for more than 3 months at time of diagnosis.
    - Pain is continuous, intermittent, and/or "throbbing" and often worse at night
    - Pain is unrelated to motion or position (non-mechanical)
    - Localized stiffness
    - Elevated ESR/CRP
- Atypical presentations: as many as 15% of affected patients
    - Little or no fever
    - Little or no back or neck pain
    - Little or no local tenderness
    - Cervical osteomyelitis may present with headache, dysphagia, sore throat rather than febrile neck pain
    - Vertebral osteomyelitis of the thoracic and lumbar spine may present with pain in the chest, shoulder, abdominal, hip or leg.
    - Risk factors: IV drug use, DM, history of septicemia, spinal trauma, pulmonary tuberculosis, urinary tract infections, surgery, older men

Major differential diagnoses:
- Benign neck or back pain
- Degenerative disc disease
- Tumor
- Fracture
- Spondyloarthropathies: In particular, reactive arthritis is a difficult differential in this situation because of the concomitant infection (perhaps with fever and systemic symptoms) and back pain. Differentiation may be difficult, but is generally possible based on the severity of the systemic manifestations and local examination findings. Patients with *focal pain*—particularly that which is exacerbated by vertebral percussion—should be further evaluated/treated for osteomyelitis.

[257] Strausbaugh LJ. Vertebral osteomyelitis. How to differentiate it from other causes of back and neck pain. *Postgrad Med* 1995 Jun;97(6):147-8, 151-4
[258] Macnab I, McCulloch J. Backache. Second Edition. Williams and Wilkins: Baltimore, 1990

Clinical assessment:
- **History/subjective:**
  - o Spinal pain
  - o Malaise: may or may not have systemic symptoms
- **Physical examination/objective:**
  - o Mild local tenderness
  - o Paravertebral muscle spasm with limited ROM
  - o Fever (50%)
  - o Neurologic signs (20-40%)
  - o Spinal percussion is positive for pain
  - o May have painful and limited SLR due to hamstring spasm
- **Imaging & laboratory assessments:**
  - o High ESR—elevated to 20-100 mm/hr in 90% of patients. ESR was considered "the most useful test for monitoring the disease activity and the efficacy of treatment." [259]
  - o 50% have slight elevation of WBC.
  - o The disc space is the first structure destroyed—the clinician and radiologist must not misinterpret early signs of infection with "degenerative disc disease."
  - o **MRI has a sensitivity and specificity of >90% and also helps to assess epidural abscess.**
  - o Radiographs are positive in 80% after the condition has been present for at least 10-14 days.
  - o Bone scan is diagnostic in 90% of cases.
  - o "Computed tomography is the imaging study of choice for preoperative evaluation and biopsy procedures. It is not a good screening test..."[260] and is generally used after routine radiographs and/or bone scan.

Establishing the diagnosis:
- Diagnosis is established based on a consistent spectrum of clinical signs and symptoms and is confirmed with imaging and/or biopsy, aspiration, and/or blood cultures

Complications:
- Abscesses
- Meningitis
- Vertebral collapse, fracture
- Neurologic injury: paralysis
- Septicemia and death

Clinical management:
- Immediate/urgent referral for diagnostic procedures, IV and oral antimicrobials, and surgery if needed.

Treatments:
- **Antimicrobial drugs: Organism-specific IV/oral antimicrobials are generally administered on an in-patient basis.**
- Rest: Bed rest, bracing, activity limitation
- Surgery: Surgery for debridement and complications such as cord compression, vertebral collapse or instability.
- **Immunonutrition:** Immunonutritional considerations are listed below; doses listed are for adults. Although studies have not been performed specifically in patients with bone/joint infections, general benefits derived from the use of immunonutrition are reductions in severity/frequency/duration of major infections, abbreviated hospitalization (i.e., early discharge due to expedited healing and recovery), reductions in the need for medications, significant improvements in survival, and hospital savings.[261,262,263,264,265,266,267]

[259] Macnab I, McCulloch J. Backache. Second Edition. Williams and Wilkins: Baltimore, 1990

[260] Strausbaugh LJ. Vertebral osteomyelitis. How to differentiate it from other causes of back and neck pain. Postgrad Med 1995 Jun;97(6):147-8, 151-4

[261] "To evaluate the metabolic and immune effects of dietary arginine, glutamine and omega-3 fatty acids (fish oil) supplementation, we performed a prospective study... CONCLUSIONS: The feeding of Neomune in critically injured patients was well tolerated as Traumacal and significant improvement was observed in serum protein. Shorten ICU stay and wean-off respirator day may benefit from using the immunonutrient formula." Chuntrasakul C, Siltham S, Sarasombath S, Sittapairochana C, Leowattana W, Chockvivatanavanit S, Bunnak A. Comparison of a immunonutrition formula enriched arginine, glutamine and omega-3 fatty acid, with a currently high-enriched enteral nutrition for trauma patients. J Med Assoc Thai. 2003 Jun;86(6):552-6

[262] "CONCLUSIONS: In conclusion, arginine-enhanced formula improves fistula rates in postoperative head and neck cancer patients and decreases length of stay." de Luis DA, Izaola O, Cuellar L, Terroba MC, Aller R. Randomized clinical trial with an enteral arginine-enhanced formula in early postsurgical head and neck cancer patients. Eur J Clin Nutr. 2004;58(11):1505-8

- o Paleo-Mediterranean diet: As detailed later in this text and elsewhere.[268,269]
- o Vitamin and mineral supplementation: Anti-infective benefits shown in elderly diabetics.[270]
- o High-dose vitamin A: Vitamin A shows potent immunosupportive benefits, and vitamin A stores are depleted by the stress of infection and injury. Consider 200,000-300,000 IU per day of retinol palmitate for 1-4 weeks, then taper; reduce dose or discontinue with onset of toxicity symptoms such as skin problems (dry skin, flaking skin, chapped or split lips, red skin rash, hair loss), joint pain, bone pain, headaches, anorexia (loss of appetite), edema (water retention, weight gain, swollen ankles, difficulty breathing), fatigue, and/or liver damage.
- o Arginine: Dose for adults is in the range of 5-10 grams daily.
- o Fatty acid supplementation: In contrast to the higher doses used to provide an anti-inflammatory effect in patients with autoimmune/inflammatory disorders, doses used for immunosupportive treatments should be kept rather modest to avoid the *relative* immunosuppression that has been controversially reported in patients treated with EPA and DHA. Reasonable doses are in the following ranges for adults: EPA+DHA: 500-1,500, and GLA: 300-500 mg.
- o Glutamine: **Glutamine enhances bacterial killing by neutrophils**[271], and **administration of 18 grams per day in divided doses to patients in intensive care units was shown to improve survival, expedite hospital discharge, and reduce total healthcare costs.**[272] Another study using glutamine 12-18 grams per day showed no benefit in overall mortality but significant benefits in terms of reduced healthcare costs (-30%) and significantly reduced need for medical interventions.[273] After administering glutamine 26 grams/d to severely burned patients, Garrel et al[274] concluded that **glutamine reduced the risk of infection by 3-fold and that oral glutamine "may be a life-saving intervention" in patients with severe burns**. A dose of 30 grams/d was used in a recent clinical trial showing hemodynamic benefit in patients with sickle cell anemia.[275] The highest glutamine dose that the current author is aware of is the

---

[263] "In this prospective, randomised, double-blind, placebo-controlled study, we randomly assigned 50 patients who were scheduled to undergo coronary artery bypass to receive either an oral immune-enhancing nutritional supplement containing L-arginine, omega3 polyunsaturated fatty acids, and yeast RNA (n=25), or a control (n=25) for a minimum of 5 days... Intake of an oral immune-enhancing nutritional supplement for a minimum of 5 days before surgery can improve outlook in high-risk patients who are undergoing elective cardiac surgery." Tepaske R, Velthuis H, Oudemans-van Straaten HM, Heisterkamp SH, van Deventer SJ, Ince C, Eysman L, Kesecioglu J. Effect of preoperative oral immune-enhancing nutritional supplement on patients at high risk of infection after cardiac surgery: a randomised placebo-controlled trial. *Lancet*. 2001 Sep 1;358(9283):696-701

[264] "The feeding of IMMUNE FORMULA was well tolerated and significant improvement was observed in nutritional and immunologic parameters as in other immunoenhancing diets. Further clinical trials of prospective double-blind randomized design are necessary to address the so that the necessity of using immunonutrition in critically ill patients will be clarified." Chuntrasakul C, Siltharm S, Sarasombath S, Sittapairochana C, Leowattana W, Chockvivatanavanit S, Bunnak A. Metabolic and immune effects of dietary arginine, glutamine and omega-3 fatty acids supplementation in immunocompromised patients. *J Med Assoc Thai*. 1998 May;81(5):334-43

[265] "enteral diet supplemented with arginine, dietary nucleotides, and omega-3 fatty acids (IMPACT, Sandoz Nutrition, Bern, Switzerland) " Senkal M, Mumme A, Eickhoff U, Geier B, Spath G, Wulfert D, Joosten U, Frei A, Kemen M. Early postoperative enteral immunonutrition: clinical outcome and cost-comparison analysis in surgical patients. *Crit Care Med* 1997;25(9):1489-96

[266] "supplemented diet with glutamine, arginine and omega-3-fatty acids... It was clearly established in this trial that early postoperative enteral feeding is safe in patients who have undergone major operations for gastrointestinal cancer. Supplementation of enteral nutrition with glutamine, arginine, and omega-3-fatty acids positively modulated postsurgical immunosuppressive and inflammatory responses." Wu GH, Zhang YW, Wu ZH. Modulation of postoperative immune and inflammatory response by immune-enhancing enteral diet in gastrointestinal cancer patients. *World J Gastroenterol*. 2001 Jun;7(3):357-62 http://www.wjgnet.com/1007-9327/7/357.pdf

[267] "using a formula supplemented with arginine, mRNA, and omega-3 fatty acids from fish oil (Impact)... CONCLUSIONS: Immune-enhancing enteral nutrition resulted in a significant reduction in the mortality rate and infection rate in septic patients admitted to the ICU. These reductions were greater for patients with less severe illness." Galban C, Montejo JC, Mesejo A, Marco P, Celaya S, Sanchez-Segura JM, Farre M, Bryg DJ. An immune-enhancing enteral diet reduces mortality rate and episodes of bacteremia in septic intensive care unit patients. *Crit Care Med*. 2000 Mar;28(3):643-8

[268] Vasquez A. A Five-Part Nutritional Protocol that Produces Consistently Positive Results. *Nutritional Wellness* 2005 September http://www.nutritionalwellness.com/archives/2005/sep/09_vasquez.php

[269] Vasquez A. Implementing the Five-Part Nutritional Wellness Protocol for the Treatment of Various Health Problems. *Nutritional Wellness* 2005 November. http://www.nutritionalwellness.com/archives/2005/nov/11_vasquez.php

[270] "CONCLUSIONS: A multivitamin and mineral supplement reduced the incidence of participant-reported infection and related absenteeism in a sample of participants with type 2 diabetes mellitus and a high prevalence of subclinical micronutrient deficiency." Barringer TA, Kirk JK, Santaniello AC, Foley KL, Michielutte R. Effect of a multivitamin and mineral supplement on infection and quality of life. A randomized, double-blind, placebo-controlled trial. *Ann Intern Med*. 2003 Mar 4;138(5):365-71 http://www.annals.org/cgi/reprint/138/5/365

[271] Furukawa S, Saito H, Fukatsu K, Hashiguchi Y, Inaba T, Lin MT, Inoue T, Han I, Matsuda T, Muto T. Glutamine-enhanced bacterial killing by neutrophils from postoperative patients. *Nutrition* 1997;13(10):863-9. *In vitro* study.

[272] Griffiths RD, Jones C, Palmer TE. Six-month outcome of critically ill patients given glutamine-supplemented parenteral nutrition. *Nutrition* 1997 Apr;13(4):295-302

[273] "There was no mortality difference between those patients receiving glutamine-containing enteral feed and the controls. However, there was a significant reduction in the median postintervention ICU and hospital patient costs in the glutamine recipients $23 000 versus $30 900 in the control patients." Jones C, Palmer TE, Griffiths RD. Randomized clinical outcome study of critically ill patients given glutamine-supplemented enteral nutrition. *Nutrition*. 1999 Feb;15(2):108-15

[274] The glutamine dose in this study was "a total of 26 g/day" administered in four divided doses. CONCLUSION: "The results of this prospective randomized clinical trial show that enteral G reduces blood culture positivity, particularly with P. aeruginosa, in adults with severe burns and may be a life-saving intervention." Garrel D, Patenaude J, Nedelec B, Samson L, Dorais J, Champoux J, D'Elia M, Bernier J. Decreased mortality and infectious morbidity in adult burn patients given enteral glutamine supplements: a prospective, controlled, randomized clinical trial. *Crit Care Med*. 2003 Oct;31(10):2444-9

[275] Niihara Y, Matsui NM, Shen YM, Akiyama DA, Johnson CS, Sunga MA, Magpayo J, Embury SH, Kalra VK, Cho SH, Tanaka KR. L-glutamine therapy reduces endothelial adhesion of sickle red blood cells to human umbilical vein endothelial cells. *BMC Blood Disord*. 2005 Jul 25;5:4 http://www.biomedcentral.com.proxy.hsc.unt.edu/1471-2326/5/4

study by Scheltinga et al[276] who used 0.57 gm/kg/day in cancer patients following chemotherapy administration; for a 220-lb-pt, this would be approximately 57 grams of glutamine per day.

o <u>Melatonin</u>: 20-40 mg hs (*hora somni*—Latin: sleep time). Immunostimulatory anti-infective action of melatonin was demonstrated in a small clinical trial wherein **septic newborns administered 20 mg melatonin showed significantly increased survival over nontreated controls.**[277]

---

[276] "Subjects with hematologic malignancies in remission underwent a standard treatment of high-dose chemotherapy and total body irradiation before bone marrow transplantation. After completion of this regimen, they were randomized to receive either standard parenteral nutrition (STD, n = 10) or an isocaloric, isonitrogenous nutrient solution enriched with crystalline L-glutamine (0.57 g/kg/day, GLN, n = 10)." Scheltinga MR, Young LS, Benfell K, Bye RL, Ziegler TR, Santos AA, Antin JH, Schloerb PR, Wilmore DW. Glutamine-enriched intravenous feedings attenuate extracellular fluid expansion after a standard stress. *Ann Surg.* 1991 Oct;214(4):385-93; discussion 393-5 http://www.pubmedcentral.nih.gov/articlerender.fcgi?tool=pubmed&pubmedid=1953094 For additional review, see Ziegler TR. Glutamine supplementation in cancer patients receiving bone marrow transplantation and high dose chemotherapy. J Nutr. 2001 Sep;131(9 Suppl):2578S-84S http://jn.nutrition.org/cgi/content/full/131/9/2578S

[277] Gitto E, Karbownik M, Reiter RJ, Tan DX, Cuzzocrea S, Chiurazzi P, Cordaro S, Corona G, Trimarchi G, Barberi I. Effects of melatonin treatment in septic newborns. *Pediatr Res.* 2001 Dec;50(6):756-60 http://www.pedresearch.org/cgi/content/full/50/6/756

Additional orthopedic problems of the cervical spine

Problem & presentation	Assessment & Management
Atlantoaxial instability: excess mobility between the atlas and axis (commonly due to lesion of the dens or transverse ligament) makes the spinal cord vulnerable to compressive injury when the atlas translates anteriorly on the axis especially during cervical flexion; may progress to neurologic compromise including paralysis • Os odontoidium: congenital failure of ossification of the dens such that the osseous tip of the dens is connected to the body of C2 by connective tissue rather than bone • Agenesis or hypoplasia of the dens (odontoid process): the dens may be too short or completely absent • Fracture of the odontoid: fracture of the dens may occur after cervical or head trauma • Rupture of the transverse ligament of the atlas at the axis: this may occur after trauma but is more commonly seen in patients with inflammatory arthropathy, especially rheumatoid arthritis • Down's syndrome: patients with Down's syndrome have a high prevalence of atlantoaxial and atlantooccipital instability, especially due to os odontoidium and dens hypoplasia	• Clinical suspicion is followed by lateral cervical and APOM (anteroposterior open mouth) radiographs to assess ADI (atlantodental interval) and dens • MRI should be performed in patients with suspected myelopathy • Neurologic examination of the upper and lower extremities • Do not force neck flexion; do not perform the Soto-Hall test • Onset of myelopathy or recent fracture mandates referral to ER and/or neurosurgeon; immobilize with spine board or hard cervical collar and transport appropriately • Surgical correction of atlantoaxial instability is the best option for the prevention of neurologic deficits[278] • Patients with atlantoaxial or atlantooccipital instability are at increased risk of serious neurologic compromise following minor cervical trauma and should therefore avoid contact sports and other activities that increase the risk for head and neck trauma
Klippel-Feil Syndrome: defined as congenital fusion of two or more cervical vertebrae; malformations of the urinary tract and lumbar spine are also seen. Less than 50% of patients with this syndrome show the classic clinical triad of short neck, low hairline, and restricted neck motion. Chronic neck pain and headaches are a common presentation of this disorder	• **Cervical spine exam with neurologic exam** • **Radiographs of the cervical spine are essential** to assess for malformed vertebrae and vertebral fusion • Obtain radiographs of the lumbar spine before performing lumbar spinal manipulation • Educate patient about the condition and emphasize the importance of avoiding cervical trauma and contact sports: *"As persons with Klippel-Feil syndrome may be at increased risk of sustaining a neurologic deficit in the setting of spinal stenosis after minor trauma, they should be provided appropriate guidance to alter their behavior if they experience an episode of neurologic compromise."*[279] • Low-velocity low-amplitude spinal manipulation to the levels above and below anomalous vertebrae was used in conjunction with physiotherapy (diathermy and ultrasound) to reduce chronic symptomatology in a single case report[280] • Referral for orthopedic evaluation is recommended

[278] Moon MS, Choi WT, Moon YW, Moon JL, Kim SS. Brooks' posterior stabilization surgery for atlantoaxial instability: review of 54 cases. *J Orthop Surg* (Hong Kong). 2002 Dec;10(2):160-4.

[279] Vaidyanathan S, Hughes PL, Soni BM, Singh G, Sett P. Klippel-Feil syndrome - the risk of cervical spinal cord injury: a case report. *BMC Fam Pract.* 2002;3(1):6

[280] Chorny SB, Smith RP, Matheny DA. Clinical management of multiple congenital spinal anomalies: a case report. *Chiropractic Technique* 1993; 5: 65-67

INTEGRATIVE ORTHOPEDICS – THIRD EDITION

Chapter 6:
Thoracic spine, ribs, and chest wall

Introduction
The thoracic cage is a biomechanically complex region comprised of almost innumerable muscles, fascial planes, articulations, important arteries and veins, and dermatomes—all of which overlie important visceral structures such as the heart, lungs, arteriovenous structures, lymphatics, and upper abdominal viscera. When the patient presents with complaints involving the thoracic spine, ribs, and chest wall, the clinician's chief tasks are the exclusion of underlying visceral disease, identification of the painful structures, and provision of effective treatment.

- **Assessments and differential diagnoses**
- **Thoracic spine**
  - Scoliosis
  - Vertebral osteomyelitis
  - Thoracic and thoracolumbar compression fractures
  - Thoracic disc herniation
  - Scheuermann's disease
  - Thoracic segmental dysfunction
  - T4 syndrome
- **Rib cage and chest wall**
  - Costochondritis: Tietze's syndrome
  - Intercostal strain
  - Intercostal neuralgia
  - Rib fracture
  - Pectoralis muscle strain
  - Rib subluxation, costovertebral syndrome
- **Lungs**
  - Pleurisy & Pleuritis

Key Concepts and Core Competencies:

- Work through the following cases to determine the top diagnostic considerations and the proper assessment and management of each differential diagnoses:
  1. In a patient with fever and focal back pain exacerbated by spinal percussion, what is the most likely diagnosis and how will you assess/manage this problem?
  2. If the back pain were not midline, but rather unilateral at the lower costovertebral junction, what would be the most obvious diagnostic consideration and its appropriate assessment and treatment?
  3. Pain in the midline anterior chest wall during exertion and relieved by rest in an overweight middle-aged smoker with acute elevation of serum AST, ALT, and CRP.
  4. Pain in the midline anterior chest wall during exertion and relieved by rest in a young athlete who demonstrates palpatory point tenderness.
  5. Unilateral pain in the anterolateral chest wall in a dermatomal distribution preceded by paresthesia and hypersensitivity and followed by a erythematous blistering rash in a dermatomal distribution along the rib.
- How do you differentiate chest/back pain resulting from a "benign" musculoskeletal condition from pain that is a manifestation of intrathoracic pathology?
- Since "chest pain" and "back pain" can be the clinical presentations of many conditions—some benign, others lethal—clearly we need to have a thorough understanding of how to assess the thorax and to render proper care or referral. History and physical examination are essential, and a chest radiograph is commonly ordered if the doctor has suspicion of lung disease (e.g., pneumonia, pneumothorax, atelectasis) or other intra-thoracic pathology (e.g., mediastinal lymphadenopathy in lymphoma). The most common and important challenge in dealing with pain in the chest and thoracic wall is in the distinction between benign musculoskeletal pain and viscerosomatic pain referral from underlying cardiac, circulatory, pulmonary, hepatobiliary, pancreatic, infectious, or malignant disease.
- Even if a doctor is specializing in "musculoskeletal medicine", he/she must have the clinical diagnostic skills to determine when the presentation of what appears to be musculoskeletal pain is actually the presentation of underlying pathology—bone infection, bone cancer, lymphoma, cardiovascular disease, or pulmonary disease such as pneumonia.

Thoracic spine, ribs, and chest wall: diagnostic and clinical considerations

	DDX Category	Examples
V	Vascular	Dissecting aortic aneurysm
	Visceral referral	Angina
		Pancreatic disease/cancer
		Pulmonary embolism
		Cholecystitis
I	Infectious	Empyema, pneumonia, lung infections
	Inflammatory	Ankylosing spondylitis
	Immunologic	Lymphoma
		Bone/ tissue infections
		Pleurisy
		Gastroesophageal reflux
N	Neurologic	Metastatic disease
	Nutritional	Primary bone tumors
	New growth: neoplasia or pregnancy	Multiple myeloma
		Herpes zoster
D	Deficiency	Degenerative joint/spine disease
	Degenerative	Congenital malformations of bones/ viscera
	Developmental	Scoliosis
		Postural syndromes
		Scheuermann's disease
I	Iatrogenic (drug related)	Drug reactions
	Intoxication	
	Idiosyncratic	
C	Congenital	Myocardial infarction
	Cardiac or circulatory	Cardiac disease: valve disease, etc.
		Congenital malformations of bones/ viscera
A	Allergy	Ankylosing spondylitis
	Autoimmune	Fractures, injuries
	Abuse	
T	Trauma	Fractures, injuries to vertebrae, ribs, muscles
E	Endocrine	Hypothyroidism
	Exposure	Asbestosis, mesothelioma
S	Subluxation	Segmental dysfunction of spine and ribs
	Structural	Muscle tension
	Stress	Costochondritis
	Secondary gain	
M	Mental	Lung tumors
	Malpractice compensation	Anxiety
	Mental disorder	Preexisting injury or disease
	Malignancy	Secondary gain
	Metabolic disease	
	Malingering	

Clinical assessments for the thoracic spine, ribs, and chest wall

Selected assessments[1]	Positive finding and Implications
1. <u>History</u>	<ul><li><u>S</u>ystemic symptoms and signs</li><li><u>C</u>omplications</li><li><u>I</u>ndicators from the history (trauma, risk factors)</li><li><u>Non-mechanical</u> pain</li></ul> **Positive findings in the history suggest increased risk for serious pathology and potential complications. Obtain laboratory and imaging studies as indicated. Defer or modify physical examination based on your assessment of the situation.**
2. <u>Cervical spine regional assessment</u> *if indicated*:	<ul><li>trauma to the thoracic spine necessitates evaluation of the cervical spine for associated injuries</li><li>*See Cervical Spine and Neck notes*</li></ul>
3. <u>General observation</u>: appearance and posture	Abnormalities and asymmetries may indicate:<ul><li>Scoliosis</li><li>Shoulder girdle deformity/asymmetry</li><li>Hyperkyphosis: compression fracture, osteoporosis, Scheuermann's disease, poor posture</li></ul>
4. <u>Active patient rage of motion</u>: (ROM), extension, flexion, rotation, side bending	Decreased or painful ROM or asymmetry may be caused by:<ul><li>Muscle spasm, contracture</li><li>Scoliosis</li><li>Soft tissue contracture</li><li>Disc herniation, disc inflammation</li><li>Fracture: vertebra, rib</li></ul>
5. <u>Assessment of the sternum</u>: this is only necessary in patients with chest pain	<ul><li>Abnormalities and asymmetries include pectus excavatum, pectus carinatum, fracture, or infection</li></ul>
6. <u>Spinal percussion</u>[2]	<ul><li><u>**Deep and intense pain with percussion of the spine with a reflex hammer or with the fingertips**</u>**: Strongly consider obtaining radiographs or other imaging in any patient with exacerbation of pain following spinal percussion, as this indicates the possibility of a bone lesion: spinal fracture, spinal tumor, or vertebral osteomyelitis. Other considerations are herniated disc and joint or ligament injury**</li></ul>
7. <u>Rib/sternum percussion</u>: percussion of the rib or sternum with a reflex hammer	<ul><li>Intense pain in the rib following benign percussion with a reflex hammer or with the fingertips suggests a rib fracture or costochondral or costovertebral sprain: correlate the location of pain with the anatomical structures that are likely involved and the mechanism of injury</li></ul>
8. <u>Tuning fork</u>: 128 Hz tuning fork is placed near suspected fracture location *on the bone*	<ul><li>Pain with vibration suggests a fractured or broken rib</li></ul>

---

[1] Review relevant information in Magee DJ. <u>Orthopedic Physical Assessment. Third edition</u>. Philadelphia: WB Saunders, 1997 and Bates B. <u>A Guide to Physical Examination and History Taking. 6th Edition</u>. Philadelphia; J. B. Lippincott Company, 1995
[2] Gatterman MI (Ed.). <u>Chiropractic Management of Spine-Related Disorders</u>. Baltimore; Williams and Wilkins, 1990. page 187. Clinicians need to remember that the characteristics of the pain pattern seen with spinal percussion are not diagnostic (i.e., dull versus acute pain; rapid or slow relief of pain following the percussion). The finding of ***any*** pain with benign spinal percussion is abnormal and mandates investigation.

Clinical assessments for the thoracic spine, ribs, and chest wall—*continued*

Selected assessments	*Positive finding and Implications*
9. **Sternal compression**: patient supine, doctor places firm pressure on the sternum	▪ Pain in the ribs distant from the site of compression suggests rib fracture
10. **Assessment of the lungs and heart**[3]	▪ **Abnormalities include decreased breath sounds, fremitus, rhonchi, rales, crepitus, clicks, murmurs, etc. and suggest pathology/abnormality of the lungs or heart**
11. **Chest wall expansion**: assessed with tape measure (around 4th intercostal space), or with doctor's hands on thoracolumbar region during patient's inspiration	Normal excursion at the 4th intercostal space is 1.5 – 3 inches. Reduced excursion or asymmetry requires assessment for: ▪ Ankylosing spondylitis ▪ Lung pathology ▪ Paralysis of diaphragm or intercostal nerves ▪ Scoliosis
12. **Neurologic assessment**: strength, sensation, reflexes	▪ Weakness, spasticity, loss of function, loss of sensation, hyporeflexia, or hyperreflexia suggest neurologic compromise at the cord, nerve root, or peripheral nerve or may indicate muscle disease such as myopathy or muscle injury
13. **Palpation**: ribs, spine, scapula, muscles	▪ Pain, mass, or enlargement may indicate any of several problems: functional/biomechanical subluxation, abscess, muscle spasm, fracture, tumor, etc
14. **Motion palpation**: thoracic spine and ribs	▪ Hypermobility and/or hypomobility are seen with segmental dysfunction, degenerative changes, and congenital anomalies. ▪ Functional musculoskeletal disorders are treated with mobilization, massage, myofascial techniques, and manipulation of ribs and spine
15. **Assessment of neighboring regions**: functional-anatomical-biomechanical relationships	▪ Altered lumbar or pelvic biomechanics may contribute to lumbar, thoracic, and cervical dysfunction by altering the "foundation" upon which the spinal column stands
16. **Adam's test**: patient is standing and then bends forward at the waist; doctor observes from behind or in front to look for asymmetry of rib heights characteristic of the asymmetry and spinal twisting of scoliosis	▪ Asymmetric "rib hump" suggests angular rotation and structural changes consistent with scoliosis
17. **Imaging**: radiographs are routine for patients with pain after trauma and when underlying disease is suspected	Abnormal radiographs may demonstrate: ▪ Cancer ▪ Ankylosing spondylitis ▪ Scoliosis ▪ Pneumonia ▪ Pneumothorax, atelectasis ▪ Mediastinal lymphadenopathy ▪ Fracture ▪ Infection ▪ Other imaging assessments may also be used such as MRI, CT, and bone scan depending on the type of lesion that is suspected

---

[3] Cardiopulmonary examinations are detailed in Bates B. A Guide to Physical Examination and History Taking. 6th Edition. Philadelphia; J. B. Lippincott Company, 1995 and in Beers MH, Berkow R (eds). The Merck Manual. Seventeenth Edition. Whitehouse Station; Merck Research Laboratories 1999

Scoliosis

<u>Description/pathophysiology</u>:

1. **Idiopathic scoliosis**: Approximately 90% of all scoliosis has no known cause. Idiopathic scoliosis is primarily characterized by progressive lateral curvatures of the spinal column with resultant compensatory musculoskeletal changes, pulmonary compromise, and biomechanical stress. This appears to be a disorder of neuromuscular coordination rather than a primary structural disorder because the development and shape of the spinal elements—discs and vertebrae—are normal. Family history of scoliosis is present in up to 30%. Neurologic abnormalities including morphologic abnormalities in the brain stem and altered proprioception, posture, and equilibrium have been reported[4] along with perturbations in platelets, muscle tissue, collagen synthesis, and melatonin secretion.[5,6] These findings indicate that scoliosis is much more than a "spine problem"—it is a poorly understood *systemic condition* with *manifestations in the spine*.

2. **Idiopathic infantile scoliosis**: a generally mild form with a spontaneous resolution rate of 70%.[7]

3. **Congenital scoliosis due to spinal malformation**: (up to 7%); due to abnormalities in the formation of the spine, such as malformed vertebrae. Concomitant renal, cardiac, and genitourinary abnormalities are common.

4. **Neuromuscular scoliosis**: due to disorders of the nervous system and/or muscles.

5. **Pathologic scoliosis**: pathologic changes in the bones (e.g., osteoid osteoma), nerves, or muscles of the spinal column can result in a secondary scoliosis.

<u>Complications</u>:

- Cardiopulmonary insufficiency
- Pain due to degenerative changes in adults
- Skeletal-cosmetic deformity
- Social awkwardness and isolation
- Curves of greater than 60 degrees are associated with reduced life expectancy[8]

<u>Clinical presentations</u>:

- Patients with mild idiopathic scoliosis are often asymptomatic or have "normal" complaints. Scoliosis is often detected during routine examinations performed for other purposes
- Patients with more severe disease are generally aware of their condition and may have the aforementioned complications

<u>Major differential diagnoses</u>:

- Pathologic causes include cancer, osteoid osteoma, neuromusculoskeletal disease, neurofibromatosis, Marfan's syndrome, cerebral palsy, muscular dystrophy, polio, myelodysplasia[9]
- Structural causes include leg length inequality, and vertebral or pelvic malformation or anomaly

<u>Clinical assessment</u>:

- History:
    - Determine age of onset and speed of progression
    - Inquire about history of pneumonia, pain, or difficulty breathing
- Physical examination:
    - Assess range of motion, thoracic excursion, and pulmonary function (as indicated).
    - Adam's test: standing patient bends forward so that doctor can assess for asymmetric rib hump.
    - Note side, number, and severity of curves

---

[4] Geissele AE, Kransdorf MJ, Geyer CA, Jelinek JS, Van Dam BE. Magnetic resonance imaging of the brain stem in adolescent idiopathic scoliosis. *Spine* 1991 Jul;16(7):761-3
[5] Worthington V, Shambaugh P. Systemic abnormalities in idiopathic scoliosis. *J Manipulative Physiol Ther*. 1991 Oct;14(8):467-71
[6] Ahn UM, Ahn NU, Nallamshetty L, Buchowski JM, Rose PS, Miller NH, Kostuik JP, Sponseller PD. The etiology of adolescent idiopathic scoliosis. *Am J Orthop*. 2002 Jul;31(7):387-95
[7] Hay WW, Groothuis JR, Hayward AR, Levin ML. <u>Current Pediatric Diagnosis and Treatment, 13th edition</u>. Stamford: Appleton and Lange, 1997 page 709-10
[8] Hay WW, Groothuis JR, Hayward AR, Levin ML. <u>Current Pediatric Diagnosis and Treatment, 13th edition</u>. Stamford: Appleton and Lange, 1997 page 709-10
[9] Hay WW, Groothuis JR, Hayward AR, Levin ML. <u>Current Pediatric Diagnosis and Treatment, 13th edition</u>. Stamford: Appleton and Lange, 1997 page 709-10

Imaging & laboratory assessments:

- Radiographic assessment of the thoracic and lumbar spine is the *standard of care* for patients with moderate-severe scoliosis to accurately measure the degree of curvature and number of curves, and to monitor rate of progression

Clinical management:

- **Search for underlying cause. "Idiopathic scoliosis" is a diagnosis of exclusion and can be made only after reasonably excluding other causes**
- Treatment and management must be individualized based on the patient's functional status, age, and speed of progression. The progression tends to be more rapid in females, in young patients who have not reached skeletal maturity, and in patients with more severe scoliotic curves. Less than 10% of cases are severe enough to require interventional treatment[10]
- Referral if clinical outcome is unsatisfactory or if serious complications become evident. Referral for orthopedic evaluation is recommended[11,12] for the following:
    1. Curvatures greater than 20 degrees in children
    2. Rapidly progressing curves which advance more than 6 degrees per year in pre-pubertal children.
    3. Organ/functional/cardiopulmonary compromise
    4. Curves greater than 40-60 degrees in adolescents or adults
- **Since pain is uncommon in children with scoliosis, further evaluation is indicated if pain is significant/severe.[13] This is especially true if both the pain and the onset of scoliosis are acute or subacute.**
    - **"It is imperative to seek the underlying cause in any case where there is pain, since in these instances the scoliosis is almost always secondary to some other disorder such as a bone or spinal cord tumor."[14]**

Treatment considerations:

- **Allopathic management of scoliosis includes:**
    - Bracing with spinal orthosis for curves of 20-40 degrees[15]
    - Surgery for curves greater than 40-60 degrees[16]
- **Goal: reduction in pain, maintenance of respiratory and musculoskeletal function:**
    - Massage
    - Manipulation
    - Mobilization
    - Moist heat to help with relaxation and stretching of muscles
- **Specific exercises:**
    - Studies have shown that exercises[17,18] can improve respiratory function and to reduce the progression of curves. In some cases, the curves have been reduced; but individual results vary, and some participants have experienced a progression of the condition when treated with exercise
    - A recent article by Blum[19] describes the successful management of a female patient with debilitating scoliosis who was able to regain daily activities at home and work with a multifaceted treatment program that included SOT orthopedic block placement, cranial manipulation, and Pilates rehabilitative exercises
    - Proprioceptive training and rehabilitation
- **Relieve pain and inflammation and promote healing with nutrition and botanical medicines**: Doses listed are for average-sized, healthy adults. Proportionately lower doses may be used in children, small adults, persons with medical illness, and when several treatments are used simultaneously. A multiple-intervention therapeutic approach is necessary to achieve maximum benefit because of the multifaceted nature of pain and inflammation. Risk-to-benefit ratios and drug interactions need to be considered per patient. **See Chapter 3 for review of therapeutic interventions.** Specifically consider the following:

[10] Beers MH, Berkow R (eds). The Merck Manual. Seventeenth Edition. Whitehouse Station; Merck Research Laboratories 1999, page 2429
[11] Hay WW, Groothuis JR, Hayward AR, Levin ML. Current Pediatric Diagnosis and Treatment. 13th edition. Stamford: Appleton and Lange, 1997 page 709-10
[12] Brier S. Primary Care Orthopedics. St. Louis: Mosby, 1999 page 204
[13] Beers MH, Berkow R (eds). The Merck Manual. Seventeenth Edition. Whitehouse Station; Merck Research Laboratories 1999, page 2429
[14] Hay WW, Groothuis JR, Hayward AR, Levin ML. Current Pediatric Diagnosis and Treatment. 13th edition. Stamford: Appleton and Lange, 1997 page 709-10
[15] Hay WW, Groothuis JR, Hayward AR, Levin ML. Current Pediatric Diagnosis and Treatment. 13th edition. Stamford: Appleton and Lange, 1997 page 709-10
[16] Hay WW, Groothuis JR, Hayward AR, Levin ML. Current Pediatric Diagnosis and Treatment. 13th edition. Stamford: Appleton and Lange, 1997 page 709-10
[17] Brier S. Primary Care Orthopedics. St. Louis: Mosby, 1999
[18] Basmajian JV (ed). Therapeutic Exercise. Fourth Edition. Baltimore: Williams and Wilkins. 1984
[19] Blum CL. Chiropractic and pilates therapy for the treatment of adult scoliosis. J Manipulative Physiol Ther. 2002 May;25(4):E3

- o **Combination fatty acid supplementation: Fish oil:** common therapeutic doses are 1,000-3,000 mg of combined EPA and DHA. Much higher doses have been used (e.g., 10,000 mg EPA with 3,333 mg DHA for 6 weeks[20]) in clinical trials with no adverse effects. **GLA** (from evening primrose oil, borage seed oil, black currant seed oil, and hemp oil); approximately 500 mg per day is the common anti-inflammatory dose[21]

- o <u>**Vitamin E**</u>: 400-1200 IU per day of mixed tocopherols with a relatively high concentration (~40%) of gamma-tocopherol

- o <u>**Vitamin C**</u>: Doses of 1-2 grams per day have been suggested to reduce back pain and the need for surgery in patients with low back pain[22]

- o <u>**Vitamin D**</u>: Always remember the importance and prevalence of correctable vitamin D deficiency in patients with back pain. Just because a patient has scoliosis and back pain does not mean that the cause of the back pain is the scoliosis. Search for an underlying cause of the pain—pathologic, functional, or nutritional. Vitamin D deficiency is common in the general population and is even more common in patients with musculoskeletal pain and back pain; treatment with 4,000-10,000 IU per day corrects the nutritional deficiency and results in complete alleviation of pain in the majority of affected patients[23]

- o *Harpagophytum procumbens* (**Devil's claw**): The safety and effectiveness of *Harpagophytum* has been established in patients with hip pain, **low-back pain**[24,25,26] Products are generally standardized for the content of harpagosides, with a target dose of 60 mg harpagoside per day[27]

- o **Ginger:** Anti-inflammatory via inhibition of 5-lipoxygenase and cyclooxygenase[28,29] and relieves musculoskeletal pain[30,31], osteoarthritis of the knees[32] and migraine headaches[33]

- o *Boswellia serrata*: Anti-inflammatory via inhibition of 5-lipoxygenase.[34] The target dose is approximately 150 mg of boswellic acids TID; dose and number of capsules/tablets will vary depending upon the concentration found in differing products

- o *Uncaria* ("**Cat's claw**"): *Uncaria* inhibits NF-κB, TNFα, COX-2, and thus PGE-2 production and has proven clinical benefit in knee osteoarthritis[35] Most products are between 250-500 mg and are standardized to 3.0% alkaloids and 15% total polyphenols; QD-TID po dosing should be sufficient as *part* of a comprehensive plan. This herb should probably not be used during pregnancy based on its historical use as a contraceptive

- o <u>**Glucosamine**</u>: helps to rebuild articular cartilage and is thus used in the treatment of joint degeneration and joint pain seen with osteoarthritis.[36,37,38] 500 mg TID is the standard dose for adults.

- o <u>**Topical application of *Capsicum annuum*, *Capsicum frutescens* (Cayenne pepper, hot chili pepper):**</u> Proven effective in reducing the pain associated with chronic low back pain[39] and chronic neck pain.[40] Apply as needed according to manufacturer's directions and patient tolerance

[20] "In this study eicosapentaenoic acid (EPA) and docosahexaenoic acid (DHA) were given in a cumulative manner, every 6 weeks, starting with 10 mg, then 100 mg, 1000 mg and 10,000 mg EPA daily... The corresponding DHA doses were 3, 33, 333 and 3333 mg." Du Plooy WJ, Venter CP, Muntingh GM, Venter HL, Glatthaar II, Smith KA. The cumulative dose response effect of eicosapentaenoic and docosahexaenoic acid on blood pressure, plasma lipid profile and diet pattern in mild to moderate essential hypertensive black patients. *Prostaglandins Leukot Essent Fatty Acids* 1992 Aug;46(4):315-21
[21] "Forty patients with rheumatoid arthritis and upper gastrointestinal lesions due to non-steroidal anti-inflammatory drugs entered a prospective 6-month double-blind placebo controlled study of dietary supplementation with gamma-linolenic acid 540 mg/day..." Brzeski M, Madhok R, Capell HA. Evening primrose oil in patients with rheumatoid arthritis and side-effects of non-steroidal anti-inflammatory drugs. *Br J Rheumatol.* 1991 Oct;30(5):370-2
[22] Greenwood J. Optimum vitamin C intake as a factor in the preservation of disc integrity. *Med Ann Dist Columbia.* 1964 Jun;33:274-6
[23] Al Faraj S, Al Mutairi K. Vitamin D deficiency and chronic low back pain in Saudi Arabia. *Spine.* 2003 Jan 15;28(2):177-9
[24] Chrubasik S, Thanner J, Kunzel O, Conradt C, Black A, Pollak S. Comparison of outcome measures during treatment with the proprietary Harpagophytum extract doloteffin in patients with pain in the lower back, knee or hip. *Phytomedicine* 2002 Apr;9(3):181-94
[25] "However, subsidiary analyses, concentrating on the current pain component of the Arhus index, painted a slightly different picture, with the benefits seeming, if anything, to be greatest in the H600 group and in patients without more severe pain, radiation or neurological deficit." Chrubasik S, Junck H, Breitschwerdt H, Conradt C, Zappe H. Effectiveness of Harpagophytum extract WS 1531 in the treatment of exacerbation of low back pain: a randomized, placebo-controlled, double-blind study. *Eur J Anaesthesiol* 1999 Feb;16(2):118-29
[26] Chrubasik S, Model A, Black A, Pollak S. A randomized double-blind pilot study comparing Doloteffin and Vioxx in the treatment of low back pain. *Rheumatology* (Oxford). 2003 Jan;42(1):141-8
[27] "They took an 8-week course of Doloteffin at a dose providing 60 mg harpagoside per day... Doloteffin is well worth considering for osteoarthritic knee and hip pain and nonspecific low back pain." Chrubasik S, Thanner J, Kunzel O, Conradt C, Black A, Pollak S. Comparison of outcome measures during treatment with the proprietary Harpagophytum extract doloteffin in patients with pain in the lower back, knee or hip. *Phytomedicine* 2002 Apr;9(3):181-94
[28] Kiuchi F, Iwakami S, Shibuya M, Hanaoka F, Sankawa U. Inhibition of prostaglandin and leukotriene biosynthesis by gingerols and diarylheptanoids. *Chem Pharm Bull* (Tokyo) 1992 Feb;40(2):387-91
[29] Tjendraputra E, Tran VH, Liu-Brennan D, Roufogalis BD, Duke CC. Effect of ginger constituents and synthetic analogues on cyclooxygenase-2 enzyme in intact cells. *Bioorg Chem* 2001 Jun;29(3):156-63
[30] "In all 56 patients (28 with rheumatoid arthritis, 18 with osteoarthritis and 10 with muscular discomfort) used powdered ginger against their afflictions. Amongst the arthritis patients more than three-quarters experienced, to varying degrees, relief in pain and swelling." Srivastava KC, Mustafa T. Ginger (Zingiber officinale) in rheumatism and musculoskeletal disorders. *Med Hypotheses.* 1992 Dec;39(4):342-8
[31] "Ginger is reported in Ayurvedic and Tibb systems of medicine to be useful in rheumatic disorders. Seven patients suffering from such disorders reported relief in pain and associated symptoms on ginger administration." Srivastava KC, Mustafa T. Ginger (Zingiber officinale) and rheumatic disorders. *Med Hypotheses.* 1989 May;29(1):25-8
[32] Altman RD, Marcussen KC. Effects of a ginger extract on knee pain in patients with osteoarthritis. *Arthritis Rheum.* 2001 Nov;44(11):2531-8
[33] Mustafa T, Srivastava KC. Ginger (Zingiber officinale) in migraine headache. *J Ethnopharmacol.* 1990 Jul;29(3):267-73
[34] Wildfeuer A, Neu IS, Safayhi H, Metzger G, Wehrmann M, Vogel U, Ammon HP. Effects of boswellic acids extracted from a herbal medicine on the biosynthesis of leukotrienes and the course of experimental autoimmune encephalomyelitis. *Arzneimittelforschung* 1998 Jun;48(6):668-74
[35] Piscoya J, Rodriguez Z, Bustamante SA, Okuhama NN, Miller MJ, Sandoval M.Efficacy and safety of freeze-dried cat's claw in osteoarthritis of the knee: mechanisms of action of the species Uncaria guianensis. *Inflamm Res.* 2001 Sep;50(9):442-8
[36] Braham R, Dawson B, Goodman C. The effect of glucosamine supplementation on people experiencing regular knee pain. *Br J Sports Med.* 2003;37(1):45-9
[37] Nguyen P, Mohamed SE, Gardiner D, Salinas T. A randomized double-blind clinical trial of the effect of chondroitin sulfate and glucosamine hydrochloride on temporomandibular joint disorders: a pilot study. *Cranio.* 2001 Apr;19(2):130-9
[38] "...oral glucosamine therapy achieved a significantly greater improvement in articular pain score than ibuprofen, and the investigators rated treatment efficacy as 'good' in a significantly greater proportion of glucosamine than ibuprofen recipients." Matheson AJ, Perry CM. Glucosamine: a review of its use in the management of osteoarthritis. *Drugs Aging.* 2003; 20(14): 1041-60
[39] Keitel W, Frerick H, Kuhn U, Schmidt U, Kuhlmann M, Bredehorst A. Capsicum pain plaster in chronic non-specific low back pain. *Arzneimittelforschung.* 2001 Nov;51(11):896-903
[40] Mathias BJ, Dillingham TR, Zeigler DN, Chang AS, Belandres PV. Topical capsaicin for chronic neck pain. A pilot study. *Am J Phys Med Rehabil* 1995 Jan-Feb;74(1):39-44

Vertebral Osteomyelitis
Infectious Discitis

<u>Description/pathophysiology</u>:
- Bacterial or fungal infection of the spine
- Back pain is common; spinal infection is relatively rare. Spinal infections are "a rare cause of common symptoms."[41]

<u>Clinical presentations</u>:
- <u>Classic presentation</u>: "...the diagnosis is suggested by the clinical findings: a sick patient with severe pain, a rigid back, fever, and a raised WBC and sedimentation rate."[42]
  - Patient generally appears sick with systemic manifestations: fatigue, sweats, anorexia, fever
  - Back/neck/spine pain (90%): Most common region for spinal osteomyelitis is the lumbar spine, followed by the thoracic spine, then the cervical spine. Cervical spine infections are more common in IV drug abusers
  - Pain may be acute, subacute, or chronic:
    - 30% of patients with vertebral osteomyelitis have had pain for 3 weeks to 3 months at time of diagnosis
    - 50% of patients with vertebral osteomyelitis have had pain for more than 3 months at time of diagnosis
  - Pain is continuous, intermittent, and/or "throbbing" and often worse at night
  - Pain is unrelated to motion or position (non-mechanical)
  - Localized stiffness
  - Elevated ESR/CRP
- <u>Atypical presentations</u>: as many as 15% of affected patients
  - Little or no fever
  - Little or no back or neck pain
  - Little or no local tenderness
  - Cervical osteomyelitis may present with headache, dysphagia, sore throat rather than febrile neck pain
  - Vertebral osteomyelitis of the thoracic and lumbar spine may present with pain in the chest, shoulder, abdominal, hip or leg.
  - Risk factors: IV drug use, DM, history of septicemia, spinal trauma, pulmonary tuberculosis, urinary tract infections, surgery, older men

<u>Major differential diagnoses</u>:
- Benign neck or back pain
- Degenerative disc disease
- Tumor
- Fracture
- Spondyloarthropathies: In particular, reactive arthritis is a difficult differential in this situation because of the concomitant infection (perhaps with fever and systemic symptoms) and back pain. Differentiation may be difficult, but is generally possible based on the severity of the systemic manifestations and local examination findings. Patients with *focal pain*—particularly that which is exacerbated by vertebral percussion—should be further evaluated/treated for osteomyelitis

<u>Clinical assessment</u>:
- <u>History/subjective</u>:
  - Spinal pain
  - Malaise: may or may not have systemic symptoms

---

[41] Strausbaugh LJ. Vertebral osteomyelitis. How to differentiate it from other causes of back and neck pain. *Postgrad Med* 1995 Jun;97(6):147-8, 151-4
[42] Macnab I, McCulloch J. Backache. Second Edition. Williams and Wilkins: Baltimore, 1990

- **Physical examination/objective**:
  - Mild local tenderness
  - Paravertebral muscle spasm with limited ROM
  - Fever (50%)
  - Neurologic signs (20-40%)
  - Spinal percussion is positive for pain
  - May have painful and limited SLR due to hamstring spasm
- **Imaging & laboratory assessments**:
  - High ESR—elevated to 20-100 mm/hr in 90% of patients. ESR was considered "the most useful test for monitoring the disease activity and the efficacy of treatment." [43]
  - 50% have slight elevation of WBC
  - The disc space is the first structure destroyed—the clinician and radiologist must not misinterpret early signs of infection with "degenerative disc disease."
  - **MRI has a sensitivity and specificity of >90% and also helps to assess epidural abscess.**
  - Radiographs are positive in 80% after the condition has been present for at least 10-14 days.
  - Bone scan is diagnostic in 90% of cases
  - "Computed tomography is the imaging study of choice for preoperative evaluation and biopsy procedures. It is not a good screening test…"[44] and is generally used after routine radiographs and/or bone scan

Establishing the diagnosis:
- Diagnosis is established based on a consistent spectrum of clinical signs and symptoms and is confirmed with imaging and/or biopsy, aspiration, and/or blood cultures

Complications:
- Abscesses
- Meningitis
- Vertebral collapse, fracture
- Neurologic injury: paralysis
- Septicemia and death

> **"Up to 10-15% of patients with vertebral osteomyelitis will develop neurologic findings or frank spinal-cord compression."**
>
> King RW, Johnson D. Osteomyelitis.
> Updated July 13, 2006. *eMedicine*
> http://www.emedicine.com/emerg/topic349.htm
> Accessed December 24, 2006

Clinical management:
- **Immediate/urgent referral for diagnostic procedures, IV and oral antimicrobials**, and surgery if needed

Treatments:
- **Antimicrobial drugs: Organism-specific IV/oral antimicrobials are generally administered on an in-patient basis.**
- Rest: Bed rest, bracing, activity limitation
- Surgery: Surgery for debridement and complications such as cord compression, vertebral collapse or instability
- **Immunonutrition:** Immunonutritional considerations are listed below; doses listed are for adults. Although studies have not been performed specifically in patients with bone/joint infections, general benefits derived from the use of immunonutrition are reductions in severity/frequency/duration of major infections, abbreviated hospitalization (i.e., early discharge due to expedited healing and recovery), reductions in the need for medications, significant improvements in survival, and hospital savings.[45,46,47,48,49,50,51]

[43] Macnab I, McCulloch J. Backache. Second Edition. Williams and Wilkins: Baltimore, 1990
[44] Strausbaugh LJ. Vertebral osteomyelitis. How to differentiate it from other causes of back and neck pain. Postgrad Med 1995 Jun;97(6):147-8, 151-4
[45] "To evaluate the metabolic and immune effects of dietary arginine, glutamine and omega-3 fatty acids (fish oil) supplementation, we performed a prospective study... CONCLUSIONS: The feeding of Neomune in critically injured patients was well tolerated as Traumacal and significant improvement was observed in serum protein. Shorten ICU stay and wean-off respirator day may benefit from using the immunonutrient formula." Chuntrasakul C, Siltham S, Sarasombath S, Sittapairochana C, Leowattana W, Chockvivatanavanit S, Bunnak A. Comparison of a immunonutrition formula enriched arginine, glutamine and omega-3 fatty acid, with a currently high-enriched enteral nutrition for trauma patients. J Med Assoc Thai. 2003 Jun;86(6):552-6
[46] "CONCLUSIONS: In conclusion, arginine-enhanced formula improves fistula rates in postoperative head and neck cancer patients and decreases length of stay." de Luis DA, Izaola O, Cuellar L, Terroba MC, Aller R. Randomized clinical trial with an enteral arginine-enhanced formula in early postsurgical head and neck cancer patients. Eur J Clin Nutr. 2004;58(11):1505-8
[47] "In this prospective, randomised, double-blind, placebo-controlled study, we randomly assigned 50 patients who were scheduled to undergo coronary artery bypass to receive either an oral immune-enhancing nutritional supplement containing L-arginine, omega3 polyunsaturated fatty acids, and yeast RNA (n=25), or a control (n=25) for a minimum of 5 days... Intake of an oral immune-enhancing nutritional supplement for a minimum of 5 days before surgery can improve outlook in high-risk patients who are undergoing elective cardiac surgery." Tepaske R, Velthuis H, Oudemans-van Straaten HM, Heisterkamp SH,

- o Paleo-Mediterranean diet: As detailed later in this text and elsewhere[52,53]
- o Vitamin and mineral supplementation: anti-infective benefits shown in elderly diabetics[54]
- o High-dose vitamin A: Vitamin A shows potent immunosupportive benefits, and vitamin A stores are depleted by the stress of infection and injury. Consider 200,000-300,000 IU per day of retinol palmitate for 1-4 weeks, then taper; reduce dose or discontinue with onset of toxicity symptoms such as skin problems (dry skin, flaking skin, chapped or split lips, red skin rash, hair loss), joint pain, bone pain, headaches, anorexia (loss of appetite), edema (water retention, weight gain, swollen ankles, difficulty breathing), fatigue, and/or liver damage
- o Arginine: Dose for adults is in the range of 5-10 grams daily
- o Fatty acid supplementation: In contrast to the higher doses used to provide an anti-inflammatory effect in patients with autoimmune/inflammatory disorders, doses used for immunosupportive treatments should be kept rather modest to avoid the *relative* immunosuppression that has been controversially reported in patients treated with EPA and DHA. Reasonable doses are in the following ranges for adults: EPA+DHA: 500-1,500, and GLA: 300-500 mg
- o Glutamine: Glutamine enhances bacterial killing by neutrophils[55], and administration of 18 grams per day in divided doses to patients in intensive care units was shown to improve survival, expedite hospital discharge, and reduce total healthcare costs.[56] Another study using glutamine 12-18 grams per day showed no benefit in overall mortality but significant benefits in terms of reduced healthcare costs (-30%) and significantly reduced need for medical interventions.[57] After administering glutamine 26 grams/d to severely burned patients, Garrel et al[58] concluded that glutamine reduced the risk of infection by 3-fold and that oral glutamine "may be a life-saving intervention" in patients with severe burns. A dose of 30 grams/d was used in a recent clinical trial showing hemodynamic benefit in patients with sickle cell anemia.[59] The highest glutamine dose that the current author is aware of is the study by Scheltinga et al[60] who used 0.57 gm/kg/day in cancer patients following chemotherapy administration; for a 220-lb-pt, this would be approximately 57 grams of glutamine per day
- o Melatonin: 20-40 mg hs (*hora somni*—Latin: sleep time). Immunostimulatory anti-infective action of melatonin was demonstrated in a small clinical trial wherein septic newborns administered 20 mg melatonin showed significantly increased survival over nontreated controls[61]

van Deventer SJ, Ince C, Eysman L, Kesecioglu J. Effect of preoperative oral immune-enhancing nutritional supplement on patients at high risk of infection after cardiac surgery: a randomised placebo-controlled trial. *Lancet*. 2001 Sep 1;358(9283):696-701

[48] "The feeding of IMMUNE FORMULA was well tolerated and significant improvement was observed in nutritional and immunologic parameters as in other immunoenhancing diets. Further clinical trials of prospective double-blind randomized design are necessary to address the so that the necessity of using immunonutrition in critically ill patients will be clarified." Chuntrasakul C, Siltharm S, Sarasombath S, Sittapairochana C, Leowattana W, Chockvivatanavanit S, Bunnak A. Metabolic and immune effects of dietary arginine, glutamine and omega-3 fatty acids supplementation in immunocompromised patients. *J Med Assoc Thai*. 1998 May;81(5):334-43

[49] "enteral diet supplemented with arginine, dietary nucleotides, and omega-3 fatty acids (IMPACT, Sandoz Nutrition, Bern, Switzerland)" Senkal M, Mumme A, Eickhoff U, Geier B, Spath G, Wulfert D, Joosten U, Frei A, Kemen M. Early postoperative enteral immunonutrition: clinical outcome and cost-comparison analysis in surgical patients. *Crit Care Med* 1997;25(9):1489-96

[50] "supplemented diet with glutamine, arginine and omega-3-fatty acids... It was clearly established in this trial that early postoperative enteral feeding is safe in patients who have undergone major operations for gastrointestinal cancer. Supplementation of enteral nutrition with glutamine, arginine, and omega-3-fatty acids positively modulated postsurgical immunosuppressive and inflammatory responses." Wu GH, Zhang YW, Wu ZH. Modulation of postoperative immune and inflammatory response by immune-enhancing enteral diet in gastrointestinal cancer patients. *World J Gastroenterol*. 2001 Jun;7(3):357-62 http://www.wjgnet.com/1007-9327/7/357.pdf

[51] "using a formula supplemented with arginine, mRNA, and omega-3 fatty acids from fish oil (Impact)... CONCLUSIONS: Immune-enhancing enteral nutrition resulted in a significant reduction in the mortality rate and infection rate in septic patients admitted to the ICU. These reductions were greater for patients with less severe illness." Galban C, Montejo JC, Mesejo A, Marco P, Celaya S, Sanchez-Segura JM, Farre M, Bryg DJ. An immune-enhancing enteral diet reduces mortality rate and episodes of bacteremia in septic intensive care unit patients. *Crit Care Med*. 2000 Mar;28(3):643-8

[52] Vasquez A. A Five-Part Nutritional Protocol that Produces Consistently Positive Results. *Nutritional Wellness* 2005 September http://www.nutritionalwellness.com/archives/2005/sep/09_vasquez.php

[53] Vasquez A. Implementing the Five-Part Nutritional Wellness Protocol for the Treatment of Various Health Problems. *Nutritional Wellness* 2005 November. http://www.nutritionalwellness.com/archives/2005/nov/11_vasquez.php

[54] "CONCLUSIONS: A multivitamin and mineral supplement reduced the incidence of participant-reported infection and related absenteeism in a sample of participants with type 2 diabetes mellitus and a high prevalence of subclinical micronutrient deficiency." Barringer TA, Kirk JK, Santaniello AC, Foley KL, Michielutte R. Effect of a multivitamin and mineral supplement on infection and quality of life. A randomized, double-blind, placebo-controlled trial. *Ann Intern Med*. 2003 Mar 4;138(5):365-71 http://www.annals.org/cgi/reprint/138/5/365

[55] Furukawa S, Saito H, Fukatsu K, Hashiguchi Y, Inaba T, Lin MT, Inoue T, Han I, Matsuda T, Muto T. Glutamine-enhanced bacterial killing by neutrophils from postoperative patients. *Nutrition* 1997;13(10):863-9. *In vitro* study.

[56] Griffiths RD, Jones C, Palmer TE. Six-month outcome of critically ill patients given glutamine-supplemented parenteral nutrition. *Nutrition* 1997 Apr;13(4):295-302

[57] "There was no mortality difference between those patients receiving glutamine-containing enteral feed and the controls. However, there was a significant reduction in the median postintervention ICU and hospital patient costs in the glutamine recipients $23 000 versus $30 900 in the control patients." Jones C, Palmer TE, Griffiths RD. Randomized clinical outcome study of critically ill patients given glutamine-supplemented enteral nutrition. *Nutrition*. 1999 Feb;15(2):108-15

[58] The glutamine dose in this study was "a total of 26 g/day" administered in four divided doses. CONCLUSION: "The results of this prospective randomized clinical trial show that enteral G reduces blood culture positivity, particularly with P. aeruginosa, in adults with severe burns and may be a life-saving intervention." Garrel D, Patenaude J, Nedelec B, Samson L, Dorais J, Champoux J, D'Elia M, Bernier J. Decreased mortality and infectious morbidity in adult burn patients given enteral glutamine supplements: a prospective, controlled, randomized clinical trial. *Crit Care Med*. 2003 Oct;31(10):2444-9

[59] Niihara Y, Matsui NM, Shen YM, Akiyama DA, Johnson CS, Sunga MA, Magpayo J, Embury SH, Kalra VK, Cho SH, Tanaka KR. L-glutamine therapy reduces endothelial adhesion of sickle red blood cells to human umbilical vein endothelial cells. *BMC Blood Disord*. 2005 Jul 25;5:4 http://www.biomedcentral.com.proxy.hsc.unt.edu/1471-2326/5/4

[60] "Subjects with hematologic malignancies in remission underwent a standard treatment of high-dose chemotherapy and total body irradiation before bone marrow transplantation. After completion of this regimen, they were randomized to receive either standard parenteral nutrition (STD, n = 10) or an isocaloric, isonitrogenous nutrient solution enriched with crystalline L-glutamine (0.57 g/kg/day, GLN, n = 10)." Scheltinga MR, Young LS, Benfell K, Bye RL, Ziegler TR, Santos AA, Antin JH, Wilmore DW. Glutamine-enriched intravenous feedings attenuate extracellular fluid expansion after a standard stress. *Ann Surg*. 1991 Oct;214(4):385-93; discussion 393-5 http://www.pubmedcentral.nih.gov/articlerender.fcgi?tool=pubmed&pubmedid=1953094 For additional review, see Ziegler TR. Glutamine supplementation in cancer patients receiving bone marrow transplantation and high dose chemotherapy. *J Nutr*. 2001 Sep;131(9 Suppl):2578S-84S http://jn.nutrition.org/cgi/content/full/131/9/2578S

[61] Gitto E, Karbownik M, Reiter RJ, Tan DX, Cuzzocrea S, Chiurazzi P, Cordaro S, Corona G, Trimarchi G, Barberi I. Effects of melatonin treatment in septic newborns. *Pediatr Res*. 2001 Dec;50(6):756-60 http://www.pedresearch.org/cgi/content/full/50/6/756

Selected orthopedic problems of the thoracic spine

Problem	Presentation	Assessment	Treatment
Thoracic and thoracolumbar fractures	**Acute, subacute, or chronic mid-back pain**, generally associated with: ■ Trauma ■ Infection or positive HIV status ■ Drug or medication use, especially prednisone ■ Alcoholism ■ Diabetes ■ Cancer: metastasis or primary bone tumor such as multiple myeloma	■ Patient generally assumes antalgic posturing ■ Pain from new fractures is associated with intense pain with minimal motion. Pain is acutely increased with spinal percussion ■ Hyperreflexia and muscle weakness strongly suggest myelopathy due to retropulsed bone fragments or swelling—**medical emergency** ■ Image with CT and radiography: radiography assesses degree and level(s) of compression. CT is used to assess for retropulsed bone fragments which may have entered the spinal canal and which could promote spinal cord injury	■ **Referral to surgical orthopedist is recommended** to limit liability and to ensure proper care and evaluation for myelopathy ■ **"Acute back pain from vertebral crush fracture should be treated with an orthopedic support, analgesics, and …heat and massage."**[62] ■ "Bone support" and treatment of the underlying problem ■ Patient is advised about signs and symptoms of myelopathy and urgency of immediate treatment if myelopathy develops
Thoracic disc herniation	■ **Acute, subacute, or chronic mid-back pain, generally associated with trauma or heavy lifting**	■ Patient generally assumes antalgic posturing ■ Neurologic examination: hyperreflexia and/or muscle weakness strongly suggest myelopathy due disc herniation—**medical emergency** ■ Image with CT, radiography, and/or MRI for disc herniation	■ **Referral to medical orthopedist is recommended to limit liability and to ensure proper care and evaluation for myelopathy** ■ **Patient is advised about signs and symptoms of myelopathy and urgency of immediate treatment if myelopathy develops**

---

[62] Beers MH, Berkow R (eds). The Merck Manual. 17th Edition. Whitehouse Station; Merck Research Laboratories 1999 page 472

Selected orthopedic problems of the thoracic spine—*continued*

Problem	Presentation	Assessment	Treatment
Scheuermann's disease • An idiopathic spinal condition (probably autosomal dominant[63]) affecting adolescents which results in marked thoracic hyperkyphosis	• **Painless onset of progressive thoracic hyperkyphosis**	• Clinical assessment and routine labs to rule out infection or metabolic bone disease • Assessment for cardiopulmonary and neurologic compromise in severe cases • Radiographs are diagnostic, showing: vertebral end plate deformity, disk space narrowing, and anterior wedging of vertebral bodies	• *"Early treatment may be limited to observation and exercises, whereas patients who have kyphosis of up to 75 degrees and who have growth remaining may benefit from bracing. Surgical correction is reserved for severe cases that are symptomatic and refractory to conservative management."*[64]
Thoracic segmental dysfunction	• **Thoracic spine pain or discomfort**	• Neuro-orthopedic assessment reveals no evidence of neurologic deficit or fracture • Labs, if taken, are normal • Consider viscerosomatic referral (e.g., MI, pancreatitis, mesothelioma) • Determine location and type of dysfunction by static or motion palpation	• Spinal manipulation, preferably followed by icing and massage and corrective exercises and ergonomics • See example and *reminder* of thoracic spinal manipulation in following section
T4 Syndrome • A functional clinical entity and diagnosis of exclusion characterized by nondermatomal upper extremity paresthesia that responds to thoracic spinal manipulation[65]	• Upper back stiffness associated with upper extremity pain (arm and hand) paresthesias, or numbness • May have associated headache	• Spinal and paraspinal tenderness may be present • Patient appears healthy without evidence of underlying disease • No evidence of muscle weakness change in reflex, or other neurologic signs	• Joint manipulation, stretching, and strengthening exercises directed at the upper thoracic dysfunctional segments: intervertebral and costovertebral • Condition responds rapidly to thoracic spine manipulation

[63] Lowe TG. Scheuermann's disease. *Orthop Clin North Am*. 1999 Jul;30(3):475-87, ix
[64] Ali RM, Green DW, Patel TC. Scheuermann's kyphosis. *Curr Opin Pediatr*. 1999 Feb;11(1):70-5
[65] "Paresthesias, numbness, or upper extremity pains associated with or without headaches and upper back stiffness characterize the T4 syndrome. In addition, no hard neurological signs are present. " DeFranca GG, Levine LJ. The T4 syndrome. *J Manipulative Physiol Ther* 1995 Jan;18(1):34-7

Selected orthopedic problems of the rib cage

Problem	Presentation	Assessment	Treatment
<u>Costochondritis (Tietze's syndrome)</u> ▪ Inflammation of the rib cartilage at the costosternal junction	▪ **<u>Peristernal pain with point tenderness</u>, with or without preceding trauma**	▪ Increased pain with hyperabduction of the ipsilateral arm which stretches muscles that attach to the peristernal structures ▪ Increased pain with deep inspiration ▪ **Increased pain with palpation-provocation of the peristernal costal cartilage or costosternal junction** ▪ Moderate-severe trauma suggests the need to assess for anterior rib fracture with radiographs ▪ Cardiopulmonary assessment and vitals to exclude cardiopulmonary disease and viscerosomatic referral of pain ▪ Laboratory tests and imaging assessments exclude infection[66,67] and cancer[68,69]	▪ Conservative care, especially with ice and anti-inflammatory treatments during the acute phase ▪ Treat underlying causes (e.g., infection or cancer) as indicated
<u>Intercostal strain</u> ▪ Strain of the intercostal muscles	▪ **Intercostal pain with point tenderness following exertion, twisting motions, throwing, swinging a bat or racket, etc**	▪ Tenderness-pain with palpation-provocation of the rib interspace ▪ Increased pain with hyperabduction of the ipsilateral arm and deep inspiration ▪ Cardiopulmonary assessment and vitals to exclude cardiopulmonary disease and viscerosomatic referral of pain	▪ Conservative care, especially with ice and anti-inflammatory treatments during the acute phase
<u>Intercostal neuralgia</u> ▪ Inflammation of the intercostal nerve	▪ **<u>Intercostal pain along the distribution of the intercostal nerve</u>**	▪ Assess for: Infection (herpes zoster), rib fracture, intercostal strain ▪ Cardiopulmonary assessment and vitals to exclude cardiopulmonary disease and viscerosomatic referral of pain	▪ Treat the cause of the problem: see notes on rib fracture and intercostal strain if applicable ▪ Antiviral and analgesic treatments for **herpes zoster** include oral ascorbate, NAC, lipoic acid, licorice and (for post-herpetic neuralgia) topical capsaicin, and high-dose cobalamin

[66] Alvarez F, Chocarro A, Garcia I, De Castro M, Gonzalez A. Primary costochondritis due to Escherichia coli. *Scand J Infect Dis* 2000;32(4):430-1
[67] Heckenkamp J, Helling HJ, Rehm KE. Post-traumatic costochondritis caused by Candida albicans. Aetiology, diagnosis and treatment. *Scand Cardiovasc* J 1997;31(3):165-7
[68] Thongngarm T, Lemos LB,Lawhon N,Harisdangkul V. Malignant tumor with chest wall pain mimicking Tietze's syndrome. *Clin Rheumatol* 2001;20(4):276-8
[69] Cocco R, Galieni P, Bellan C, Fioravanti A. [Lymphomas presenting as Tietze's syndrome: a report of 4 clinical cases] [Article in Italian] *Ann Ital Med Int* 1999 Apr-Jun;14(2):118-23

Selected orthopedic problems of the rib cage—*continued*

Problem & Presentation	Assessment	Treatment
<u>Rib fracture</u> ▪ Pain in the thoracic wall following trauma ▪ Stress fractures of the ribs can occur after prolonged illness with excessive coughing ▪ Acute focal thoracic wall pain with deep breathing, coughing, or sneezing	▪ **Compression of the sternum** while the patient is lying supine may exacerbate pain at fracture site ▪ **Percussion** or application of **tuning fork** *along the affected rib* near site of fracture should exacerbate pain ▪ **Radiographs** are the fist imaging assessment to assess the number and severity of fractures as well as for the presence of pneumothorax; radiographs may reveal evidence of fracture only 2-3 weeks following injury when callus formation is visible. Radiographs can be followed by **bone scan** if necessary ▪ Direct trauma severe enough to cause rib fracture warrants evaluation for visceral injury—orthopedic referral is recommended. Fracture of ribs 1-3 is associated with risk for aortic laceration[70] and requires advanced assessment	▪ Anything other than a very simple nondisplaced fracture should be referred for orthopedic evaluation. Small single fractures and "cracked ribs" can be managed conservatively with rest and analgesics.[71] [72] Patients must avoid sudden motions and additional trauma. Healing takes 6-8 weeks ▪ Patient is educated about pneumothorax and pneumonia and advised to seek immediate care with any shortness of breath, fever, or dyspnea ▪ Pain management is important to avoid hypoventilation that predisposes to respiratory failure and pneumonia
<u>Pectoralis muscle strain</u> ▪ **Similar presentation as costochondritis** ▪ **Anterior-lateral chest pain with point tenderness,** with preceding trauma or exertion	▪ Increased pain with hyperabduction of the ipsilateral arm which stretches pectoralis muscles ▪ NO significantly increased pain with deep inspiration ▪ **Increased pain with palpation-provocation of the pectoralis muscles** ▪ Cardiopulmonary assessment and vitals are normal	▪ Conservative care, especially with rest, ice and anti-inflammatory treatments during the acute phase
<u>Rib head subluxation</u> ▪ **Posterior paraspinal pain often exacerbated by motions (such as breathing) and associated with chronically poor or static posturing**	▪ Palpation of the rib heads reveals one or two rib heads that are "prominent and tender"; may be bilateral ▪ Posterior lung auscultation to evaluate for lung disease	▪ Manipulation of rib heads after excluding lung disease and osteoporosis

[70] Brier S. <u>Primary Care Orthopedics</u>. St. Louis: Mosby, 1999 page 19
[71] Souza TA. <u>Differential Diagnosis for the Chiropractor: Protocols and Algorithms</u>. Gaithersburg: Aspen. 1997 page 607-608
[72] Gatterman MI (Ed.). <u>Chiropractic Management of Spine-Related Disorders</u>. Baltimore; Williams and Wilkins, 1990. page 183

Thoracic Spine: Supine Thoracic Flexion, "Anterior Thoracic"

Patient position:	• Supine on table; to facilitate positioning, patient's leg opposite doctor may be flexed at hip and knee with foot flat on table • Patient is instructed to place right hand on right trapezius and left hand on left trapezius; the patient is instructed, "Do not place your hands behind your neck and do not interlace your fingers."
Doctor position:	• Facing table at 45° angle in fencer stance with feet apart and knees bent • Doctor must be midline and balanced at time of impulse in order to provide symmetric force
Assessment:	• <u>Subjective</u>: mechanical midback pain • <u>Motion palpation</u>: flexion restriction • <u>Static palpation</u>: extension malposition; focal loss of thoracic kyphosis; focal approximation of spinous processes consistent with extension malposition; vertebra may feel anteriorly displaced • <u>Soft tissue</u>: local paravertebral myohypertonicity is common; local paresthesia is very common, and patients are often exquisitely sensitive to the lightest touch
Treatment contact:	• Closed fist contact with spinous processes between doctor's distal interphalangeal joints and thenar eminence; the trust is delivered from the doctor's chest through the patient's arms which compress the patient's chest; Dr Harris (pictured as patient) prefers to use a forearm contact to reduce wear-and-tear on his hands and wrists
Supporting contact:	• The supporting contact is the hand-arm that supports the patient's upper torso; the supporting contact pulls toward the doctor and superiorly at time of impulse
Pretreatment positioning:	• Patient lifts head from table; doctor uses supporting hand and arm to lift patient off table to allow placement of contact hand and to facilitate spinal flexion
Therapeutic action:	• Doctor uses **body drop thrust** technique at 45° toward ground and toward the head of the table; the trust should simultaneously generate compression and long-axis traction; the contact hand remains tense to provide solid leverage *inferior* to the targeted motion segment; the supporting hand and arm pull toward doctor at time of impulse to accentuate traction and spinal flexion; patient is instructed to breath deeply then relax and exhale; upon exhalation, the doctor establishes and maintains premanipulative tension to achieve joint flexion, then applies HVLA thrust; the thrust must be fast and shallow; slow and deep impulses can sprain the interspinous ligaments
Image:	

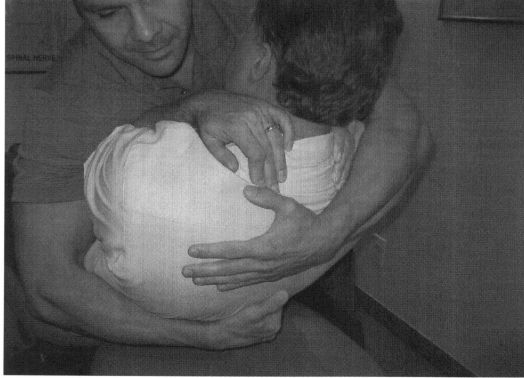

Resources:	• <u>States Manual, Second Edition</u>[73] page 67 • <u>Kimberly Manual, 2006 Edition</u>[74] page 93-94 • <u>Chiropractic Technique</u>[75] page 349

[73] Kirk CR, Lawrence DJ, Valvo NL. <u>States Manual of Spinal, Pelvic, and Extravertebral Technics, Second Edition</u>. Lombard, Illinois: National College of Chiropractic; 1985
[74] Kimberly PE. <u>Outline of Osteopathic Manipulative Procedures, The Kimberly Manual 2006</u>. Kirksville College of Osteopathic Medicine. Walsworth Publishing , Marceline, Mo
[75] Bergmann TF, Peterson DH, Lawrence DJ. <u>Chiropractic Technique</u>. New York; Churchill Livingstone: 1993

Pleurisy & Pleuritis

<u>Description/pathophysiology</u>:
- Painful inflammation of the parietal pleura usually with pleural effusion[Ψ]

<u>Clinical presentations</u>:
- Sudden onset of chest pain
- **Exacerbated by respiration: breathing, coughing, sneezing**
- Stabbing sensation
- Mild to severe
- May cause referred pain to the abdomen or pain to the neck and shoulder
- Rapid and shallow breathing

<u>Major differential diagnoses</u>:
- Infection: viral or bacterial respiratory infection, osteomyelitis
- Myocardial infarction
- Intra-abdominal disease
- Intercostal neuritis; herpes zoster
- Pneumothorax or other pulmonary disorder
- Musculoskeletal lesion such as costochondritis, intercostal strain, pectoralis muscle strain, rib fracture

<u>Clinical assessment</u>:
- **<u>History/subjective</u>:**
  - See clinical presentations
- **<u>Physical examination/objective</u>:**
  - Pleural friction rub heard with auscultation of the chest is considered pathognomonic[76], yet occurs infrequently; varies from faint crackles to harsh grating
- **<u>Imaging & laboratory assessments</u>:**
  - Routine labs: chemistry panel, CBC, CRP are performed to assess for infection, inflammation, CO_2 concentration and other possible abnormalities which will help identify the severity and underlying cause of the problem
  - Radiographs may be used to rule out other conditions, establish the cause, assess for effusion, and confirm the diagnosis
- **<u>Establishing the diagnosis</u>:**
  - Radiographs can be diagnostic; exclude other causes of similar clinical presentations

<u>Complications</u>:
- Depends on underlying cause

<u>Clinical management</u>:
- *Medical standard*: "Treatment of pleuritis consists of treating the underlying disease."[77]
- <u>**The underlying cause must always be sought. Consider the following causes:**</u>
  - **Pulmonary infection, such as bacterial pneumonia, tuberculosis, or coxsackievirus B**
  - **Myocardial infarction**
  - **Malignant plural effusion, asbestos-related pleural disease**
  - **Rib fracture**
  - **Medication side-effect**
- Referral if clinical outcome is unsatisfactory or if serious complications are possible/evident.
- Pain will diminish when significant effusion develops. Thus, decreased pain may signify a worsening of the patient's condition. Monitor for dyspnea, tachypnea, and tachycardia
- Important to avoid shallow breathing and cough suppression, which may predispose to fluid accumulation and pneumonia

<u>Treatments</u>:
- **Treat the underlying cause and implement pain relief:** Wrap chest with wide elastic bandages to reduce pain, but not to excessively limit respiratory excursion. Botanical and nutritional antiinflammatories for symptomatic relief: fish oil, GLA, vitamin E, ginger and other natural treatments may also be used.

[Ψ] I have included this information on pleurisy/pleuritis for the sake of completeness. Pleuritis is a condition that involves the chest wall and may present challenges in differentiating from truly musculoskeletal conditions such as chostochondritis, even though pleuritis is not a true musculoskeletal/orthopedic condition.
[76] Beers MH, Berkow R (eds). <u>The Merck Manual. Seventeenth Edition</u>. Whitehouse Station; Merck Research Laboratories 1999 page 643
[77] Tierney ML. McPhee SJ, Papadakis MA (eds). <u>Current Medical Diagnosis and Treatment 2002, 41st Edition</u>. New York: Lange Medical Books; 2002. Page 350

Chapter 7:
Shoulder

Introduction
Disorders of the shoulder are common, especially due to overuse injuries and trauma. Because of the joint's inherent bony instability and its dependency upon soft tissues, overuse and post-traumatic injuries to muscles, ligaments, and tendons are commonplace. Occasionally, autoimmune/inflammatory and endocrinologic disorders make their first clinical presentation in this region. Malignant disease of the lungs and breast are also important regional considerations.

<u>Topics</u>:
- **Clinical assessments**
- **General considerations and common conditions of the shoulder**
    - o Shoulder impingement syndrome
    - o Supraspinatus tendonitis
    - o Biceps tendonitis
    - o Shoulder bursitis
    - o Rotator cuff tendonitis/injuries
    - o Deltoid strain
- **Adhesive capsulitis and frozen shoulder syndrome**
- **Calcific tendonitis of the rotator cuff**
- **Additional orthopedic problems of the shoulder region**
    - o Clavicle fractures
    - o Thoracic outlet syndrome
    - o Acromioclavicular joint sprain, AC separation

<u>Focus</u>:
- Since rotator cuff injuries are a potentially serious cause of pain and disability, you need to be able to distinguish rotator cuff disease from the more benign problems of the biceps tendon, deltoid, pectorals, etc. Which problems are associated with injury? Overuse? Idiopathic onset? How are these common problems managed?

<u>Introduction</u>:
- The "shoulder" is a region of the body that correlates anatomically with the **trapezius, deltoid(s), rotator cuff (supraspinatus, infraspinatus, teres minor, subscapularis), and other muscles and tendons of the proximal arm (coracobrachialis, long heads of the biceps and triceps),** as well as the bones of the **humerus, clavicle, and scapula** and their functional and anatomic articulations with the thorax, including the **spine and rib cage.** The high degree of functional mobility of the shoulder is afforded by the lack of bony apposition and the dependence upon soft tissues for joint support. While this allows for much biomechanical freedom, the cost for this polydirectional freedom is the common soft-tissue disorders that characteristically plague this region of the body and can ultimately impair function and quality of life.

<u>Core Competencies</u>:
- Differentially diagnose and treat rotator cuff tendonitis from proximal biceps tendonitis.
- Differentially diagnose overuse bursitis from septic bursitis.
- Differentiate thoracic outlet syndrome from fibromyalgia and the musculoskeletal manifestations of hypothyroidism.
- Describe how to clinically distinguish fibromyalgia from polymyalgia rheumatica.
- How are clavicle fractures managed?
- Describe the sequential application of the Spencer technique[1] for in-office shoulder manipulation and myofascial release.
- Be able to explain how thoracic hyperkyphosis and/or scapulothoracic restrictions can cause and perpetuate rotator cuff injuries at the shoulder.

---

[1] The "seven stages of Spencer" is an organized technique of range-of-motion exercises and post-isometric stretching to improve functionality of the shoulder. This clinical trial showed improved shoulder function in a group of elderly patients treated with this technique. Knebl JA, Shores JH, Gamber RG, Gray WT, Herron KM. Improving functional ability in the elderly via the Spencer technique, an osteopathic manipulative treatment: a randomized, controlled trial. *J Am Osteopath Assoc.* 2002 Jul;102(7):387-96 http://www.jaoa.org/cgi/reprint/102/7/387 See also "CONCLUSION: Manipulative therapy for the shoulder girdle in addition to usual medical care accelerates recovery of shoulder symptoms." Bergman GJ, Winters JC, Groenier KH, Pool JJ, Meyboom-de Jong B, Postema K, van der Heijden GJ. Manipulative therapy in addition to usual medical care for patients with shoulder dysfunction and pain: a randomized, controlled trial. *Ann Intern Med.* 2004 Sep 21;141(6):432-9 http://www.annals.org/cgi/reprint/141/6/432.pdf

Conceptual Algorithm for the Assessment of Shoulder Complaints

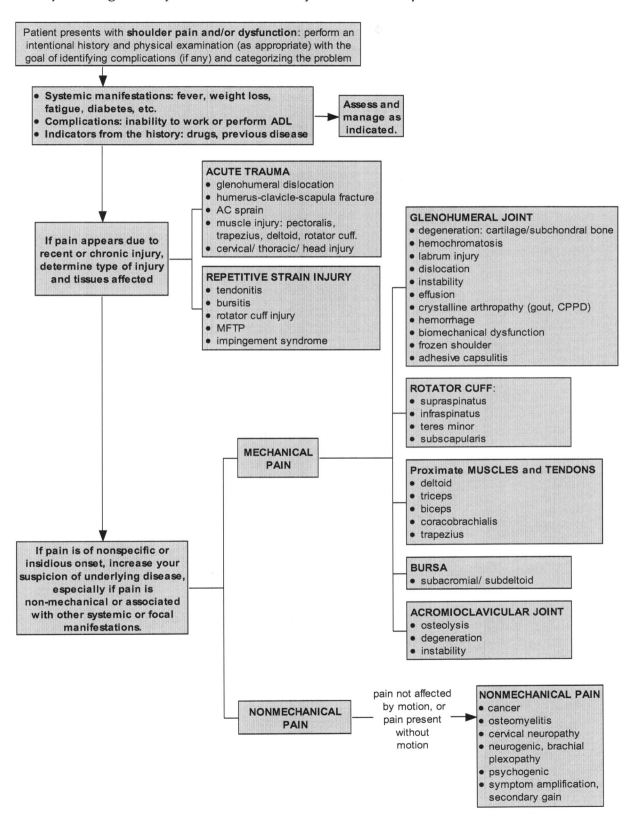

Clinical Examination of the Shoulder: Many Tests, Many Names, and Many Methods

With its polydirectional motions and numerous structures, the shoulder lends itself to a plethora of assessments and provocative tests. Unfortunately for doctors and students, many of these clinical assessments have formal names as well as trivial names. Further complicating the memorization and documentation of these tests are the variations in performance of these tests as described in authoritative references from different authors. In the sections that follow, I have described and referenced each test. For the sake of direction and clarity, I have **bolded** and/or <u>underlined</u> preferred names and procedures when variations were present in the reference texts and articles. However, for the sake of charting and documentation, description of clinical examination procedures and patient responses is more accurate and is preferred to the use of formal names of tests when charting clinical findings, for example, "left shoulder pain w/ max flexion" is more clear and comprehensible than "positive left Neer."

Clinical examination of the shoulder

Selected assessments	*Positive finding and Implications*
1. <u>**History**</u>	▪ **Indicators from the history (trauma, risk factors), systemic manifestations, neuromuscular compromise, nonmechanical pain:** these suggest increased risk for serious pathology and potential complications. Defer or modify physical examination based on your assessment of the situation
2. **Observation**: Assess overall appearance as well as details	Search for evidence of: ▪ Dislocation ▪ Muscle atrophy ▪ AC (acromioclavicular) separation ▪ Ecchymosis ▪ Hyperkyphosis ▪ Poor posture ▪ Congenital anomaly ▪ Asymmetric development due to asymmetric use ▪ Muscle atrophy may be due to neurologic deficit or disuse (secondary to injury or pain) ▪ Ecchymosis is seen after fractures, contusions, and AC separations ▪ Hyperkyphosis (possibly secondary to compression fractures, poor posture, or Scheuermann's disease) will alter the biomechanics of the glenohumeral (GH) joint predisposing the patient to impingement syndrome
3. <u>**Range of motion (ROM)**</u>: Should be "full and painless": • Abduction, adduction • Internal rotation at 0° and 90° of abduction • External rotation at 0° and 90° of abduction • Flexion, extension • Elevation, depression • Protraction, retraction	▪ Limitation ▪ Pain ▪ Injury ▪ Muscle spasm ▪ Pain ▪ Contracture/adhesion of soft tissues: muscles, joint capsule ▪ Nerve injury: suggested by *painless weakness*

Clinical examination of the shoulder—*continued*

Clinical assessments	Positive finding and Implications
4. **Apley scratch test**: Patient reaches above and behind head to touch contralateral scapula[2]	▪ Pain or restricted motion indicates impaired external rotation and abduction which may be due to muscular restrictions, joint pathology, or impingement syndrome
5. **Internal rotation and adduction, "Apley bra test"**: Patient maximally internally rotates arm with forearm behind back, then raises hand up the spine.[3] *This test is considered the "opposite" of the Apley test and requires a similar motion to that used when fastening a bra with the clasp behind the back; hence the nickname "Apley bra test"*	▪ Assess level of reach up the spine (T5-T10) and compare to other shoulder ▪ Pain or restricted motion indicates impaired internal rotation and adduction
6. **Palpation and provocation:** *Compare with opposite shoulder*	▪ Pain, tenderness, mass, enlargement, abnormality are seen with recent injury, inflammation, muscle spasm/strain, joint dysfunction, and other causes
7. **Palpation of the greater tubercle of the humerus**: The greater tubercle is exposed from under the acromion by adduction of the arm in front of the thorax, such as when the patient places the hand on the opposite shoulder with the elbow on the sternum	▪ Pain at the site of attachment of the rotator cuff with deep palpation by the doctor suggests rotator cuff tendonitis, especially the supraspinatus
8. **Biceps tendon palpation**: This is best performed with the shoulder in the neutral position or slightly extended; when performed at 90° of shoulder flexion this has been referred to as Lippman's test[4]	▪ Tenderness with palpation of the biceps tendon at the anterior proximal humerus suggests irritation and inflammation: biceps tendonitis
9. **Scapulothoracic motion:** Decreased motion of the scapula mandates increased motion of the glenohumeral joint to maintain ROM. Therefore decreased motion of the scapula on the thorax predisposes to shoulder impingement and degeneration	▪ Scapula should rotate 60° with full shoulder abduction to 180°; thus with full shoulder abduction scapulothoracic motion contributes 1/3 and glenohumeral motion contributes 2/3 of total abduction.[5] Reduced scapulothoracic motion in a patient who is neuromuscularly intact suggests adhesions between the scapula and posterior thorax or simply tight muscles—rhomboids, trapezius, and perhaps latissimus dorsi. Conversely or additionally, the serratus anterior may be weak. Adhesions and tight muscles can be released and lengthened with manipulation and stretching, respectively, to improve scapulothoracic motion and thus glenohumeral function

[2] Hoppenfeld S. Physical examination of the spine and extremities. Norwalk: Appleton and Lange, 1976, p. 21. This is a commonly performed and well-known test, but it is of limited clinical value.
[3] Hoppenfeld S. Physical examination of the spine and extremities. Norwalk: Appleton and Lange, 1976, p. 21
[4] Magee DJ. Orthopedic Physical Assessment. Third edition. Philadelphia: WB Saunders, 1997 page 216
[5] Norkin CC, Levangie PK. Joint Structure and Function: A Comprehensive Analysis. Second Edition. Philadelphia: FA Davis Publishers; 1992, page 229

Clinical assessments	Positive finding and Implications
10. **Scapular winging**: Elevation of the vertebral border of the scapula when anteroposterior pressure is applied to the 90° forward flexed arm (as in the "push-up" position)	<ul><li>Mild elevation: muscle imbalance, muscle weakness, muscle fatigue</li><li>Moderate/severe elevation: Injury to the serratus anterior and/or long thoracic nerve</li></ul>
11. **Muscle testing and provocation**:<ul><li>Trapezius</li><li>Deltoid(s)</li><li>Biceps</li><li>Triceps</li><li>Pectoralis major</li><li>Teres major, latissimus dorsi</li><li>Supraspinatus</li><li>Infraspinatus, teres minor</li><li>Subscapularis</li><li>Serratus anterior</li></ul>	<ul><li>Pain: muscle injury, tendonitis</li><li>Weakness: may be secondary to pain, may indicate neuropathy</li></ul>
12. **"Empty can" test**, supraspinatus isolation test[6]: Patient's straight arm is abducted 90° and brought slightly forward so that wrist is anterior to the body and arm is in scapular plane	<ul><li>Weakness and pain when patient resists downward force applied to the distal forearm when shoulder is 90° abducted, internally rotated, with the arm in the scapular plane, with the elbow extended suggests injury and/or inflammation of the **supraspinatus tendon** but may also be seen with deltoid injury, bursitis, and biceps tendonitis</li></ul>
13. **Hawkins test**, Hawkins-Kennedy impingement test, the "pour can" test: Patient's arm is bent at the elbow 90°, then 90° abducted[7] and then forcefully internally rotated. This test is also performed in 90° of flexion[8] [9] rather than abduction, again with internal rotation	<ul><li>The purpose of this test is to bring the greater tubercle of the humerus into contact with the acromion process to compress the subacromial structures, especially of the supraspinatus tendon and subacromial bursa leading to a diagnosis of **subacromial impingement syndrome**, which characteristically involves either or both of the biceps tendon and the supraspinatus tendon and may also include the subacromial bursa</li></ul>
14. **"Glass half full" test**[10]: Patient's shoulder is 90° forward flexed and thumb points upward, doctor then pushes arm downward; similar to Speed's test except for forearm position	<ul><li>Pain and/or weakness at the supraspinatus tendon when patient resists downward motion of the doctor's force on the distal forearm when shoulder is flexed to 90° and thumb is pointing up indicates **supraspinatus muscle injury or tendonitis**: this test produces the greatest amount of supraspinatus EMG activity [11]</li></ul>

[6] Magee DJ. Orthopedic Physical Assessment. Third edition. Philadelphia: WB Saunders, 1997 page 216

[7] Pearsall AW, Speer KP. Frozen shoulder syndrome: diagnostic and treatment strategies in the primary care setting. *Med Sci Sports Exerc* 1998 Apr;30(4 Suppl):S33-9

[8] Clarnette RG, Miniaci A. Clinical exam of the shoulder. *Med Sci Sports Exerc* 1998 Apr;30(4 Suppl):S1-6

[9] Howard TM, O'Connor FG. The injured shoulder. Primary care assessment. *Arch Fam Med.* 1997 Jul-Aug;6(4):376-84

[10] Pearsall AW, Speer KP. Frozen shoulder syndrome: diagnostic and treatment strategies in the primary care setting. *Med Sci Sports Exerc* 1998 Apr;30(4 Suppl):S33-9

[11] Pearsall AW, Speer KP. Frozen shoulder syndrome: diagnostic and treatment strategies in the primary care setting. *Med Sci Sports Exerc* 1998 Apr;30(4 Suppl):S33-9

Clinical examination of the shoulder—*continued*

Clinical assessments	Positive finding and Implications
15. <u>Drop arm test</u>[12], <u>Codman's test,</u> <u>arm drop test</u>[13]: Doctor supports patient arm at 90° abduction, then suddenly removes support	• Patient is unable to maintain shoulder at 90° abduction when doctor removes support, suggesting **rotator cuff tendonitis, especially of the supraspinatus** • Inability to provide any resistance is highly suggestive of a complete supraspinatus tear or nerve lesion, especially of C5
16. <u>Lift off test</u>[14]	• Inability to elevate the dorsum of the hand from the sacrum is considered sensitive and indicative of subscapularis pathology, namely a "complete tear of the subscapularis."[15]
17. <u>Speed's test</u>: Patient begins with arm forward flexed to 90° with elbow straight and thumb or palm up; doctor applies downward force to distal arm.[16] [17] Less common method, "Reverse Speed's test": Patient's arm begins in extension and then is resisted while swinging forward to full flexion[18]	• Pain at the long head of the biceps tendon in bicipital groove with this test indicates **biceps tendonitis** but may also suggest biceps injury, irritation of the superior labrum of the glenohumeral joint, or injury of the anterior deltoid
18. <u>Yergason's test</u>: Patient begins with neutral shoulder, 90° flexed elbow and pronated forearm; doctor provides resistance to forearm while patient attempts to forcefully flex the elbow, supinate the forearm (i.e., maximal activity of the biceps)[19]	• Pain at the long head of the biceps tendon in bicipital groove with resisted forearm supination, external rotation of the shoulder and elbow flexion suggests **biceps tendonitis with possible associated instability of the biceps tendon in the bicipital groove**
19. <u>Supination abduction test</u>: With the forearm in supination, the shoulder is brought to ≥90° of abduction to assess for painful displacement of the biceps tendon; can be performed with biceps tendon palpation	• Pain at the long head of the biceps tendon in bicipital groove with resisted abduction while forearm is in supination suggests biceps tendonitis and probable associated instability of the biceps tendon in the bicipital groove; doctor can palpate and provoke the biceps tendon while performing this test by providing transverse friction to the long biceps tendon
20. <u>Maximal shoulder abduction,</u> <u>shoulder impingement test</u>: Starting from the neutral position, the doctor brings the patient's shoulder into abduction while applying pressure on the acromion process to "sandwich" the subacromial structures between the acromion and the humerus.	• "Positive impingement sign" at 60°-120 indicates inflammation of the supraspinatus tendon, subacromial bursa, and/or biceps tendon • Pain at the AC joint at 120-180° of motion suggests AC arthropathy; assess for AC separation • *This is a quick and easy procedure for assessing subacromial bursitis and supraspinatus tendonitis*

[12] Howard TM, O'Connor FG. The injured shoulder. Primary care assessment. *Arch Fam Med.* 1997 Jul-Aug;6(4):376-84
[13] Magee DJ. <u>Orthopedic Physical Assessment. Third edition</u>. Philadelphia: WB Saunders, 1997 page 216
[14] Magee DJ. <u>Orthopedic Physical Assessment. Third edition</u>. Philadelphia: WB Saunders, 1997 page 217
[15] Belzer JP, Durkin RC. Common disorders of the shoulder. *Prim Care* 1996 Jun;23(2):365-88
[16] Magee DJ. <u>Orthopedic Physical Assessment. Third edition</u>. Philadelphia: WB Saunders, 1997 page 215
[17] Howard TM, O'Connor FG. The injured shoulder. Primary care assessment. *Arch Fam Med.* 1997 Jul-Aug;6(4):376-84
[18] Clarnette RG, Miniaci A. Clinical exam of the shoulder. *Med Sci Sports Exerc* 1998 Apr;30(4 Suppl):S1-6
[19] Howard TM, O'Connor FG. The injured shoulder. Primary care assessment. *Arch Fam Med.* 1997 Jul-Aug;6(4):376-84

Clinical examination of the shoulder—*continued*

Clinical assessments	Positive finding and Implications
21. **Neer's test**[20], maximal shoulder flexion: Begin with internal rotation of arm and elbow extension; flex shoulder by raising arm forward to 180°[21]	▪ Grimace or shoulder pain while arm is arcing forward suggests impingement at the acromion or the coracoacromial arch ▪ "Positive impingement sign" at 60°-120° indicates inflammation of the supraspinatus, subacromial bursa, and/or biceps tendon ▪ Positive result at full flexion with arm traction suggests overuse injury of the supraspinatus or biceps
22. **Load and shift test**[22]: Doctor stabilizes scapula and then anteriorly and posteriorly translates the humerus to assess laxity of the joint capsule; this is the horizontal (anterior-posterior) version of the sulcus test, which assesses for inferior translation of the humerus relative to the glenoid fossa	▪ Excess motion indicates laxity and instability of the glenohumeral joint Grades of instability: [23] Grade 0. Normal: minimal translation Grade 1. Mild: <1 cm Grade 2. Moderate: 1-2 cm Grade 3. Severe: >2 cm
23. **Sulcus test**, sulcus sign[24]: With the patient's arm in neutral, the doctor applies downward force (inferior traction) on the arm while looking at the lateral deltoid for evidence of inferior translation of the humerus	▪ Subacromial/deltoid indentation appears when humerus is tractioned inferiorly; estimate the amount of laxity Grades of instability: [25] Grade 0. Normal: minimal translation Grade 1. Mild: <1 cm Grade 2. Moderate: 1-2 cm Grade 3. Severe: >2 cm
24. **Anterior apprehension test for glenohumeral instability**: External rotation is applied to 90° abducted shoulder, posteroanterior pressure can be added to humeral head by doctor[26]	▪ Pain or apprehension suggests anterior glenohumeral instability, which is often associated with a history of dislocation, trauma, impingement syndrome and rotator cuff disease
25. **Anterior apprehension *suppression* test for anterior glenohumeral instability**, relocation test: Anteroposterior pressure on the head of the humerus during the anterior apprehension test	▪ Relief of pain or apprehension with a previously positive anterior apprehension test confirms anterior glenohumeral instability

[20] Magee DJ. Orthopedic Physical Assessment. Third edition. Philadelphia: WB Saunders, 1997 page 217
[21] Howard TM, O'Connor FG. The injured shoulder. Primary care assessment. *Arch Fam Med.* 1997 Jul-Aug;6(4):376-84
[22] Clarnette RG, Miniaci A. Clinical exam of the shoulder. *Med Sci Sports Exerc* 1998 Apr;30(4 Suppl):S1-6
[23] Howard TM, O'Connor FG. The injured shoulder. Primary care assessment. *Arch Fam Med.* 1997 Jul-Aug;6(4):376-84
[24] Magee DJ. Orthopedic Physical Assessment. Third edition. Philadelphia: WB Saunders, 1997 page 210-211
[25] Howard TM, O'Connor FG. The injured shoulder. Primary care assessment. *Arch Fam Med.* 1997 Jul-Aug;6(4):376-84
[26] Magee DJ. Orthopedic Physical Assessment. Third edition. Philadelphia: WB Saunders, 1997 page 202-203

Clinical examination of the shoulder—*continued*

Clinical assessments	*Positive finding and Implications*
26. **Posterior apprehension test** for posterior glenohumeral instability: Patient is in the supine position, patient's shoulder is 90° abducted and horizontally adducted to 60° while doctor applies anteroposterior pressure on the elbow while continuing to horizontally adduct the arm[27]	▪ The production of pain or apprehension with this maneuver indicates posterior shoulder instability
27. **Clunk test**: Patient's arm is brought into full flexion/abduction while posteroanterior pressure is applied at humeral head and anteroposterior pressure is applied to the distal posterior arm, promoting anterior translation of the humeral head and thus pressure on the glenoid labrum[28] ▪ Modified version: Patient's arm begins in extension and then is resisted while swinging forward to full flexion[29]	▪ Clunk or grinding sensation suggests a tear of the glenohumeral labrum, which may be seen with pain or instability associated with anterior glenohumeral instability
28. **Adson test**: Assess for thoracic outlet syndrome (TOS); patient stands with arms in neutral position, doctor assesses radial pulse of patient, then extends and externally rotates patient's arm; patient takes a deep breath, with head turned to opposite side, then same side	Diminution of pulse accompanied by shoulder/arm pain or paresthesia suggests: ▪ **Thoracic outlet syndrome**: underlying causes include cervical rib, scalene hypertrophy, poor posture, and hypertonic cervical musculature. A positive Adson test has been suggested to indicate **compression of the subclavian artery by a cervical rib and/or hypertonic scalene muscles**[30] ▪ Consider also pathology in the region of the supraclavicular fossa ▪ Cervical rib
29. **Wright test**: Patient is seated with arms down; from behind patient, the doctor holds the patient's wrist and assess the radial pulse while the arm is straight and brought into full abduction; repeat bilaterally[31]	▪ Diminution of pulse accompanied by shoulder/arm pain or paresthesia suggests **thoracic outlet syndrome**: underlying causes include cervical rib, scalene hypertrophy, poor posture, and hypertonic cervical musculature. Thought to indicate neurovascular compression due to tight pectoralis minor
30. **Roos test**: Patient abducts both shoulders to 90° and externally rotates arm; patient then opens and closes hands for 2 minutes while the doctor simply observes.[32] Some consider this to be the best test for thoracic outlet syndrome	▪ This test attempts to provoke ischemia that manifests as shoulder/arm pain or paresthesia and suggests **thoracic outlet syndrome**: underlying causes include cervical rib, scalene hypertrophy, poor posture, and hypertonic cervical musculature ▪ Some *normal* people cannot perform this test without significant discomfort

[27] Magee DJ. Orthopedic Physical Assessment. Third edition. Philadelphia: WB Saunders, 1997 page 207
[28] Magee DJ. Orthopedic Physical Assessment. Third edition. Philadelphia: WB Saunders, 1997 page 212-213
[29] Clarnette RG, Miniaci A. Clinical exam of the shoulder. *Med Sci Sports Exerc* 1998 Apr;30(4 Suppl):S1-6
[30] Hoppenfeld S. Physical examination of the spine and extremities. Norwalk: Appleton and Lange, 1976, p. 127
[31] Gatterman MI (Ed.). Chiropractic Management of Spine-Related Disorders. Baltimore; Williams and Wilkins, 1990. Page 222-223
[32] Howard TM, O'Connor FG. The injured shoulder. Primary care assessment. *Arch Fam Med*. 1997 Jul-Aug;6(4):376-84

Clinical examination of the shoulder—*continued*

Clinical assessments	*Positive finding and Implications*
31. **Eden's test**, costoclavicular maneuver: Patient places chin on chest; from behind the patient, doctor pulls patient's arms into extension while palpating radial pulse[33]	▪ Diminution of pulse accompanied by shoulder/arm pain or paresthesia suggests **thoracic outlet syndrome**: underlying causes include costoclavicular compression of the subclavicular neurovascular bundle
32. **Motion palpation of the shoulder**: This is the chiropractic/osteopathic assessment of the shoulder for subtle alterations and restrictions in motion [34]	▪ Hypermobility or hypomobility
33. **Cervical spine regional assessment**:	*See Cervical Spine and Neck notes*
34. **Neurologic assessment**: Assess muscle strength, reflexes, and sensation	▪ Abnormal findings include: weakness, loss of function, loss of sensation, hyperreflexia, hyporeflexia, and pain Common indications include the following: ▪ Neurologic compromise: cord, nerve root, peripheral nerve, double crush syndrome, myopathy ▪ Muscle lesion: tendonitis, myopathy, myositis, strain
35. **Radiographs**: For bone lesions and to quickly and inexpensively assess joint space, osteophytes, degeneration, tumor, and other problems	▪ Degeneration ▪ Calcification of tendons ▪ Fracture ▪ **Cancer, including apical lung tumor, Pancoast tumor**, which may present with shoulder, arm, or scapular pain that is misdiagnosed as musculoskeletal in origin[35] ▪ "When a patient has sustained an injury, radiographs are necessary."[36]
36. **MRI**: For soft tissue lesions	▪ **MRI is generally the imaging test of choice for the visualization of soft tissue lesions**: "…shoulder MR imaging rapidly is becoming the study of choice in the evaluation of soft-tissue pathologies of the shoulder, such as rotator cuff tears or injuries to the anterior ligaments of the shoulder."[37]

[33] Gatterman MI (Ed.). Chiropractic Management of Spine-Related Disorders. Baltimore; Williams and Wilkins, 1990. Page 222
[34] Motion Palpation Institute information is available at www.motionpalpation.com as of January 10, 2004
[35] "Ten patients diagnosed with Pancoast tumor were studied retrospectively… Five patients had previously been diagnosed with degenerative, inflammatory, or infectious diseases of the cervical spine or shoulder. In the remaining five patients, the diagnosis was made during the first clinical visit." Villas C, Collia A, Aquerreta JD, Aristu J, Torre W, Diaz De Rada P, Gocci S. Cervicobrachialgia and pancoast tumor: value of standard anteroposterior cervical radiographs in early diagnosis. *Orthopedics*. 2004 Oct;27(10):1092-5
[36] Belzer JP, Durkin RC. Common disorders of the shoulder. *Prim Care* 1996 Jun;23(2):365-88
[37] Belzer JP, Durkin RC. Common disorders of the shoulder. *Prim Care* 1996 Jun;23(2):365-88

Practical Examination Flow for the Shoulder

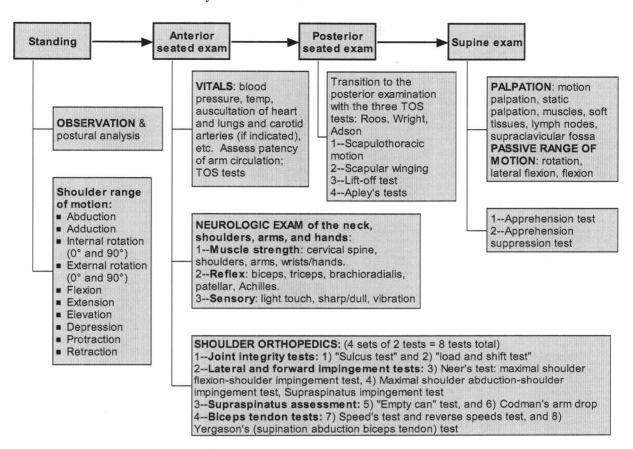

Standing	Anterior	Posterior	Supine
1. Observation 2. Squat and rise 3. Toe walk 4. Heel walk 5. Thoracic and shoulder range of motion is easiest tested when the patient is standing	6. Vital signs: temperature, blood pressure, pulse, respiratory rate, auscultation of heart and lungs. 7. Complete shoulder ROM assessment (if not previously completed). 8. Begin tests for TOS and shoulder orthopedics tests	9. Orthopedics (up—traction, down—compression, diagonal—lateral bending with contralateral shoulder depression) 10. Percussion and palpation of spine, ribs and thorax 11. Finish tests for TOS and shoulder orthopedics tests 12. Thoracic spine and cardiopulmonary examination	13. Additional shoulder tests, such as shoulder apprehension 14. Neck flexion and motion palpation

Common Shoulder Problems:

- **General considerations and common conditions**
- **Shoulder impingement syndrome**
- **Supraspinatus tendonitis**
- **Biceps tendonitis**
- **Shoulder bursitis**
- **Rotator cuff injury**
- **Deltoid strain**

Description/pathophysiology:

- **Shoulder impingement syndrome**: Inflammation of the subacromial structures (supraspinatus tendon, biceps tendon, subacromial bursa) leads to pain experienced with full abduction or full flexion of the shoulder. This is a potentially serious problem as it can progress to rotator cuff or biceps tendon rupture.
- **Supraspinatus tendonitis**: The tendon of the supraspinatus is compressed with overhead motions and with many midrange motions of the shoulder. The tendon of the supraspinatus is noted to have a very poor blood supply, and the combination of *frequent compression* (which means *frequent injury*) with a *poor blood supply* greatly predisposes this tendon to inflammation, degeneration, and ultimate rupture. The supraspinatus also works with the deltoid to resist inferior dislocation of the humerus when a heavy load is carried while the shoulder is in adduction, e.g., when carrying a heavy suitcase.[38]
- **Shoulder bursitis, subdeltoid bursitis, subacromial bursitis**: The bursa of the shoulder lies over the rotator cuff and separates it from the deltoid and the acromion. Inflammation/irritation of this bursa, most commonly from overuse, is often the first manifestation of impingement syndrome.[39]
- **Biceps tendonitis**: Irritation and inflammation of the proximal tendon of the long head of the biceps due to any of several factors: lack of stabilization by the transverse ligament of the humerus, compression under the acromion, and/or overuse.
- **Rotator cuff injury**: Irritation and inflammation of the muscles and tendons that make up the rotator cuff (supraspinatus, infraspinatus, teres minor, subscapularis) due to compression under the acromion and/or overuse.
- **Deltoid strain**: Injury to the deltoid—anterior, middle, or posterior aspect can resemble impingement syndrome and rotator cuff disease.

Typical causes of shoulder irritation and injury: the spectrum of common problems from irritation to complete tear of tendons

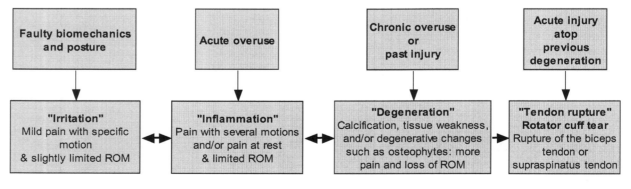

---

[38] Moore KL. Clinically Oriented Anatomy, Third Edition. Baltimore: Williams and Wilkins. 1992 page 537
[39] Belzer JP, Durkin RC. Common disorders of the shoulder. *Prim Care* 1996 Jun;23(2):365-88

Complications:
- Pain
- Limited motion and ability to engage in activities of daily living (ADL)
- Permanent disability with rupture of the rotator cuff

Clinical presentations:
- **Pain with full abduction or full flexion of the shoulder—i.e., worse with overhead motions and positions.**
  - Pain at night is common with repetitive strain injuries, especially rotator cuff injuries.[40] Night pain is also common with cancer—this is important to remember in the differential diagnosis.
  - Pain upon waking suggests that the patient is sleeping in an awkward position such as with full shoulder flexion, thus promoting long-term impingement of the subacromial structures.
  - Pain is generally local but may radiate proximally to the neck or distally to the arm (not past the elbow).
- Occurs following acute injury or repetitive overuse

Major differential diagnoses:
- Some patients may have an "anterior acromial spur," which is an osteophyte projecting inferiorly from the acromion that contributes to their impingement syndrome.[41] This can be viewed radiographically.
- Referred pain:
  - Liver/gall bladder problems
  - Cardiac/ angina
  - Lung tumor
- Cancer: primary (e.g., osteosarcoma), or metastatic (especially breast and lung), local lung tumor such as Pancoast tumor causing referred pain, local pain due to spread into nearby ribs and vertebrae, or compression of the brachial plexus
- Cervical radiculopathy
- Brachial plexus neuropathy
- Systemic disease process, e.g., hemochromatosis and CPPD

> **Lung cancer can cause shoulder pain**
>
> "Ten patients diagnosed with Pancoast tumor were studied retrospectively... Five patients had previously been diagnosed with degenerative, inflammatory, or infectious diseases of the cervical spine or shoulder. In the remaining five patients, the diagnosis was made during the first clinical visit."
>
> Villas C, et al. Cervicobrachialgia and pancoast tumor: value of standard anteroposterior cervical radiographs in early diagnosis. *Orthopedics* 2004;27:1092-5

Clinical assessment:
- History
- Physical examination:
  - **Tenderness with palpation of the affected structures.**
  - **Pain with compression of the various subacromial structures:** Perform the aforementioned physical examination procedures to <u>identify injured structures</u> and to <u>quantify specific deficits</u>.
  - Limited range of motion
  - "*A painful arc*" is noted with shoulder abduction from 90° to 160°

Imaging & laboratory assessments:
- Lab results should be normal.
- Radiographs can be used for the detection of gross degeneration, fracture, etc.
- MRI is considered the best assessment for soft-tissue complaints of the shoulder.[42]

[40] Belzer JP, Durkin RC. Common disorders of the shoulder. *Prim Care* 1996 Jun;23(2):365-88
[41] Belzer JP, Durkin RC. Common disorders of the shoulder. *Prim Care* 1996 Jun;23(2):365-88
[42] Belzer JP, Durkin RC. Common disorders of the shoulder. *Prim Care* 1996 Jun;23(2):365-88

Clinical management:

- The persistence of symptoms for more than 3-4 months despite adequate conservative care indicates the need for investigational imaging: radiographs and/or MRI. Surgery is necessary to repair a full-thickness tear of the rotator cuff, to debride joints with osteocartilaginous debris, and to remove hypertrophic osteophytes that contribute to tissue injury.[43]

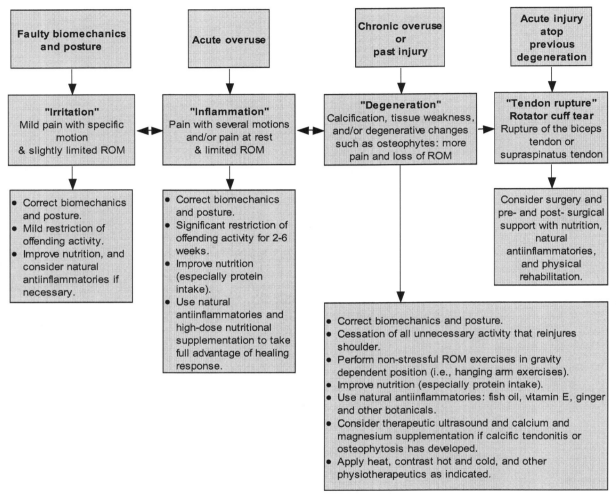

Treatment:

- **Review therapeutic concepts and interventions discussed in Chapter 3**
- Protect & prevent re-injury: Maintain proper spinal posture and neutral positioning as much as possible to promote proper scapulothoracic motion. Avoid overhead lifting and reaching. Patients with impingement syndrome should avoid overhead activities and postures, such as chin-ups, certain swimming strokes, and prone and supine sleeping positions where the arms are placed above shoulder level. Use a brace or sling as needed.
- Relative rest: Avoid motions and activities that cause significant pain. This means the athletes need to take some time off from their activities and reduce the amount of weight lifted. **Reduce frequency, duration, and amount** of weight lifting, repetitions, laps, etc.
- Ice/heat: Until 48-72 hours after injury: apply ice or cold pack for 10-20 minutes each 1-2 hours for reduction in pain and inflammation. Avoid "frostbite" and cold injuries to skin. After 48-72 hours post-injury: apply gentle heat as needed for the relief of pain and reduction in muscle spasm. Avoid exacerbating inflammation and/or creating dynamic instability by inducing excessive muscle relaxation. Avoid burns and heat injuries to skin. Use caution in patients with decreased skin

---

[43] "The arthroscope can be used to review and document the status of the joint and cuff, assess the tear pattern, debride damaged tissues, and smooth the acromion. In addition, a trained shoulder arthroscopist can mobilize the available tissues and repair any viable tendon to bone..." Millstein ES, Snyder SJ. Arthroscopic evaluation and management of rotator cuff tears. *Orthop Clin North Am.* 2003 Oct;34(4):507-20

sensitivity and/or suboptimal ability to follow directions and employ good judgment. In the subacute and chronic phases, ice may be used to reduce inflammation and pain, while heat can be applied to increase circulation.

- **Educate**: *Give the injury plenty of time to heal.*
- **Treat the whole problem**: **Rotator cuff injuries are notorious for becoming chronic problems, and this chronicity is directly caused by four main factors:**
    1. Lack of biomechanical correction:
        a. ***Intrinsic biomechanical faults***: Muscle imbalances, myofascial restrictions, scapulothoracic adhesions, thoracic hyperkyphosis; correctable with doctor-applied intervention and patient-implemented stretching and exercises.
        b. ***Extrinsic biomechanical faults***: Ergonomics and posture; correctable through conscious attention and re-habituation.
    2. Noncompliance: Patient's refusal to take time off from the specific activities and habits that contribute to chronic tissue irritation,
    3. Lack of overall health improvement and creation of an optimized internal healing environment: If patients are allowed to remain deficient in vitamins, minerals, and amino acids required for healing, then healing will be incomplete and retarded at best.
    4. Intrinsic properties of the shoulder histology and anatomy: Lack of direct/sufficient blood supply to tendons of the rotator cuff; development of acromial osteophytes will present a constant threat to the proximal biceps tendon (long head) and the supraspinatus tendon.
- **Rehabilitative exercises, stretching, and manipulation:** Assess and correct impaired scapulothoracic motion by observation during active abduction and manipulation/mobilization/stretching, respectively. Educate patient on ways to avoid re-injury and to decrease likelihood of recurrence. Rehabilitative exercise with minimal resistance in a comfortable/reasonable range of motion to improve/maintain flexibility of joint capsules, ligaments, and other soft tissues and to maintain muscle strength. Isometric exercises can be used to maintain muscle strength in patients for whom range-of-motion exercises are painful or contraindicated. Motion is important to prevent the development of intra-articular adhesions or "frozen shoulder." **When out of the acute inflammatory stage, patient should perform exercises to strengthen and balance the musculature of the shoulder and rotator cuff. Resisted internal and external rotation can strengthen the pectorals/subscapularis and infraspinatus/teres minor, respectively.** Biceps tendonitis may be relieved with strengthening of the posterior deltoid. Modify behavior and home/occupational workstations to minimize strain and stress on injured tissues. Use tools/machines to work efficiently and to reduce unnecessary lifting and straining motions. Normal activities can be fully resumed when symptoms have decreased, when physical examination findings (e.g., strength, range of motion, segmental function, trigger points) are within normal limits, when there is no residual complication that leaves the patient excessively vulnerable to serious re-injury. **Utilize the Spencer technique[44] for in-office mobilization and manipulation and myofascial release of the shoulder; see full-text article for description of procedures:** http://www.jaoa.org/cgi/reprint/102/7/387; if additional details are necessary, see procedural review in *Outline of Osteopathic Manipulative Procedures* by Kimberly.[45]

> **Spencer technique for shoulder rehabilitation**
>
> Post-isometric stretching and passive gymnastics in the following directions and vectors:
> 1. Extension,
> 2. Flexion,
> 3. Compression,
> 4. Traction,
> 5. Abduction,
> 6. Internal rotation,
> 7. Pump.
>
> Knebl JA, Shores JH, Gamber RG, Gray WT, Herron KM. Improving functional ability in the elderly via the Spencer technique, an osteopathic manipulative treatment: a randomized, controlled trial. *J Am Osteopath Assoc* 2002;102:387-96

---

[44] The "seven stages of Spencer" is an organized technique of range-of-motion exercises and post-isometric stretching to improve functionality of the shoulder. This clinical trial showed improved shoulder function in a group of elderly patients treated with this technique. Knebl JA, Shores JH, Gamber RG, Gray WT, Herron KM. Improving functional ability in the elderly via the Spencer technique, an osteopathic manipulative treatment: a randomized, controlled trial. *J Am Osteopath Assoc.* 2002 Jul;102(7):387-96 http://www.jaoa.org/cgi/reprint/102/7/387 See also "CONCLUSION: Manipulative therapy for the shoulder girdle in addition to usual medical care accelerates recovery of shoulder symptoms." Bergman GJ, Winters JC, Groenier KH, Pool JJ, Meyboom-de Jong B, Postema K, van der Heijden GJ. Manipulative therapy in addition to usual medical care for patients with shoulder dysfunction and pain: a randomized, controlled trial. *Ann Intern Med.* 2004 Sep 21;141(6):432-9 http://www.annals.org/cgi/reprint/141/6/432.pdf

[45] Kimberly PE. *Outline of Osteopathic Manipulative Procedures. The Kimberly Manual 2006.* Kirksville College of Osteopathic Medicine. Walsworth Publishing Company Marceline, Mo

Adhesive capsulitis
Frozen shoulder
Frozen shoulder syndrome (FSS)

<u>Description/pathophysiology</u>:[46,47]

- Conditions associated with inflammation of the glenohumeral synovium with the propensity for resultant motion-limiting and painful adhesions; adhesions may also arise secondary to limitations in motion due to pain; may be self-limiting (within 2 years) or may be chronic and unresolving without aggressive intervention.
  - o <u>Primary adhesive capsulitis (primary FSS)</u>: *"idiopathic"* inflammation of the glenohumeral joint leading to painful and restricted active and passive range of motion of the shoulder. Often separated into three phases:[48]
    1. <u>Painful</u>—generally acute onset of pain without injury (after waking); lasts weeks to months.
    2. <u>Stiffening</u>—less pain, but ROM is limited due to contracture and adhesions in the glenohumeral joint; lasts weeks to months to one year.
    3. <u>Thawing</u>—slow regain of motion; lasts weeks to months.
  - o <u>Secondary adhesive capsulitis (secondary FSS)</u>: resultant from other problems, such as impingement syndrome (see notes on impingement syndrome) or disuse due to other injury such as forearm or elbow injury.

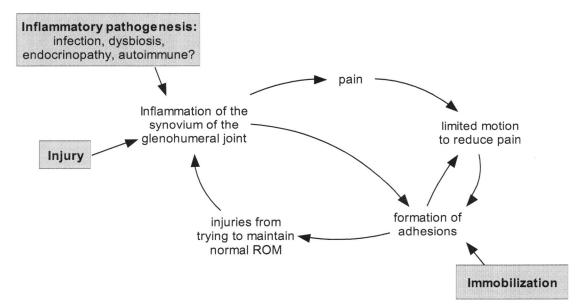

<u>Complications</u>:

- Pain, particularly with attempted motion.
- Limited motion and ability to engage in activities of daily living (ADL).

<u>Clinical presentations</u>:

- **Painful and restricted active and passive range of motion of the shoulder**
- Bilateral in 34% of cases
- Most common in women age 30-60 years
- <u>Often associated with</u>:
  - o <u>Diabetes mellitus</u>

---

[46] After much consideration, I decided to merge the information on frozen shoulder and adhesive capsulitis. Even though these entities are commonly named in the research literature as if they were two different conditions, their overlap and similarities make them clinically, diagnostically, and therapeutically indistinguishable. I tend to think of the idiopathic form as "adhesive capsulitis" and problems secondary to injury or immobilization as "frozen shoulder."
[47] Pearsall AW, Speer KP. Frozen shoulder syndrome: diagnostic and treatment strategies in the primary care setting. *Med Sci Sports Exerc* 1998 Apr;30(4 Suppl):S33-9
[48] Belzer JP, Durkin RC. Common disorders of the shoulder. *Prim Care* 1996 Jun;23(2):365-88

- o Previous shoulder injury and/or immobilization
- o Thoracic hyperkyphosis: increases compression of the supraspinatus tendon at the acromion when performing shoulder abduction
- o Thyroid disease: hyperthyroidism and hypothyroidism[49]
- o Hypoparathyroidism[50]
- o Increased prevalence of HLA-B27: according to one study[51] (refuted[52])
- o Cervical spine problems
- o Ischemic heart disease

Major differential diagnoses:
- Impingement syndrome
- Rotator cuff tear
- Neuropathy, radiculitis
- Brachial plexopathy, including Pancoast syndrome

Clinical assessment:
- History: patient reports limited shoulder motion *with* or *without* history of inciting event
- Physical examination and diagnosis: **Limited ROM:** the most consistent finding is reduced external rotation at 0° and 90° of abduction. The diagnosis can be made based on **history** and **characteristic findings on physical examination** (*significant and polydirectional* ROM limitations at the shoulder) and **exclusion of other causes.** Significant loss of motion at the glenohumeral joint has been defined as ❶ 50% loss of external rotation, ❷ less than 135° of flexion, and ❸ less than 90° of abduction.[53]

Imaging & laboratory assessments:
- Radiographs should be grossly normal. Pearsall and Speer[54] recommend the following 3 views:
  1) AP view: Rotator cuff arthropathy is suggested by an acromion-humerus distance of less than 6 cm
  2) Axillary view
  3) Supraspinatus "outlet view"
- Arthrography: May provide additional information and is considered the "diagnostic test of choice" as it demonstrates the decreased volume and other findings associated with adhesive capsulitis.[55]
- CRP/ESR: May be elevated
- Thyroid disease: Assess with TSH, free T4, and anti-TPO antibodies. Recall that TSH values greater than 2-3 suggest present or impending thyroid dysfunction[56,57] and that many patients with positive anti-TPO antibodies will have normal TSH and free T4 but should still receive thyroid hormone treatment to prevent future hypothyroidism.[58] Hypothyroidism is a cause of adhesive capsulitis. [59]
- Diabetes mellitus: Greatly increased incidence among IDEM patients and often the FSS is bilateral. *"It is imperative...that any new patient presenting with suspected frozen shoulder syndrome be screened for diabetes."*[60]

Establishing the diagnosis:
- The diagnosis of FSS is established in a patient with **painful limitation of shoulder motion for 1 month** *after radiographs and other assessments have ruled out another cause for the shoulder dysfunction.*[61]

[49] Bowman CA, Jeffcoate WJ, Pattrick M, Doherty M. Bilateral adhesive capsulitis, oligoarthritis and proximal myopathy as presentation of hypothyroidism. *Br J Rheumatol* 1988 Feb;27(1):62-4

[50] "CONCLUSION: Our cases suggest that there may be a common immunological or genetic basis for primary hypoparathyroidism and adhesive capsulitis." Harzy T, Benbouazza K, Amine B, Rahmouni R, Guedira N, Hajjaj-Hassouni N. Idiopathic hypoparathyroidism and adhesive capsulitis of the shoulder in two first-degree relatives. *Joint Bone Spine.* 2004 May;71(3):234-6

[51] "HLA-B27 was significantly more common in patients with frozen shoulder (42%) than in the controls (10%)." Bulgen DY, Hazleman BL, Voak D. HLA-B27 and frozen shoulder. *Lancet.* 1976 May 15;1(7968):1042-4

[52] "In 50 patients who had frozen shoulder unassociated with a primary illness, HLA-B27 was detected in only two (4%), a frequency which did not differ significantly from controls." Rizk TE, Pinals RS. Histocompatibility type and racial incidence in frozen shoulder. *Arch Phys Med Rehabil.* 1984 Jan;65(1):33-4

[53] Belzer JP, Durkin RC. Common disorders of the shoulder. *Prim Care* 1996 Jun;23(2):365-88

[54] "...a reliable sign of long-standing rotator cuff arthropathy is an acromial-humeral head distance of less than 6 cm [six centimeters] as viewed on a anteroposterior shoulder radiograph." Pearsall AW, Speer KP. Frozen shoulder syndrome: diagnostic and treatment strategies in the primary care setting. *Med Sci Sports Exerc* 1998 Apr;30(4 Suppl):S33-9

[55] Brier S. Primary Care Orthopedics. St. Louis: Mosby, 1999 page 62

[56] "Now American Association of Clinical Endocrinologists encourages doctors to consider treatment for patients who test outside the boundaries of a narrower margin based on a target TSH level of 0.3 to 3.04. AACE believes the new range will result in proper diagnosis for millions of Americans who suffer from a mild thyroid disorder, but have gone untreated until now." Available at http://www.aace.com/pub/tam2003/press.php as of August 24, 2003.

[57] Weetman AP. Hypothyroidism: screening and subclinical disease. *BMJ.* 1997 Apr 19;314(7088):1175-8. Available at http://bmj.com/cgi/content/full/314/7088/1175 as of August 24, 2003.

[58] Beers MH, Berkow R (eds). The Merck Manual. 17th Edition. Whitehouse Station; Merck Research Laboratories 1999 page 96

[59] Bowman CA, Jeffcoate WJ, Pattrick M, Doherty M. Bilateral adhesive capsulitis, oligoarthritis and proximal myopathy as presentation of hypothyroidism. *Br J Rheumatol* 1988 Feb;27(1):62-4

[60] Pearsall AW, Speer KP. Frozen shoulder syndrome: diagnostic and treatment strategies in the primary care setting. *Med Sci Sports Exerc* 1998 Apr;30(4 Suppl):S33-9

[61] Pearsall AW, Speer KP. Frozen shoulder syndrome: diagnostic and treatment strategies in the primary care setting. *Med Sci Sports Exerc* 1998 Apr;30(4 Suppl):S33-9

Clinical management:
- Conservative treatments are generally used
- Hypothyroid patients may experience clinical exacerbation with the initiation of thyroxin treatment; this exacerbation is followed by clinical and biochemical improvement.[62]

Treatment options:
- **Review therapeutic concepts and interventions discussed in Chapter 3**
- Treatment of underlying autoimmune or endocrinologic disorder (e.g., diabetes, hypothyroidism): Recall that both autoimmune thyroid disease and diabetes are inflammatory disorders and that the adhesive capsulitis may simply be a *focal manifestation* of a *systemic inflammatory process*. The solution then, is to address the underlying problem—the cause of the inflammation.
  - **Find and treat *the cause* of *the cause* of the problem:** A patient may have adhesive capsulitis due to thyroid disease.[63] A patient may have thyroid disease due to iron overload[64] or celiac disease.[65] In this situation, the problem (adhesive capsulitis) may be caused by a secondary disorder (thyroid disease) that is caused by a primary disorder (iron overload or celiac disease). This example speaks not only to the need to screen all musculoskeletal patients for iron overload[66] as suggested in Chapter 1, but it also demonstrates the need to remain astute with regard to clinical pathophysiology and to remain vigilant in the search for underlying problems that prevent patients from attaining optimal health.
- Exercise and Mobilization: Passive and active exercise/mobilization for the preservation of mobility; motion must be kept within patient's pain tolerance and should not induce additional injury which will exacerbate inflammation and additional adhesions.
- Anti-inflammatory and analgesic botanicals and nutraceuticals: **Assume that the inflammation is right; it is correct. The inflammation is to be understood and its cause** *addressed*—**not merely** *suppressed*. **Do not simply mask an inflammatory response with phytonutraceuticals without simultaneously searching for and addressing the underlying cause of the disease.** Vitamin D at 2,000 – 4,000 IU per day along with ALA, EPA, DHA, GLA, and mixed tocopherols (e.g., 1,000 IU per day) can be followed by *Uncaria, Boswellia*, and NF-kappaB inhibitors as described later in this text. **Yes, address the underlying fatty acid imbalances and nutritional deficiencies. Yes, alleviate the pain and inflammation with nutritional and botanical medicines; but always remember that the inflammation is there for a reason, that reason is the true problem (not the inflammation), and your job as a true healer is to find and address the problem, not the body's response to the problem.**
- Search for and eradicate occult infections: The association of HLA-B27 with adhesive capsulitis[67] raises the possibility of dysbiosis as a precipitating factor for adhesive capsulitis in some patients. In these patients, adhesive capsulitis may simply be a variant of **reactive arthritis**—localized joint inflammation as a manifestation of a systemic inflammatory response to occult infection with microorganisms possessing antigens similar to those of their human host (i.e., "molecular mimicry"). Gastrointestinal microorganisms associated with inducing a systemic inflammatory response that leads to a diagnosis of reactive arthritis include *Endolimax nana*[68], *Entamoeba histolytica*[69], *Giardia lamblia*[70], *Klebsiella pneumoniae*[71], *Proteus mirabilis*[72,73,74], *Helicobacter pylori*[75], *Salmonella typhimurium*[76], *Campylobacter jejuni*.[77] HLA-B27 is strongly and consistently

---

[62] Bowman CA, Jeffcoate WJ, Pattrick M, Doherty M. Bilateral adhesive capsulitis, oligoarthritis and proximal myopathy as presentation of hypothyroidism. *Br J Rheumatol* 1988 Feb;27(1):62-4

[63] Bowman CA, Jeffcoate WJ, Pattrick M, Doherty M. Bilateral adhesive capsulitis, oligoarthritis and proximal myopathy as presentation of hypothyroidism. *Br J Rheumatol.* 1988 Feb;27(1):62-4

[64] Edwards CQ, Kelly TM, Ellwein G, Kushner JP. Thyroid disease in hemochromatosis. Increased incidence in homozygous men. *Arch Intern Med.* 1983 Oct;143(10):1890-3

[65] Collin P, Kaukinen K, Valimaki M, Salmi J. Endocrinological disorders and celiac disease. *Endocr Rev.* 2002 Aug;23(4):464-83 http://edrv.endojournals.org/cgi/content/full/23/4/464

[66] Vasquez A. Musculoskeletal disorders and iron overload disease: comment on the American College of Rheumatology guidelines for the initial evaluation of the adult patient with acute musculoskeletal symptoms. *Arthritis Rheum.* 1996 Oct;39(10):1767-8

[67] "HLA-B27 was significantly more common in patients with frozen shoulder (42%) than in the controls (10%)." Bulgen DY, Hazleman BL, Voak D. HLA-B27 and frozen shoulder. *Lancet.* 1976 May 15;1(7968):1042-4

[68] "Endolimax nana grew on stool culture. Both the patient's diarrhea and arthritis responded effectively to therapy with metronidazole. The diagnosis of parasitic rheumatism was made in retrospect." Burnstein SL, Liakos S. Parasitic rheumatism presenting as rheumatoid arthritis. *J Rheumatol.* 1983 Jun;10(3):514-5

[69] Galland L. Intestinal protozoan infection is a common unsuspected cause of chronic illness. *J Advancement Med.* 1989;2: 539-552

[70] Galland L. Intestinal protozoan infection is a common unsuspected cause of chronic illness. *J Advancement Med.* 1989;2: 539-552

[71] Ahmadi K, Wilson C, Tiwana H, Binder A, Ebringer A. Antibodies to Klebsiella pneumoniae lipopolysaccharide in patients with ankylosing spondylitis. *Br J Rheumatol.* 1998 Dec;37(12):1330-3

[72] Ebringer A, Rashid T, Wilson C. Rheumatoid arthritis: proposal for the use of anti-microbial therapy in early cases. *Scand J Rheumatol* 2003;32(1):2-11

[73] Rashid T, Darlington G, Kjeldsen-Kragh J, Forre O, Collado A, Ebringer A. Proteus IgG antibodies and C-reactive protein in English, Norwegian and Spanish patients with rheumatoid arthritis. *Clin Rheumatol* 1999;18(3):190-5

[74] Wilson C, Rashid T, Tiwana H, Beyan H, Hughes L, Bansal S, Ebringer A, Binder A. Cytotoxicity responses to Peptide antigens in rheumatoid arthritis and ankylosing spondylitis. *J Rheumatol* 2003 May;30(5):972-8

[75] "Four cases of reactive arthritis (ReA) related to Helicobacter pylori (HP) are presented." Melby KK, Kvien TK, Glennas A. Helicobacter pylori--a trigger of reactive arthritis? *Infection.* 1999;27(4-5):252-5

[76] "Four were positive for HLA-B27, 6 were HLA-B7 positive, and 1 had HLA-Bw60. Of the 4 B27 positive patients, 3 were DR1 positive; of the 6 B7 positive patients, 5 were DR2 positive." Inman RD, Johnston ME, Hodge M, Falk J, Helewa A. Postdysenteric reactive arthritis. A clinical and immunogenetic study following an outbreak of salmonellosis. *Arthritis Rheum.* 1988 Nov;31(11):1377-83

associated with increased inflammatory reactivity to microbial antigens, particularly lipopolysaccharides from enteric and genitourinary colonization/infection with *Klebsiella pneumoniae*. In patients with otherwise refractory adhesive capsulitis and/or those patients with a compelling clinical picture (e.g., history of gastroenteritis or positive stool results), appropriate antimicrobial therapy directed toward enteric, genitourinary and possibly intraarticular[78] and cutaneous[79] microbes should be implemented following comprehensive parasitology analysis and other culture and sensitivity techniques. Inclusion of patients with antigens other than HLA-B27 for this treatment approach is likewise warranted, as previous research has associated HLA-B7, HLA-DR1, and HLA-DR2 with reactive arthritis following *Salmonella typhimurium* gastroenteritis[80], for example. By logical extension, **all patients with idiopathic inflammatory disorders are candidates for assessment for occult infection and appropriate immune supportive and antimicrobial therapy—this is a very safe and effective approach that is extensively detailed in Chapter 4 of *Integrative Rheumatology*.** A survey of the literature suggests that essentially any gastrointestinal, cutaneous, respiratory, or genitourinary colonization with inciting microorganisms may precipitate a systemic inflammatory response in susceptible individuals.[81]

- <u>Manipulation under anesthesia</u>: Can be considered for patients refractory to improvement for 4-6 months of conservative care.[82]
- <u>Surgery</u>: May be recommended for patients who do not experience improvement after 3 months of conservative care.

Report of two cases: the author's experience in using synthetic thyroid hormone and nutritional supplementation in the treatment of idiopathic adhesive capsulitis:

o *Presentations*: Two middle-aged female patients presented with multi-year histories of idiopathic, spontaneous adhesive capsulitis (frozen shoulder). Both patients had previous medical histories of autoimmune hypothyroidism evidenced by persistent elevation of antithyroid antibodies, particularly anti-TPO[83], and both patients had already been treated for several years with bovine/porcine-sourced thyroid hormone such as Armour thyroid. Both patients had painful restriction of motion at the shoulder, which was bilateral in one patient and unilateral in the other.

o *Interventions*: Both patients were treated with general dietary improvement (including wheat exclusion) and nutritional supplementation with a high-potency multivitamin/multimineral supplement, mixed tocopherols with a high concentration of gamma tocopherol, and modest doses of fatty acids, particularly EPA and DHA. In both cases, their bovine/porcine-sourced thyroid hormone was replaced with synthetic "hypoallergenic" thyroid hormone, either L-thyroxine/Synthroid (synthetic T4 only) or Liotrix/Thyrolar (synthetic T3 and T4). When Synthroid was used, only the 50 mcg pill was used because it is the only reasonable dose that does not contain tartrazine, a known allergen and inflammatory irritant for some patients. No musculoskeletal manipulation, therapeutic exercise, or ergonomic modifications were used.

o *Rationale*: The advantage of the synthetic source of T4 and T3 is that it does not perpetuate the antigenic stimulation that is commonly seen with bovine- or porcine-sourced thyroid replacement; for this reason, Armour thyroid or other bovine- or porcine-sourced thyroid replacement is generally contraindicated in patients with thyroid autoimmunity. Many patients with thyroid autoimmunity have occult celiac disease ("wheat allergy"), and their thyroid status normalizes and autoimmunity can completely disappear following implementation of a wheat-free gluten-free diet. Fish oil[84], gamma-tocopherol[85], and multivitamin/multimineral supplementation (containing 200 mcg of selenium) all provide health-promoting and anti-inflammatory benefits; several studies have shown that selenium can ameliorate thyroid autoimmunity.[86]

o *Results*: Both patients responded within 7-14 days dramatic reductions in pain and increased range of motion. In one case, her shoulder disease returned with discontinuation of thyroid treatment and the disease again remitted with reinstatement of thyroid treatment. With the combination of diet improvement, nutritional supplementation, and the use of hypoallergenic/hypoimmunogenic thyroid hormone, both patients appear to have been rapidly cured of their idiopathic adhesive capsulitis that had persisted for years under allopathic management. Both patients remained free of adhesive capsulitis years later.

---

[77] "A severe attack of acute polyarthritis following a verified Campylobacter jejuni enteritis is described in a 12-year-old boy. The patient possesses the HLA-B27 antigen--often found in postinfectious arthritis following acute enteric infections." Bekassay AN, Enell H, Schalen C. Severe polyarthritis following Campylobacter enteritis in a 12-year-old boy. *Acta Paediatr Scand.* 1980 Mar;69(2):269-71

[78] "Current evidence supports the concept that reactive arthritis (ReA) is an immune-mediated synovitis resulting from slow bacterial infections and showing intra-articular persistence of viable, non-culturable bacteria and/or immunogenetic bacterial antigens synthesized by metabolically active bacteria residing in the joint and/or elsewhere in the body." Colmegna I, Cuchacovich R, Espinoza LR. HLA-B27-associated reactive arthritis: pathogenetic and clinical considerations. *Clin Microbiol Rev.* 2004 Apr;17(2):348-69

[79] "To our knowledge, this is the first demonstration of the efficacy of prolonged antibiotic therapy on the joint manifestations of chronic rheumatism associated with acne." Delyle LG, Vittecoq O, Bourdel A, Duparc F, Michot C, Le Loet X. Chronic destructive oligoarthritis associated with Propionibacterium acnes in a female patient with acne vulgaris: septic-reactive arthritis? *Arthritis Rheum.* 2000 Dec;43(12):2843-7

[80] "Four were positive for HLA-B27, 6 were HLA-B7 positive, and 1 had HLA-Bw60. Of the 4 B27 positive patients, 3 were DR1 positive; of the 6 B7 positive patients, 5 were DR2 positive." Inman RD, Johnston ME, Hodge M, Falk J, Helewa A. Postdysenteric reactive arthritis. A clinical and immunogenetic study following an outbreak of salmonellosis. *Arthritis Rheum.* 1988 Nov;31(11):1377-83

[81] **Vasquez A. Reducing Pain and Inflammation Naturally. Part 6: Nutritional and Botanical Treatments Against "Silent Infections" and Gastrointestinal Dysbiosis, Commonly Overlooked Causes of Neuromusculoskeletal Inflammation and Chronic Health Problems. *Nutritional Perspectives* 2006; January** http://optimalhealthresearch.com/part6.html

[82] Kivimaki J, Pohjolainen T. Manipulation under anesthesia for frozen shoulder with and without steroid injection. *Arch Phys Med Rehabil.* 2001 Sep;82(9):1188-90

[83] Beers MH, Berkow R (eds). The Merck Manual. 17th Edition. Whitehouse Station; Merck Research Laboratories 1999 page 96

[84] Simopoulos AP. Essential fatty acids in health and chronic disease. *Am J Clin Nutr.* 1999 Sep;70(3 Suppl):560S-569S

[85] Jiang Q, Christen S, Shigenaga MK, Ames BN. gamma-tocopherol, the major form of vitamin E in the US diet, deserves more attention. *Am J Clin Nutr* 2001;74(6):714-22

[86] "Group I (Gr I) (n=34) was treated with selenomethionine (Seme) 200 microg, plus L-thyroxine (LT(4)) to maintain TSH levels between 0.3-2.0 mU/l... In Gr I, antibodies against thyroid peroxidase (anti-TPO) levels showed an overall decrease of 46% at 3 months and of 55.5% at 6 months..." Duntas LH, Mantzou E, Koutras DA. Effects of a six-month treatment with selenomethionine in patients with autoimmune thyroiditis. *Eur J Endocrinol.* 2003 Apr;148(4):389-93

Tendonitis of the rotator cuff
Calcific tendonitis of the rotator cuff

Description/pathophysiology:
- Inflammation of the tendons of the muscles that comprise the rotator cuff:
  - Supraspinatus: The tendon of this muscle is most often affected, often in isolation (i.e., without injury to the other tendons of the rotator cuff)[87]
  - Infraspinatus, Teres minor, Subscapularis: Tendons of these muscles may also be affected, but this is less common and more often associated with direct injury
- Deposition of calcium in the tendons of the rotator cuff is initially asymptomatic. Later as the calcium is resorbed, pain and inflammation become problematic

Complications:
- Painful and limited ROM and ADL.
- May ultimately culminate in lysis of the inflamed tendon(s)

Clinical presentations:
- An achy sensation of deep pressure in superior-lateral shoulder unrelated to motion
- Impingement may exacerbate pain
- Symptoms may last for days to months
- Pain may be mild or severe
- Bilateral presentation is common (46%) and suggests a systemic/metabolic disturbance (no associations have been identified in the research)

Major differential diagnoses:
- Referred pain:
  - Liver/gall bladder problems
  - Cardiac/ angina
  - Lung tumor
- Local cancer: primary (e.g., osteosarcoma), or metastatic (especially breast and lung)
- Cervical radiculopathy
- Brachial plexus neuropathy
- Systemic disease process[88]
  - Hemochromatosis: test serum ferritin
  - Calcium pyrophosphate dihydrate (CPPD) crystal deposition: assess for hyperparathyroidism, hypophosphatasia, Wilson's disease, acromegaly, gout, hypothyroidism
  - Hypomagnesemia
  - Hypothyroidism

Clinical assessment:
- History: may have a normal history or past trauma to shoulder
- Physical examination: pain with pressure on the involved structures

Imaging & laboratory assessments:
- Radiographs demonstrate deposition of calcium in the tendons of the rotator cuff.
- MRI and ultrasound are used to image the tendons, especially for signs of rupture or partial tears

---

[87] Belzer JP, Durkin RC. Common disorders of the shoulder. *Prim Care* 1996 Jun;23(2):365-88

[88] "If young people develop CPPD crystal deposition disease, it may be associated with metabolic diseases such as hemochromatosis, hyperparathyroidism, hypophosphatasia, hypomagnesemia, Wilson's disease, hypothyroidism, gout, acromegaly, and X-linked hypophosphatemic rickets." Ahn JK, Kim HJ, Kim EH, Jeon CH, Cha HS, Ha CW, Ahn JM, Koh EM. Idiopathic calcium pyrophosphate dihydrate (CPPD) crystal deposition disease in a young male patient: a case report. *J Korean Med Sci.* 2003 Dec;18(6):917-20 See OptimalHealthResearch.com/articles.htm for the complete text.

Clinical management:
- Assess for and treat any underlying problems
- Assist self-resolution
- Referral if clinical outcome is unsatisfactory or if serious complications are evident

Treatment:
- **Review therapeutic concepts and interventions discussed in Chapter 3**
- Magnesium supplementation to bowel tolerance or 600 mg per day, which ever comes first
- Exercise and ROM maintenance to tolerance
- **Cross fiber friction massage: deep for tendonitis, while only light pressure is used in the treatment of *calcific* tendonitis to address the overlying bursitis**[89]
- **Therapeutic ultrasound with cortisone cream for calcific tendonitis**[90]
- Acupuncture for pain relief[91]
- Invasive decompression or surgery for severe and recalcitrant cases

Additional orthopedic problems of the shoulder region

Problem and Presentation	Assessment and Management
Clavicle fracture • Pain in the "shoulder" or anterior upper thorax following either direct trauma to the clavicle or shoulder or a fall on an outstretched arm • The clavicle is the most commonly fractured bone in the body	Assessment: • Increased pain with application of tuning fork or local percussion on clavicle • Assess for related injuries to arm, wrist, hand, neck, sternoclavicular (SC) joints, acromioclavicular (AC) joints, subclavian artery, brachial plexus, cephalic vein, and other local and adjacent structures • Radiographs Management: • Because of the diversity of complications including non-union, cosmetic deformity, AC separation, functional disability, and risk to underlying neurovascular structures, orthopedic consultation is recommended

[89] Gimblett PA, Saville J, Ebrall P. A conservative management protocol for calcific tendonitis of the shoulder. *J Manipulative Physiol Ther*. 1999 Nov-Dec;22(9):622-7
[90] "...10 sessions of phonophoresis with... a topical cream containing cortisone, and 7 minutes of 10% pulsed ultrasound at 1.7 W/cm2. This was combined with cross-friction techniques to the supraspinatus tendon and range of motion exercises... ...cortisone would appear to be an integral part of the treatment protocol." Gimblett PA, Saville J, Ebrall P. A conservative management protocol for calcific tendonitis of the shoulder. *J Manipulative Physiol Ther*. 1999 Nov-Dec;22(9):622-7
[91] "Acupuncture with penetration of the skin was shown to be more effective than a similar therapeutic setting with placebo needling in the treatment of pain. ... This study showed that needling is an important part of the acupuncture effect in the treatment of chronic shoulder pain in athletes." Kleinhenz J, Streitberger K, Windeler J, Gussbacher A, Mavridis G, Martin E. Randomised clinical trial comparing the effects of acupuncture and a newly designed placebo needle in rotator cuff tendinitis. *Pain*. 1999 Nov;83(2):235-41

Problem and Presentation	Assessment and Management
Thoracic outlet syndrome (TOS) • Signs and symptoms resultant from neurovascular compression of the brachial plexus and/or subclavian artery generally due to hypertonic or imbalanced musculoskeletal structures • Periodic or constant pain, numbness, or paresthesia in the neck, shoulder or arm • Symptoms are typically mechanical and reproducible with specific postures and positions of the upper extremity	**Assessment:** • Clinical assessments are sufficient for diagnosis and include Wrights, Roos, and Adson's tests. • Assessment for underlying disease with history, physical examination (i.e., palpation for supraclavicular and axillary lymph nodes, auscultation of carotid and subclavian arteries, auscultation of lungs) is performed to exclude underlying disease. • Palpation/radiographs may reveal the presence of a cervical rib, which can cause or exacerbate neurovascular compression leading to TOS. **Management:** • Conservative care,[92] including modification of posture to avoid the "head forward" position common to many desk workers is important along with stretching procedures for the cervical musculature, especially the anterolateral and lateral muscles such as the scalenes. Thrice daily stretching of the scalenes with the head moved laterally or laterally-posteriorly often produces dramatic results within a few days for most patients who are compliant. • Additional treatments, assessment for underlying disease and/or referral is indicated for patients who do not improve within 2-3 weeks.
Acromioclavicular joint sprain, AC separation, "shoulder separation" • Shoulder pain at the acromion-clavicular junction • Visible and palpable "step defect" or lack of alignment between the distal clavicle and the acromion process following trauma to the upper extremity or shoulder • Results from trauma resulting in damage to acromioclavicular ligament and the coracoclavicular ligaments	**Assessment:** • Assess function, strength, and pain with the customary active and passive range-of-motion and physical examination assessments. • Anteroposterior radiograph of the shoulder is used to accurately quantify the degree of separation and to assess for local fracture. **Management:** • **Type/grade #1**: pain, swelling, and injury at the AC joint, but no evidence of separation; treat with ice, rest, and analgesics. • **Type/grade #2—partially torn AC ligament**: visible and palpable separation at the AC joint with moderate to severe pain; treatment may include immobilization with Kenney-Howard sling for 2-6 weeks. Elbow is always supported to maintain AC contact. Referral for orthopedic co-management is recommended since some of these patients require surgical intervention.[93] • **Type/grade #3—completely torn AC and coracoclavicular ligaments**: obvious separation at the AC joint with visible deformity. Some patients may be treated conservatively with immobilization with Kenney-Howard sling for 4-6 weeks[94]; however orthopedic referral is strongly advised to ensure proper care and to limit practitioner liability. Some authors use a 3-point evaluation system while most specialists use a 5- or 6-point evaluation system. My judgment is that the 3-point classification is more clinically useful for non-specialist general practitioners who simply need to decide whether or not to make a referral to a medical orthopedist. Clinicians who are specialists in advanced techniques of bracing, casting, and rehabilitating these injuries can use the more detailed 5-point system to guide treatment.[95] For the majority of clinicians, simply knowing when to use conservative care and when to refer is all that is clinically essential. All patients should receive supportive diet, nutritional and botanical antiinflammatories and analgesics, and rehabilitation whether or not surgical repair is pursued.

[92] Liebenson CS. Thoracic outlet syndrome: diagnosis and conservative management. *J Manipulative Physiol Ther*. 1988 Dec;11(6):493-9
[93] Winkel D, et al. Diagnosis and Treatment of the Upper Extremities: Nonoperative Orthopaedic Medicine and Manual Therapy. Gaithersburg: Aspen Publications. 1997; page 92
[94] Souza TA. Differential Diagnosis for the Chiropractor: Protocols and Algorithms. Gaithersburg: Aspen Publications. 1997 page 169
[95] Bradley JP, Elkousy H. Decision making: operative versus nonoperative treatment of acromioclavicular joint injuries. *Clin Sports Med*. 2003;22(2):277-90

Chapter 8:
Arm, Elbow, and Forearm

Introduction
This section reviews common problems of the arm, elbow, and forearm. These disorders are frequently encountered in clinical practice among athletic and sedentary patients alike. An understanding of the clinical assessments can lead to a precise diagnosis and to an effective treatment plan—not just routine treatment with antiinflammatory drugs for every problem regardless of its etiology and nuances.

Overview:
- Compared with that required for the shoulder, the essential clinical information for the arm, elbow, and forearm is much easier to learn and much shorter in length. While individual consideration must be made for each patient and for each separate condition, generally speaking: if it is a muscle injury or mild joint injury, then treat it with nutrition and rest; if it is a significant injury to the joint, intracapsular joint degeneration, or bone fracture, then refer the patient to a medical orthopedist for casting and/or surgery unless you are a specialist in this field. Peripheral nerve compression/entrapment syndromes often respond to conservative treatments; but progressive functional loss indicates the need for orthopedic or neurologic referral.

Core competencies:
1. You must know how to diagnose and manage supracondylar fractures of the humerus.
2. You must know how to diagnose and manage lateral epicondylitis.
3. Know that acute compartment syndrome can also occur in the forearm just as it more commonly occurs in the lower leg. Be able to describe the mechanism by which acute compartment syndrome can lead to local paralysis, muscle necrosis, renal failure, and death (as discussed in Chapter 1).
4. When treating bursitis, as a matter of course you should generally consider the possibility of bursa infection and perform a basic screening assessment for infection—temperature, pulse rate, CBC and CRP—even if the problem appears routine and noninfectious. Infection with multidrug-resistant *Staphylococcus aureus* (MRSA) is not an uncommon cause of bursitis, and patients may have no systemic complaints.

> *Author's experience*: A 28-year-old pregnant woman presented with shoulder pain consistent with subdeltoid bursitis. Blood pressure, pulse rate, and respiratory rate were normal; the patient was afebrile and had no systemic complaints. This case appeared straightforward, and I decided to treat her nutritionally; however, before she left the office I decided to order a CBC. The CBC returned the next day showing leukocytosis; the patient was referred to the emergency department for aspiration, which showed purulent bursitis, and she was admitted to the hospital and treated with intravenous antibiotics.

Clinical assessments of the arm, elbow, and forearm

Clinical assessments[1]	Positive finding and Implications
1. **History**: *See Chapter 1 for additional information*	<ul><li>**Indicators from the history (trauma, risk factors)**</li><li>**Systemic manifestations**</li><li>**Complications**</li><li>**Mechanical/ Nonmechanical**</li></ul> Increased risk for serious pathology and potential complications. Defer or modify physical examination based on your assessment of the situation
2. **Observation**	Search for: <ul><li>Asymmetry, dislocation</li><li>Muscle atrophy</li><li>Ecchymosis</li><li>Inflammation</li><li>Scars</li><li>*Other findings…*</li></ul> Possible implications: <ul><li>Injury, congenital anomaly, asymmetric development due to asymmetric use.</li><li>Muscle atrophy may be due to neurologic deficit or disuse (secondary to injury or pain)</li><li>Ecchymosis is seen after fractures and soft tissue injuries</li></ul>
3. **Range of motion**: ROM should be "full and painless" in all directions: <ul><li>Flexion</li><li>Extension</li><li>Pronation</li><li>Supination</li></ul>	Search for: <ul><li>Limitation</li><li>Pain</li></ul> Possible implications: <ul><li>Injury</li><li>Muscle spasm</li><li>Contracture/adhesion of soft tissues: muscles, joint capsule</li><li>Swelling</li></ul>
4. **Muscle testing and provocation** <ul><li>Biceps</li><li>Triceps</li><li>Brachioradialis</li><li>Wrist flexors</li><li>Wrist extensors</li></ul>	<ul><li>Pain—muscle injury, tendonitis</li><li>Weakness—may be secondary to pain, may indicate neuropathy</li><li>Pain *and* weakness may indicate myopathy, as seen with polymyositis, dermatomyositis, or adverse drug effect</li></ul>
5. **Palpation and provocation**: compare with opposite side	<ul><li>Pain, tenderness, mass, enlargement, or other abnormality may indicate recent injury, inflammation, myofascial trigger points, or other problem. Be aware of subcutaneous swelling, tissue edema, and enlarged lymph nodes</li></ul>
6. **Biceps tendon palpation**: When performed at 90° of shoulder flexion this has been referred to as Lippman's test[2]	<ul><li>Tenderness with palpation of the biceps tendon at the anterior proximal humerus suggests irritation, inflammation, and biceps tendonitis, which may be secondary to anterior impingement syndrome</li></ul>

---

[1] Review relevant information in Magee DJ. Orthopedic Physical Assessment. Third edition. Philadelphia: WB Saunders, 1997 and Bates B. A Guide to Physical Examination and History Taking. 6th Edition. Philadelphia; J. B. Lippincott Company, 1995
[2] Magee DJ. Orthopedic Physical Assessment. Third edition. Philadelphia: WB Saunders, 1997 page 216

Clinical assessments of the arm, elbow, and forearm—*continued*

Selected assessments	Positive finding and Implications
7. **Valgus testing**: Flex elbow to 25° then add lateral pressure to elbow and assess for excessive motion	▪ Excessive motion and/or pain suggest injury to the medial collateral ligament; may be associated with articular or osseous injury at the radial head
8. **Varus testing**: Flex elbow to 25° then add medial pressure to elbow and assess for excessive motion	▪ Excessive motion and/or pain suggest injury to the lateral collateral ligament
9. **Mill's test**: Patient's elbow is extended with forearm pronated; doctor induces passive wrist flexion to stretch the wrist extensors[3]	▪ Pain at lateral epicondyle and/or wrist extensor group suggests **lateral epicondylitis**, injury to the wrist extensors, or possibly radial nerve injury ▪ *Recall that* <u>Mill's</u> *test stretches* <u>Muscle</u>, *while* <u>Cozen's</u> *test requires* <u>Contraction</u> *of muscle*
10. **Reverse Mill's test**: Patient's elbow is extended; doctor induces passive wrist extension to stretch the wrist flexors[4]	▪ Pain at medial epicondyle and/or wrist flexor group suggests **medial epicondylitis** or injury to the wrist flexors
11. **Cozen's test**: Patient's elbow is extended or flexed, forearm pronated with wrist extended, patient resists wrist flexion force by doctor[5]	▪ Pain at the lateral epicondyle or weakness due to pain suggests **lateral epicondylitis** and/or injury to the wrist extensors. Painless weakness suggests nerve lesion: C7 or radial nerve ▪ *Recall that* <u>Mill's</u> *test stretches* <u>Muscle</u>, *while* <u>Cozen's</u> *test requires* <u>Contraction</u> *of muscle*
12. **Reverse Cozen's test**: With the wrist flexed, patient resists wrist extension	▪ Pain in the anterior forearm or medial epicondyle suggests **medial epicondylitis** and/or injury to the wrist flexors
13. **Cervical spine regional assessment**	▪ Pain felt in the upper extremity may originate in the cervical spine or structures of the neck ▪ *See Cervical Spine and Neck notes*
14. **Neurologic assessment**	▪ Weakness, loss of function, loss of sensation, hyporeflexia, hyperreflexia, paresthesia suggest neurologic compromise—cord, nerve root, peripheral nerve, double crush syndrome. Painful weakness suggests muscle injury or myopathy
15. **Radiographs**	Assess for: ▪ Degeneration ▪ Calcification ▪ Fracture ▪ Infection

---

[3] Magee DJ. <u>Orthopedic Physical Assessment. Third edition</u>. Philadelphia: WB Saunders, 1997 page 258
[4] Souza TA. <u>Differential Diagnosis for the Chiropractor: Protocols and Algorithms</u>. Gaithersburg: Aspen Publications. 1997 page 179
[5] Magee DJ. <u>Orthopedic Physical Assessment. Third edition</u>. Philadelphia: WB Saunders, 1997 page 258.

Algorithm for the Assessment and Management of Elbow Complaints

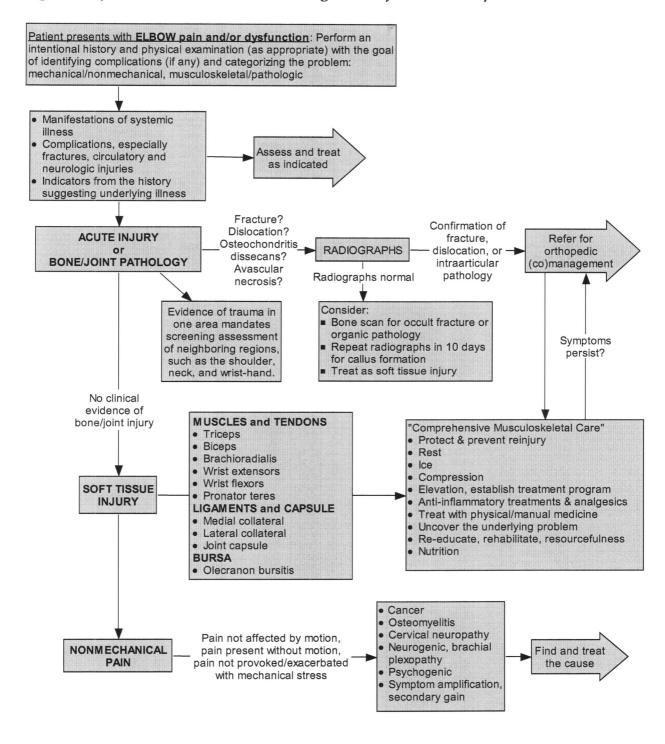

Selected Orthopedic Problems of the Arm, Elbow, and Forearm

Regarding elbow injuries in children: "**Unless you have considerable training and experience in pediatric musculoskeletal trauma, do not get involved with managing elbow injuries. They are notorious for related neurovascular damage and for malunions and nonunions that cause pain, stiffness, and deformities. Every swollen elbow requires high-quality AP and lateral radiographs.**"[6]

Problem	Presentation	Assessment	Management
Humerus fracture: May result in neurovascular compromise[7]; in children, humeral fractures can result in permanent deformity if not treated quickly[8] Fractures involving the middle or distal humerus commonly result in neurovascular lesions and must therefore be assessed and managed as potential neurovascular emergencies.	▪ **Arm/humerus pain following fall on outstretched arm, hyperextension injury, or direct trauma** ▪ Most common in children younger than 10 years ▪ **Clinical assessment for fracture neurovascular injury: cautious physical examination followed by radiographs** ▪ **Bone fracture may sever nearby nerves and arteries and may present with pulselessness, pallor, or muscle weakness**	▪ **Midshaft fracture:** Test for lesion of radial nerve (extensor weakness) and profunda brachii artery and radial collateral artery: myalgia, ecchymosis, blood accumulation ▪ **Supracondylar fracture of humerus:** Test for radial nerve lesion (forearm extensor weakness) or median nerve lesion (forearm flexor weakness); assess brachial artery (distal pulselessness) ▪ **Medial epicondyle fracture:** Test for lesion of ulnar nerve (flexor carpi ulnaris and interossei)	▪ Surgical correction is generally necessary. Nerve and vascular injuries are common[9] ▪ **Emergency surgery for neurovascular injuries. Urgent orthopedic referral for fractures; when managing pediatric trauma, consider working with an orthopedist who specializes in pediatric trauma/orthopedics**
Fracture of the olecranon	▪ Elbow pain and possible deformity after trauma involving the upper extremity, including direct trauma to elbow	▪ Radiographs ▪ Clinical assessment for concomitant humeral fracture, neurovascular injury, and distal extremity injury ▪ Proximal displacement of olecranon due to tension from triceps is common	▪ Orthopedic referral followed by integrative care is recommended
Fracture of radial head: 20% of acute elbow injuries include a fracture of the radial head (proximal end of radius at elbow); may occur during treatment for radial head subluxation	▪ Elbow pain or restricted motion following trauma to the elbow (direct) or upper extremity (indirect)	▪ Physical examination may reveal local tenderness and restricted motion ▪ Radiographs demonstrate overt or minor/chip fracture	▪ Orthopedic referral followed by integrative care is recommended

---

[6] Shaw BA, Gerardi JA, Hennrikus WL. How to avoid orthopedic pitfalls in children. *Patient Care* 1999; Feb 28: 95-116
[7] Wu J, Perron AD, Miller MD, Powell SM, Brady WJ. Orthopedic pitfalls in the ED: pediatric supracondylar humerus fractures. *Am J Emerg Med.* 2002 Oct;20(6):544-50
[8] Shaw BA, Gerardi JA, Hennrikus WL. How to avoid orthopedic pitfalls in children. *Patient Care* 1999; Feb 28: 95-116
[9] Gosens T, Bongers KJ. Neurovascular complications and functional outcome in displaced supracondylar fractures of the humerus in children. *Injury.* 2003 May;34(4):267-73

Selected Orthopedic Problems of the Arm, Elbow, and Forearm—*continued*

Problem	Presentation	Assessment	Management
Midshaft fracture of ulna	▪ Midshaft pain perhaps accompanied by deformity following complex trauma or direct blow to ulna ("nightstick fracture")	▪ Local pain following injury exacerbated by local percussion or vibration ▪ Radiographs show fracture	▪ Casting or orthopedic referral followed by integrative care is recommended
Fracture of distal radius near wrist: These are common fractures following a fall on an outstretched hand, and the fracture frequently extends into the joint, thus increasing risk for chronic pain and functional compromise	▪ Distal radius pain following direct trauma ▪ Posterior displacement of radial fragments is termed "Colle's fracture"	▪ Pain is generally exacerbated by careful local percussion and application of 128 Hz tuning fork ▪ Radiographs	▪ Due to increased risk for chronic complications—especially for injuries that extend into the joint—orthopedic surgical consultation is required
Elbow dislocation: 10% of elbow dislocations have a concomitant fracture of the radius	▪ Elbow pain and possible deformity after trauma involving the upper extremity	▪ **Detailed clinical assessment for neurovascular injury**[10,11] ▪ Radiographs	▪ Orthopedic referral is recommended followed by conservative care
Valgus injury to elbow: Sprain of the medial collateral ligament and/or compression injury to radial head	▪ Injury to elbow with valgus force ▪ Throwing injury ▪ Injury from swinging racket, bat, or golf club	▪ **Valgus stress shows laxity** ▪ **Palpation and provocation of affected structures** ▪ **Consider radiographs if concerned about fracture or avascular necrosis**	▪ Conservative care emphasizing rest and anti-inflammation ▪ If laxity is significant and/or functional compromise is a concern, refer for orthopedic consultation
Radial head subluxation, "Nursemaid's elbow": The colloquial name is derived from occasions when a child's guardian would forcibly pull the child by the wrist, thus inducing a traction dislocation of the radius from the capitulum and annular ligament	▪ Traction force on distal forearm ▪ Most common in children, due to laxity of ligaments	▪ Palpation and provocation of affected structures ▪ Radiographs to exclude fracture, especially if swelling is present[12]	▪ "Reduction is accomplished by elbow flexion and rotation. Radiographic confirmation of reduction should be performed."[13] ▪ Since manual reduction can result in fracture of the radial head, recommend orthopedic referral unless the practitioner is uniquely skilled in this maneuver

[10] Squires NA, Tomaino MM. Brachial artery rupture without median nerve dysfunction after closed elbow dislocation. *Am J Orthop*. 2003 Jun;32(6):298-300
[11] Akansel G, Dalbayrak S, Yilmaz M, Bekler H, Arslan A. MRI demonstration of intra-articular median nerve entrapment after elbow dislocation. *Skeletal Radiol*. 2003 Sep;32(9):537-41. Epub 2003 Jul 31
[12] Shaw BA, Gerardi JA, Hennrikus WL. How to avoid orthopedic pitfalls in children. *Patient Care* 1999; Feb 28: 95-116
[13] Souza TA. Differential Diagnosis for the Chiropractor: Protocols and Algorithms. Gaithersberg: Aspen Publications. 1997 page 187

Problem	Presentation	Assessment	Management
Triceps tendonitis "Posterior tennis elbow"	▪ Injury ▪ Overuse ▪ Pain at posterior elbow	▪ Pain with contraction of triceps and deep palpation of distal/olecranon insertion	▪ Rest, anti-inflammatory treatments, ergonomic improvements, and other appropriate interventions (review Chapter 3)
Biceps tendonitis	▪ Chronic irritation, overuse, and compression under the acromion are generally the cause of *proximal* biceps tendonitis ▪ Injury and acute overuse are generally the cause of *distal* biceps tendonitis	▪ Pain with contraction of biceps and deep palpation of insertion	▪ Rest, anti-inflammatory treatments, ergonomic improvements, and other appropriate interventions (review Chapter 3) ▪ In chronic cases of proximal biceps tendonitis, encourage strengthening of the teres minor, teres major, posterior deltoid, and latissimus dorsi to establish muscle balance about the glenohumeral joint; test for and treat myofascial restrictions of the shoulder with Spencer technique[14]
Rupture of the biceps tendon	▪ Pain/weakness with biceps contraction ▪ Usually acute onset after heavy lifting or sports activity	▪ Lack of biceps strength and tissue deficit suggests tear of biceps tendon and the need for orthopedic referral	▪ Orthopedic referral for surgical reattachment for complete tears.
Anterior capsule strain	▪ Pain after trauma or hyperextension of elbow	▪ Pain with hyperextension and deep palpation	▪ Rest, anti-inflammatory treatments, ergonomic improvements, and other appropriate interventions (review Chapter 3)
Lateral epicondylitis: "Tennis elbow"	▪ Following trauma or overuse of the brachioradialis or the lateral wrist extensors	▪ Cozen's test ▪ Mill's test ▪ Tenderness with local palpation at the lateral epicondyle	▪ Rest, anti-inflammatory treatments, ergonomic improvements, and other appropriate interventions (review Chapter 3) ▪ Joint manipulation of the elbow can be helpful[15,16] ▪ Repetitive mobilization of the scaphoid bone in the palmar direction while the wrist is in extension has also been shown effective[17]

[14] The "seven stages of Spencer" is an organized technique of range-of-motion exercises and post-isometric stretching to improve functionality of the shoulder. This clinical trial showed improved shoulder function in a group of elderly patients treated with this technique. Knebl JA, Shores JH, Gamber RG, Gray WT, Herron KM. Improving functional ability in the elderly via the Spencer technique, an osteopathic manipulative treatment: a randomized, controlled trial. *J Am Osteopath Assoc.* 2002 Jul;102(7):387-96 http://www.jaoa.org/cgi/reprint/102/7/387 See also "CONCLUSION: Manipulative therapy for the shoulder girdle in addition to usual medical care accelerates recovery of shoulder symptoms." Bergman GJ, Winters JC, Groenier KH, Pool JJ, Meyboom-de Jong B, Postema K, van der Heijden GJ. Manipulative therapy in addition to usual medical care for patients with shoulder dysfunction and pain: a randomized, controlled trial. *Ann Intern Med.* 2004 Sep 21;141(6):432-9 http://www.annals.org/cgi/reprint/141/6/432.pdf

[15] Kaufman RL. Conservative chiropractic care of lateral epicondylitis. *J Manipulative Physiol Ther.* 2000 Nov-Dec;23(9):619-22

[16] Kirk C, Lawrence DJ, Valvo NL. States Manual of Spinal, Pelvic, and Extravertebral Technics. Second Edition. Lombard; National College of Chiropractic. 1985; page 194

[17] Struijs PA, Damen PJ, Bakker EW, Blankevoort L, Assendelft WJ, van Dijk CN. Manipulation of the wrist for management of lateral epicondylitis: a randomized pilot study. *Phys Ther.* 2003 Jul;83(7):608-16 http://www.ptjournal.org/cgi/content/full/83/7/608

Selected Orthopedic Problems of the Arm, Elbow, and Forearm—*continued*

Problem	*Presentation*	*Assessment*	*Management*
Olecranon bursitis: Accumulation of synovial, inflammatory, or purulent material in the olecranon bursa	▪ Pain after trauma at tip of elbow: overuse, prolonged resting on elbow, fall onto tip of elbow ▪ Whether traumatic or not, consider bursa infection	▪ "Goose egg" swelling at the elbow ▪ Differentially diagnose olecranon bursitis from subcutaneous nodules seen with rheumatoid arthritis ▪ Test CBC and CRP for infection	▪ Rest, anti-inflammatory treatments, ergonomic improvements, and other appropriate interventions (review Chapter 3); if infected, use antibiotics ▪ Consider allergy treatment in chronic "idiopathic" cases, especially when accompanied by other allergic problems like eczema[18]
Medial epicondylitis: "Golfer's elbow"	▪ Following trauma or overuse of the medial wrist flexors and pronators (hammering, golfing, throwing) ▪ Throwing injury	▪ Reverse Mill's test ▪ Reverse Cozen's test ▪ Palpatory tenderness at medial epicondyle ▪ Evaluate for fracture with history of direct trauma	▪ Rest, anti-inflammatory treatments, ergonomic improvements, and other appropriate interventions (review Chapter 3)
Joint effusion: accumulation of intraarticular fluid	▪ Limited ROM ▪ Effusion may be palpable	▪ Determine cause ▪ Joint aspiration if necessary to exclude gout or septic arthritis	▪ Rest, anti-inflammatory treatments, ergonomic improvements, and other appropriate interventions (review Chapter 3) ▪ IV/oral antibiotics if infected
Inflammatory arthropathy	▪ Elbow may be affected along with other joints and structures	▪ Lab tests: CRP, ANA, CCP, ferritin and other tests as indicated ▪ Radiographs, imaging	▪ Treat per disease ▪ If autoimmune disease is confirmed, see *Integrative Rheumatology* for therapeutic and management guidelines
Septic arthritis	▪ **Acute febrile non-traumatic arthritis**	▪ Lab tests ▪ Radiographs, imaging ▪ **Joint aspiration**	▪ **Emergency antibiotics**
Osteochondrosis of the elbow or radial head, Panner's disease, avascular necrosis of the capitellum, osteochondrosis deformans, osteochondritis dissecans of the elbow: This condition probably represents a continuum of disorders characterized by necrosis of the proximal radius.	▪ Classic presentation is elbow pain and stiffness in dominant arm in a young athlete ▪ May have locking, clicking, and intermittent swelling	▪ Clinical examination of the elbow. ▪ Radiographic examination should include standard AP and lateral views with oblique and radial head views.[19] "It represents a major threat to the elbow joint integrity, and it is important to diagnose early."[20]	▪ Conservative care with rest and splinting for 2-3 weeks followed by stretching and strengthening has been advocated for uncomplicated cases without evidence of intraarticular degeneration[21,22]; however, given the potential seriousness of the condition, orthopedic referral is recommended at time of diagnosis to ensure timely and proper treatment and to avoid the complications seen in improperly managed cases[23,24]

[18] "Onset of bursitis in all cases coincided with flaring of dermatitis." Nassif A, Smith DL, Hanifin JM. Olecranon and pretibial bursitis in atopic dermatitis: coincidence or association? *J Am Acad Dermatol*. 1994 May;30(5 Pt 1):737-42

[19] Souza TA. Differential Diagnosis for the Chiropractor: Protocols and Algorithms. Gaithersberg: Aspen Publications. 1997 page 188-189

[20] Stoane JM, Poplausky MR, Haller JO, Berdon WE. Panner's disease: X-ray, MR imaging findings and review of the literature. *Comput Med Imaging Graph*. 1995 Nov-Dec;19(6):473-6

[21] "If there is no loose body formation, children who develop osteochondritis dissecans when younger than the age of 13 years generally recover uneventfully with rest and physiotherapy to reduce pain and swelling." Brier S. Primary Care Orthopedics. St. Louis: Mosby, 1999 page 87

[22] Souza TA. Differential Diagnosis for the Chiropractor: Protocols and Algorithms. Gaithersberg: Aspen Publications. 1997 page 188-189

[23] "Residual limitations were highest in the type 2 lesions that were treated either nonsurgically or surgically after a long delay." Mitsunaga MM, Adishian DA, Bianco AJ Jr. Osteochondritis dissecans of the capitellum. *J Trauma*. 1982 Jan;22(1):53-5

[24] Byrd JW, Elrod BF, Jones KS. Elbow arthroscopy for neglected osteochondritis dissecans of the capitellum. *J South Orthop Assoc*. 2001 Spring;10(1):12-6

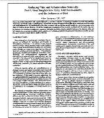

Vasquez A. Reducing Pain and Inflammation Naturally - Part 1: New Insights into Fatty Acid Biochemistry and the Influence of Diet. *Nutritional Perspectives* 2004; October: 5, 7-10, 12, 14

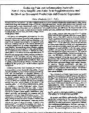

Vasquez A. Reducing Pain and Inflammation Naturally - Part 2: New Insights into Fatty Acid Supplementation and Its Effect on Eicosanoid Production and Genetic Expression. *Nutritional Perspectives* 2005; January: 5-16

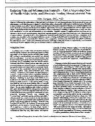

Vasquez A. Reducing Pain and Inflammation Naturally - Part 3: Improving overall health while safely and effectively treating musculoskeletal pain. *Nutritional Perspectives* 2005; 28: 34-38, 40-42

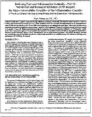

Vasquez A. Reducing Pain and Inflammation Naturally - Part 4: Nutritional and Botanical Inhibition of NF-kappaB, the Major Intracellular Amplifier of the Inflammatory Cascade. A Practical Clinical Strategy Exemplifying Anti-Inflammatory Nutrigenomics. *Nutritional Perspectives* 2005; July: 5-12

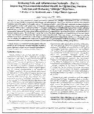

Vasquez A. Reducing Pain and Inflammation Naturally - Part 5: Improving neuromusculoskeletal health by optimizing immune function and reducing allergic reactions: a review of 16 treatments and a 3-step clinical approach. *Nutritional Perspectives* 2005; October: 27-35, 40

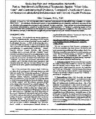

Vasquez A. Reducing Pain and Inflammation Naturally - Part 6: Nutritional and Botanical Treatments Against "Silent Infections" and Gastrointestinal Dysbiosis, Commonly Overlooked Causes of Neuromusculoskeletal Inflammation and Chronic Health Problems. *Nutritional Perspectives* 2006; January

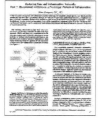

Vasquez A. Reducing Pain and Inflammation Naturally - Part 7: Rheumatoid Arthritis as a Prototypic Pattern of Inflammation. *Nutritional Perspectives* 2009 July

Chapter 9:
Hand/Wrist Pain and Carpal Tunnel Syndrome

Introduction
Carpal tunnel syndrome affects 4-10 million Americans and surely tens of millions if not hundreds of millions of people worldwide. Other mechanical and degenerative disorders of the wrist and hand are also common, resulting in huge decrements in quality of life and occupational productivity. Systemic disorders such as hemochromatosis (this author's first publishable research interest[1]), rheumatoid arthritis, psoriasis, scleroderma, and systemic lupus erythematosus commonly have their first clinical manifestations in the bones, soft tissues, skin and nails of the hands.

---

[1] Vasquez A. Musculoskeletal disorders and iron overload disease: comment on the American College of Rheumatology guidelines for the initial evaluation of the adult patient with acute musculoskeletal symptoms. *Arthritis & Rheumatism*: Official Journal of the American College of Rheumatology 1996; 39:1767-8

Topics:

1. Clinical assessments and differential diagnoses
2. De Quervain's tenosynovitis
3. Dupuytren's contracture
4. Fracture of the scaphoid
5. Boxer's fracture: fracture of the 4th or 5th metacarpal
6. Carpal tunnel syndrome, CTS

Core Competencies:

1. You must know how to differentially diagnose and treat rheumatoid arthritis, osteoarthritis, and hemochromatosis by 1) physical examination of the hands/wrists and 2) laboratory tests.
2. You must know how to properly administer high-dose pyridoxine, riboflavin, and magnesium as a component of the treatment plan for a patient with carpal tunnel syndrome.
3. You must know how to diagnose and manage fracture of the scaphoid.
4. You must know how to manage a hand/bone injury that has been contaminated with human saliva, such as a hand injury resulting from a fist fight.

Algorithm for the Assessment and Management of Wrist and Hand Complaints

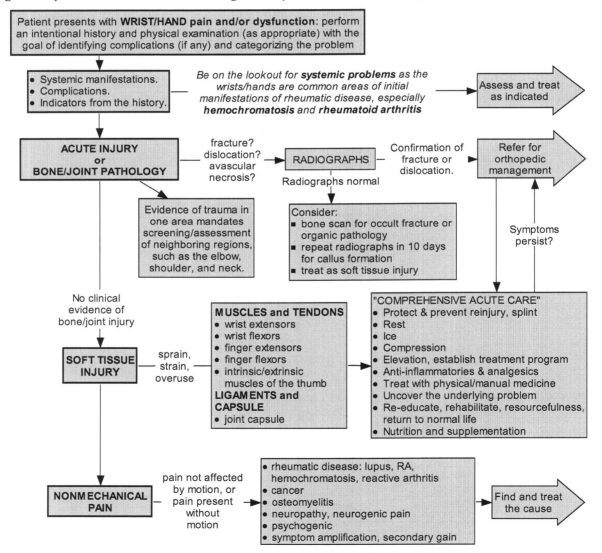

Selected Clinical Assessments for the Wrist and Hands

Clinical assessments	*Positive finding and Implications*
1. <u>History</u>: *See Chapter 1 for additional information*	▪ **Indicators from the history (trauma, risk factors)** ▪ **Systemic manifestations** ▪ **Complications** ▪ **Mechanical/ Nonmechanical** **Be on the lookout for systemic manifestations of disease as the wrists/hands are common areas of involvement with rheumatic diseases, especially hemochromatosis and rheumatoid arthritis**
2. <u>Observation</u>: Visually scan for obvious and subtle abnormalities	▪ Asymmetry ▪ Dislocation or deformity ▪ Injury, congenital anomaly, asymmetric development due to asymmetric use ▪ Muscle atrophy may be due to neurologic deficit or disuse (secondary to injury or pain) ▪ Ecchymosis is seen after fractures and soft tissue injuries
3. <u>ROM should be "full and painless"</u>; Motion of wrist, fingers, and thumb ▪ Flexion / extension ▪ Pronation / supination ▪ Thumb opposition ▪ Radial deviation ▪ Ulnar deviation	▪ Limitation in motion or pain (from joints or muscles) may indicate recent or previous injury, muscle spasm, contracture/adhesion of soft tissues: muscles, joint capsule ▪ In posttraumatic cases, pain may be severely limited due to fracture or dislocation: assess and treat as appropriate
4. <u>Muscle testing</u>: To assess neuromuscular integrity	▪ Pain—muscle injury, tendonitis ▪ Weakness—may be secondary to pain, may indicate neuropathy
5. <u>Palpation and provocation</u>: Compare with opposite wrist/hand	▪ Pain, tenderness, mass, enlargement, abnormality ▪ Pain with manual compression of the "anatomical snuff box" in a patient with a recent fall on the wrist suggests fracture of the scaphoid
6. <u>Finkelstein's test</u>: Ulnar deviation with thumb in hyperadduction and held under fingers of same hand	▪ Wrist pain (radial side) suggests De Quervain's tenosynovitis—inflammation of the abductor pollicis longus and the extensor pollicis brevis; treat conservatively
7. <u>Phalen's test</u>: Forced wrist flexion	▪ Reproduction of carpal tunnel syndrome (CTS) manifestations (i.e., paresthesia) with forced wrist <u>f</u>lexion held for up to 1 minute suggests carpal tunnel syndrome ▪ *Recall that <u>Phalen's</u> test places the wrists into forced flexion*

Selected clinical assessments of the wrist and hands—*continued*

Clinical assessments	Positive finding and Implications
8. **Reverse Phalen's test**: Forced wrist extension	▪ Reproduction of CTS manifestations (i.e., paresthesia) with forced wrist <u>extension</u> held for up to 1 minute suggests carpal tunnel syndrome
9. **Tinel's test**: Doctor taps over the transverse carpal ligament	▪ Reproduction of CTS paresthesia with tapping over the carpal tunnel suggests hyperirritability of the median nerve consistent with carpal tunnel syndrome
10. **Carpal tunnel compression test, the "pressure-provocative test"**: Dr applies pressure directly over the carpal tunnel for 30 seconds[2]	▪ Reproduction or exacerbation of manifestations of carpal tunnel syndrome with compression of the median nerve suggests carpal tunnel syndrome
11. **Cervical spine regional assessment**: Especially important after trauma	▪ *See Cervical Spine and Neck notes*
12. **Shoulder and elbow regional assessment**: Especially important after trauma	▪ *See Shoulder and Elbow notes*
13. **Neurologic exam**: Sensory, strength, and reflexes	Assess for: ▪ Weakness, loss of function, loss of sensation, hyporeflexia, hyperreflexia Which may suggest: ▪ Neurologic compromise: cord, nerve root, peripheral nerve, double crush syndrome ▪ Muscle injury, myopathy
14. **Radiographs**: Other imaging assessments are generally used after radiographs have been performed	▪ Degeneration: recall that degenerative arthritis (osteoarthritis) cannot be diagnosed until rheumatic diseases such as lupus, rheumatoid arthritis, and hemochromatosis have been excluded ▪ Calcification ▪ Fracture ▪ Infection ▪ Rheumatic disease
15. **Electromyography**: Most commonly used in the assessment of median nerve defects seen in carpal tunnel syndrome; this assessment is generally not necessary in routine clinical practice	▪ Abnormalities of nerve conduction suggest compressive, autoimmune or metabolic neuropathy

---

[2] Souza TA. <u>Differential Diagnosis for the Chiropractor: Protocols and Algorithms</u>. Gaithersburg: Aspen Publications. 1997 page 211

Selected problems of the wrist and hand* All conditions on this page are highly popular on licensing examinations for all professions.

Problem and Presentation	Assessment and Management
Boxer's fracture, Fracture of the 4th or 5th metacarpal • Pain, with or without deformity affecting the **4th or 5th metacarpals** after direct trauma	• Brief clinical assessment followed by radiographs. • Although all open fractures require surgical consultation, some smaller and less severe fractures can be treated nonsurgically with splinting. Recommend referral to orthopedist • Irrigation and debridement are the standard of care, and **intravenous antibiotics** are used for fractures with open wounds contaminated with human saliva to avoid recalcitrant infections with oral bacteria such as *Eikenella corrodens*[3]
De Quervain's tenosynovitis • Inflammation of the abductor pollicis longus and the extensor pollicis brevis • Wrist pain (radial side) especially with overuse of the thumb and/or ulnar deviation • Some patients with De Quervans have underlying RA as a cause of the synovitis	• Pain with resisted thumb extension • **Finkelstein's test:** Ulnar deviation with thumb in hyperadduction and held under fingers of same hand • Conservative care for 3 weeks, if no improvement immobilize with brace or cast for 2-3 weeks, if no improvement refer to orthopedist
Dupuytren's contracture, palmar fibromatosis • Contraction of the palmar fascia leading to flexion deformities of the fingers; may be hereditary (autosomal dominant) in many patients • **Flexion deformities of the 4th and 5th fingers** *Associated with:* • Heredity (autosomal dominant) • Diabetes • Alcoholism • Down's syndrome • Epilepsy • Peyronie's disease • Hypothyroidism	• **Flexion deformities of the fingers, usually 4th and 5th fingers** • **Tender nodule in the ulnar side of the palm** • Heat, massage, therapeutic ultrasound, mobilization • High-dose antioxidant supplementation: Emphasize mixed tocopherols and lipoic acid • Assess for and treat underlying contributors: diabetes, alcoholism, hypothyroidism, etc • Acetyl-carnitine 1,000 mg twice daily: Therapeutic trial based on results seen with Peyronie's disease[4] • Oral supplementation with proteolytic enzymes and antioxidants • Consider injection of clostridial collagenase[5]
Fracture of the scaphoid • **May result in permanent disability and the need for extensive surgery (bone grafting and internal fixation) if not promptly diagnosed and effectively treated;** the two main pathophysiologic considerations are 1) that the scaphoid directly articulates with the radius and therefore fractures to the scaphoid can affect articular surfaces, and 2) the **proximal pole of the scaphoid may become necrotic if a waist-line fracture of the scaphoid separates the proximal pole from the distal pole which receives blood and nutrient supply** • Pain at the **"anatomic snuff box"** following a fall on the palm with an extended wrist • Clinical findings such as swelling limited ROM are often minimal	• **Pain at the "anatomic snuff box" with direct pressure, tapping, and/or ulnar deviation** • **(Oblique) scaphoid radiographic view** • **Potentially false-negative radiographs may be followed by bone scan or MRI, or repeat radiographs at approximately 2 weeks to visualize callus formation** • **Since 20% of scaphoid fractures are predisposed to avascular necrosis, and since repeated casting and radiographic evaluation are often necessary, referral to orthopedist is strongly recommended** • If initial radiographs are normal but clinical suspicion is high, cast the wrist for 2 weeks then repeat radiographs

[3] "Clinicians must have a high index of suspicion when evaluating any hand injury and clenched fist injuries of the hand should be treated by early adequate surgical debridement followed by IV penicillin given until operative cultures confirm or deny contamination with Eikenella corrodens." Schmidt DR, Heckman JD. Eikenella corrodens in human bite infections of the hand. *J Trauma.* 1983 Jun;23(6):478-82
[4] "These results suggest that acetyl-L-carnitine is significantly more effective and safe than tamoxifen in the therapy of acute and early chronic Peyronie's disease." Biagiotti G, Cavallini G. Acetyl-L-carnitine vs tamoxifen in the oral therapy of Peyronie's disease: a preliminary report. *BJU Int.* 2001 Jul;88(1):63-7
[5] Pending further placebo, double-blind studies, collagenase injection to treat Dupuytren's disease may be a safe and effective alternative to surgical fasciectomy. Badalamente MA, Hurst LC. Enzyme injection as nonsurgical treatment of Dupuytren's disease. *J Hand Surg* [Am]. 2000 Jul;25(4):629-36

Carpal tunnel syndrome, CTS

Description/pathophysiology:
- Symptoms resultant from compression of the median nerve in the osteofibrous tunnel bordered by the carpal bones and the transverse carpal ligament. This compression may be due to:
  - Inflammatory edema of the finger flexor tendons and their associated synovial sheaths as they traverse the carpal tunnel; inflammation/edema may be due to overuse, injury, systemic edema (e.g., secondary to estrogen excess, pregnancy), hypothyroidism, or inflammatory process such as RA
  - May be exacerbated by external compression due to poor ergonomics, posture, or habits, such as sleeping prone on wrists, working with wrist on edge of desk/table, working with wrists in extreme flexion or extension
  - Rarely caused by congenital stenosis of the carpal tunnel
  - Specific nutritional deficiencies responsive to nutritional supplementation in many patients[6]
  - The median nerve can be compressed anywhere from its origin at the nerve roots all the way to the carpal tunnel. The concept of the "double crush" holds that two or more areas of minor compression to a nerve can result in a functional lesion similar to what would be expected with a single major compression; these compressive locations and their clinical assessment will be reviewed later in this section on CTS.

Complications:
- Loss of strength, muscle atrophy (intrinsic thenar muscles), and compromise of function of the hand; in severe cases, patients lose function of one or both hands and may be largely unable to work and function in their daily lives.
- Pain, paresthesia in the distribution of the median nerve

Clinical presentations:
- Pain-numbness-tingling in the thumb, index and middle fingers, and radial surface of the palm
- Symptoms are often worse at night
- May also have weakness of grip strength and loss of coordination of fine motor skills of the hand

Major differential diagnoses and contributing conditions:
- Double crush syndrome[7]
- Hypothyroidism
- Diabetes mellitus
- Acromegaly
- Amyloidosis
- Estrogen excess
- Pregnancy
- Nutritional deficiency or nutritional dependency, especially pyridoxine and riboflavin

Clinical assessments:
- History:
  - Pain, numbness, tingling in the median nerve distribution
  - Symptoms are worse at night.
  - May also have weakness of grip strength
- Physical examination:
  - Intrinsic thumb muscles may be weak
  - Assess for atrophy of the thenar eminence by observation and bilateral comparison

---

[6] Folkers K, Wolaniuk A, Vadhanavikit S. Enzymology of the response of the carpal tunnel syndrome to riboflavin and to combined riboflavin and pyridoxine. *Proc Natl Acad Sci* U S A. 1984 Nov;81(22):7076-8

[7] "Results supported the DSC hypothesis. DSC evaluation requires both structural and functional diagnosis of peripheral neurones using MRI and electrophysiological examination." Flak M, Durmala J, Czernicki K, Dobosiewicz K. Double crush syndrome evaluation in the median nerve in clinical, radiological and electrophysiological examination. *Stud Health Technol Inform.* 2006;123:435-41

- o Positive neuro-orthopedic assessment:
  - Phalen's test
  - Reverse Phalen's test
  - Tinel's test
  - Direct pressure at the carpal tunnel reproduces symptoms, i.e., numbness or tingling of the thenar palm
- o Assessment for compression of the median nerve and its contributory nerve roots:

Location	Screening assessments	Therapeutic considerations
Intervertebral disc of any level from C5-T1	▪ Cervical compression tests ▪ MRI if clinically warranted	▪ Consider traction for disc decompression
Intervertebral foramina on the affected side	▪ Provocative positioning to exacerbate hand paresthesia: combinations of ipsilateral side-bending and extension to exacerbate foraminal compression of nerve root ▪ Cervical oblique radiographs to assess IVFs	▪ Osseous and soft-tissue manipulation as indicated per patient to cervical and shoulder region ▪ Improve spinal health and posture ▪ Ergonomic and workstation improvements
Compression of brachial plexus due to thoracic outlet compression at anterior-middle scalenes, costoclavicular space, or secondary to tight pectoralis major	▪ Tests for TOS (see Chapter on shoulder)	▪ Stretch scalenes and pectoralis minor to relieve chronic compression of neurovascular bundle ▪ Improve posture ▪ Ergonomic and workstation improvements
Compression of median nerve at pronator teres	▪ Palpation and provocation at dual origin of pronator teres: proximal medial ulna and medial epicondyle	▪ Osseous and soft-tissue manipulation as indicated per patient to elbow region and pronator teres

Imaging & laboratory assessments:

- Assessment for hypothyroidism with TSH, free T4, free T3, and anti-TPO antibodies: **Hypothyroidism is relatively common among patients with CTS.**[8] **Musculoskeletal complaints are common in patients with thyroid problems, particularly hypothyroidism.**[9] With a suggestive or compelling clinical presentation, treatment of overt or subclinical hypothyroidism with thyroid hormone replacement is justified unless specifically contraindicated when the TSH value is greater than 2 μIU/mL[10], greater than 3 μIU/mL[11], or when antithyroid antibodies are present.[12] For most patients, treatment of hypothyroidism is best accomplished with a natural glandular source of thyroid hormone (such as a "nutritional" glandular product or Armour thyroid) or a hypoallergenic synthetic bioidentical combination of both T3 and T4[13] (such as Liotrix/Thyrolar) and should also be accompanied by general nutritional supplementation with a

[8] Palumbo CF, Szabo RM, Olmsted SL. The effects of hypothyroidism and thyroid replacement on the development of carpal tunnel syndrome. *J Hand Surg* [Am]. 2000 Jul;25(4):734-9
[9] Cakir M, Samanci N, Balci N, Balci MK. Musculoskeletal manifestations in patients with thyroid disease. *Clin Endocrinol* (Oxf). 2003 Aug;59(2):162-7
[10] Weetman AP. Hypothyroidism: screening and subclinical disease. *BMJ*. 1997 Apr 19;314(7088):1175-8. Available at http://bmj.com/cgi/content/full/314/7088/1175 as of January 11, 2004.
[11] "Now American Association of Clinical Endocrinologists encourages doctors to consider treatment for patients who test outside the boundaries of a narrower margin based on a target TSH level of 0.3 to 3.04. AACE believes the new range will result in proper diagnosis for millions of Americans who suffer from a mild thyroid disorder, but have gone untreated until now." Available at http://www.aace.com/pub/tam2003/press.php as of January 11, 2004.
[12] Beers MH, Berkow R (eds). The Merck Manual of Diagnosis and Therapy, 17th Edition. Whitehouse Station; Merck Research Laboratories 1999 page 96
[13] Bunevicius R, Kazanavicius G, Zalinkevicius R, Prange AJ Jr. Effects of thyroxine as compared with thyroxine plus triiodothyronine in patients with hypothyroidism. *N Engl J Med*. 1999 Feb 11;340(6):424-9

high-potency broad-spectrum multivitamin/multimineral supplement that contains 200-600 mcg of selenium[14,15] and 15-25 mg of zinc.[16] Zinc, selenium, and iron are required for peripheral conversion and function of thyroid hormones; corresponding mineral deficiencies can precipitate a mild functional hypothyroidism.

- <u>Basic routine laboratory assessment with CBC, CRP, CCP, and chemistry/metabolic panel</u>: This approach is sufficient to screen for diabetes and rheumatoid arthritis, both of which are more common in patients with CTS.[17,18]
- <u>Assessment of vitamin levels and functional enzyme status</u>: This is generally not necessary; consider assessment of vitamin B6 status with erythrocyte glutamic oxaloacetic transaminase (EGOT) and/or serum P5P levels.
- <u>Electromyography</u>: EMG can be used to objectively quantify impaired nerve conduction
- <u>Serum ferritin</u>: Assess for iron overload or iron deficiency.

Clinical management: Referral if clinical outcome is unsatisfactory.

Treatments:
- **<u>Pyridoxine (vitamin B-6; concomitant administration with magnesium)</u>**: Many patients with CTS have serum and biochemical evidence of pyridoxine deficiency[19] which remit along with the CTS following supplementation with pyridoxine, thus helping to obviate the need for surgery.[20,21,22,23,24,25] *The Merck Manual of Diagnosis and Therapy, 17th Edition Manual* advocates a trial of 50 mg twice daily[26] while others have recommended a dose of 200 mg per day.[27] A recent clinical trial[28] showed that enzyme saturation proceeds from 83% with 30 mg of pyridoxine to 93% with 200 mg of pyridoxine, thus proving again that dose-responsiveness is not maximized until higher *supranutritional* doses are used; this precept was previously reviewed in a brilliant required-reading article by Bruce Ames et al.[29] In my practice I commonly use at least 250 mg daily with breakfast for a *loading dose* trial period of 2-12 weeks before tapering down to a maintenance dose of 50-250 mg/day. Long-term ultrahigh-dose administration of pyridoxine HCL can be neurotoxic, producing a peripheral neuropathy that is not unlike the presentation of carpal tunnel syndrome. One of the problems with supplementation with vitamin B-6 in the form of pyridoxine HCL is that this particular synthetic form of vitamin B-6 appears to be mildly neurotoxic and must be converted to the active form(s) of the vitamin before becoming harmless and physiologically functional. The phosphorylation of pyridoxine HCL into its active phosphorylated forms (e.g., pyridoxal-5-phosphate, P5P) requires the presence of magnesium. Many people are deficient in magnesium and therefore may not respond to supplementation with pyridoxine HCL because of deficiency-induced biochemical inability to convert the vitamin to its active form in sufficient quantities to achieve a therapeutic effect. Obviously, either using an activated form of pyridoxine such as the commercially available pyridoxal-5-phosphate would

[14] Duntas LH, Mantzou E, Koutras DA. Effects of a six month treatment with selenomethionine in patients with autoimmune thyroiditis. *Eur J Endocrinol.* 2003 Apr;148(4):389-93

[15] Olivieri O, Girelli D, Stanzial AM, Rossi L, Bassi A, Corrocher R. Selenium, zinc, and thyroid hormones in healthy subjects: low T3/T4 ratio in the elderly is related to impaired selenium status. *Biol Trace Elem Res.* 1996 Jan;51(1):31-41

[16] Nishiyama S, Futagoishi-Suginohara Y, Matsukura M, Nakamura T, Higashi A, Shinohara M, Matsuda I. Zinc supplementation alters thyroid hormone metabolism in disabled patients with zinc deficiency. *J Am Coll Nutr.* 1994 Feb;13(1):62-7

[17] Van Dijk MA, Reitsma JB, Fischer JC, Sanders GT. Indications for requesting laboratory tests for concurrent diseases in patients with carpal tunnel syndrome: a systematic review. *Clin Chem.* 2003 Sep;49(9):1437-44

[18] Solomon DH, Katz JN, Bohn R, Mogun H, Avorn J. Nonoccupational risk factors for carpal tunnel syndrome. *J Gen Intern Med.* 1999 May;14(5):310-4

[19] Fuhr JE, Farrow A, Nelson HS Jr. Vitamin B6 levels in patients with carpal tunnel syndrome. *Arch Surg.* 1989 Nov;124(11):1329-30

[20] Ellis JM, Kishi T, Azuma J, Folkers K. Vitamin B6 deficiency in patients with a clinical syndrome including the carpal tunnel defect. Biochemical and clinical response to therapy with pyridoxine. *Res Commun Chem Pathol Pharmacol.* 1976 Apr;13(4):743-57

[21] Ellis J, Folkers K, Watanabe T, Kaji M, Saji S, Caldwell JW, Temple CA, Wood FS. Clinical results of a cross-over treatment with pyridoxine and placebo of the carpal tunnel syndrome. *Am J Clin Nutr.* 1979 Oct;32(10):2040-6

[22] Ellis J, Folkers K, Levy M, Takemura K, Shizukuishi S, Ulrich R, Harrison P. Therapy with vitamin B6 with and without surgery for treatment of patients having the idiopathic carpal tunnel syndrome. *Res Commun Chem Pathol Pharmacol.* 1981 Aug;33(2):331-44

[23] Ellis JM, Folkers K, Levy M, Shizukuishi S, Lewandowski J, Nishii S, Schubert HA, Ulrich R. Response of vitamin B-6 deficiency and the carpal tunnel syndrome to pyridoxine. *Proc Natl Acad Sci U S A.* 1982 Dec;79(23):7494-8

[24] Kasdan ML, Janes C. Carpal tunnel syndrome and vitamin B6. *Plast Reconstr Surg.* 1987 Mar;79(3):456-62

[25] Ellis JM. Treatment of carpal tunnel syndrome with vitamin B6. *South Med J.* 1987 Jul;80(7):882-4

[26] Beers MH, Berkow R (eds). The Merck Manual of Diagnosis and Therapy, 17th Edition. Whitehouse Station; Merck Research Laboratories 1999 Page 492

[27] "Current treatment for carpal tunnel syndrome should include NSAIDs, nighttime splinting, ergonomic workstation review, and vitamin B6 200 mg per day." Holm G, Moody LE. Carpal tunnel syndrome: current theory, treatment, and the use of B6. *J Am Acad Nurse Pract.* 2003 Jan;15(1):18-22

[28] "The in vivo study showed increasing aspartate aminotransferase saturation with increasing pyridoxine doses. 83% saturation was reached with 30 mg daily, 88% with 100 mg, and 93% with 200 mg after 20 days of oral supplementation." Oshiro M, Nonoyama K, Oliveira RA, Barretto OC. Red cell aspartate aminotransferase saturation with oral pyridoxine intake. *Sao Paulo Med J.* 2005 Mar 2;123(2):54-7 http://www.scielo.br/scielo.php?script=sci_arttext&pid=S1516-31802005000200004&lng=es&lng=en&nrm=iso

[29] Ames BN, Elson-Schwab I, Silver EA. High-dose vitamin therapy stimulates variant enzymes with decreased coenzyme binding affinity (increased K(m)): relevance to genetic disease and polymorphisms. *Am J Clin Nutr.* 2002 Apr;75(4):616-58 http://www.ajcn.org/cgi/content/full/75/4/616

obviate this problem; gastrointestinal absorption of P5P appears to be limited. Coadministration of magnesium is advised with the use of pyridoxine HCL, and generally long-term high-dose (i.e., bowel tolerance) supplementation is necessary to replenish body magnesium levels. If necessary, assessment of magnesium status is performed by measuring either RBC or WBC intracellular magnesium levels; serum levels of magnesium are generally meaningless from a nutritional standpoint. Furthermore, magnesium supplementation should occur along with concomitant urinary alkalinization so that supplemented magnesium will be retained. Failure to alkalinize the urine with either diet[30] or alkalinization therapy such as sodium bicarbonate and/or potassium citrate[31], or alkaline minerals[32] allows for facilitated excretion of magnesium and subsequent "failure" of pyridoxine therapy due to insufficient magnesium-dependent phosphorylation and activation of the vitamin. Vitamin B6 probably exerts its beneficial effects in the treatment of CTS via several mechanisms, including:

o Facilitating biosynthesis of pain-relieving serotonin
o Reducing excitatory glutamate levels
o Diuretic effect: perhaps via inhibition of anti-diuretic hormone (ADH) secretion
o Diuretic effect via estrogen-lowering[33]: probably effected via upregulation of hepatic transaminases but possibly also via a direct pituitary effect[34]

Likewise, magnesium supplementation appears to provide some analgesic benefit which is at least partially due to its role in inhibiting activation of NMDA receptors and reducing/normalizing neuronal transmission. Magnesium is a required co-factor for tissue alkaline phosphatase, the enzyme required for pyridoxine dephosphorylation prior to tissue uptake of pyridoxal-5-phosphate; thus, magnesium deficiency appears to cause tissue/cellular deficiency of vitamin B6 by reducing cellular uptake of the vitamin.[35]

o **Drug-nutrient interactions**: High doses of **vitamin B6** can reduce blood levels and effectiveness of **barbiturate drugs** such as pentobarbital [Nembutal], phenobarbital [Phenobarbitone], secobarbital [Seconal], and thiopental [Pentothal]
o **Drug-nutrient interactions**: High doses of **magnesium** may decrease the absorption or effectiveness of several drugs, including: Azithromycin (Zithromax), Cimetidine (Tagamet), Ciprofloxacin (Ciloxan, Cipro), Doxycycline (Atridox, Doryx, Doxy, Monodox, Periostat, Vibramycin), Famotidine (Mylanta-AR, Pepcid, Pepcid AC), Hydroxychloroquine (Plaquenil), Levofloxacin (Levaquin), Nitrofurantoin (Furadantin, Macrobid, Macrodantin), Nizatidine (Axid, Axid AR), Ofloxacin (Floxin, Ocuflox), Tetracycline (Achromycin, Sumycin, Helidac), Warfarin (Coumadin). Misoprostol (Cytotec, Arthrotec) with magnesium may result in diarrhea. Spironolactone (Aldactone, Aldactazide) or Amiloride (Midamor, Moduretic) may cause dangerously high levels of magnesium

Before moving on to the next section readers should have crystalline clarity with regard to the following:

o Most patients consuming an American/Western-style diet have subtle chronic metabolic acidosis, which results in many adverse effects, one of which is increased urinary excretion of magnesium and reduced tissue/intracellular levels of magnesium.

---

[30] Cordain L. <u>The Paleo Diet: Lose Weight and Get Healthy by Eating the Food You Were Designed to Eat</u>. Indianapolis; John Wiley and Sons, 2002
[31] Maurer M, Riesen W, Muser J, Hulter HN, Krapf R. Neutralization of Western diet inhibits bone resorption independently of K intake and reduces cortisol secretion in humans. *Am J Physiol Renal Physiol*. 2003 Jan;284(1):F32-40. Epub 2002 Sep 24
[32] Vormann J, Worlitschek M, Goedecke T, Silver B. Supplementation with alkaline minerals reduces symptoms in patients with chronic low back pain. *J Trace Elem Med Biol*. 2001;15(2-3):179-83
[33] "Administration of vitamin B6 at doses of 200-800 mg/day reduces blood estrogen, increases progesterone and results in improved symptoms under double-blind conditions." Abraham GE. Nutritional factors in the etiology of the premenstrual tension syndromes. *J Reprod Med*. 1983 Jul;28(7):446-64
[34] "These results indicate that pharmacological doses of PLP inhibit pituitary cell proliferation and hormone secretion, in part mediated through PLP-induced cell-cycle arrest and apoptosis. Pyridoxine may therefore be appropriate for testing as a relatively safe drug for adjuvant treatment of hormone-secreting pituitary adenomas." Ren SG, Melmed S. Pyridoxal phosphate inhibits pituitary cell proliferation and hormone secretion. *Endocrinology*. 2006 Aug;147(8):3936-42 http://www.pubmedcentral.nih.gov/articlerender.fcgi?tool=pubmed&pubmedid=16690808
[35] "Mg deficiency impairs vitamin B6 status by depleting intracellular Mg and thus inhibits the activity of alkaline phosphatase, a metalloenzyme required for the uptake of pyridoxal phosphate by tissues." Planells E, Lerma A, Sanchez-Morito N, Aranda P, LLopis J. Effect of magnesium deficiency on vitamin B2 and B6 status in the rat. *J Am Coll Nutr*. 1997 Aug;16(4):352-6

o This acidotic predisposition toward magnesium deficiency is exacerbated by low dietary intake of magnesium, as well as other factors such as overconsumption of caffeine, sugar, and also by chronic mental/emotional stress.

o The resultant magnesium deficiency thus impairs activation/phosphorylation of pyridoxine HCL into the active form pyridoxal-5-phosphate via magnesium-dependent pyridoxal kinase; this results in a simultaneous diminution of effectiveness and enhancement of pyridoxine HCL-mediated neurotoxicity. Cofactors for various tissue-specific isoforms of pyridoxal kinase include magnesium, zinc, cobalt, and manganese; of these, zinc appears most important, particularly in the liver and brain. The final production of active P5P requires a (ribo)flavin-dependent oxidase; thus, *B2 insufficiency precipitates B6 insufficiency.*[36]

o Furthermore, magnesium deficiency impairs alkaline phosphatase, the enzyme required for cellular uptake of pyridoxal-5-phosphate; in this way, magnesium deficiency causes tissue insufficiency of pyridoxine.

o Additionally, chronic metabolic acidosis further impairs intracellular accumulation of magnesium, apparently because the elevated intracellular concentration of hydrogen ions creates an electrochemically repulsive force, given that both hydrogen and magnesium are positively-charged cations.

o In this situation, if a patient is supplemented with pyridoxine HCL *without magnesium* and *without systemic alkalinization*, we should not expect that optimal clinical responsiveness will be observed even if the patient is functionally vitamin B6 deficient and if the condition is pyridoxine responsive. Thus, the *correct treatment* in the *correct patient* **fails** not because of failure of the treatment *per se*, but rather due failure to create an internal milieu wherein vitamin B6 can function optimally.

  ▪ Readers should now understand the inherent bias of the medical studies that have "proved" the "ineffectiveness" of vitamin B6 supplementation. Why did so many of these studies fail to show positive benefit? *The supplementation failed because the doctors had no training in nutrition and thus implemented a treatment that had little hope for optimal success because the researchers failed to improve the diet, correct the diet-induced metabolic acidosis, and provide co-factors necessary for B6 function.*

  ▪ Readers should now understand how to reduce B6 toxicity while increasing its effectiveness. *Alkalinization followed by supplementation with zinc, magnesium, and riboflavin.*

  ▪ Readers should now understand why an alkalinizing Paleo-Mediterranean diet is *primarily* essential for creating an internal environment wherein the *secondary* addition of high-dose nutritional supplements can function.

- <u>Riboflavin (vitamin B-2)</u>: Patients with CTS may respond to riboflavin therapy alone, and the combination of B-2 with B-6 appears more efficacious than the use of either B-6 or B-2 alone.[37] Recall from our discussion of migraine headaches that doses of riboflavin of 400 mg per day have been used safely[38]; thus, in patients with CTS, we may safely proceed with riboflavin 400 mg, preferably administered with breakfast.

- <u>Yoga</u>: Yoga postures and relaxation showed superior results compared to use of a night splint in the treatment of CTS.[39] In contrast to surgical lesion of the transverse carpal ligament, yoga is fun, feels good, and can improve aspects of overall health[40] and socioemotional wellbeing.

[36] Holman P. Pyridoxine - Vitamin B6. *Journal of the Australasian College of Nutritional & Environmental Medicine*, Vol. 14, No. 1, July 1995, pages 5-16 http://www.acnem.org/journal/14-1_july_1995/pyridoxine-vitamin_b6.htm Kudos to Mr. Holman for his excellent summation of pyridoxine metabolism.
[37] Folkers K, Wolaniuk A, Vadhanavikit S. Enzymology of the response of the carpal tunnel syndrome to riboflavin and to combined riboflavin and pyridoxine. *Proc Natl Acad Sci U S A*. 1984 Nov;81(22):7076-8
[38] Schoenen J, Jacquy J, Lenaerts M. Effectiveness of high-dose riboflavin in migraine prophylaxis. A randomized controlled trial. *Neurology* 1998 Feb;50(2):466-70
[39] Garfinkel MS, Singhal A, Katz WA, Allan DA, Reshetar R, Schumacher HR Jr. Yoga-based intervention for carpal tunnel syndrome: a randomized trial. *JAMA*. 1998 Nov 11;280:1601-3
[40] "It is likely that the yoga practices of controlling body, mind, and spirit combine to provide useful psychophysiological effects for healthy people and for people compromised by musculoskeletal and cardiopulmonary disease." Raub JA. Psychophysiologic effects of Hatha Yoga on musculoskeletal and cardiopulmonary function: a literature review. *J Altern Complement Med*. 2002 Dec;8(6):797-812

- <u>Mobilization and manipulation of the carpal bones, myofascial release</u>: Symptoms of CTS may be effectively reduced simply by a mobilization technique of squeezing the metacarpal heads together and also stretching the third and fourth digits into extension.[41] Osteopathic-type manipulation (similar to chiropractic manipulation) of the wrist has shown clinical, electromyographic, and MRI evidence of efficacy[42,43], and the technique is intuitive and commonly known among clinicians with training in manipulation. Additional effectiveness can be obtained when patients are taught to regularly perform stretching maneuvers with the forearm in supination, wrist in forced extension, and the thumb brought firmly back toward the body with the use of the contralateral hand.
- <u>Trial of anti-inflammatory botanicals</u>: Particularly bromelain and proteolytic enzymes.
- <u>Reduce intake of dietary salt</u>: Excess sodium ingestion promotes water retention and magnesium excretion (among many other adverse effects).
- <u>Deep tissue massage to the muscles of the forearm</u>: The median nerve can be compressed proximal to the carpal tunnel at its relationships to the flexor digitorum superficialis, pronator teres[44], and/or the lacertus fibrosus extension from the biceps tendon.[45] Soft-tissue manipulative treatments should be used as part of the comprehensive treatment plan for CTS before any patient is considered a surgical candidate.
- <u>Behavioral and occupational ergonomic modifications</u>: Improve work station functionality, avoid overuse of the hands and wrists, and particularly avoid direct compression of the wrist while working.
- <u>Treatment of endocrine abnormalities and concomitant disease</u>: Diabetes mellitus, thyroid disease, rheumatoid arthritis, in women: assess for high estrogen/ low progesterone, or the use of estrogen supplementation.[46]
- <u>Weight loss</u>: If the patient is overweight, the patient should lose weight.
- <u>Use of a wrist splint at night</u>: A commonly advocated treatment in allopathic textbooks.
- <u>Surgery</u>: For non-responsive cases only as a last resort after nutrition, diet, weight loss, ergonomics, and competent manipulation, mobilization, and massage have been utilized *in combination* along with assessment for and treatment of endocrinologic contributions.

---

[41] Manente G, Torrieri F, Pineto F, Uncini A. A relief maneuver in carpal tunnel syndrome. *Muscle Nerve*. 1999 Nov;22(11):1587-9
[42] "All participants who were treated improved clinically, with decrease in both symptoms and palpatory restriction." Sucher BM. Palpatory diagnosis and manipulative management of carpal tunnel syndrome. *J Am Osteopath Assoc*. 1994 Aug;94(8):647-63
[43] Sucher BM. Myofascial manipulative release of carpal tunnel syndrome: documentation with magnetic resonance imaging. *J Am Osteopath Assoc*. 1993 Dec;93(12):1273-8
[44] Olehnik WK, Manske PR, Szerzinski J. Median nerve compression in the proximal forearm. *J Hand Surg* [Am]. 1994 Jan;19(1):121-6
[45] Wertsch JJ, Melvin J. Median nerve anatomy and entrapment syndromes: a review. *Arch Phys Med Rehabil*. 1982 Dec;63(12):623-7
[46] "Recent weight gain and use of estrogen replacement therapy were identified as possible risk factors; this provides some support for the theory that fluid retention in the soft tissues of the carpal tunnel is etiologically involved, although these results are preliminary and further research must be carried out to refute or support these findings." Dieck GS, Kelsey JL. An epidemiologic study of the carpal tunnel syndrome in an adult female population. *Prev Med*. 1985 Jan;14(1):63-9

Myofascial Release Techniques for the Treatment of Carpal Tunnel Syndrome:
Respectfully attributed to and adapted from the work of Benjamin Sucher, D.O.[47,48,49]

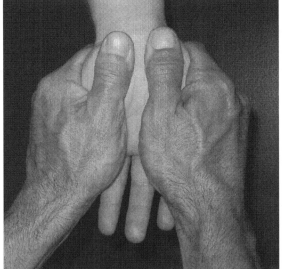

In this demonstration, the doctor is working on the patient's right wrist. In the doctor's right hand, the patient's pisiform, triquetral, and hamate bones are grasped and rolled externally, in a clockwise direction. In the doctor's left hand, the patient's scaphoid and trapezium bones are grasped and rolled externally from midline, in a counterclockwise direction. The combination of these two motions generates strong tension in the transverse carpal ligament (flexor retinaculum) that eventually leads to relaxation of the ligament and allows for increased cross-sectional area within the carpal tunnel, thus relieving pressure on its contents, particularly the median nerve. This maneuver is generally referred to as the **opponens roll**, and the following techniques are variations of same.

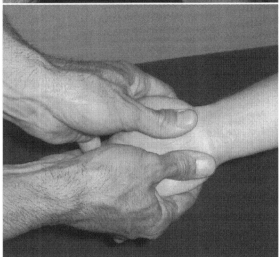

In this maneuver, the doctor's contacts and motions are the same as above, except that in this case the doctor's fingers are interposed between those of the patient. This positioning provides for greater control of the patient's distal palm, allowing the doctor to force the patient's wrist into extension while applying tension to the transverse carpal ligament. The addition of wrist extension appears to increase the clinical efficacy of the maneuver.

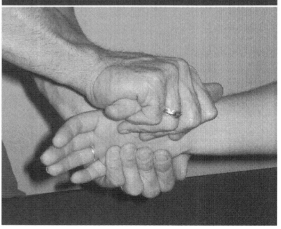

In this positioning, the actions are the same as above, but the doctor is using his fingers rather than thumbs to apply the mobilizing force. In the doctor's right hand, the patient's scaphoid and trapezium bones are grasped and rolled externally from the palmar surface, in a counterclockwise direction. In the doctor's left hand, the patient's pisiform, triquetral, and hamate bones are grasped and rolled externally from the palmar surface, in a clockwise direction. The action and concept are to "open" the carpal tunnel by tractioning the transverse carpal ligament.

---

[47] Sucher BM. Palpatory diagnosis and manipulative management of carpal tunnel syndrome. *J Am Osteopath Assoc*. 1994 Aug;94(8):647-63
[48] Sucher BM. Myofascial manipulative release of carpal tunnel syndrome: documentation with magnetic resonance imaging. *J Am Osteopath Assoc*. 1993 Dec;93(12):1273-8
[49] Sucher BM, Hinrichs RN, Welcher RL, Quiroz LD, St Laurent BF, Morrison BJ. Manipulative treatment of carpal tunnel syndrome: biomechanical and osteopathic intervention to increase the length of the transverse carpal ligament: part 2. Effect of sex differences and manipulative "priming". *J Am Osteopath Assoc*. 2005 Mar;105(3):135-43
http://www.jaoa.org/cgi/content/full/105/3/135

Chapter 10:
Lumbar Spine and Low Back Pain

Introduction
Low back pain is pandemic throughout the world; it is a major cause of pain, suffering, disability, lost productivity and wages, as well as medical and surgical expense. The cause is often considered to be enigmatic, particularly by a healthcare system filled with doctors untrained in nutrition, biomechanics, and manual assessment and treatment. Low back pain commonly responds very positively to manipulative and nutritional interventions. However, each clinician must always remain vigilant for those cases of low back pain caused by visceral referral and serious neurologic compromise.

<u>Topics</u>:
1. Clinical assessments and differential diagnoses
2. Low back pain—general considerations
3. Lumbar intervertebral disc herniation, "Slipped disc", and Sciatica—lumbar radiculitis and lumbar radiculopathy
4. Lumbar (Central) Spinal Stenosis and Lateral Recess Stenosis/Syndrome
5. Cauda equina syndrome
6. Vertebral osteomyelitis and infectious discitis

Why an epidemic of low back pain?
- Sedentary lifestyles combined with bipedalism, periodic trauma, untrained neuromuscular systems (lack of strength and coordination[1]), and lack of sun exposure producing epidemic vitamin D deficiency, which directly results in low back pain.[2] Complicating this is the diet-induced chronic metabolic acidosis which also promotes enhanced pain perception and magnesium loss.

How much?
- More than 14% of new patient visits to physicians are for low back complaints.[3]
- Surgery for low back problems is the third most common type of surgery performed, although most low back pain is benign, self-limiting, and remarkably responsive to manipulative and nutritional interventions.

What are the most important considerations in the assessment of low back pain?
- Assess each patient for organic causes of low back pain (infection, cancer, viscerosomatic referral, insufficiency fracture, etc.) and for neurologic compromise.

Core competencies:
1. You must know how to diagnose cauda equina syndrome *by history and physical examination alone* (e.g., without CT or MRI results). Know the appropriate management of cauda equina syndrome.
2. You must know how to diagnose and manage vertebral osteomyelitis and infectious discitis.
3. Be able to explain the mechanism by which vitamin D deficiency causes low back pain (reviewed in Chapter 1); know the indications, contraindications, dosing, and monitoring involved with vitamin D supplementation at doses of 2,000-10,000 IU/d for adults.
4. Provide the diagnostic criteria and management strategy of each of the following:

Disorders	*Typical Presentation, Diagnosis*	*Management Strategy*
Rheumatoid arthritis		
Psoriatic arthritis		
Ankylosing spondylitis		
Reactive arthritis		
Enteropathic spondyloarthropathy		
Osteitis condensans ilii		

5. List at least four ways to improve proprioceptive/sensorimotor function in patients with low back pain.
6. Differentially diagnose a bladder infection from a kidney infection; describe appropriate management strategies for both problems.

---

[1] "Gluteal activation and pelvic stability often are decreased in chronic low back pain sufferers..." Bullock-Saxton JE, Janda V, Bullock MI. Reflex activation of gluteal muscles in walking. An approach to restoration of muscle function for patients with low back pain. *Spine.* 1993 May;18(6):704-8
[2] "Vitamin D deficiency is a major contributor to chronic low back pain in areas where vitamin D deficiency is endemic. Screening for vitamin D deficiency and treatment with supplements should be mandatory in this setting." Al Faraj S, Al Mutairi K. Vitamin D deficiency and chronic low back pain in Saudi Arabia. *Spine.* 2003 Jan 15;28(2):177-9
[3] Brier S. <u>Primary Care Orthopedics</u>. St. Louis: Mosby, 1999, page 213

Low Back pain: Differential Diagnostic Considerations

	DDX Category	Examples:
V	Vascular Visceral referral	Aortic aneurysm Pancreatic disease/cancer
I	Infectious Inflammatory Immunologic	Ankylosing spondylitis, Reiter's syndrome Rheumatoid arthritis Psoriatic arthritis Enteropathic spondyloarthropathy Lymphoma, leukemia Bone/ tissue infections Gastrointestinal disease Kidney infection Psoriatic arthritis Herpes zoster
N	Neurologic Nutritional New growth: neoplasia or pregnancy	Metastatic disease Primary bone tumors Multiple myeloma Herpes zoster Cauda equina syndrome
D	Deficiency Degenerative Developmental	Degenerative joint/spine disease Congenital malformations of bones/ viscera Scoliosis Postural syndromes Disc herniation Varicose veins in the leg mimicking sciatica
I	Iatrogenic (drug related) Intoxication Idiosyncratic	Anticoagulants predispose to epidural or spinal cord bleeding[4] Prednisone use promotes osteoporosis and spinal fractures Excess alcohol consumption[5]
C	Congenital	Congenital malformations of bones: hemivertebrae, leg length inequality, etc.
A	Allergy Autoimmune Abuse	Ankylosing spondylitis Fractures, injuries
T	Trauma	Fractures: injuries to vertebrae, ribs, muscles
E	Endocrine Exposure	Diabetes mellitus
S	Subluxation Structural Stress Secondary gain	Segmental dysfunction of lumbar spine and pelvis Muscle tension
M	Mental Malpractice Mental disorder Malignancy Metabolic disease Menstrual Myofascial	Anxiety Depression Endometriosis, hematocolpos[6] Ovarian tumor Nephrolithiasis Metastasis to spine Myofascial trigger points in quadratus lumborum, piriformis, iliacus, psoas

[4] Souza TA. <u>Differential Diagnosis for the Chiropractor: Protocols and Algorithms</u>. Gaithersburg: Aspen Publications. 1997 page 110
[5] "Alcohol abuse was significantly more frequent among the male low back patients." Sandstrom J, Andersson GB, Wallerstedt S. The role of alcohol abuse in working disability in patients with low back pain. *Scand J Rehabil Med*. 1984;16(4):147-9
[6] London NJ, Sefton GK. Hematocolpos. An unusual cause of sciatica in an adolescent girl. *Spine*. 1996 Jun 1;21(11):1381-2

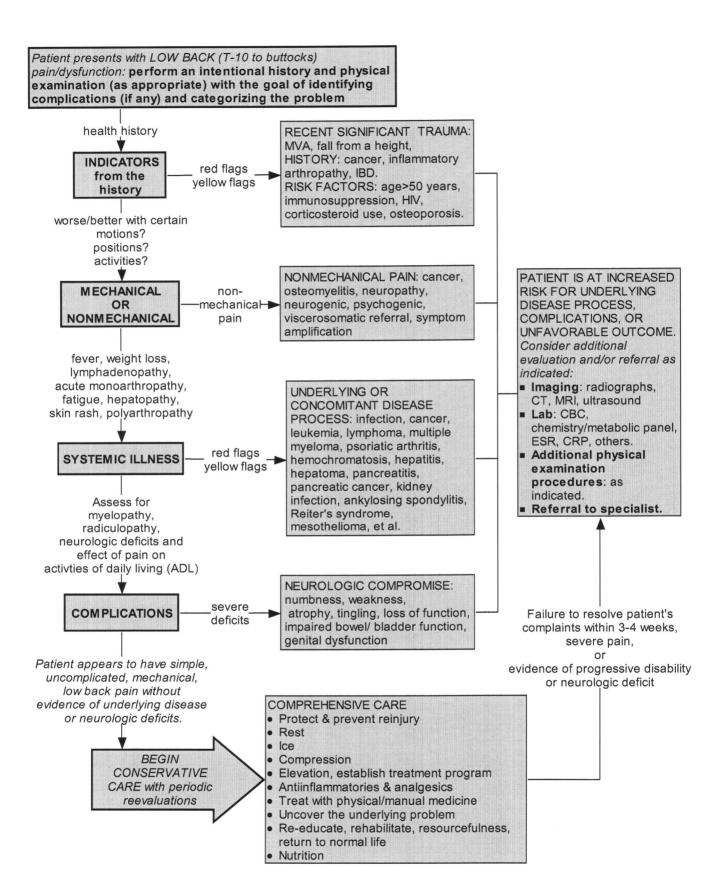

Patient presents with LOW BACK (T-10 to buttocks) pain/dysfunction: **perform an intentional history and physical examination (as appropriate) with the goal of identifying complications (if any) and categorizing the problem**

health history

INDICATORS from the history

red flags
yellow flags

RECENT SIGNIFICANT TRAUMA: MVA, fall from a height, HISTORY: cancer, inflammatory arthropathy, IBD. RISK FACTORS: age>50 years, immunosuppression, HIV, corticosteroid use, osteoporosis.

worse/better with certain motions? positions? activities?

MECHANICAL OR NONMECHANICAL

non-mechanical pain

NONMECHANICAL PAIN: cancer, osteomyelitis, neuropathy, neurogenic, psychogenic, viscerosomatic referral, symptom amplification

fever, weight loss, lymphadenopathy, acute monoarthropathy, fatigue, hepatopathy, skin rash, polyarthropathy

SYSTEMIC ILLNESS

red flags
yellow flags

UNDERLYING OR CONCOMITANT DISEASE PROCESS: infection, cancer, leukemia, lymphoma, multiple myeloma, psoriatic arthritis, hemochromatosis, hepatitis, hepatoma, pancreatitis, pancreatic cancer, kidney infection, ankylosing spondylitis, Reiter's syndrome, mesothelioma, et al.

Assess for myelopathy, radiculopathy, neurologic deficits and effect of pain on activties of daily living (ADL)

COMPLICATIONS

severe deficits

NEUROLOGIC COMPROMISE: numbness, weakness, atrophy, tingling, loss of function, impaired bowel/ bladder function, genital dysfunction

PATIENT IS AT INCREASED RISK FOR UNDERLYING DISEASE PROCESS, COMPLICATIONS, OR UNFAVORABLE OUTCOME. *Consider additional evaluation and/or referral as indicated:*
- **Imaging**: radiographs, CT, MRI, ultrasound
- **Lab**: CBC, chemistry/metabolic panel, ESR, CRP, others.
- **Additional physical examination procedures**: as indicated.
- **Referral to specialist.**

Failure to resolve patient's complaints within 3-4 weeks, severe pain, or evidence of progressive disability or neurologic deficit

Patient appears to have simple, uncomplicated, mechanical, low back pain without evidence of underlying disease or neurologic deficits.

BEGIN CONSERVATIVE CARE with periodic reevaluations

COMPREHENSIVE CARE
- Protect & prevent reinjury
- Rest
- Ice
- Compression
- Elevation, establish treatment program
- Antiinflammatories & analgesics
- Treat with physical/manual medicine
- Uncover the underlying problem
- Re-educate, rehabilitate, resourcefulness, return to normal life
- Nutrition

Algorithm for the Assessment and Management of Low Back Complaints: Low back pain can be the presenting manifestation of serious illness; therefore, the careful consideration and exclusion of serious problems must be the clinician's first consideration, followed by the provision of symptomatic relief by addressing the underling problem or imbalance.

High-Risk Pain Patients

When a patient has musculoskeletal pain and any of the following characteristics, radiographs should be considered as an appropriate component of comprehensive evaluation. These considerations are particularly—though not exclusively—relevant for spine and low back pain.[7]

1.   **More than 50 years of age**
2.   **Physical trauma** (accident, fall, etc.)
3.   **Pain at night**
4.   **Back pain not relieved by lying supine**
5.   **Neurologic deficits** (motor or sensory)
6.   **Unexplained weight loss**
7.   **Documentation or suspicion of inflammatory arthropathy**[8]
     - **Ankylosing spondylitis**
     - **Lupus**
     - **Rheumatoid arthritis**
     - **Juvenile rheumatoid arthritis**
     - **Psoriatic arthritis**
8.   **Drug or alcohol abuse** (increased risk of infection, nutritional deficiencies, anesthesia)
9.   **History of cancer**
10. **Intravenous drug use**
11. **Immunosuppression, due to illness (e.g., HIV) or medications (e.g., steroids or cyclosporine)**
12. **History of corticosteroid use** (causes osteoporosis and increased risk for infection)
13. **Fever above 100° F or suspicion of septic arthritis or osteomyelitis**
14. **Diabetes** (increased risk of infection, nutritional deficiencies, anesthesia)
15. **Hypertension** (abdominal aneurysm: low back pain, nausea, pulsatile abdominal mass)
16. **Recent visit for same problem and not improved**
17. **Patient seeking compensation for pain/ injury** (increased need for documentation)
18. **Skin lesion** (psoriasis, melanoma, dermatomyositis, the butterfly rash of lupus, scars from previous surgery, accident, etc....)
19. **Deformity or immobility**
20. **Lymphadenopathy** (suggests cancer or infection)
21. **Elevated ESR/CRP** (cancer, infection, inflammatory disorder)
22. **Elevated WBC count**
23. **Elevated alkaline phosphatase** (bone lesions, metabolic bone disease, hepatopathy)
24. **Elevated acid phosphatase** (occasionally used to monitor prostate cancer)
25. **Positive rheumatoid factor and/or CCP—cyclic citrullinated protein antibodies**
26. **Positive HLA-B27** (propensity for inflammatory arthropathies)
27. **Serum gammopathy** (multiple myeloma is the most common primary bone tumor)
28. **High-risk for disease:** *examples:*
     - Long-term heavy smoking of cigarettes
     - Long-term exposure to radiation
     - Obesity
29. **Strong family history of inflammatory, musculoskeletal, or malignant disease**

> Strongly consider the possibility of **osteoporotic fracture** in any patient—regardless of age or gender—who presents with spinal pain following multi-year use of **corticosteroids/prednisone** as treatment for a chronic inflammatory disorder.
>
> This applies both to *new patients with a previous history of long-term* pain as well as *long-term patients with new pain.*
>
> This continues to apply to patients for months and a few years after they have stopped multi-year use of **corticosteroids/prednisone.**

---

[7] Remember that metastasis often travel first from the primary site to bone, therefore bone pain may be an early manifestation of occult cancer. Most of the above are from "Table 1: The high-risk patient: clinical indications for radiography in low back pain patients." J Taylor, DC, DACBR, D Resnick, MD. Imaging decisions in the management of low back pain. Advances in Chiropractic. Mosby Year Book. 1994; 1-28

[8] Radiographs are often essential for diagnosis or to rule out complications of the disease. For example, in patients with inflammatory arthropathies such as these, spontaneous rupture of the transverse ligament (at the odontoid process) has been reported; although rare, this complication could be life-threatening if mismanaged or undiagnosed.

Clinical Assessments of the Low Back

Selected assessments	Positive finding and Implications	
1. **History**: *See Chapter 1 for additional information*	<ul><li>Indicators from the history (trauma, risk factors)</li><li>Systemic manifestations</li><li>Complications, especially numbness or weakness</li><li>Nonmechanical pain, night pain</li></ul>	"Red flags" in the history indicate increased risk for serious pathology and potential complications. Defer or modify physical examination as indicated.
2. **Radiation of pain** to buttocks, thigh, leg, and/or foot	<u>Radiation of pain *above the knee* (buttocks or thigh) suggests:</u><ul><li>**Facet irritation**</li><li>**MFTP**</li><li>**SIJ dysfunction**</li><li>**Mild radiculitis due to disc herniation**</li></ul><u>Radiation of pain to *below the knee* or to the foot suggests:</u><ul><li>**Radiculitis or radiculopathy due to disc herniation**</li><li>Herpes zoster</li><li>Lateral recess stenosis</li></ul>	
3. **Dejerine's triad/sign, Valsalva test**:	<ul><li>Increased radicular or dermatomal pain with coughing, sneezing, straining— "bear down like you are trying to have a bowel movement."</li><li>Increased radicular or dermatomal pain provoked by increased intrathecal pressure suggests a SOL (space-occupying lesion, e.g., tumor, disc herniation) compressing the spinal cord or nerve root</li></ul>	
4. **Observation** of structures and overlying skin	<ul><li>Scars: previous injury or surgery</li><li>Injury, congenital anomaly, asymmetric development due to asymmetric use.</li><li>Muscle atrophy may be due to neurologic deficit (radiculopathy or other CNS or PNS injury) or disuse (due to injury or pain).</li><li>Ecchymosis is seen after fractures and soft tissue injuries.</li><li>Systemic illness, infection—*Does the patient appear ill or in a state of declining health?*</li><li>Dermatitis, psoriasis, genital mucosal lesions</li><li>Poor posture, gait abnormalities, pes planus</li><li>Obesity</li></ul>	

Clinical Assessments of the Low Back—*continued*

Selected assessments	Positive finding and Implications
5. **Active motion from patient**: ROM should be "full and painless"	**Assess the following active motions**: A large portion of your examination and history should be complete before you ever lay hands on the patient. ▪ Walk on heels: Tests tibialis anterior, fibularis/peroneus longus and brevis, deep and superficial fibular/peroneal nerves, cerebellum, dorsal columns, and nerve roots L4-L5 ▪ Walk on toes: Tests gastrocnemius, soleus, tibial nerve, cerebellum, dorsal columns, and S1 nerve root ▪ Squat and rise: This is a valuable screening test for quickly assessing the lumbosacral junction, SI joints, hips, knees, ankles, gluteus and quadriceps strength, neurologic integrity (quadriceps are innervated mostly by L3 and L4[9]), and balance, which relies on cerebellum, dorsal columns, and vestibular input ▪ Full lumbar flexion / extension: Helps in the evaluation of flexibility and spinal integrity; acute pain may reveal an occult fracture or recently injured disc ▪ Rotation: Helps in the evaluation of spinal integrity and range of motion ▪ Lateral bending: Helps in the evaluation of spinal integrity and range of motion **Limitation or pain may suggest any of the following**: ▪ Muscle disease, myopathy, myositis, muscle spasm, or simple muscle tightness ▪ Contracture/adhesion of soft tissues: muscles, joint capsule ▪ Fracture ▪ Disc herniation ▪ Neurologic compromise: lesion of the brain, spinal cord, peripheral nerve, neuromuscular junction
Notice that by this point in the examination—if the patient was able to complete all of the above without revelation of major problem—we have already assessed range of motion of major lower body joints and strength of all major lower extremity muscles and have made significant progress in excluding systemic illness, fracture, myelopathy, nerve lesions, and other major considerations.	
6. **Muscle testing and provocation**: ▪ Toe walk ▪ Heel walk ▪ Squat and rise ▪ Trunk rotation ▪ Trunk lateral flexion ▪ Hip flexion ▪ Hip extension ▪ Knee flexion ▪ Knee extension ▪ Ankle inversion ▪ Ankle eversion	▪ Pain: muscle injury, tendonitis, joint injury ▪ Weakness: may be secondary to pain, may indicate nerve compromise

---

[9] Moore KL. Clinically Oriented Anatomy. Third Edition. Baltimore; Williams and Wilkins: 1992, page 387

Selected assessments	Positive finding and Implications

7. <u>Muscle testing and provocation</u>:
  ▪ Toe walk
  ▪ Heel walk
  ▪ Squat and rise
  ▪ Trunk rotation
  ▪ Trunk lateral flexion
  ▪ Hip flexion
  ▪ Hip extension
  ▪ Knee flexion
  ▪ Knee extension
  ▪ Ankle inversion
  ▪ Ankle eversion
	▪ Pain: muscle injury, tendonitis, joint injury
	▪ Weakness: may be secondary to pain, may indicate nerve compromise

8. <u>Bechterew's test</u>: patient seated with flexion of spine, patient then extends knee; first the non-sciatic leg is tested, then the affected leg, then both legs.[10][11] This is an excellent test, similar to the standard straight leg-raising (SLR) test; however this test also includes mild spinal compression due to gravity and allows for greater flexion of the spine and thus more traction on the spinal cord and nerve roots, thus making the test more sensitive	**Radiation of pain <u>above the knee</u> (buttocks, thigh) suggests:** ▪ **Facet irritation** ▪ **MFTP in the lumbar/gluteal region** ▪ **SIJ dysfunction** ▪ **Disc herniation (mild)** **Radiation of pain to <u>below the knee</u> or to the foot suggests:** ▪ **Radiculitis or radiculopathy due to disc herniation** ▪ Herpes zoster, a cause of radiculitis ▪ Lateral recess stenosis
9. <u>Kemp's test, axial compression test</u>: Patient seated, then lumbar spine is passively moved into extension, lateral flexion, and ipsilateral rotation; doctor is behind patient and adds vertical compression to spinal column by pushing down with forearm rested across patient's shoulders. The doctor also applies force to lumbar spine to accentuate and focus the stress to the lumbar spine.[12]	Local, paraspinal pain: ▪ Facet irritation ▪ Mild disc injury Sacroiliac pain: ▪ Sprain or lesion of the sacroiliac joints Pain radiating into leg and foot in dermatomal pattern: ▪ Discogenic radiculopathy ▪ Lateral stenosis

[10] Gatterman MI (Ed.). <u>Chiropractic Management of Spine-Related Disorders</u>. Baltimore; Williams and Wilkins, 1990. Page 139-140
[11] Souza TA. <u>Differential Diagnosis for the Chiropractor: Protocols and Algorithms</u>. Gaithersburg: Aspen Publications. 1997 page 113, 116
[12] Gatterman MI (Ed.). <u>Chiropractic Management of Spine-Related Disorders</u>. Baltimore; Williams and Wilkins, 1990. Page 141

Clinical Assessments of the Low Back—*continued*

Selected assessments	Positive finding and Implications
10. **Palpation and provocation** of spine and soft tissues: *compare with opposite side.*	Pain, tenderness, mass, enlargement, abnormality may indicate: • Injury • Inflammation • Muscle spasm • Muscle hypertrophy or muscle atrophy • Lipoma
11. **Spinal percussion:** Percussion of the spine with a reflex hammer or with the fingertips[13]	• **Pain with percussion of the spine with a reflex hammer or with the fingertips** • **Strongly consider obtaining radiographs or other imaging in any patient with exacerbation of pain following spinal percussion, as this indicates the possibility of a bone lesion: spinal fracture, spinal tumor, or vertebral osteomyelitis. Other considerations are herniated disc and joint or ligament injury.**
12. **Assessment of the lungs and heart**[14] as indicated	• Abnormalities: decreased breath sounds, fremitus, crepitus, murmurs, etc. • Pathology/abnormality of the lungs, heart
13. **Motion palpation** of the lumbar spine	• Hypermobility and/or hypomobility • **Segmental dysfunction** • Degenerative changes • Congenital anomalies
14. **Straight leg raising (SLR):** Passive leg raising with patient supine; especially reliable for disc herniation when pain is experienced below 45° of SLR; pain beginning at 60° of SLR is considered to provide "little diagnostic information."[15]	Dermatomal radiation of pain below knee or to the foot indicates nerve root compression (radiculopathy), which may be due to: • **Disc herniation** • Stenosis • Tumor • Fracture 95% sensitivity and 40% specificity for disc herniations at L4-L5 or L5-S1; less sensitive for herniations above this level[16]
15. **Well leg raise:** Supine patient lifts straight leg not affected by radiculopathy	• Exacerbation of radicular pain upon raising the "non-radicular leg" is considered a strong confirmation of discogenic sciatica
16. **Braggard's test:** Ankle dorsiflexion with SLR	• Radiation of pain in a dermatomal pattern confirms assessment of discogenic radiculopathy

[13] Gatterman MI (Ed.). Chiropractic Management of Spine-Related Disorders. Baltimore; Williams and Wilkins, 1990. Page 187
[14] Cardiopulmonary examinations are detailed in Bates B. A Guide to Physical Examination and History Taking. 6th Edition. Philadelphia; J. B. Lippincott Company, 1995
[15] Souza TA. Differential Diagnosis for the Chiropractor: Protocols and Algorithms. Gaithersburg: Aspen Publications. 1997 page 113
[16] Tierney ML. McPhee SJ, Papadakis MA (eds). Current Medical Diagnosis and Treatment 2006, 45th Edition. Lange Medical; page 817

Selected assessments	Positive finding and Implications
17. **Neurologic assessment**: Ideally, neurologic function is assessed at the start of every visit (to discover new problems) and after each manipulative treatment (to confirm safety of treatment)	Abnormal findings: ▪ Weakness, loss of function ▪ Loss of sensation ▪ Hyporeflexia, hyperreflexia Possible causes: ▪ **Neurologic compromise**: compression or other lesion of the spinal cord, nerve root, peripheral nerve, double crush syndrome, brain injury ▪ Muscle injury, myopathy
18. **Abdominal and/or pelvic examination**: Remember that low back and pelvic pain may arise from structures and organs in the abdomen and pelvis	Perform palpation and assessments with consideration for the following: ▪ Pain ▪ Mass ▪ Tenderness, guarding, rebound tenderness ▪ Kidney infection ▪ Tumor ▪ Abdominal aortic aneurysm ▪ In women, consider fibroid tumors, endometriosis, ectopic or normal pregnancy, dermoid tumor, ovarian cyst and tumors, pelvic inflammatory disease, and other problems
19. **SIJ gapping test, SIJ distraction test**: Patient supine, doctor applies outward (posterolateral) force on anterior superior iliac spine (ASIS) bilaterally and simultaneously: this test is performed to gap and stress the anterior aspect of the sacroiliac joints	▪ Pain in the SIJ with posterolateral forces applied to the ASIS suggests SIJ dysfunction or strain of the anterior SI ligaments
20. **SIJ compression test**: *Version 1*: Patient in side posture position, doctor applies downward force on iliac crest; *Version 2*: Patient supine, doctor applies posteromedial pressure to anterior superior iliac spine (ASIS) bilaterally and simultaneously. The goal is to apply a compressive force to the sacroiliac joints	▪ Pain provoked in the sacroiliac joints when this test is performed suggests SIJ dysfunction or lesion

Clinical Assessments of the Low Back—*continued*

Selected assessments	Positive finding and Implications
21. **Thomas test**: Supine patient brings unaffected thigh to abdomen (hip hyperflexion) while affected/tested leg remains on table. When the pelvis is rotated posteriorly with forced hyperflexion of the hip, the opposite hip should have sufficient flexibility to remain in extension on the surface of the table[17]	• The test result is considered positive/abnormal when the thigh that should remain on table lifts off the table due to joint hypomobility, capsular restriction, or tightness of the hip flexors—the iliacus, psoas, rectus femoris • This is a valuable test to include in the evaluation of low back pain because many patient have tight hip flexors which cause strain on the low back and which promote anterior pelvic rotation and thus lumbar hyperlordosis, which promotes lumbar facet syndrome • This test is very similar to Gaenslen's test. The subtle difference is that Thomas test assess the extensibility of the hip flexors whereas Gaenslen test assesses the ability of the sacroiliac joints to handle an extension force
22. **Radiographs**: Generally used to image problems related to bones and calcified tissues, which are visible with radiography. **Astute radiologists will take lumbar radiographs with the patient standing barefoot** and will **include the femoral heads in the visual field** for the assessment of leg length inequality	Abnormal findings may include: • Degeneration • Fracture • Infection • Tumor • Inflammatory arthropathy such as ankylosing spondylitis or reactive arthritis • Aneurysm of the abdominal aorta • Congenital anomaly such as hemivertebrae, lumbarization, sacralization • Leg length inequality <u>Important points to remember about the use of radiographs in patients with low back pain</u>: • Degenerative changes are common in the asymptomatic population and that the finding of degenerative changes in a patient with low back pain does not necessarily imply that the degenerative changes are the *cause* of the low back pain[18] • Most patients with low back pain do not need to be radiographed for the first 3-4 weeks of care unless they have specific indicators from their history or physical examination that suggest fracture, bone lesion, or other changes *that will be visible radiographically* • Do not use radiography for lesions that would be better assessed with ultrasound, CT, MRI, or laboratory tests
23. **Diagnostic ultrasound (US)**: Generally not used to assess low back pain unless a specific abdominal lesion is suspected	• Calcification and enlargement of the outline of the abdominal aorta; physical examination may reveal a larger-than-expected pulsatile mass, which represents the enlarging aorta. If an aneurysm of the abdominal aorta (AAA) is found, refer patient to surgeon; AAA is more common in patients over 40 years of age with a history of smoking, diabetes and/or hypertension

[17] Brier S. <u>Primary Care Orthopedics</u>. St. Louis: Mosby, 1999 page 287
[18] Tierney ML. McPhee SJ, Papadakis MA (eds). <u>Current Medical Diagnosis and Treatment 2006, 45th Edition</u>. Lange Medical; page 817

Clinical Assessments of the Low Back—*continued*

Selected assessments	*Positive finding and Implications*
24. **MRI**: Mostly used for the assessment of soft tissues, such as discs and nerves	Possible findings: ▪ Disc herniation ▪ Nerve compression ▪ Degeneration ▪ Other pathology such as osteomyelitis or cancer
25. **CT**: Used to image bone and the diameter and patency of the spinal canal; also able to image soft tissues and viscera. Resolution is poor compared to MRI	Possible findings: ▪ Fracture of vertebra or pelvis ▪ Impingement of the spinal canal due to degeneration, disc herniation, or other process. ▪ Disease of bone, soft-tissue, or viscera ▪ Degeneration ▪ Other pathology such as osteomyelitis or cancer
26. **Bone scan**: Primarily used for the detection of occult fractures, infections, and malignant disease	Possible findings: ▪ Fracture ▪ Infection ▪ Malignancy: Bone scans are typically **normal** in **multiple myeloma**; lytic lesions do not show increased uptake of radioactive isotope[19]

---

[19] Tierney ML. McPhee SJ, Papadakis MA (eds). Current Medical Diagnosis and Treatment 2006, 45th Edition. Lange Medical; page 817

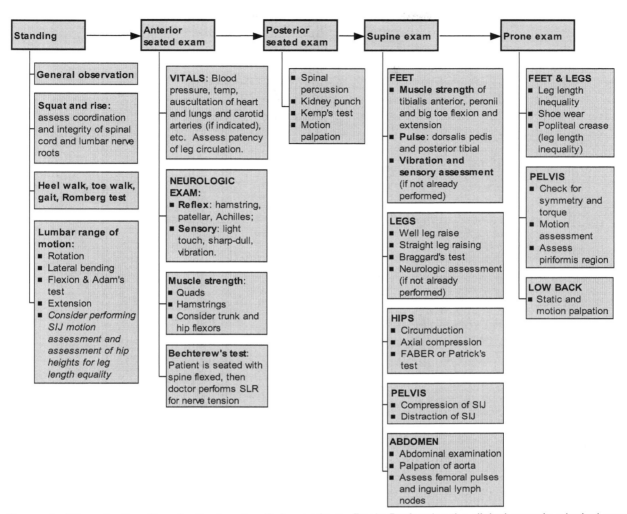

| Standing | Anterior seated exam | Posterior seated exam | Supine exam | Prone exam |

General observation

Squat and rise: assess coordination and integrity of spinal cord and lumbar nerve roots

Heel walk, toe walk, gait, Romberg test

Lumbar range of motion:
- Rotation
- Lateral bending
- Flexion & Adam's test
- Extension
- *Consider performing SIJ motion assessment and assessment of hip heights for leg length equality*

VITALS: Blood pressure, temp, auscultation of heart and lungs and carotid arteries (if indicated), etc. Assess patency of leg circulation.

NEUROLOGIC EXAM:
- **Reflex:** hamstring, patellar, Achilles;
- **Sensory:** light touch, sharp-dull, vibration.

Muscle strength:
- Quads
- Hamstrings
- Consider trunk and hip flexors

Bechterew's test: Patient is seated with spine flexed, then doctor performs SLR for nerve tension

- Spinal percussion
- Kidney punch
- Kemp's test
- Motion palpation

FEET
- **Muscle strength** of tibialis anterior, peronii and big toe flexion and extension
- **Pulse:** dorsalis pedis and posterior tibial
- **Vibration and sensory assessment** (if not already performed)

LEGS
- Well leg raise
- Straight leg raising
- Braggard's test
- Neurologic assessment (if not already performed)

HIPS
- Circumduction
- Axial compression
- FABER or Patrick's test

PELVIS
- Compression of SIJ
- Distraction of SIJ

ABDOMEN
- Abdominal examination
- Palpation of aorta
- Assess femoral pulses and inguinal lymph nodes

FEET & LEGS
- Leg length inequality
- Shoe wear
- Popliteal crease (leg length inequality)

PELVIS
- Check for symmetry and torque
- Motion assessment
- Assess piriformis region

LOW BACK
- Static and motion palpation

Suggested Examination Flow for the Lumbar Spine and Low Back: Performing the clinical exam in a logical sequence allows the exam to flow easily for the doctor and the patient.

Standing	Anterior Seated	Posterior Seated	Supine	Prone
1. Observation 2. Squat and rise 3. Toe walk, heel walk, gait, Romberg 4. Range of motion 5. Motion palpation of the sacroiliac joints 6. Check for leg length inequality by assessing femoral trochanter and iliac crest heights	7. Vital signs 8. Neurologic examination, including cranial nerves (if indicated) 9. Reflexes 10. Sensory 11. Muscle strength 12. Bechterew's test: this is a seated version of straight leg raising for radiculitis; the patient is seated on table with flexed back and neck, doctor then extends knee	13. Spinal percussion 14. Kidney punch 15. Kemp's test: exacerbate foraminal encroachment by applying simultaneous axial compression, lateral flexion, and slight rotation 16. Motion palpation of spine and SI joints	17. Complete the assessment of neurologic function and motor strength if not already completed 18. Nerve tension tests: straight leg raising (SLR), Braggard's test, "well leg raise" for nerve tension as well as the accompanying increase in intrathecal pressure 19. Screen hip 20. Screen SIJ 21. Screen abdomen	22. Check torque and symmetry of pelvis 23. Motion palpation of lumbar spine and SI joints 24. Assess piriformis region for tightness, especially if sciatica is present 25. Leg length inequality 26. Static and deep palpation including the quadratus lumborum

Low Back Pain: General Considerations

<u>Description/pathophysiology</u>:
- Low back pain is a common ailment and a frequent cause for patients to seek healthcare. While the cause of the pain in a minority of patients is due to serious problems such as metastatic disease, viscerosomatic referral, osteomyelitis/discitis, or recent fracture which need to be diagnosed and treated on an urgent basis, the majority of patients with low back pain have no serious disease and no dysfunction that is readily apparent with standard medical evaluation. Recall, however, that *no disease is rare to the person who has it*, and each patient has to be evaluated fully before the low back pain is ascribed to a benign cause.
- Patients with low back pain can be categorized based on the underlying cause. Of the following five categories, the fifth category of relatively benign musculoskeletal disorders will be the emphasis of this chapter:
  1. <u>**Serious organic diseases requiring immediate attention**</u>: metastatic disease, viscerosomatic referral, osteomyelitis/discitis, etc.
  2. <u>**Serious musculoskeletal disorders requiring immediate attention**</u>: recent fracture (pathologic fracture, osteoporosis, compression fracture, fall from a height, major motor vehicle accident), cauda equina syndrome, and severe radiculopathy (i.e., severe pain or progressive muscular deficits).
  3. <u>**Rheumatologic diseases affecting the low back and pelvis**</u>: ankylosing spondylitis, Reiter's syndrome, enteropathic spondyloarthropathy.[20]
  4. <u>**Psychogenic**</u>: emotional overlay, symptom amplification, secondary gain, depression.
  5. <u>**Benign functional/musculoskeletal disorders requiring conservative treatment and monitoring**</u>: muscle spasm, facet irritation, segmental dysfunction, myofascial trigger points (MFTP), disc injuries causing radiculitis or mild radiculopathy, self-limiting inflammation due to mild injury, vitamin D deficiency.

---

[20] See <u>Integrative Rheumatology</u> from <u>www.OptimalHealthResearch.com</u> for detailed information on the integrative treatments for rheumatic diseases.

Description/pathophysiology—*continued*

- Chronic low back pain has been enigmatic from the pharmacosurgical allopathic perspective, and the condition has been largely described as "idiopathic" in most medical journal descriptions. However, at least two discoveries within the past few years have shed *paradigm-shifting* light on this once-enigmatic and now largely curable problem that afflicts millions of sufferers worldwide.

  1. <u>Vitamin D deficiency is a major cause of musculoskeletal pain and low back pain</u>: In the early years of this new millennium, we experienced an incontrovertible paradigm shift with regard to our understanding and appreciation about the many clinical benefits of vitamin D. Several articles are particularly noteworthy in this regard and deserve appropriate attention:

     - <u>Review: Vitamin D supplementation, 25-hydroxyvitamin D concentrations, and safety *(Am J Clin Nutr* 1999 May[21])</u>: In this review, Dr Vieth provides a bulletproof summary of the literature proving that vitamin D3 is safe in doses that far exceed the 400-800 IU/d doses that are advocated for daily intake and supplementation, and he subtly yet boldly challenges anyone to refute his findings. Because of the boldness of his tact, Dr Vieth's article was a powerful push in the right direction for researchers and clinicians to become more confident in their clinical use of vitamin D supplementation. Armed with evidence that 15-minutes of full-body sunbathing could produce at least 10,000 IU of vitamin D3 and that populations with higher vitamin D levels had improved health outcomes, clinicians were empowered to use doses of vitamin D that were more consistent with what would be acquired if we lived in a more natural environment—namely outdoors and not "protected" from roofs, clothes, umbrellas, and sunscreen for 98% of our lives. Download at: http://www.ajcn.org/cgi/content/full/69/5/842

       > **All patients with low back pain—or any chronic musculoskeletal pain—must be tested and treated for vitamin D deficiency**
       >
       > "Vitamin D deficiency is a major contributor to chronic low back pain in areas where vitamin D deficiency is endemic. Screening for vitamin D deficiency and treatment with supplements should be **mandatory** in this setting."
       >
       > Al Faraj S, Al Mutairi K. Vitamin D deficiency and chronic low back pain in Saudi Arabia. *Spine* 2003;28:177-9

     - <u>Clinical intervention: Vitamin D deficiency and chronic low back pain in Saudi Arabia *(Spine* 2003[22])</u>: **This is a "must have" article for doctors who use nutrition in their practice.** Authors of this research found that 83% of the study patients (n = 299) were vitamin D deficient, and that **essentially all patients were relieved of their low back pain following supplementation with vitamin D at doses of 5,000 IU/d or 10,000 IU/d for three months.**

     - <u>Clinical study: Prevalence of severe hypovitaminosis D in patients with persistent, nonspecific musculoskeletal pain *(Mayo Clin Proc* 2003[23])</u>: These authors found that 140 out of 150 (93% of total) patients with persistent, nonspecific musculoskeletal pain were vitamin D deficient. Note that "persistent, nonspecific musculoskeletal pain" is very similar to the clinical presentation of *so-called* fibromyalgia, and Holick[24] later commented that "**Vitamin D deficiency is often misdiagnosed as fibromyalgia.**"

     - <u>Review of the research literature: Vitamin D in preventive medicine: are we ignoring the evidence? *(Br J Nutr* 2003[25])</u>: The pioneering aspect of this review by Dr Zittermann is that his was the first review article to advocate that vitamin D3 had major health-promoting systemic benefits in conditions other than osteoporosis. Until his review, we only had individual articles showing systemic benefit of vitamin D, but these had not been sufficiently organized to create a paradigm shift. To my knowledge, Dr Zittermann's review was the first to connect vitamin D to potential benefits in such diverse conditions as inflammation, autoimmunity, infectious

---

[21] Vieth R. Vitamin D supplementation, 25-hydroxyvitamin D concentrations, and safety. *Am J Clin Nutr*. 1999 May;69(5):842-56

[22] Al Faraj S, Al Mutairi K. Vitamin D deficiency and chronic low back pain in Saudi Arabia. *Spine*. 2003;28:177-9

[23] Plotnikoff GA, Quigley JM. Prevalence of severe hypovitaminosis D in patients with persistent, nonspecific musculoskeletal pain. *Mayo Clin Proc*. 2003;78(12):1463-70

[24] Holick MF. Vitamin D: importance in the prevention of cancers, type 1 diabetes, heart disease, and osteoporosis. *Am J Clin Nutr* 2004;79:362-71
http://www.ajcn.org/cgi/content/full/79/3/362

[25] Zittermann A. Vitamin D in preventive medicine: are we ignoring the evidence? *Br J Nutr* 2003;89:552-72

disease, hypertension, cardiovascular disease, diabetes mellitus, and cancer. One shortcoming to this article—perhaps—is the lack of strong advocation (note that the title of his article is written as a question) for doctor's to take direct action on the available research and begin testing and treating their patients for vitamin D deficiency with physiologic doses in the range of 4,000-10,000 IU per day. Dr Zittermann's article can be downloaded at the publisher's website.[26]

All patients with low back pain—or any chronic musculoskeletal pain—must be tested and treated for vitamin D deficiency

"All patients with persistent, nonspecific musculoskeletal pain are at high risk for the consequences of unrecognized and untreated severe hypovitaminosis D. ... Because osteomalacia is a known cause of persistent, nonspecific musculoskeletal pain, **screening all outpatients with such pain for hypovitaminosis D should be standard practice in clinical care.**"

Plotnikoff GA, Quigley JM. Prevalence of severe hypovitaminosis D in patients with persistent, nonspecific musculoskeletal pain. *Mayo Clin Proc* 2003;78:1463-70

- **Literature review with clinical applications:** The clinical importance of vitamin D (cholecalciferol): a paradigm shift with implications for all healthcare providers (*Altern Ther Health Med* 2004[27]): The important contributions of this article were the emphases on clinical relevance and action. This article was a call to arms, and before the first paragraph was over, I was telling doctors that they need to start testing their patients for vitamin D deficiency and to ensure that their patients have serum 25-hydroxy-vitamin D levels within our optimal range; importantly we advocated the use of 4,000 IU/d for virtually all adult patients (excluding those few patients with relative contraindications). We reviewed the clinical benefits of cholecalciferol in the treatment/prevention of cardiovascular disease, hypertension, depression, type-2 diabetes, type-1 diabetes, multiple sclerosis, migraine headaches, osteoarthritis, osteoarthritis, polycystic ovary syndrome, cancer, inflammation and musculoskeletal pain; importantly, we gave doctors clear guidelines for the clinical use and monitoring of vitamin D therapy. **Download at:** http://optimalhealthresearch.com/cholecalciferol.html Soon thereafter, I published shorter versions of these diagnostic and treatment conclusions in *The Lancet*[28], *JMPT*[29], and *British Medical Journal*.[30] Our letter published in *JAMA*[31] on vitamin D was so severely edited that by the time it was published I hardly recognized it; the editors were careful to excise any meaning from our rebuttal so that the status quo would be maintained and nutritional interventions would appear inefficacious.

2. **The majority of patients with low back pain (and spine pain including neck pain) have proprioceptive defects**: The increasingly widespread realization that patients with chronic joint pain and recurrent injuries have proprioceptive defects is a paradigm shift of its own right, and it obviously sheds new light on therapy and prevention of musculoskeletal pain and recurrent injuries. **Spinal manipulation, skin taping,** and **specific exercises** have all been shown to improve sensorimotor coordination. Very interestingly, **vitamin D supplementation** also improves sensorimotor coordination and thereby helps prevent falls and subsequent musculoskeletal injuries, particularly in the elderly.[32] Thus, vitamin D3 supplementation helps prevent fractures (especially in elderly patients) by at least two different mechanisms: ❶ vitamin D3 increases calcium absorption in the gut and helps preserve bone strength, and ❷ it also improves balance and coordination so that falls are avoided.

---

[26] http://ingentaconnect.com/content/cabi/bjn/2003/00000089/00000005/art00002?token=00421040644a467b4d616d3f4e4b34496e5865462440256f3b74675d3e786a775c
[27] **Vasquez A,** Manso G, Cannell J. The clinical importance of vitamin D (cholecalciferol): a paradigm shift with implications for all healthcare providers. *Altern Ther Health Med* 2004;10:28-36 http://optimalhealthresearch.com/cholecalciferol.html
[28] Vasquez A. Subphysiologic Doses of Vitamin D are Subtherapeutic. [Letter]. *The Lancet* 2005 Published on-line May 6 http://optimalhealthresearch.com/lancet.html
[29] Vasquez A. Health care for our bones: a practical nutritional approach to preventing osteoporosis. *J Manipulative Physiol Ther.* 2005 Mar-Apr;28(3):213
[30] Vasquez A, Cannell J. Calcium and vitamin D in preventing fractures: data are not sufficient to show inefficacy. *BMJ.* 2005 Jul 9;331(7508):108-9
[31] Muanza DN, Vasquez A, Cannell J, Grant WP. Isoflavones and postmenopausal women. *JAMA.* 2004 Nov 17;292(19):2337
[32] Dhesi JK, Jackson SH, Bearne LM, Moniz C, Hurley MV, Swift CG, Allain TJ. Vitamin D supplementation improves neuromuscular function in older people who fall. *Age Ageing.* 2004 Nov;33(6):589-95

Complications of low back pain:

- Chronic back pain: Patients may also have pain radiating to buttock or leg.
- Neuromuscular compromise: Weakness, incontinence, sexual dysfunction.
- Inability to engage in ADL: Asking questions about ADL (activities of daily living) is an important way to gain somewhat objective information about the patient's subjective pain. Severe pain causes restrictions and limitations in normal ADL, unless the patient has had pain for so long that he/she has adapted activities and overall lifestyle to accommodate the problem. If a patient complains of acute pain but then does not note limitations in ADL, then the doctor has uncovered an inconsistency that suggests stoicism, symptom amplification, or malingering.
- Medication toxicities and adverse surgical results: Liver and kidney damage are more common among patients who use acetaminophen and NSAIDs; NSAID hepatotoxicity and nephrotoxicity are dose-related. More than 17,000 Americans per year die from NSAID use.[33] The COX-2 inhibitor Vioxx reportedly killed as many as 55,000 patients and injured up to 139,000 Americans who took the drug.[34] Low back pain, like osteoarthritis, is a benign condition except when medically managed; then it becomes a life-threatening condition, by virtue of its pharmaceutical treatment. Drugs and surgery are more dangerous than manipulative therapy for the treatment of spinal pain.[35]

Major differential diagnoses:

- Cancer, metastatic disease: Malignant neoplasms account for approximately 1% of all low back pain and are most often associated with at least one of the following four patient characteristics:[36]
  - o Patient older than age 50 years
  - o Previous history of cancer[37]
  - o Unexplained weight loss
  - o Failure to respond to conservative care within one month

> **Correction of vitamin D deficiency improves muscle strength and neuromuscular coordination**
>
> "Vitamin D supplementation, in fallers with vitamin D insufficiency, has a **significant beneficial effect on functional performance, reaction time and balance**… This suggests that **vitamin D supplementation improves neuromuscular or neuroprotective function**, which may in part explain the mechanism whereby vitamin D reduces falls and fractures."
>
> Dhesi JK, et al. Vitamin D supplementation improves neuromuscular function in older people who fall. *Age Ageing.* 2004;33:589-95

- Viscerosomatic referral: Nephrolithiasis, stomach ulcer, etc.
- Renal infection: Costovertebral tenderness and fever; test urinalysis, CBC, chemistry/metabolic panel.
- Osteomyelitis and discitis: More common in diabetics and patients with recurrent urinary tract infections.
- Vitamin D deficiency: a common cause of low back pain.[38,39]
- Fracture: Compression fractures are more common in elderly persons, especially after age 70 years. Compression fractures are more common in patients with a history of chronic corticosteroid use and may arise spontaneously with minimal exertion or trauma.
- Cauda equina syndrome: Back pain may be mild-moderate while neurologic deficits progress; the classic presentation of sacral nerve root compression includes anogenital numbness ("saddle anesthesia"), bowel/bladder incontinence, and sexual dysfunction—penile numbness and erectile dysfunction in men, and clitoral numbness and vaginal weakness/numbness in women.
- Rheumatologic diseases: ankylosing spondylitis, Reiter's syndrome, enteropathic spondyloarthropathy
- Psychogenic pain: emotional overlay, symptom amplification, secondary gain, depression.
- Anatomic and biomechanical anomalies:

---

[33] Singh G. Recent considerations in nonsteroidal anti-inflammatory drug gastropathy. *Am J Med.* 1998 Jul 27; 105(1B): 31S-38S

[34] http://www.commondreams.org/views05/0223-35.htm and http://www.fda.gov/cder/drug/infopage/vioxx/vioxxgraham.pdf Accessed July 26, 2006

[35] Rosner AL. Evidence-based clinical guidelines for the management of acute low-back pain: response to the guidelines prepared for the Australian Medical Health and Research Council. *J Manipulative Physiol Ther.* 2001;24(3):214-20

[36] Souza TA. Differential Diagnosis for the Chiropractor: Protocols and Algorithms. Gaithersburg: Aspen Publications. 1997 page 105, 108

[37] Jenner JR, Barry M. ABC of rheumatology. Low back pain. *BMJ* 1995 Apr 8;310(6984):929-32

[38] Plotnikoff GA, Quigley JM. Prevalence of severe hypovitaminosis D in patients with persistent, nonspecific musculoskeletal pain. *Mayo Clin Proc.* 2003;78(12):1463-70

[39] Al Faraj S, Al Mutairi K. Vitamin D deficiency and chronic low back pain in Saudi Arabia. *Spine.* 2003 Jan 15;28(2):177-9

- o Facet tropism: asymmetry of the orientation of the lumbar or lumbosacral facets seen in 20-40% of the population and is generally not considered a cause of low back pain.[40]
- o Leg length inequalities[41]
- o Hemivertebrae and other vertebral anomalies
- o Scoliosis: Scoliosis is not generally painful, and the presence of pain with scoliosis—particularly recent-onset scoliosis—indicates the need for investigation for a pathologic underlying cause.
- Miscellaneous concerns:
  - o Consider that a combination of different problems may synergize to create a clinical presentation that resembles lumbar radiculitis and sciatica. For example, in my clinical practice a patient presented with a **classic picture of lumbar radiculopathy**: low back pain, leg pain, and foot pain and numbness; however in her case these symptoms turned out to be due to several different problems such as obesity (back pain), varicose veins (leg pain), and tarsal tunnel syndrome (foot pain), respectively.

The five most important considerations in the initial evaluation of low back pain
During the initial evaluation of low back pain, the most important problems to consider and exclude are:
1. Infection
2. Malignancy, cancer
3. Fracture
4. Rheumatic disease
5. Abdominal-pelvic disease such as aortic aneurysm, pancreatic cancer, endometriosis, uterine cancer, or ectopic pregnancy
6. Neurologic deficits, including cauda equina syndrome which may present only with bowel and bladder deficits while lower extremity strength remains intact
Mnemonic acronym: "I'm Fran"

Clinical assessment:

- History: Low back pain, may also have radiating pain to buttocks, thigh, leg and foot.
  - o Risk factors and predisposing factors:
    - Compression, weight lifting, carrying heavy loads or equipment, etc.
    - Compression *with flexion*—i.e., bending over to lift a heavy object
    - Compression with flexion *and rotation*—i.e., bending *and twisting* to lift a heavy object
    - Exaggerated flexion and/or rotation: creates tears in the annulus fibrosis
    - Shearing forces: common in motor vehicle accidents
    - Repetitive vibration: such as with machine operators or truck drivers
    - Sedentary lifestyle, lack of exercise: altered center of gravity, excess weight, muscle atrophy
    - Obesity
    - Cigarette/tobacco smoking
    - Depression, psychoemotional problems, secondary gain
  - o During the evaluation of spinal pain and low back pain, the doctor must ask about signs and symptoms of myelopathy, cauda equina syndrome, and radiculopathy. Recall that the spinal cord is only present in the cervical and thoracic spine to the level of approximately L1-L2. In the lumbar spine, the spinal cord ends and is replaced, so to speak, by the cauda equina; with regard to motor deficits, compression of the spinal cord presents with upper motor neuron signs of spasticity and hyperreflexia whereas compression of the cauda equina presents with lower motor neuron signs such as flaccid weakness and hyporeflexia. Cauda equina syndrome is a medical emergency that must be considered and evaluated by history and/or physical examination before the patient is treated and released from care.

Clinical assessment—*continued*

- History—*continued*: **Three screening questions** to ask when evaluating for myelopathy, cauda equina syndrome, and radiculopathy:
  1. **"Do you notice any pain, numbness, weakness or tingling in your arms, hands, legs or feet?"**
  2. **"Have you noticed any difficulty controlling your bowels or bladder (incontinence), or have you had any difficulty going to the bathroom (urinary retention)?"**
  3. **"Have you noticed any numbness or change in sensation near your anus or genitals?"**

---

[40] Souza TA. Differential Diagnosis for the Chiropractor: Protocols and Algorithms. Gaithersburg: Aspen Publications. 1997 page 107
[41] Jenner JR, Barry M. ABC of rheumatology. Low back pain. *BMJ* 1995 Apr 8;310(6984):929-32

- Physical examination: For the evaluation of neurologic competence during the routine evaluation of a typical patient with low back pain, see Physical Examination notes in Chapter 1 as well as your notes and text from your Neurology and Physical Exam courses. Some pertinent reminders are provided here:
  - o Start your neuromusculoskeletal examination with **observation** and **active patient motion**: *Squat and rise, heel walk, toe walk, gait assessment, Romberg, thoracic and lumbar range of motion in flexion, extension, rotation, and side-bending.* These tests are performed to provide the doctor with a quick overview of the patient's overall "intactness", biomechanics, lower extremity muscle strength, and neurologic status. Patients with occult fractures or acute disc lesions will generally not be able to perform these basic maneuvers without being stopped by pain, and thus the doctor can be alerted to the probability of a major problem *before the doctor ever touches the patient.*
  - o The second part of the exam is generally the completion of the neurologic examination: Complete your assessment of sensory challenges (vibration, sharp/dull, light touch, and proprioception), muscle strength testing, and reflexes. Early in the exam, the patient is still becoming acquainted with the doctor, and so the doctor starts with these more gentle procedures in order to ease into the examination and build rapport; in most situations, it would be a mistake to begin the exam with aggressive orthopedic tests when the doctor has not yet won the trust and confidence of the patient. More importantly, diving into the exam with overly aggressive orthopedic challenge exams such as forced neck flexion or compressive hip circumduction could be devastating if the patient has an occult fracture; this is why the recommendation is made here to start with observation, active patient motion, and gentle physical examination procedures so that the more aggressive tests are left toward the end of the examination, by which time the patient has been largely screened for major problems
  - o The third and final portion of the exam includes your orthopedic tests, biomechanical and myofascial assessments: These were reviewed earlier in this chapter, in Chapter 1, and other courses. Be sure to assess the **quadratus lumborum** for myofascial trigger points—a common and easily treatable cause of low back pain.[42,43,44]

Imaging & laboratory assessments:

- Radiographs: Generally not indicated in most patients who present with acute low back pain, unless indicators from the history or physical examination raise a cautionary *red flag* and/or a combination of *yellow flags* that lead the doctor to think that the patient has a problem that needs to be screened *and which will be demonstrable on plain radiography.* "**If pain appears mechanical, reserve the use of radiographs for 3 to 4 weeks** unless a radiographic evaluation is likely to change the treatment approach to the patient."[45] Radiographs may show fracture, degeneration, loss of disc height, anomalies, and gross bone lesions.
  - o "**Most patients with simple mechanical low back pain without peripheralization of pain do not need radiologic examination immediately**… If the diagnosis remains in question and the patient's condition does not respond to therapy, a radiologic evaluation is appropriate."[46]
- Abdominal ultrasound: Used for the assessment of abdominal aneurysms, tumors, masses, including uterine fibroids
- Bone scan: Assessment for occult fracture, occult metastatic disease
- CT scan: Lesions within the spinal canal, disc herniations, spinal stenosis
- MRI: Disc herniations, nerve compression, osteomyelitis, cancer, soft tissue assessment

---

[42] "The quadratus lumborum should be examined in patients presenting with flank pain as well as low back, buttock and lateral hip pain." de Franca GG, Levine LJ. The quadratus lumborum and low back pain. *J Manipulative Physiol Ther.* 1991 Feb;14(2):142-9

[43] "Trigger points (TPs) in muscles of the lower torso associated with the spine are an important cause of low back pain. The quadratus lumborum is the muscle most commonly involved..." Simons DG, Travell JG. Myofascial origins of low back pain. 2. Torso muscles. *Postgrad Med.* 1983 Feb;73(2):81-92

[44] "Successful treatment of myofascial pain requires the identification of TrPs by manual examination, identification of mechanical or systemic perpetuating factors, treatment of the specific TrPs, and corrective action to prevent their recurrence." Gerwin RD. Myofascial aspects of low back pain. *Neurosurg Clin N Am.* 1991 Oct;2(4):761-84

[45] Souza TA. Differential Diagnosis for the Chiropractor: Protocols and Algorithms. Gaithersburg: Aspen Publications. 1997 page 106

[46] Brier S. Primary Care Orthopedics. St. Louis: Mosby, 1999 page 213

Clinical management:

- Mechanical low back pain should be managed conservatively-yet-assertively for approximately 1 month. Failure to achieve significant resolution of pain after 3-4 weeks indicates the need for additional evaluation or referral to a specialist.[47]
- Referral if clinical outcome is unsatisfactory or if serious complications become evident.

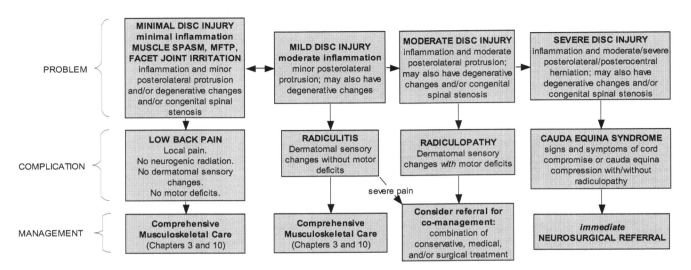

Management Algorithm Based on Underlying Injury and Clinical Presentation: Noted above.

Treatment Considerations:

- Rest: Bed rest has been and continues to be commonly recommended by medical physicians. While this may be appropriate for a very small minority of patients, the vast majority of patients do better to avoid prolonged bed rest and to engage in early rehabilitative exercise.
- Soft lumbar support belts: More effective for behavioral modification than they are for actually providing direct biomechanical support for the low back. The use of these support belts restricts motion in the lumbar spine and thereby reduces the hydrodynamic variations and osmotic gradients necessary for disc and cartilage nutrition; in this way, immobilization and excess restrictions in motion can retard the healing process. Furthermore, the relative motion restriction would serve to perpetuate sensorimotor coordination deficits. Behavioral modification can be important however, especially for reducing forward flexion and for promoting body/postural awareness.
- Massage: Research indicates that massage can improve flexibility, reduce pain, and increase serotonin and dopamine in patients with low back pain.[48]
- Spinal manipulation: Clearly effective, safe, and cost-effective for the treatment of low back pain.[49] Spinal manipulation can be safe and effective for the management of lumbar intervertebral disc herniation.[50] See *samples* of manipulative procedures that follow.
- Treatment of myofascial trigger points: Treatment of associated muscle spasm and myofascial trigger points can increase range of motion and decrease pain; see Chapter 3 for review.
- Vitamin C: Former Clinical Professor of Neurosurgery at Baylor University College of Medicine James Greenwood, MD, FACS reported his experience with over 500 patients with low back pain. Patients were administered up to 1,000 milligrams of vitamin C, either with or without surgical treatment for low back pain. "It can be stated with reasonable assurance that a significant percentage of patients with early disc

---

[47] Souza TA. <u>Differential Diagnosis for the Chiropractor: Protocols and Algorithms</u>. Gaithersburg: Aspen Publications. 1997 page 106

[48] Hernandez-Reif M, Field T, Krasnegor J, Theakston H.Lower back pain is reduced and range of motion increased after massage therapy. *Int J Neurosci* 2001;106(3-4):131-45

[49] Magna P, Angus DE, Swan WR. Findings and recommendations from an independent review of chiropractic management of low back pain. *JNMS: Journal of the Neuromusculoskeletal System* 1994; 2: 1-8

[50] Quon JA, Cassidy JD, O'Connor SM, Kirkaldy-Willis WH. Lumbar intervertebral disc herniation: treatment by rotational manipulation. *J Manipulative Physiol Ther* 1989 Jun;12(3):220-7

lesions were able to avoid surgery by the use of large doses of vitamin C... The number of reoperations on the same patients for recurrent at the same level or a new disc lesion at a different level has been greatly reduced."[51] Obviously, we can use more than 1,000 mg of vitamin C per day, and we can combine supplemental vitamin C (dose range from 3,000 mg to bowel tolerance) with bioflavonoids for an improved tissue-healing, anti-inflammatory, and antioxidant benefit.

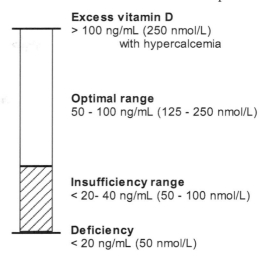

Excess vitamin D
> 100 ng/mL (250 nmol/L) with hypercalcemia

Optimal range
50 - 100 ng/mL (125 - 250 nmol/L)

Insufficiency range
< 20- 40 ng/mL (50 - 100 nmol/L)

Deficiency
< 20 ng/mL (50 nmol/L)

Interpretation of serum 25(OH) vitamin D levels. Modified from Vasquez et al, *Alternative Therapies in Health and Medicine* 2004 and Vasquez A. *Musculoskeletal Pain: Expanded Clinical Strategies* (Institute for Functional Medicine) 2008.

- Vitamin D: Vitamin D deficiency is common in patients with low back pain[52], limb pain[53], chronic persistent musculoskeletal pain[54], and in general medical patients.[55,56] In our review of the literature[57], we concluded that optimal serum 25(OH)-vitamin D levels should be defined as 50 – 100 ng/mL (125 - 250 nmol/L) and that, "Until proven otherwise, the balance of the research clearly indicates that oral supplementation in the range of 1,000 IU per day for infants, 2,000 IU per day for children and 4,000 IU per day for adults is safe and reasonable to meet physiologic requirements, to promote optimal health, and to reduce the risk of several serious diseases. Safety and effectiveness of supplementation are assured by periodic monitoring of serum 25(OH)D and serum calcium." For additional research on the importance and safety of vitamin D, see the articles by Vieth[58], Heaney et al[59], Holick[60], and Vasquez, Manso, and Cannell.[61] Vitamin D3 supplementation at 5,000–10,000 IU/d for 3 months was shown to alleviate low back pain in all adults with initially low serum levels of vitamin D.[62]

- Exercise, proprioceptive rehabilitation, stretching: The exercise plan should emphasize strengthening of abdominal and lumbar paraspinal muscles, as well as rehabilitating poor sensorimotor function as reviewed in Chapter 3. Stretching and post-isometric stretching—especially of the iliopsoas and piriformis—are particularly important to establish muscle tension balance, correct faulty biomechanics, and alleviate pain from myofascial trigger points.

- Dextrose prolotherapy: Due to its ability to promote proliferation of connective tissue, dextrose prolotherapy may provide benefit for patients with ligamentous laxity and disc degeneration, as demonstrated in studies of patients with back pain, knee pain, and hand osteoarthritis.[63, 64,65,66,67]

[51] Greenwood J. Optimum vitamin C intake as a factor in the preservation of disc integrity. *Med Ann Dist Columbia*. 1964 Jun;33:274-6

[52] Al Faraj S, Al Mutairi K. Vitamin D deficiency and chronic low back pain in Saudi Arabia. *Spine*. 2003 Jan 15;28(2):177-9

[53] Masood H, Narang AP, Bhat IA, Shah GN. Persistent limb pain and raised serum alkaline phosphatase the earliest markers of subclinical hypovitaminosis D in Kashmir. *Indian J Physiol Pharmacol*. 1989 Oct-Dec;33(4):259-61

[54] Plotnikoff GA, Quigley JM. Prevalence of severe hypovitaminosis D in patients with persistent, nonspecific musculoskeletal pain. *Mayo Clin Proc*. 2003 Dec;78(12):1463-70

[55] Thomas MK, Lloyd-Jones DM, Thadhani RI, Shaw AC, Deraska DJ, Kitch BT, Vamvakas EC, Dick IM, Prince RL, Finkelstein JS. Hypovitaminosis D in medical inpatients. *N Engl J Med*. 1998 Mar 19;338(12):777-83

[56] Kauppinen-Makelin R, Tahtela R, Loyttyniemi E, Karkkainen J, Valimaki MJ. A high prevalence of hypovitaminosis D in Finnish medical in- and outpatients. *J Intern Med*. 2001 Jun;249(6):559-63

[57] Vasquez A, Manso G, Cannell J. The Clinical Importance of Vitamin D (Cholecalciferol): A Paradigm Shift with Implications for All Healthcare Providers. *Alternative Therapies in Health and Medicine* and *Integrative Medicine: A Clinician's Journal* www.optimalhealthresearch.com/monograph04

[58] Vieth R. Vitamin D supplementation, 25-hydroxyvitamin D concentrations, and safety. *Am J Clin Nutr*. 1999 May;69(5):842-56

[59] Heaney RP, Davies KM, Chen TC, Holick MF, Barger-Lux MJ. Human serum 25-hydroxycholecalciferol response to extended oral dosing with cholecalciferol. *Am J Clin Nutr*. 2003 Jan;77(1):204-10

[60] Holick MF. Vitamin D: importance in the prevention of cancers, type 1 diabetes, heart disease, and osteoporosis. *Am J Clin Nutr*. 2004 Mar;79(3):362-71

[61] Vasquez A, Manso G, Cannell J. The Clinical Importance of Vitamin D (Cholecalciferol): A Paradigm Shift with Implications for All Healthcare Providers. *Alternative Therapies in Health and Medicine* and *Integrative Medicine: A Clinician's Journal* www.optimalhealthresearch.com/monograph04

[62] Al Faraj S, Al Mutairi K. Vitamin D deficiency and chronic low back pain in Saudi Arabia. *Spine*. 2003 Jan 15;28(2):177-9

[63] "Prolotherapy injection with 10% dextrose resulted in clinically and statistically significant improvements in knee osteoarthritis. Preliminary blinded radiographic readings (1-year films, with 3-year total follow-up period planned) demonstrated improvement in several measures of osteoarthritis severity. ACL laxity, when present in these osteoarthritic patients, improved. " Reeves KD, Hassanein K. Randomized prospective double-blind placebo-controlled study of dextrose prolotherapy for knee osteoarthritis with or without ACL laxity. *Altern Ther Health Med* 2000 Mar;6(2):68-74, 77-80

[64] Mooney V. Prolotherapy at the fringe of medical care, or is it the frontier? *Spine J*. 2003 Jul-Aug;3(4):253-4

- Intravenous colchicine: Michael Rask MD has been the strongest advocate of the use of intravenous colchicine for the treatment of herniated spinal discs, and his monograph "*Colchicine use in 6,000 patients with disk disease and other related resistantly-painful spinal disorders*"[68] is required reading for any physician interested in using this technique clinically—the details of his protocol are much too extensive to review here, and clinicians will be better served by reading the original article. Notably, as part of the protocol for patients with disc herniation, in addition to intravenous colchicine, Rask advocates 1) treatment of myofascial trigger points, 2) weight loss, 3) cessation of alcohol, tobacco, and caffeine, 4) avoidance of *Solanaceae* plants such as eggplant, potato, tomato, and green and red peppers, 5) avoidance of sugars and junk foods, and 6) a strict vegan diet, especially for patients who are overweight. Although Rask[69] notes that colchicine is "extremely effective" and "an exceedingly safe medication", other authors[70] have been less optimistic noting that the benefit was "often of short duration." Given that intravenous colchicine has been associated with complications such as pancytopenia, organ failure, and death[71], it is not a treatment to be taken lightly nor should inexperienced physicians administer it. Colchicine can be administered orally, but its low therapeutic efficacy in relation to its moderate gastrointestinal toxicity limits its applicability. In a poorly designed study by Schnebel and Simmons[72], orally administered colchicine was no better yet was more toxic than placebo; this study appears to have been designed specifically to show inefficacy and toxicity of colchicine since the patients were either given *no treatment* alternating with a *gastroirritative toxic dose* of colchicine.
- Anti-inflammatory & analgesic diet, nutrients, and botanicals:
  - Anti-inflammatory healing-supportive diet: Pro-inflammatory foods and food components such as arachidonic acid (high in cow's milk, beef, liver, pork, and lamb)[73,74], saturated fats[75,76], corn oil[77,78], high glycemic foods[79,80], white bread[81], high-fat high-carbohydrate fast-food breakfast[82] should be

---

[65] This study used intradiscal injection therapy with glucosamine, chondroitin sulfate, hypertonic dextrose and DMSO. "Although the results were statistically significant for the 30 patients as a whole, 17 of the 30 patients (57%) improved markedly with an average of 72% improvement in disability scores and 76% in visual analogue scores. The other 13 patients (43%) had little or no improvement." Klein RG, Eek BC, O'Neill CW, Elin C, Mooney V, Derby RR. Biochemical injection treatment for discogenic low back pain: a pilot study. *Spine J.* 2003 May-Jun;3(3):220-6

[66] "Dextrose prolotherapy was clinically effective and safe in the treatment of pain with joint movement and range limitation in osteoarthritic finger joints." Reeves KD, Hassanein K. Randomized, prospective, placebo-controlled double-blind study of dextrose prolotherapy for osteoarthritic thumb and finger (DIP, PIP, and trapeziometacarpal) joints: evidence of clinical efficacy. *J Altern Complement Med.* 2000 Jun;6(4):311-20

[67] "RESULTS: Each patient was injected an average of 3.5 times. Overall, 43.4% of patients fell into the sustained improvement group with an average improvement in numeric pain scores of 71%, comparing pretreatment and 18 month measurements." Miller MR, Mathews RS, Reeves KD. Treatment of painful advanced internal lumbar disc derangement with intradiscal injection of hypertonic dextrose. *Pain Physician.* 2006 Apr;9(2):115-21 http://www.painphysicianjournal.com/linkout_vw.php?issn=1533-3159&vol=9&page=115

[68] Rask MR. Colchicine use in 6,000 patients with disk disease and other related resistantly-painful spinal disorders. *Journal of Neurological and Orthopaedic Medicine and Surgery* 1989; 10: 291-298 Contact Information: The American Academy of Neurological and Orthopaedic Surgeons; 10 Cascade Creek Lane. Las Vegas, NV 89113 phone: (702) 388-7390 fax: (702) 388-7395 aanos@aanos.org

[69] Rask MR. Colchicine use in 6,000 patients with disk disease and other related resistantly-painful spinal disorders. *Journal of Neurological and Orthopaedic Medicine and Surgery* 1989; 10: 291-298

[70] "Results indicate a significant difference between the two groups, the intravenous colchicine group showing improvement in symptoms for a few hours or days over a 3-week course of treatment. However, the relief was often of short duration." Simmons JW, Harris WP, Koulisis CW, Kimmich SJ. Intravenous colchicine for low back pain: a double-blind study. *Spine.* 1990 Jul;15(7):716-7

[71] "Bone marrow depression has been reported, primarily in cases of acute colchicine intoxication, and intravenous administration of the drug has been associated with severe pancytopenia and death." Levy M, Spino M, Read SE. Colchicine: a state-of-the-art review. *Pharmacotherapy.* 1991;11(3):196-211

[72] Schnebel BE, Simmons JW. The use of oral colchicine for low back pain. A double-blind study. *Spine.* 1988 Mar;13(3):354-7 Use of colchicine in this study varied from abstinence for 3 days followed by a toxic dose on day 4; therefore patients in the treatment group were subjected to no treatment for 75% of the time, followed by a dose that caused gastrointestinal toxicity—vomiting and diarrhea—the other 25% of the time. At neither phase of the study were patients exposed to a treatment that had any possibility of being effective in relation to the potential toxicity. This study was so poorly designed that its publication brings into question the editorial quality of *Spine* during this era.

[73] Vasquez A. Reducing Pain and Inflammation Naturally. Part 2: New Insights into Fatty Acid Supplementation and Its Effect on Eicosanoid Production and Genetic Expression. *Nutritional Perspectives* 2005; January: 5-16 www.optimalhealthresearch.com/part2

[74] Evans AR, Junger H, Southall MD, Nicol GD, Sorkin LS, Broome JT, Bailey TW, Vasko MR. Isoprostanes, novel eicosanoids that produce nociception and sensitize rat sensory neurons. *J Pharmacol Exp Ther.* 2000 Jun;293(3):912-20

[75] Lee JY, Sohn KH, Rhee SH, Hwang D. Saturated fatty acids, but not unsaturated fatty acids, induce the expression of cyclooxygenase-2 mediated through Toll-like receptor 4. *J Biol Chem.* 2001 May 18;276(20):16683-9. Epub 2001 Mar 2 http://www.jbc.org/cgi/content/full/276/20/16683

[76] "CONCLUSIONS: Both fat and protein intakes stimulate ROS generation. The increase in ROS generation lasted 3 h after cream intake and 1 h after protein intake. Cream intake also caused a significant and prolonged increase in lipid peroxidation." Mohanty P, Ghanim H, Hamouda W, Aljada A, Garg R, Dandona P. Both lipid and protein intakes stimulate increased generation of reactive oxygen species by polymorphonuclear leukocytes and mononuclear cells. *Am J Clin Nutr.* 2002 Apr;75(4):767-72 http://www.ajcn.org/cgi/content/full/75/4/767

[77] Rusyn I, Bradham CA, Cohn L, Schoonhoven R, Swenberg JA, Brenner DA, Thurman RG. Corn oil rapidly activates nuclear factor-kappaB in hepatic Kupffer cells by oxidant-dependent mechanisms. *Carcinogenesis.* 1999 Nov;20(11):2095-100 http://carcin.oxfordjournals.org/cgi/content/full/20/11/2095

[78] "Exposing endothelial cells to 90 micromol linoleic acid/L for 6 h resulted in a significant increase in lipid hydroperoxides that coincided wih an increase in intracellular calcium concentrations." Hennig B, Toborek M, Joshi-Barve S, Barger SW, Barve S, Mattson MP, McClain CJ. Linoleic acid activates nuclear transcription factor-kappa B (NF-kappa B) and induces NF-kappa B-dependent transcription in cultured endothelial cells. *Am J Clin Nutr.* 1996 Mar;63(3):322-8 http://www.ajcn.org/cgi/reprint/63/3/322

[79] Mohanty P, Hamouda W, Garg R, Aljada A, Ghanim H, Dandona P. Glucose challenge stimulates reactive oxygen species (ROS) generation by leucocytes. *J Clin Endocrinol Metab.* 2000 Aug;85(8):2970-3 http://jcem.endojournals.org/cgi/content/full/85/8/2970 Glucose/carbohydrate and saturated fat consumption appear to be the two biggest offenders in the food-stimulated production of oxidative stress. The effect by protein is much less. "CONCLUSIONS: Both fat and protein intakes stimulate ROS generation. The increase in ROS generation lasted 3 h after cream intake and 1 h after protein intake. Cream intake also caused a significant and prolonged increase in lipid peroxidation." Mohanty P, Ghanim H, Hamouda W, Aljada A, Garg R, Dandona P. Both lipid and protein intakes stimulate increased generation of reactive oxygen species by polymorphonuclear leukocytes and mononuclear cells. *Am J Clin Nutr.* 2002 Apr;75(4):767-72 http://www.ajcn.org/cgi/content/full/75/4/767

avoided generally and especially during times of musculoskeletal inflammation. The Paleo-Mediterranean diet is based on abundant consumption of fruits, vegetables, seeds, nuts, berries, omega-3 and monounsaturated fatty acids, and lean sources of protein such as lean meats, fatty cold-water fish, soy and whey proteins.[83,84,85,86,87] The American/Western style of eating results in subclinical pathogenic chronic diet-induced metabolic acidosis[88,89] which can be corrected with a Paleo-Mediterranean diet[90,] or alkalinizing supplements[91] for the alleviation of musculoskeletal pain in general and low back pain in particular.[92] Ensure adequate fluid intake; teas—especially green teas—provide anti-inflammatory and antioxidant benefits that are clinically significant. Adequate/increased protein intake expedites recovery following injury and shows numerous other benefits[93,94]; in otherwise healthy patients with no liver, renal, or other metabolic disorders, ensure adequate intake of 0.5-0.9 gram of protein per pound of body weight.[95] Physiologically, the body's limit for handling nitrogenous groups from dietary protein is reached when protein intake is greater than 200-300 grams/d; as long as protein intake is kept below this level or below 30-40% of daily calories and/or combined with a *whole foods* fruit- and vegetable-rich diet, patients and doctors need not worry about the familiar myth of "too much protein."[96]

o   <u>Fatty acid supplementation for eicosanoid and genomic modulation</u>: Combination therapy with EPA-DHA (fish oil) and GLA (borage oil) is preferred for optimal results.[97]

▪   <u>Fish oil, EPA with DHA</u>: Up to three grams per day (3,000 mg/d) of combined EPA and DHA is a reasonable therapeutic dose.[98,99,100,101] In a recent open trial with data from 125 patients with

[80] Koska J, Blazicek P, Marko M, Grna JD, Kvetnansky R, Vigas M. Insulin, catecholamines, glucose and antioxidant enzymes in oxidative damage during different loads in healthy humans. *Physiol Res*. 2000;49 Suppl 1:S95-100 http://www.biomed.cas.cz/physiolres/pdf/2000/49_S95.pdf

[81] "Conclusion - The present study shows that high GI carbohydrate, but not low GI carbohydrate, mediates an acute proinflammatory process as measured by NF-kappaB activity." Dickinson S, Hancock DP, Petocz P, Brand-Miller JC..High glycemic index carbohydrate mediates an acute proinflammatory process as measured by NF-kappaB activation. *Asia Pac J Clin Nutr*. 2005;14 Suppl:S120

[82] Aljada A, Mohanty P, Ghanim H, Abdo T, Tripathy D, Chaudhuri A, Dandona P. Increase in intranuclear nuclear factor kappaB and decrease in inhibitor kappaB in mononuclear cells after a mixed meal: evidence for a proinflammatory effect. *Am J Clin Nutr*. 2004 Apr;79(4):682-90 http://www.ajcn.org/cgi/content/full/79/4/682

[83] Eaton SB, Shostak M, Konner M. The Paleolithic Prescription: A program of diet & exercise and a design for living, New York: Harper & Row, 1988

[84] O'Keefe JH Jr, Cordain L. Cardiovascular disease resulting from a diet and lifestyle at odds with our Paleolithic genome: how to become a 21st-century hunter-gatherer. *Mayo Clin Proc*. 2004;79(1):101-8

[85] Cordain L. The Paleo Diet: Lose Weight and Get Healthy by Eating the Food You Were Designed to Eat. Indianapolis; John Wiley and Sons, 2002

[86] Vasquez A. A Five-Part Nutritional Protocol that Produces Consistently Positive Results. *Nutritional Wellness* 2005 September Available in the printed version and on-line at http://www.nutritionalwellness.com/archives/2005/sep/09_vasquez.php and http://optimalhealthresearch.com/protocol

[87] Vasquez A. Implementing the Five-Part Nutritional Wellness Protocol for the Treatment of Various Health Problems. *Nutritional Wellness* 2005 November. Available on-line at http://www.nutritionalwellness.com/archives/2005/nov/11_vasquez.php and http://optimalhealthresearch.com/protocol

[88] "As a result, healthy adults consuming the standard US diet sustain a chronic, low-grade pathogenic metabolic acidosis that worsens with age as kidney function declines." Cordain L, Eaton SB, Sebastian A, Mann N, Lindeberg S, Watkins BA, O'Keefe JH, Brand-Miller J. Origins and evolution of the Western diet: health implications for the 21st century. *Am J Clin Nutr*. 2005 Feb;81(2):341-54 http://www.ajcn.org/cgi/content/full/81/2/341

[89] "An acidogenic Western diet results in mild metabolic acidosis in association with a state of cortisol excess, altered divalent ion metabolism, and increased bone resorptive indices." Maurer M, Riesen W, Muser J, Hulter HN, Krapf R. Neutralization of Western diet inhibits bone resorption independently of K intake and reduces cortisol secretion in humans. *Am J Physiol Renal Physiol*. 2003 Jan;284(1):F32-40. Epub 2002 Sep 24. http://ajprenal.physiology.org/cgi/content/full/284/1/F32

[90] Cordain L. The Paleo Diet: Lose Weight and Get Healthy by Eating the Food You Were Designed to Eat. Indianapolis; John Wiley and Sons, 2002

[91] For long-term out-patient treatment of patients who do not achieve alkalinization with diet alone, oral administration of potassium citrate and/or sodium bicarbonate can be implemented. See the following article for concepts: "Urine alkalinization is a treatment regimen that increases poison elimination by the administration of intravenous sodium bicarbonate to produce urine with a pH > or = 7.5." Proudfoot AT, Krenzelok EP, Vale JA. Position Paper on urine alkalinization. *J Toxicol Clin Toxicol*. 2004;42:1-26 http://www.eapcct.org/publicfile.php?folder=congress&file=PS_UrineAlkalinization.pdf Also see: Vormann J, Worlitschek M, Goedecke T, Silver B. Supplementation with alkaline minerals reduces symptoms in patients with chronic low back pain. *J Trace Elem Med Biol*. 2001;15(2-3):179-83 Also see: Maurer M, Riesen W, Muser J, Hulter HN, Krapf R. Neutralization of Western diet inhibits bone resorption independently of K intake and reduces cortisol secretion in humans. *Am J Physiol Renal Physiol*. 2003 Jan;284(1):F32-40. Epub 2002 Sep 24. http://ajprenal.physiology.org/cgi/content/full/284/1/F32

[92] "The results show that a disturbed acid-base balance may contribute to the symptoms of low back pain. The simple and safe addition of an alkaline multimineral preparate was able to reduce the pain symptoms in these patients with chronic low back pain." Vormann J, Worlitschek M, Goedecke T, Silver B. Supplementation with alkaline minerals reduces symptoms in patients with chronic low back pain. *J Trace Elem Med Biol*. 2001;15(2-3):179-83

[93] Vegetarians and healing. *JAMA* 1995; 273: 910

[94] Castaneda C, Charnley JM, Evans WJ, Crim MC. Elderly women accommodate to a low-protein diet with losses of body cell mass, muscle function, and immune response. *Am J Clin Nutr* 1995 Jul;62(1):30-9

[95] Nancy Clark, MS, RD. The Power of Protein. *The Physician and Sportsmedicine* 1996, volume 24, number 4. http://www.physsportsmed.com/issues/1996/04_96/protein.htm

[96] "I can assure you that as long as you eat plenty of fresh fruits and vegetables, there is no such thing as too much protein." (page 41). Cordain L. The Paleo Diet: Lose Weight and Get Healthy by Eating the Food You Were Designed to Eat. Indianapolis; John Wiley and Sons: 2002, pages 41, 67, 101

[97] Vasquez A. Reducing Pain and Inflammation Naturally. Part 2: New Insights into Fatty Acid Supplementation and Its Effect on Eicosanoid Production and Genetic Expression. *Nutritional Perspectives* 2005; January: 5-16 www.optimalhealthresearch.com/part2

[98] "…clinical benefits of the n-3 fatty acids were not apparent until they were consumed for > or =12 wk. It appears that a minimum daily dose of 3 g eicosapentaenoic and docosahexaenoic acids is necessary to derive the expected benefits [in patients with rheumatoid arthritis]." Kremer JM. n-3 fatty acid supplements in rheumatoid arthritis. *AmJ Clin Nutr*.2000;71(1S):349S-51S

[99] Rubin D, Laposata M. Cellular interactions between n-6 and n-3 fatty acids: a mass analysis of fatty acid elongation/desaturation, distribution among complex lipids, and conversion to eicosanoids. *J Lipid Res*. 1992 Oct;33(10):1431-40.

[100] The recent GISSI (Gruppo Italiano per lo Studio della Sopravvivenza nell'Infarto miocardico)-Prevention study of 11,324 patients showed a 45% decrease in risk of sudden cardiac death and a 20% reduction in all-cause mortality in the group taking 850 mg/d of omega-3 fatty acids. These fatty acids have potent anti-inflammatory effects and may also be antiatherogenic." O'Keefe JH Jr, Harris WS. From Inuit to implementation: omega-3 fatty acids come of age. *Mayo Clin Proc*. 2000 Jun;75(6):607-14

[101] "Many of the placebo-controlled trials of fish oil in chronic inflammatory diseases reveal significant benefit, including decreased disease activity and a lowered use of anti-inflammatory drugs." Simopoulos AP. Omega-3 fatty acids in inflammation and autoimmune diseases. *J Am Coll Nutr*. 2002 Dec;21(6):495-505

discogenic low back pain in a neurosurgical practice, a daily dose of 1,200-2,400 mg EPA and DHA was shown to alleviate low back pain. Further, 59% of patients were able to discontinue NSAID use due to pain relief from fish oil supplementation; 80% of patients were satisfied with their improvement, and 88% chose to continue treatment.[102]

- GLA, Gamma-linolenic acid: Approximately 500 mg per day is the common anti-inflammatory dose[103] although higher doses of 2.8 grams per day have been safely used in patients with rheumatoid arthritis.[104]

o Botanical medicines and nutritional supplements: Tailor the selection, dose, and combinations to the patient's size, age, and other clinical characteristics.

- Topical application of *Capsicum annuum, Capsicum frutescens* (Cayenne pepper, hot chili pepper): Controlled clinical trials have conclusively demonstrated capsaicin's ability to deplete sensory fibers of substance P to thus reduce pain in diabetic neuropathy, chronic low back pain[105], chronic neck pain[106], osteoarthritis[107], rheumatoid arthritis, notalgia paresthetica, reflex sympathetic dystrophy, and cluster headache (intranasal).

- *Boswellia serrata*: Boswellia inhibits 5-lipoxygenase with no apparent effect on cyclooxygenase and has been shown effective in the treatment of osteoarthritis of the knees[108] as well as asthma and ulcerative colitis. When used as monotherapy, the target dose is approximately 150 mg of boswellic acids TID (thrice daily).

- *Zingiber officinale* (Ginger): Ginger is a well known spice and food with a long history of use as an anti-inflammatory, anti-nausea, and gastroprotective agent, and components of ginger have been shown to reduce production of the leukotriene LTB4 by inhibiting 5-lipoxygenase and to reduce production of the prostaglandin PGE2 by inhibiting cyclooxygenase. Ginger has been shown to safely reduce nonspecific musculoskeletal pain[109,110] and to provide relief from osteoarthritis of the knees, migraine headaches, and nausea/vomiting of pregnancy.[111]

- Pancreatic/proteolytic enzymes: Orally-administered pancreatic and proteolytic enzymes are absorbed from the gastrointestinal tract into the systemic circulation to exert analgesic, anti-inflammatory, anti-edematous benefits with therapeutic relevance for acute and chronic musculoskeletal disorders.[112,113]

- *Harpagophytum procumbens* (Devil's claw): The safety and analgesic effectiveness of Harpagophytum has been established in patients with hip pain, low back pain, and knee pain.[114,115,116,117,118,119,120]

[102] Maroon JC, Bost JW. Omega-3 fatty acids (fish oil) as an anti-inflammatory: an alternative to nonsteroidal anti-inflammatory drugs for discogenic pain. *Surg Neurol.* 2006 Apr;65(4):326-31

[103] "Forty patients with rheumatoid arthritis and upper gastrointestinal lesions due to non-steroidal anti-inflammatory drugs entered a prospective 6-month double-blind placebo controlled study of dietary supplementation with gamma-linolenic acid 540 mg/day..." Brzeski M, Madhok R, Capell HA. Evening primrose oil in patients with rheumatoid arthritis and side-effects of non-steroidal anti-inflammatory drugs. *Br J Rheumatol.* 1991 Oct;30(5):370-2

[104] Zurier RB, Rossetti RG, Jacobson EW, DeMarco DM, Liu NY, Temming JE, White BM, Laposata M. gamma-Linolenic acid treatment of rheumatoid arthritis. A randomized, placebo-controlled trial. *Arthritis Rheum.* 1996 Nov;39(11):1808-17

[105] Keitel W, Frerick H, Kuhn U, Schmidt U, Kuhlmann M, Bredehorst A. Capsicum pain plaster in chronic non-specific low back pain. *Arzneimittelforschung.* 2001 Nov;51(11):896-903

[106] Mathias BJ, Dillingham TR, Zeigler DN, Chang AS, Belandres PV. Topical capsaicin for chronic neck pain. A pilot study. *Am J Phys Med Rehabil* 1995 Jan-Feb;74(1):39-44

[107] McCarthy GM, McCarty DJ. Effect of topical capsaicin in the therapy of painful osteoarthritis of the hands. *J Rheumatol.* 1992;19(4):604-7

[108] Kimmatkar N, Thawani V, Hingorani L, Khiyani R. Efficacy and tolerability of Boswellia serrata extract in treatment of osteoarthritis of knee--a randomized double blind placebo controlled trial. *Phytomedicine.* 2003 Jan;10(1):3-7

[109] Srivastava KC, Mustafa T. Ginger (Zingiber officinale) in rheumatism and musculoskeletal disorders. *Med Hypotheses.* 1992 Dec;39(4):342-8

[110] Srivastava KC, Mustafa T. Ginger (Zingiber officinale) and rheumatic disorders. *Med Hypotheses.* 1989 May;29(1):25-8

[111] "...oral ginger 1 g per day... No adverse effect of ginger on pregnancy outcome was detected." Vutyavanich T, Kraisarin T, Ruangsri R. Ginger for nausea and vomiting in pregnancy: randomized, double-masked, placebo-controlled trial. *Obstet Gynecol* 2001 Apr;97(4):577-82.

[112] Trickett P. Proteolytic enzymes in treatment of athletic injuries. *Appl Ther.* 1964;30:647-52

[113] Walker AF, Bundy R, Hicks SM, Middleton RW. Bromelain reduces mild acute knee pain and improves well-being in a dose-dependent fashion in an open study of otherwise healthy adults. *Phytomedicine.* 2002; 9: 681-6

[114] Chantre P, Cappelaere A, Leblan D, Guedon D, Vandermander J, Fournie B. Efficacy and tolerance of Harpagophytum procumbens versus diacerhein in treatment of osteoarthritis. *Phytomedicine* 2000 Jun;7(3):177-83

[115] Leblan D, Chantre P, Fournie B. Harpagophytum procumbens in the treatment of knee and hip osteoarthritis. Four-month results of a prospective, multicenter, double-blind trial versus diacerhein. *Joint Bone Spine* 2000;67(5):462-7

[116] Whitehouse LW, Znamirowska M, Paul CJ. Devil's Claw (Harpagophytum procumbens): no evidence for anti-inflammatory activity in the treatment of arthritic disease. *Can Med Assoc J* 1983 Aug 1;129(3):249-51

[117] Moussard C, Alber D, Toubin MM, Thevenon N, Henry JC. A drug used in traditional medicine, harpagophytum procumbens: no evidence for NSAID-like effect on whole blood eicosanoid production in human. *Prostaglandins Leukot Essent Fatty Acids* 1992 Aug;46(4):283-6

[118] Chrubasik S, Model A, Black A, Pollak S. A randomized double-blind pilot study comparing Doloteffin and Vioxx in the treatment of low back pain. *Rheumatology* (Oxford). 2003 Jan;42(1):141-8

[119] "The majority of responders' were patients who had suffered less than 42 days of pain, and subgroup analyses suggested that the effect was confined to patients with more severe and radiating pain accompanied by neurological deficit... There was no evidence for Harpagophytum-related side-effects, except possibly for mild and infrequent

- Willow bark (*Salix* spp): Numerous studies—especially among patients with low back pain—have validated the analgesic and anti-inflammatory benefits of willow bark extract.[121,122,123] Contraindications to the use of willow include aspirin/salicylate allergy and perhaps pregnancy, use of anticoagulant medication, or impending surgery.[124,125] The daily dose is generally kept below 240 mg of salicin, and products should include other components of the whole plant.

- Niacinamide: Niacinamide alleviates osteoarthritis pain.[126,127] The standard dose of 500 mg given orally 6 times per day is more effective than 1,000 mg 3 times per day. Hepatic dysfunction is rare when daily doses are kept below 3,000 mg per day; measure liver enzymes after 3 months of treatment and yearly thereafter.

- *Uncaria guianensis* and *Uncaria tomentosa* ("cat's claw", "una de gato"): Analgesic and anti-inflammatory benefits have been shown in osteoarthritis[128] and rheumatoid arthritis.

- Glucosamine sulfate and chondroitin sulfate: Glucosamine and chondroitin are the "building blocks" from which cartilage is built and oral supplementation is intended to enhance cartilage anabolism and to thus counteract the enhanced cartilage catabolism seen in destructive arthritic processes. The adult dose of glucosamine sulfate is generally 1500-2000 mg per day in divided doses, and the dose of chondroitin sulfate is approximately 1000 mg daily; these treatments can be used singly, in combination, and with other treatments.

- Vitamin E, with an emphasis on gamma-tocopherol: The gamma form of vitamin E inhibits cyclooxygenase and thus has anti-inflammatory activity that appears clinically significant in conditions such as rheumatoid arthritis, spondylosis and back pain[129], osteoarthritis, and several autoimmune diseases.

- Yoga: A recent clinical trial showed yoga to be superior to aerobic and strengthening exercises which were superior to an educational self-care booklet for the treatment of low back pain.[130] A sample of yoga-like postures and low-back exercises is provided on the following page.

---

gastrointestinal symptoms." Chrubasik S, Junck H, Breitschwerdt H, Conradt C, Zappe H. Effectiveness of Harpagophytum extract WS 1531 in the treatment of exacerbation of low back pain: a randomized, placebo-controlled, double-blind study. *Eur J Anaesthesiol* 1999 Feb;16(2):118-29

[120] "They took an 8-week course of Doloteffin at a dose providing 60 mg harpagoside per day... Doloteffin is well worth considering for osteoarthritic knee and hip pain and nonspecific low back pain." Chrubasik S, Thanner J, Kunzel O, Conradt C, Black A, Pollak S. Comparison of outcome measures during treatment with the proprietary Harpagophytum extract doloteffin in patients with pain in the lower back, knee or hip. *Phytomedicine* 2002 Apr;9(3):181-94

[121] Chrubasik S, Eisenberg E, Balan E, Weinberger T, Luzzati R, Conradt C. Treatment of low back pain exacerbations with willow bark extract: a randomized double-blind study. *Am J Med.* 2000;109:9-14

[122] Chrubasik S, Kunzel O, Model A, Conradt C, Black A. Treatment of low back pain with a herbal or synthetic anti-rheumatic: a randomized controlled study. Willow bark extract for low back pain. *Rheumatology* (Oxford). 2001;40:1388-93

[123] Hare LG, Woodside JV, Young IS. Dietary salicylates. *J Clin Pathol* 2003 Sep;56(9):649-50 http://jcp.bmj.com/cgi/content/full/56/9/649

[124] **Vasquez A, Muanza DN. Evaluation of Presence of Aspirin-Related Warnings with Willow Bark: Comment on the Article by Clauson et al. *Ann Pharmacotherapy* 2005 Oct;39:1763**

[125] Clauson KA, Santamarina ML, Buettner CM, Cauffield JS. Evaluation of Presence of Aspirin-Related Warnings with Willow Bark (July/August). *Ann Pharmacother* 2005;39(7-8):1234-7

[126] Kaufman W. Niacinamide therapy for joint mobility. Therapeutic reversal of a common clinical manifestation of the "normal" aging process. *Conn State Med J* 1953;17:584-591

[127] Jonas WB, Rapoza CP, Blair WF. The effect of niacinamide on osteoarthritis: a pilot study. *Inflamm Res* 1996 Jul;45(7):330-4

[128] Piscoya J, Rodriguez Z, Bustamante SA, Okuhama NN, Miller MJ, Sandoval M. Efficacy and safety of freeze-dried cat's claw in osteoarthritis of the knee: mechanisms of action of the species Uncaria guianensis. *Inflamm Res.* 2001 Sep;50(9):442-8

[129] "Vitamin E administration at a dose of 100 mg daily for three weeks resulted in a significant increase in serum vitamin E level accompanied by complete relief of pain... The results therefore strongly indicate that vitamin E is effective in curing spondylosis and most probably due to its antioxidant activity." Mahmud Z, Ali SM. Role of vitamin A and E in spondylosis. *Bangladesh Med Res Counc Bull.* 1992 Apr;18(1):47-59

[130] "CONCLUSIONS: Yoga was more effective than a self-care book for improving function and reducing chronic low back pain, and the benefits persisted for at least several months." Sherman KJ, Cherkin DC, Erro J, Miglioretti DL, Deyo RA. Comparing yoga, exercise, and a self-care book for chronic low back pain: a randomized, controlled trial. *Ann Intern Med.* 2005 Dec 20;143(12):849-56 http://www.annals.org/cgi/reprint/143/12/849.pdf

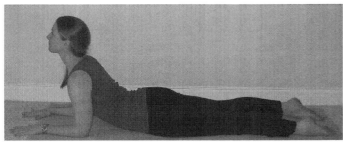

Prone Extension on Elbows: The purpose of this posture is to bring the spine into extension and begin stretching the psoas by virtue of lumbar and hip extension. Intradiscal pressure is reduced by 50% relative to standing intradiscal pressure (0.50 MPa) but remains positive at 0.25 MPa; i.e., intradiscal pressure does not become negative.[131] This posture is best suited for patients with disc injuries and is relatively contraindicated for patients with facet irritation and either central or lateral stenosis. This is an early phase of the extension/McKenzie protocol.[132] Except perhaps for passive traction, no postures or positions result in negative intradiscal pressure[133]; however, full spinal extension with the upper body supported (shown right) has not been measured and may result in reduced and perhaps negative pressure due to facet loading and mechanical leverage.

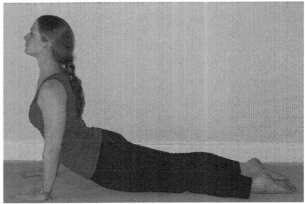

Full Extension on Elbows (press up; upward facing dog): A more advanced form of the previous exercise, with greater traction and a deeper stretch of the psoas and iliacus via lumbopelvic and hip extension. Patients can raise and lower for sets of 10+ repetitions; repetition also helps 'pump' and rehydrate the disc, as does any oscillating and noncompressive motion. Exacerbation of pain should be avoided; sciatic patients who centralize with this or other postures have improved prognosis over patients who do not centralize.[134]

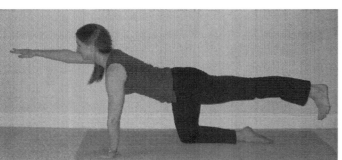

Hip Extensions: Starting from a position on hands and knees, the hip and knee of one leg are extended directly posteriorly. This exercise strengthens and conditions the low back erectors, glutei, and hamstrings while also providing a gentle undulating motion in the lumbar spine. Repeated for 20-50 repetitions on one side before switching to the opposite side. More advanced patients can use variations such as: ❶ holding the leg in the air for 5-10 seconds before lowering, ❷ raising the opposite arm with each repetition (above), ❸ alternately directing the lower extremity medially, then posteriorly, then laterally; using combinations of all three directions to stress different muscle fibers and increase proprioceptive feedback and variation, ❹ bringing the knee of the active leg more anterior during repetitions to accentuate lumbar flexion, which increases hydrodynamic oscillations in the disc to facilitate nutrition.

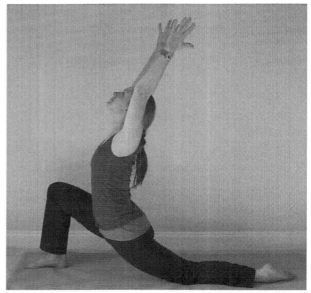

Lunge with Extension: This is a deeper version of the yoga posture Warrior 1 and is an excellent stretch for the hip flexors, particularly the iliopsoas.

---

[131] Wilke HJ, Neef P, Caimi M, Hoogland T, Claes LE. New in vivo measurements of pressures in the intervertebral disc in daily life. *Spine*. 1999 Apr 15;24(8):755-62

[132] Kuritzky L, White J. Extend Yourself for Low-Back Pain Relief. *Physician and Sportsmedicine* 1997, January http://www.physsportsmed.com/issues/1997/01jan/back_pa.htm

[133] Rohlmannt A, Claes LE, Bergmannt G, Graichen F, Neef P, Wilke HJ. Comparison of intradiscal pressures and spinal fixator loads for different body positions and exercises. *Ergonomics*.2001;44:781-94

[134] Skytte L, May S, Petersen P. Centralization: its prognostic value in patients with referred symptoms and sciatica. *Spine*. 2005 Jun 1;30(11):E293-9

Lumbar Spine: Side-Posture Segmental Rotation (Lumbar "Push-Pull")

Patient position:
- Lateral recumbent (side-posture) with no/minimal lateral flexion and minimal thoracic rotation; upper leg is flexed at hip and knee, with foot placed/locked behind the calf that is on the table; the patient grasps his/her own forearms and maintains modest tension to provide anchoring for the doctor's caudad arm, which is placed under the patient's superior arm; the lower leg is straight

Doctor position:
- Doctor is facing the table standing on the cephalad leg while the caudad leg is flexed at the hip and knee and placed atop the patient's flexed upper leg to provide leverage at the time of thrust
- Regarding the doctor's cephalad arm, the humerus is directed toward the patient's shoulder, and the elbow is bent allowing the forearm to push into the sulcus formed by the pectoralis major and deltoid; doctors forearm emerges under patient's elbow, so that fingertips are on the superior/lateral aspect of the lumbar spinous process of the superior vertebra of the targeted motion segment.
- Regarding the doctor's caudad arm, the elbow is flexed and the forearm is placed along the posterior aspect of the patient's superior ilium; fingers hook the inferior/lateral aspect of the lumbar spinous process of the inferior vertebra of the targeted motion segment

Assessment:
- <u>Subjective</u>: asymptomatic or lumbar pain, which may not be at the affected segment
- <u>Motion palpation</u>: rotational restriction
- <u>Static palpation</u>: may have rotational malposition
- <u>Soft tissue</u>: may have muscle spasm at nearby area of hypermobility

Treatment contact:
- The doctor's cephalad contacts are at the patient's deltopectoral sulcus and directly on the superior/lateral aspect of the lumbar spinous process of the superior vertebra of the motion segment
- Three caudad contacts: 1) doctor's fingertips pull directly on the inferior/lateral aspect of the lumbar spinous process of the inferior vertebra of the targeted motion segment; 2) doctor's forearm on patient's ilium; 3) doctors caudad lower leg is atop patient's flexed leg. All contacts are active

Pretreatment positioning:
- Rotational tension is applied and focused at the lumbar spinal segment being treated
- Thoracic rotation and lateral flexion are minimized to the extent possible
- Modest lumbar lateral flexion toward the table helps to gap the inferior articular process of the superior segment from the superior articular process of the inferior segment

Therapeutic action:
- 1) Doctor's cephalad elbow thrusts toward patient's shoulder to create simultaneous rotation and long-axis traction; 2) cephalad fingertips push toward the ground while atop the superior/lateral aspect of the lumbar spinous process of the superior vertebra of the targeted motion segment; 3) doctor's caudad fingertips hook and pull the inferior vertebra; 4) forearm pushes patient's ilium into rotation; 5) extension "kick" of doctor's knee quickly creates rotational force. All five actions must occur simultaneously

Image:

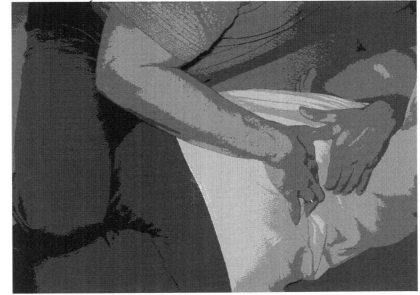

	Lumbar Side-Posture Rotational Manipulation/Mobilization, "Lumbar Roll"

Patient position:	• Side-posture, lateral recumbent; lower leg is straight; upper leg is flexed at hip and knee with foot behind calf of the leg that is straight on the table
Doctor position:	• Facing table at 45° angle in fencer stance with feet apart and knees bent • Notice in the photograph how Dr Harris approximates his center of gravity and biomechanical leverage directly over his therapeutic contact
Assessment:	• <u>Subjective</u>: asymptomatic or with lumbar pain; lumbar disc herniation[135], use a cautious and gentle technique if the patient has radicular symptoms, and as a rule of thumb the patient should be positioned with the symptomatic leg down on the table (e.g., "good leg *up*, bad leg *down*")[136] • <u>Motion palpation</u>: focal restrictions with focal pain are perhaps better treated with a lesion-specific technique such as the "push-pull" maneuver; this is an excellent technique if the patient has general discomfort without localization, or has pain and will benefit from rotational manipulation for its muscle stretching and afferent-stimulating analgesic benefits • <u>Static palpation</u>: minor displacements and malpositions may be noted; if specific biomechanical lesions are found, use a more specific technique such as the "push-pull" maneuver • <u>Soft tissue</u>: palpate for hypertonicity/spasm with or without relative muscle atrophy; patients with chronic low back pain tend to have weaker extensor muscles than the general population; however, during an acutely painful episode, their otherwise weakened muscles will be hypertonic thus leading to a paradoxical combination of atrophy and spasm—atrophic hypertonicity
Treatment contact:	• Doctor uses a palmar/calcaneal contact over the lumbar facet joints • Rotation and traction are provided at the time of impulse with the doctor's thigh which is compressed and providing long-axis traction against the patient's upper leg, which is flexed at the hip and knee
Support:	• Doctor's cephalad hand applies rotational resistance to patient's shoulder as shown
Pretreatment positioning:	• Premanipulative tension is attained and maintained prior to **body drop thrust** • The premanipulative tension and the therapeutic impulse are established and delivered through the contact hand and the doctor's caudad leg which has compressive contact with the patient's flexed leg
Therapeutic action:	• Drop thrust impulse with rotational emphasis • Notice how Dr Harris has the forearm of his contact hand perpendicular to the patient's coronal plane to direct his impulse in a posterior-to-anterior direction
Image:	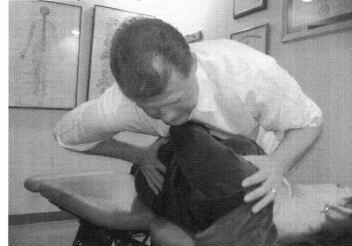

---

[135] Quon JA, Cassidy JD, O'Connor SM, Kirkaldy-Willis WH. Lumbar intervertebral disc herniation: treatment by rotational manipulation. *J Manipulative Physiol Ther*. 1989 Jun;12(3):220-7
[136] Brier S. <u>Primary Care Orthopedics</u>. St. Louis: Mosby, 1999 page 257

Lumbar Intervertebral Disc Herniations
"Slipped Disc"
Sciatica: Lumbar Radiculitis and Lumbar Radiculopathy

<u>Description/pathophysiology</u>:

- <u>Lumbar disc herniation</u>: Acute injuries and/or degenerative changes affecting the intervertebral disc predisposes to protrusion or extrusion of the nucleus pulposus and/or diametric enlargement of the annulus fibrosis, thus resulting in inflammatory and/or compressive effects on nearby structures, such as nerve roots and/or the cauda equina. The primary mechanisms of injury are: 1) loading of the spine while in the flexed position (i.e., bending over at the waist to lift a heavy object), and 2) degenerative failure of the annulus. Conservative management is appropriate for patients without severe pain and those without severe

> **Acute disc herniations are unsettling and painful, but they largely self-resolve over time**
> "A high proportion of intervertebral disc herniations have the potential to resolve spontaneously."
>
> Bush K, Cowan N, Katz DE, Gishen P. The natural history of sciatica associated with disc pathology. *Spine* 1992 Oct;17(10):1205-12

  or progressive neurologic deficits, as the condition tends to remit both in terms of clinical manifestations and radiologic abnormalities.[137] Approximately 35% of asymptomatic people have CT/MRI evidence of disc protrusions or mild herniations, and the vast majority of lumbar disc herniations occur at L4-L5 or L5-S1 and thus affects the L5 or S1 nerve roots, respectively. Three types of disc injury that can be considered subtypes of disc herniation are: ❶ disc bulge: circumferential symmetric enlargement of the disc, may result in nerve root irritation or compression especially when combined with another compressive lesion such as degenerative facet hypertrophy or congenital spinal stenosis, ❷ disc protrusion: focal lesion of the annulus fibrosis resulting in a wide-based area of the disc protruding from the normal circumference, and ❸ disc extrusion: "the base against the parent disk is narrower than the diameter of the extruded material itself, or there is no connection with the parent disk."[138] Officially recognized terminology and classification for lumbar disc pathology are updated periodically and are available on the internet.[139]
- <u>Lumbar radiculitis</u>: Inflammation of or near the nerve root that results in *dermatomal* **sensory changes**. Causes include local inflammation due to injury to the intervertebral disc, infections (e.g., herpes zoster) and others.
  - Here I use the term "**radiculitis**" to indicate **inflammation-induced or "irritative" changes** that result in sensory changes without motor disturbances. I use the term "**radiculopathy**" to denote primarily **compressive mechanisms of injury** that result in *both* sensory and motor changes. This conceptualization of "biochemical" vs. "compressive" and thus "sensory changes only" vs. "sensory changes and motor deficits" has support from the research literature.[140,141] Many articles and texts do not distinguish radiculitis from radiculopathy; however, I find the differentiation both conceptually and clinically valuable.
- <u>Lumbar radiculopathy</u>: Compression of the nerve root that results in *dermatomal* **sensory** changes as well as **deficits in muscle strength**. Causes include 1) protrusion or extrusion of the nucleus pulposus and/or extension of the annulus fibrosis in the posterolateral direction toward the nerve root, 2) foraminal encroachment, and 3) pathology, such as space-occupying lesion (SOL) due to infection or metastasis.

<u>Complications</u>:

- Nerve compression with resultant loss of neuromuscular function
- Pain, numbness, tingling

---

[137] Bush K, Cowan N, Katz DE, Gishen P. The natural history of sciatica associated with disc pathology. *Spine* 1992 Oct;17(10):1205-12
[138] Milette PC. The proper terminology for reporting lumbar intervertebral disk disorders.
AJNR Am J Neuroradiol. 1997 Nov-Dec;18(10):1859-66 http://www.ajnr.org/cgi/reprint/18/10/1859 and http://www.theassr.org/pdf/nomenclature.pdf
[139] American Society of Neuroradiology, American Society of Spine Radiology
and North American Spine Society. "Nomenclature and Classification of Lumbar Disc Pathology" http://www.asnr.org/spine_nomenclature/glossary.shtml Accessed January 2007
[140] Quon JA, Cassidy JD, O'Connor SM, Kirkaldy-Willis WH. Lumbar intervertebral disc herniation: treatment by rotational manipulation. *J Manipulative Physiol Ther* 1989 Jun;12(3):220-7
[141] Souza TA. <u>Differential Diagnosis for the Chiropractor: Protocols and Algorithms</u>. Gaithersburg: Aspen Publications. 1997 page 130

Clinical presentations:

- Acute or subacute onset of pain
- Sensory changes: Numbness, tingling, paresthesias
- Motor lesions: flaccid weakness with hyporeflexia
- Pain in the back, buttocks, thigh, leg, foot: Pain that extends beyond the knee is more likely to be radiculitis/radiculopathy than is pain that stays regional to the buttocks and thigh; such regional pain is commonly due to referred pain from joint irritation of the lumbar facets or sacroiliac joints or due to myofascial trigger points
- Often exacerbated with coughing, straining, or sneezing: Coughing, straining, and sneezing all result in increased intrathecal pressure which specifically amplifies pain due to an intrathecal lesion (e.g., cauda equina tumor) or pain due to compression of the thecal sac (e.g., disc herniation, epidural abscess)
- Paraspinal muscle spasm
- Risk factors: lifting heavy objects, cigarette smokers, use of vibrating equipment such as jackhammers, occupational drivers, sedentary lifestyle, obesity
- Classic presentation: patient age 30-50 years with a history of chronic/recurrent low back pain notices an exacerbation of low back pain or the onset of leg pain associated with a bending and/or twisting motion; leg pain typically predominates over the severity of the low back pain in patients with acute disc herniation

Major differential diagnoses:

- Infection
- Malignancy
- Fracture
- Rheumatic disease such as reactive arthritis or ankylosing spondylitis (see *Integrative Rheumatology*[142])
- Abdominal disease such as pancreatitis, pancreatic cancer, renal infection, renal colic
- Neurologic lesions including cauda equina syndrome
- Musculoskeletal lesions such as myofascial trigger points, disc herniation, facet/joint irritation

Clinical assessment:

- History: remarkable or unremarkable, generally positive for low back pain exacerbated by heavy lifting or combination of bending and twisting
- Physical examination: *see clinical assessments*

---

[142] Vasquez A. *Integrative Rheumatology*. Fort Worth, Texas; Integrative and Biological Medicine Research and Consulting, 2006: http://OptimalHealthResearch.com

Differential Assessment of Low back Pain and Leg Pain

	Disc herniation causing nerve compression	Facet irritation, SIJ dysfunction, MFTP in lumbar-buttock region
Pain pattern	• Dermatomal	• Non-dermatomal, regional
Radiation	• Often buttocks, thigh, leg, and foot • 50% of patients with lumbar spinal stenosis have radiating pain below the knee[143]	• Buttocks and thigh, rarely lower leg with SIJ[144] or myofascial lesions[145]; *pain generally does not extend to foot unless the lesion is radicular*
Weakness	• Probable—related to nerve root compression; sensory/motor deficits correlate with specific level of nerve root compression	• No neurologic weakness; weakness if any is due to pain
Reflexes	• May be diminished	• Normal
History	• Acute or chronic onset	• Acute or chronic onset
Assessment	• SLR is almost always abnormal • Positive nerve tension tests • May have positive Kemp's test • Myofascial provocation is not specific and does not reproduce presenting symptomatology	• SLR almost always normal • Normal nerve tension tests • Should have positive Kemp's test with facet irritation • Myofascial provocation is positive with MFTP • Sacroiliac provocation tests and/or pelvic manipulation are positive with SIJ dysfunction

Imaging & laboratory assessments:
- **Lab**: Should be normal; any laboratory abnormality requires investigation; recommended screening tests for *disease exclusion* and *holistic health assessment* include
  - **Chemistry/metabolic panel**:
  - **CBC**: Screen for infection
  - **CRP**: Screen for infection or inflammation
  - **ESR**: May be more reliable than CRP for multiple myeloma[146]
  - **Serum 25-hydroxy-vitamin (25-OH-D)**: The currently recommended standard of care includes testing low back pain patients for vitamin D deficiency; in patients with vitamin D deficiency supplementation with 5,000 – 10,000 IU/d for adults was shown to alleviate low back pain in nearly all patients after 3 months.[147] In the absence of laboratory confirmation, properly selected adult patients should be treated with vitamin D3 supplementation at 2,000-4,000 IU/d; this is safe and reasonable empiric treatment for low back pain and correction of vitamin D deficiency.[148]

[143] Tierney ML. McPhee SJ, Papadakis MA (eds). Current Medical Diagnosis and Treatment 2006, 45th Edition. Lange Medical; page 820
[144] Hendler N, Kozikowski JG, Morrison C, Sethuraman G. Diagnosis and management of sacroiliac joint disease. *JNMS: Journal of the Neuromuscuuloskeletal System* 1995; 3: 169-74
[145] Jenner JR, Barry M. ABC of rheumatology. Low back pain. *BMJ* 1995 Apr 8;310(6984):929-32
[146] "We conclude that ESR, a simple and easily performed marker, was found to be an independent prognostic factor for survival in patients with multiple myeloma." Alexandrakis MG, Passam FH, Ganotakis ES, Sfiridaki K, Xilouri I, Perisinakis K, Kyriakou DS. The clinical and prognostic significance of erythrocyte sedimentation rate (ESR), serum interleukin-6 (IL-6) and acute phase protein levels in multiple myeloma. *Clin Lab Haematol.* 2003 Feb;25(1):41-6
[147] Al Faraj S, Al Mutairi K. Vitamin D deficiency and chronic low back pain in Saudi Arabia. *Spine.* 2003 Jan 15;28(2):177-9
[148] Vasquez A, Manso G, Cannell J. The Clinical Importance of Vitamin D (Cholecalciferol): A Paradigm Shift with Implications for All Healthcare Providers. *Alternative Therapies in Health and Medicine* and *Integrative Medicine: A Clinician's Journal* www.optimalhealthresearch.com/monograph04

- o Additional tests: Also consider testing thyroid, cholesterol/lipids, and ferritin; if inflammatory arthropathy is confirmed, perform stool testing for gastrointestinal dysbiosis and implement management protocols detailed in *Integrative Rheumatology*[149]
- Radiographs: May show degeneration and loss of disc height; excellent initial evaluation, especially for the exclusion of fracture and gross bone lesions
- CT: Good for imaging disc herniation
- MRI: Allows for visualization of neural as well as soft-tissue musculoskeletal elements

Clinical management:

- **Lumbar disc protrusion/herniation**: Monitor for complications such as radiculopathy and cauda equina syndrome. Provide good nutrition, massage, manipulation (as appropriate), ergonomic improvements, and other treatments as indicated and as outlined previously in this chapter and reviewed in Chapter 3. The major problems/complications arise from 1) neurologic compromise, and 2) unremitting severe pain. Many asymptomatic people have MRI evidence of disc protrusion; once the acute inflammation has subsided the pain will greatly diminish and the disc will typically show a trend toward regression back to normal size. Although spinal manipulation is often of significant benefit to patients with nerve root compression due to disc herniation, both the doctor and the patient need to be aware that spinal manipulation may exacerbate injury to the disc. Spinal manipulation for the treatment of patients with disc herniation should be performed only by experienced doctors trained in manipulation and only after obtaining informed consent from the patient.
- **Lumbar radiculitis (dermatomal sensory changes only):** Comprehensive musculoskeletal care (Chapter 3 and previous) is appropriate: prevent further injury, limit activities, reduce inflammation, reduce muscle spasm, relieve pain, manipulation (as appropriate), etc.
- **Cauda equina syndrome: immediate referral to orthopedist, neurosurgeon, or emergency room**
- **Lumbar radiculopathy (sensory and motor deficits):** Comprehensive musculoskeletal care (Chapter 3 and previous) is appropriate for the vast majority of cases. Referral if clinical outcome is unsatisfactory or if serious complications such as *persistent* or *progressive* motor deficits become evident.
- Severe pain and/or motor deficits indicate the need for patient education, PAR discussion (see Chapter 1), and **informed consent** for patients who *choose* conservative/non-surgical management. An aggressive course of comprehensive therapy may be undertaken if *both* **doctor** *and* **patient** are willing; however the physician must realize the great significance of motor deficits and must refer the patient for neurosurgical evaluation if the deficits do not improve quickly and/or if they worsen. To be on the safe side, Gatterman et al[150] advised, "Sensory and motor deficits with asymmetric reflexes should be referred for a neurological evaluation." In one study of discogenic sciatica, 95% of patients with "neurologic signs" made partial or complete recovery: "The presence of neurologic signs was certainly not an absolute indication for surgery... Only a small portion of patients needed surgical decompression."[151] Moderate-severe motor deficits indicate the need for neurosurgical referral. Re-evaluate symptoms and neurologic function before and after each treatment.

---

[149] Vasquez A. *Integrative Rheumatology*. Fort Worth, Texas; Integrative and Biological Medicine Research and Consulting, 2006: http://OptimalHealthResearch.com
[150] Chapter 10 in Gatterman MI (Ed.). Chiropractic Management of Spine-Related Disorders. Baltimore; Williams and Wilkins, 1990.
[151] Bush K, Cowan N, Katz DE, Gishen P. The natural history of sciatica associated with disc pathology. A prospective study with clinical and independent radiologic follow-up. *Spine* 1992;17(10):1205-12

Lumbar radiculopathy with <u>severe pain</u> and/or <u>motor deficits</u>: managing the risk-benefit ratio for both doctor and patient
A wise strategy for both the treating doctor and the patient who has significant radiculopathy is for the holistic physician to refer the patient to a neurosurgeon/orthopedist for evaluation and consultation. This allows for ❶ physician-physician communication, and ❷ complete patient education, thus allowing for the patient to ❸ <u>give informed consent</u> based on the risks and benefits of conservative treatment versus surgical treatment. This referral also demonstrates that ❹ <u>the conservative physician was aware of the potential complications</u> of unsuccessful treatment and that ❺ <u>the doctor acted in the best interest of the patient</u> by providing an appropriate and timely referral.

<u>Treatment considerations</u>:

- <u>Limit strenuous/damaging activities</u>
- <u>Manipulation/mobilization</u>: Gentle thrust with premanipulative positioning is advised.
  - "Present knowledge indicates that the risk-benefit factors are such that spinal manipulation that is not too vigorous is a justified, alternative, nonsurgical, treatment for low back pain and sciatica."[152]
  - The disc-protective and rotation-limiting benefits provided by the facet joints are realized only when the spine is in the extended position, and the rotational amplitude of the manipulative thrust must be strictly controlled by the physician[153]
- <u>Proprioceptive retraining</u>
- <u>Muscle strengthening</u> for the low back and abdominal muscles
- <u>Anti-inflammatory diet, nutritional supplementation, and botanical medicines</u>: Supplemented Paleo-Mediterranean diet, supplemental emphasis on proteolytic enzymes[154], *Harpagophytum*[155,156,157] and willow bark[158,159]
- <u>Intravenous colchicine</u>: See previous discussion in this chapter and the article by Rask[160]
- <u>Allopathic/medical treatments include</u>: Anti-inflammatory drugs, prescription analgesics (e.g., narcotics and opioids), epidural injections of analgesics, corticosteroid injections, decompressive surgery

[152] Quon JA, Cassidy JD, O'Connor SM, Kirkaldy-Willis WH. Lumbar intervertebral disc herniation: treatment by rotational manipulation. *J Manipulative Physiol Ther* 1989 Jun;12(3):220-7

[153] Souza TA. <u>Differential Diagnosis for the Chiropractor: Protocols and Algorithms</u>. Gaithersburg: Aspen Publications. 1997 page 108, 130

[154] Trickett P. Proteolytic enzymes in treatment of athletic injuries. *Appl Ther*. 1964;30:647-52

[155] Chrubasik S, Model A, Black A, Pollak S. A randomized double-blind pilot study comparing Doloteffin and Vioxx in the treatment of low back pain. *Rheumatology* (Oxford). 2003 Jan;42(1):141-8

[156] "The majority of responders' were patients who had suffered less than 42 days of pain, and subgroup analyses suggested that the effect was confined to patients with more severe and radiating pain accompanied by neurological deficit... There was no evidence for Harpagophytum-related side-effects, except possibly for mild and infrequent gastrointestinal symptoms." Chrubasik S, Junck H, Breitschwerdt H, Conradt C, Zappe H. Effectiveness of Harpagophytum extract WS 1531 in the treatment of exacerbation of low back pain: a randomized, placebo-controlled, double-blind study. *Eur J Anaesthesiol* 1999 Feb;16(2):118-29

[157] "They took an 8-week course of Doloteffin at a dose providing 60 mg harpagoside per day... Doloteffin is well worth considering for osteoarthritic knee and hip pain and nonspecific low back pain." Chrubasik S, Thanner J, Kunzel O, Conradt C, Black A, Pollak S. Comparison of outcome measures during treatment with the proprietary Harpagophytum extract doloteffin in patients with pain in the lower back, knee or hip. *Phytomedicine* 2002 Apr;9(3):181-94

[158] Chrubasik S, Eisenberg E, Balan E, Weinberger T, Luzzati R, Conradt C. Treatment of low back pain exacerbations with willow bark extract: a randomized double-blind study. *Am J Med*. 2000;109:9-14

[159] Chrubasik S, Kunzel O, Model A, Conradt C, Black A. Treatment of low back pain with a herbal or synthetic anti-rheumatic: a randomized controlled study. Willow bark extract for low back pain. *Rheumatology* (Oxford). 2001;40:1388-93

[160] Rask MR. Colchicine use in 6,000 patients with disk disease and other related resistantly-painful spinal disorders. *Journal of Neurological and Orthopaedic Medicine and Surgery* 1989; 10: 291-298 Contact Information: The American Academy of Neurological and Orthopaedic Surgeons; 10 Cascade Creek Lane. Las Vegas, NV 89113 phone: (702) 388-7390 fax: (702) 388-7395 aanos@aanos.org

Lumbar (Central) Spinal Stenosis
Lateral Recess Stenosis/Syndrome

<u>Description/pathophysiology</u>:

- <u>Lumbar (Central) Spinal Stenosis</u>: Narrowing of the central spinal canal due to one or more factors, including ❶ congenital stenosis, which may be present in persons of normal stature, but is particularly common in achondroplastic patients, ❷ anterior compression: disc bulge/herniation, ❸ posterior compression: facet hypertrophy due to degenerative enlargement of the facet joints; hypertrophy of the ligamentum flavum. Nerves may be compressed directly or the arterial supply to the nerves may be compressed; in either case the nerves are injured and cause pain and loss of function, which manifests as numbness and motor deficits; since spinal flexion increases the diameter of the spinal canal, the neurogenic pain and the neurologic deficits are often transient, dependent on spinal positioning, and absent during the neurologic exam, especially if the patient is seated. The observation that injected epidural corticosteroids can provide some relief of pain for ≤50% of patients[161] suggests that the pathophysiology involves an inflammatory mechanism—one that might be favorably influenced with the dietary, nutritional, and botanical interventions outlined previously and reviewed in Chapter 3
- <u>Lateral Recess Stenosis</u>: Narrowing of the intervertebral foramen (IVF) leading to intermittent nerve compression. Ciric et al[162] wrote that the diagnosis could be made radiographically by finding an IVF height of less than 2 mm in height, and that a lateral recess height of 5 mm or more "rules out the possibility of a lateral recess stenosis"; a more recent study by Strojnik[163] used CT imaging with surgical confirmation and found that "A CT scan height of 3.6 mm or less is also indicative of stenosis."

<u>Complications</u>:

- Pain and neuromuscular compromise; increased risk for cauda equina syndrome

<u>Clinical presentations</u>:

- Generally older patient, though may be present in younger patients especially with a combination of disc degeneration and congenital stenosis[164]
- Diffuse pain, classically exacerbated by extension and standing/walking and relieved by flexion
- Leg pain may be unilateral or bilateral and is often referred to as "neurogenic claudication" in contrast to the leg pain due to arterial insufficiency—vascular claudication
- Exertional pain (neurogenic claudication) is often relieved with 15 minutes rest or lumbar flexion

<u>Major differential diagnoses</u>:

- <u>Piriformis syndrome</u>
- <u>Vascular claudication</u>: Check for diminished foot/ankle pulses; distal pain *in the calves* worse with exertion, relieved with rest; although vascular claudication typically affects the calves, vascular insufficiency to the gluteus will result in proximal pain in the buttock-hip region exacerbated with the exertion of walking uphill or climbing stairs
- <u>Pathologic nerve compression</u>: Cauda equina syndrome, or compression due to infection or metastasis
- <u>Peripheral neuropathy</u>: Vitamin B-12 deficiency (test serum methylmalonic acid or begin oral vitamin B-12 at 2,000-4,000 mcg per day for a 3-month therapeutic trial), diabetes mellitus, toxic metal or xenobiotic exposure, Guillain-Barre syndrome, and others

---

[161] Tierney ML. McPhee SJ, Papadakis MA (eds). <u>Current Medical Diagnosis and Treatment 2006, 45th Edition</u>. Lange Medical; page 820

[162] "The diagnosis is assured when the lateral recess measures less than 2 mm in height. A lateral recess of 5 mm or more rules out the possibility of a lateral recess stenosis." Ciric I, Mikhael MA, Tarkington JA, Vick NA. The lateral recess syndrome. A variant of spinal stenosis. *J Neurosurg.* 1980 Oct;53(4):433-43

[163] "A CT scan height of 3.6 mm or less is also indicative of stenosis." Strojnik T. Measurement of the lateral recess angle as a possible alternative for evaluation of the lateral recess stenosis on a CT scan. *Wien Klin Wochenschr.* 2001;113 Suppl 3:53-8

[164] Epstein NE, Epstein JA, Carras R, Murthy VS, Hyman RA. Coexisting cervical and lumbar spinal stenosis: diagnosis and management. *Neurosurgery 1984;15(4):489-96*

Clinical assessment:

- <u>History</u>: Aching, numbness, and transient neurologic deficits in the lower extremities; often bilateral. In contrast to vascular claudication in which the pain is classically localized distally to the calves, the ache and numbness of lumbar neuroclaudication is generally localized proximally in the buttocks and thighs. After prolonged walking or standing (both of which generally result in spinal extension which exacerbates stenosis), loss of coordination may become manifest, resulting in unsteady gait, leg weakness, imbalance and what might be described as "spaghetti legs" or "drunken sailor gait"[165]—obviously, these symptoms would need to be differentiated from cerebellar lesions and lesions of the peripheral nerves and dorsal columns

- <u>Physical examination</u>: *See clinical assessments detailed previously in this chapter*
  - o Kemp's test and spinal extension exacerbate symptoms in lateral and central stenosis, respectively; in patients with peripheral vascular claudication, movement of the spine should have no effect on leg symptoms
  - o Ankle pulses should be normal in patients with neurogenic claudication, and this is a major finding to distinguish neurogenic from vascular claudication (in addition to the *proximal* rather than *distal* location of the pain)
  - o Findings on the neurologic exam may be completely normal, especially if the patient is seated (i.e., spine in flexion) during the exam; symptoms and neurologic deficits may be provoked by performing the neurologic exam after the patient has been positioned either prone or supine with lumbar hyperextension

Imaging & laboratory assessments:

- <u>Lab tests</u> : To exclude organic disease; perform screening lab tests as previously outlined
- <u>Radiographs</u>: Lateral lumbar radiographs demonstrate decreased distance between posterior aspect of vertebral body and/or disc and the spinolaminar junction; 12 mm or less is considered evidence of stenosis. Improved techniques have made **MRI** the best imaging assessment for **central stenosis** due to either bone or soft tissues; whereas **CT imaging with contrast myelography** appears best for **lateral recess stenosis**[166]

Clinical management/ treatment:

- <u>Dietary and phytonutraceutical anti-inflammation</u>: Dietary modification with phytonutraceutical interventions as discussed previously and in Chapter 3
- <u>Manipulative treatment</u>: Carefully applied spinal manipulation can be effective in the treatment of **lateral stenosis**[167] but **practitioners should refrain from using rotational manipulation in patients with central spinal stenosis**—especially achrondroplastic patients.[168] **Flexion-distraction technique** has been used successfully in patients with severe back and leg symptoms due to spinal stenosis.[169,170] A study completed in 2006 by Murphy et al[171] showed remarkable safety and high efficacy of **flexion-distraction mobilization**, neural mobilization, and low back exercises for patients with lumbar spinal stenosis; access the full-text at http://www.biomedcentral.com/1471-2474/7/16
- <u>Epidural corticosteroid injection</u>: Provides quick *partial* relief in 50% of patients and lasting relief in 25% of patients[172]
- <u>Neurosurgical referral</u>: For severe/progressive neurologic deficits or pain; surgical benefits may only last for short duration in 80% of patients[173]

---

[165] Tierney ML. McPhee SJ, Papadakis MA (eds). <u>Current Medical Diagnosis and Treatment 2006, 45th Edition</u>. Lange Medical; page 820
[166] Bartynski WS, Lin L. Lumbar root compression in the lateral recess: MR imaging, conventional myelography, and CT myelography comparison with surgical confirmation. *AJNR Am J Neuroradiol*. 2003 Mar;24(3):348-60 http://www.ajnr.org/cgi/content/full/24/3/348
[167] "The Lateral Recess Syndrome (LRS) represents stenosis of the lateral subarticular gutter that will often lead to nerve root compression... Recent studies indicate that spinal manipulation can provide relief and should be considered before surgical referral is made for decompression." Ben-Eliyahu DJ, Rutili MM, Przybysz JA. Lateral recess syndrome: diagnosis and chiropractic management. *J Manipulative Physiol Ther*. 1983 Mar;6(1):25-31
[168] Haldeman S, Rubinstein SM. Cauda equina syndrome in patients undergoing manipulation of the lumbar spine. *Spine* 1992 Dec;17(12):1469-73
[169] "Flexion-distraction manipulation of the lumbar spine was performed... He experienced a decrease in the frequency and intensity of his leg symptoms and a resolution of his low back pain. These improvements were maintained at a 5-month follow-up visit." Snow GJ. Chiropractic management of a patient with lumbar spinal stenosis. *J Manipulative Physiol Ther*. 2001 May;24(4):300-4
[170] "A 76-yr-old male with a chief complaint of low back pain and left lower extremity pain ... A diagnosis of lumbar spinal stenosis secondary to spondylosis was made. ... Twelve treatments of flexion-distraction manipulation, deep tissue massage, ultrasound, therapeutic exercise, heel lift, and modification of activities of daily living. He was discharged from care asymptomatic in 3 wk." DuPriest CM. Nonoperative management of lumbar spinal stenosis. *J Manipulative Physiol Ther*. 1993 Jul-Aug;16(6):411-4
[171] Murphy DR, Hurwitz EL, Gregory AA, Clary R. A non-surgical approach to the management of lumbar spinal stenosis: a prospective observational cohort study. *BMC Musculoskelet Disord*. 2006 Feb 23;7:16 http://www.biomedcentral.com/1471-2474/7/16
[172] Tierney ML. McPhee SJ, Papadakis MA (eds). <u>Current Medical Diagnosis and Treatment 2006, 45th Edition</u>. Lange Medical; page 820
[173] Tierney ML. McPhee SJ, Papadakis MA (eds). <u>Current Medical Diagnosis and Treatment 2006, 45th Edition</u>. Lange Medical; page 820

Cauda Equina Syndrome (CES)
Cauda Equina Compression Syndrome

> "Serious legal implications about emergency room and doctor office management of this problem exist."[174]

> "Cauda equina syndrome is an absolute indication for surgery. ...it is generally recommended that surgical decompression be executed within 6 hours after the onset of acute symptoms."[175]

Description/pathophysiology:
- Compression of the cauda equina; most commonly caused by compression from intervertebral disc herniation/protrusion, especially if accompanied by hypertrophic/degenerative osseous changes and/or congenital spinal stenosis; may also be caused by impingement due to tumor, infection or trauma[176]
- Most common levels of discogenic CES are L4-L5, L5-S1, and L3-L4.
- Long-term complications due to nerve compression are common; one study[177] reported that 56% of patients suffered permanent neurologic deficits: 28% had chronic pain and numbness; 28% had persistent incontinence and weakness. Surgery within 6-48 hours of clinical onset appears highly beneficial for the restoration and maintenance of continence.

Complications:
- Loss of neuromuscular function in regions supplied by the cauda equina: Loss of bowel/bladder control and function; numbness and loss of function in the anogenital regions: erectile dysfunction in men; loss of vaginal muscle tone and/or vaginal numbness in women[178]

Clinical presentations:
- Onset is typically acute or subacute; 76% of cases fully develop within 24 hours
- Bilateral sciatica and bilateral leg/foot weakness are seen in nearly all CES patients; 86% are unable to walk due to pain and/or weakness.
- **Importantly, a small proportion of CES patients may not have leg weakness and will have only urinary retention and perineal numbness** (saddle anesthesia)[179]
- **Urinary obstruction leading to overflow incontinence** or **fecal incontinence** is seen in 93% of patients. Since urinary incontinence has a high sensitivity (90%) for CES, the absence of urinary obstruction/incontinence suggests against the presence of CES[180]
- Risk factors include ❶ male gender, ❷ history of back pain, ❸ previous disc herniations, ❹ age > 40 years (range 22-67 years), ❺ congenital or acquired spinal stenosis

Major differential diagnoses:
- Benign low back pain
- Radiculopathy or radiculitis
- Peripheral neuropathy
- Non-neurogenic urinary incontinence

---

[174] Shapiro S. Cauda equina syndrome secondary to lumbar disc herniation. *Neurosurgery* 1993 May;32(5):743-6; discussion 746-7

[175] Quon JA, Cassidy JD, O'Connor SM, Kirkaldy-Willis WH. Lumbar intervertebral disc herniation: treatment by rotational manipulation. *J Manipulative Physiol Ther* 1989 Jun;12(3):220-7

[176] Brier S. Primary Care Orthopedics. St. Louis: Mosby, 1999 page 237

[177] Shapiro S. Cauda equina syndrome secondary to lumbar disc herniation. *Neurosurgery* 1993 May;32(5):743-6; discussion 746-7

[178] Haldeman S, Rubinstein SM. Cauda equina syndrome in patients undergoing manipulation of the lumbar spine. *Spine* 1992 Dec;17(12):1469-73

[179] Haldeman S, Rubinstein SM. Cauda equina syndrome in patients undergoing manipulation of the lumbar spine. *Spine* 1992 Dec;17(12):1469-73

[180] Souza TA. Differential Diagnosis for the Chiropractor: Protocols and Algorithms. Gaithersburg: Aspen Publications. 1997 page 108

Clinical assessment:

- <u>History</u>: Ask about radiculopathy, sciatica, bowel/bladder dysfunction, and perineal/anogenital numbness.
    1. "Do you notice any **pain, numbness, weakness or tingling** in your legs or feet?"
    2. "Have you noticed any **difficulty controlling your bowels or bladder** (incontinence), or have you had any difficulty going to the bathroom (urinary retention)?"
    3. "Have you noticed any **numbness or change in sensation near your anus or genitals**?"
- <u>Physical examination</u>: neurologic examination of lower extremities and anogenital region:
    o Bilateral sciatica (nearly 100%).
    o Bilateral leg/foot weakness (nearly 100%); 86% unable to walk due to pain and/or weakness.
    o Urine and/or fecal incontinence (93%).
    o Saddle hypesthesia or numbness.
    o **Assess reflex and strength of anal sphincter.**

Imaging & laboratory assessments:

- **Clinical evaluation followed by MRI** or surgical consult.
- Lab tests are not necessary for initially evaluating this condition and would cause an unacceptable delay in treatment.

Clinical **management**:

- Make <u>immediate</u> arrangements for patient to be transported for imaging and/or surgery
- **Obviously, if the patient has lower extremity weakness, he/she will need to be transported for imaging/surgery via ambulance, taxi, or other means.**

Treatment:

- **Surgery (laminectomy and discectomy):** Emergency surgery (within 6 hours of onset) has been generally recommended; however two relatively recent articles have shown that performing surgery for CES on an emergency basis (within 6 hours of presentation) does not improve long-term outcome compared to performing surgery on an urgent basis (within 24 hours) especially if the patient already has urinary retention and overflow incontinence.[181,182]
- Regardless of these nuances in surgical management, **the diagnosing clinician who first encounters the clinical presentation of cauda equina syndrome has an absolute obligation to treat the condition as an emergency and ensure that the patient receives imaging and/or neurosurgical consultation immediately.**[183] Speaking in more practical terms, if a doctor diagnoses cauda equina syndrome in his/her office, the appropriate action is to have the patient transported immediately by taxi or ambulance to the nearest hospital; calling 911 is reasonable and appropriate if rapid transport by other means is not available.

> **Cauda equina syndrome is a medicolegal urgency and a surgical emergency**
>
> "Cauda equina syndrome secondary to a disc herniation has resulted in numerous law suits. These are based on delay in diagnosis, failure to diagnose, and inappropriate surgical treatment."
>
> Kostuik JP. Point of View. *Spine*. 2000 Feb 1;25(3):352

---

[181] "Where urinary retention with overflow incontinence exists at presentation we believe that urgent decompression confers no benefit." Gleave JR, Macfarlane R. Cauda equina syndrome: what is the relationship between timing of surgery and outcome? *Br J Neurosurg*. 2002 Aug;16(4):325-8

[182] "No difference was found between urgently operated patients and those operated on the next available list when urological outcome and quality of life assessments were made using a validated questionnaire at a mean time of 16 months after surgery... Emergency decompressive surgery did not significantly improve outcome in CES compared with a delayed approach." Hussain SA, Gullan RW, Chitnavis BP. Cauda equina syndrome: outcome and implications for management. *Br J Neurosurg*. 2003 Apr;17(2):164-7

[183] "The data strongly support the management of cauda equina syndrome from lumbar disc herniation as a diagnostic and surgical emergency." Shapiro S. Medical realities of cauda equina syndrome secondary to lumbar disc herniation. *Spine*. 2000 Feb 1;25(3):348-51

Vertebral Osteomyelitis
Infectious Discitis

Description/pathophysiology:
- Bacterial or fungal infection of the spine
- Back pain is common; spinal infection is relatively rare. Spinal infections are "a rare cause of common symptoms."[184]

Clinical presentations:
- Classic presentation: "...the diagnosis is suggested by the clinical findings: a sick patient with severe pain, a rigid back, fever, and a raised WBC and sedimentation rate."[185]
  - o Patient generally appears sick with systemic manifestations: fatigue, sweats, anorexia, fever
  - o Back/neck/spine pain (90%): Most common region for spinal osteomyelitis is the lumbar spine, followed by the thoracic spine, then the cervical spine. Cervical spine infections are more common in IV drug abusers
  - o Pain may be acute, subacute, or chronic:
    - 30% of patients with vertebral osteomyelitis have had pain for 3 weeks to 3 months at time of diagnosis
    - 50% of patients with vertebral osteomyelitis have had pain for more than 3 months at time of diagnosis
  - o Pain is continuous, intermittent, and/or "throbbing" and often worse at night
  - o Pain is unrelated to motion or position (non-mechanical)
  - o Localized stiffness
  - o Elevated ESR/CRP
  - o Vertebral osteomyelitis is more common in patients with a history of recurrent urinary tract infections and diabetes mellitus
- Atypical presentations: as many as 15% of affected patients
  - o Little or no fever
  - o Little or no back or neck pain
  - o Little or no local tenderness
  - o Cervical osteomyelitis may present with headache, dysphagia, sore throat rather than febrile neck pain
  - o Vertebral osteomyelitis of the thoracic and lumbar spine may present with pain in the chest, shoulder, abdominal, hip or leg
  - o Risk factors: IV drug use, DM, history of septicemia, spinal trauma, pulmonary tuberculosis, urinary tract infections, surgery, older men

Major differential diagnoses:
- Benign neck or back pain
- Degenerative disc disease
- Tumor
- Fracture
- Spondyloarthropathies: In particular, reactive arthritis is a difficult differential in this situation because of the concomitant infection (perhaps with fever and systemic symptoms) and back pain. Differentiation may be difficult, but is generally possible based on the severity of the systemic manifestations and local examination findings. Patients with *focal pain*—particularly that which is exacerbated by vertebral percussion—should be further evaluated for osteomyelitis, fracture, or acute disc herniation

---

[184] Strausbaugh LJ. Vertebral osteomyelitis. How to differentiate it from other causes of back and neck pain. *Postgrad Med* 1995 Jun;97(6):147-8, 151-4
[185] Macnab I, McCulloch J. Backache. Second Edition. Williams and Wilkins: Baltimore, 1990

Clinical assessment:

- **History/subjective**:
  - Spinal pain
  - Malaise: may or may not have systemic symptoms
- **Physical examination/objective**:
  - Mild local tenderness
  - Paravertebral muscle spasm with limited ROM
  - Fever (50%)
  - Neurologic signs (20-40%)
  - Spinal percussion is positive for pain
  - May have painful and limited SLR due to hamstring spasm
- **Imaging & laboratory assessments**:
  - High ESR—elevated to 20-100 mm/hr in 90% of patients. ESR was considered "the most useful test for monitoring the disease activity and the efficacy of treatment."[186]
  - 50% have slight elevation of WBC.
  - The disc space is the first structure destroyed—the clinician and radiologist must not misinterpret early signs of infection with "degenerative disc disease."
  - **MRI has a sensitivity and specificity of >90% and also helps to assess epidural abscess.**
  - Radiographs are positive in 80% after the condition has been present for at least 10-14 days.
  - Bone scan is diagnostic in 90% of cases.
  - "Computed tomography is the imaging study of choice for preoperative evaluation and biopsy procedures. It is not a good screening test…"[187] and is generally used after routine radiographs and/or bone scan.

Establishing the diagnosis:

- Diagnosis is established based on a consistent spectrum of clinical signs and symptoms and is confirmed with imaging and/or biopsy, aspiration, and/or blood cultures

Complications:

- Abscesses
- Meningitis
- Vertebral collapse, fracture
- Neurologic injury: paralysis
- Septicemia and death

> "Up to 10-15% of patients with vertebral osteomyelitis will develop neurologic findings or frank spinal-cord compression."
>
> King RW, Johnson D. Osteomyelitis. Updated July 13, 2006. *eMedicine*
> http://www.emedicine.com/emerg/topic349.htm

Clinical management:

- Immediate/urgent referral for diagnostic procedures, IV and oral antimicrobials, and surgery if needed

Treatments:

- **Antimicrobial drugs: Organism-specific IV/oral antimicrobials are generally administered on an in-patient basis.**
- Rest: Bed rest, bracing, activity limitation
- Surgery: Surgery for debridement and complications such as cord compression, vertebral collapse or instability.
- **Immunonutrition considerations:** Immunonutritional considerations are listed below; doses listed are for adults. Although studies have not been performed specifically in patients with bone/joint infections, general benefits derived from the use of immunonutrition are reductions in severity/frequency/duration of major infections, abbreviated hospitalization (i.e., early discharge due to expedited healing and

[186] Macnab I, McCulloch J. Backache. Second Edition. Williams and Wilkins: Baltimore, 1990
[187] Strausbaugh LJ. Vertebral osteomyelitis. How to differentiate it from other causes of back and neck pain. Postgrad Med 1995 Jun;97(6):147-8, 151-4

recovery), reductions in the need for medications, significant improvements in survival, and hospital savings.[188,189,190,191,192,193,194]

- o Paleo-Mediterranean diet: As detailed later in this text and elsewhere[195,196]

- o Vitamin and mineral supplementation: anti-infective benefits shown in elderly diabetics[197]

- o High-dose vitamin A: Vitamin A shows potent immunosupportive benefits, and vitamin A stores are depleted by the stress of infection and injury. Consider 200,000-300,000 IU per day of retinol palmitate for 1-4 weeks, then taper; reduce dose or discontinue with onset of toxicity symptoms such as skin problems (dry skin, flaking skin, chapped or split lips, red skin rash, hair loss), joint pain, bone pain, headaches, anorexia (loss of appetite), edema (water retention, weight gain, swollen ankles, difficulty breathing), fatigue, and/or liver damage.

- o Arginine: Dose for adults is in the range of 5-10 grams daily

- o Fatty acid supplementation: In contrast to the higher doses used to provide an anti-inflammatory effect in patients with autoimmune/inflammatory disorders, doses used for immunosupportive treatments should be kept rather modest to avoid the *relative* immunosuppression that has been controversially reported in patients treated with EPA and DHA. Reasonable doses are in the following ranges for adults: EPA+DHA: 500-1,500, and GLA: 300-500 mg.

- o Glutamine: Glutamine enhances bacterial killing by neutrophils[198], and administration of 18 grams per day in divided doses to patients in intensive care units was shown to improve survival, expedite hospital discharge, and reduce total healthcare costs.[199] Another study using glutamine 12-18 grams per day showed no benefit in overall mortality but significant benefits in terms of reduced healthcare costs (-30%) and significantly reduced need for medical interventions.[200] After administering glutamine 26 grams/d to severely burned patients, Garrel et al[201] concluded that glutamine reduced

---

[188] "To evaluate the metabolic and immune effects of dietary arginine, glutamine and omega-3 fatty acids (fish oil) supplementation, we performed a prospective study... CONCLUSIONS: The feeding of Neomune in critically injured patients was well tolerated as Traumacal and significant improvement was observed in serum protein. Shorten ICU stay and wean-off respirator day may benefit from using the immunonutrient formula." Chuntrasakul C, Siltham S, Sarasombath S, Sittapairochana C, Leowattana W, Chockvivatanavanit S, Bunnak A. Comparison of a immunonutrition formula enriched arginine, glutamine and omega-3 fatty acid, with a currently high-enriched enteral nutrition for trauma patients. *J Med Assoc Thai*. 2003 Jun;86(6):552-6

[189] "CONCLUSIONS: In conclusion, arginine-enhanced formula improves fistula rates in postoperative head and neck cancer patients and decreases length of stay." de Luis DA, Izaola O, Cuellar L, Terroba MC, Aller R. Randomized clinical trial with an enteral arginine-enhanced formula in early postsurgical head and neck cancer patients. *Eur J Clin Nutr*. 2004;58(11):1505-8

[190] "In this prospective, randomised, double-blind, placebo-controlled study, we randomly assigned 50 patients who were scheduled to undergo coronary artery bypass to receive either an oral immune-enhancing nutritional supplement containing L-arginine, omega3 polyunsaturated fatty acids, and yeast RNA (n=25), or a control (n=25) for a minimum of 5 days... Intake of an oral immune-enhancing nutritional supplement for a minimum of 5 days before surgery can improve outlook in high-risk patients who are undergoing elective cardiac surgery." Tepaske R, Velthuis H, Oudemans-van Straaten HM, Heisterkamp SH, van Deventer SJ, Ince C, Eysman L, Kesecioglu J. Effect of preoperative oral immune-enhancing nutritional supplement on patients at high risk of infection after cardiac surgery: a randomised placebo-controlled trial. *Lancet*. 2001 Sep 1;358(9283):696-701

[191] "The feeding of IMMUNE FORMULA was well tolerated and significant improvement was observed in nutritional and immunologic parameters as in other immunoenhancing diets. Further clinical trials of prospective double-blind randomized design are necessary to address the so that the necessity of using immunonutrition in critically ill patients will be clarified." Chuntrasakul C, Siltharm S, Sarasombath S, Sittapairochana C, Leowattana W, Chockvivatanavanit S, Bunnak A. Metabolic and immune effects of dietary arginine, glutamine and omega-3 fatty acids supplementation in immunocompromised patients. *J Med Assoc Thai*. 1998 May;81(5):334-43

[192] "enteral diet supplemented with arginine, dietary nucleotides, and omega-3 fatty acids (IMPACT, Sandoz Nutrition, Bern, Switzerland) " Senkal M, Mumme A, Eickhoff U, Geier B, Spath G, Wulfert D, Joosten U, Frei A, Kemen M. Early postoperative enteral immunonutrition: clinical outcome and cost-comparison analysis in surgical patients. *Crit Care Med* 1997;25(9):1489-96

[193] "supplemented diet with glutamine, arginine and omega-3-fatty acids... It was clearly established in this trial that early postoperative enteral feeding is safe in patients who have undergone major operations for gastrointestinal cancer. Supplementation of enteral nutrition with glutamine, arginine, and omega-3-fatty acids positively modulated postsurgical immunosuppressive and inflammatory responses." Wu GH, Zhang YW, Wu ZH. Modulation of postoperative immune and inflammatory response by immune-enhancing enteral diet in gastrointestinal cancer patients. *World J Gastroenterol*. 2001 Jun;7(3):357-62 http://www.wjgnet.com/1007-9327/7/357.pdf

[194] "using a formula supplemented with arginine, mRNA, and omega-3 fatty acids from fish oil (Impact)... CONCLUSIONS: Immune-enhancing enteral nutrition resulted in a significant reduction in the mortality rate and infection rate in septic patients admitted to the ICU. These reductions were greater for patients with less severe illness." Galban C, Montejo JC, Mesejo A, Marco P, Celaya S, Sanchez-Segura JM, Farre M, Bryg DJ. An immune-enhancing enteral diet reduces mortality rate and episodes of bacteremia in septic intensive care unit patients. *Crit Care Med*. 2000 Mar;28(3):643-8

[195] Vasquez A. A Five-Part Nutritional Protocol that Produces Consistently Positive Results. *Nutritional Wellness* 2005 September http://www.nutritionalwellness.com/archives/2005/sep/09_vasquez.php

[196] Vasquez A. Implementing the Five-Part Nutritional Protocol for the Treatment of Various Health Problems. *Nutritional Wellness* 2005 November. http://www.nutritionalwellness.com/archives/2005/nov/11_vasquez.php

[197] "CONCLUSIONS: A multivitamin and mineral supplement reduced the incidence of participant-reported infection and related absenteeism in a sample of participants with type 2 diabetes mellitus and a high prevalence of subclinical micronutrient deficiency." Barringer TA, Kirk JK, Santaniello AC, Foley KL, Michielutte R. Effect of a multivitamin and mineral supplement on infection and quality of life. A randomized, double-blind, placebo-controlled trial. *Ann Intern Med*. 2003 Mar 4;138(5):365-71 http://www.annals.org/cgi/reprint/138/5/365

[198] Furukawa S, Saito H, Fukatsu K, Hashiguchi Y, Inaba T, Lin MT, Inoue T, Han I, Matsuda T, Muto T. Glutamine-enhanced bacterial killing by neutrophils from postoperative patients. *Nutrition* 1997;13(10):863-9. *In vitro* study.

[199] Griffiths RD, Jones C, Palmer TE. Six-month outcome of critically ill patients given glutamine-supplemented parenteral nutrition. *Nutrition* 1997;13(4):295-302

[200] "There was no mortality difference between those patients receiving glutamine-containing enteral feed and the controls. However, there was a significant reduction in the median postintervention ICU and hospital patient costs in the glutamine recipients $23 000 versus $30 900 in the control patients." Jones C, Palmer TE, Griffiths RD. Randomized clinical outcome study of critically ill patients given glutamine-supplemented enteral nutrition. *Nutrition*. 1999 Feb;15(2):108-15

[201] The glutamine dose in this study was "a total of 26 g/day" administered in four divided doses. CONCLUSION: "The results of this prospective randomized clinical trial show that enteral G reduces blood culture positivity, particularly with P. aeruginosa, in adults with severe burns and may be a life-saving intervention." Garrel D, Patenaude J, Nedelec B, Samson L, Dorais J, Champoux J, D'Elia M, Bernier J. Decreased mortality and infectious morbidity in adult burn patients given enteral glutamine supplements: a prospective, controlled, randomized clinical trial. *Crit Care Med*. 2003 Oct;31(10):2444-9

the risk of infection by 3-fold and that oral glutamine "may be a life-saving intervention" in patients with severe burns. A dose of 30 grams/d was used in a recent clinical trial showing hemodynamic benefit in patients with sickle cell anemia.[202] The highest glutamine dose that the current author is aware of is the study by Scheltinga et al[203] who used 0.57 gm/kg/day in cancer patients following chemotherapy administration; for a 220-lb-pt, this would be approximately 57 grams of glutamine per day.

- o **Melatonin**: 20-40 mg hs (*hora somni*—Latin: sleep time). Immunostimulatory anti-infective action of melatonin was demonstrated in a small clinical trial wherein septic newborns administered 20 mg melatonin showed significantly increased survival over nontreated controls.[204]

[202] Niihara Y, Matsui NM, Shen YM, Akiyama DA, Johnson CS, Sunga MA, Magpayo J, Embury SH, Kalra VK, Cho SH, Tanaka KR. L-glutamine therapy reduces endothelial adhesion of sickle red blood cells to human umbilical vein endothelial cells. *BMC Blood Disord*. 2005 Jul 25;5:4 http://www.biomedcentral.com.proxy.hsc.unt.edu/1471-2326/5/4

[203] "Subjects with hematologic malignancies in remission underwent a standard treatment of high-dose chemotherapy and total body irradiation before bone marrow transplantation. After completion of this regimen, they were randomized to receive either standard parenteral nutrition (STD, n = 10) or an isocaloric, isonitrogenous nutrient solution enriched with crystalline L-glutamine (0.57 g/kg/day, GLN, n = 10)." Scheltinga MR, Young LS, Benfell K, Bye RL, Ziegler TR, Santos AA, Antin JH, Schloerb PR, Wilmore DW. Glutamine-enriched intravenous feedings attenuate extracellular fluid expansion after a standard stress. *Ann Surg*. 1991 Oct;214(4):385-93; discussion 393-5 http://www.pubmedcentral.nih.gov/articlerender.fcgi?tool=pubmed&pubmedid=1953094 For additional review, see Ziegler TR. Glutamine supplementation in cancer patients receiving bone marrow transplantation and high dose chemotherapy. *J Nutr*. 2001 Sep;131(9 Suppl):2578S-84S http://jn.nutrition.org/cgi/content/full/131/9/2578S

[204] Gitto E, Karbownik M, Reiter RJ, Tan DX, Cuzzocrea S, Chiurazzi P, Cordaro S, Corona G, Trimarchi G, Barberi I. Effects of melatonin treatment in septic newborns. *Pediatr Res*. 2001 Dec;50(6):756-60 http://www.pedresearch.org/cgi/content/full/50/6/756

BACK PAIN PROTOCOL:

History & Exam:

Diagnosis/DDX:

Laboratory/imaging:

Standard of care:

5-part nutrition protocol:	
Benefits/mechanism:	
Dose/frequency:	
Risks/contraindications:	
Monitoring/duration:	
Vitamin D:	
Benefits/mechanism:	
Dose/frequency:	
Risks/contraindications:	
Monitoring/duration:	
Botanicals:	
Benefits/mechanism:	
Dose/frequency:	
Risks/contraindications:	
Monitoring/duration:	
Exercises:	
Benefits/mechanism:	
Dose/frequency:	
Risks/contraindications:	
Monitoring/duration:	
Manipulation:	
Benefits:	
Dose:	
Risks/contraindications:	
Monitoring/duration:	

Chapter 11:
Pelvis and Sacroiliac Joints

Introduction
Very few clinicians have the ability to skillfully assess the pelvis and sacroiliac joints for biomechanical aberrancies that result in acute and chronic pain and either complete or partial disability. The sacroiliac joints' contribution to chronic low back pain should be appreciated; assessment and manipulative treatment of the pelvis can result in rapid alleviation of pain otherwise unresponsive to pharmacologic symptomatic treatment. Disorders such as ankylosing spondylitis, rheumatoid arthritis, and osteitis condensans ilii should also be within the clinician's range of differential diagnoses.

Concepts:

- The bony pelvis is comprised of the sacrum and the right and left ilia, which are formed by the fusion of the ilium, ischium, and pubis. Bilateral sacroiliac joints posteriorly and the pubic symphysis anteriorly are the intrinsic articulations of the pelvis that allow for multiplanar motions that occur with activities such as walking, running, squatting/rising, and — for women — childbirth.

- From the viewpoint of functional biomechanics, the pelvis serves as the interface between the spinal column and the lower extremity, which interacts primarily with the ground, i.e., the environment. Therefore any chronic biomechanical imbalances of the lower extremities that are not properly compensated for by the time these forces are transmitted to the hip joints will be transferred into the bones and soft tissues of the pelvis and will then be directly transmitted to the spinal column, which must then either compensate for or bear the brunt of these imbalances. For example, we see some evidence that leg length inequalities are associated with low-back pain[1] and lumbar disc herniation[2] and that a functional relationship may exist between the pelvis, neck, and temporomandibular structures.[3] Musculoskeletal assessment and treatment of the pelvis may prove valuable for patients with chronic *non-pelvic* or *extra-pelvic* pain.

Core Competencies:

- You must know how to distinguish benign sacroiliac and pelvic pain from that which results from rheumatic diseases such as the spondyloarthropathies and infections.

- Review your material from gastroenterology and gynecology so that you are familiar with gastrointestinal and pelvic-genitourinary disorders and diseases that can cause pain and nerve compression from their origin in the pelvic-abdominal cavity.

- *Bonus*: Know how to perform genitourinary microbial assessments for the occult "infections" that can cause systemic inflammation[4] and variants of reactive arthritis such as ankylosing spondylitis and rheumatoid arthritis[5] — review Chapter 4 of *Integrative Rheumatology*[6] for details.

> "Urogenital swab culture is the only useful diagnostic method for the detection of the arthritogenic infection in extra-articularly asymptomatic patients with undifferentiated oligoarthritis."
>
> Erlacher et al. Reactive arthritis: urogenital swab culture is the only useful diagnostic method for the detection of the arthritogenic infection in extra-articularly asymptomatic patients with undifferentiated oligoarthritis. *Br J Rheumatol*. 1995 Sep;34(9):838-42

---

[1] "Patients with low back pain who were found to have a leg length discrepancy were treated with a lift to the shoe on the short side. A small group of such patients with longstanding pain had major or total relief over a long period of follow-up." Gofton JP. Persistent low back pain and leg length disparity. *J Rheumatol*. 1985 Aug;12(4):747-50

[2] "The results of this study showed a statistically significant association between leg length discrepancy and the side of radiating pain in a case series of patients with lumbar herniated discs. The relation was more pronounced and statistically significant in women only." ten Brinke A, van der Aa HE, van der Palen J, Oosterveld F. Is leg length discrepancy associated with the side of radiating pain in patients with a lumbar herniated disc? *Spine*. 1999 Apr 1;24(7):684-6

[3] Fink M, Wahling K, Stiesch-Scholz M, Tschernitschek H. The functional relationship between the craniomandibular system, cervical spine, and the sacroiliac joint: a preliminary investigation. *Cranio*. 2003 Jul;21(3):202-8

[4] "Urogenital swab culture is the only useful diagnostic method for the detection of the arthritogenic infection in extra-articularly asymptomatic patients with undifferentiated oligoarthritis." Erlacher L, Wintersberger W, Menschik M, Benke-Studnicka A, Machold K, Stanek G, Soltz-Szots J, Smolen J, Graninger W. Reactive arthritis: urogenital swab culture is the only useful diagnostic method for the detection of the arthritogenic infection in extra-articularly asymptomatic patients with undifferentiated oligoarthritis. *Br J Rheumatol*. 1995 Sep;34(9):838-42

[5] **Vasquez A. Reducing Pain and Inflammation Naturally. Part 6: Nutritional and Botanical Treatments Against "Silent Infections" and Gastrointestinal Dysbiosis, Commonly Overlooked Causes of Neuromusculoskeletal Inflammation and Chronic Health Problems.** *Nutr Perspect* 2006; Jan http://optimalhealthresearch.com/part6

[6] **Vasquez A.** Integrative Rheumatology. http://www.optimalhealthresearch.com/rheumatology.html

Lumbar-Pelvis-Hip Pain: Differential Diagnostic Considerations

	DDX Category	Examples:
V	Vascular	Aortic aneurysm
	Visceral referral	Pancreatic disease/cancer
I	Infectious	Ankylosing spondylitis
	Inflammatory	Lymphoma, leukemia
	Immunologic	Bone/ tissue infections
		Pelvic inflammatory disease
		Sexually transmitted infections
		Gastrointestinal disease
		Kidney infection
		Osteitis condensans ilii
N	Neurologic	Ovarian cancer
	Nutritional	Endometriosis
	New growth: neoplasia or	Metastatic disease
	pregnancy	Primary bone tumors
		Multiple myeloma
		Herpes zoster
		Cauda equina syndrome
D	Deficiency	Degenerative joint/spine disease
	Degenerative	Congenital malformations of bones/ viscera
	Developmental	Scoliosis
		Postural syndromes
		Disc herniation
		Hip "osteoarthritis" after the exclusion of hemochromatosis
		Slipped capital femoral epiphysis
		Avascular necrosis of the femoral head
I	Iatrogenic (drug related)	Anticoagulants predispose to epidural or spinal cord bleeding
	Intoxication	Use of antidepressants suggests previous diagnosis of clinical
	Idiosyncratic	depression
		Alcoholism
C	Congenital	Congenital malformations of bones: hemivertebrae, leg length inequality,
A	Allergy	Ankylosing spondylitis
	Autoimmune	Fractures, injuries
	Abuse	Rheumatoid arthritis
T	Trauma	Fractures: injuries to vertebrae, ribs, muscles
E	Endocrine	Diabetes
	Exposure	
S	Subluxation	Segmental dysfunction of lumbar spine and pelvis
	Structural	Muscle tension
	Stress	Somatoform disorder, conversion disorder
	Secondary gain	Leg length inequality
M	Mental	Anxiety
	Malpractice seeker	Depression
	Mental disorder	Endometriosis
	Malignancy	Ovarian tumor
	Metabolic disease	Nephrolithiasis
	Menstrual	Osteoporosis, osteoporotic fractures

High-Risk Pain Patients

When a patient has musculoskeletal pain and any of the following characteristics, radiographs should be considered as an appropriate component of comprehensive evaluation. These considerations are particularly—though not exclusively—relevant for spine and low-back pain.[7]

1. **More than 50 years of age**
2. **Physical trauma** (accident, fall, etc.)
3. **Pain at night**
4. **Back pain not relieved by lying supine**
5. **Neurologic deficits** (motor or sensory)
6. **Unexplained weight loss**
7. **Documentation or suspicion of inflammatory arthropathy**[8]
   - **Ankylosing spondylitis**
   - **Lupus**
   - **Rheumatoid arthritis**
   - **Juvenile rheumatoid arthritis**
   - **Psoriatic arthritis**
8. **Drug or alcohol abuse** (increased risk of infection, nutritional deficiencies, anesthesia)
9. **History of cancer**
10. **Intravenous drug use**
11. **Immunosuppression, due to illness (e.g., HIV) or medications (e.g., steroids or cyclosporine)**
12. **History of corticosteroid use** (causes osteoporosis and increased risk for infection)
13. **Fever above 100° F or suspicion of septic arthritis or osteomyelitis**
14. **Diabetes** (increased risk of infection, nutritional deficiencies, anesthesia)
15. **Hypertension** (abdominal aneurysm: low back pain, nausea, pulsatile abdominal mass)
16. **Recent visit for same problem and not improved**
17. **Patient seeking compensation for pain/ injury** (increased need for documentation)
18. **Skin lesion** (psoriasis, melanoma, dermatomyositis, the butterfly rash of lupus, scars from previous surgery, accident, etc....)
19. **Deformity or immobility**
20. **Lymphadenopathy** (suggests cancer or infection)
21. **Elevated ESR/CRP** (cancer, infection, inflammatory disorder)
22. **Elevated WBC count**
23. **Elevated alkaline phosphatase** (bone lesions, metabolic bone disease, hepatopathy)
24. **Elevated acid phosphatase** (occasionally used to monitor prostate cancer)
25. **Positive rheumatoid factor and/or CCP—cyclic citrullinated protein antibodies**
26. **Positive HLA-B27** (propensity for inflammatory arthropathies)
27. **Serum gammopathy** (multiple myeloma is the most common primary bone tumor)
28. **High-risk for disease:** *examples:*
   - Long-term heavy smoking of cigarettes
   - Long-term exposure to radiation
   - Obesity
29. **Strong family history of inflammatory, musculoskeletal, or malignant disease**

---

[7] Remember that metastasis often travel first from the primary site to bone, therefore bone pain may be an early manifestation of occult cancer. Most of the above are from "Table 1: The high-risk patient: clinical indications for radiography in low back pain patients." J Taylor, DC, DACBR, D Resnick, MD. Imaging decisions in the management of low back pain. Advances in Chiropractic. Mosby Year Book. 1994; 1-28

[8] Radiographs are often essential for diagnosis or to rule out complications of the disease. For example, in patients with inflammatory arthropathies such as these, spontaneous rupture of the transverse ligament (at the odontoid process) has been reported; although rare, this complication could be life-threatening if mismanaged or undiagnosed.

Clinical Assessments for the Sacroiliac Joints

Selected Assessments[9,10]	*Positive Finding and Implications*
1. **History, observation, and neurologic examination**: *See Chapter 1 for additional information*	▪ **Indicators from the history (trauma, risk factors)** ▪ **Systemic manifestations** ▪ **Complications: neurologic deficits** ▪ **Mechanical/ Nonmechanical**
2. **Active range of motion**: aROM should be "full and painless" ▪ Walk on heels (L4 and L5) ▪ Walk on toes (S1) ▪ Squat and rise: this is a valuable screening test for quickly assessing quadriceps strength, neurologic integrity (mostly L3 and L4[11]) and balance ▪ Lumbar flexion ▪ Lumbar extension ▪ Rotation ▪ Lateral bending ▪ Hip circumduction	Limitation or pain may suggest any of the following: ▪ Pain ▪ Injury ▪ Muscle spasm ▪ Tight muscles ▪ Contracture/adhesion of soft tissues: muscles, joint capsule ▪ Fracture ▪ Disc herniation/injury
3. **Static palpation of the pelvis**: Manually and visually assess bony landmarks for symmetry	▪ Side-to-side comparison of the major bony landmarks (e.g., PSIS, ASIS, iliac crest, maleoli) suggests pelvic torque when these landmarks are not positioned symmetrically and when the findings are consistent, such as a functional short leg associated with a posteriorly rotated ilium ▪ Static palpation also includes assessment for myofascial trigger points, edema, muscle hypertrophy and atrophy, and general tissue tone
4. **Abdominal and/or pelvic examination**: Remember that low back and pelvic pain may arise from structures and organs in the abdomen and pelvis ▪ Pain ▪ Mass ▪ Tenderness ▪ Guarding ▪ Rebound tenderness	Perform palpation and assessments with consideration for the following: ▪ Mass ▪ Kidney infection ▪ Tumor: colon, ovarian, endometrial, prostatic, metastatic ▪ Abdominal aneurysm ▪ Infection ▪ In women, consider fibroid tumors, endometriosis, ectopic or normal pregnancy, dermoid tumor, ovarian cyst and tumors, and pelvic inflammatory disease
5. **SIJ gapping test, SIJ distraction test**: Patient **supine**, doctor applies outward (posterolateral) force on anterior superior iliac spine (ASIS) bilaterally and simultaneously: this test is performed to gap and stress the anterior aspect of the sacroiliac joints	▪ Pain in the SIJ with posterolateral forces applied to the ASIS suggests SIJ dysfunction or strain of the anterior SI ligaments

---

[9] Review relevant information in Magee DJ. Orthopedic Physical Assessment. Third edition. Philadelphia: WB Saunders, 1997 and Bates B. A Guide to Physical Examination and History Taking. 6th Edition. Philadelphia; J. B. Lippincott Company, 1995
[10] Laslett M, Williams M. The reliability of selected pain provocation tests for sacroiliac joint pathology. Spine 1994 Jun 1;19(11):1243-9
[11] Moore KL. Clinically Oriented Anatomy. Third Edition. Baltimore; Williams and Wilkins: 1992, page 387

Clinical Assessments for the Sacroiliac Joints—*continued*

Clinical Assessments	*Positive Finding and Implications*
6. **SIJ compression test**: • *Version 1*: Patient in *side posture* position, doctor applies downward compressive force on iliac crest • *Version 2*: Patient *supine*, doctor applies posteromedial pressure to anterior superior iliac spine (ASIS) bilaterally and simultaneously	• Pain provoked in the sacroiliac joints when this test is performed suggests SIJ dysfunction or lesion
7. **Thomas test**: *Supine* patient brings unaffected thigh to abdomen (hip hyperflexion) while affected/tested leg remains on table. When the pelvis is rotated posteriorly with forced hyperflexion of the hip, the opposite hip should have sufficient flexibility to remain in extension on the surface of the table[12]	• The test result is considered positive/abnormal when the thigh that should remain on table lifts off the table due to joint hypomobility, capsular restriction, or tightness of the hip flexors—the iliacus, psoas, rectus femoris • This test is very similar to Gaenslen's test. The subtle difference is that Thomas test assess the extensibility of the hip flexors whereas Gaenslen test assesses the ability of the sacroiliac joints to handle an extension force
8. **Gaenslen's test**: *Supine* patient brings unaffected thigh to abdomen (hip hyperflexion) while affected/tested leg is allowed to come off the side of the table so that the affected/tested side can fall into extension; this allows stress to be applied to the sacroiliac joint[13]	• The test result is considered positive/abnormal when pain is produced in the sacroiliac joint on the side that is in extension, suggesting a lesion or sprain of the sacroiliac joint
9. **Posterior shear test, posterior glide test, thigh thrust test**: Patient *supine* close to table edge with hip flexed on same side as SI joint to be assessed. Doctor grasps the patient's flexed knee with cephalad hand and rolls patient toward doctor to allow caudad hand to be placed behind patient's sacrum. Patient's pelvis is then replaced on top of doctor's caudad hand. Doctor then pushes axially through the patient's femur to produce a shearing force at the sacroiliac joint. *Use caution to avoid hip adduction that could promote hip dislocation.* Repeat on opposite side. As with all tests and examinations near the pelvis, use social awareness and clear communication when performing this test; consider having your assistant enter the room as a witness	• A normal result is that the doctor feels a slight motion in the joint that this bilaterally symmetrical and painless; an abnormal result shows either asymmetric motion (suggesting fixation or hypo- or hypermobility) or pain (suggesting joint sprain or lesion such as infection)

---

[12] Brier S. <u>Primary Care Orthopedics</u>. St. Louis: Mosby, 1999 page 287
[13] Brier S. <u>Primary Care Orthopedics</u>. St. Louis: Mosby, 1999 page 426

Clinical Assessments for the Sacroiliac Joints—*continued*

Clinical Assessments	*Positive Finding and Implications*
10. <u>Patrick's test, FABER, figure four test</u>: This is a common ROM and joint provocation maneuver; *supine* patient, doctor passively moves thigh into <u>f</u>lexion, <u>ab</u>duction, <u>e</u>xternal <u>r</u>otation with ipsilateral ankle placed at contralateral knee	▪ Pain or limited motion suggest **hip joint pathology such as osteoarthritis** or **regional muscle tightness**, particularly of the iliopsoas and adductors ▪ Toward the end of the maneuver, when the ipsilateral ankle is placed at contralateral knee, the doctor can stabilize the opposite ASIS while placing downward pressure on the knee of the leg being tested; pain posteriorly at the PSIS is consistent with **lesion of the SIJ**, such as osteitis condensans ilii[14]
11. <u>Myofascial assessments</u>: Beginning with the patient *supine* and then transitioning to the *prone* position, the doctor palpates muscles (especially iliopsoas, quadratus lumborum, and piriformis), tendons, and fascial structures such as the iliotibial band for restriction, tightness, myofascial trigger points (discussed in Chapter 3), muscle spasm, muscle imbalance and atrophy	▪ By the time the history, physical examination, and screening laboratory tests (all reviewed in Chapter 1) have suggested against the presence of acute trauma or underlying disease such as cancer and infection, then the clinician can make a provisional assessment that the patient's pain-dysfunction is a "functional" *rather than pathologic or traumatic* problem. These problems arise from myofascial and musculoskeletal structures, each of which will reveal its character and severity only though the doctor's skilled palpation and provocation. Recall and review the anatomy of the region, and develop your own stepwise process of assessing *each* of the myofascial and muscular structures of the region
12. <u>Sacral thrust test</u>: Patient is *prone*, doctor applies posteroanterior force on sacrum	▪ Pain in the SIJ suggests SIJ dysfunction or lesion ▪ This test can be performed with more stress on one side than the other to emphasize either joint and to make the assessment more meaningful
13. <u>Cranial shear test</u>: Patient is *prone* on a low table, doctor applies cephalad force on sacral apex while inferiorly tractioning leg on affected side by holding patient's lower leg and ankle between the doctor's legs; test is repeated on other side. This test produces an axial shearing force through the sacroiliac joint when the sacrum is pushed superiorly while the leg is tractioned inferiorly	▪ Pain in the SIJ suggests SIJ dysfunction or lesion
14. <u>Motion palpation of the sacroiliac joints, Gillett's test, march test</u>: Doctor sits behind patient while patient marches in place. Doctor assesses SIJ motion by making manual contact on pelvic landmarks such as the posterior superior iliac spine and sacral apex. Motion of the sacroiliac joint is determined by visual and kinesthetic assessment of joint motion[15]	▪ Hypermobility and/or hypomobility suggest biomechanical dysfunction that may respond to manipulation. Although a recent radiographic study of sacroiliac joint mobility showed no difference between the mobility of symptomatic and asymptomatic joints[16], some patients still derive symptomatic benefit from manipulation

[14] Vadivelu R, Green TP, An uncommon cause of back pain in pregnancy. *Postgrad Med J.* 2005 Jan;81(951):65-7 http://pmj.bmj.com/cgi/content/full/81/951/65
[15] Bergmann TF, Peterson DH, Lawrence DJ. <u>Chiropractic Technique: Principles and Procedures</u>. New York, Churchill Livingstone: 1993, pages 495-496
[16] Laslett M, Williams M. The reliability of selected pain provocation tests for sacroiliac joint pathology. *Spine* 1994 Jun 1;19(11):1243-9

Suggested Examination Flow for the Pelvis and SIJ

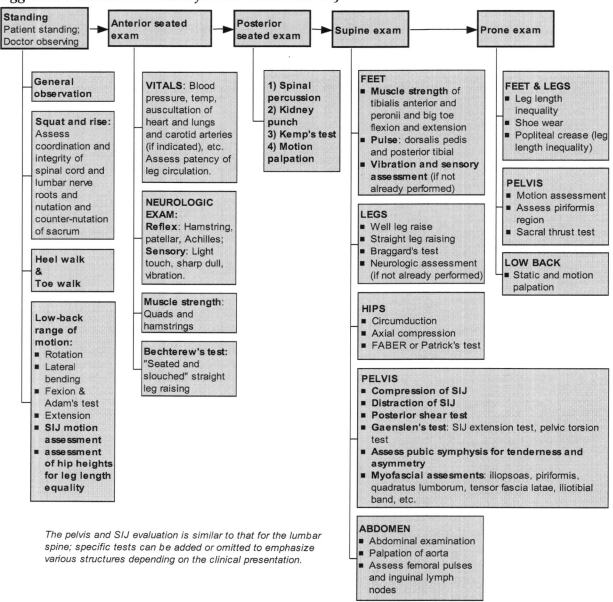

The pelvis and SIJ evaluation is similar to that for the lumbar spine; specific tests can be added or omitted to emphasize various structures depending on the clinical presentation.

Standing	Anterior Seated	Posterior Seated	Supine	Prone
1. Observation 2. Squat and rise 3. Toe walk, heel walk, gait, Romberg 4. Range of motion 5. Motion palpation of sacroiliac joints 6. Leg length inequality	7. Vital signs 8. Neurologic examination 9. Reflexes 10. Sensory 11. Muscle strength 12. Bechterew's test	13. Spinal percussion 14. Kidney punch 15. Kemp's test 16. Motion palpation of spine and SI joints	17. Nerve tension tests: straight leg raising (SLR), Braggard's test, "well leg raise" 18. Hip assessment 19. SIJ compression and distraction tests 20. Abdominal examination 21. Pelvic and genitourinary exams as indicated—pelvic or abdominal ultrasound or CT for follow-up 22. Myofascial assessments of pelvis and hip region	23. Torque and symmetry of pelvis 24. Motion palpation of lumbar spine and SI joints 25. Assess piriformis and gluteal region 26. Leg length equality 27. Static and deep palpation including the quadratus lumborum

Pelvis and Sacroiliac Joints (SIJ)—*General Considerations*

"The conditions affecting the SI joint include those that affect any joint... rheumatoid arthritis, degenerative osteoarthritis, infection, ligamentous strain, and subluxation.... inflammatory bowel diseases, postsurgical enteropathies, renal osteodystrophy, ankylosing spondylitis, Reiter's syndrome, psoriasis, gout, diffuse idiopathic skeletal hyperostosis, and neoplasms such as Ewing's sarcoma...."[17]

Data and Concepts:

- Eight true articulations of the pelvis:
  - 2 sacroiliac joints: Some clinicians and researchers further divide each sacroiliac joint into an upper (fibrocartilagenous) and lower (synovial diarthrodial) joint.
  - 2 hip joints: connection of the acetabulum and the femoral head
  - 1 symphysis pubis
  - 3 joints of the lumbosacral junction: comprised of 2 facet joints and 1 intervertebral disc
- Lesions of the sacroiliac joints can be tripartitely categorized:
  1. Acute and chronic functional problems: Subtle biomechanical dysfunction of the SIJ as assessed with motion and static palpation and treated with manipulation and other "physical medicine" techniques.
  2. Gross orthopedic problems: Symphysis pubis diastasis, major instability of the SIJ and symphysis pubis, gross/severe dislocation of the SIJ, symphysis pubis, with/without fracture of the ilium or sacrum, including the relatively common sacral insufficiency fractures seen in osteoporotic patients.
  3. Systemic problems, particularly musculoskeletal infections: Cancer and metastasis, infection and septic arthritis, systemic disease, autoimmune diseases, and other problems. Apparently because of the proximity to the anogenital region, the musculoskeletal structures comprising the pelvis and hip region seem to show an increased tendency toward infection.
- Clinical considerations:
  - Presentations of sacroiliac joint problems are commonly similar to those of mechanical low back problems. In other words, anytime a patient presents with "low-back pain", they should be assessed for sacroiliac dysfunction or lesion.
  - Clinical assessments for SIJ problems are many, yet different studies report varying levels of clinical validity for these tests[18,19] As always, the physician uses a wide range of reasonably valid assessments and then mentally summarizes the results of these tests in combination with the patient's history and other data to arrive at a clinical diagnosis, which is then addressed empirically. Pain directly over the SIJ is characteristic of SIJ dysfunction, and the localization of pain to the SIJ with the use of 2 or more orthopedic tests helps to confirm the presence of an SIJ lesion.[20]
  - Treatment of SIJ or other musculoskeletal pain begins first with excluding underlying pathology—particularly infection in younger adults and fractures in older osteoporotic patients and in any post-trauma patient. Non-pathogenic and non-surgical musculoskeletal problems generally respond well to musculoskeletal interventions as partly reviewed in Chapter 3: systemic de-inflammation[21,22], therapeutic anti-inflammation[23,24], and proprioceptive rehabilitation, musculoskeletal work directed toward the joints, fascia, and muscles. Degenerative SIJs can be treated with glucosamine, niacinamide, willow, and the other nutritional and botanical medicines reviewed in Chapter 3. Hypermobile joints that do not respond to stabilizing exercise and the use of a trochanter belt may be stabilized with dextrose prolotherapy.[25,26] Acupuncture and topical capsaicin can be used to alleviate pain. Medicosurgical management for recalcitrant cases may include anti-inflammatory pharmaceuticals and analgesics, injected nerve blocks (etc), and surgical interventions including fusion for chronic joint instability and pain.[27]

[17] Hendler N, Kozikowski JG, MorrisonC, Sethuraman G. Diagnosis and management of sacroiliac joint disease.*JNMS:Journal of the Neuromusculoskeletal System* 1995;3:169-74
[18] Laslett M, Williams M. The reliability of selected pain provocation tests for sacroiliac joint pathology. *Spine* 1994 Jun 1;19(11):1243-9
[19] Paydar D, Thiel H, Gemmell H. Intra- and interexaminer reliability of certain pelvic palpatory procedures and the sitting flexion test for sacroiliac joint mobility and dysfunction. *JNMS: Journal of the Neuromusculoskeletal System* 1994; 2: 65-9
[20] McKenzie-Brown AM, Shah RV, Sehgal N, Everett CR.A systematic review of sacroiliac joint interventions. *Pain Physician.* 2005 Jan;8(1):115-25 http://www.painphysicianjournal.com/linkout_vw.php?issn=1533-3159&vol=8&page=115
[21] Vasquez A. Reducing Pain and Inflammation Naturally. Part 1: New Insights into Fatty Acid Biochemistry and the Influence of Diet. *Nutritional Perspectives* 2004; October: 5, 7-10, 12, 14
[22] Vasquez A. Reducing Pain and Inflammation Naturally. Part 2: New Insights into Fatty Acid Supplementation and Its Effect on Eicosanoid Production and Genetic Expression. *Nutr Perspectives*2005;Jan: 5-16
[23] Vasquez A. Reducing pain and inflammation naturally - Part 3: Improving overall health while safely and effectively treating musculoskeletal pain. *Nutritional Perspectives* 2005; 28: 34-38, 40-42
[24] Vasquez A. Reducing pain and inflammation naturally - Part 4: Nutritional and Botanical Inhibition of NF-kappaB, the Major Intracellular Amplifier of the Inflammatory Cascade. A Practical Clinical Strategy Exemplifying Anti-Inflammatory Nutrigenomics. *Nutritional Perspectives* 2005;July: 5-12 http://www.optimalhealthresearch.com/part4
[25] Forst SL, Wheeler MT, Fortin JD, Vilensky JA. The sacroiliac joint: anatomy, physiology and clinical significance. *Pain Physician.* 2006 Jan;9(1):61-7 http://www.painphysicianjournal.com/linkout_vw.php?issn=1533-3159&vol=9&page=61
[26] Chakraverty R, Dias R. Audit of conservative management of chronic low back pain in a secondary care setting--part I: facet joint and sacroiliac joint interventions. *Acupunct Med.* 2004 Dec;22(4):207-13 http://www.acupunctureinmedicine.org.uk/servearticle.php?artid=546
[27] Slipman CW, Whyte Ii WS, Chow DW, Chou L, Lenrow D, Ellen M. Sacroiliac joint syndrome. *Pain Physician.* 2001 Apr;4(2):143-52 http://www.painphysicianjournal.com/linkout_vw.php?issn=1533-3159&vol=4&page=143

Selected Orthopedic and Functional Problems of the Pelvis and SIJ—*Musculoskeletal Lesions*

Problem &Typical Presentation	Assessment & Treatment Considerations
Osteitis condensans ilii (OCI) • Considered a rare and benign cause of low-back and SIJ pain, classically presenting in women who are or have recently been pregnant[28] • This condition is benign and self-limiting	• Tests for the lumbar spine should be more unremarkable than those specific for the SIJ: Patrick/FABER test, Gaenslen test, sacral thrust, cranial shear and posterior sheer tests should direct attention to the SIJ; bilateral lesions are common • Anteroposterior lumbopelvic radiograph shows well-defined triangular sclerosis on the iliac side of the lower sacroiliac joints; OCI is distinguished from inflammatory sacroiliitis: ❶ absence of joint space irregularity, ❷ only the iliac side of the joint is affected (rather than iliac *and sacral*), ❸ lack of serologic evidence of inflammation—CRP is normal in OCI • Phytonutritional pain relief, muscular stabilization (strength and proprioception); use caution when using phytonutritional inventions in women who are pregnant or nursing

Sacroiliac Syndrome: SIJ sprain, SIJ functional subluxation and/or dysfunction[29]
• Acute onset of sharp or dull pain in the SIJ following overexertion, minor trauma, or "straightening up from a stooped position" [30]
• Referred pain from the SIJs may radiate into the following regions:
   ♦ Abdomen
   ♦ Low back
   ♦ Thigh
   ♦ Groin
   ♦ Trochanter and lateral thigh
   ♦ Leg and calf
   ♦ Ankle and foot[31,32]
	• History and physical examination including stress tests of the SIJ, motion and static palpation
	• Trochanteric/SIJ support belt for hypermobility
	• Mobilization and manipulation for hypomobility
	• Always look at lower extremity biomechanics *in toto*, especially when working with pelvic and lumbar problems
	• See Comprehensive Musculoskeletal Care in Chapter 3; myofascial and manipulative work, muscle stretching-strengthening-balancing, proprioceptive retraining, MFTP identification and treatment; pharmacosurgical consultation for recalcitrant cases

SIJ orthopedic subluxation • Intense severe acute-onset continuous pain with associated muscle spasm • Pain is not relieved by positioning	• History and physical examination • CT scan is more sensitive than radiography • Immediate and dramatic relief with manipulation[33] • Severe trauma mandates assessment for fracture and visceral complications
Symphysis pubis diastasis Separation of the symphysis pubis from rupture of the connecting soft tissues • Low back, SIJ, and/or pubic pain and dysfunction associated with pregnancy and/or vaginal delivery; seen in 1 per 600-3,400 deliveries[34]	• Joint widening and increased motion • Radiographs reveal dislocation of the symphysis pubis • "Conservative management is usually effective."[35] • Massage to alleviate pain and muscle spasm • Trochanteric-SIJ support belt • Surgical/orthopedic referral for gross instability that does not respond to conservative care • **All cases of <u>post-traumatic</u> symphysis pubis diastasis warrant immediate assessment and management of visceral and genitourinary complications**

[28] Vadivelu R, Green TP, An uncommon cause of back pain in pregnancy. *Postgrad Med J.* 2005 Jan;81(951):65-7 http://pmj.bmj.com/cgi/content/full/81/951/65
[29] Slipman CW, Whyte Ii WS, Chow DW, Chou L, Lenrow D, Ellen M. Sacroiliac joint syndrome. *Pain Physician.* 2001 Apr;4(2):143-52 http://www.painphysicianjournal.com/linkout_vw.php?issn=1533-3159&vol=4&page=143
[30] Hendler N, Kozikowski JG, MorrisonC, Sethuraman G. Diagnosis and management of sacroiliac joint disease.*JNMS:Journal of the Neuromusculoskeletal System* 1995;3:169-74
[31] Hendler N, Kozikowski JG, MorrisonC, Sethuraman G. Diagnosis and management of sacroiliac joint disease.*JNMS:Journal of the Neuromusculoskeletal System* 1995;3:169-74
[32] McKenzie-Brown AM, Shah RV, Sehgal N, Everett CR.A systematic review of sacroiliac joint interventions. *Pain Physician.* 2005 Jan;8(1):115-25 http://www.painphysicianjournal.com/linkout_vw.php?issn=1533-3159&vol=8&page=115
[33] Hendler N, Kozikowski JG, MorrisonC, Sethuraman G. Diagnosis and management of sacroiliac joint disease.*JNMS:Journal of the Neuromusculoskeletal System* 1995;3:169-74
[34] "The incidence of symphysis pubis separation is reported to be between 1:600 and 1:3400 obstetric patients. Treatment should generally be conservative and symptomatic." Senechal PK. Symphysis pubis separation during childbirth. *J Am Board Fam Pract.* 1994 Mar-Apr;7(2):141-4
[35] Stern PJ, Cote P, O'Connor SM, Mior SA. Symphysis pubis diastasis: a complication of pregnancy. *JNMS: Journal of the Neuromusculoskeletal System* 1993; 1: 74-8

Selected Orthopedic and Functional Problems of the Pelvis and SIJ—*Infections*

Problem &Typical Presentation	Assessment & Treatment
Osteitis pubis Inflammatory destruction of the symphysis pubis due to infection or mechanical irritation ▪ Pain at the pubic symphysis ▪ Osteitis pubis is more common in males, especially athletes, especially soccer players	▪ Pain with palpation of the symphysis pubis and insertions of the adductors ▪ Assess for pelvic torque ▪ Radiographs reveal sclerosis, symphysis pubis widening ▪ Assess for infection: CBC, CRP, physical examination and history ▪ For non-infectious cases, implement Comprehensive Musculoskeletal Care (Chapter 3) ▪ Conservative management of osteitis pubis includes antiinflammatories and analgesics; "daily application of therapeutic modalities (cryomassage, laser, ultrasound, or electric stimulation) for 14 days" and progressive rehabilitation[36] ▪ Effective treatment for joint infections must be implemented expeditiously
Pyogenic sacroiliitis ▪ Usually unilateral ▪ May have fever ▪ Inability to bear weight on the affected side ▪ May also have back, flank, or thigh pain ▪ May present as "acute abdomen" with lower quadrant pain, tenderness, guarding[37] ▪ Acute presentation is rare, common presentation is chronic[38]	▪ Pain increased with weight-bearing and SIJ compression and provocation tests ▪ May have redness, local tenderness, and swelling ▪ Elevated WBC and CRP ▪ MRI is the imaging technique of choice ▪ Acute infection warrants immediate and aggressive antimicrobial treatment; some patients will require surgical debridement[39] ▪ Follow-up medical treatment with Comprehensive Musculoskeletal Care (Chapter 3), immunonutrition, and probiotics
Septic arthritis of the pubic symphysis All joint infections require aggressive antimicrobial treatment ▪ "Typical features of **pubic symphysis infection** included fever (74%), pubic pain (68%), painful or waddling gait (59%), pain with hip motion (45%), and groin pain (41%). Risk factors included female incontinence surgery (24%); sports, especially soccer (19%); pelvic malignancy (17%); and intravenous drug use (15%)."[40]	▪ Pain with palpation of the symphysis pubis and insertions of the adductors ▪ Abnormal CBC and CRP ▪ May have systemic manifestations of infection: fever, weight loss, anorexia, etc. ▪ "Since osteomyelitis is present in 97% of patients, we recommend **antibiotic courses of 6 weeks' duration. Surgical debridement is required in 55% of patients.**"[41] ▪ Follow-up medical treatment with Comprehensive Musculoskeletal Care, immunonutrition, and probiotics as reviewed in Chapter 3

[36] Rodriguez C, Miguel A, Lima H, Heinrichs K. Osteitis Pubis Syndrome in the Professional Soccer Athlete: A Case Report. *J Athl Train*. 2001 Dec;36(4):437-440
[37] Hendler N, Kozikowski JG, MorrisonC, Sethuraman G. Diagnosis and management of sacroiliac joint disease.*JNMS:Journal of the Neuromusculoskeletal System* 1995;3:169-74
[38] Hendler N, Kozikowski JG, MorrisonC, Sethuraman G. Diagnosis and management of sacroiliac joint disease.*JNMS:Journal of the Neuromusculoskeletal System* 1995;3:169-74
[39] Doita M, Yoshiya S, Nabeshima Y, Tanase Y, Nishida K, Miyamoto H, Watanabe Y, Kurosaka M. Acute pyogenic sacroiliitis without predisposing conditions. *Spine*. 2003 Sep 15;28(18):E384-9
[40] Ross JJ, Hu LT. Septic arthritis of the pubic symphysis: review of 100 cases. *Medicine* (Baltimore). 2003 Sep;82(5):340-5
[41] Ross JJ, Hu LT. Septic arthritis of the pubic symphysis: review of 100 cases. *Medicine* (Baltimore). 2003 Sep;82(5):340-5

Chapter 12:
Hip and Thigh

Introduction

Disorders of the hip and thigh can be musculoskeletal, inflammatory, degenerative, malignant, infectious, and neurologic in origin. The clinician must be astute and efficient in his/her evaluation of the patient in order to avoid missing an important diagnosis.

---

1. Clinical assessments and differential diagnoses of hip and thigh pain and dysfunction
2. Selected orthopedic problems of the hip seen in *infants, children, and adolescents*
    o   Developmental dysplasia of the hip
    o   Septic arthritis of the hip
    o   Avascular necrosis of the femoral head, Perthe's disease, Legg-Calve-Perthe's disease
    o   Apophysitis, apophyseal fracture
    o   Transient synovitis, irritable hip
    o   Slipped capital femoral epiphysis
3. Suggested flow algorithm for the assessment & management of hip pain in young patients
4. Common serious hip problems in infants, children, and adolescents: general expectation of prevalence and probability by age in weeks to years
5. Orthopedic problems of the hip and thigh seen in mostly *in adults*
    o   Avascular necrosis (AVN) of the femoral head, osteonecrosis
    o   Bursitis
    o   Femoral neuropathy
    o   Fracture: Femoral neck, Intertrochanteric, Subtrochanteric
    o   Hernia, "sports hernia"
    o   Iron overload, hemochromatosis
    o   Joint pain due to leg length inequality
    o   Meralgia paresthetica
    o   Muscle strain, overuse injury, tendonitis
    o   Osteoarthrosis, osteoarthritis
    o   Snapping tendon, internal snapping hip, iliopsoas tendonitis
    o   Stress fracture of the femur
    o   Tear of the acetabular labrum
    o   Traumatic synovitis

Core competencies:

1. You must know how to diagnose developmental dysplasia of the hip in a newborn.
2. Describe the initial evaluation and management of fractures of the femur.
3. Describe the differential diagnosis and management of slipped capital femoral epiphysis, avascular necrosis, and septic arthritis.
4. Differentially diagnose and manage meralgia paresthetica from femoral neuropathy. What metabolic disease is associated with femoral neuropathy?
5. Since differentiation based on physical examination and history is impossible, you must know which lab tests are used to distinguish hip osteoarthritis from hemochromatoic arthropathy and how the tests are correlatively interpreted.

Lumbar-pelvis-hip pain: differential diagnostic considerations

	DDX Category	Examples:
V	**Vascular**	**Avascular necrosis of the hip**
	Visceral referral	Aortic aneurysm
		Nephrolithiasis
I	Infectious	**Rheumatoid arthritis of the hip: a leading cause of protrusio**
	Inflammatory	**acetabuli**
	Immunologic	Ankylosing spondylitis
		Lymphoma, leukemia
		Bone/ tissue/joint infections
		Gastrointestinal disease
		Kidney infection
N	Neurologic	Metastatic disease
	Nutritional	Primary bone tumors
	New growth	Herpes zoster
D	Deficiency	**Developmental dysplasia of the hip**
	Degenerative	Degenerative joint/spine disease
	Developmental	Congenital malformations of bones/ viscera
		Leg length inequalities and scoliosis
		Postural syndromes
		Disc herniation
		Hip osteoarthritis *after the exclusion of* **hemochromatosis**[1]
		Slipped capital femoral epiphysis
		Avascular necrosis of the femoral head
I	Iatrogenic (drug related)	Anticoagulants predispose to epidural or spinal cord bleeding
	Intoxication	Use of antidepressants suggests previous diagnosis of clinical
	Idiosyncratic	depression
		Alcoholism
C	**Congenital**	Congenital malformations of bones: hemivertebrae, leg length
		inequality
		Congenital hip dysplasia: this term has been officially replaced
		by "developmental dysplasia of the hip"
A	Allergy	Ankylosing spondylitis
	Autoimmune	Fractures, injuries
	Abuse	Rheumatoid arthritis
T	Trauma	Fractures: injuries to vertebrae, ribs, muscles
E	Endocrine	Diabetes
	Exposure	
S	Subluxation	Segmental dysfunction of lumbar spine and pelvis
	Structural	Muscle tension
	Stress	Somatoform disorder, conversion disorder
	Secondary gain	Meralgia paresthetica: associated with obesity
M	Mental	Anxiety
	Malpractice seeker	Depression
	Mental disorder	Nephrolithiasis
	Malignancy	Osteoporosis, osteoporotic fractures
	Metabolic disease	Iron overload[2]
	Menstrual	Femoral neuropathy: closely associated with diabetes mellitus

---

[1] Axford JS, Bomford A, Revell P, Watt I, Williams R, Hamilton EBD. Hip arthropathy in genetic hemochromatosis: radiographic and histologic features. *Arthritis Rheum* 1991; 34: 357-61
[2] Vasquez A. Musculoskeletal disorders and iron overload disease: comment on the American College of Rheumatology guidelines for the initial evaluation of the adult patient with acute musculoskeletal symptoms. *Arthritis Rheum* 1996 Oct; 39(10):1767-8

Hip Joint and Thigh

"Pathologic conditions ranging from a benign muscle or tendon strain to a potentially catastrophic femoral neck stress fracture can have similar clinical presentations."[3]

Clinical assessments for the hips

Selected assessments	Positive finding and Implications
1. **History**: *see Chapter 1 for additional information*	▪ **Indicators from the history (trauma, risk factors)** ▪ **Systemic manifestations** ▪ **Complications** ▪ **Mechanical/ Nonmechanical** Systemic manifestations, nonmechanical pain, and other "red flags" and "yellow flags" *suggest* increased risk for serious pathology and potential complications and therefore indicate the need for additional investigation by history, examination, laboratory, imaging and/or post-treatment observation
2. **Active motion from patient**: ROM should be "full and painless" ▪ Walk on heels (L4 and L5) ▪ Walk on toes (S1) ▪ Squat and rise: this is a valuable screening test for quickly assessing quadriceps strength, neurologic integrity (mostly L3 and L4[4]) and balance ▪ Flexion ▪ Extension ▪ Internal rotation ▪ External rotation ▪ Circumduction	Limitation or pain may suggest any of the following: ▪ Pain ▪ Injury ▪ Muscle spasm ▪ Tight muscles ▪ Contracture/adhesion of soft tissues: muscles, joint capsule ▪ Fracture ▪ Disc herniation ▪ Neurologic compromise: lesion of the brain, spinal cord, or peripheral nerve Notice that by this point in the examination we have already tested gross range of motion, lower extremity muscle strength, and integrity of most joints and bones
3. **Observation**: Posture, ease of motion, and overlying skin	Search for evidence of the following: ▪ Scars ▪ Injury, congenital anomaly, asymmetric development due to asymmetric use. ▪ Muscle atrophy may be due to neurologic deficit (radiculopathy or other CNS or PNS injury) or disuse (due to injury or pain). ▪ Ecchymosis is seen after fractures and soft tissue injuries. ▪ Systemic illness ▪ Previous surgery ▪ Infection ▪ Dermatitis ▪ Poor posture ▪ Gait abnormalities ▪ Obesity

[3] O'Kane JW. Anterior hip pain. *Am Fam Physician* 1999 Oct 15;60(6):1687-96
[4] Moore KL. Clinically Oriented Anatomy. Third Edition. Baltimore; Williams and Wilkins: 1992, page 387

Clinical assessments for the hips—*continued*

Selected assessments	Positive finding and Implications
4. <u>Walking, gait analysis</u>: Observe for symmetry, flow, balance and biomechanics	Search for: • Excessive internal/external rotation of the lower extremity • Excessive supination/pronation • Leg length inequality *Treat what you find; aim to restore symmetry and balance*
5. <u>Gaenslen's test</u>: Supine patient brings thigh to abdomen (hip hyperflexion) while affected/tested leg is allowed to come off the side of the table so that the affected/tested side can fall into extension	• This test allows hyperextension stress to be applied to the sacroiliac joint.[5] The test result is considered positive/abnormal when pain is produced in the sacroiliac joint on the side that is in extension, **suggesting a lesion or sprain of the sacroiliac joint**
3. <u>**Thomas test**</u>: Supine patient brings unaffected thigh to abdomen (hip hyperflexion) while affected/tested leg remains on table	• When the pelvis is rotated posteriorly with forced hyperflexion of the hip, the opposite hip should have sufficient flexibility to remain in extension on the surface of the table.[6] The test result is considered positive/abnormal when the thigh that should remain on table lifts off the table due to joint hypomobility, capsular restriction, or **tightness of the hip flexors—the iliacus, psoas, and rectus femoris**. • Remember: <u>T</u>homas test for <u>t</u>ightness of hip flexors • Positioning is very similar to **Gaenslen's test** (used to assess the sacroiliac joint[7]); tests can be performed in succession by switching emphasis to opposite limb
6. <u>Ober's test</u>: Patient is on the table in side posture position, with superior leg extended off table posteriorly, with or without knee flexion	• When the superior leg remains suspended in air without support (i.e., restricted motion toward adduction) this suggests **tightness of the iliotibial band (ITB)** or abductors, possibly including the tensor fasciae latae and the gluteus medius. The test is relatively insensitive, and many patients with functional tightness of the ITB will have a normal result but should be treated nonetheless
7. <u>Patrick's test, FABER, figure four test</u>: This is a common ROM and joint provocation maneuver; supine patient, Dr passively moves thigh into <u>f</u>lexion, <u>ab</u>duction, <u>e</u>xternal <u>r</u>otation with ipsilateral ankle placed at contralateral knee	• Pain or limited motion suggest **hip joint pathology such as osteoarthritis** or **regional muscle tightness**, particularly of the iliopsoas and adductors • Toward the end of the maneuver, when the ipsilateral ankle is placed at contralateral knee, the doctor can stabilize the opposite ASIS while placing downward pressure on the knee of the leg being tested; pain posteriorly at the PSIS is consistent with **lesion of the SIJ**, such as osteitis condensans ilii[8]
8. <u>Inspect patient's shoes</u>: Examination of *well worn* shoes	Analyze for wear, distribution, and symmetry: • Look for symmetry between the left and right shoe to assess for possible biomechanical faults, including unequal leg length which may result in excess wear at the heel of the longer leg • Look for excess wear on the outer posterior sole, which often correlates with tight gluteus and piriformis and unequal leg length • Excess wear on the outer sole and stress on the outer shoe correlates with a high arch and rigid foot, which may benefit from a shoe with extra shock absorption • Excess wear on the inner sole and stress on the inner shoe correlates with a hypermobile foot, fallen longitudinal arch, and foot pronation which often needs arch support and a more rigid shoe • Assess for other biomechanical faults

[5] Brier S. <u>Primary Care Orthopedics</u>. St. Louis: Mosby, 1999 page 426
[6] Brier S. <u>Primary Care Orthopedics</u>. St. Louis: Mosby, 1999 page 287
[7] Brier S. <u>Primary Care Orthopedics</u>. St. Louis: Mosby, 1999 page 426
[8] Vadivelu R, Green TP, An uncommon cause of back pain in pregnancy. *Postgrad Med J*. 2005 Jan;81(951):65-7 http://pmj.bmj.com/cgi/content/full/81/951/65

Selected orthopedic problems of the hip seen in <u>infants</u>, <u>children</u>, and <u>adolescents</u>

Problem & Presentation	Assessment & Management
<u>Developmental dysplasia of the hip</u> • Previously called congenital hip dislocation[9]: congenital-developmental acetabular deformity; completely reversible if detected early but can otherwise lead to permanent deformity, impaired function, and the need for arthroplasty • Usually diagnosed in infants before age 6 weeks • Most common in first-born females delivered from a breech position[10] • Delays in diagnosis are often attributed to 1) inadequate examination by the physician, or 2) discontinuous healthcare for the child, i.e.: lack of regular health assessments by the same physician	• <u>Ortolani test</u> ["anterior-<u>o</u>pen"]: supine infant with flexed and aBducted hip, the physician gently pulls the femur anteriorly while palpating at the trochanter for hints of anterior glide/dislocation • <u>Barlow test</u> ["<u>b</u>ackwards-closed"]: supine infant with flexed and aDDucted hip; physician gently pushes the femur posteriorly while palpating at the gluteus maximus for hints of posterior glide/dislocation • <u>Allis's sign</u> ["<u>a</u>ltitude"]: supine infant with flexed hips and knees; the inferior knee has the dislocated hip • Confirm your suspicion of congenital hip dysplasia with diagnostic ultrasound imaging before progressing to radiography[11] • Treatment is with splinting of the hip in flexion and moderate abduction (with a Pavlik harness) and is best supervised by a pediatric orthopedic surgeon[12]
<u>Septic arthritis of the hip</u> • Acute onset of painful hip and limp If the patient has new onset of non-traumatic joint pain along with fever, the clinician should assume the joint is septic and ensure that joint aspiration is performed urgently	• Classically, the patient has elevated WBC and ESR • CRP • Patient has <u>fever</u> and appears <u>ill</u> • "...joint aspiration should be performed."[13] • Emergency referral for oral/IV antimicrobials • Immune support and comprehensive musculoskeletal care • "Septic arthritis is still a life-threatening disease with a mortality of 2–5% and high morbidity."[14]
<u>Avascular necrosis (AVN) of the femoral head, Perthe's disease, Legg-Calve-Perthe's disease</u> • Idiopathic ischemic necrosis of the femoral head • 80% of affected children are between ages 4-9 y • More common in boys • Unilateral hip pain • May have knee pain • May have limp • History of lower extremity trauma is common • Hip pain in children that lasts longer than 7 days is suspicious for AVN and should generally be assessed radiographically and/or with bone scan	• Radiographs; if radiographs are normal and clinical suspicion is high order MRI or bone scan • Crutches should be used to prevent physical damage to the vulnerable necrotic tissue • **Orthopedic referral is recommended** although not all patients will require surgery and some may be managed conservatively[15] In the majority of cases, **femoral head AVN must be managed early in order to prevent later deformity and degeneration**; radiographs are a reasonable first evaluation and can be followed by bone scan[16]
<u>Apophysitis, avulsion fracture</u>[17] • Adolescent with hip pain following sudden or forceful hip muscle contraction • Localized pain and swelling • Muscle weakness	• Radiographs • Treatment may be conservative or surgical depending on severity of displacement as visualized radio-graphically; nonsurgical treatment and rest are generally sufficient

---

[9] The term "developmental dysplasia of the hip" (DDH) has officially replaced the previous term "congenital dislocation of the hip." Shaw BA, Gerardi JA, Hennrikus WL. How to avoid orthopedic pitfalls in children. *Patient Care* 1999; Feb 28: 95-116

[10] Shaw BA, Gerardi JA, Hennrikus WL. How to avoid orthopedic pitfalls in children. *Patient Care* 1999; Feb 28: 95-116

[11] Hay WW, Groothuis JR, Hayward AR, Levin ML. <u>Current Pediatric Diagnosis and Treatment, 13th edition</u>. Stamford: Appleton and Lange; 1997, pages 705-6

[12] Hay WW, Groothuis JR, Hayward AR, Levin ML. <u>Current Pediatric Diagnosis and Treatment, 13th edition</u>. Stamford: Appleton and Lange; 1997, pages 705-6

[13] Maroo S. Diagnosis of hip pain in children. *Hosp Med* 1999 Nov;60(11):788-93

[14] Zacher J, Gursche A. Regional musculoskeletal conditions: 'hip' pain. *Best Pract Res Clin Rheumatol*. 2003 Feb;17(1):71-85

[15] Souza TA. <u>Differential Diagnosis for the Chiropractor: Protocols and Algorithms</u>. Gaithersburg, Maryland: Aspen Publications. 1997 page 263

[16] "A scan should be performed in all patients with a suggestive presentation in routine roentgenograms and in cases of transient synovitis with unusual features or that fail to subside rapidly or that recur." Paterson D, Savage JP. The nuclide bone scan in the diagnosis of Perthes' disease. *Clin Orthop Relat Res*. 1986 Aug;(209):23-9

[17] "In the adolescent, acute muscle contraction about the hip can result in avulsion of an apophysis (an ossification center at the attachment of tendon to bone)." O'Kane JW. Anterior hip pain. *Am Fam Physician* 1999 Oct 15;60(6):1687-96

Selected orthopedic problems of the hip seen in <u>infants</u>, <u>children</u>, and <u>adolescents</u>—*continued*

Problem & Presentation	*Assessment & Management*
<u>Transient synovitis, irritable hip</u> ▪ Non-specific short-term inflammation and effusion of the hip joint; patient may have recent history of viral infection, and up to 10% of patients may eventually be diagnosed with RA or AVN[18] ▪ Acute onset of painful hip and limp ▪ Decreased pain with hip in flexion, abduction, and internal rotation ▪ More common in boys, age 3-6 years and generally younger than 10 years ▪ Transient synovitis (benign) must be distinguished from septic arthritis "Transient synovitis is the most common cause of acute hip pain in children three to 10 years of age."[19]	▪ The child appears *healthy* with NO FEVER; if fever is present the clinician must exclude septic arthritis with joint aspiration ▪ May have slight elevation of ESR but WBC should be normal ▪ "Radiography is indicated to exclude osseous pathological conditions"[20] and MRI may be used to help exclude septic arthritis; do not use ultrasound to differentiate transient synovitis from septic arthritis[21] ▪ Joint aspiration is indicated when septic arthritis is suspected[22] ▪ Comprehensive musculoskeletal care (described in Chapter 3), restricted exertion and weight-bearing for several weeks; continue to monitor until symptoms are resolved, generally within 2 weeks ▪ Refer for co-management or aggressively reassess if clinical presentation is unclear or if condition does not improve within 7-10 days
<u>Slipped capital femoral epiphysis (SCFE)</u> ▪ Fracture through the epiphyseal growth plate resulting in dislocation of the femoral head from the neck of the femur ▪ Seen in adolescents generally 8-17 years of age ▪ Painful non-traumatic hip pain; patient may keep the lower extremity in external rotation[23] ▪ Classic presentation is a tall overweight boy with hip pain, medial knee pain, and a painful limp ▪ *"Slipped femoral capital epiphysis is a developmental injury that must be considered in any adolescent who presents with hip pain."*[24] SCFE is the most common cause of hip pain in adolescents[25]	▪ Any hip pain or limited motion in an adolescent (8-15 years of age) warrants radiographic evaluation[26] ▪ Radiographs of both hips (bilateral SCFE in 20-40%)—"AP and frog lateral views are recommended in all children over age of 9 years with hip pain."[27] ▪ Urgent orthopedic referral: *"...the patient should be referred immediately to an orthopedist for surgical stabilization."*[28] ▪ Outpatient surgery is followed by months of limited activity SCFE can result in deformity that can progress to joint destruction if not identified and treated early

As a general rule, when a child or adolescent presents with hip pain, **most diagnoses and exclusions require radiographs**; septic arthritis must always be considered, but is less likely if the patient as no fever or other systemic manifestations and if the CBC and CRP/ESR are normal. **Blood samples for basic lab tests for infection and inflammation should be drawn on the first day of evaluation unless the diagnosis is crystal clear and the problem is managed completely;** *lab tests help ensure that you will never miss a smoldering subclinical infection that is presenting as benign musculoskeletal pain.* If what appears to be "transient synovitis" has not resolved within 10 days, the clinical reevaluation should exclude AVN and septic arthritis.

[18] Souza TA. <u>Differential Diagnosis for the Chiropractor: Protocols and Algorithms</u>. Gaithersburg, Maryland: Aspen Publications. 1997 page 265
[19] Hart JJ. Transient synovitis of the hip in children. *Am Fam Physician.* 1996 Oct;54(5):1587-91, 1595-6
[20] Maroo S. Diagnosis of hip pain in children. *Hosp Med* 1999 Nov;60(11):788-93
[21] "Ultrasound cannot be used safely to distinguish between pediatric septic hip and transient synovitis." Zamzam MM. The role of ultrasound in differentiating septic arthritis from transient synovitis of the hip in children. *J Pediatr Orthop B.* 2006 Nov;15(6):418-22
[22] Maroo S. Diagnosis of hip pain in children. *Hosp Med* 1999 Nov;60(11):788-93
[23] Shaw BA, Gerardi JA, Hennrikus WL. How to avoid orthopedic pitfalls in children. *Patient Care* 1999; Feb 28: 95-116
[24] O'Kane JW. Anterior hip pain. *Am Fam Physician* 1999 Oct 15;60(6):1687-96
[25] Maroo S. Diagnosis of hip pain in children. *Hosp Med* 1999 Nov;60(11):788-93
[26] Shaw BA, Gerardi JA, Hennrikus WL. How to avoid orthopedic pitfalls in children. *Patient Care* 1999; Feb 28: 95-116
[27] Maroo S. Diagnosis of hip pain in children. *Hosp Med* 1999 Nov;60(11):788-93
[28] O'Kane JW. Anterior hip pain. *Am Fam Physician* 1999 Oct 15;60(6):1687-96

Suggested Algorithm for the Assessment & Management of Hip Pain in Young Patients

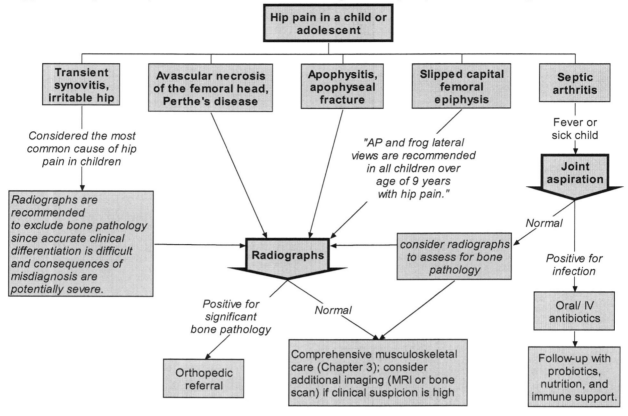

Common Serious Hip Problems in Infants, Children, and Adolescents: General Expectation of Prevalence and Probability by Age in Weeks to Years

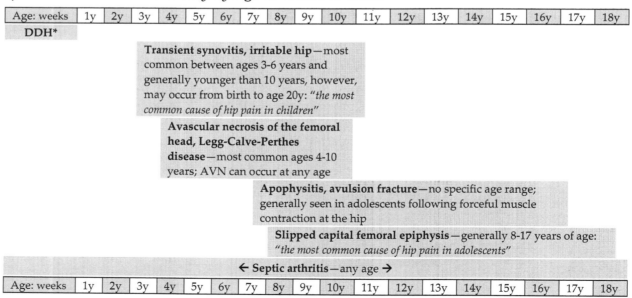

* **DDH: Developmental Dysplasia of the Hip** (previously "congenital hip dysplasia") should be diagnosed and treated before age 6 weeks.

Orthopedic Problems of the Hip and Thigh Seen Mostly in Adults

Problem & Presentation	Assessment & Management
Avascular necrosis (AVN) of the femoral head, osteonecrosis: ischemic necrosis of the femoral head ▪ Ages 20-40 years ▪ Most common in young men ▪ Unilateral hip pain ▪ Onset is generally subacute ▪ May have knee pain and/or groin pain ▪ May have limp ▪ History of trauma is common Disorders associated with AVN: Corticosteroid use, hemoglobinopathies, smoking, hyperlipidemia, alcoholism, pancreatitis, liver disease and "fat globules from the liver"[29]	▪ Limited ROM ▪ Painful hip examination with limited motion ▪ **Radiographs** ▪ Crutches ▪ **Orthopedic referral is recommended** although not all patients will require surgery and some may be managed conservatively.[30]
Fracture ▪ Femoral neck ▪ Inter-trochanteric ▪ Sub-trochanteric Predisposing factors: Elderly, history of cancer especially multiple myeloma, renal osteodystrophy, young male, hemochromatosis[31], bone cyst, osteoporosis, vitamin D deficiency, trauma, erosive joint disease (RA), alcoholism, corticosteroid use	▪ Painful hip examination, especially with weight-bearing and fulcrum-type tests—take care not to exacerbate the fracture or cause additional tissue-neurovascular injury when performing the physical examination ▪ Attempted ROM is generally painful; weight bearing is painful and/or impossible ▪ **Radiographs** ▪ Referral to orthopedic surgeon
Stress fracture ▪ *"Femoral stress fractures, particularly those of the femoral <u>neck</u>, are worrisome because of the possibility of progression to displacement and osteonecrosis of the femoral head."*[32] ▪ Overtraining athlete with deep pain in anterior hip and proximal thigh ▪ Risk is increased with malnutrition, overtraining, corticosteroid treatment, postmenopausal, hypoestrogenism **When patient safety or long-term outcome are questionable, refer the patient for evaluation by a medical specialist; better to err on the side of caution than to have the patient suffer a negative outcome and the doctor suffer unnecessary stress and liability**	▪ Pain with weight-bearing, jumping ▪ Evaluate initially with radiographs, reassess at 2-4 weeks if initial radiographs are negative ▪ Bone scan has been the assessment of choice, but MRI is now recognized as having a similar sensitivity with greater specificity[33] ▪ **Orthopedic referral is generally advised[34] since the many different types of stress fractures require specific and often surgical treatment** ▪ Stress fractures of the **femoral <u>shaft</u>** can be treated conservatively with crutches for 1 to 4 weeks and progressive resumption of activity over the next 3 months; "Stress fractures of the femoral shaft are less common and have a low complication rate … Treatment consists of protected weight-bearing for 1 to 4 weeks, followed by gradual resumption of activity."[35] ▪ Supplementation with protein, calcium, magnesium, vitamin D (2,000-4,000 IU/d), vitamin K and other nutrients for bone support is advised; systemic alkalinization[36,37,38] to promote mineral retention as discussed in Chapter 2

[29] Skinner HB, Scherger JE. Identifying structural hip and knee problems. Patient age, history, and limited examination may be all that's needed. *Postgrad Med* 1999;106(7):51-2, 55-6, 61-4
[30] Souza TA. Differential Diagnosis for the Chiropractor: Protocols and Algorithms. Gaithersburg, Maryland: Aspen Publications. 1997 page 263
[31] Eyres KS, McCloskey EV, Fern ED, et al. Osteoporotic fractures: an unusual presentation of hemochromatosis. *Bone* 1992; 13: 431-3
[32] O'Kane JW. Anterior hip pain. *Am Fam Physician* 1999 Oct 15;60(6):1687-96
[33] O'Kane JW. Anterior hip pain. *Am Fam Physician* 1999 Oct 15;60(6):1687-96
[34] O'Kane JW. Anterior hip pain. *Am Fam Physician* 1999 Oct 15;60(6):1687-96
[35] Browning KH, Donley BG. Evaluation and management of common running injuries. *Cleve Clin J Med* 2000 Jul;67(7):511-20
[36] Sebastian A, Harris ST, Ottaway JH, Todd KM, Morris RC Jr. Improved mineral balance and skeletal metabolism in postmenopausal women treated with potassium bicarbonate. *N Engl J Med.* 1994;330(25):1776-81
[37] Tucker KL, Hannan MT, Chen H, Cupples LA, Wilson PW, Kiel DP. Potassium, magnesium, and fruit and vegetable intakes are associated with greater bone mineral density in elderly men and women. *Am J Clin Nutr.* 1999;69(4):727-36
[38] Whiting SJ, Boyle JL, Thompson A, Mirwald RL, Faulkner RA. Dietary protein, phosphorus and potassium are beneficial to bone mineral density in adult men consuming adequate dietary calcium. *J Am Coll Nutr.* 2002;21(5):402-9

Femur Fractures: Overview of Assessment and Management

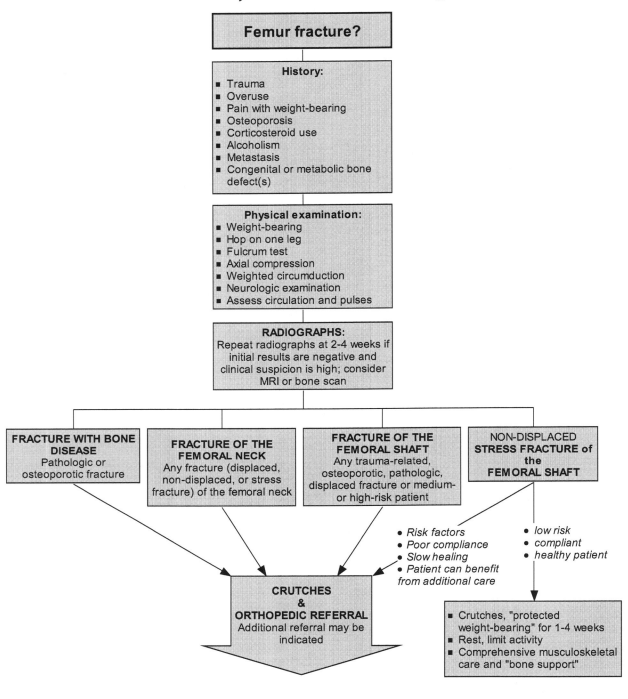

When patient safety and/or long-term outcome are in doubt, refer the patient for evaluation by an allopathic/osteopathic specialist; better to err on the side of caution than to have the patient suffer a negative outcome and the doctor suffer unnecessary stress and liability.

Rationale for referral: *protecting the patient* and/or *protecting the practitioner*—either way, referral is often good for the patient and the doctor.

Orthopedic Problems of the Hip and Thigh Seen Mostly in Adults—*continued*

Problem & Typical presentation	*Assessment & Management*
Bursitis[39] • Ischial bursitis • Subtrochanteric bursitis • Iliopectineal and iliopsoas bursitis Caused by • Compression • Direct injury • Overuse	• Pain with palpation and provocation of the affected bursa • Clinical assessment, lab tests, and monitoring to exclude infection: perform CBC and CRP, measure vital signs especially temperature • Comprehensive musculoskeletal care as described in Chapter 3 (mnemonics: "price a turn" and "bend stems"): avoid direct compression, stretch the IT band, improve lower extremity biomechanics; natural anti-inflammatory treatments, especially proteolytic enzymes
Femoral neuropathy • Neurogenic anterior thigh pain • Most commonly seen in diabetics • May also have manifestations of lumbar radiculopathy which mimic lumbar disc herniation and present with severe pain, muscle weakness, and decreased reflexes[40]	• Fasting serum glucose • Assess for intraabdominal and intrapelvic mass or pathology if no other cause for the problem can be found: consider radiographs, CT scan, ultrasound, and laboratory studies • Treat the underlying problem (e.g., diabetes) and help the nerves to heal: lipoic acid, GLA, vitamin E, vitamin B-12, etc
Hernia, "sports hernia" • "Sports hernia" refers to non-palpable hernias • Patient presents with lower abdominal soft tissue bulge, worse with heavy lifting, bearing down, Valsalva, etc. • May present as exercise-related groin pain	• Hernia examination: generally femoral in women, and inguinal in men • Herniography: radiography with contrast medium • Ultrasound imaging • Consider strangulated avascular intestine if severe; treat as medical emergency if suspected or confirmed • Comprehensive Musculoskeletal Care as described in Chapter 3, with emphasis on anti-inflammation and tissue healing • Surgery for severe, complicated, or recalcitrant cases
Iron overload, hemochromatosis • Iron overload diseases are among the most common hereditary disorders in the human population[41] • Adult patient • Pain with walking and weight-bearing • Bilateral or unilateral • Restricted motion • Mimics osteoarthritis *See diagnosis and management algorithm for iron overload in Chapter 1*	• Clinically and radiographically indistinguishable from osteoarthritis[42] • Pain and limited range of motion: weighted circumduction and anvil test • Radiographic changes: degeneration, perhaps chondrocalcinosis • Lab tests: normal ESR, CRP, with ferritin > 200 and percent saturation of transferrin greater than 45%* • **Therapeutic phlebotomy is the treatment of choice**; deferoxamine is an expensive, cumbersome, and less effective alternative • All first-degree relatives must be screened, since the condition is frequently autosomal recessive • **Iron removal therapy via phlebotomy or deferoxamine chelation is mandatory**
Joint pain due to leg length inequality • Increased compressive forces on the hip joint due to anatomic leg length inequality • Usually the "shorter" leg is the one with the painful hip because it receives more impact	• Use your tape measure from trochanter to lateral maleoli and compare to opposite side. Alternatively, order a "scanogram" (short sequential radiographic views of feet, ankle, knees, hips) or weight-bearing acetabulum-in-view hip/low back radiograph • Foot lift, heel lift; consider custom orthoses

[39] Souza TA. Differential Diagnosis for the Chiropractor: Protocols and Algorithms. Gaithersburg: Aspen Publications. 1997 page 263-4
[40] Naftulin S, Fast A, Thomas M. Diabetic lumbar radiculopathy: sciatica without disc herniation. *Spine* 1993 Dec;18(16):2419-22
[41] **Vasquez A. Musculoskeletal disorders and iron overload disease: comment on the American College of Rheumatology guidelines for the initial evaluation of the adult patient with acute musculoskeletal symptoms. *Arthritis Rheum* 1996 Oct; 39(10):1767-8**
[42] Axford JS, Bomford A, Revell P, Watt I, Williams R, Hamilton EBD. Hip arthropathy in genetic hemochromatosis: radiographic and histologic features. *Arthritis Rheum* 1991; 34: 357-61

Problem & Typical presentation	*Assessment & Management*
Meralgia paresthetica ▪ Compression of the lateral femoral cutaneous nerve, often at the inguinal ligament ▪ Patient presents with numbness and tingling in the lateral thigh ▪ Often due to prolonged sitting ▪ Associated with obesity	▪ Direct compression on lateral femoral cutaneous nerve, 1 inch inferior to ASIS ▪ Sensory changes on anterolateral thigh ▪ Abdominal examination to exclude intraabdominal pathology ▪ Comprehensive musculoskeletal care as described in Chapter 3 ▪ Avoid prolonged sitting ▪ Lose weight if necessary
Muscle strain, overuse injury, tendonitis ▪ Recent history of physical activity or overuse	▪ Pain is worse with active contraction or passive stretching of the affected muscle/tendon ▪ Comprehensive musculoskeletal care as described in Chapter 3 with an emphasis on rest, sufficient dietary protein, ice, and anti-inflammatory treatments
Osteoarthrosis, osteoarthritis ▪ Generally older patient or history of trauma ▪ Pain with walking and weight-bearing ▪ Bilateral or unilateral ▪ Restricted motion	▪ Pain and limited range of motion: weighted circumduction, anvil test ▪ Bilateral or unilateral ▪ Radiographic changes typical for degeneration but not exclusive of hemochromatosis; **rule out hemochromatosis by assessing ferritin and transferrin saturation.[43] ESR/CRP, and ferritin must be normal before osteoarthritis is diagnosed** ▪ Comprehensive musculoskeletal care as described in Chapter 3 with emphasis on the following: ▪ Glucosamine-chondroitin: 1,000-2,000 mg/d in divided doses ▪ *Uncaria guianensis/ tomentosa* ("cat's claw"): Benefits shown in knee osteoarthritis[44] ▪ Topical application of *Capsicum*: Benefits osteoarthritis[45] ▪ *Zingiber officinale* (Ginger): Reduces musculoskeletal pain[46,47] and provides relief from osteoarthritis of the knees[48] ▪ *Harpagophytum procumbens* (Devil's claw): Safety and analgesic effective for hip pain, low-back pain, and knee pain[49,50] ▪ Niacinamide: Niacinamide alleviates osteoarthritis.[51] 500 mg orally 4-6 times per day; measure liver enzymes after 3 months and yearly thereafter[52] ▪ Vitamin E, with an emphasis on gamma-tocopherol: Often benefits osteoarthritis ▪ Pancreatic/proteolytic enzymes: Analgesic, anti-inflammatory, anti-edematous benefits[53,54,55] ▪ Vitamin D3: 2,000-4,000 IU/d; periodically monitor for hypercalcemia; use extreme caution with coadministered hydrochlorothiazide or preexisting sarcoidosis or hypercalcemia

[43] Vasquez A. Musculoskeletal disorders and iron overload disease: comment on the American College of Rheumatology guidelines for the initial evaluation of the adult patient with acute musculoskeletal symptoms. *Arthritis Rheum* 1996 Oct; 39(10):1767-8

[44] Piscoya J, Rodriguez Z, Bustamante SA, Okuhama NN, Miller MJ, Sandoval M. Efficacy and safety of freeze-dried cat's claw in osteoarthritis of the knee: mechanisms of action of the species Uncaria guianensis. *Inflamm Res.* 2001 Sep;50(9):442-8

[45] McCarthy GM, McCarty DJ. Effect of topical capsaicin in the therapy of painful osteoarthritis of the hands. *J Rheumatol.* 1992;19(4):604-7

[46] Srivastava KC, Mustafa T. Ginger (Zingiber officinale) in rheumatism and musculoskeletal disorders. *Med Hypotheses* 1992 Dec;39(4):342-8

[47] Srivastava KC, Mustafa T. Ginger (Zingiber officinale) and rheumatic disorders. *Med Hypotheses.* 1989 May;29(1):25-8

[48] Altman RD, Marcussen KC. Effects of a ginger extract on knee pain in patients with osteoarthritis. *Arthritis Rheum.* 2001 Nov;44(11):2531-8

[49] Chrubasik S, Thanner J, Kunzel O, Conradt C, Black A, Pollak S. Comparison of outcome measures during treatment with the proprietary Harpagophytum extract doloteffin in patients with pain in the lower back, knee or hip. *Phytomedicine* 2002 Apr;9(3):181-94

[50] Leblan D, Chantre P, Fournie B. Harpagophytum procumbens in the treatment of knee and hip osteoarthritis. Four-month results of a prospective, multicenter, double-blind trial versus diacerhein. *Joint Bone Spine* 2000;67(5):462-7

[51] Kaufman W. Niacinamide therapy for joint mobility. Therapeutic reversal of a common clinical manifestation of the "normal" aging process. *Conn State Med J* 1953;17:584-591

[52] Gaby AR. Literature review and commentary: Niacinamide for osteoarthritis. *Townsend Letter for Doctors and Patients.* 2002: May; 32

[53] Trickett P. Proteolytic enzymes in treatment of athletic injuries. *Appl Ther.* 1964;30:647-52

[54] Walker AF, Bundy R, Hicks SM, Middleton RW. Bromelain reduces mild acute knee pain and improves well-being in a dose-dependent fashion in an open study of otherwise healthy adults. *Phytomedicine.* 2002; 9: 681-6

[55] Brien S, Lewith G, Walker A, Hicks SM, Middleton D. Bromelain as a Treatment for Osteoarthritis: a Review of Clinical Studies. *Evidence-based Complementary and Alternative Medicine.* 2004;1(3)251–257

Orthopedic Problems of the Hip and Thigh Seen Mostly in Adults—*continued*

Problem & Typical presentation	Assessment & Management
Snapping tendon, internal snapping hip, iliopsoas tendonitis ▪ Sound made by the tendon of the iliopsoas as it slides over the femoral head or iliopectineal eminence ▪ **Snap or deep clunk at the hip or flexor crease with extension of the hip** ▪ Most patients do not have pain	▪ **Snap or deep clunk at the hip or flexor crease with extension of hip** ▪ Localize and reproduce snapping sensation by contraction of the problematic muscle/tendon ▪ DDX with an intra-articular osteophyte which is radiographically visible and which is characteristically reproducible with passive joint motion ▪ Comprehensive musculoskeletal care as described in Chapter 3, also improve lower extremity biomechanics; natural anti-inflammatory treatments, especially proteolytic enzymes; begin with strengthening and stretching of the affected muscle-tendon[56]
Tear of the acetabular labrum ▪ Activity-related pain worse with extension associated with deep "clicking" and subjective joint instability	▪ Palpation of clicking with motion of hip into extension ▪ Failure of conservative treatment for 6 months in association with characteristic clinical presentation suggests diagnosis ▪ Specialized MR imaging is 90% accurate for the diagnosis ▪ Conservative treatment can be attempted; surgical arthroscopic assessment and treatment is recommended if severe or recalcitrant
Traumatic synovitis **Viral synovitis** ▪ Inflammation of the hip joint, often following trauma or viral infection ▪ Painful hip after direct injury or systemic infection ▪ Cause unknown in many cases	▪ **History with clinical assessment with palpation, ROM tests** ▪ Consider radiographs to evaluate for possible fracture, especially with history of trauma ▪ Lab tests to exclude septic arthritis ▪ Comprehensive musculoskeletal care as described in Chapter 3 (mnemonics: "price a turn" and "bend stems"): natural anti-inflammatory treatments, especially proteolytic enzymes

---

[56] Souza TA. Differential Diagnosis for the Chiropractor: Protocols and Algorithms. Gaithersburg, Maryland: Aspen Publications. 1997 page 265

Chapter 13:
Leg, Ankle, and Foot

Introduction
Degenerative and traumatic disorders of the knee are commonplace among athletes and with all populations exposed to aging (i.e., everyone). Septic and malignant disorders—as well as other differential considerations—are less common but need to be considered with each patient evaluation. Systemic disorders such as iron overload, rheumatoid arthritis, and reactive arthritis can also cause knee pain.

Topics:

1. **Knee Structures: Clinical Evaluation**
2. **Clinical Assessments and Examination Flow for the Knee**
3. **Knee Pain and Dysfunction—Regional Considerations with Clinical Implications**
4. **Trauma—Fractures and Dislocations**
   - Fracture of the femoral condyles
   - Fracture of the patella
   - Fracture of the tibial plateau
   - Patellar dislocation, patellar subluxation
5. **Trauma (acute or recurrent)—Soft Tissue Injuries and Disorders**
   - Anterior cruciate ligament sprain or rupture
   - Fibular nerve neuropraxia, peroneal neuropraxia
   - Infrapatellar bursitis
   - Lateral collateral ligament sprain or rupture
   - Medial collateral ligament sprain or rupture
   - Meniscus injuries
   - Pes anserine bursitis
   - Popliteal cyst
   - Posterior cruciate ligament sprain or rupture
   - Prepatellar bursitis
   - Traumatic bursitis
6. **Degenerative, Developmental, and Metabolic Conditions**
   - Chondromalacia patellae
   - Iron overload, hemochromatosis
   - Osgood-Schlatter disease
   - Osteoarthrosis, osteoarthritis
   - Osteochondral fragments and "joint mice"
   - Osteochondritis dissecans
   - Patellar malalignment syndrome, patellofemoral arthralgia, lateral patellar compression syndrome
   - Slipped capital femoral epiphysis
7. **Lower Extremity Biomechanical Dysfunction**

<u>**Core competencies**</u>:

- Name the two best and most commonly used tests for assessing the anterior cruciate ligament (ACL). Which test is better and why?
- McMurray's test is one of the most commonly used tests for assessing menisci. How is the test performed, and what is the sensitivity and specificity of a positive finding? Is the test clinically valuable?
- If you think your patient may have a meniscus injury, how do you decide *for* or *against* ordering an expensive MRI?
- Why must you examine the hip of an adolescent patient who presents with knee pain?

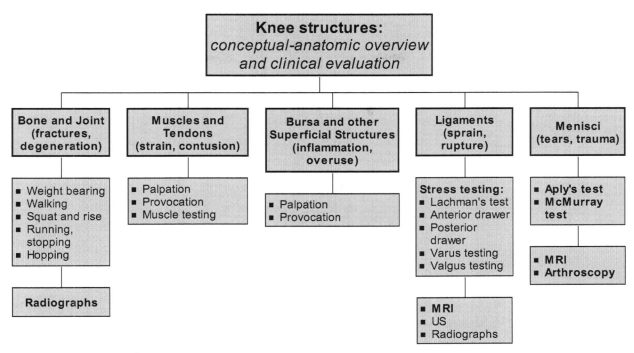

Clinical Assessments for the Knee

Selected assessments	Positive Finding and Implications
1. **History**: *See Chapter 1 for additional information*	▪ Indicators from the history (trauma, risk factors), systemic manifestations, complications, and mechanical-nonmechanical characteristics ▪ **Ask about limited motion, pain, joint locking, instability**
2. **Walking, gait analysis**: Observe for symmetry, flow, balance and biomechanics	▪ Excessive internal or external rotation of the lower extremity ▪ Excessive supination or pronation ▪ Leg length inequality ▪ Pelvic torque ▪ *Treat what you find*
3. **Squat and rise**: In the case of the knee examination, we use this test to stress the articular surfaces of the femorotibial and patellofemoral articulations, and the menisci are compressed with full knee flexion. The test requires full range of motion of the knee and full ankle dorsiflexion	Inability to perform this test may suggest the following: ▪ Patellofemoral arthritis or joint degeneration: full flexion of the knee pushes the patella into the medial femoral condyle ▪ Osteochondritis ▪ Tight quadriceps ▪ Knee effusion: inflammation, hemarthrosis, infection ▪ Meniscus injury ▪ Quadriceps weakness or lesion ▪ Neurologic deficit ▪ Tightness of the gastrosoleus and tendocalcaneus
4. **Waddle test**: From the standing position, the patient squats down onto the toes with the heels off the ground and in contact with the buttocks; the patient then waddles forward with small steps; this test provides repetitive compressive stress to the menisci and requires full knee flexion	▪ Posteromedial pain and clicking and inability to fully flex knee suggests torn posterior horn of medial meniscus ▪ Inability to fully flex the knee may be due to compression of the calf with the posterior thigh, tightness in the quads, restriction in the anterior capsule of the knee, joint effusion, intraarticular fragments of bone or cartilage

Selected assessments	Positive finding and Implications
5. **Reflexes and sensory neurologic exam**: Strength, reflexes, vibration and sensory	• Assess for neurologic injury or peripheral neuropathy which may cause altered biomechanics or proprioception • Neurogenic arthropathy (Charcot joint) • Neuropathy, radiculopathy, peroneal neuropraxia • Sensory deficit (loss of 2-point discrimination) is the single most common physical examination finding in patients with acute compartment syndrome: "...the most reliable physical finding in compartment syndrome is sensory deficit." [1]
6. **Peripheral vascular examination**: Assess distal pulses and capillary refill	• Assess for vascular injury or atherosclerosis (intermittent claudication), popliteal artery aneurysm, or the *rare* pulselessness of compartment syndrome • If peripheral vascular disease is found, assess for diabetes, hyperhomocysteinemia, hypothyroidism, hypercholesterolemia and other risk factors; manage as indicated
7. **Inspection, observation, palpation**: Look for deviations from what you know is normal, as well as asymmetry and differences between the left and right knees	• Follow-up on abnormal findings: swelling, bruising, scars, joint laxity, deformity, muscle hypertrophy or muscle atrophy
8. **Ober's test**: Patient is on the table in side posture position, with superior leg extended off table posteriorly, with or without knee flexion	• When the superior leg remains suspended in air without support (i.e., restricted motion toward adduction) this suggests **tightness of the iliotibial band (ITB)** or abductors, possibly including the tensor fasciae latae and the gluteus medius. **The test is relatively insensitive, and many patients with functional tightness of the ITB will have a normal result but should be treated nonetheless**
9. **Ballottement test**: Patient is supine with knee extended and relaxed; doctor applies anteroposterior force to patella to assess if it is floating from the surface of the femur due to joint effusion	• Application of pressure produces a tapping sensation as the floating patella contacts the femur and indicates joint effusion (accumulation of fluid within the joint capsule). Common etiologies include trauma, inflammatory arthritis, osteoarthritis, gout, infection (emergency), blood (hemarthrosis—hemophilia, torn cruciate ligaments, fracture); use patient history and joint aspiration to assess as indicated
10. **Patella grinding test**: Patient is supine with knee extended and relaxed; doctor applies anteroposterior force to the patella while either 1) the doctor moves the patella in different directions, or 2) the patient contracts the quadriceps	• Pain or crepitus suggests cartilage degeneration at the patellofemoral joint
11. **Valgus stress**: Patient's knee is slightly flexed as the doctor applies stress to the lateral aspect of the knee while stabilizing the ankle	• Valgus motion at the knee indicates sprain/rupture of the medial collateral ligaments; concomitant injury of the medial meniscus may be present, perhaps with tear of the anterior cruciate ("unhappy triad")
12. **Varus stress**: Patient's knee is slightly flexed as the doctor applies stress to the medial aspect of the knee while stabilizing the ankle	• Varus motion at the knee indicates sprain/rupture of the lateral collateral ligaments and/or iliotibial band: may have injury to common peroneal nerve—test anterior and lateral muscles and toe extensors

---

[1] Edwards S. Acute compartment syndrome. *Emerg Nurse*. 2004 Jun;12(3):32-8 http://www.nursing-standard.co.uk/archives/en_pdfs/envol12-03/env12n3p3238.pdf

Clinical assessments for the knee—*continued*

Clinical assessments	*Positive finding and Implications*
13. **Bounce test**: Patient supine with knee flexed and heel in doctor's hand; doctor allows knee to drop into extension. The purpose of the test is to assess for intraarticular lesions	Inability to achieve complete knee extension and hyperextension: ▪ Meniscus injury ▪ Joint effusion ▪ Osteocartilaginous fragments ("joint mice") such as with osteochondritis dissecans ▪ False positive results will be seen in patients with tight hamstrings, capsular restrictions, or muscle guarding
14. **Thomas test**: Supine patient brings unaffected thigh to abdomen (hip hyperflexion) while affected/tested leg remains on table. When the pelvis is rotated posteriorly with forced hyperflexion of the hip, the opposite hip should have sufficient extensibility to remain in extension on the surface of the table[2]	▪ The test result is considered positive/abnormal when the thigh that should remain on table lifts off the table due to joint hypomobility, capsular restriction, or tightness of the hip flexors—the iliacus, psoas, rectus femoris. The relevance of this test when assessing knee pain is that biomechanical faults at the hip may induce compensatory biomechanical problems at the knee (especially in athletes) and *vice versa* ▪ This test is very similar to Gaenslen's test, which is performed for sacroiliac joint problems. In Gaenslen's test, the thigh of the affected/tested leg is allowed to come off the table and fall into hyperextension, allowing stress to be applied to the sacroiliac joint[3]
15. **Anterior drawer tests**: Supine patient with knee flexed to 90° and foot flat on table; doctor pulls straight at proximal tibia with vector parallel with femur. Assesses anterior cruciate ligament (ACL); always compare side-to-side	▪ In patients with intact ligaments, anterior translation of the tibia under the femoral condyles is tightly controlled by the ACL ▪ Anterior glide of tibia of more than 1 cm is positive test and is highly suggestive of ACL injury ▪ May have false negative with hamstring spasm
16. **Slocum test**: Essentially the same as the anterior drawer test, just with the addition of external or internal rotation to assess the medial and lateral collateral ligaments (MCL and LCL), respectively	Compare right knee to left knee; asymmetric anterior glide of tibia indicates injury to the: ▪ ACL with anterior translation greater than 1 cm ▪ MCL with increased translation of the tibia and external rotation of the leg ▪ LCL with increased translation of the tibia and internal rotation of the leg
17. **Lachman's test**: Essentially the same as the anterior drawer test, yet with less knee flexion (only 10-20° rather than 90°); may need to stabilize femur by placing anteroposterior pressure at distal femur Always compare sides.	▪ Anterior glide of tibia is indicative of ACL injury; may also have injury to the MCL and ITB ▪ Less likely than the anterior drawer test to have false negative with hamstring spasm ▪ **Considered the best test for the ACL and is superior to the anterior drawer test[4]**
18. **Posterior drawer test**: Supine patient with knee flexed to 90° and foot on the table; doctor pushes straight posteroanterior at proximal tibia. Always compare sides	▪ Posterior glide of tibia indicates posterior cruciate ligament injury ▪ May have false negative result with excess tightness of the quadriceps

[2] Brier S. Primary Care Orthopedics. St. Louis: Mosby, 1999 page 287
[3] Brier S. Primary Care Orthopedics. St. Louis: Mosby, 1999 page 426
[4] Magee DJ. Orthopedic Physical Assessment. Third edition. Philadelphia: WB Saunders, 1997 page 542

Clinical assessments for the knee—*continued*

Selected assessments	Positive finding and Implications
19. **Sag sign**[5], **"Gravity sign near extension" with "active reduction"**: Patient supine on table with 15 cm object under distal femur to create 20-40° of knee flexion[6]; this is basically a reverse Lachman's test with the posterior force on the tibia being provided by gravity	▪ A positive result with this test indicates a tear/lesion of the posterior cruciate ligament ▪ Proximal tibia will be abnormally posterior (compare to opposite knee) and the lower surface of the knee will be concave (rather than the normal convex); abnormalities will normalize with quadriceps contraction
20. **McMurray test**: Patient supine, ❶ begin test with knee and hip fully flexed so that heel touches buttock; ❷ **doctor then extends the hip and knee while** *internally* **rotating the leg and placing** *valgus* **stress at the knee to stress the** *lateral* **meniscus**; ❸ return to flexed hip and knee position; ❹ **doctor then extends the hip and knee while** *externally* **rotating the leg and placing** *varus* **stress at the knee to stress the** *medial* **meniscus**[7]; the procedure can be repeated multiple times[8] ▪ *Remember: the heel points to the injured meniscus* ▪ *VaLgus stress for Lateral meniscus*	▪ Pain, clicking, or locking as the knee is being extended suggests meniscal injury ▪ Even though this is a commonly performed test, clinicians should be aware that *"there is no adequate clinical test available"* for the diagnosis of meniscus injuries.[9] **The McMurray test has a sensitivity of only 53 percent and a specificity of only 59 percent**[10]; thus negative result does not exclude meniscal injury and a positive result does not necessarily imply that the patient has a meniscal injury
21. **Apley grinding test**: Distraction and compression of the knee when the patient is prone with knee is 90° flexed	▪ Pain exacerbated by distraction suggests ligament injury ▪ Pain exacerbated by compression and rotational grinding suggests meniscus injury or damage to articular surface
22. **Inspect patient's shoes**: Examination of *well worn* shoes; analyze for wear distribution and symmetry	▪ Look for symmetry between the left and right shoe to assess for possible biomechanical faults, including unequal leg length which may result in excess wear at the heel of the longer leg ▪ Look for excess wear on the outer posterior sole, which often correlates with tight gluteus and piriformis and unequal leg length ▪ Excess wear on the outer sole and stress on the outer shoe correlates with a high arch and rigid foot, which may benefit from a shoe with extra shock absorption ▪ Excess wear on the inner sole and stress on the inner shoe correlates with a fallen longitudinal arch and hypermobile foot, which often needs arch support and a more rigid shoe ▪ Assess for other biomechanical faults

---

[5] Magee DJ. Orthopedic Physical Assessment. Third edition. Philadelphia: WB Saunders, 1997 page 546
[6] Tandeter HB, Shvartzman P. Acute knee injuries: use of decision rules for selective radiograph ordering. *Am Fam Physician* 1999 Dec;60(9):2599-608
[7] Calmbach WL, Hutchens M. Evaluation of patients presenting with knee pain: Part I. History, physical examination, radiographs, and laboratory tests. *Am Fam Physician.* 2003 Sep 1;68(5):907-12 http://www.aafp.org/afp/20030901/907.html
[8] Johnson MW. Acute Knee Effusions: A Systematic Approach to Diagnosis. *American Family Physician* 2000 Apr; 61:2391-400. http://www.aafp.org/afp/20000415/2391.html
[9] Smith BW, Green GA. Acute knee injuries: Part II. Diagnosis and management. *Am Fam Physician* 1995 Mar;51(4):799-806
[10] "The McMurray test had a sensitivity of 53 percent and a specificity of 59 percent." Huffman GB. Reliability of Clinical Examination of a Painful Knee. *American Family Physician* 2002; March 15 http://www.aafp.org/afp/20020315/tips/2.html

Suggested examination flow for the knee

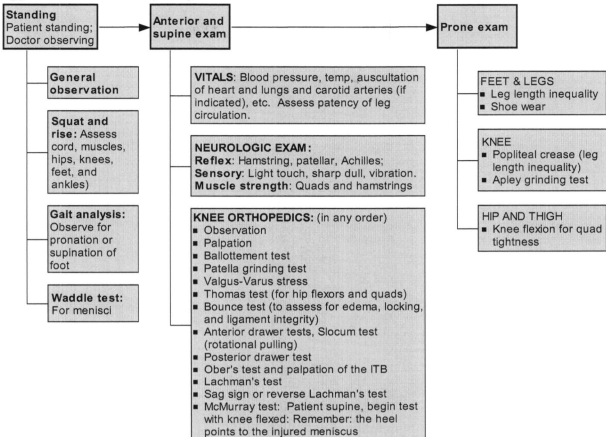

Standing	*Anterior-supine*	*Prone*

1. General observation
2. Squat and rise
3. Gait analysis: observe for pronation or supination of foot
4. Waddle test for menisci
	1. *Vital signs*: Blood pressure, temp, auscultation of heart and lungs and carotid arteries (if indicated), etc. Assess patency of leg circulation
	2. *Neurologic exam*: Reflex, sensory, muscle strength
	3. *Knee orthopedics*:
	  1) Observation
	  2) Palpation
	  3) Ballottement test
	  4) Patella grinding test
	  5) Valgus stress
	  6) Varus stress
	  7) **Thomas test** (for hip flexors and quads)
	  8) **Bounce test** (to assess for edema, locking, and ligament integrity)
	  9) **Anterior drawer tests,** Slocum test (rotational pulling)
	  10) **Posterior drawer test**
	  11) **Lachman's test**
	  12) **Sag sign or reverse Lachman's test**
	  13) **McMurray test**: Patient supine, begin test with knee flexed: *Remember: the heel points to the injured meniscus*
		1. *Feet and legs*: Leg length inequality, Shoe wear
		2. *Knee*: Popliteal crease (leg length inequality), **Apley grinding test**
		3. *Hip and thigh*: knee flexion for quad tightness

Knee Pain and Dysfunction—*Regional Considerations with Clinical Implications*

Description/pathophysiology:

- Injuries to the osseous, cartilaginous, meniscal, ligamentous, muscular, and soft tissues are briefly surveyed:
  - **Bones**: **Fractures** are assessed with radiographs and generally referred for orthopedic co-management unless the clinician is skilled in casting and willing to accept the associated medicolegal risks; nutritional supplementation with calcium, magnesium, vitamin D, vitamin K, and other "bone supporting nutrients" expedites healing and helps prevent recurrence.
  - **Cartilage**: For most degenerative disorders of cartilage such as the prototype—**osteoarthritis**, Comprehensive Musculoskeletal Care (Chapter 3) is generally sufficient, especially with emphasis on physiologic doses of vitamin D3 to retard cartilage degeneration, glucosamine and chondroitin to support glycosaminoglycan synthesis, niacinamide to promote chondrocyte rejuvenation, proteolytic enzymes for anti-inflammation, and phytomedicinals such as willow and *Uncaria* for symptomatic relief. A more severe form of osteocartilaginous degeneration known as **osteochondritis dissecans** may be managed surgically or nonsurgically depending on location and severity; orthopedic surgical consultation is reasonable to ensure patient care and minimize professional liability. Clinicians must exclude **life-threatening hemochromatosis** by measuring serum ferritin (reviewed in Chapter 1) before making a diagnosis of osteoarthritis. Other metabolic disorders such as **gout, pseudogout** (**CPPD, calcium pyrophosphate dihydrate deposition disease**), **iron overload**, and the **iatrogenic acute hyperuricemic gout** precipitated classically by the use of diuretics in a diabetic patient with renal insufficiency.
  - **Menisci**: Menisci are unfortunately easy to injure and difficult to heal; they are particularly difficult and/or expensive to diagnose, since no adequate clinical examinations exist and since the best diagnostic tool—MRI—can easily cost several hundred or a few thousand dollars. Pain along the joint line is the most consistent finding in patients with **meniscal injuries**; the famous McMurray tests appears to have a sensitivity and specificity that barely exceed 50%, thus making its clinical usefulness perhaps not much better than that of a coin flip. Comprehensive Musculoskeletal Care (with an emphasis on proprioceptive retraining, glucosamine sulfate, and *Uncaria*/niacinamide) may be sufficient if the disability is mild and the patient is not a competitive athlete; otherwise, surgery may provide some benefit. *Meniscal repair* appears superior to *meniscectomy* for preserving function and reducing pain and degeneration.[11]
  - **Ligaments**: Injury or rupture of the extraarticular ligaments (MCL and LCL) can generally be nonsurgically managed; rupture of the intraarticular ACL and PCL may require surgery, especially for athletic and active patients.
  - **Muscles**: Muscles of the quadriceps affect knee function, and muscles proximal and distal to the knee may be affected by injury or various disorders culminating in muscle necrosis. The majority of mild-moderate **muscle tears and contusions** are managed non-surgically. If *muscle injury* progresses to the point of *muscle destruction* (**rhabdomyolysis**) then the patient must be monitored for the **renal failure** that can result from excess myoglobin, which is directly nephrotoxic especially if the patient is dehydrated or if the urine is acidic.[12] Elevations of serum creatine kinase may be used to estimate the presence and severity of muscle injury; elevated myoglobin in urine causes the urine to become dark and suggests the need to have the patient immediately evaluated for rhabdomyolysis and impending renal failure, which may be treated with forced diuresis and hemodialysis.[13] In outpatient settings, lab tests should generally *not* be performed because by the time results are available the patient with acute compartment syndrome will have already suffered permanent injury; surgical intervention should occur within six hours of onset. Causes of muscle damage other than direct trauma include dermatomyositis, polymyositis, ischemic infarction as with myocardial infarction or compartment syndrome, extreme overexertion, hypothyroid myopathy, acute alcohol intoxication, anticoagulant drugs (predisposing to intracompartmental bleeding), specific insect and snake bites, tourniquet use, compression due to a tight-fitting bandage, brace, or cast, and drug effects—particularly the statin

---

[11] "Medial meniscal repair offers a better chance than partial meniscectomy to preserve the articular cartilage of the medial compartment." Aglietti P, Zaccherotti G, De Biase P, Taddei I. A comparison between medial meniscus repair, partial meniscectomy, and normal meniscus in anterior cruciate ligament reconstructed knees. *Clin Orthop.* 1994 Oct;(307):165-73
[12] "The diagnosis of rhabdomyolysis was made through clinical and laboratory findings (creatine kinase activity of 26320 IU/l). The initial treatment consisted of fluid replacement and forced diuresis... Partial recovery of renal function was recorded, after ten hemodialysis sessions." Daher Ede F, Silva Junior GB, Brunetta DM, Pontes LB, Bezerra GP. Rhabdomyolysis and acute renal failure after strenuous exercise and alcohol abuse: case report and literature review. *Sao Paulo Med J.* 2005 Jan 2;123(1):33-7. http://www.scielo.br/pdf/spmj/v123n1/a08v1231.pdf
[13] "The diagnosis of rhabdomyolysis was made through clinical and laboratory findings (creatine kinase activity of 26320 IU/l). The initial treatment consisted of fluid replacement and forced diuresis... Partial recovery of renal function was recorded, after ten hemodialysis sessions." Daher Ede F, Silva Junior GB, Brunetta DM, Pontes LB, Bezerra GP. Rhabdomyolysis and acute renal failure after strenuous exercise and alcohol abuse: case report and literature review. *Sao Paulo Med J.* 2005 Jan 2;123(1):33-7. http://www.scielo.br/pdf/spmj/v123n1/a08v1231.pdf

drugs.[14] **Muscle imbalances**—most commonly characterized by a relatively weak vastus medialis and a relatively overdeveloped vastus lateralis—can cause knee pain by placing excess lateral force on the patella and promoting cartilage degeneration at the lateral aspect of the patellofemoral joint, and by creating excess tension in the iliotibial band (ITB) ; typically seen in runners and cyclists, **lateral patellar compression syndrome** can easily be treated with a combination of vastus medialis strengthening, ITB stretching, and botanical and nutritional support for damaged cartilage.

- o **Other soft tissues, bursa, etc**: Assess for infection and systemic disease; otherwise treat nutritionally, botanically, manually, and with appropriate and multifaceted exercise, ergonomic, and proprioceptive interventions.

Complications:
- Secondary injury due to biomechanical compensation
- Social and athletic isolation
- Degeneration
- Chronic disability and pain

Clinical presentations:
- Knee pain
- Subjective instability
- Locking
- Weakness due to pain or instability
- Swelling, effusion

Major differential diagnoses:
- CPPD: calcium pyrophosphate dihydrate deposition disease: pseudogout
- Gout
- Hemochromatosis
- Rheumatic disease: rheumatoid arthritis, lupus, ankylosing spondylitis, others
- Septic arthritis

Clinical assessment:
- History: Get the major attributes, assess for systemic manifestations, complications, indicators from the history, and the mechanical or nonmechanical nature of the problem.
  - o *What exactly is the problem? Other than pain, what other symptoms are present that will help guide the diagnosis and therefore treatment?*
    - **Pain, stiffness, grinding**—these are mechanical symptoms consistent with cartilage degeneration
    - **Locking, catching**—suggests osteocartilaginous fragments (osteochondritis dissecans: OD) or meniscus injury
    - **Snapping**—suggests tendonitis or suggests osteocartilaginous fragments (OD) or meniscus injury
    - **Swelling, joint effusion**—excess synovial fluid can be removed with a large-bore needle; chemical or microscopic analysis helps to distinguish inflammation from crystalline arthropathy from infection. "Knee swelling within four to six hours of injury is indicative of hemarthrosis."[15]
    - **Instability or weakness or "knee giving out from under you"**—suggests osteocartilaginous fragments (OD) or meniscus injury, but also consider transient ischemic attacks (TIA), hypoglycemia, or neuromuscular problem
    - **Numbness, tingling**—suggests neuropathy or nerve compression
  - o *Where is the pain felt?*
    - Internal / External: Inside the joint, or in the surrounding tendons ligaments, bursa, muscles?
    - Anterior / Posterior
    - Lateral / Medial

---

[14] Edwards S. Acute compartment syndrome. *Emerg Nurse*. 2004 Jun;12(3):32-8 http://www.nursing-standard.co.uk/archives/en_pdfs/envol12-03/env12n3p3238.pdf
[15] Johnson MW. Acute knee effusions: a systematic approach to diagnosis. *Am Fam Physician*. 2000 Apr 15;61(8):2391-400

- ▪ Radiating pain, pain elsewhere in body
  - ○ **Indicators from the history:** Past injuries and mechanism of injury: *examples*
    - ▪ **Hyperextension, sudden deceleration or cutting move**—ACL tear, patella injury
    - ▪ **Valgus force**—MCL injury, also consider ACL and medial menisci
    - ▪ **Repetitive overuse**—Chondromalacia patella, degeneration, soft tissue injury, bursitis, patellar tracking problems
    - ▪ **Frequent kneeling, squatting, hyperflexion**—bursitis, injury to posterior aspect of menisci, chondromalacia patella
    - ▪ Other diagnoses or health problems such as diabetes, asthma, hypothyroidism, hypercholesterolemia?
    - ▪ Chronic analgesic use may mask pain and cause patient and doctor to underestimate the amount of impairment and tissue damage.
- Physical examination: May be difficult to interpret in the acute knee due to generalized pain and factors which obstruct mechanical evaluation of the knee, such as joint effusion and muscle spasm. **See clinical assessments outlined previously.** As mentioned previously, the most chronic and troublesome of knee injuries—injuries to the menisci—are the most difficult to assess clinically, and yet the most accurate imaging assessment—MRI— is prohibitively expensive for many patients.

Imaging & laboratory assessments:

- **Radiographic considerations** include the following:
  - ○ Acute trauma with probability of fracture
  - ○ Do not rely on regular "straight" anteroposterior (AP) weight-bearing radiographs to demonstrate degenerative arthritis of the knees. The regular AP view will often be normal even in patients with moderately severe activity-limiting knee degeneration. Non-weightbearing views will only show severe long-standing arthritis, fractures, tumors, but are often useless when evaluating knee pain. The best standard radiographic views of the knee are ❶ lateral, ❷ AP with 30 degrees of knee flexion, ❸ skyline (previously "sunrise") view of the patellofemoral articulation with 30 degrees of knee flexion.[16]
  - ○ Use stress views in children to differentiate ligament injuries from (epi)physeal fractures
  - ○ **Criteria for the selection of patients to undergo radiographic evaluation for fracture include:**[17]
    - ✓ **Local tenderness at the head of fibula or patella**
    - ✓ **Inability to flex the knee to 90°**
    - ✓ **Age >55 years**
    - ✓ **Inability to bear weight or walk >4 steps**
    - ✓ **Blunt trauma or fall with age <12 years or >50 years**
- **MRI** is used for the evaluation of meniscus injuries and ligament injuries
  - ❖ Additional considerations with the use of MRI are: 1) The cost: $600-$1,200, and 2) the usefulness of the information: What are to going to do if you get a "positive" finding—surgery or simply more conservative care? Recall that orthoscopic surgery for knee osteoarthritis is no better than placebo[18] despite its overuse and billion-dollar expense.[19]
- **Ultrasound** can provide accurate imaging for some ligament injuries and is less expensive than MRI and less radioactive than radiography.[20]

Clinical management:

- Referral if clinical outcome is unsatisfactory or if serious complications rise.
- For acute injury to the knee with hemarthrosis, joint aspiration is recommended to reduce the painful pressure and to lessen possible intraarticular damage and adhesions that may result from accumulation of blood and resultant free-radical damage.

---

[16] "...we recommend that a single skyline view in 30 degrees flexion is adequate and should be a standard investigation in knee disorders. We also stress the importance of weight-bearing PA radiograph in 30 degrees knee flexion for adequate assessment in all patients with suspected arthritis." Bhatnagar S, Carey-Smith R, Darrah C, Bhatnagar P, Glasgow MM. Evidence-based practice in the utilization of knee radiographs-A survey of all members of the British Orthopaedic Association. Int Orthop. 2006 Oct;30(5):409-11
[17] Tandeter HB, Shvartzman P. Acute knee injuries: use of decision rules for selective radiograph ordering. *Am Fam Physician* 1999 Dec;60(9):2599-608
[18] Moseley JB, O'Malley K, Petersen NJ, Menke TJ, Brody BA, Kuykendall DH, Hollingsworth JC, Ashton CM, Wray NP. A controlled trial of arthroscopic surgery for osteoarthritis of the knee. *N Engl J Med* 2002 Jul 11;347(2):81-8
[19] Gina Kolata. A Knee Surgery for Arthritis Is Called Sham. *The New York Times*, July 11, 2002
[20] "We established a method of diagnosing pathologic conditions of both the anterior cruciate ligament (ACL) and the posterior cruciate ligament (PCL) by using ultrasound... This is a safe and an effective method of determining the rupture of ACL and PCL." Suzuki S, Kasahara K, Futami T, Iwasaki R, Ueo T, Yamamuro T. Ultrasound diagnosis of pathology of the anterior and posterior cruciate ligaments of the knee joint. *Arch Orthop Trauma Surg.* 1991;110(4):200-3

Therapeutic considerations:

- Treatment must be based on the underlying disorder, a few of which were mentioned previously and more of which are listed in the following sections. Use the concepts listed under Comprehensive Musculoskeletal Care in Chapter 3 as appropriate.

- Avoid activities and exercises that create significant biomechanical stress. For example, use cycling (midrange motion with no impact) instead of running (repetitive impact). Many yoga postures involve extreme knee flexion in squatting and kneeling positions and may promote damage to the menisci.

- Bracing, wraps and crutches[21] with "physical therapy" are sufficient treatment for grade 3 sprains of the collateral ligaments.[22] Posterolateral injuries, complex/combined injuries, and other injuries are subject to orthopedic medical consultation and possible surgical reconstruction. Snug bandages/wraps may help to reduce swelling and can help to provide support for injured tissues. Care must be utilized to avoid induction of arterial, venous, or lymphatic obstruction.

- Ice and warmth: Until 48-72 hours after injury: apply ice or cold pack for 10 minutes each 30-60 minutes for reduction in pain and inflammation. After 48-72 hours post-injury: apply gentle heat as needed for the relief of pain and reduction in muscle spasm.

- Look for leg length inequalities and biomechanical faults.

- Dextrose prolotherapy may provide benefit for degenerative knees and ligamentous laxity.[23,24]

- Proprioceptive rehabilitation: Proprioceptive defects are common in patients with chronic low-back pain, neck pain, knee pain and arthritis[25], and ankle instability. Prophylactic proprioceptive rehabilitation programs have been proven to reduce the incidence of knee and ankle injuries and should be utilized by all athletes desiring to remain or become injury-free.

- Optimize hormonal balance in women: Women are 4-6 times more likely to sustain knee injuries than are men when participating in athletic activities. The increased incidence of knee injuries may be due to any combination of predisposing factors, including biomechanical/structural issues (e.g., increased Q angle) and hormonal fluctuations.[26] Progesterone appears to impair neuromuscular coordination while estrogen increases ligamentous laxity; sports-induced knee injuries occur more often in women during the premenstrual phase (rise in progesterone) and are less common during menses (when progesterone and estradiol are both lower and more stable). Attention to optimizing hormonal function with dietary, botanical, lifestyle, or pharmaceutical interventions may thereby reduce the risk for recurrent knee problems in women.

- Botanical medicines and nutritional supplementation: Tailor the selection, dose, and combinations to the patient's size, age, and other clinical characteristics.
    - Niacinamide: Niacinamide alleviates osteoarthritis pain.[27,28,29,30] The standard dose of 500 mg given orally 6 times per day is more effective than 1,000 mg 3 times per day. Hepatic dysfunction is rare when daily doses are kept below 3,000 mg per day; measure liver enzymes after 3 months of treatment and yearly thereafter.[31]
    - Glucosamine sulfate and chondroitin sulfate: Glucosamine and chondroitin are the "building blocks" from which cartilage is built and oral supplementation is intended to enhance cartilage anabolism and to thus counteract the enhanced cartilage catabolism seen in destructive arthritic processes. The adult dose of glucosamine sulfate is generally 1500-2000 mg per day in divided doses, and the dose of chondroitin sulfate is approximately 1000 mg daily; these treatments can be used singly, in combination, and with other treatments.
    - Vitamin C: Doses of 1-2 grams per day have been suggested to reduce pain and the need for surgery in patients with low-back pain by improving disc integrity, and increased vitamin C

[21] Joyce BM, Kirby RL. Canes, crutches and walkers. *Am Fam Physician* 1991 Feb;43(2):535-42
[22] "We recommend nonoperative, conservative management of isolated grade III collateral ligament sprains for four to eight weeks, with emphasis on physical therapy and bracing during the rehabilitative period." Smith BW, Green GA. Acute knee injuries: Part II. Diagnosis and management. *Am Fam Physician* 1995 Mar;51(4):799-806
[23] Reeves KD, Hassanein KM. Long-term effects of dextrose prolotherapy for anterior cruciate ligament laxity. *Altern Ther Health Med*. 2003 May-Jun;9(3):58-62
[24] Reeves KD, Hassanein K. Randomized prospective double-blind placebo-controlled study of dextrose prolotherapy for knee osteoarthritis with or without ACL laxity. *Altern Ther Health Med*. 2000 Mar;6(2):68-74, 77-80
[25] Callaghan MJ, Selfe J, Bagley PJ, Oldham JA. The Effects of Patellar Taping on Knee Joint Proprioception. *J Athl Train*. 2002 Mar;37(1):19-24
[26] Hewett TE. Neuromuscular and hormonal factors associated with knee injuries in female athletes. Strategies for intervention. *Sports Med* 2000;29(5):313-27
[27] Kaufman W. Niacinamide therapy for joint mobility. Therapeutic reversal of a common clinical manifestation of the "normal" aging process. *Conn State Med J* 1953;17:584-591
[28] Kaufman W. The use of vitamin therapy to reverse certain concomitants of aging. *J Am Geriatr Soc* 1955;3:927-936
[29] Jonas WB, Rapoza CP, Blair WF. The effect of niacinamide on osteoarthritis: a pilot study. *Inflamm Res* 1996 Jul;45(7):330-4
[30] McCarty MF, Russell AL. Niacinamide therapy for osteoarthritis--does it inhibit nitric oxide synthase induction by interleukin 1 in chondrocytes? *Med Hypotheses*. 1999;53(4):350-60
[31] Gaby AR. Literature review and commentary: Niacinamide for osteoarthritis. *Townsend Letter for Doctors and Patients*. 2002: May; 32

intake is also associated with improved joint health and musculoskeletal function; "**A 3-fold reduction in risk of OA progression was found for both the middle tertile and highest tertile of vitamin C intake. This related predominantly to a reduced risk of cartilage loss. Those with high vitamin C intake also had a reduced risk of developing knee pain.**"[32]

o *Uncaria guianensis* and *Uncaria tomentosa* ("cat's claw", "una de gato"): Analgesic and anti-inflammatory benefits have been shown in knee osteoarthritis[33] and rheumatoid arthritis.[34]

o Topical application of *Capsicum annuum*, *Capsicum frutescens* (Cayenne pepper, hot chili pepper): Controlled clinical trials have conclusively demonstrated capsaicin's ability to deplete sensory fibers of substance P to thus reduce pain in diabetic neuropathy, chronic low back pain, chronic neck pain, osteoarthritis, rheumatoid arthritis, notalgia paresthetica, reflex sympathetic dystrophy, and cluster headache (intranasal application).

o *Boswellia serrata*: Boswellia inhibits 5-lipoxygenase with no apparent effect on cyclooxygenase[35] and has been shown effective in the treatment of knee osteoarthritis[36] as well as asthma and ulcerative colitis. When used as monotherapy, the target dose is approximately 150 mg of boswellic acids TID (thrice daily).

o *Zingiber officinale* (Ginger): Ginger is a well known spice and food with a long history of use as an anti-inflammatory, anti-nausea, and gastroprotective agent[37], and components of ginger have been shown to reduce production of the leukotriene LTB4 by inhibiting 5-lipoxygenase and to reduce production of the prostaglandin PGE2 by inhibiting cyclooxygenase.[38,39] Ginger has been shown to safely reduce nonspecific musculoskeletal pain[40,41] and to provide relief from knee osteoarthritis[42], migraine headaches, and nausea/vomiting of pregnancy.

o *Harpagophytum procumbens* (Devil's claw): The safety and analgesic effectiveness of Harpagophytum has been established in patients with hip pain, low-back pain, and knee pain.[43,44,45]

o Willow bark (*Salix* spp): Numerous studies—especially among patients with low-back pain—have validated the analgesic and anti-inflammatory benefits of willow bark extract.[46,47,48] Contraindications to the use of willow include aspirin/salicylate allergy and perhaps pregnancy, use of anticoagulant medication, or impending surgery.[49,50] The daily dose is generally kept below 240 mg of salicin, and products should include other components of the whole plant.

o Vitamin E, with an emphasis on gamma-tocopherol: Vitamin E as mixed tocopherols has anti-oxidant and anti-inflammatory benefits; clinically, vitamin E supplementation appears to reduce pain and inflammation in patients with joint disorders including knee osteoarthritis.

o Pancreatic/proteolytic enzymes: Orally-administered pancreatic and proteolytic enzymes are absorbed from the gastrointestinal tract into the systemic circulation[51,52] to exert analgesic, anti-inflammatory, anti-edematous benefits with therapeutic relevance for acute and chronic musculoskeletal disorders, especially knee osteoarthritis.[53,54,55,56]

[32] "A 3-fold reduction in risk of OA progression was found for both the middle tertile and highest tertile of vitamin C intake. This related predominantly to a reduced risk of cartilage loss. Those with high vitamin C intake also had a reduced risk of developing knee pain." McAlindon TE, Jacques P, Zhang Y, Hannan MT, Aliabadi P, Weissman B, Rush D, Levy D, Felson DT. Do antioxidant micronutrients protect against the development and progression of knee osteoarthritis? *Arthritis Rheum*. 1996 Apr;39(4):648-56

[33] Piscoya J, Rodriguez Z, Bustamante SA, Okuhama NN, Miller MJ, Sandoval M. Efficacy and safety of freeze-dried cat's claw in osteoarthritis of the knee: mechanisms of action of the species Uncaria guianensis. *Inflamm Res*. 2001 Sep;50(9):442-8

[34] "This small preliminary study demonstrates relative safety and modest benefit to the tender joint count of a highly purified extract from the pentacyclic chemotype of UT in patients with active RA taking sulfasalazine or hydroxychloroquine." Mur E, Hartig F, Eibl G, Schirmer M. Randomized double blind trial of an extract from the pentacyclic alkaloid-chemotype of uncaria tomentosa for the treatment of rheumatoid arthritis. *J Rheumatol*. 2002 Apr;29(4):678-81

[35] Safayhi H, Mack T, Sabieraj J, Anazodo MI, Subramanian LR, Ammon HP. Boswellic acids: novel, specific, nonredox inhibitors of 5-lipoxygenase. *J Pharmacol Exp Ther* 1992 Jun;261(3):1143-6

[36] Kimmatkar N, Thawani V, Hingorani L, Khiyani R. Efficacy and tolerability of Boswellia serrata extract in treatment of osteoarthritis of knee--a randomized double blind placebo controlled trial. *Phytomedicine*. 2003 Jan;10(1):3-7

[37] Langner E, Greifenberg S, Gruenwald J. Ginger: history and use. *Adv Ther* 1998 Jan-Feb;15(1):25-44

[38] Kiuchi F, Iwakami S, Shibuya M, Hanaoka F, Sankawa U. Inhibition of prostaglandin and leukotriene biosynthesis by gingerols and diarylheptanoids. *Chem Pharm Bull* (Tokyo) 1992 Feb;40(2):387-91

[39] Tjendraputra E, Tran VH, Liu-Brennan D, Roufogalis BD, Duke CC. Effect of ginger constituents and synthetic analogues on cyclooxygenase-2 enzyme in intact cells. *Bioorg Chem* 2001 Jun;29(3):156-63

[40] Srivastava KC, Mustafa T. Ginger (Zingiber officinale) in rheumatism and musculoskeletal disorders. *Med Hypotheses*. 1992 Dec;39(4):342-8

[41] Srivastava KC, Mustafa T. Ginger (Zingiber officinale) and rheumatic disorders. *Med Hypotheses*. 1989 May;29(1):25-8

[42] Altman RD, Marcussen KC. Effects of a ginger extract on knee pain in patients with osteoarthritis. *Arthritis Rheum*. 2001 Nov;44(11):2531-8

[43] Chantre P, Cappelaere A, Leblan D, et al. Efficacy and tolerance of Harpagophytum procumbens versus diacerhein in treatment of osteoarthritis. *Phytomedicine* 2000 Jun;7(3):177-83

[44] Leblan D, Chantre P, Fournie B. Harpagophytum procumbens in the treatment of knee and hip osteoarthritis. Four-month results of a prospective, multicenter, double-blind trial versus diacerhein. *Joint Bone Spine* 2000;67(5):462-7

[45] "They took an 8-week course of Doloteffin at a dose providing 60 mg harpagoside per day... Doloteffin is well worth considering for osteoarthritic knee and hip pain and nonspecific low back pain." Chrubasik S, Thanner J, Kunzel O, Conradt C, Black A, Pollak S. Comparison of outcome measures during treatment with the proprietary Harpagophytum extract doloteffin in patients with pain in the lower back, knee or hip. *Phytomedicine* 2002 Apr;9(3):181-94

[46] Chrubasik S, Eisenberg E, Balan E, Weinberger T, Luzzati R, Conradt C. Treatment of low-back pain exacerbations with willow bark extract: a randomized double-blind study. *Am J Med*. 2000;109:9-14

[47] Chrubasik S, Kunzel O, Model A, Conradt C, Black A. Treatment of low-back pain with a herbal or synthetic anti-rheumatic: a randomized controlled study. Willow bark extract for low-back pain. *Rheumatology* (Oxford). 2001;40:1388-93

[48] Hare LG, Woodside JV, Young IS. Dietary salicylates. *J Clin Pathol* 2003 Sep;56(9):649-50 http://jcp.bmj.com/cgi/content/full/56/9/649

[49] **Vasquez A, Muanza DN. Evaluation of Presence of Aspirin-Related Warnings with Willow Bark: Comment on the Article by Clauson et al. *Ann Pharmacotherapy* 2005 Oct;39:1763**

[50] Clauson KA, Santamarina ML, Buettner CM, Cauffield JS. Evaluation of Presence of Aspirin-Related Warnings with Willow Bark (July/August). *Ann Pharmacother* 2005;39(7-8):1234-7

[51] Gotze H, Rothman SS. Enteropancreatic circulation of digestive enzymes as a conservative mechanism. *Nature* 1975; 257(5527): 607-609

[52] Liebow C, Rothman SS. Enteropancreatic Circulation of Digestive Enzymes. *Science* 1975; 189(4201): 472-474

[53] Trickett P. Proteolytic enzymes in treatment of athletic injuries. *Appl Ther*. 1964;30:647-52

[54] Walker JA, Cerny FJ, Cotter JR, Burton HW. Attenuation of contraction-induced skeletal muscle injury by bromelain. *Med Sci Sports Exerc*. 1992 Jan;24(1):20-5

[55] Walker AF, Bundy R, Hicks SM, Middleton RW. Bromelain reduces mild acute knee pain and improves well-being in a dose-dependent fashion in an open study of otherwise healthy adults. *Phytomedicine*. 2002; 9: 681-6

[56] Brien S, Lewith G, Walker A, Hicks SM, Middleton D. Bromelain as a Treatment for Osteoarthritis: a Review of Clinical Studies. *Evidence-based Complementary and Alternative Medicine*. 2004;1(3)251–257

Selected orthopedic problems of the knee

Problem & Typical Presentation	Assessment & Management
Fracture of the femoral condyles • Knee pain following a direct injury to the knee, (e.g., falling onto a flexed knee, fall from a height)	• Radiographs • **Orthopedic referral** followed by Comprehensive Musculoskeletal Care (Chapter 3)
Fracture of the patella • Many different types of fractures • Knee pain following a direct injury to the anterior knee, especially when flexed (e.g., seated patient with dashboard injury during MVA, falling onto a flexed knee)	• "**Radiographs** are essential to assess traumatic patellar injury."[57] • **Orthopedic referral** followed by Comprehensive Musculoskeletal Care (Chapter 3)
Fracture of the tibial plateau • Knee pain following a direct injury to the knee, (e.g., fall from a height, valgus injuries)	• Radiographs • **Orthopedic referral** followed by Comprehensive Musculoskeletal Care (Chapter 3)
Patellar dislocation, patellar subluxation • Following deceleration (in running) with twisting with a ripping or tearing sensation • May not have direct impact to knee • May have history of joint laxity and "knee cap" dislocations • Subjective instability	• "**Radiographs** are essential in the case of traumatic patellar injury. Studies indicate that **28 to 52 percent of patients with patellar dislocation have an associated osteochondral fracture.**"[58] • Conservative care if no fracture • Referral for orthopedic surgery consultation for fractures and failure to respond to conservative care within 6 months
Anterior cruciate ligament sprain or rupture • Can be caused by knee hyperextension or valgus injury • Unhappy triad consists of injury to medial collateral ligament, ACL, and medial meniscus • Immediate hemorrhagic effusion (hemarthrosis) is seen in 75% of patients	• **Positive anterior drawer test, Lachman's test** • Arthroscopy is considered the gold standard for diagnosis; MRI is 90% accurate compared to arthroscopy; US imaging is also considered clinically valuable and is safe and less expensive • For patients with significant symptoms that are directly ascribed to the ligament injury and patients with multiple knee injuries, **referral for orthopedic surgical consultation** is recommended to assess possibility of surgical reconstruction • Some patients with mild injuries will respond adequately to **nonsurgical care including muscle strengthening, bracing, and activity modification**. Patients treated non-surgically may not be able resume previous levels of activity and may have increased risk for joint degeneration and meniscal injury due to joint laxity; paradoxically, surgical correction may increase functional capacity at the expense of increased degeneration[59], perhaps *because of increased functional capacity* • **Dextrose prolotherapy**[60,61]
Fibular nerve neuropraxia, peroneal neuropraxia • Injury to the fibular nerve (formerly: common peroneal nerve) near the fibular head • Foot drop after acute injury or chronic compression (i.e., crossed legs) near the fibular head	• Foot drop, weak foot dorsiflexion and toe extension • Per patient, refer for management of associated injuries and nerve injury if severe due to recent acute injury • Conservative management is appropriate for long-term and chronic cases: consider supplementation with vitamin B-12, EPA, DHA, GLA, and vitamin E and *Panax Ginseng*

---

[57] Tandeter HB, Shvartzman P. Acute knee injuries: use of decision rules for selective radiograph ordering. *Am Fam Physician* 1999 Dec;60(9):2599-608

[58] Smith BW, Green GA. Acute knee injuries: Part II. Diagnosis and management. *Am Fam Physician* 1995 Mar;51(4):799-806

[59] "Compared with the conservative group (12%), surgical treatment evolved to a higher osteoarthritic morbidity." Casteleyn PP. Management of anterior cruciate ligament lesions: surgical fashion, personal whim or scientific evidence? Study of medium- and long-term results. *Acta Orthop Belg.* 1999 Sep;65(3):327-39

[60] Reeves KD, Hassanein KM. Long-term effects of dextrose prolotherapy for anterior cruciate ligament laxity. *Altern Ther Health Med.* 2003 May-Jun;9(3):58-62

[61] Reeves KD, Hassanein K. Randomized prospective double-blind placebo-controlled study of dextrose prolotherapy for knee osteoarthritis with or without ACL laxity. *Altern Ther Health Med.* 2000 Mar;6(2):68-74, 77-80

Selected orthopedic problems of the knee—*continued*

Problem & Typical Presentation	*Assessment & Management*
Infrapatellar bursitis, clergyman's knee • Commonly seen with intraarticular swelling • Swelling at anterior knee on both sides of patellar ligament near tibial tuberosity • History of trauma to inferior patellar region	• Subcutaneous swelling on both sides of patellar ligament near tibial tuberosity • **Rule out infection** • Consider hemarthrosis, degenerative arthritis, and systemic inflammatory disease • Comprehensive Musculoskeletal Care (Chapter 3) • Treat underlying disease (if any) as indicated.
Lateral collateral ligament (LCL) sprain or rupture • Lateral knee pain following varus injury	• **Varus stress test** • MRI if necessary • Conservative management for patients with mild-moderate injuries and those who refuse surgery • Dextrose prolotherapy • Orthopedic referral for patients with severe injures and those who are willing/able to undergo surgery, although isolated ligament tears are best treated non-operatively
Medial collateral ligament sprain or rupture • Sprain or rupture; more common than injuries to the LCL • Medial knee pain following valgus injury • Patient may have noted tearing sensation at time of injury	• **Valgus stress test:** there should be no abduction at the extended knee • **Pain with palpation at the medial knee at and proximal to the joint line** • MRI if necessary • Conservative management for patients with mild-moderate injuries and those who refuse surgery • Consider dextrose prolotherapy[62,63,64] • Orthopedic referral is recommended for patients with severe injures and those who are willing/able to undergo surgery, although isolated ligament tears are often treated non-operatively
Meniscus injuries • More than 33% of meniscus injuries in adults present with tear of the ACL; in younger patients the percentage of concomitant injury is as high as 92%[65] • **Pain at joint line,** May have **locking,** crepitus, **subjective instability,** "the knee gives out"; may have **swelling** • Severe injury may occur even with minimal trauma, especially those which involve knee flexion and rotation, such as yoga postures, sitting on lower leg	• **Local pain with palpation at the joint line** • **McMurray's test** • **Apley's test** • **Inability to waddle (duck walk)** • **Bounce test** • *"Meniscal injuries have always been a diagnostic challenge because there is no adequate clinical test available."*[66] • MRI is the imaging test of choice for patients for whom the additional information will change the course of treatment • **Orthopedic referral** for patients with significant disability, immobility, or pain who are willing to undergo surgery. Complete surgical removal of a damaged meniscus deprives the knee of stabilization and shock absorption and can lead to premature degeneration of the knee; partial meniscectomy may improve functional status with minimal increase in degeneration • **Crutches during acute exacerbations** to avoid additional joint damage • **Comprehensive Musculoskeletal Care (Chapter 3)** for mild injuries and/or mild symptoms, especially peripheral tears of the lateral meniscus, which may heal spontaneously or become asymptomatic

[62] Reeves KD, Hassanein KM. Long-term effects of dextrose prolotherapy for anterior cruciate ligament laxity. *Altern Ther Health Med.* 2003 May-Jun;9(3):58-62

[63] Reeves KD, Hassanein K. Randomized prospective double-blind placebo-controlled study of dextrose prolotherapy for knee osteoarthritis with or without ACL laxity. *Altern Ther Health Med.* 2000 Mar;6(2):68-74, 77-80

[64] Reeves KD, Hassanein K. Randomized, prospective, placebo-controlled double-blind study of dextrose prolotherapy for osteoarthritic thumb and finger (DIP, PIP, and trapeziometacarpal) joints: evidence of clinical efficacy. *J Altern Complement Med.* 2000 Aug;6(4):311-20

[65] Smith BW, Green GA. Acute knee injuries: Part II. Diagnosis and management. *Am Fam Physician* 1995 Mar;51(4):799-806

[66] Smith BW, Green GA. Acute knee injuries: Part II. Diagnosis and management. *Am Fam Physician* 1995 Mar;51(4):799-806

Selected orthopedic problems of the knee — *continued*

Problem & Typical Presentation	Assessment & Management
<u>Pes anserine bursitis</u> ▪ Inflammation of the bursa located at the collective insertion of the sartorius, gracilis, and semitendinosus muscles at the anteromedial aspect of the proximal tibia	▪ The bursa may become inflamed from overuse or direct trauma ▪ Clinically pes anserine bursitis presents with medial knee pain, which may mimic medial meniscus injury or sprain of the medial collateral ligament ▪ Resisted knee flexion and direct palpation generally exacerbate the pain ▪ Infection is excluded with clinical assessment and lab tests (Chapter 1) ▪ Comprehensive Musculoskeletal Care (Chapter 3) emphasizing rest and anti-inflammation
<u>Popliteal cyst</u>, baker's cyst ▪ The most common synovial cyst of the knee; located posteriorly ▪ Commonly associated with meniscal injuries	▪ Palpation reveals palpable fullness at medial posterior knee ▪ Clinical assessment may begin and end with palpation; other assessments ranging from transillumination, aspiration, US imaging, MRI and arthrography may be used if necessary ▪ Infection and systemic inflammatory disease are assessed clinically and with lab tests (Chapter 1) ▪ Comprehensive Musculoskeletal Care (Chapter 3) emphasizing rest and anti-inflammation
<u>Posterior cruciate ligament sprain or rupture</u> ▪ Knee pain following direct force to proximal tibia, such as with dashboard injury in a motor vehicle accident	▪ **Clinical findings include positive posterior drawer test, sag sign** ▪ If the injury is acute and traumatic, radiographs should be performed to assess for fracture and gross instability ▪ Arthroscopic examination is considered the gold standard for diagnosis and allows assessment for meniscal injuries and hemarthrosis; MRI is 90% accurate compared to arthroscopy ▪ For patients with significant symptoms that are directly ascribed to the ligament injury and patients with multiple knee injuries, **referral for orthopedic surgical consultation is recommended** to assess feasibility of surgical reconstruction ▪ Some patients with mild injuries will respond adequately to **conservative care including quadriceps strengthening, bracing, and activity modification**
<u>Prepatellar bursitis</u>, housemaid's knee ▪ Swelling at anterior knee ▪ Periodic ▪ History of acute or recurrent trauma to inferior patellar region	▪ Subcutaneous swelling covering patella ▪ Rule out infection and systemic inflammatory disease ▪ Comprehensive Musculoskeletal Care (Chapter 3)
<u>Traumatic bursitis</u> ▪ Pain and swelling following direct impact to anterior knee	▪ Swollen bursa found with clinical examination ▪ Rule out infection ▪ Comprehensive Musculoskeletal Care (Chapter 3)

Selected orthopedic problems of the knee—*continued*

Problem & Typical Presentation	Assessment & Management
Chondromalacia patellae • A condition characterized by retropatellar cartilage disorganization, degeneration, and eventual replacement with fibrous tissue • *Chondromalacia* is an overused term clinically, as some doctors use it to describe any retropatellar pain; indeed some researchers have used *chondromalacia patellae* as if it were synonymous with *patellofemoral pain syndrome*, when clearly this is not the case	• In contrast to other forms of retropatellar pain, *chondromalacia patellae* is a rather specific histologic condition, somewhat similar clinically, histologically, and microscopically to osteoarthritis except that—unlike osteoarthritis which is generally progressive—*chondromalacia patellae* tends to be self-resolving, perhaps due to fibrous metaplasia of affected chondrocytes[67] • Requires visual-histologic evaluation of joint cartilage for diagnosis of "cartilage softening" — such invasive diagnostic procedures are by-and-large unnecessary for a condition that simply presents as benign knee pain • The condition presents with an osteoarthritis-like pain which eventually remits as cartilage is replaced with fibrous tissue • Patients should be treated with cartilage-supporting, anti-inflammatory, and analgesic nutrients and botanical medicines described in Chapter 3 and reassured that the condition is benign; muscle imbalances, muscle weakness, and patellar tracking problems should be vigilantly pursued and corrected
Iron overload, hemochromatosis • Iron accumulation disorders are among the most common genetic traits in the human population • Clinically and radiographically, the manifestations are virtually indistinguishable from osteoarthritis[68] • Metacarpophalangeal joints, wrists, hips and knees are most common affected	• Pain and limited range of motion; increased pain with weighted circumduction and anvil test • Radiographic changes very similar to osteoarthritis • Normal ESR, CRP, with **high ferritin** possibly with an elevated transferrin saturation • Therapeutic phlebotomy is the treatment of choice; deferoxamine is an expensive cumbersome and less effective alternative • Iron-removal therapy with therapeutic phlebotomy and serologic testing of all first-degree relatives is mandatory • See Chapter 1 for more details on diagnosis and management
Osgood-Schlatter disease • Partial avulsion of the apophysis of the infrapatellar ligament • Anterior infrapatellar knee pain in athletic adolescent	• Prominent tibial tuberosity • Assess for other causes of pain, e.g., meniscus injuries, ligament injuries • Comprehensive Musculoskeletal Care (Chapter 3)
Osteoarthrosis, osteoarthritis, • Degenerative arthritis • Generally older patient or history of trauma • Pain with walking and weight-bearing • Bilateral or unilateral • Restricted motion	• Pain and limited range of motion: weighted circumduction and anvil test • Bilateral or unilateral • Restricted motion • Radiographic changes • Normal ESR, CRP, and ferritin. • Rule out hemochromatosis by assessing ferritin and transferrin saturation[69] • Comprehensive Musculoskeletal Care (Chapter 3) • Dextrose prolotherapy[70] • Injection of hyaluronate[71]

[67] Bentley G. Articular cartilage changes in chondromalacia patellae. *J Bone Joint Surg Br.* 1985 Nov;67(5):769-74 http://www.jbjs.org.uk/cgi/reprint/67-B/5/769
[68] Axford JS, Bomford A, Revell P, Watt I, Williams R, Hamilton EBD. Hip arthropathy in genetic hemochromatosis: radiographic and histologic features. *Arthritis Rheum* 1991; 34: 357-61
[69] **Vasquez A. Musculoskeletal disorders and iron overload disease: comment on the American College of Rheumatology guidelines for the initial evaluation of the adult patient with acute musculoskeletal symptoms. *Arthritis Rheum* 1996 Oct; 39(10):1767-8**
[70] Reeves KD, Hassanein K. Randomized prospective double-blind placebo-controlled study of dextrose prolotherapy for knee osteoarthritis with or without ACL laxity. *Altern Ther Health Med* 2000 Mar;6(2):68-74, 77-80
[71] Wen DY. Intra-articular hyaluronic acid injections for knee osteoarthritis. *Am Fam Physician* 2000 Aug 1;62(3):565-70, 572

Selected orthopedic problems of the knee—*continued*

Problem & Typical Presentation	*Assessment & Management*
Osteochondral fragments, "joint mice" • History of knee injury, ACL or PCL tear, or joint degeneration is typical	• Radiographs or MRI can be used to visualize fragments • Arthroscopic debridement may be followed by Comprehensive Musculoskeletal Care (Chapter 3)
Osteochondritis dissecans[72] • A disorder of unclear etiology (trauma and/or avascular necrosis) that results in the death and subsequent fragmentation of subchondral bone • Primarily affects ages 10-30 years • Knee pain, swelling, locking, and crepitus due to intraarticular loose bodies (joint mice) • Some patients are almost asymptomatic, while others have acute pain	• Radiographs: consider to assess both knees as the condition is bilateral in 30% • MRI is used to assess severity and need for surgical intervention • May heal spontaneously; may require surgery to remove osteocartilaginous fragments • Orthopedic referral is recommended, particularly as surgical revascularization can promote recovery and may lessen extent of damage
Patellar malalignment syndrome, patellofemoral arthralgia, lateral patellar compression syndrome • Pain with forceful knee extension, as with climbing stairs • Pain with prolonged sitting with knees bent is known as "movie sign" or "movie theater knee" • No or minimal swelling • Most common in young women with knee valgus	• Patellofemoral tenderness with compression and lateral subluxation • Radiographs—skyline view (sunrise view) • Conservative care emphasizing activity modification) avoid prolonged knee hyperflexion) and supplements to support cartilage health • Exercise and bracing and attention to biomechanical function[73]; exercises should be performed with the goal of balancing the medial and lateral forces on the patella • Knee brace with patella cutout • Correct foot hyperpronation with orthoses/orthotics
Slipped capital femoral epiphysis • Classic presentation is a tall overweight boy with hip pain, **knee pain**, and/or a painful limp • *Remember that knee pain is a common initial complaint from hip disease due to irritation of the obturator nerve*	• Radiographs of both hips show diagnostic findings • Physical examination should be limited to avoid exacerbation of fracture displacement; loss of internal rotation starting from 90° hip flexion is the characteristic finding • Orthopedic referral for surgical consultation followed by Comprehensive Musculoskeletal Care (Chapter 3) • See Chapter 12 on the Hip and Thigh for more details and differential diagnosis and management
Lower extremity biomechanical dysfunction • Excessive foot pronation or supination • Functional or anatomical leg length inequality • Pelvic torque • Proprioceptive defects at the ankle, knee, hips-pelvis, and/or low-back • Assess biomechanics and ergonomics "in action" if this is feasible	• Assess gait, posture, ergonomics • Clinically assess muscle strength, balance, proprioception • Assess shoes for wear—distribution and symmetry • Intervene with any and all appropriate treatments, including dietary, nutritional, botanical, strengthening, stretching, and coordinating interventions as indicated • Use orthoses and "shoe inserts" as needed to provide additional shock absorption and/or correct leg length discrepancies and/or hyperpronation problems
	Remember that when you are assessing and treating nonpathologic *functional* conditions of the knee, you need to also assess regional tissues such as the ITB but also the biomechanics of the hip *proximally* and the foot and ankle *distally* since the foot-ankle-knee-hip-pelvis complex is all part of the same kinematic chain. Furthermore, in those instances when the clinician is available to observe the patient during (simulated) performance of work-related or recreational tasks, additional biomechanical and ergonomic data can be obtained to refine the diagnosis and implement an effective treatment plan

[72] Tatum R. Osteochondritis dissecans of the knee: a radiology case report. *J Manipulative Physiol Ther* 2000 Jun;23(5):347-51
[73] Dryburgh DR. Chondromalacia patellae. *J Manipulative Physiol Ther*. 1988 Jun;11(3):214-7

Chapter 14:
Leg, Ankle, and Foot

Introduction
Twisted, sprained, kicked and injured ankles and shins are common; therefore, clinicians must have the ability to assess these and exclude important complications—such as acute compartment syndrome—before releasing the patient from care. Disorders of the foot, forefoot, and toes are also common, important, and disabling if not treated properly.

Topics:

1. **Clinical assessments and differential diagnoses**
2. **Leg, ankle, and foot—general considerations**
3. **Selected orthopedic problems of the leg**
   - Acute and chronic compartment syndromes
   - Fracture of the tibia or fibula
   - Stress fracture of the tibia or fibula
   - Peroneal neuropraxia
   - Shin splints
   - Tibial periostitis
   - Tibialis posterior strain/ tendonitis
4. **Ankle sprain and "twisted ankle"**
5. **Additional problems of the ankle and foot**
   - Achilles' tendonitis
   - Fractures
     - Fracture of ankle or foot
     - Avulsion fracture of the 5th metatarsal
     - Jones fracture
     - Metatarsal stress fracture
   - Metatarsalgia
   - Morton's neuroma
   - Plantar fasciitis
   - Tarsal tunnel syndrome

> **Ankle injuries are very common**
>
> "Ten percent of emergency department (ED) visits are related to ankle injury, and approximately 75% of these injuries are sprains."
>
> Eisenhart AW, Gaeta TJ, Yens DP. Osteopathic manipulative treatment in the emergency department for patients with acute ankle injuries. *J Am Osteopath Assoc.* 2003 Sep;103(9):417-21
> http://www.jaoa.org/cgi/reprint/103/9/417

Focus:

- Be able to differentiate shin splints, tibial stress fracture, and compressive compartment syndromes since they are similar in etiology and presentation yet they involve different assessments, treatments, and complications.

Core competencies:

1. Know how to identify and manage acute compartment syndrome.
2. Know how to differentiate gout from septic arthritis.
3. Know how to grade ankle sprains; know the management of the each grade of ankle sprain.
4. Appreciate the "orthopedic" implications of diabetes mellitus with regard to complications that have a proclivity for the foot and ankle.

> **Foot complications in diabetics need to be taken seriously**
>
> "Foot ulcers develop in approximately 15% of people with diabetes and are a preceding factor in approximately 85% of lower limb amputations."
>
> Delmas L. Best practice in the assessment and management of diabetic foot ulcers. *Rehabil Nurs.* 2006 Nov-Dec;31(6):228-34

Clinical assessments for the leg and ankle

Clinical Assessments	*Positive Finding and Implications*
1. <u>History</u>: See Chapter 1	▪ **Indicators from the history (trauma, risk factors)** ▪ **Systemic manifestations** ▪ **Complications** ▪ **Mechanical/ Nonmechanical**
2. <u>Observation</u>: Overall posture, specific structures, overlying skin	▪ Scars ▪ Injury, congenital anomaly, asymmetric development due to asymmetric use ▪ Muscle atrophy may be due to neurologic deficit (radiculopathy or other CNS or PNS injury) or disuse (due to injury or pain) ▪ Ecchymosis is seen after fractures and soft tissue injuries ▪ Systemic illness ▪ Previous surgery ▪ Infection ▪ Dermatitis ▪ Poor posture ▪ Gait abnormalities ▪ Obesity
3. <u>Walking, gait analysis</u>: Observe for symmetry, flow, balance and biomechanics	Search for: ▪ Excessive internal/external rotation of the lower extremity ▪ Leg length inequality ▪ Genu varus/valgus ▪ Supination/pronation *Treat what you find*

4.   <u>Reflexes and sensory neurologic exam</u>:
  ▪   Walk on heels (L4 and L5)
  ▪   Walk on toes (S1)
  ▪   Squat and rise: this is a valuable screening test for quickly assessing quadriceps strength (including L3 and L4[1]), neurologic integrity, balance, and the ability of joints and bones to withstand stress
  ▪   Reflexes and sensory tests
	Limitation or pain may suggest any of the following:
	▪ Pain
	▪ Muscle strain or tightness
	▪ Contracture/adhesion of soft tissues: muscles, joint capsule
	▪ Fracture: femur, patella, tibia, fibula, tarsals, metatarsals, phalanges
	▪ Disc herniation causing radiculopathic weakness
	▪ Neurologic compromise: lesion of the brain, spinal cord, or peripheral nerve

5. <u>Peripheral vascular examination</u>: Assess pulses and capillary refill; look for trophic changes in hair and nails	▪ Absent or grossly asymmetric posterior tibial and/or dorsalis pedis pulses suggests peripheral vascular disease, vascular injury (including acute compartment syndrome), or congenital agenesis; clinical correlation is required

6.   <u>Active and passive range of motion</u>:
  ▪   Plantar flexion, dorsiflexion
  ▪   Inversion, eversion
  ▪   Toe flexion and extension
	▪ Assess for symmetry and smoothness of motion
	▪ Excess motion suggests joint laxity and/or ligament injury
	▪ Restrictions to passive and active motion can arise from muscles, fascia, joint capsules, intra-articular debris and damage to articular surfaces; active motion may be prematurely limited by pain

---

[1] Moore KL. <u>Clinically Oriented Anatomy. Third Edition</u>. Baltimore; Williams and Wilkins: 1992, page 387

Clinical assessments for the leg and ankle—*continued*

Clinical Assessments	Positive Finding and Implications
7. **Observation, palpation, provocation**: Skin, bones, muscles, ligaments, and other structures	<ul><li>Scars from previous injury or surgery</li><li>Injury, congenital anomaly, asymmetric development due to asymmetric use</li><li>Muscle atrophy may be due to neurologic deficit (radiculopathy or other CNS or PNS injury) or disuse (due to injury or pain)</li><li>Ecchymosis is generally seen after fractures, ligament ruptures, and soft tissue injuries</li><li>Infection: red indurated tissue should be evaluated for infection, particularly if accompanied by systemic manifestations of infection or a predisposing history such as immunosuppression or diabetes</li><li>Poor posture</li><li>Gait abnormalities</li></ul>
8. **Anterior and posterior drawer tests of the ankle**: Doctor grips patient's foot and lower leg and applies anterior and posterior stress to assess integrity of ligaments connecting the talus and calcaneus of the foot with the fibula and tibia of the leg	<ul><li>Increased or asymmetric motion indicates ligament sprain or rupture</li><li>Anterior displacement of the talus becomes possible with rupture of the anterior talofibular ligament—the most commonly injured ligament with inversion sprains of the ankle[2]; the anterior drawer test may be weakly positive if the ligament is sprained or stretched (grade 2) and will become more obviously abnormal with complete rupture of the ligament (grade 3)</li><li>Posterior drawer test becomes positive with rupture of the calcaneofibular ligament; this injury is seen in more severe ankle injuries (grade 3); concomitant lesion of the anterior talofibular ligament is common</li></ul>
9. **Thompson test**: Patient prone on examination table; doctor squeezes patient's calf to induce ankle plantar flexion	<ul><li>Lack of foot plantar flexion indicates ruptured Achilles' tendon; most patients will be aware of this problem before they come into your office. The test simply allows for the objective assessment of the tendocalcaneous integrity while eliminating complicating factors such as pain, malingering, or nerve injury that might otherwise obfuscate the diagnosis</li></ul>
10. **Motion palpation**: Proximal tibiofibular joint, the talocrural articulation, and the articulations between the tarsals, metatarsals, and phalanges	<ul><li>Hypermobility: treated with bracing, orthoses, restricted movement (including stiff hard-soled shoes), nutritional support to help strengthen connective tissues, taping, possibly prolotherapy</li><li>Hypomobility: addressed with manipulation, mobilization, and stretching</li></ul>
11. **Inspect patient's shoes**: Examination of worn shoes	Analyze for wear, distribution, and symmetry:<ul><li>Look for symmetry between the left and right shoe to assess for possible biomechanical faults, including unequal leg length which may result in excess wear at the heel of the longer leg</li><li>Look for excess wear on the outer posterior sole, which often correlates with tight gluteus and piriformis and unequal leg length</li><li>Excess wear on the outer sole and stress on the outer shoe correlates with a high arch and rigid foot, which may benefit from a shoe with extra shock absorption</li><li>Excess wear on the inner sole and stress on the inner shoe correlates with a fallen longitudinal arch and hypermobile foot, which often needs arch support and a more rigid shoe</li><li>Assess for other biomechanical faults</li></ul>

---

[2] Beers MH, Berkow R (eds). The Merck Manual. Seventeenth Edition. Whitehouse Station; Merck Research Laboratories 1999 page 483-484

Leg, Ankle, Foot: *General Considerations*

Description/pathophysiology:

- Problems of the leg, ankle, and foot deserve our attention and are not less important than problems of the neck, hands, or low-back despite the fact that we can easily overlook problems of the lower extremity because they are generally ❶ out of our field of vision, ❷ covered by clothes and shoes, and ❸ distal to the cerebrocentric vantage point from which people typically view themselves; these three influences often conspire to encourage patients to ignore their leg, foot, and ankle problems until these problems have progressed from mild to moderate or severe. As the prevalence of diabetes mellitus continues to spread like wildfire across so-called modernized societies, **doctors will need to keep lower extremity problems higher on their list of daily considerations since diabetes mellitus is a major cause of peripheral neuropathy as well as lower extremity degeneration that eventually necessitates amputation**[3]; diabetic patients also show an increased incidence of foot **osteomyelitis**.[4]

- Critical lower extremity problems can also develop in patients who are healthy and athletic. Stress fractures of the metatarsals are not uncommon in long-distance runners, and **acute compartment syndrome can develop within hours and can be a life-threatening emergency if muscle necrosis precipitates myoglobinuric renal failure**.[5]

- For these and other reasons provided in the sections that follow, distal lower extremity problems need to be approached with care and diligence, especially when the onset is acute following trauma or exertion or when the patient's overall condition includes risk factors such as diabetes mellitus or corticosteroid use that increase the likeliness for complications. The approach to the patient begins with history and a physical examination that emphasizes peripheral neurovascular status (to exclude arteriovenous insufficiency, neuropathy, and compartment syndromes) as part of the four-part anatomy-based examination as outlined below.

Lesion	Leg, Ankle & Foot
Bone	<ul><li>Fracture of tibia or fibula, talus, calcaneus, cuboid, cuneiforms, navicular, metatarsals, phalanges; including stress fractures and avulsion fracture of ligamentous insertion</li><li>Osteomyelitis</li><li>Bone tumor, especially osteosarcoma and Ewing's sarcoma</li><li>Osteomalacia of vitamin D deficiency</li><li>Heel spur from the calcaneus</li></ul>
Joints	<ul><li>Proximal tibiofibular joint hypermobility or hypomobility</li><li>Systemic and degenerative conditions: gout, osteoarthritis, hemochromatosis</li><li>Rheumatic disease and inflammatory arthropathies such as rheumatoid arthritis, lupus, and reactive arthritis</li><li>Segmental dysfunction, biomechanical aberrations, and subluxations</li></ul>
Soft tissue	<ul><li>Ligament sprain</li><li>Muscle or tendon strain, tendonitis</li><li>Compartment syndromes</li><li>Bursitis</li><li>Pretibial edema of hypothyroidism</li><li>Edema associated with renal or cardiovascular disease</li><li>Plantar fasciitis</li></ul>
Neuro-vascular	<ul><li>Peripheral neuropathy: diabetes, vitamin B-12 deficiency, Guillain-Barre syndrome</li><li>Arterial or venous insufficiency</li><li>Morton's neuroma</li><li>Neurovascular compression associated with compartment syndromes</li><li>Fibular nerve neuropraxia, due to direct trauma or compartment syndrome</li></ul>

---

[3] "Foot ulcers develop in approximately 15% of people with diabetes and are a preceding factor in approximately 85% of lower limb amputations." Delmas L. Best practice in the assessment and management of diabetic foot ulcers. *Rehabil Nurs.* 2006 Nov-Dec;31(6):228-34

[4] "Osteomyelitis (OM) in adults usually involves the digits of the feet and is most often associated with diabetes mellitus (DM)." Henke PK, Blackburn SA, Wainess RW, Cowan J, Terando A, Proctor M, Wakefield TW, Upchurch GR Jr, Stanley JC, Greenfield LJ. Osteomyelitis of the foot and toe in adults is a surgical disease: conservative management worsens lower extremity salvage. *Ann Surg.* 2005 Jun;241(6):885-92; discussion 892-4 http://www.pubmedcentral.nih.gov/articlerender.fcgi?tool=pubmed&pubmedid=15912038

[5] "Compartment syndrome (CS) is a limb-threatening and life-threatening condition observed when perfusion pressure falls below tissue pressure in a closed anatomic space. The current body of knowledge unequivocally reflects that untreated CS leads to tissue necrosis, permanent functional impairment, and, if severe, renal failure and death. " Paula R. Compartment Syndrome, Extremity. *eMedicine* June 22, 2006 http://www.emedicine.com/emerg/topic739.htm Accessed January 11, 2007

Clinical presentations:

- Pain, restricted motion, and limited weight bearing are the most common presenting complaints, followed by weakness and numbness; the clinician's task is to determine the identity of the involved structures, the nature of the problem, and its underlying cause; serious life- and limb-threatening conditions need to be considered and excluded before the patient is treated and released from care.

Major differential diagnoses:

- Systemic arthropathy or arthritis from rheumatic or metabolic disease
- Neuropathic pain and peripheral neuropathies
- **Septic arthritis and osteomyelitis — medical emergency**
- Tissue/bone injury from acute trauma or repetitive strain injury
- **Compartment syndromes affecting the anterior, posterior or lateral compartments — surgical emergency**
- Cancer such as osteosarcoma and Ewing's sarcoma

Clinical assessment:

- History: Get the major attributes, assess for systemic manifestations, complications, indicators from the history, and the mechanical/nonmechanical nature of the problem. Ask about injury and/or overuse: If the patient is athletic, ask about specific activities, intensity, duration, frequency, age of shoes, orthoses, etc; ask athletes about type of running surface, changes of direction and routine, *coronal* and *sagittal* angle of surface.
- Physical examination:
  - Assess the area of complaint *and the neighboring regions*
  - Examine the shoes worn for *work* and *athletics*
  - Assess structures according to their respective properties and functions:
    - Bones — percussion, vibration, torsion, functional stress testing such as fulcrum tests and weight-bearing
    - Fascia — light and deep palpation, stretching, restricted motion, fascial adhesions
    - Joints — palpate for swelling, effusion, local bursitis and tenosynovitis; assess range of motion and palpatory quality of motion
    - Ligaments — tension and torsion tests
    - Muscles — palpation, stretching, strength testing

Imaging & laboratory assessments:

- As detailed in Chapter 1, screening laboratory tests — *minimally including CBC, CRP, and metabolic/chemistry panel* — should be performed to uncover occult or concomitant disease processes and to facilitate comprehensive patient assessment for overall health evaluation and intervention.
- Radiographs are generally all that are needed, particularly when evaluating for fracture, avulsion, dislocation, and cancers and most chronic infections; films that are initially negative for suspected fracture can be repeated at 2-4 weeks after the injury to assess for callus formation.
- CT, MRI, and ultrasound can be used for more complicated lesions, particularly those involving intraarticular lesions and soft tissues.

Clinical management:

- Treat the underlying problem(s); co-manage or refer as indicated.

Treatment:

- **Treatment must be based on identifying and then effectively addressing the underlying disorder or cause of the problem**
- Common therapeutic interventions will be outlined here; review Chapter 3 for additional considerations and details.
- Protect, and prevent re-injury: Avoid motions and activities that cause significant pain, as pain indicates that damaged/inflamed tissues are being stressed. **Use bracing, casting, taping, bandages, wrapping, canes, crutches, and walkers as needed to support and take weight off of injured tissues during the acute phase of healing and until fractured and broken bones (if any) are sufficiently healed.**[6,7] Use orthoses ("orthotics") and new or better-fitting shoes as indicated.

---

[6] Van Hook FW, Demonbreun D, Weiss BD. Ambulatory devices for chronic gait disorders in the elderly. *Am Fam Physician*. 2003 Apr 15;67(8):1717-24 http://www.aafp.org/afp/20030415/1717.html and http://www.aafp.org/afp/20030415/1717.pdf Accessed July 23, 2006
[7] Joyce BM, Kirby RL. Canes, crutches and walkers. *Am Fam Physician*. 1991 Feb;43(2):535-42

- Relative or complete rest: Take time away from the activities that promote additional injury or that unnecessarily drain energies which could otherwise be used for healing and recuperation.

- Ice/heat: **During the acute phase, apply ice or cold pack for 10 minutes each 30-60 minutes for reduction in pain and inflammation**. During the subacute and chronic phase, apply gentle heat as needed for the relief of pain and reduction in muscle spasm and to promote healing by increasing circulation.

- Individualize treatment: The cornerstone of effective holistic and integrative treatment is to design treatment plans that simultaneously 1) address "the problem" while also 2) improving the patient's overall health.

- Compression: Snug bandages/wraps may help to reduce swelling and can provide support for injured tissues and weakened joints. Care must be utilized to avoid arterial, venous, or lymphatic obstruction.

- Educate, establish treatment program, elevation of injured limb (as applicable), exercise, ergonomic improvements: Educate about the need for appropriate follow-up office visits for reexamination, reassessment, and treatment. Educate patient on ways to avoid re-injury and to decrease likelihood of recurrence. Therapeutic exercise can include strength training, stretching, improving endurance, and functional training specific to the patient's occupational or athletic activities; these can be tailored to great detail to the patient's condition and goals. **Proprioceptive retraining/rehabilitation is especially important** for the long-term functional improvement of patients with proprioceptive deficits, commonly seen in patients with chronic low-back pain, neck pain, knee arthritis, and **ankle instability**.[8] Exercise promotes loss of superfluous body fat; thus the short-term myokine-mediated anti-inflammatory benefits of exercise are extended by adipose reduction and the associated reduction in pro-inflammatory adipokines. Modify home and occupational workstations to minimize strain and stress on injured tissues; educate patients to use tools, machines, props, and stepstools to work efficiently and to reduce unnecessary lifting and straining motions. **Elevate the injured limb to minimize swelling and edema.**

- Anti-inflammatory healing-supportive diet: **Pro-inflammatory foods** and food components such as arachidonic acid (high in cow's milk, beef, liver, pork, and lamb) , saturated fats , corn oil , high glycemic foods, white bread, high-fat high-carbohydrate fast-food breakfast should be avoided generally and especially during times of musculoskeletal inflammation. The **Paleo-Mediterranean diet** is based on abundant consumption of fruits, vegetables, seeds, nuts, berries, omega-3 and monounsaturated fatty acids, and lean sources of protein such as lean meats, fatty cold-water fish, soy and whey proteins. The American/Western style of eating results in subclinical diet-induced pathogenic chronic metabolic acidosis which can be corrected with a Paleo-Mediterranean diet[9] or alkalinizing supplements[10] for the alleviation of musculoskeletal pain in general and low-back pain in particular.[11] Ensure adequate fluid intake; teas—especially green teas—provide anti-inflammatory and antioxidant benefits that are clinically significant. Adequate/increased protein intake expedites recovery following injury and shows numerous other benefits; in otherwise healthy patients with no liver, renal, or other metabolic disorders, ensure adequate intake of 0.5-0.9 gram of protein per pound of body weight.[12] Physiologically, the body's limit for handling nitrogenous groups from dietary protein is reached when protein intake is greater than 200-300 grams/d; as long as protein intake is kept below this level or below 30-40% of daily calories and/or combined with a *whole foods* fruit- and vegetable-rich diet, patients and doctors need not worry about the familiar myth of "too much protein."[13]

- Fatty acid supplementation for eicosanoid and genomic modulation: Combination therapy with EPA-DHA (fish oil) and GLA (borage oil) is preferred for optimal results.[14]
  - Fish oil, EPA with DHA: Up to three grams per day (3,000 mg/d) of combined EPA and DHA is a reasonable therapeutic dose for anti-inflammatory purposes.[15,16,17,18]

[8] Olmsted LC, Carcia CR, Hertel J, Shultz SJ. Efficacy of the Star Excursion Balance Tests in Detecting Reach Deficits in Subjects With Chronic Ankle Instability. *J Athl Train*. 2002 Dec;37(4):501-506

[9] Cordain L. The Paleo Diet: Lose Weight and Get Healthy by Eating the Food You Were Designed to Eat. Indianapolis; John Wiley and Sons, 2002

[10] For long-term out-patient treatment of patients who do not achieve alkalinization with diet alone, oral administration of potassium citrate and/or sodium bicarbonate can be implemented. See the following article for concepts: "Urine alkalinization is a treatment regimen that increases poison elimination by the administration of intravenous sodium bicarbonate to produce urine with a pH > or = 7.5." Proudfoot AT, Krenzelok EP, Vale JA. Position Paper on urine alkalinization. *J Toxicol Clin Toxicol*. 2004;42:1-26 http://www.eapcct.org/publicfile.php?folder=congress&file=PS_UrineAlkalinization.pdf Also see: Vormann J, Worlitschek M, Goedecke T, Silver B. Supplementation with alkaline minerals reduces symptoms in patients with chronic low back pain. *J Trace Elem Med Biol*. 2001;15(2-3):179-83 Also see: Maurer M, Riesen W, Muser J, Hulter HN, Krapf R. Neutralization of Western diet inhibits bone resorption independently of K intake and reduces cortisol secretion in humans. *Am J Physiol Renal Physiol*. 2003 Jan;284(1):F32-40. Epub 2002 Sep 24. http://ajprenal.physiology.org/cgi/content/full/284/1/F32

[11] "The results show that a disturbed acid-base balance may contribute to the symptoms of low back pain. The simple and safe addition of an alkaline multimineral preparate was able to reduce the pain symptoms in these patients with chronic low back pain." Vormann J, Worlitschek M, Goedecke T, Silver B. Supplementation with alkaline minerals reduces symptoms in patients with chronic low back pain. *J Trace Elem Med Biol*. 2001;15(2-3):179-83

[12] Nancy Clark, MS, RD. The Power of Protein. *The Physician and Sportsmedicine* 1996, volume 24, number 4. http://www.physsportsmed.com/issues/1996/04_96/protein.htm

[13] "I can assure you that as long as you eat plenty of fresh fruits and vegetables, there is no such thing as too much protein." (page 41). Cordain L. The Paleo Diet: Lose Weight and Get Healthy by Eating the Food You Were Designed to Eat. Indianapolis; John Wiley and Sons: 2002, pages 41, 67, 101

[14] Vasquez A. Reducing Pain and Inflammation Naturally. Part 2: New Insights into Fatty Acid Supplementation and Its Effect on Eicosanoid Production and Genetic Expression. *Nutritional Perspectives* 2005; January: 5-16 www.optimalhealthresearch.com/part2

[15] "...clinical benefits of the n-3 fatty acids were not apparent until they were consumed for > or =12 wk. It appears that a minimum daily dose of 3 g eicosapentaenoic and docosahexaenoic acids is necessary to derive the expected benefits [in patients with rheumatoid arthritis]." Kremer JM. n-3 fatty acid supplements in rheumatoid arthritis.*AmJ Clin Nutr*.2000;71(1Suppl):349S-51S

[16] Rubin D, Laposata M. Cellular interactions between n-6 and n-3 fatty acids: a mass analysis of fatty acid elongation/desaturation, distribution among complex lipids, and conversion to eicosanoids. *J Lipid Res*. 1992 Oct;33(10):1431-40.

- o GLA, Gamma-linolenic acid: Approximately 500 mg per day is the common anti-inflammatory dose[19] although higher doses of 2.8 grams per day have been safely used in patients with rheumatoid arthritis.[20]
- Nutritional supplementation: Upon the foundation of a health-promoting healing-supportive anti-inflammatory diet such as the Paleo-Mediterranean diet, a patient-tailored program of nutritional supplementation can be built to expedite restoration/optimization of tissue structure and function. Since vitamin deficiencies are common and because multivitamin/multimineral supplementation generally has a very high benefit:risk ratio, essentially all adults should take a multivitamin/multimineral supplement[21], upon which additional problem-specific nutritional supplementation can be added. Supplementation can be tailored to the type of tissue that has been injured, such as calcium, magnesium, and vitamins D and K for bone fractures, glucosamine sulfate and niacinamide for cartilage injuries, and proteolytic enzymes for muscle strains.
  - o **Pancreatic/proteolytic enzymes: Orally-administered pancreatic and proteolytic enzymes are absorbed from the gastrointestinal tract into the systemic circulation to exert analgesic, anti-inflammatory, anti-edematous benefits with therapeutic relevance for acute and chronic musculoskeletal disorders.[22,23,24,25]**
  - o Vitamin E, with an emphasis on gamma-tocopherol: The gamma form of vitamin E inhibits cyclooxygenase and thus has anti-inflammatory activity[26] that appears clinically significant in conditions such as rheumatoid arthritis, spondylosis and back pain, osteoarthritis , and some autoimmune diseases.
  - o Niacinamide: Niacinamide alleviates osteoarthritis pain and appears to have an anti-aging benefit.[27,28,29,30,31] The standard dose of 500 mg given orally 6 times per day is more effective than 1,000 mg 3 times per day. Hepatic dysfunction is rare when daily doses are kept below 3,000 mg per day; measure liver enzymes after 3 months of treatment and yearly thereafter.[32]
  - o Glucosamine sulfate and chondroitin sulfate: Glucosamine and chondroitin are the "building blocks" from which cartilage is built and oral supplementation is intended to enhance cartilage anabolism and to thus counteract the enhanced cartilage catabolism seen in destructive arthritic processes. The adult dose of glucosamine sulfate is generally 1500-2000 mg per day in divided doses, and the dose of chondroitin sulfate is approximately 1000 mg daily; these treatments can be used singly, in combination, and with other treatments.
  - o Vitamin C: Doses of 1-2 grams per day have been suggested to reduce pain and the need for surgery in patients with low-back pain by improving disc integrity[33], and increased vitamin C intake is also associated with improved joint health and musculoskeletal function.[34]
- Botanical medicines: Tailor the selection, dose, and combinations to the patient's size, age, and other clinical characteristics.
  - o _Uncaria guianensis_ and _Uncaria tomentosa_ ("cat's claw", "una de gato"): Analgesic and anti-inflammatory benefits have been shown in osteoarthritis[35] and rheumatoid arthritis.[36]

---

[17] "The recent GISSI (Gruppo Italiano per lo Studio della Sopravvivenza nell'Infarto miocardico)-Prevention study of 11,324 patients showed a 45% decrease in risk of sudden cardiac death and a 20% reduction in all-cause mortality in the group taking 850 mg/d of omega-3 fatty acids. These fatty acids have potent anti-inflammatory effects and may also be antiatherogenic." O'Keefe JH Jr, Harris WS. From Inuit to implementation: omega-3 fatty acids come of age. _Mayo Clin Proc._ 2000 Jun;75(6):607-14

[18] "Many of the placebo-controlled trials of fish oil in chronic inflammatory diseases reveal significant benefit, including decreased disease activity and a lowered use of anti-inflammatory drugs." Simopoulos AP. Omega-3 fatty acids in inflammation and autoimmune diseases. _J Am Coll Nutr._ 2002 Dec;21(6):495-505

[19] "Forty patients with rheumatoid arthritis and upper gastrointestinal lesions due to non-steroidal anti-inflammatory drugs entered a prospective 6-month double-blind placebo controlled study of dietary supplementation with gamma-linolenic acid 540 mg/day..." Brzeski M, Madhok R, Capell HA. Evening primrose oil in patients with rheumatoid arthritis and side-effects of non-steroidal anti-inflammatory drugs. _Br J Rheumatol._ 1991 Oct;30(5):370-2

[20] Zurier RB, Rossetti RG, Jacobson EW, DeMarco DM, Liu NY, Temming JE, White BM, Laposata M. gamma-Linolenic acid treatment of rheumatoid arthritis. A randomized, placebo-controlled trial. _Arthritis Rheum._ 1996 Nov;39(11):1808-17

[21] "Most people do not consume an optimal amount of all vitamins by diet alone. Pending strong evidence of effectiveness from randomized trials, it appears prudent for all adults to take vitamin supplements." Fletcher RH, Fairfield KM. Vitamins for chronic disease prevention in adults: clinical applications. _JAMA._ 2002 Jun 19;287(23):3127-9

[22] Trickett P. Proteolytic enzymes in treatment of athletic injuries. _Appl Ther._ 1964;30:647-52

[23] Walker JA, Cerny FJ, Cotter JR, Burton HW. Attenuation of contraction-induced skeletal muscle injury by bromelain. _Med Sci Sports Exerc._ 1992 Jan;24(1):20-5

[24] Walker AF, Bundy R, Hicks SM, Middleton RW. Bromelain reduces mild acute knee pain and improves well-being in a dose-dependent fashion in an open study of otherwise healthy adults. _Phytomedicine._ 2002; 9: 681-6

[25] Brien S, Lewith G, Walker A, Hicks SM, Middleton D. Bromelain as a Treatment for Osteoarthritis: a Review of Clinical Studies. _Evidence-based Complementary and Alternative Medicine._ 2004;1(3)251–257

[26] Jiang Q, Christen S, Shigenaga MK, Ames BN. gamma-tocopherol, the major form of vitamin E in the US diet, deserves more attention. _Am J Clin Nutr_ 2001 Dec;74(6):714-22

[27] Kaufman W. Niacinamide therapy for joint mobility. Therapeutic reversal of a common clinical manifestation of the "normal" aging process. _Conn State Med J_ 1953;17:584-591

[28] Kaufman W. The use of vitamin therapy to reverse certain concomitants of aging. _J Am Geriatr Soc_ 1955;3:927-936

[29] Matuoka K, Chen KY, Takenawa T. Rapid reversion of aging phenotypes by nicotinamide through possible modulation of histone acetylation. _Cell Mol Life Sci._ 2001;58(14):2108-16

[30] Jonas WB, Rapoza CP, Blair WF. The effect of niacinamide on osteoarthritis: a pilot study. _Inflamm Res_ 1996 Jul;45(7):330-4

[31] McCarty MF, Russell AL. Niacinamide therapy for osteoarthritis--does it inhibit nitric oxide synthase induction by interleukin 1 in chondrocytes? _Med Hypotheses._ 1999;53(4):350-60

[32] Gaby AR. Literature review and commentary: Niacinamide for osteoarthritis. _Townsend Letter for Doctors and Patients._ 2002: May; 32

[33] Greenwood J. Optimum vitamin C intake as a factor in the preservation of disc integrity. _Med Ann Dist Columbia._ 1964 Jun;33:274-6

[34] "A 3-fold reduction in risk of OA progression was found for both the middle tertile and highest tertile of vitamin C intake. This related predominantly to a reduced risk of cartilage loss. Those with high vitamin C intake also had a reduced risk of developing knee pain." McAlindon TE, Jacques P, Zhang Y, Hannan MT, Aliabadi P, Weissman B, Rush D, Levy D, Felson DT. Do antioxidant micronutrients protect against the development and progression of knee osteoarthritis? _Arthritis Rheum._ 1996 Apr;39(4):648-56

[35] Piscoya J, Rodriguez Z, Bustamante SA, Okuhama NN, Miller MJ, Sandoval M. Efficacy and safety of freeze-dried cat's claw in osteoarthritis of the knee: mechanisms of action of the species Uncaria guianensis. _Inflamm Res._ 2001 Sep;50(9):442-8

[36] "This small preliminary study demonstrates relative safety and modest benefit to the tender joint count of a highly purified extract from the pentacyclic chemotype of UT in patients with active RA taking sulfasalazine or hydroxychloroquine." Mur E, Hartig F, Eibl G, Schirmer M. Randomized double blind trial of an extract from the pentacyclic alkaloid-chemotype of uncaria tomentosa for the treatment of rheumatoid arthritis. _J Rheumatol._ 2002 Apr;29(4):678-81

o Topical application of *Capsicum annuum, Capsicum frutescens* (Cayenne pepper, hot chili pepper): Controlled clinical trials have conclusively demonstrated capsaicin's ability to deplete sensory fibers of substance P to thus reduce pain in diabetic neuropathy[37], chronic low back pain[38], chronic neck pain[39], osteoarthritis[40], rheumatoid arthritis[41], notalgia paresthetica[42], reflex sympathetic dystrophy[43], and cluster headache (intranasal application).[44,45,46]

o *Boswellia serrata*: Boswellia inhibits 5-lipoxygenase[47] with no apparent effect on cyclooxygenase[48] and has been shown effective in the treatment of osteoarthritis of the knees[49] as well as asthma[50] and ulcerative colitis.[51] When used as monotherapy, the target dose is approximately 150 mg of boswellic acids TID (thrice daily).

o *Zingiber officinale* (Ginger): Ginger is a well known spice and food with a long history of use as an anti-inflammatory, anti-nausea, and gastroprotective agent[52], and components of ginger have been shown to reduce production of the leukotriene LTB4 by inhibiting 5-lipoxygenase and to reduce production of the prostaglandin PGE2 by inhibiting cyclooxygenase.[53,54] Ginger has been shown to safely reduce nonspecific musculoskeletal pain[55,56] and to provide relief from osteoarthritis of the knees[57], migraine headaches,[58] and nausea/vomiting of pregnancy.[59]

o *Harpagophytum procumbens* (Devil's claw): The safety and **analgesic** effectiveness of Harpagophytum has been established in patients with hip pain, low-back pain, and knee pain.[60,61,62,63,64,65,66,67]

o Willow bark (*Salix* spp): Numerous studies—especially among patients with low-back pain—have validated the analgesic and anti-inflammatory benefits of willow bark extract.[68,69,70] Contraindications to the use of willow include aspirin/salicylate allergy and perhaps pregnancy, use of anticoagulant medication, or impending surgery.[71,72] The daily dose is generally kept below 240 mg of salicin, and products should include other components of the whole plant.

[37] "Study results suggest that topical capsaicin cream is safe and effective in treating painful diabetic neuropathy. "[No authors listed] Treatment of painful diabetic neuropathy with topical capsaicin. A multicenter, double-blind, vehicle-controlled study. The Capsaicin Study Group. *Arch Intern Med.* 1991 Nov;151(11):2225-9

[38] Keitel W, Frerick H, Kuhn U, Schmidt U, Kuhlmann M, Bredehorst A. Capsicum pain plaster in chronic non-specific low back pain. *Arzneimittelforschung.* 2001 Nov;51(11):896-903

[39] Mathias BJ, Dillingham TR, Zeigler DN, Chang AS, Belandres PV. Topical capsaicin for chronic neck pain. A pilot study. *Am J Phys Med Rehabil* 1995 Jan-Feb;74(1):39-44

[40] McCarthy GM, McCarty DJ. Effect of topical capsaicin in the therapy of painful osteoarthritis of the hands. *J Rheumatol.* 1992;19(4):604-7

[41] Deal CL, Schnitzer TJ, Lipstein E, et al. Treatment of arthritis with topical capsaicin: a double-blind trial. *Clin Ther.* 1991 May-Jun;13(3):383-95

[42] Leibsohn E. Treatment of notalgia paresthetica with capsaicin. *Cutis* 1992 May;49(5):335-6

[43] "Capsaicin is effective for psoriasis, pruritus, and cluster headache; it is often helpful for the itching and pain of postmastectomy pain syndrome, oral mucositis, cutaneous allergy, loin pain/hematuria syndrome, neck pain, amputation stump pain, and skin tumor; and it may be beneficial for neural dysfunction (detrusor hyperreflexia, reflex sympathetic dystrophy, and rhinopathy)." Hautkappe M, Roizen MF, Toledano A, Roth S, Jeffries JA, Ostermeier AM. Review of the effectiveness of capsaicin for painful cutaneous disorders and neural dysfunction. *Clin J Pain* 1998 Jun;14(2):97-106

[44] "Capsaicin application to human nasal mucosa was found to induce painful sensation, sneezing, and nasal secretion. All of these factors exhibit desensitization upon repeated applications." Sicuteri F, Fusco BM, Marabini S, Campagnolo V, Maggi CA, Geppetti P, Fanciullacci M. Beneficial effect of capsaicin application to the nasal mucosa in cluster headache. *Clin J Pain.* 1989;5(1):49-53

[45] "The efficacy of repeated nasal applications of capsaicin in cluster headache is congruent with previous reports on the therapeutic effect of capsaicin in other pain syndromes (post-herpetic neuralgia, diabetic neuropathy, trigeminal neuralgia) and supports the use of the drug to produce a selective analgesia." Fusco BM, Marabini S, Maggi CA, Fiore G, Geppetti P. Preventative effect of repeated nasal applications of capsaicin in cluster headache. *Pain.* 1994 Dec;59(3):321-5

[46] "These results indicate that intranasal capsaicin may provide a new therapeutic option for the treatment of this disease." Marks DR, Rapoport A, Padla D, Weeks R, Rosum R, Sheftell F, Arrowsmith F. A double-blind placebo-controlled trial of intranasal capsaicin for cluster headache. *Cephalalgia.* 1993 Apr;13(2):114-6

[47] Wildfeuer A, Neu IS, Safayhi H, Metzger G, Wehrmann M, Vogel U, Ammon HP. Effects of boswellic acids extracted from a herbal medicine on the biosynthesis of leukotrienes and the course of experimental autoimmune encephalomyelitis. *Arzneimittelforschung* 1998 Jun;48(6):668-74

[48] Safayhi H, Mack T, Sabieraj J, Anazodo MI, Subramanian LR, Ammon HP. Boswellic acids: novel, specific, nonredox inhibitors of 5-lipoxygenase. *J Pharmacol Exp Ther* 1992 Jun;261(3):1143-6

[49] Kimmatkar N, Thawani V, Hingorani L, Khiyani R. Efficacy and tolerability of Boswellia serrata extract in treatment of osteoarthritis of knee--a randomized double blind placebo controlled trial. *Phytomedicine.* 2003 Jan;10(1):3-7

[50] Gupta I, Gupta V, Parihar A, Gupta S, Ludtke R, Safayhi H, Ammon HP. Effects of Boswellia serrata gum resin in patients with bronchial asthma: results of a double-blind, placebo-controlled, 6-week clinical study. *Eur J Med Res.* 1998 Nov 17;3(11):511-4

[51] Gupta I, Parihar A, Malhotra P, Singh GB, Ludtke R, Safayhi H, Ammon HP. Effects of Boswellia serrata gum resin in patients with ulcerative colitis. *Eur J Med Res.* 1997 Jan;2(1):37-43

[52] Langner E, Greifenberg S, Gruenwald J. Ginger: history and use. *Adv Ther* 1998 Jan-Feb;15(1):25-44

[53] Kiuchi F, Iwakami S, Shibuya M, Hanaoka F, Sankawa U. Inhibition of prostaglandin and leukotriene biosynthesis by gingerols and diarylheptanoids. *Chem Pharm Bull* (Tokyo) 1992 Feb;40(2):387-91

[54] Tjendraputra E, Tran VH, Liu-Brennan D, Roufogalis BD, Duke CC. Effect of ginger constituents and synthetic analogues on cyclooxygenase-2 enzyme in intact cells. *Bioorg Chem* 2001 Jun;29(3):156-63

[55] Srivastava KC, Mustafa T. Ginger (Zingiber officinale) in rheumatism and musculoskeletal disorders. *Med Hypotheses.* 1992 Dec;39(4):342-8

[56] Srivastava KC, Mustafa T. Ginger (Zingiber officinale) and rheumatic disorders. *Med Hypotheses.* 1989 May;29(1):25-8

[57] Altman RD, Marcussen KC. Effects of a ginger extract on knee pain in patients with osteoarthritis. *Arthritis Rheum.* 2001 Nov;44(11):2531-8

[58] Mustafa T, Srivastava KC. Ginger (Zingiber officinale) in migraine headache. *J Ethnopharmacol.* 1990 Jul;29(3):267-73

[59] "...oral ginger 1 g per day... No adverse effect of ginger on pregnancy outcome was detected." Vutyavanich T, Kraisarin T, Ruangsri R. Ginger for nausea and vomiting in pregnancy: randomized, double-masked, placebo-controlled trial. *Obstet Gynecol* 2001 Apr;97(4):577-82.

[60] Chrubasik S, Thanner J, Kunzel O, Conradt C, Black A, Pollak S. Comparison of outcome measures during treatment with the proprietary Harpagophytum extract doloteffin in patients with pain in the lower back, knee or hip. *Phytomedicine* 2002 Apr;9(3):181-94

[61] Chantre P, Cappelaere A, Leblan D, Guedon D, Vandermander J, Fournie B. Efficacy and tolerance of Harpagophytum procumbens versus diacerhein in treatment of osteoarthritis. *Phytomedicine* 2000 Jun;7(3):177-83

[62] Leblan D, Chantre P, Fournie B. Harpagophytum procumbens in the treatment of knee and hip osteoarthritis. Four-month results of a prospective, multicenter, double-blind trial versus diacerhein. *Joint Bone Spine* 2000;67(5):462-7

[63] Whitehouse LW, Znamirowska M, Paul CJ. Devil's Claw (Harpagophytum procumbens): no evidence for anti-inflammatory activity in the treatment of arthritic disease. *Can Med Assoc J* 1983 Aug 1;129(3):249-51

[64] Moussard C, Alber D, Toubin MM, Thevenon N, Henry JC. A drug used in traditional medicine, harpagophytum procumbens: no evidence for NSAID-like effect on whole blood eicosanoid production in human. *Prostaglandins Leukot Essent Fatty Acids* 1992 Aug;46(4):283-6

[65] Chrubasik S, Model A, Black A, Pollak S. A randomized double-blind pilot study comparing Doloteffin and Vioxx in the treatment of low back pain. *Rheumatology* (Oxford). 2003 Jan;42(1):141-8

[66] "The majority of responders' were patients who had suffered less than 42 days of pain, and subgroup analyses suggested that the effect was confined to patients with more severe and radiating pain accompanied by neurological deficit... There was no evidence for Harpagophytum-related side-effects, except possibly for mild and infrequent gastrointestinal symptoms." Chrubasik S, Junck H, Breitschwerdt H, Conradt C, Zappe H. Effectiveness of Harpagophytum extract WS 1531 in the treatment of exacerbation of low back pain: a randomized, placebo-controlled, double-blind study. *Eur J Anaesthesiol* 1999 Feb;16(2):118-29

[67] "They took an 8-week course of Doloteffin at a dose providing 60 mg harpagoside per day... Doloteffin is well worth considering for osteoarthritic knee and hip pain and nonspecific low back pain." Chrubasik S, Thanner J, Kunzel O, Conradt C, Black A, Pollak S. Comparison of outcome measures during treatment with the proprietary Harpagophytum extract doloteffin in patients with pain in the lower back, knee or hip. *Phytomedicine* 2002 Apr;9(3):181-94

[68] Chrubasik S, Eisenberg E, Balan E, Weinberger T, Luzzati R, Conradt C. Treatment of low-back pain exacerbations with willow bark extract: a randomized double-blind study. *Am J Med.* 2000;109:9-14

[69] Chrubasik S, Kunzel O, Model A, Conradt C, Black A. Treatment of low-back pain with a herbal or anti-rheumatic: a randomized controlled study. Willow bark extract for low-back pain. *Rheumatology* (Oxford). 2001;40:1388-93

[70] Hare LG, Woodside JV, Young IS. Dietary salicylates. *J Clin Pathol* 2003 Sep;56(9):649-50 http://jcp.bmj.com/cgi/content/full/56/9/649

[71] **Vasquez A, Muanza DN. Evaluation of Presence of Aspirin-Related Warnings with Willow Bark: Comment on the Article by Clauson et al. *Ann Pharmacotherapy* 2005 Oct;39:1763**

[72] Clauson KA, Santamarina ML, Buettner CM, Cauffield JS. Evaluation of Presence of Aspirin-Related Warnings with Willow Bark (July/August). *Ann Pharmacother* 2005;39(7-8):1234-7

- <u>Treat with physical/manual medicine, massage, mobilization, and manipulation</u>: Gentle massage provides comfort, increases circulation, reduces edema, and promotes healing. After the acute phase, deeper massage may help restore range of motion by breaking adhesions and reducing the feeling of vulnerability that may occur after injury. Treat MFTP with post-isometric stretching and nutrition as reviewed in Chapter 3. Consider physiotherapy, if appropriate.[73] **Use manipulative therapy to patient tolerance after contraindications (e.g., fracture, infection) have been excluded; a clinical trial[74] found osteopathic manipulation to provide significant benefits to patients with acute ankle sprain, as discussed in greater detail later in this chapter.**

- <u>Uncover the underlying problem and contributing factors</u>: Congenital anomalies, underlying pathology, previous injury, and psychoemotional disorders may have been present before the "injury."[75]

- <u>Rehabilitation</u>: Pre-rehabilitation assessment has three main goals: 1) identification of the type of injury, 2) quantification of the severity of the injury, and 3) determining the appropriate interventions.[76] Rehabilitative exercises emphasizing strength, coordination, proprioception, range of motion, and functional utility (appropriate per occupation and hobbies) should be employed. Isometric exercises can be used to maintain/increase muscle strength in patients for whom range-of-motion exercises are painful or contraindicated.

- <u>Rehabilitation for lifestyle transformation</u>: Rehabilitation can become more than restorative; if the plan is comprehensive and it effects long-term improvements in overall health, then such a program can become transformative. The plan must be comprehensive and require active participation of the patient in order to attain optimal *short-term effectiveness* and *long-term sustainable success*.

- <u>Reassurance and resourcefulness</u>: Education, explanation, reassurance, and support help to address the mental and emotional aspects of injury. Books, websites, and national/local support groups and organizations may be available for emotional, physical, psychological-emotional, and legal assistance.

- <u>Referral</u>: **Patients with severe pain, serious conditions/complications, or documented noncompliance are excellent candidates for co-management or unidirectional referral.**

- <u>Proprioceptive Rehabilitation</u>: Proprioceptive deficits are common in patients with chronic low-back pain[77], neck pain[78], knee pain and arthritis[79], and **ankle instability**.[80] Means of challenging and thus developing neuromuscular coordination include use of vigorous full-body exercise, wobble board, balance shoes, foam, exercise ball, or other labile support surface.[81,82,83,84,85] Spinal manipulation may also improve proprioceptive function[86]; and skin taping appears to promote sensorimotor integration by increasing afferent input.[87]

- <u>Prolotherapy</u>: **Due to its ability to promote proliferation of connective tissue, dextrose prolotherapy may provide benefit for patients with ligamentous laxity, as demonstrated in studies of patients with back pain, knee pain, and hand osteoarthritis.**[88,89,90,91,92]

[73] Download the free notes at http://www.OptimalHealthResearch.com/physiotherapy
[74] "Ten percent of emergency department (ED) visits are related to ankle injury, and approximately 75% of these injuries are sprains." Eisenhart AW, Gaeta TJ, Yens DP.Osteopathic manipulative treatment in the emergency department for patients with acute ankle injuries. *J Am Osteopath Assoc.* 2003 Sep;103(9):417-21 http://www.jaoa.org/cgi/reprint/103/9/417
[75] Seifert S. Medical Illness Simulating Trauma (MIST) syndrome: case reports and discussion of syndrome. *Fam Med* 1993 Apr;25(4):273-6
[76] Geffen SJ. 3: Rehabilitation principles for treating chronic musculoskeletal injuries. *Med J Aust.* 2003 Mar 3;178(5):238-42
[77] Newcomer KL, Jacobson TD, Gabriel DA, Larson DR, Brey RH, An KN. Muscle activation patterns in subjects with and without low back pain. *Arch Phys Med Rehabil.* 2002;83(6):816-21
[78] McPartland JM, Brodeur RR, Hallgren RC. Chronic neck pain, standing balance, and suboccipital muscle atrophy--a pilot study. *J Manipulative Physiol Ther.* 1997 Jan;20(1):24-9
[79] Callaghan MJ, Selfe J, Bagley PJ, Oldham JA. The Effects of Patellar Taping on Knee Joint Proprioception. *J Athl Train.* 2002 Mar;37(1):19-24
[80] Olmsted LC, Carcia CR, Hertel J, Shultz SJ. Efficacy of the Star Excursion Balance Tests in Detecting Reach Deficits in Subjects With Chronic Ankle Instability. *J Athl Train.* 2002 Dec;37(4):501-506 http://www.pubmedcentral.gov/articlerender.fcgi?tool=pubmed&pubmedid=12937574
[81] Troy Blackburn J, Hirth CJ, Guskiewicz KM. Exercise Sandals Increase Lower Extremity Electromyographic Activity During Functional Activities. *J Athl Train.* 2003 Sep;38(3):198-203
[82] Bullock-Saxton JE, Janda V, Bullock MI.Reflex activation of gluteal muscles in walking. An approach to restoration of muscle function for patients with low-back pain. *Spine* 1993 May;18(6):704-8
[83] Olmsted LC, Carcia CR, Hertel J, Shultz SJ. Efficacy of the Star Excursion Balance Tests in Detecting Reach Deficits in Subjects With Chronic Ankle Instability. *J Athl Train.* 2002 Dec;37(4):501-506
[84] Troy Blackburn J, Hirth CJ, Guskiewicz KM. Exercise Sandals Increase Lower Extremity Electromyographic Activity During Functional Activities. *J Athl Train.* 2003 Sep;38(3):198-203
[85] Willems T, Witvrouw E, Verstuyft J, Vaes P, De Clercq D. Proprioception and Muscle Strength in Subjects With a History of Ankle Sprains and Chronic Instability. *J Athl Train.* 2002 Dec;37(4):487-493
[86] "RESULTS: Subjects receiving manipulation demonstrated a mean reduction in visual analogue scores of 44%, along with a 41% improvement in mean scores for the head repositioning skill." Rogers RG. The effects of spinal manipulation on cervical kinesthesia in patients with chronic neck pain: a pilot study. *J Manipulative Physiol Ther.* 1997 Feb;20(2):80-5
[87] Callaghan MJ, Selfe J, Bagley PJ, Oldham JA. The Effects of Patellar Taping on Knee Joint Proprioception. *J Athl Train.* 2002 Mar;37(1):19-24
[88] "Prolotherapy injection with 10% dextrose resulted in clinically and statistically significant improvements in knee osteoarthritis. Preliminary blinded radiographic readings (1-year films, with 3-year total follow-up period planned) demonstrated improvement in several measures of osteoarthritis severity. ACL laxity, when present in these osteoarthritic patients, improved. " Reeves KD, Hassanein K. Randomized prospective double-blind placebo-controlled study of dextrose prolotherapy for knee osteoarthritis with or without ACL laxity. *Altern Ther Health Med* 2000 Mar;6(2):68-74, 77-80
[89] Mooney V. Prolotherapy at the fringe of medical care, or is it the frontier? *Spine J.* 2003 Jul-Aug;3(4):253-4
[90] This study used intradiscal injection therapy with glucosamine, chondroitin sulfate, hypertonic dextrose and DMSO. "Although the results were statistically significant for the 30 patients as a whole, 17 of the 30 patients (57%) improved markedly with an average of 72% improvement in disability scores and 76% in visual analogue scores. The other 13 patients (43%) had little or no improvement." Klein RG, Eek BC, O'Neill CW, Elin C, Mooney V, Derby RR. Biochemical injection treatment for discogenic low back pain: a pilot study. *Spine J.* 2003 May-Jun;3(3):220-6
[91] "Dextrose prolotherapy was clinically effective and safe in the treatment of pain with joint movement and range limitation in osteoarthritic finger joints." Reeves KD, Hassanein K. Randomized, prospective, placebo-controlled double-blind study of dextrose prolotherapy for osteoarthritic thumb and finger (DIP, PIP, and trapeziometacarpal) joints: evidence of clinical efficacy. *J Altern Complement Med.* 2000 Aug;6(4):311-20
[92] "RESULTS: Each patient was injected an average of 3.5 times. Overall, 43.4% of patients fell into the sustained improvement group with an average improvement in numeric pain scores of 71%, comparing pretreatment and 18 month measurements." Miller MR, Mathews RS, Reeves KD. Treatment of painful advanced internal lumbar disc derangement with intradiscal injection of hypertonic dextrose. *Pain Physician.* 2006 Apr;9(2):115-21 http://www.painphysicianjournal.com/linkout_vw.php?issn=1533-3159&vol=9&page=115

Selected orthopedic problems of the leg

Problem & Typical Presentation	Assessment & Management
Acute compartment syndrome (ACS), chronic compartment syndrome, exertional compartment syndrome ▪ Compression of neurovascular elements within a fascia-bound compartment; compression can lead to permanent nerve death, and tissue ischemia can result in tissue necrosis, with myonecrosis liberating myoglobin which can precipitate acute renal failure and death ▪ ACS can develop without trauma following hyperemic compression or rapid muscle hypertrophy from exercise or overexertion ▪ Acute trauma can lead to bleeding and edema with subsequent compression of neurovascular structures that are contained within fascial sheaths; compression can lead to ischemia and death of muscle and nerve ▪ Compartment syndromes can also occur due to intracompartmental bleeding in patients with blood clotting disorders or following the use of restrictive bandages or tourniquets[93] ▪ The classic location for ACS is the anterolateral leg; however ACS can also occur in the posterior leg, thigh, forearm, and several other locations—anywhere that tissue swelling within a confined area can cause neurovascular injury and/or tissue ischemia Typical presentation of leg ACS ▪ Pain and sensation of pressure or "fullness" in anterior leg, especially following trauma or prolonged exertion ▪ May have numbness at dorsum of foot ▪ May have foot drop and weakness of the tibialis anterior and extensor hallucis longus **Clinicians must recognize and treat acute compartment syndrome as a surgical emergency; surgery should occur within six hours of symptom onset.**	**Typical presentation includes the "4 p's":** ▪ **Pain, Painful passive stretch, Pallor, Pulselessness**—a rare finding; indicates need for urgent referral and surgical intervention ▪ History: Trauma, exertion, bleeding disorder, alcoholism ▪ Observation: Walking and especially walking-on-heels are impaired ▪ Examination: Tenderness with provocation and palpation of the involved muscles, painful stretch, distal pallor, distal pulselessness; **sensory deficit (numbness; loss of two-point discrimination) is the most consistent physical finding**; intra-compartmental catheter can be used to measure pressure and is considered the standard diagnostic procedure[94]; if the clinical picture includes myoglobinuria (dark urine) then emergency treatment for incipient renal failure must be pursued[95]; serum creatine kinase may be elevated[96] ▪ Inability to walk, toe-walk, heel-walk and/or evidence of neurovascular lesions (numbness, cyanosis) indicates the need for immediate referral for surgical intervention (fasciotomy); **complications can include muscle necrosis and permanent neurologic impairment.[97] Surgical treatment—fasciotomy—should be performed within 6 hours of symptom onset.** ▪ Despite its milder severity, chronic/exertional compartment syndrome is described in the medical research literature as an indication for surgery[98] based on the potential risks involved with non-treatment and the failure of conservative treatment with massage and stretching to reduce intracompartmental pressures[99,100] ▪ Mild cases can be managed conservatively with massage, rest and resumption of activity only after pain is absent; cases that are conservatively managed require patient education and informed consent; aggressive massage to hypoxic or ischemic muscles might exacerbate tissue damage and myoglobinuria ▪ From both strategic and clinical viewpoints, patients with acute compartment syndrome should be referred for surgical consultation; this referral must be made on an emergency basis if neurovascular compromise is evident
	"Compartment syndrome (CS) is a limb-threatening and life-threatening condition observed when perfusion pressure falls below tissue pressure in a closed anatomic space. The current body of knowledge unequivocally reflects that untreated CS leads to tissue necrosis, permanent functional impairment, and, if severe, renal failure and death." Paula R. Compartment Syndrome, Extremity. *eMedicine* June 22, 2006 http://www.emedicine.com/emerg/topic739.htm Accessed January 11, 2007

93 Edwards S. Acute compartment syndrome. *Emerg Nurse.* 2004 Jun;12(3):32-8 http://www.nursing-standard.co.uk/archives/en_pdfs/envol12-03/env12n3p3238.pdf
94 Browning KH, Donley BG. Evaluation and management of common running injuries. *Cleve Clin J Med* 2000 Jul;67(7):511-20
95 Edwards S. Acute compartment syndrome. *Emerg Nurse.* 2004 Jun;12(3):32-8 http://www.nursing-standard.co.uk/archives/en_pdfs/envol12-03/env12n3p3238.pdf
96 "The results of our study suggest that although raised CK levels are not diagnostic, they are a useful adjunct in making a diagnosis, and hence CK estimation should be done in all patients with suspected compartment syndrome." Ihedioha U, Sinha S, Campbell AC. Do creatine kinase (CK) levels influence the diagnosis or outcome in patients with compartment syndrome? *Scott Med J.* 2005 Nov;50(4):158-9
97 "Without immediate attention to this problem, the possibility of myoneural ischemia is real... ...permanent impairment may occur in the lower leg... An early sign of anterior compartment syndrome is the presence of exquisite pain on passive stretch." Brier S. Primary Care Orthopedics. St. Louis: Mosby, 1999 page 370-2
98 "There is agreement among orthopedic surgeons on the role of ICPs for diagnosis and the choice of fasciotomy as a first-line surgical procedure." Tzortziou V, Maffulli N, Padhiar N. Diagnosis and management of chronic exertional compartment syndrome (CECS) in the United Kingdom. *Clin J Sport Med.* 2006 May;16(3):209-13
99 "Other than complete cessation of causative activities, nonoperative management of CECS is usually unsuccessful. Surgical release of the involved compartments is recommended for patients who wish to continue to exercise." Bong MR, Polatsch DB, Jazrawi LM, Rokito AS. Chronic exertional compartment syndrome: diagnosis and management. *Bull Hosp Jt Dis.* 2005;62(3-4):77-84 http://www.nyuhjdbulletin.org/Permalink.aspx?permalinkId=b1995544-b30f-4662-83cf-af93f33c0374
100 "There was no significant difference in the 3-minute postexercise compartment pressures after the treatment." Blackman PG, Simmons LR, Crossley KM. Treatment of chronic exertional anterior compartment syndrome with massage: a pilot study. *Clin J Sport Med.* 1998 Jan;8(1):14-7

Selected orthopedic problems of the leg—*continued*

Problem & Typical Presentation	Assessment & Management
Fracture of the tibia or fibula ▪ Localized bone pain following trauma ▪ Exacerbation of pain with weight-bearing, more so with the tibia than the fibula	▪ Localized bone pain ▪ Exacerbation of pain with weight-bearing, tuning fork, and/or other provocative assessment such as the fulcrum test ▪ Assessment for neurovascular compromise is mandatory ▪ **Radiographs**: consider views of the ankle and foot as indicated ▪ Crutches and casting ▪ Assess for compartment syndromes ▪ Orthopedic referral for fractures without neurovascular injury ▪ Immediate referral for fractures with neurovascular injury
Stress fracture of the tibia or fibula ▪ Localized bone pain in an endurance or overtrained athlete ▪ Exacerbation of pain with weight-bearing ▪ May have pain at night	▪ **Localized bone pain** in an endurance or overtrained athlete ▪ **Radiographs—most likely to be positive after 2-3 weeks after the onset of symptoms;** may also image with MRI or bone scan ▪ May have swelling, pain with percussion, pain with fulcrum test ▪ Conservative care emphasizing rest for up to 12 weeks ▪ Consider crutches ▪ Resumption of activity only after pain is absent ▪ Referral to an orthopedic surgeon is advised for fractures of the anterior middle third of the tibia, since these have a higher risk of complications[101] ▪ Assess for compartment syndromes
Peroneal neuropraxia, peroneal neuropathy ▪ Injury or compression to the common peroneal nerve near the fibular head ▪ Acute: Foot drop after injury near the fibular head ▪ Chronic: Foot drop following events or postures that compress the common peroneal/fibular* nerve (e.g., sitting with legs crossed)	▪ Foot drop, weak foot dorsiflexion and toe extension ▪ Assess for acute and chronic anterior compartment syndrome ▪ Acute cases warrant orthopedic consult or referral to assess injuries and feasibility ▪ Chronic non-traumatic cases will generally improve with time[102] and with "nerve support" such as with EFAs and cobalamin

* Note that the official nomenclature regarding the "peroneus" muscles has been changed to "fibularis" such that peroneus longus, peroneus brevis, and peroneus tertius are now referred to as **fibularis longus, fibularis brevis,** and **fibularis tertius**, respectively. Relatedly, what were previously the common, deep, and superficial peroneal nerves are now the **common, deep,** and **superficial fibular nerves**, respectively.

[101] Browning KH, Donley BG. Evaluation and management of common running injuries. *Cleve Clin J Med* 2000 Jul;67(7):511-20
[102] Brier S. Primary Care Orthopedics. St. Louis: Mosby, 1999 page 342-3

Selected orthopedic problems of the leg—*continued*

Problem & Typical Presentation	Assessment & Management
Blount's disease, tibia vara ▪ Developmental disorder of the proximal tibia characterized by varus deformity; femur may also be affected ▪ Etiologic factors include in utero molding of tibia and/or insufficient strength of tibia to support child's weight (i.e., biomechanical overload) ▪ More common in patients of African or Mediterranean descent[103] ▪ Not to be confused with physiologic "bowleg" or rickets	▪ Physical examination and radiographs show inward bowing (medial concavity) of tibia; 50-70% of affected patients are affected bilaterally ▪ Test for vitamin D deficiency (see Chapter 1) ▪ Occurs in two types: early onset before age 3y, and late onset after age 3y ▪ The condition often resolves by 18-24 months of age; any persistence beyond age 2 years is abnormal[104] ▪ Orthopedic consult is recommended because severe and non-resolving cases are treated with orthopedic bracing or surgical osteotomy[105]
"Shin splints" ▪ Overuse strain of the compartmentalized muscles[106] of the lower leg and/or inflammation of the tibial periosteum[107] ▪ <u>Anterolateral shin splints</u>: Overuse strain of the tibialis anterior, extensor hallucis longus, extensor digitorum longus; presents with muscular and/or periosteal pain with heel strike in an untrained or overexerting athlete ▪ <u>Posteromedial shin splints</u>: Involves the tibialis posterior, flexor hallucis longus, flexor digitorum longus; presents with pain worse with toe-off, associated with excessive pronation	▪ Tenderness with provocation, stretch, and palpation of the involved muscles and underlying periosteum ▪ Evaluate for and exclude stress fracture and acute compartment syndrome ▪ Consider screening laboratory assessments (Chapter 1) to help exclude underlying disease and to facilitate health assessment and intervention ▪ Comprehensive Musculoskeletal Care (Chapter 3 and previous), with emphasis on rest, decreased exercise, and *gradual* strengthening of the leg muscles, anti-inflammatory and tissue-healing nutritional support; patient may need new shock-absorbing shoes, a softer running surface, arch support and orthosis/orthoses
Tibial periostitis ▪ Inflammation of the periosteum surrounding the tibia due to jarring motions and muscle overuse; may precede stress fracture of the tibia, since the mechanism of injury is identical: repetitive overuse ▪ Leg pain with diffuse discomfort ▪ Often bilateral ▪ Tibial periostitis is commonly a component of shin splints	▪ No exacerbation of pain with static weight-bearing (in contrast to fractures which are more painful with weight-bearing stress) ▪ Tenderness along the shaft of the tibia, especially the distal anteromedial aspect ▪ Evaluate for and exclude stress fracture and acute compartment syndrome ▪ Test for vitamin D deficiency or use empiric vitamin D replacement for all patients with bone pain as this is commonly the presenting manifestation of vitamin-D-deficiency-induced osteomalacia[108]; measure serum 25-hydroxyvitamin D (detailed in Chapter 1) and/or implement physiologic replacement with 4,000 IU/d for adults without contraindications ▪ Comprehensive Musculoskeletal Care as above for shin splints
Tibialis posterior strain/ tendonitis ▪ An aspect of posteromedial shin splints ▪ Posterior leg pain with contraction of the tibialis posterior: toe-off, running, jumping ▪ More common in runners, jumpers	▪ Palpable diffuse tenderness at distal third posteromedial leg ▪ Comprehensive Musculoskeletal Care as above for shin splints; adapt treatment plan as needed

[103] Skinner HB, Scherger JE. Identifying structural hip and knee problems. Patient age, history, and limited examination may be all that's needed. *Postgrad Med* 1999;106(7):51-2, 55-6, 61-4
[104] Cheema J. Blount Disease. Last Updated: May 2, 2003 *eMedicine* http://www.emedicine.com/radio/topic83.htm Accessed January 14, 2007
[105] DeOrio MJ. Blount Disease. Last Updated: March 15, 2005. *eMedicine* http://www.emedicine.com/orthoped/topic369.htm Accessed January 14, 2007
[106] Beers MH, Berkow R (eds). The Merck Manual. Seventeenth Edition. Whitehouse Station; Merck Research Laboratories 1999 page 499
[107] Browning KH, Donley BG. Evaluation and management of common running injuries. *Cleve Clin J Med* 2000 Jul;67(7):511-20
[108] Holick MF. Vitamin D deficiency: what a pain it is. *Mayo Clin Proc.* 2003 Dec;78(12):1457-9

Ankle sprain, "twisted ankle"

<u>Description/pathophysiology</u>:
- Although an apparently simple disorder, ankle sprain—due to the severity of pain and accompanying injuries—is a major cause of emergency department visits. Eisenhart et al[109] wrote that "Ten percent of emergency department (ED) visits are related to ankle injury, and approximately 75% of these injuries are sprains."
- Up to 95% of ankle sprains are inversion sprains and thus affect the ligaments on the lateral aspect of the ankle and may also involve strain of the peroneal/fibular muscles. As mentioned previously, be aware that the official nomenclature regarding the "peroneus" muscles has been changed to "fibularis" such that peroneus longus, peroneus brevis, and peroneus tertius are now referred to as fibularis longus, fibularis brevis, and fibularis tertius, respectively. Relatedly, what were previously the common, deep, and superficial peroneal nerves are now the common, deep, and superficial fibular nerves, respectively.

<u>Clinical presentations</u>:
- Ankle pain after trauma or "twisting" the ankle
- Accompanying ecchymosis suggests ligament tear and is also seen with avulsion fracture

<u>Major differential diagnoses</u>:
- Most diagnoses of ankle sprain are straightforward; however keep in mind the possibility of underlying disease, especially if swelling or dysfunction appears out of proportion to what you expect, if the condition is recalcitrant to treatment, or if it is accompanied by systemic manifestations such as weight loss. *I am aware of one case report in the chiropractic literature of a 27-year-old patient presenting with ankle pain following a rigorous tennis match; the combination of his low-grade fever and the periosteal reaction noted on radiographs ultimately lead to the diagnosis of Ewing's sarcoma—an aggressive bone malignancy that commonly begins in the distal lower extremity.*
- Assess neurologic function bilaterally in the lower extremity as primary or recurrent ankle sprains may have resulted from proprioceptive defects or uncoordination secondary to neurologic conditions such as peripheral neuropathy or lesion of the dorsal column in the spinal cord. For example, a twisted ankle may be the presenting manifestation of proprioceptive defects secondary to peripheral neuropathy secondary to diabetes mellitus or vitamin B-12 deficiency.

<u>Clinical assessment</u>:
- **History/subjective**:
  - Ankle pain after trauma or "twisting" the ankle
  - *Did the ankle turn inwardly or outwardly? Was a popping sound heard at the time of injury?*
  - *What was the patient doing at the time of the accident—standing, walking, running, turning?*
  - *Was the patient bearing additional weight at the time of the injury, such as carrying a weighted object?* More weight or momentum at the time of the injury probably placed more stress on the tissues and would be expected to produce more tissue injury.
  - *Does the patient have a history of previous injuries?* Recurrent injuries are associated with additional tissue weakness, cumulative scar tissue, and more profound proprioceptive defects—all of which require consideration in the determination of the treatment plan and prognosis.
- **Physical examination/objective**:
  - Assess weight-bearing, gait, and patient's affect; ankle sprains are often very painful.
  - Local assessment includes observation, comparison for symmetry with the other ankle, observation for scars, deformity, edema, and ecchymosis.
  - Assess for tenderness, pain with palpation and provocation of bones and ligaments; use a tuning fork to assess for occult fracture; radiography is well-suited for fracture assessment.

---

[109] "Ten percent of emergency department (ED) visits are related to ankle injury, and approximately 75% of these injuries are sprains." Eisenhart AW, Gaeta TJ, Yens DP. Osteopathic manipulative treatment in the emergency department for patients with acute ankle injuries. *J Am Osteopath Assoc.* 2003 Sep;103(9):417-21 http://www.jaoa.org/cgi/reprint/103/9/417

- **Imaging & laboratory assessments**:
  - o Radiographs are reasonable for moderately and severely sprained ankles to exclude concomitant fracture, particularly of the 5th metatarsal and distal fibula; stress views are recommended to help quantify severity of joint laxity and thus guide treatment.[110]

Establishing the diagnosis:

- Ankle sprain is a clinical diagnosis based on the history and physical examination
- Grades (and treatments):[111,112]

Grade	Characteristics	Management
Grade 1	▪ Mild sprain with mild tenderness and swelling; no evidence of ligament sprain or rupture	▪ Comprehensive Musculoskeletal Care (Chapter 3) emphasizing rest, anti-inflammation, and proprioceptive retraining for 6 weeks
Grade 2	▪ Moderate sprain with moderate tenderness ▪ Functionally, the patient is able to walk but unable to run ▪ Soft tissue swelling ▪ Evidence of ligament laxity *but not rupture*: anterior drawer test indicating *partial* lesion of the anterior talofibular ligament is *weakly* positive	▪ Comprehensive Musculoskeletal Care as above ▪ Cast immobilization for 10-21 days may be recommended[113], especially for patients who are noncompliant with activity limitation and who might prolong or exacerbate injury
Grade 3	▪ Severe sprain with inability to walk due to instability and severe pain ▪ Major soft tissue swelling ▪ Hemorrhage due to ligament rupture and sometimes fracture ▪ Gross ligamentous instability, positive anterior drawer test and varus instability indicating rupture of the anterior talofibular ligament and/or the calcaneofibular ligament	▪ Comprehensive Musculoskeletal Care as above; most grade 3 sprains can be managed nonsurgically[114] ▪ Radiographs to assess for avulsion fracture ▪ Cast immobilization is often recommended[115] ▪ Recommend orthopedic consultation since reconstructive surgery is beneficial in some cases

Complications:

- Untreated nonunion fractures are predisposed to necrosis, infection, and chronic pain
- Ankle sprains result in ligament damage and ligament laxity. Lax ligaments are unable to provide structural stability to the joint, thus predisposing to future injury and recurrent microtrauma to joint surfaces. Additionally, lax ligaments fail to provide complete and accurate proprioceptive information, thus predisposing to additional injury. Lax ligaments fail to provide complete and accurate afferent proprioceptive input to block nociceptive input, thus perpetuating the perception of chronic pain.

Clinical management:

- Referral if clinical outcome is unsatisfactory or if complications arise.

Treatments:

- **Comprehensive Musculoskeletal Care:** described previously and in Chapter 3, with emphasis on:
  - o Frequent icing
  - o Assertive anti-inflammatory treatments: Many nutritionally-oriented doctors use proteolytic enzymes based on clinical experience and results of an uncontrolled open trial[116]; however, two

[110] Beers MH, Berkow R (eds). The Merck Manual. Seventeenth Edition. Whitehouse Station; Merck Research Laboratories 1999 page 484
[111] Beers MH, Berkow R (eds). The Merck Manual. Seventeenth Edition. Whitehouse Station; Merck Research Laboratories 1999 page 484
[112] Moreau W. Certified Chiropractic Sports Physician Program: Module 1, Session #2: Lower Extremity Diagnosis, Treatment, Rehabilitation. Western States Chiropractic College Division of Continuing Education, Portland, Oregon, February 10-11, 2001
[113] Beers MH, Berkow R (eds). The Merck Manual. Seventeenth Edition. Whitehouse Station; Merck Research Laboratories 1999 page 484
[114] Tierney ML. McPhee SJ, Papadakis MA (eds). Current Medical Diagnosis and Treatment 2006, 45th Edition. Lange Medical; page 826
[115] Beers MH, Berkow R (eds). The Merck Manual. Seventeenth Edition. Whitehouse Station; Merck Research Laboratories 1999 page 484
[116] **Trickett P. Proteolytic enzymes in treatment of athletic injuries.** *Appl Ther.* **1964;30:647-52**

controlled studies[117] have failed to substantiate this purported and observed benefit. At least one of these two negative studies[118] had inexcusable methodological defects that should have prevented its publication; furthermore, doses used in research studies (most of which appear to be conducted by non-clinicians) are often only 25-50% of the doses used by clinicians knowledgeable in these treatments, and this dosing inadequacy may be sufficient to explain the contrast between the clinical efficacy observed by skilled clinicians versus the lackluster response reported in the research literature.

> o Manipulative treatments emphasizing myofascial techniques as described in the Figure to the right and in the article by Eisenhart et al.[119]
> o Rest (consider crutches) and/or bracing (tape or cast).

- **Rehabilitation** with an emphasis on:
  - o Stretching the Achilles tendon.
  - o Strengthening the peroneal muscles.[120]
  - o Proprioceptive rehabilitation.[121]
    - ▪ Exercise sandals appear to be an effective rehabilitation tool for neuromuscular rehabilitation of the lower extremity and are expected to improve proprioceptive coordination, joint stability, and to reduce the recurrence of injury.[122]
    - ▪ Download the review by Mattacola and Dwyer, *Rehabilitation of the Ankle After Acute Sprain or Chronic Instability*: http://www.pubmedcentral.nih.gov/articlerender.fcgi?artid=164373

- **Stepwise therapeutic exercise and rehabilitation**: Begin within patient tolerance and increase intensity and duration as tissues heal and strengthen; examples from Moreau:[123]
  - o *Non-weight bearing phase*
    - ▪ Aquatic exercises
    - ▪ Rubber tubing
    - ▪ Isometrics
    - ▪ Skin taping to reduce swelling, provide mechanical support, and increase proprioceptive input
  - o *Weight-bearing phase*
    - ▪ Wobble board, balance sandals
    - ▪ Attentive walking, preferably barefoot
    - ▪ Heel and toe walking
  - o *Strenuous activities for functional restoration and health promotion*
    - ▪ Rope skipping
    - ▪ Jogging and running
    - ▪ Sprinting forward, running backward
    - ▪ Running in curves and circles, figure eight
    - ▪ Sports-specific training

Manipulative Treatment of Ankle Sprains

- Suitable for acute Grade 1 and Grade 2 sprains in adults, with no evidence of fracture or other contraindication
- Palpation of the tibia and fibula often reveals torsion of the interosseous ligament posterior displacement of the proximal fibula; palpation of the foot may reveal an inferiorly displaced cuboid—these are corrected with torsion, myofascial techniques, and strain-counterstrain; edema is addressed with manual lymphatic drainage
- "The results of our study indicate statistically significant reductions in edema and pain—and a trend toward increased ROM—immediately following one OMT [osteopathic manipulative therapy] intervention session."

Eisenhart AW, Gaeta TJ, Yens DP. Osteopathic manipulative treatment in the emergency department for patients with acute ankle injuries. *J Am Osteopath Assoc.* 2003 Sep;103(9):417-21 http://www.jaoa.org/cgi/reprint/103/9/417

---

[117] "No statistically significant difference in swelling, bruising and function between the 2 groups in the measurements of volume and allied parameters was found. No side effects were noted." Craig RP. The quantitative evaluation of the use of oral proteolytic enzymes in the treatment of sprained ankles. *Injury.* 1975 May;6(4):313-6

[118] Kerkhoffs GM, Struijs PA, de Wit C, Rahlfs VW, Zwipp H, van Dijk CN. A double blind, randomised, parallel group study on the efficacy and safety of treating acute lateral ankle sprain with oral hydrolytic enzymes. *Br J Sports Med.* 2004 Aug;38(4):431-5 http://bjsm.bmj.com/cgi/content/full/38/4/431

[119] Eisenhart AW, Gaeta TJ, Yens DP.Osteopathic manipulative treatment in the emergency department for patients with acute ankle injuries. *J Am Osteopath Assoc.* 2003 Sep;103(9):417-21 http://www.jaoa.org/cgi/reprint/103/9/417

[120] **Mattacola CG, Dwyer MK. Rehabilitation of the Ankle After Acute Sprain or Chronic Instability. *J Athl Train.* 2002;37(4):413-429 http://www.pubmedcentral.nih.gov/articlerender.fcgi?artid=164373**

[121] Willems T, Witvrouw E, Verstuyft J, Vaes P, De Clercq D. Proprioception and Muscle Strength in Subjects With a History of Ankle Sprains and Chronic Instability. *J Athl Train.* 2002 Dec;37(4):487-493

[122] Troy Blackburn J, Hirth CJ, Guskiewicz KM. Exercise Sandals Increase Lower Extremity Electromyographic Activity During Functional Activities. *J Athl Train.* 2003 Sep;38(3):198-203

[123] Moreau W. Certified Chiropractic Sports Physician Program: Module 1, Session #2: Lower Extremity Diagnosis, Treatment, Rehabilitation. Western States Chiropractic College Division of Continuing Education, Portland, Oregon, February 10-11, 2001

Additional orthopedic problems of the ankle and foot

Problem & Typical Presentation	Assessment & Management
Achilles' tendonitis ▪ Inflammation of the Achilles tendon from acute injury or chronic overuse; recall that rheumatoid arthritis and reactive arthritis also commonly affect this region (enthesopathy); test with CRP, CBC, and other lab tests as indicated ▪ Posterior heel pain, generally worse in morning and after exercise	▪ Pain at the Achilles' tendon exacerbated by compression and forceful plantar flexion of the foot ▪ Thompson test: to exclude complete rupture ▪ Consider lab tests for rheumatic disease especially if condition is bilateral, nontraumatic, or accompanied by systemic manifestations ▪ See Chapter 3 for Comprehensive Musculoskeletal Care ▪ Stretching, avoid high-heeled shoes ▪ Treat over-pronation of foot which is commonly present and leads to torque and bending of the Achilles' tendon ▪ Orthopedic referral for casting if unresponsive to treatment or if tendon is severed as evaluated by Thompson test
Fracture of the ankle or foot ▪ Bone fractures can occur with direct trauma or non-contact injury such as with a "twisted ankle" or sprained ankle ▪ **Ankle/foot pain associated with trauma, injury, corticosteroid use, or osteoporosis**	▪ Observation for swelling, hemorrhage, or deformity ▪ Palpation and provocation ▪ Fracture screen with ultrasound or tuning fork, fulcrum test; if fracture suspicion is high, start with radiographs before choosing 1) repeat radiographs in 2 weeks for callous formation, 2) CT, or 3) MRI or bone scan ▪ Because ankle fractures are often complex, intraarticular, or likely to be associated with chronic pain or disability, orthopedic referral for evaluation and casting are encouraged
Fracture: Avulsion fracture of the 5th metatarsal ▪ Pain at the middle lateral aspect of the foot following a "twisted ankle"	▪ Pain with palpation, provocation, and/or tuning fork ▪ Radiographs ▪ Unless the treating clinician is adept at casting and willing to accept potential liability, orthopedic referral is commonly recommended for co-management since different types of fractures (spiral, transverse) have a propensity for nonunion or delayed union and since casting may be necessary
Fracture: Jones fracture ▪ Fracture of the 5th metatarsal ▪ **Pain at the middle inferior lateral aspect of the foot following overuse or a "twisted ankle"**	▪ Pain with palpation, provocation, and/or tuning fork, fulcrum test ▪ Radiographs ▪ **"...Jones fracture has a propensity for nonunion or delayed union, and referral to an orthopedic surgeon is recommended."[124]**
Fracture: Metatarsal stress fracture ▪ **Pain in the metatarsal shaft in a runner or obese patient**	▪ Pain with palpation and provocation and toe-walking, fulcrum test ▪ Radiographs followed by bone scan if necessary ▪ A walking cast and/or crutches will remove stress and promote effective healing ▪ See Chapter 3 for Comprehensive Musculoskeletal Care, emphasizing rest and nutritional bone support

[124] Browning KH, Donley BG. Evaluation and management of common running injuries. *Cleve Clin J Med* 2000 Jul;67(7):511-20

Additional orthopedic problems of the ankle and foot—*continued*

Problem & Typical Presentation	Assessment & Management
Metatarsalgia • Pain at the metatarsal head • Pain at the 2nd or 3rd metatarsal head generally in a runner or obese patient	• Pain with palpation and provocation of affected bone • Exclude other causes such as Morton neuroma or stress fracture or plantar fascitis • Consider radiographs to exclude stress fracture • See Chapter 3 for Comprehensive Musculoskeletal Care • Metatarsal pads and/or orthosis to reestablish the transverse arch and properly distribute weight • Weight loss and wider shoes if necessary
Morton neuroma • Irritation of the interdigital nerve between the metatarsal heads, typically between the 3rd and 4th metatarsal heads • Burning or stabbing pain worse with wearing shoes, especially shoes that are too tight at the distal foot	• Exacerbation with compression of the distal foot • Exacerbation with deep pressure • A palpable mass is notable in some cases • MRI can be used for conclusive diagnosis. • Discard poorly fitting shoes, especially those that are too small • See Chapter 3 for Comprehensive Musculoskeletal Care • Metatarsal pads to reestablish the transverse arch and properly distribute weight • Orthoses • Surgery or corticosteroid injection can help recalcitrant cases
Plantar fascitis, plantar fasciitis • Inflammation of the plantar fascia which originates at the medial calcaneal tubercle and inserts into the fascia of the toes; chronic microtrauma, inflammation, and tension often preceded the formation of calcaneal osteophytes or "heel spurs" • Inferior heel pain • Diffuse pain and tenderness exacerbated by walking, prolonged standing, and point pressure applied to sole of foot especially near the origin of the plantar fascia at the calcaneus	• Physical examination of the foot; radiographs are unnecessary except for recalcitrant cases or to exclude fracture or disease • Diffuse tenderness in the plantar fascia with palpation and provocation • Heel spurs generally invoke local tenderness at the medial calcaneal tubercle and are visible radiographically • See Chapter 3 for Comprehensive Musculoskeletal Care emphasizing rest, antiinflammatories, ice, heel pads, arch support, weight loss (if indicated), reduced walking/standing, increased stretching of the Achilles' tendon, ultrasound, deep massage, myofascial stretch (ankle dorsiflexion with toe hyperextension)[125] • Manipulative therapy, strain-counterstrain[126] • Surgery may help those who fail to respond to conservative care for 6-12 months
Tarsal tunnel syndrome • Compression neuropathy of the posterior tibial nerve in the lower leg or by the flexor retinaculum, medial surface of the calcaneus, posteromedial talus, and distal posteromedial tibia • Numbness and tingling in the sole of the foot and toes	• Rule out fracture, infection or other disease • Pes planus (flat feet) is a common concomitant finding • See Chapter 3 for Comprehensive Musculoskeletal Care • The most important treatment is correction of foot hyperpronation with arch support and heel cup • Physiotherapy with underwater ultrasound has been advocated • Consider MRI of the ankle if necessary for assessment or preoperative evaluation • Many patients with tarsal tunnel syndrome may eventually need surgical decompression, which is successful in approximately 80-90% of patients

---

[125] "This study supports the use of the tissue-specific plantar fascia-stretching protocol as the key component of treatment for chronic plantar fasciitis. Long-term benefits of the stretch include a marked decrease in pain and functional limitations and a high rate of satisfaction." Digiovanni BF, Nawoczenski DA, Malay DP, Graci PA, Williams TT, Wilding GE, Baumhauer JF. Plantar fascia-specific stretching exercise improves outcomes in patients with chronic plantar fasciitis. A prospective clinical trial with two-year follow-up. *J Bone Joint Surg Am.* 2006;88(8):1775-81
[126] "Significant reductions in symptom severity were reported by subjects with plantar fasciitis immediately after counterstrain treatment. A smaller, but still significant, reduction in symptom severity persisted for more than 48 hours posttreatment." Wynne MM, Burns JM, Eland DC, Conatser RR, Howell JN. Effect of counterstrain on stretch reflexes, hoffmann reflexes, and clinical outcomes in subjects with plantar fasciitis. *J Am Osteopath Assoc.* 2006 Sep;106(9):547-56 http://www.jaoa.org/cgi/content/full/106/9/547

Chapter 15:
Iron Overload and Genetic Hemochromatosis

Introduction

In its "classic" form, homozygous genetic hemochromatosis is noted in about 1 per 200-250 Caucasian persons with a similar incidence among Hispanics. The incidence among persons of African descent is much higher. The heterozygous form of iron overload which is phenotypically milder occurs in as many as 1 per 7 (14% of total) persons; any disorder that is common in the general population will be even more common in a clinical population of symptomatic care-seeking patients, especially those with musculoskeletal disorders and complaints.[1]

Testing serum ferritin on a routine basis in clinical practice allows for the detection of iron deficiency (very common, even among non-anemic patients) and iron overload (quite common, especially among patients with joint pain, diabetes, heart failure, and liver disease as well as many other clinical manifestations—most common of which is asymptomaticity.

---

[1] Vasquez A. Musculoskeletal disorders and iron overload disease: comment on the American College of Rheumatology guidelines for the initial evaluation of the adult patient with acute musculoskeletal symptoms. *Arthritis & Rheumatism*: Official Journal of the American College of Rheumatology 1996; 39:1767-8

Iron Overload
Primary/Genetic Hemochromatosis
Secondary Hemochromatosis

<u>Description/pathophysiology</u>:

- **Hereditary iron overload disorders are now recognized as being among the most common genetic diseases in the human population.**[2,3,4,5,6,7,8]

- Iron overload is a phenotypic state to which a patient arrives by either genetic or environmental/iatrogenic routes. The severity of iron overload can range from moderate to severe.

- Excess iron catalyses oxidative stress which damages body tissues and structures in which the iron is stored. In patients with genetic hemochromatosis, two problems exist simultaneously: 1) a disproportionately large amount of iron is absorbed from the gastrointestinal tract (i.e., these patients' iron absorption is "too efficient"), and 2) iron is preferentially deposited in parenchymal tissues such as the heart, liver, pancreas, pituitary gland, and joints rather than being stored safely within the reticuloendothelial system. The deposition of excess iron in parenchymal tissues promotes destruction of these organs/tissues via oxidative mechanisms and subsequent tissue necrosis and fibrosis, leading to the protean manifestations of the disease dependent upon which organs are most affected in the individual patient: heart failure, hepatic fibrosis, hypoinsulinemic diabetes, hypopituarism, and hemochromatoic arthropathy.[9]

- Iron overload can be defined as a state of "iron toxicity" similar to mercury toxicity or poisoning with any other heavy metal or toxin, except that the mechanism is more related to the *quantity* of the iron rather than the unique characteristics or *quality* of iron itself. In other words, whereas the toxicity of mercury can be seen even when only small amounts of the metal are present, the toxicity of iron is directly related to the amount of the excess iron, rather than the inherent toxicity of the iron itself.

Iron overload disorders are common

Genetic hemochromatosis is considered one of the most common hereditary disorders in the Caucasian population with a homozygote frequency of 1 per 200-250 (approx 0.5%) and a heterozygote frequency of about 1 in 7 (approx 14%); the condition is at least as common in other ethnic groups except that this predisposition toward iron overload is more common in Africans (as high as 1 in 20) and African-Americans (as high as about 1 in 80 in some series among hospitalized patients). Of course, the expected frequency would be even higher among symptomatic patients than among the general population. **Thus, as a clinician, if you are not appreciating this condition among your patients several times per year, it is because you are not sufficiently screening your patients for it.**

Rationale for screening all patients

1. Hereditary iron-accumulation disorders occur in a large percentage of the population.
2. Persons with the disease usually have no symptoms.
3. Clinical manifestations are often indicative of irreversible organ damage or organ failure.
4. Iron overload can cause death if not treated early.
5. Early treatment ensures normal life expectancy.
6. **Therefore, early detection (before the onset of symptoms and organ damage) requires screening asymptomatic patients**.

<u>Test of choice</u>: **Serum ferritin**, shows the best correlation with body iron stores and thus prognosis and need for treatment.

---

[2] Olynyk JK, Bacon BR. Hereditary hemochromatosis: detecting and correcting iron overload. *Postgrad Med* 1994; 96: 151-65
[3] Phatak PD, Cappuccio JD. Management of hereditary hemochromatosis. *Blood Rev* 1994; 8: 193-8
[4] Rouault TA. Hereditary hemochromatosis. *JAMA* 1993; 269: 3152-4
[5] Crosby WH. Hemochromatosis: current concepts and management. Hosp Pract 1987; 22:173-92
[6] Bloom PD, Gordeuk VR, MacPhail AP. HLA-linked hemochromatosis and other forms of iron overload. *Dermatol Clin* 1995; 13: 57-63
[7] Barton JC, Bertoli LF. Hemochromatosis: the genetic disorder of the twenty-first century. *Nat Med* 1996; 2: 394-5
[8] Lauffer, RB. <u>Iron and Your Heart</u>. New York: St. Martin's Press, 1991
[9] **Vasquez A. Musculoskeletal disorders and iron overload disease: comment on the American College of Rheumatology guidelines for the initial evaluation of the adult patient with acute musculoskeletal symptoms. *Arthritis Rheum* 1996 Oct;39(10):1767-8**

Clinical presentations:

- **Many patients are asymptomatic.**
- **Most patients eventually present with a problem that is attributed to another disorder:**
  - Patients may present with diabetes, which is erroneously attributed to metabolic syndrome or type-2 diabetes.[10]
  - Patients may present with joint pain that is erroneously attributed to osteoarthritis[11], rheumatoid arthritis[12], or some other musculoskeletal syndrome.[13]
  - Patients may present with heart failure that is written off as "idiopathic cardiomyopathy."[14]
- Fatigue, lethargy, weakness
- Chronic abdominal pain
- Liver damage: hepatomegally, elevated serum levels of liver enzymes and alkaline phosphatase, fibrosis and cirrhosis, hepatocellular carcinoma, or other findings such as hematemesis and melena, ascites, hyperbilirubenemia and jaundice, hypoalbuminemia, hepatic encephalopathy, clotting dysfunction, anemia, liver abscess, increased incidence of esophageal carcinoma.
- Abnormal glucose metabolism or diabetes mellitus: elevated glucose levels. Usually asymptomatic, yet can cause weight loss, polyuria, polyphagia, polydypsia.
- Musculoskeletal disorders: arthritis and arthralgia, generalized osteoporosis, bone pain, myalgia. Especially arthropathy of the hands and wrists, hips, and knees.
- Cardiac dysfunction: cardiomyopathy, arrhythmia, fibrillation, congestive heart failure; shortness of breath or dyspnea on exertion, fatigue.

Conditions causally associated with iron overload
Primary/genetic disorders
1. Homozygous genetic hemochromatosis
2. Heterozygous genetic hemochromatosis
3. African iron overload
4. African-American hemochromatosis (African-American iron overload)
5. Non-HLA-linked hemochromatosis
6. Juvenile hemochromatosis
7. Neonatal hemochromatosis
Secondary and metabolic disorders
8. Dietary excess of iron
9. Parenteral administration of iron in the form of iron injections and blood transfusions
10. Porphyria cutanea tarda
11. Portacaval shunt
12. Hepatic cirrhosis, portal hypertension, and splenomegally
13. AIDS
14. Sudden infant death syndrome
15. Alcoholism
16. Metabolic syndrome
Inherited red blood cell abnormalities ("iron-loading anemias", hemoglobinopathies)
17. Alpha-thalassemia
18. Beta-thalassemia
19. Thalassemia intermedia
20. Sideroblastic anemia
21. Aplastic anemia
22. Anemia associated with pyruvate kinase deficiency
23. AC hemoglobinopathy
24. AS hemoglobinopathy
25. X-linked hypochromic anemia
26. Pyridoxine-responsive anemia
27. Atransferrinemia

- Cutaneous manifestations: 'slate-gray' or ashen coloration, increased pigmentation ('tan') of the skin, atrophy of the skin, ichthyosis, koilonychia, loss of body hair, increased incidence of malignant melanoma.
- Endocrine disorders: hypogonadotrophic hypogonadism, (autoimmune) hypothyroidism, hyperthyroidism; manifest as decreased libido, impotence, testicular atrophy, or sterility in males, amenorrhea or difficulty conceiving in females, loss of body hair.

---

[10] "Most of the patients (95%) had one or more of the following conditions; obesity, hyperlipidaemia, abnormal glucose metabolism, or hypertension. INTERPRETATION: We have found a new non-HLA-linked iron-overload syndrome which suggests a link between iron excess and metabolic disorders." Moirand R, Mortaji AM, Loreal O, Paillard F, Brissot P, Deugnier Y. A new syndrome of liver iron overload with normal transferrin saturation. *Lancet*. 1997 Jan 11;349(9045):95-7

[11] Axford JS, Bomford A, Revell P, Watt I, Williams R, Hamilton EBD. Hip arthropathy in genetic hemochromatosis: radiographic and histologic features. *Arthritis Rheum* 1991; 34: 357-61

[12] Bensen WG, Laskin CA, Little HA, Fam AG. Hemochromatoic arthropathy mimicking rheumatoid arthritis. A case with subcutaneous nodules, tenosynovitis, and bursitis. *Arthritis Rheum* 1978; 21: 844-8

[13] Olynyk J, Hall P, Ahern M, Kwiatek R, Mackinnon M. Screening for genetic hemochromatosis in a rheumatology clinic. *Australian and New Zealand Journal of Medicine* 1994; 24: 22-25

[14] [No authors listed] Case records of the Massachusetts General Hospital. Weekly clinicopathological exercises. Case 31-1994. A 25-year-old man with the recent onset of diabetes mellitus and congestive heart failure. *N Engl J Med*. 1994 Aug 18;331(7):460-6

- <u>Susceptibility to increased frequency and severity of infections</u>, especially infections due to *Yersinia enterocolitica, Vibrio vulnificus, HIV,* and *Mycobacterium tuberculosis.*
- <u>Neurologic symptoms</u>: blurred vision, sensorineural hearing loss, hyperactivity, dementia, attention deficit disorder, ataxia, lightheadedness, dizziness, anxiety, depression, tinnitus, confusion, lethargy, memory loss, disorientation, headaches and migraine headaches, personality changes, hallucinations, paranoia, chronic treatment-resistant psychiatric illness such as schizophrenia, compulsive disorders, bipolar affective disorder.
- <u>'Alcoholism'</u>: Alcoholism can cause elevated liver enzymes and liver damage, and many iron overload patients are erroneously diagnosed as alcoholics despite their abstinence from alcohol when the clinician fails to consider iron overload as the cause for the hepatopathy.
- <u>Any race, nationality, or ethnic background</u>: Hereditary iron overload conditions have been identified in people of all ethnic backgrounds and nationalities. Secondary iron overload conditions can occur irrespective of genetic predisposition.
- <u>Either gender</u>: Iron overload conditions occur in both men and women
- <u>A family history of, or suggestive of, a hereditary iron overload condition</u>: family history of iron overload, hereditary anemia or iron-loading anemia, cardiac disorders or "heart disease", arthritis, diabetes, neurologic disorders, liver disease, impotence, amenorrhea, sterility.

Musculoskeletal manifestations of iron overload
Clinical findings may include:
▪ **Joint pain**
▪ **Bone pain**
▪ Joint swelling
▪ Loss of motion
▪ Bursitis
▪ Tendonitis
▪ Tenosynovitis
▪ Subcutaneous nodules
Sites of involvement
▪ **Metacarpophalangeal joints**
▪ **Wrist**
▪ **Hip**
▪ **Knee**
▪ Shoulder
▪ Ankle
▪ Metatarsophalangeal joints
▪ Elbow
▪ Spine
▪ Symphysis pubis
▪ Achilles tendon
▪ Plantar fascia
Radiographic findings
▪ **Joint space narrowing**
▪ **Sclerosis**
▪ Cysts
▪ Pseudocysts
▪ Osteophytes
▪ **Hook-like osteophytes at the metacarpal heads (high specificity)**
▪ Flattened or "squared-off" metacarpal heads
▪ Generalized osteopenia
▪ Generalized osteoporosis
▪ Chondrocalcinosis
▪ Subchondral cysts
▪ Carpal erosions
▪ Calcific tendonitis

<u>Differential diagnoses</u>:
- <u>Diabetes mellitus</u>: Remember that the classic presentation of hemochromatosis is "bronze diabetes with cirrhosis." **All patients with diabetes should be tested for iron overload**.[15,16]
- <u>Cardiomyopathy</u>:
- <u>Hepatopathy</u>: **Iron overload is one of the most important rule-outs in patients with liver disease**.[17] Liver biopsy is often indicated to assess condition and disease co-existence.
- <u>Musculoskeletal disorders</u>: **Patients with polyarthropathy should be tested for iron overload**.[18,19]
  - Degenerative arthritis or osteoarthritis
  - Pseudogout, calcium pyrophosphate dihydrate deposition disease
  - Rheumatoid arthritis[20]

[15] Czink E, Tamas G. Screening for idiopathic hemochromatosis among diabetic patients. *Diabetes Care* 1991; 14: 929-30
[16] Phelps G, Chapman I, Hall P, Braund W, Mackinnon M. Prevalence of genetic haemochromatosis among diabetic patients. *Lancet* 1989; 2: 233-4
[17] Herrera JL. Abnormal liver enzyme levels: clinical evaluation in asymptomatic patients. *Postgrad Med* 1993; 93: 119-32
[18] M'Seffar AM, Fornasier VL, Fox IH. Arthropathy as the major clinical indicator of occult iron storage disease. *JAMA* 1977; 238: 1825-8
[19] Vasquez A. Musculoskeletal disorders and iron overload disease: comment on the American College of Rheumatology guidelines for the initial evaluation of the adult patient with acute musculoskeletal symptoms [letter/ comment]. *Arthritis Rheum* 1996;39:1767-8

- o Ankylosing spondylitis: The resemblance here is only superficial, related primarily to calcification of the intervertebral discs and ligaments.[21]
- • <u>Hypogonadotrophic hypogonadism</u>: impotence in men, subfertility in women[22]
- • <u>Hyperthyroidism and hypothyroidism</u>[23,24]
- • <u>Porphyria cutanea tarda</u>: "Virtually all patients have increased iron stores; serum iron, iron saturation, and ferritin values."[25] **All patients with porphyria cutanea tarda must be tested for iron overload.**

Clinical assessment:
- • <u>History/subjective</u>:
  - o The manifestations of the condition are so protean that history is generally non-sensitive and non-specific for the disorder. Rarely, a patient will mention that a relative was diagnosed with iron overload or that a relative had an unusual heart or liver disease, and this clue may lead to a diagnosis of iron overload in unsuspecting family members.
- • <u>Physical examination/objective</u>:
  - o The classic presentation of the fully developed disease is "bronze diabetes with arthritis and cirrhosis."
  - o Physical examination should be specific for the patient's complaint(s) of arthritis, cardiomyopathy, diabetes, etc.
- • <u>Imaging & laboratory assessments</u>:
  - o **Routine screening with serum ferritin for iron overload among all patients should be the standard of care in clinical practice**.
    - ▪ "In view of the high prevalence of hereditary hemochromatosis, its dire consequences when untreated, and its treatability, screening for the disorder should be performed routinely."[26]
    - ▪ "Screening for hemochromatosis is both feasible and cost-effective, and we recommend its use in patients seeking medical care."[27]
    - ▪ "The high gene frequency in the general population warrants routine screening tests in asymptomatic healthy young adults."[28]
    - ▪ "CONCLUSIONS: Primary iron overload occurs in African Americans... Clinicians should look for this condition."[29]
  - o <u>Imaging</u>: The radiographic findings are nearly identical to those of osteoarthritis, except more joints are typically involved and that the distribution is typically symmetric (both due to the systemic/metabolic nature of the disease). Hook-like osteophytes at the metacarpal heads—with the "hooks" pointing proximally (rather than distally, as in rheumatoid arthritis) may be the only finding that could be called pathognomonic. Flattened or "squared-off" metacarpal heads are also seen. See previous table labeled *"Musculoskeletal manifestations of iron overload"* for more details.

---

[20] Bensen WG, Laskin CA, Little HA, Fam AG. Hemochromatoic arthropathy mimicking rheumatoid arthritis. A case with subcutaneous nodules, tenosynovitis, and bursitis. *Arthritis Rheum* 1978; 21: 844-8

[21] Bywaters EGL, Hamilton EBD, Williams R. The spine in idiopathic hemochromatosis. *Ann Rheum Dis* 1971; 30: 453-65

[22] Tweed MJ, Roland JM. Haemochromatosis as an endocrine cause of subfertility. *BMJ*. 1998 Mar 21;316(7135):915-6 http://bmj.bmjjournals.com/cgi/content/full/316/7135/915

[23] Edwards CQ, Kelly TM, Ellwein G, Kushner JP. Thyroid disease in hemochromatosis. Increased incidence in homozygous men. *Arch Intern Med* 1983 Oct;143(10):1890-3

[24] Phillips G Jr, Becker B, Keller VA, Hartman J 4th. Hypothyroidism in adults with sickle cell anemia. *Am J Med* 1992 May;92(5):567-70

[25] "Virtually all patients have increased iron stores; serum iron, iron saturation, and ferritin values." Rich MW. Porphyria cutanea tarda. Don't forget to look at the urine. *Postgrad Med*. 1999;105: 208-10, 213-4

[26] Fairbanks VF. Laboratory testing for iron status. *Hosp Pract* (Off Ed) 1991 Suppl 3:17-24

[27] Balan V, Baldus W, Fairbanks V, Michels V, Burritt M, Klee G. Screening for hemochromatosis: a cost-effectiveness study based on 12, 258 patients. *Gastroenterology* 1994; 107: 453-9

[28] Gushusrt TP, Triest WE. Diagnosis and management of precirrhotic hemochromatosis. *W Virginia Med J* 1990; 86: 91-5

[29] Wurapa RK, Gordeuk VR, Brittenham GM, Khiyami A, Schechter GP, Edwards CQ. Primary iron overload in African Americans. *Am J Med*. 1996 Jul;101(1):9-18

- o Laboratory evaluation: Serum ferritin is the test of choice when looking for primary iron overload, secondary iron overload, and/or iron deficiency and should be a component of each new patient's evaluation, just as are CBC and the chemistry/metabolic panel.
  - **Ferritin: Routine use of serum ferritin is the most reasonable and cost-effective means for diagnosing this condition in symptomatic and asymptomatic patients.** Elevations of ferritin (i.e., >200 mcg/L in women and >300 mcg/L in men) need to be retested along with CRP (to rule out false elevation due to excessive inflammation) before making the presumptive diagnosis of iron overload. **In the absence of significant inflammation, ferritin values >200 mcg/L in women and >300 mcg/L in men indicate iron overload and the need for treatment/phlebotomy regardless of the absence of symptoms or end-stage complications.**[30] Another benefit to the use of serum ferritin is the frequent detection of iron deficiency.
  - Transferrin saturation: good test for detecting genetic hemochromatosis before iron overload has occurred; values greater than 40% should be repeated *in conjunction with a measurement of serum ferritin.*
  - CRP: should be relatively normal as iron overload is not inflammatory, per se. If the ferritin is elevated and the CRP is markedly elevated, then inflammatory and hepatocentric diseases must be considered, namely advanced cancer, viral hepatitis or other hepatopathy, and alcoholic liver disease. If the ferritin is elevated and the CRP is normal, then the most likely diagnosis is iron overload, which should be confirmed either with liver biopsy or diagnostic/therapeutic phlebotomy.
  - CBC: may show anemia, but the findings here are nonspecific
  - Chemistry panel: may show evidence of diabetes and hepatopathy
  - Thyroid assessment: may show hyperthyroidism or hypothyroidism, both of which are more common in patients with iron overload.
  - Bone marrow biopsy: unnecessary and archaic in this setting, now that serum ferritin is widely available.
  - Liver biopsy: traditionally considered the "gold standard" for diagnosing iron overload but is now clearly unnecessary for the diagnosis, which can be established by monitoring the response to therapeutic phlebotomy, which is the treatment of choice.[31] **Life-saving diagnostic and therapeutic phlebotomy should never be denied or delayed for lack of liver biopsy in patients with laboratory indicators of iron overload.**[32]
  - Genetic testing, such as for the HFE mutation is a waste of time and money in most clinical situations; these tests should be reserved for research purposes. The only value these tests may have in clinical practice is that of supporting a diagnosis in a patient with elevated serum ferritin who refuses biopsy, liver MRI, or phlebotomy; however, a negative result is meaningless if the ferritin is high and the clinical picture is compatible with iron overload. If the diagnosis is established, genetic relatives must be tested.

---

[30] Barton JC, McDonnell SM, Adams PC, Brissot P, Powell LW, Edwards CQ, Cook JD, Kowdley KV. Management of hemochromatosis. Hemochromatosis Management Working Group. *Ann Intern Med.* 1998 Dec 1;129(11):932-9

[31] "Therapeutic phlebotomy is used to remove excess iron and maintain low normal body iron stores, and it should be initiated in men with serum ferritin levels of 300 microg/L or more and in women with serum ferritin levels of 200 microg/L or more, regardless of the presence or absence of symptoms." Barton JC, McDonnell SM, Adams PC, Brissot P, Powell LW, Edwards CQ, Cook JD, Kowdley KV. Management of hemochromatosis. Hemochromatosis Management Working Group. *Ann Intern Med.* 1998 Dec 1;129(11):932-9

[32] Sullivan JL, as quoted in Crawford R, ed. "The debate." In: *Ironic Blood: information on iron overload.* West Palm Beach: Iron Overload Diseases Association, Inc. 1996; 16 (2)

Guide to Patient Management Based on Iron Status

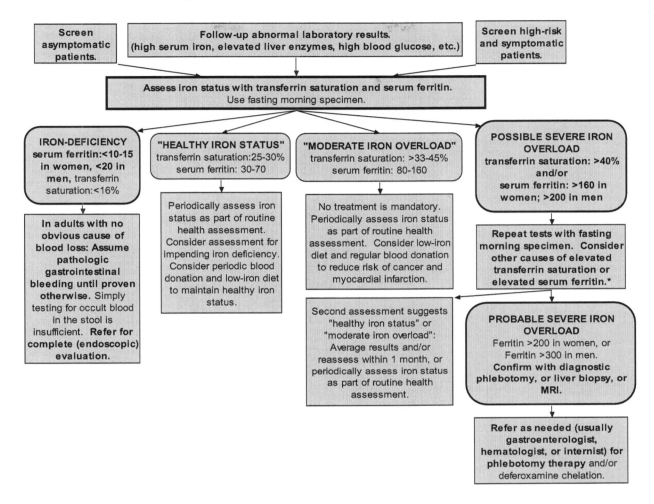

Establishing the diagnosis: Any *one* of the following three is sufficient:
- Diagnostic liver biopsy shows heavy iron deposits.
- Characteristic laboratory findings (ferritin >200 in women or >300 in men) *and* the ability to resist intractable anemia with serial/weekly phlebotomies.
- Characteristic MRI of liver *and* the ability to tolerate serial/weekly phlebotomies.

Complications:
- Patients diagnosed *and effectively treated* before the onset of signs and symptoms have normal life expectancy.
- The most common causes of premature mortality in undiagnosed and untreated patients are related to heart failure, liver failure, infections and/or complications of diabetes.

Clinical management:
- Treatment for severe iron overload is iron-removal therapy. Since blood is high in iron, the removal of blood—therapeutic phlebotomy—is the treatment of choice. Deferoxamine chelation can be administered to patients who refuse or cannot withstand phlebotomy (i.e., patients with cardiomyopathy, severe anemia, hypoproteinemia) but is much less effective, much more expensive, and with side effects such as neurotoxicity. Adjunctive nutritional and lifestyle

modifications are no substitute for iron-removal therapy, and weekly phlebotomy is the treatment of choice.

<u>Treatments:</u>

- *Medical standard*: Iron-removal is accomplished by weekly phlebotomy of 1-2 units (250-500 mL of blood, each of which removes 250 mg of iron), and deferoxamine chelation is used in patients who cannot tolerate phlebotomy. Complications of the disease, such as arthritis, heart failure, hypogonadism, and diabetes are treated appropriately. Cirrhotic patients must be monitored for hepatoma with twice-yearly liver ultrasound and measurement of serum alpha-fetoprotein. Always, when a hereditary iron overload disorder is diagnosed, all (first-degree) blood relatives must be screened for iron overload.

- <u>Diet modifications</u>: These are no substitute for iron-removal therapy with phlebotomy and are weak in their effectiveness by comparison.
    - o Decrease consumption of foods and nutritional supplements which are significant sources of iron: Iron supplements, iron-fortified foods and supplements, liver, beef, pork, lamb.
    - o Increase consumption of foods that will decrease intestinal absorption of iron from ingested food: tannins in tea, phytates (in whole-grain products, bran, legumes, nuts, and seeds), soy protein, egg, calcium supplements.
    - o Ensure adequate protein intake to replace protein lost during phlebotomy.
    - o Decrease consumption of excess ascorbic acid (vitamin C); high-dose vitamin C supplementation is clearly contraindicated.[33]
    - o Alcohol consumption should be avoided because ethanol exacerbates liver damage and increases iron absorption from the gut.

- <u>Silymarin</u>: Milk thistle has proved benefit in an animal model of iron overload[34] and is probably suitable for use in patients with iron overload, particularly given its ability to reverse cirrhosis.[35]

- <u>Antioxidant supplementation (excluding high-dose ascorbate)</u>: Oxidative stress is increased and antioxidant reserves are decreased in patients with iron overload.

- <u>Coenzyme Q10</u>: CoQ-10 probably has a role in the treatment of hemochromatoic cardiomyopathy given its safety and efficacy in other cardiomyopathies.[36,37,38,39,40,41,42,43]

[33] Mclarlan CJ, et al. Congestive cardiomyopathy and hemochromatosis: rapid progression possibly accelerated by excessive ingestion of ascorbic acid. *Aust NZ J Med* 1982; 12: 187-8

[34] "CONCLUSIONS: Oral administration of silybin protects against iron-induced hepatic toxicity in vivo. This effect seems to be caused by the prominent antioxidant activity of this compound." Pietrangelo A, Borella F, Casalgrandi G, et al. Antioxidant activity of silybin in vivo during long-term iron overload in rats. *Gastroenterology*. 1995 Dec;109(6):1941-9

[35] Salmi HA, Sarna S. Effect of silymarin and chemical, functional, and morphological alterations of the liver. A double-blind controlled study. *Scand J Gastroenterol* 1982; 17: 517-21

[36] Greenberg S, Frishman WH. Co-enzyme Q-10: a new drug for cardiovascular disease. *J Clin Pharmacol* 1990; 30: 596-608

[37] Langsjoen PH, Langsjoen PH, Folkers K. Long-term efficacy and safety of coenzyme Q-10 therapy for idiopathic dilated cardiomyopathy. *Am J Cardiol* 1990; 65: 521-3

[38] Manzoli U, Rossi E, Littarru GP, et al. Coenzyme Q-10 in dilated cardiomyopathy. *Int J Tiss Reac* 1990; 12: 173-8

[39] Langsjoen PH, Folkers K, Lyson K, Muratsu K, Lyson T, Langsjoen P. Pronounced increase of survival of patients with cardiomyopathy when treated with coenzyme Q-10 and conventional therapy. *Int J Tiss Reac* 1990; 12: 163-8

[40] Folkers K. Heart failure is a dominant deficiency of coenzyme Q-10 and challenges for future clinical research on CoQ-10. *Clin Investig* 1993; 71: s51-s54

[41] Folkers K, Langsjoen P, Langsjoen PH. Therapy with coenzyme Q-10 of patients in heart failure who are eligible or ineligible for a transplant. *Biochem Biophys Res Commun* 1992;182:247-53

[42] Mortensen SA, et al. Coenzyme Q-10: clinical benefits with biochemical correlates suggesting a scientific breakthrough.... *Int J Tiss Reac* 1990;12:155-62

[43] Langsjoen PH, Langsjoen PH, Folkers K. A six-year clinical study of therapy of cardiomyopathy with coenzyme Q-10. *Int J Tiss Reac* 1990; 12: 169-71

Chapter 16:
Fibromyalgia

Introduction:
Fibromyalgia—also referred to as fibromyalgia syndrome (FMS)—is a clinical entity that has remained enigmatic to the medical profession despite the consistent publication of research that delineates its cause and its effective treatments. This chapter summarizes clinical assessments, treatments, and essential background information that should provide empowering knowledge for clinicians and for the patients suffering with this condition.

Fibromyalgia (FM), Fibromyalgia Syndrome (FMS)

Introduction

- Fibromyalgia is commonly described as an idiopathic syndrome principally characterized by widespread body pain and numerous myofascial tender points at specific locations. The condition is most common in women 20 to 50 years old and often presents with associated complaints of fatigue, headaches, subjective numbness, altered sleep patterns, and gastrointestinal disturbances. Fibromyalgia in children and adolescents presents similarly to fibromyalgia in adults except for the comparatively higher prevalence of sleep disturbance and the finding of fewer tender points.[1]

  Until recently, fibromyalgia was considered a diagnosis of exclusion after infection, autoimmunity, or other primary causes were ruled out by clinical and laboratory assessment. However, current criteria base the diagnosis on positive findings of chronic, widespread musculoskeletal pain in characteristic locations; these criteria will be described below. Fibromyalgia shares several clinical and demographic features with chronic fatigue syndrome (CFS) and irritable bowel syndrome (IBS); the reason for these overlaps is not generally understood by most clinicians and researchers but will be made plain here.

  The prevailing medical view, expressed by clinicians and the authors of widely cited articles, is that fibromyalgia is idiopathic with strong neuropsychogenic influences and that, since the underlying causes of the condition have not been identified, the best therapeutic approach is symptom suppression via perpetual pharmacotherapy with adjunctive use of psychotherapy and limited exercise.[2,3,4] The term *syndrome* connotes that a cluster of symptoms is of a nonorganic, psychogenic, or idiopathic nature, whereas *disease* validates the organic and pathophysiological nature of an illness. This author advocates the use of *disease* rather than *syndrome* when describing fibromyalgia in appreciation of the real, organic, biochemical, and histopathological findings which clearly indicate that fibromyalgia is a specific disease entity and not simply a psychogenic or enigmatic cluster of symptoms. If fibromyalgia is a real, organic clinical entity (as will be documented here), then the appropriate designation is *fibromyalgia disease* (FMD) rather than *fibromyalgia syndrome* (FMS), as previously and commonly used in the biomedical literature. For consistency and clarity within this section, the general term "fibromyalgia" (FM) will be used.

Clinical Presentation

- Fibromyalgia is common, affecting approximately 2% of the U.S. population, and 10% of affected patients have severe symptoms resulting in partial or total disability. Affected patients report chronic aches, pains, and stiffness, with a proclivity for localization near the neck, shoulders, low back, and hips. Pain and fatigue are typically exacerbated following physical exertion or psychological stress. Associated manifestations include fatigue, sleep disorders (including insomnia, unrestful sleep, and objective abnormalities such as an increase in stage 1 sleep, a reduction in delta sleep, and alpha-delta sleep anomaly), subjective numbness, headaches, and IBS-like gastrointestinal disturbances. Clinical findings shared between fibromyalgia and IBS include abdominal pain and discomfort, changed frequency of stool including diarrhea and/or constipation, abdominal bloating and distention, dyspepsia, heartburn, headaches (including migraine), fatigue, myalgias, restless leg syndrome, anxiety, and depression. The **high prevalence (>50%) of migraine-type headaches in fibromyalgia patients** suggests an underlying pathogenesis shared between cephalgia (*ceph*=head, *algia*=pain) and widespread myalgia (*myo*=muscle, *algia*=pain), namely impaired mitochondrial function.[5] Cognitive symptoms such as "brain fog" and difficulty with memory and word retrieval, as well as **environmental intolerance and multiple chemical sensitivity**, are seen in both fibromyalgia and CFS[6]; again, this overlap of shared symptoms suggests a common etiopathogenesis. Routine physical examination and laboratory

[1] Siegel DM, Janeway D, Baum J. Fibromyalgia syndrome in children and adolescents: clinical features at presentation and status at follow-up. *Pediatrics.* 1998;101(3 Pt 1):377-82
[2] Chakrabarty S, Zoorob R. Fibromyalgia. *Am Fam Physician.* 2007 Jul 15;76(2):247-54
[3] Tierney ML. McPhee SJ, Papadakis MA (eds). Current Medical Diagnosis and Treatment 2006, 45th Edition. New York: Lange Medical Books, pages 820-821
[4] Simms RW. Nonarticular soft tissue disorders. In Andreoli TE, Carpenter CCJ, Griggs RC, and Benjamin IJ (eds). Cecil Essentials of Medicine. Seventh Edition. Philadelphia; Saunders Elsevier, 2007: 851-2
[5] Pieczenik SR, Neustadt J. Mitochondrial dysfunction and molecular pathways of disease. *Exp Mol Pathol.* 2007 Aug;83(1):84-92
[6] Brown MM, Jason LA. Functioning in individuals with chronic fatigue syndrome: increased impairment with co-occurring multiple chemical sensitivity and fibromyalgia. *Dyn Med.* 2007 May 31;6:6 http://www.dynamic-med.com/content/6/1/6

findings are generally normal, with the exception of fibromyalgia tender points (described and diagramed below).

Pathophysiology

- **Biochemical and histologic abnormalities consistent with mitochondrial dysfunction**: Muscle biopsies from patients with fibromyalgia show numerous histological, ultrastructural, and biochemical abnormalities, including defects in mitochondrial structure and function, reduced numbers of capillaries in skeletal muscle, thickened capillary endothelium, and ragged red fibers consistent with the development of mitochondrial myopathy (*myo*=muscle, *pathos*=disease). The histological finding of "rubber-band morphology" with reticular threads connecting neighboring cells in muscle biopsies of fibromyalgia patients is associated with prolonged contractions in adjacent muscle fibers; these abnormalities result in and perpetuate a low-energy state within myocytes (*myo*=muscle, *cytes*=cells).[7] Other studies have shown disorganization of actin filaments, accumulation of lipofuscin bodies consistent with premature muscle aging, accumulation of glycogen and lipid accumulation consistent with **mitochondrial impairment, significant reductions in the number of mitochondria**, increased DNA fragmentation, and focal areas of chronic muscle contraction.[8] These histological abnormalities are important and support the view that **fibromyalgia is a *disease of metabolic dysfunction*** rather than an *emotional disorder of psychogenic origin*.

- Ultrastructural and biochemical abnormalities appear to be more pathologically significant and clinically relevant than the noted histological changes in skeletal muscle biopsy samples. **Numerous mitochondrial enzyme defects are seen**, including reduced activity of 3-hydroxy-CoA dehydrogenase, citrate synthase, and cytochrome oxidase. Levels of free magnesium have been shown to be reduced by 31%, and levels of complexed ATP-magnesium are reduced

> **Objective "organic" abnormalities noted in patients with fibromyalgia**
>
> - Histologic and functional abnormalities in muscle tissue: Disorganization of actin filaments, accumulation of lipofuscin bodies consistent with premature muscle aging, increased DNA fragmentation, and focal areas of chronic muscle contraction, reduced perfusion of muscle tissue during exercise,
> - Mitochondrial defects: Accumulation of glycogen and lipid accumulation consistent with mitochondrial impairment, significant reductions in the number of mitochondria, reduced activity of 3-hydroxy-CoA dehydrogenase, citrate synthase, and cytochrome oxidase, CoQ-10 deficiency which promotes mitochondrial dysfunction (thus promoting mitophagy, which results in reduced numbers of mitochondria and perpetuates and aggravates muscle fatigue, pain, and neurocognitive dysfunction) and increased mitochondrial production of reactive oxygen radicals thus further depleting CoQ-10 levels,
> - Oxidative stress: Increased oxidative stress
> - Neuroendocrine abnormalities: HPA disturbance: hypothalamic-pituitary-adrenal disturbance,
> - Low-grade immune activation: Increased cytokine production,
> - Bacterial overgrowth in the intestines: Laboratory evidence of occult bacterial overgrowth in the small bowel,
> - Vitamin D deficiency: Common in the general population but more common in patients with chronic pain,
> - Low plasma levels of L-tryptophan: Probably caused by increased bacterial tryptophanase activity associated with bacterial overgrowth of the small intestine; without L-tryptophan the body cannot make enough serotonin for mood maintenance and pain alleviation, nor can it make melatonin for normal sleep and support of mitochondrial function and anti-oxidation.

by 12% in muscle from fibromyalgia patients compared with levels seen in healthy controls; these biochemical and bioenergetic defects contribute to rapid-onset fatigue and muscle pain. From a neurophysiological perspective, magnesium deficiency promotes hypersensitivity to pain due to a reduction in the partial blockade of N-methyl-D-aspartate (NMDA) neurotransmitter receptor sites.[9] Reduced perfusion of muscle tissue during exercise results in relative tissue hypoxia, reduced muscle healing after the microtrauma of exercise, and promotion of muscle soreness due to accumulation of lactate.[10] Increased oxidative stress is also seen in fibromyalgia patients,[11] providing additional objective evidence of the systemic, organic, and non-psychogenic nature of the illness. Evidence of hypothalamic-pituitary-adrenal disturbance and **increased cytokine production (particularly interleukin-8, which promotes sympathetic**

[7] Olsen NJ, Park JH. Skeletal muscle abnormalities in patients with fibromyalgia. *Am J Med Sci*. 1998 Jun;315(6):351-8
[8] Sprott H, Salemi S, Gay RE, et al. Increased DNA fragmentation and ultrastructural changes in fibromyalgic muscle fibres. *Ann Rheum Dis*. 2004 Mar;63(3):245-51
[9] Park JH, Niermann KJ, Olsen N. Evidence for metabolic abnormalities in the muscles of patients with fibromyalgia. *Curr Rheumatol Rep*. 2000 Apr;2(2):131-40
[10] Elvin A, Siosteen AK, Nilsson A, Kosek E. Decreased muscle blood flow in fibromyalgia patients during standardised muscle exercise: a contrast media enhanced colour Doppler study. *Eur J Pain*. 2006 Feb;10(2):137-44
[11] Altindag O, Celik H. Total antioxidant capacity and the severity of the pain in patients with fibromyalgia. *Redox Rep*. 2006;11(3):131-5

pain, and interleukin-6, which induces hyperalgesia (increased perception of pain), fatigue, and depression[12]) further characterizes the systemic and organic nature of this condition and are well documented in the research literature. **The majority of fibromyalgia patients demonstrate laboratory evidence of occult bacterial overgrowth in the small bowel**, and the details and important implications of this will be discussed below. Vitamin D deficiency, a recognized cause of chronic widespread pain, is also common in fibromyalgia patients.[13] These objective and reproducible abnormalities of biochemical, histological, nutritional, and microbiological/gastrointestinal status force clinicians to appreciate the valid and organic nature of fibromyalgia; likewise, this evidence refutes promulgations espoused within standard allopathic/pharmaceutical medicine that fibromyalgia is an idiopathic condition warranting lifelong medicalization with expensive and potentially hazardous analgesic and antidepressant drugs.

Diagnosis

- **Clinical findings:** Per guidelines by the American College of Rheumatology, a diagnosis of fibromyalgia can be made in a patient with inexplicable, widespread myofascial pain of at least 3 months' duration; *inexplicable* denotes normalcy of routine laboratory and physical examination findings and failure to find an alternate explanation or diagnosis, while *widespread* denotes bilateral pain above and below the waist not attributable to trauma or rheumatic disease and with pain at 11 of 18 classic tender points (see Figure 1). Fibromyalgia tender points are assessed bilaterally at 9 paired sites: (sub)occiput, low cervical spine, trapezius, supraspinatus, second rib (anterior, near costosternal junction), lateral epicondyle, gluteal region, greater trochanter, and medial fat pad of the knees. Tender points are provoked by the clinician's application of approximately 9 pounds of fingertip pressure, which is sufficient to cause blanching of the clinician's nail bed. The tender points of fibromyalgia are distinguished from myofascial trigger points (MFTP, described by Travell[14]) and strain-counterstrain tender points (described in the osteopathic literature by Jones[15]). In contrast to MFTP, which are located toward the center of the muscle fiber and which refer pain and show spontaneous electrocontractile activity[16], tender points of fibromyalgia are located near the tendinous insertions of muscle to bone and cause local pain only, without pain referral or contractile activity.

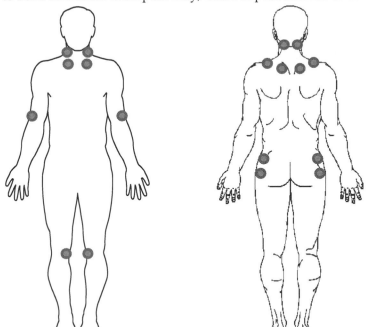

Clinical findings: Pain, on digital palpation, must be present in at least 11 of the following 18 tender point sites:
1. Occiput: at the suboccipital muscle insertions.
2. Low cervical: at the anterior aspects of the intertransverse spaces at C5-C7.
3. Trapezius: at the midpoint of the upper border.
4. Supraspinatus: at origins, above the scapula spine near the medial border.
5. Second rib: upper lateral to the second costochondral junction.
6. Lateral epicondyle: 2 cm distal to the epicondyles.
7. Gluteal: in upper outer quadrants of buttocks in anterior fold of muscle.
8. Greater trochanter: posterior to the trochanteric prominence.
9. Knee: at the medial fat pad proximal to the joint line.

Digital palpation should be performed with an approximate force of 4 kg. A tender point has to be painful at palpation, not just "tender."[17]

Illustration showing the 9 paired locations of fibromyalgia tender points: The diagnosis of fibromyalgia is supported when at least 11 out of 18 of these locations are painful following digital compression by the clinician.

[12] Wallace DJ, Linker-Israeli M, Hallegua D, Silverman S, Silver D, Weisman MH. Cytokines play an aetiopathogenetic role in fibromyalgia: a hypothesis and pilot study. *Rheumatology* (Oxford). 2001 Jul;40(7):743-9

[13] Huisman AM, White KP, Algra A, et al. Vitamin D levels in women with systemic lupus erythematosus and fibromyalgia. *J Rheumatol*. 2001 Nov;28(11):2535-9

[14] Simons DG, Travell JG, Simons LS. Travell & Simons' Myofascial Pain and Dysfunction. The Trigger Point Manual. Baltimore: Lippincott Williams & Wilkins; 1999

[15] Jones L, Kusunose R, Goering E. Jones Strain-Counterstrain. Carlsbad, Jones Strain Counterstrain Incorporated, 1995. [ISBN 0964513544]

[16] Hubbard DR, Berkoff GM. Myofascial trigger points show spontaneous needle EMG activity. *Spine*. 1993 Oct 1;18(13):1803-7

[17] The American College of Rheumatology 1990 Criteria for the Classification of Fibromyalgia. http://www.nfra.net/Diagnost.htm Accessed Nov 2011

- **Clinical profile and findings on common laboratory tests**: New-onset fibromyalgia is unlikely over age 50, and the condition never causes fever, significant weight loss, or other objective signs of acute or subacute illness. Hypothyroidism is common and can produce widespread myofascial pain similar in initial presentation to fibromyalgia; thus, a complete thyroid evaluation is essential during the initial evaluation of any fibromyalgia-like condition. Common rheumatic conditions such as rheumatoid arthritis and systemic lupus erythematosus are excluded by the lack of other clinical manifestations and the lack of positive laboratory findings such as anti-cyclic citrullinated protein (CCP) antibodies and antinuclear antibodies (ANA), respectively. C-reactive protein (CRP) and erythrocyte sedimentation rate (ESR) should be essentially normal in fibromyalgia patients; abnormalities with these or other common laboratory assessments suggest inflammatory disease, infection, or other concomitant illness. Hypophosphatemia must be excluded via demonstration of normal serum phosphate level.

Standard Medical Treatment

- Mild exercise and the use of antidepressants, especially those of the tricyclic class, are mainstays of standard medical treatment; **these interventions are only partially effective and offer little to no hope of actually curing the disease.** In July 2007, the FDA approved pregabalin (Lyrica®) for symptomatic treatment of fibromyalgia[18]; however, because the drug does not address the primary cause(s) of the disease, patients must continue treatment indefinitely. Adverse effects of pregabalin include dizziness, sleepiness, blurred vision, **weight gain**, dry mouth, swelling of hands and feet, impairment of motor function, and problems with concentration and attention. The most widely used drug for symptomatic treatment of fibromyalgia is amitriptyline (a tricyclic antidepressant), which is used "off label" for fibromyalgia and which has low efficacy and high potential for adverse effects; up to 20% of patients suffer from **weight gain**, constipation, orthostatic hypotension, and agitation as a result of the drug. Only 25% to 30% of fibromyalgia patients experience clinically significant improvement with amitriptyline.[19] Cyclobenzaprine, like most other drug treatments such as Tramadol (a nontypical opioid and centrally acting narcotic analgesic) and acetaminophen (centrally acting analgesic), shows low efficacy, has little research supporting its use, has several important adverse effects, and does not favorably alter the course of the disease over the long-term.[20] Low-intensity aerobic exercise may initially exacerbate symptoms but can result in very modest mental and physical improvement. Cognitive-behavioral therapy helps patients deal with and adapt to the impact of the illness.

Functional Medicine Considerations, Assessments, and Interventions

- Two fundamental premises of functional medicine are: (1) chronic diseases are a manifestations of chronic dysfunctions, and (2) dysfunction can result from a wide range of interconnected genotropic, metabolic, nutritional, microbial, inflammatory, toxic, environmental, and psychological influences. Many of these dysfunctions lie outside the narrow pathology-based and *pharmacocentric* view of standard medicine. The functional medicine approach to each individual fibromyalgia patient is based on the presumption that the condition has an underlying primary cause and that this cause can be identified and addressed. The cause(s) may be manifold and multifaceted and may differ among patients with the same diagnostic label. The functional medicine approach includes the diagnostic and therapeutic considerations of standard medicine but extends far beyond these in assessment, treatment, and understanding. Functional medicine clinicians appreciate that as a diagnostic label, fibromyalgia is commonly applied to any patient with chronic, widespread pain and that the current trend to limit diagnostic evaluation in such patients will clearly result in failure to identify and address readily diagnosable and treatable problems that can result in widespread pain. Clinicians must consider chronic infections (such as with hepatitis C virus and *Borrelia burgdorferi* [a bacteria strongly associated with Lyme disease]), malignant conditions such as multiple myeloma and metastatic disease, and autoimmune/rheumatic diseases such as polymyositis and polymyalgia rheumatica. A few of the other more exemplary conditions to consider in patients with widespread pain are vitamin D deficiency,

---

[18] FDA Approves First Drug for Treating Fibromyalgia. http://www.fda.gov/bbs/topics/NEWS/2007/NEW01656.html
[19] Leventhal LJ. Management of fibromyalgia. *Ann Intern Med*. 1999 Dec 7;131(11):850-8
[20] Goldenberg DL, Burckhardt C, Crofford L. Management of fibromyalgia syndrome. *JAMA*. 2004 Nov 17;292(19):2388-95

hypothyroidism, iron overload, and chronic exposure to and accumulation of xenobiotics, perhaps most importantly mercury and lead.

Conditions that May Mimic or Contribute to Fibromyalgia

- **Functional/metabolic hypothyroidism:** Both subclinical and overt hypothyroidism are well known in the rheumatology literature as causes of diffuse body pain. Hypothyroidism can mimic fibromyalgia and IBS, and it can contribute to the development of these conditions by causing impaired digestion and delayed intestinal transit, which promotes development of small intestine bacterial overgrowth (SIBO)[21], the most consistent cause of both fibromyalgia and IBS. Detailed thyroid assessment should include measurements of TSH, free T4, free T3, total T3, reverse T3 (rT3), and antithyroid peroxidase and antithyroglobulin antibodies.

```
FREE T3/REVERSE T3 RATIO
    FREE T3/REVERSE T3 RATIO                         0.93 L          1.05-1.91**
    FREE T3                              325                         230-420 pg/dL
    REVERSE T3                                        350 H          100-340*** pg/mL
            **Ratio= Free T3 in pg/dL : reverse T3 in pg/mL. Ratio for reference
            range is calculated by dividing the lower and upper end of free T3
            with the mean of reverse T3 (220 pg/mL).

            ***Observed reference range is reported for reverse T3 per client
            request.

            This test was performed using a kit that has not been approved or
            cleared by the FDA. The analytical performance characteristics of this
            test have been determined by Quest Diagnostics Nichols Institute, San
            Juan Capistrano. This test should not be used for diagnosis without
            confirmation by other medically established means.
```

A 42yo male with fatigue and elevated rT3 levels indicating functional hypothyroidism: This is an example of a case of functional hypothyroidism or metabolic hypothyroidism, which is due to impaired peripheral conversion of thyroxine (T4) into mostly its active form triiodothyronine (T3) and an excess production of reverse T3 (rT3). Patients with this condition typically benefit from receiving prescription T3 rather than the more commonly used T4; the goal is to temporarily suppress endogenous T4 production so that enzymes in the converting pathway are temporarily downregulated and thus peripheral thyroid metabolism has an opportunity to recalibrate and remain normal following the withdrawal of thyroid hormone supplementation.[22,23]

- **Vitamin D deficiency:** Chronic widespread pain associated with mental depression, headaches, low-grade systemic inflammation, and numerous other physiological and functional abnormalities can result from vitamin D deficiency.[24] Fibromyalgia patients are commonly deficient in vitamin D, and indeed, **vitamin D deficiency is often misdiagnosed as fibromyalgia**, as reported by Holick.[25] Increased severity of the deficiency correlates with worsening depression and anxiety in these patients.[26] Correction of vitamin D deficiency by administration of vitamin D3 (cholecalciferol) in doses of 5,000-10,000 IU/day for several months has resulted in a dramatic alleviation of pain; such intervention among patients with low back pain has resulted in cure rates greater than 95%.[27] Other studies with vitamin D3 doses ranging from 400 to 4000 IU/day have shown that vitamin D3 supplementation for the correction of vitamin D deficiency alleviates depression and enhances sense of well-being. Vitamin D3 supplementation—or adequate endogenous production from ultraviolet light exposure (approximately 10-30 minutes per day of full-body exposure)—to meet physiological requirements of approximately 4,000 IU/day is safe and results in numerous major health

[21] Lauritano EC, Bilotta AL, Gabrielli M, Scarpellini E, Lupascu A, Laginestra A, Novi M, Sottili S, Serricchio M, Cammarota G, Gasbarrini G, Pontecorvi A, Gasbarrini A. Association between hypothyroidism and small intestinal bacterial overgrowth. *J Clin Endocrinol Metab*. 2007 Nov;92(11):4180-4
[22] McDaniel AB. Thyroid Assessment: Controversies and Conundrums. Institute for Functional Medicine Fourteenth International Symposium. Tucson, AZ. May 23-26, 2007
[23] Friedman M, Miranda-Massari JR, Gonzalez MJ. Supraphysiological cyclic dosing of sustained release T3 in order to reset low basal body temperature. *P R Health Sci J*. 2006 Mar;25(1):23-9
[24] Plotnikoff GA, Quigley JM. Prevalence of severe hypovitaminosis D in patients with persistent, nonspecific musculoskeletal pain. *Mayo Clin Proc*. 2003;78(12):1463-70
[25] Holick MF. Vitamin D: importance in the prevention of cancers, type 1 diabetes, heart disease, and osteoporosis. *Am J Clin Nutr*. 2004 Mar;79(3):362-71
[26] Armstrong DJ, Meenagh GK, Bickle I, Lee AS, Curran ES, Finch MB. Vitamin D deficiency is associated with anxiety and depression in fibromyalgia. *Clin Rheumatol*. 2007 Apr;26(4):551-4
[27] Al Faraj S, Al Mutairi K. Vitamin D deficiency and chronic low back pain in Saudi Arabia. *Spine*. 2003;28:177-9

benefits.[28,29,30] Because use of thiazide diuretics (which promote retention of calcium by the kidney) or presence of granulomatous disease (e.g., lymphoma and sarcoidosis) predispose to hypercalcemia (high levels of calcium in the blood, a potentially dangerous condition), caution and more frequent laboratory monitoring must be employed when using physiological doses of vitamin D3 in these situations. Diagnosis of vitamin D3 deficiency is simple and is based upon measurement of serum 25-hydroxy vitamin D3 (25[OH]D) levels. Supplementation efficacy and safety are monitored by measuring 25(OH)D levels and serum calcium, respectively.

- **Occult infections, especially with *Mycoplasma* species and *Chlamydia/Chlamydophila pneumoniae***: Clinicians are increasingly appreciating the role of occult intracellular infections in the genesis and/or perpetuation of chronic health problems, including some previously perplexing problems such as chronic fatigue syndrome (CFS) and inflammatory arthritis. For chronic *Chlamydophila pneumoniae* infection, testing for serum levels of antibodies is useful followed by treatment with antibacterial drugs such as azithromycin in appropriately selected patients; for chronic *Mycoplasma* infections, because of the various subspecies involved, polymerase chain reaction (PCR) testing appears to be preferred followed by treatment with doxycycline in adults.

  o Clinical investigation: High prevalence of Mycoplasmal infections in symptomatic (chronic fatigue syndrome) family members of *Mycoplasma*-positive Gulf War illness patients (*Journal of Chronic Fatigue Syndrome* 2003[31]): The authors state, "...a relatively common finding in Gulf War Illness patients is a bacterial infection due to *Mycoplasma* species, we examined military families (149 patients: 42 veterans, 40 spouses, 32 other relatives and 35 children with at least one family complaint of illness) selected from a group of 110 veterans with Gulf War Illness who tested positive (~41%) for at least one of four *Mycoplasma* species: *M. fermentans, M. hominis, M. pneumoniae* or *M. genitalium*. Consistent with previous results, over 80% of Gulf War Illness patients who were positive for blood mycoplasmal infections had only one *Mycoplasma* species, in particular *M. fermentans* (Odds ratio = 17.9, P <0.001). In healthy control subjects the incidence of mycoplasmal infection was ~8.5% and none were found to have multiple mycoplasmal species."

  o Review: *Mycoplasma* blood infection in chronic fatigue and **fibromyalgia** syndromes (*Rheumatology International* 2003 Sep[32]): The author notes that "**Chronic fatigue syndrome (CFS) and fibromyalgia syndrome (FMS)** are characterized by a lack of consistent laboratory and clinical abnormalities. Although they are distinguishable as separate syndromes based on established criteria, a great number of patients are diagnosed with both." He goes on to say, "In studies using **polymerase chain reaction [PCR] methods, mycoplasma blood infection has been detected in about 50% of patients with CFS and/or FMS**, including patients with Gulf War illnesses and symptoms that overlap with one or both syndromes. **Such infection is detected in only about 10% of healthy individuals**, significantly less than in patients. Most patients with CFS/FMS who have mycoplasma infection appear to recover and reach their pre-illness state after **long-term antibiotic therapy with doxycycline**, and the infection can not be detected after recovery. ... It is not clear whether mycoplasmas are associated with CFS/FMS as causal agents, cofactors, or opportunistic infections in patients with immune disturbances. Whether mycoplasma infection can be detected in about 50% of all patient populations with CFS and/or FMS is yet to be determined."

  o Clinical investigation: Prevalence of antibodies to *Chlamydia pneumoniae* in persons without clinical evidence of respiratory infection (*Journal of Clinical Pathology* 2002 May[33]): "Serum samples from 402 subjects (172 children and 230 adults), without known respiratory symptoms, were collected. Antibodies to *C pneumoniae* (IgG, IgA, and IgM) were evaluated using the microimmunofluorescence (MIF) assay. ...

[28] Holick MF. Vitamin D: importance in the prevention of cancers, type 1 diabetes, heart disease, and osteoporosis. *Am J Clin Nutr*. 2004 Mar;79(3):362-71
[29] Vieth R. Vitamin D supplementation, 25-hydroxyvitamin D concentrations, and safety. *Am J Clin Nutr*. 1999 May;69(5):842-56
[30] Zittermann A. Vitamin D in preventive medicine: are we ignoring the evidence? *Br J Nutr*. 2003 May;89(5):552-72
[31] Nicolson GL, Nasralla MY, Nicolson NL. High prevalence of Mycoplasmal infections in symptomatic (chronic fatigue syndrome) family members of *Mycoplasma*-positive Gulf War illness patients. *Journal of Chronic Fatigue Syndrome* 2003; 11(2): 21-36 http://www.immed.org/GulfWarIllness/10.01.11update/GWIfamilyJCFS_.pdf
[32] Endresen GK. Mycoplasma blood infection in chronic fatigue and fibromyalgia syndromes. *Rheumatol Int*. 2003 Sep;23(5):211-5
[33] Ben-Yaakov M, Eshel G, Zaksonski L, Lazarovich Z, Boldur I. Prevalence of antibodies to Chlamydia pneumoniae in an Israeli population without clinical evidence of respiratory infection. *J Clin Pathol*. 2002 May;55(5):355-8 http://jcp.bmj.com/content/55/5/355.long

Persistent infection was indicated in three young children, in six teenagers, and in 24 adults, with a significantly higher frequency (p = 0.012) in men (18 of 117) than in women (six of 113). No seasonal differences could be detected." The authors go on to say in the text of their article that "Because there is as yet no standardization of serological criteria for persistent infection, we considered antibody titers of > 1/20 in the IgA fraction, together with **IgG titers of 1/64 to 1/256**, to be indicative of persistent infection." This article supports clinical experience and post-graduate presentations[34] showing that in persons with fatigue (and/or perhaps chronic pain and inflammatory disorders), the measurement of antibodies against *Chlamydia/Chlamydophila pneumoniae* and the finding of IgG antibody titers >1:64 suggests that the patient has a persistent *Chlamydia/Chlamydophila pneumoniae* infection which may be alleviated by the administration of—for example—azithromycin (adult dose 250 mg every other day due to the drug's long half-life, given for several weeks or months until symptoms are resolved and/or antibody titers are normalized) and N-acetyl-cysteine (NAC: 500-1,200 mg 1-3 times per day by mouth between meals). Positive antibody titers are common because the infection itself is common *as a transient condition*; the issue here is the determination of which patients have a chronic and persistent low-grade infection. The finding of an elevated antibody titer—that is a level greater than 1:64—indicates the need to consider long-term antimicrobial intervention. A brief case report from the author's experience is provided below:

			08/29/11
Chlamydia pneumoniae IgG	>1:256	High	Neg:<1:16
Chlamydia pneumoniae IgM	<1:10		Neg:<1:10

Elevated titers to *Chlamydia/Chlamydophila pneumoniae* suggesting chronic persistent infection in a 40yo male physician *without pulmonary symptoms* but with a positive history of chronic sinus congestion and low-grade fatigue—improvement with azithromycin and NAC: This patient experienced years of severe psychologic and physiologic stress during medical school to then have an acute upper respiratory illness onset in September 2010 while working in a Family Medicine residency program; recurrent bouts of upper respiratory illness—attributed to viral infections—persisted for five months until February 2011. By the summer of 2011, the patient was relatively asymptomatic except for persistent sinus congestion and low-grade fatigue. No pulmonary symptoms such as shortness of breath were ever present. Following detection of the elevated antibody titer, the patient started on azithromycin and NAC as described above, which resulted in a short-term (12-hour) exacerbation of symptoms followed by complete and sustained resolution of sinus congestion and improved energy levels and exercise endurance.[35]

- **Hemochromatosis and iron overload**: Genetic hemochromatosis is a common inherited disease among Caucasians, with a homozygote frequency of approximately 1 in 200 to 250 and a heterozygote frequency of approximately 1 in 7. Various other hereditary iron overload disorders affect all races, with the highest prevalence in persons of African descent (as high as 1 in 80 according to some small studies among hospitalized African-American patients).[36,37] Eighty percent of hemochromatosis patients have chronic musculoskeletal pain, which is commonly the earliest or only presenting complaint.[38] In contrast to the clinical presentation of fibromyalgia, the musculoskeletal manifestations of iron overload are classically arthritic (i.e., in the joints) rather than muscular, with the joints of the hands, wrists, hips, and knees most commonly affected. However, due to the widespread distribution of pain and the normalcy of routine laboratory results, iron overload can mimic fibromyalgia. Given the high population prevalence of iron overload and the high frequency with which it presents with musculoskeletal manifestations, **all patients with chronic, nontraumatic musculoskeletal pain must be tested for iron overload.** Serum ferritin, which can be used alone or with transferrin saturation, is the best single laboratory test; confirmed results greater than 200 mcg/L in women and 300 mcg/L in men necessitate treatment with diagnostic and therapeutic

---

[34] Stratton C. The Role of Chlamydophila in Autoimmune Disease. 2011 International Symposium -"The Challenge of Emerging Infections in the 21st Century: Terrain, Tolerance, and Susceptibility" hosted by The Institute for Functional Medicine www.functionalmedicine.org in Seattle, Washington in May 2011
[35] Appreciation is given to Bill Beakey DOM of Professional Co-Op Services http://professionalcoop.com/ for provision of this laboratory assessment.
[36] Wurapa RK, Gordeuk VR, Brittenham GM, Khiyami A, Schechter GP, Edwards CQ. Primary iron overload in African Americans. *Am J Med.* 1996 Jul;101(1):9-18
[37] Barton JC, Edwards CQ, Bertoli LF, Shroyer TW, Hudson SL. Iron overload in African Americans. *Am J Med.* 1995 Dec;99(6):616-23
[38] Vasquez A. Musculoskeletal disorders and iron overload disease: comment on the American College of Rheumatology guidelines for the initial evaluation of the adult patient with acute musculoskeletal symptoms. *Arthritis Rheum.* 1996 Oct;39(10):1767-8

phlebotomy.[39] Additional details about the etiologies, diagnosis, and comprehensive treatment of iron overload are available online.[40]

- **Accumulation of xenobiotics (including mercury and lead):** Xenobiotic accumulation may occasionally cause widespread pain resembling fibromyalgia, and xenobiotic detoxification (depuration) can alleviate pain in affected patients. Eight percent of American women of childbearing age have sufficiently high levels of mercury in their blood to increase the risk of neurological damage in their children.[41] Americans in general show alarmingly high concentrations and combinations of neurotoxic, carcinogenic, diabetogenic, and immunotoxic xenobiotics.[42] Adverse effects of toxic chemicals (e.g., pesticides, herbicides, solvents, plastics, formaldehyde, petroleum byproducts) and heavy metals (especially lead and mercury) are well described throughout the biomedical literature and have been clinically reviewed by Crinnion.[43,44,45,46] Among toxins with the ability to produce chronic muscle pain, mercury may deserve special recognition given its ubiquitous distribution in the human population and the scientific evidence detailing its numerous adverse effects.[47,48] Whether by metabolic, neurological, or endocrinologic means, occult mercury toxicity may manifest as a syndrome of widespread muscle pain that resembles fibromyalgia.[49] Acrodynia is a subacute peripheral pain syndrome due to mercury toxicity classically seen in children.[50] Acute mercury intoxication can result in severe skeletal muscle damage (rhabdomyolysis).[51] Mercury in organic and inorganic forms interferes with acetylcholine reception and several crucial aspects of the sarcoplasmic reticulum, including calcium-magnesium-ATPase and calcium transport; these adverse effects establish a scientific and molecular basis for a *mercurial myopathy*.[52,53] The toxicity of mercury is greatly increased by simultaneous overaccumulation of lead, elevated levels of which are also common in the U.S. population. Demonstration of high mercury and lead levels in urine following administration of a chelating agent such as dimercaptosuccinic acid (DMSA) can be used to diagnose chronic mercury or lead overload, and orally administered DMSA is also used for treatment.[54,55,56,57] Failure to preadminister a chelating agent prior to measurement of urine mercury renders the test insensitive for chronic accumulation and can thus give the false impression that mercury is not contributory to fibromyalgia, as concluded by Kotter et al.[58] Orally administered selenium, phytochelatins, a high-fiber diet, and potassium citrate can be used to augment mercury excretion.[59]

> **Potential benefits of reducing the body burden of mercury in patients with chronic pain and fatigue**
>
> "We suggest that **metal-driven inflammation** may affect the hypothalamic-pituitary-adrenal axis (HPA axis) and indirectly trigger psychosomatic multisymptoms characterizing **chronic fatigue syndrome, fibromyalgia**, and other diseases of unknown etiology."
>
> Sterzl I, et al. Mercury and nickel allergy: risk factors in fatigue and autoimmunity. *Neuro Endocrinol Lett.* 1999;20(3-4):221-228

---

[39] Barton JC, McDonnell SM, Adams PC, Brissot P, Powell LW, Edwards CQ, Cook JD, Kowdley KV. Management of hemochromatosis. Hemochromatosis Management Working Group. *Ann Intern Med.* 1998 Dec 1;129(11):932-9

[40] Vasquez A. *Integrative Rheumatology: Second Edition 2007*. Fort Worth, Texas; Integrative and Biological Medicine Research and Consulting, 2007. See excerpted Chapter 18 available at: http://optimalhealthresearch.com/hemochromatosis.html

[41] Schober SE, Sinks TH, Jones RL, Bolger PM, McDowell M, Osterloh J, Garrett ES, Canady RA, Dillon CF, Sun Y, Joseph CB, Mahaffey KR. Blood mercury levels in US children and women of childbearing age, 1999-2000. *JAMA.* 2003 Apr 2;289(13):1667-74

[42] Kristin S. Schafer, Margaret Reeves, Skip Spitzer, Susan E. Kegley. Chemical Trespass: Pesticides in Our Bodies and Corporate Accountability. Pesticide Action Network North America. May 2004 Available at http://www.panna.org/campaigns/docsTrespass/chemicalTrespass2004.dv.html on August 1, 2004 See also: Body Burden: The Pollution in People. http://ewg.org/issues/siteindex/issues.php?issueid=5004 Accessed February 6, 2006

[43] Crinnion WJ. Environmental medicine, part one: the human burden of environmental toxins and their common health effects. *Altern Med Rev.* 2000 Feb;5(1):52-63

[44] Crinnion WJ. Environmental medicine, part 2 - health effects of and protection from ubiquitous airborne solvent exposure. *Altern Med Rev.* 2000 Apr;5(2):133-43

[45] Crinnion WJ. Environmental medicine, part three: long-term effects of chronic low-dose mercury exposure. *Altern Med Rev.* 2000 Jun;5(3):209-23

[46] Crinnion WJ. Environmental medicine, part 4: pesticides - biologically persistent and ubiquitous toxins. *Altern Med Rev.* 2000 Oct;5(5):432-47

[47] Elemental Mercury Vapor Poisoning -- North Carolina, 1988. http://www.cdc.gov/mmwr/preview/mmwrhtml/00001499.htm

[48] Shih H, Gartner JC Jr. Weight loss, hypertension, weakness, and limb pain in an 11-year-old boy. *J Pediatr.* 2001 Apr;138(4):566-9

[49] Sterzl I, Prochazkova J, Hrda P, Bartova J, Matucha P, Stejskal VD. Mercury and nickel allergy: risk factors in fatigue and autoimmunity. *Neuro Endocrinol Lett.* 1999;20:221-8

[50] Padlewska KK. Acrodynia. Last Updated: February 15, 2007 eMedicine http://www.emedicine.com/derm/topic592.htm Accessed october 25, 2007

[51] Chugh KS, Singhal PC, Uberoi HS. Rhabdomyolysis and renal failure in acute mercuric chloride poisoning. *Med J Aust.* 1978 Jul 29;2(3):125-6

[52] Chiu VC, Mouring D, Haynes DH. Action of mercurials on the active and passive transport properties of sarcoplasmic reticulum. *J Bioenerg Biomembr.* 1983 Feb;15(1):13-25

[53] Shamoo AE, Maclennan DH, Elderfrawi ME. Differential effects of mercurial compounds on excitable tissues. *Chem Biol Interact.* 1976 Jan;12(1):41-52

[54] Kalra V, Dua T, Kumar V, Kaul B. Succimer in Symptomatic Lead Poisoning. *Indian Pediatrics* 2002; 39:580-585 http://www.indianpediatrics.net/june2002/june-580-585.htm

[55] Bradstreet J, Geier DA, Kartzinel JJ, Adams JB, Geier MR. A case-control study of mercury burden in children with autistic spectrum disorders. *Journal of American Physicians and Surgeons* 2003; 8: 76-79 http://www.jpands.org/vol8no3/geier.pdf

[56] Forman J, Moline J, Cernichiari E, Sayegh S, Torres JC, Landrigan MM, Hudson J, Adel HN, Landrigan PJ. A cluster of pediatric metallic mercury exposure cases treated with meso-2,3-dimercaptosuccinic acid (DMSA). *Environ Health Perspect.* 2000 Jun;108(6):575-7 http://ehp.niehs.nih.gov/docs/2000/108p575-577forman/abstract.html

[57] Miller AL. Dimercaptosuccinic acid (DMSA), a non-toxic, water-soluble treatment for heavy metal toxicity. *Altern Med Rev.* 1998 Jun;3(3):199-207

[58] Kotter I, Durk H, Saal JG, Kroiher A, Schweinsberg F. Mercury exposure from dental amalgam fillings in the etiology of primary fibromyalgia: a pilot study. *J Rheumatol.* 1995 Nov;22(11):2194-5

[59] Vasquez A. *Musculoskeletal Pain: Expanded Clinical Strategies*: published in 2008 by the Institute for Functional Medicine www.FunctionalMedicine.org

- **Small intestine bacterial overgrowth (SIBO):** SIBO provides a model for explaining the clinical and pathophysiological manifestations of fibromyalgia. Although commonly underappreciated by many clinicians, SIBO is common in clinical practice, affecting approximately 40% of patients with rheumatoid arthritis, 84% of patients with IBS, and 90% to 100% of patients with fibromyalgia. **In a study of 42 fibromyalgia patients, all 42 of them showed evidence of SIBO, and the severity of the bacterial overgrowth correlated positively with the severity of the fibromyalgia**, thus indicating the plausibility of a causal relationship.[60] The links between fibromyalgia and IBS are also strong; **most IBS patients meet strict diagnostic criteria for fibromyalgia, and most fibromyalgia patients meet strict criteria for IBS**. Lubrano et al[61] showed that fibromyalgia severity correlated with IBS severity among patients who met strict diagnostic criteria for both conditions. The high degree of overlap between these two diagnostic labels suggests that these conditions are two variations of a common pathophysiological process—SIBO.[62] SIBO causes altered bowel function, immune activation, and visceral hypersensitivity, and it is

> **Hypothesis presented in 2008 is validated in 2009: Patients with "chronic fatigue" and the associated neurologic dysfunction and muscle dysfunction have intestinal overgrowth of bacteria that produce D-lactic acid, a known neurotoxin and metabolic poison**
>
> In 2007 and 2008, the current author (AV) wrote and published _Musculoskeletal Pain: Expanded Clinical Strategies_* with the Institute for Functional Medicine; this chapter on fibromyalgia is derived and updated from that work. In that publication, I reviewed evidence that fibromyalgia—at that time considered mysterious, idiopathic, chronic, relentless, and treatable only by pain-relieving drugs—was most likely caused by small intestine bacterial overgrowth (SIBO) and the resultant absorption of metabolic toxins and immunogenic debris. This perspective has been supported by numerous publications, particularly the article published by Sheedy et al** in 2009, which showed for the first time that patients with chronic fatigue syndrome—a condition tightly correlated with and which often overlaps with fibromyalgia—have SIBO with various bacteria that are high-output producers of D-lactic acid, a known neurotoxin and metabolic poison which likely contributes to some of the main clinical, biochemical, and histologic manifestations of FM, namely the mental fatigue and dyscognition, muscle fatigue and pain, biochemical evidence of mitochondrial impairment, and histologic evidence of mitochondrial myopathy.
>
> *Vasquez A. Musculoskeletal Pain: Expanded Clinical Strategies. Institute for Functional Medicine, 2008.
> **Sheedy JR, Wettenhall RE, Scanlon D, et al. Increased d-lactic acid intestinal bacteria in patients with chronic fatigue syndrome. _In Vivo_. 2009 Jul-Aug;23(4):621-8

one causative explanation for the clinical and pathophysiological manifestations of IBS; for more details and citations, see the excellent review by Lin.[63] IBS is characterized by visceral hyperalgesia, just as fibromyalgia is characterized by skeletal muscle hyperalgesia. Given that strong evidence indicates that IBS is caused by SIBO and that IBS and fibromyalgia are variations of the same pathophysiological process, then fibromyalgia may therefore be caused by SIBO. However, these links and interconnections require substantiation, as provided below.

- o *What is the evidence linking fibromyalgia with SIBO? What are the molecular mechanisms by which absorbed toxins and metabolites from SIBO can contribute to muscle pain and the bioenergetic-mitochondrial defects seen in fibromyalgia patients?*
  1. Small intestine bacterial overgrowth is highly prevalent in fibromyalgia: Several studies (cited previously) have shown that 90% to 100% of fibromyalgia patients have evidence of SIBO; such a strong correlation and the dose-response relationship imply causality and must be integrated into any science-based model of fibromyalgia.
  2. Fibromyalgia is tightly correlated with irritable bowel syndrome, a condition caused by small intestine bacterial overgrowth: Fibromyalgia and IBS are strongly convergent, and the evidence indicates that IBS is caused largely or completely by SIBO; again, for more details and citations, see Lin, cited previously.
  3. Small intestine bacterial overgrowth leads to systemic absorption of toxins that impair brain/nerve and muscle/mitochondrial function: SIBO is associated with overproduction and absorption of bacterial cellular debris (e.g., lipopolysaccharide [LPS], bacterial DNA, peptidoglycans, teichoic acid,

[60] Pimentel M, Wallace D, Hallegua D, Chow E, Kong Y, Park S, Lin HC. A link between irritable bowel syndrome and fibromyalgia may be related to findings on lactulose breath testing. _Ann Rheum Dis_. 2004 Apr;63(4):450-2

[61] Lubrano E, Iovino P, Tremolaterra F, Parsons WJ, Ciacci C, Mazzacca G. Fibromyalgia in patients with irritable bowel syndrome. An association with the severity of the intestinal disorder. _Int J Colorectal Dis_. 2001 Aug;16(4):211-5

[62] Veale D, Kavanagh G, Fielding JF, Fitzgerald O. Primary fibromyalgia and the irritable bowel syndrome: different expressions of a common pathogenetic process. _Br J Rheumatol_. 1991 Jun;30(3):220-2

[63] Lin HC. Small intestinal bacterial overgrowth: a framework for understanding irritable bowel syndrome. _JAMA_. 2004 Aug 18;292(7):852-8

exotoxins) and antimetabolites (e.g., D-lactic acid, tyramine, tartaric acid) that are known to impair cellular energy production in ways that accord with the myopathic metabolic defects seen in skeletal muscle biopsies of fibromyalgia patients. Intestinal gram-negative bacteria produce endotoxin (LPS), which impairs skeletal muscle energy production by stimulating skeletal muscle sodium-potassium-ATPase; endotoxin also raises blood lactate under aerobic conditions in humans.[64] **Thus, via direct and indirect effects on mitochondria, chronic low-dose bacterial LPS/endotoxin exposure can result in impaired muscle metabolism and reduced ATP synthesis via impairment of mitochondrial function.** Intestinal bacteria also produce D-lactate, a well-known metabolic toxin in humans; SIBO often results in variable levels of D-lactate acidosis, severe cases of which can progress from fatigue and malaise to encephalopathy (e.g., confusion, ataxia, slurred speech, altered mental status) and death.[65] Supporting the proposal that bacterial overgrowth with D-lacate-producing bacteria is a contributor to the chronic fatigue syndromes including fibromyalgia is an excellent study published in 2009 showing that patients with chronic fatigue syndrome have intestinal overgrowth of bacteria that produce D-lactate; specifically the research showed these fatigue patients to have **a 7-fold increase in D-lactate producing *Enterococcus* and 1,100-fold increase in D-lactate producing *Streptococcus***. Energy/ATP underproduction and lactate overproduction cause muscle fatigue and muscle pain. An additional cellular toxin produced by intestinal bacteria is hydrogen sulfide, which causes DNA damage[66] (noted previously to be increased in fibromyalgia patients) and which impairs cellular energy production, a finding relevant to but not necessarily limited to the pathogenesis of ulcerative colitis.[67,68]

> □ Experimental study: Effect of *E. coli* endotoxin on mitochondrial form and function. (*Annals of Surgery* 1971 Dec[69]): Authors of this paper show that treatment of normal rat liver mitochondria with *E. coli* endotoxin results in mitochondrial impairment. They note previous research showing that animal exposure to *E. coli* endotoxin causes inhibition of mitochondrial respiration and uncoupling of oxidative phosphorylation. Near their conclusion, the authors write, "Thus we have evidence to show that topical *E. coli* endotoxin has pathologic effects on both membrane integrity and internal mechanochemical systems of isolated mitochondria." Readers

---

A practical summary of SIBO: small intestine bacterial overgrowth

1. Definition: Generalized nonspecific overpopulation of bacteria in the small intestine (and large intestine, too).
2. Frequency: Very common in clinical practice and the general population.
3. Primary symptoms: Gas and bloating, especially after carbohydrate consumption; may also have constipation and/or diarrhea.
4. Secondary symptoms: Fatigue, muscle aches, difficulty with concentration and cognition ("brain fog"), nutritional deficiencies due to malabsorption, immune activation due to absorption of microbial debris and metabolites.
5. Diagnosis: ❶ Based on the symptoms above, ❷ jejunal aspiration is the gold standard but is expensive, cumbersome, and potentially hazardous, ❸ measurement of fermentation products (hydrogen and methane) in breath following consumption of a carbohydrate such as glucose, sucrose, or lactulose; the amount of "gas" produced is proportional to the bacterial population, ❹ may find elevated short chain fatty acids (SCFA) in stool or elevated folate in blood, but not all cases of SIBO produce SCFA or folate, ❺ clinical response to low-carbohydrate diet and/or antibiotic drugs or antimicrobial herbs. The current author (AV) uses #1 in conjunction with #5 most commonly.
6. Treatments: Low-carbohydrate diet and/or antibiotic drugs (e.g., rifamixin (200 or 550 mg each) 400-550 mg tid po [1,200-1,650 mg daily] for 10-30 days) or antimicrobial herbs (e.g., time-released emulsified oregano oil 600 mg daily for 4-6 weeks, and/or berberine 400-1,000 mg daily for 4 weeks).

---

[64] Bundgaard H, Kjeldsen K, Suarez Krabbe K, van Hall G, Simonsen L, Qvist J, Hansen CM, Moller K, Fonsmark L, Lav Madsen P, Klarlund Pedersen B. Endotoxemia stimulates skeletal muscle Na+-K+-ATPase and raises blood lactate under aerobic conditions in humans. *Am J Physiol Heart Circ Physiol*. 2003 Mar;284(3):H1028-34

[65] Vella A, Farrugia G. D-lactic acidosis: pathologic consequence of saprophytism. *Mayo Clin Proc*. 1998 May;73(5):451-6

[66] Attene-Ramos MS, Wagner ED, Gaskins HR, Plewa MJ. Hydrogen sulfide induces direct radical-associated DNA damage. *Mol Cancer Res*. 2007 May;5(5):455-9

[67] Magee EA, Richardson CJ, Hughes R, Cummings JH. Contribution of dietary protein to sulfide production in the large intestine: an in vitro and a controlled feeding study in humans. *Am J Clin Nutr*. 2000 Dec;72(6):1488-94

[68] Babidge W, Millard S, Roediger W. Sulfides impair short chain fatty acid beta-oxidation at acyl-CoA dehydrogenase level in colonocytes: implications for ulcerative colitis. *Mol Cell Biochem*. 1998 Apr;181(1-2):117-24

[69] White RR 4th, Mela L, Miller LD, Berwick L. Effect of E. coli endotoxin on mitochondrial form and function: inability to complete succinate-induced condensed-to-orthodox conformational change. *Ann Surg*. 1971 Dec;174(6):983-90

should appreciate that *E. coli* is a common inhabitant of the gastrointestinal tract of humans and that its population is quantitatively increased during states of bacterial overgrowth of the small bowel, as is commonly seen in most patients with fibromyalgia. More recently, research has shown that impairment of mitochondrial function (noted in patients with fibromyalgia) can lead to destruction of mitochondria by a process termed "mitophagy" (noted in patients with fibromyalgia); over time, loss of mitochondria via mitophagy leads to reduced numbers of mitochondria in muscle and other tissues (noted in patients with fibromyalgia) and contributes to the fatigue and other symptoms which characterize FM.

□ Clinical study: Increased d-lactic acid intestinal bacteria in patients with chronic fatigue syndrome (*In Vivo* 2009 Jul-Aug[70]): This excellent clinical research fully supports the pathoetiologic model presented in this chapter, which is derived and updated from a previous publication by this author: Vasquez A. *Musculoskeletal Pain: Expanded Clinical Strategies* published by the Institute for Functional Medicine in 2008. The authors of this 2009 study state in the summary of their research, "Patients with chronic fatigue syndrome (CFS) are affected by symptoms of cognitive dysfunction and neurological impairment, the cause of which has yet to be elucidated. However, these symptoms are strikingly similar to those of patients presented with D-lactic acidosis. A significant increase of Gram-positive facultative anaerobic fecal microorganisms in 108 CFS patients as compared to 177 control subjects (p<0.01) is presented in this report. The viable count of D-lactic acid producing *Enterococcus* and *Streptococcus* spp. in the fecal samples from the CFS group (3.5 x 10(7) cfu [colony forming units]/L and 9.8 x 10(7) cfu/L respectively) were significantly higher than those for the control group (5.0 x 10(6) cfu/L and 8.9 x 10(4) cfu/L respectively). [**Note: This is approximately a 7x increase in D-lactate producing *Enterococcus* and 1,100x increase in D-lactate producing *Streptococcus*.**] Analysis of exometabolic profiles of *Enterococcus faecalis* and *Streptococcus sanguinis*, representatives of *Enterococcus* and *Streptococcus* spp. respectively, by NMR and HPLC showed that these organisms produced significantly more lactic acid (p<0.01) from (13)C-labeled glucose, than the Gram negative *Escherichia coli*. Further, **both E. faecalis and S. sanguinis secrete more D-lactic acid than E. coli.** This study suggests a probable link between intestinal colonization of Gram-positive facultative anaerobic D-lactic acid bacteria and symptom expressions in a subgroup of patients with CFS. Given the fact that **this might explain not only neurocognitive dysfunction in CFS patients but also mitochondrial dysfunction, these findings may have important clinical implications.**"

4. Bacterial LPS and other antigens absorbed from the intestine during SIBO contribute to a subclinical inflammatory state that results in pain hypersensitivity and increased cytokine release, both of which are characteristics of fibromyalgia: In animal models and in human research studies, exposure to bacterial endotoxin/LPS has been shown to increase the brain's sensitivity to and perception of pain. Immune-mediated and inflammation-mediated pathways that promote pain sensitivity and perception are reduced production of nitric oxide with increased production of prostaglandins and

---

Mitophagy: Autophagy of mitochondria

"The removal of damaged mitochondria that could contribute to cellular dysfunction or death is achieved through process of mitochondrial autophagy, i.e. mitophagy."*

"Mitochondrial number and health are regulated by mitophagy, a process by which excessive or damaged mitochondria are subjected to autophagic degradation."**

"Autophagy can be beneficial for the cells by eliminating dysfunctional mitochondria, but massive autophagy can promote cell injury and may contribute to the pathophysiology of FM (fibromyalgia)."**

*Novak I. Mitophagy: a complex mechanism of mitochondrial removal. *Antioxid Redox Signal.* 2011 Nov 12
**Rambold AS, Lippincott-Schwartz J. Mechanisms of mitochondria and autophagy crosstalk. *Cell Cycle.* 2011;10(23)
***Cordero MD, De Miguel M, Moreno Fernández AM, et al. Mitochondrial dysfunction and mitophagy activation in blood mononuclear cells of fibromyalgia patients: implications in the pathogenesis of the disease. *Arthritis Res Ther.* 2010;12(1):R17

---

[70] Sheedy JR, Wettenhall RE, Scanlon D, Gooley PR, Lewis DP, McGregor N, Stapleton DI, Butt HL, DE Meirleir KL. Increased d-lactic acid intestinal bacteria in patients with chronic fatigue syndrome. *In Vivo.* 2009 Jul-Aug;23(4):621-8

cytokines, resulting in the sensitization of peripheral and/or central neurons to pain perception/transmission. In support of this concept, Lin[71] wrote in 2004, "The immune response to bacterial antigen in SIBO provides a framework for understanding the hypersensitivity in both fibromyalgia and IBS." A later paper by Othmanm, Agüero, and Lin[72] in 2008 stated, "...a recent animal study demonstrated that exposure to endotoxin increased the production of prostaglandins and simultaneously decreased nitrous oxide production, resulting in inflammatory hyperalgesia" and "These observations suggest that SIBO is a common feature in both [IBS and FM] disorders and that altered gut microbiota in SIBO may play a role in the induction of

> **Exposure to the bacterial endotoxin lipopolysaccharide (LPS) causes increased sensitivity to painful stimuli (hyperalgesia) and a reduction in opioid analgesia (anti-analgesia)**
>
> "Intraperitoneal injection of toxins, such as the bacterial endotoxin lipopolysaccharide (LPS), is associated with a well-characterized increase in sensitivity to painful stimuli (hyperalgesia) and a longer-lasting reduction in opioid analgesia (anti-analgesia) when pain sensitivity returns to basal levels."
>
> Johnston IN, Westbrook RF. Inhibition of morphine analgesia by LPS: role of opioid and NMDA receptors and spinal glia. *Behav Brain Res*. 2005 Jan 6;156(1):75-83

somatic or visceral hypersensitivity, with affected patients meeting the diagnostic criteria for IBS, fibromyalgia or both disorders."

5. <u>Central sensitization (enhanced and autonomous pain hypersensitivity) seen in FM can be caused by bacterial LPS</u>: Somewhat independent from the immune/inflammation-mediated hyperalgesia induced by LPS is the hyperalgesia mediated by central nervous system responses. The central sensitization seen with fibromyalgia[73] might be explained as being caused by intestinally-derived endotoxinemia. Bacterial LPS promote central sensitization via direct activation of NMDA receptors and by inducing hyperalgesia and anti-analgesia.[74] Accumulated evidence suggests that fibromyalgia may be a disorder of somatic hypersensitivity induced by bacterial toxins derived from quantitative excess or qualitative abnormalities in gut bacteria.[75]

6. <u>SIBO causes nutrient malabsorption</u>: SIBO causes nutrient malabsorption[76] and can thereby contribute to the vitamin D and magnesium deficiencies that promote pain and mitochondrial dysfunction, respectively, and which are common in fibromyalgia.

7. <u>SIBO can be triggered or exacerbated by emotional stress</u>: SIBO can be triggered in humans by reduced mucosal immunity following stressful life events, and this helps explain the link between IBS, fibromyalgia, and psychoemotional stress.

8. <u>Oxidative stress triggers exaggerated pain perception: hyperalgesia [hypersensitivity to pain] and allodynia [perception of pain from normal stimuli]</u>: Patients with fibromyalgia show evidence of increased free radical (oxidant) production and reduced antioxidant defenses. Increased oxidative stress can be caused by immune activation and mitochondrial dysfunction; immune activation and mitochondrial dysfunction also promote oxidative stress and depletion of antioxidants, resulting in a vicious cycle. In the excellent review by Cordero et al[77], the authors note that recent studies have shown that oxidative stress can cause peripheral and central sensitization and alter nerve sensitivity to pain (nociception), resulting in hyperalgesia—hypersensivity to normal stimuli. The free radical (oxidant) superoxide promotes the development of pain through direct peripheral sensitization and the release of various cytokines (such as TNF-α, IL-1β, and IL-6), the formation of peroxynitrite (ONOO-), and PARP activation. PARP—poly-ADP-ribose-polymerase—is a nuclear enzyme activated by superoxide/peroxynitrite radicals; activation of PARP promotes the development of pain syndromes, including the components of small sensory fiber neuropathy, thermal and mechanical

---

[71] Lin HC. Small intestinal bacterial overgrowth: a framework for understanding irritable bowel syndrome. *JAMA*. 2004 Aug 18;292(7):852-8

[72] Othman M, Agüero R, Lin HC. Alterations in intestinal microbial flora and human disease. *Curr Opin Gastroenterol*. 2008 Jan;24(1):11-6

[73] Meeus M, Nijs J. Central sensitization: a biopsychosocial explanation for chronic widespread pain in patients with fibromyalgia and chronic fatigue syndrome. *Clin Rheumatol*. 2007 Apr;26(4):465-73

[74] Johnston IN, Westbrook RF. Inhibition of morphine analgesia by LPS: role of opioid and NMDA receptors and spinal glia. *Behav Brain Res*. 2005;156(1):75-83

[75] Othman M, Agüero R, Lin HC. Alterations in intestinal microbial flora and human disease. *Curr Opin Gastroenterol*. 2008 Jan;24(1):11-6

[76] Elphick HL, Elphick DA, Sanders DS. Small bowel bacterial overgrowth. An underrecognized cause of malnutrition in older adults. Geriatrics. 2006 Sep;61(9):21-6

[77] Cordero MD, De Miguel M, Moreno Fernández AM, et al. Mitochondrial dysfunction and mitophagy activation in blood mononuclear cells of fibromyalgia patients: implications in the pathogenesis of the disease. *Arthritis Res Ther*. 2010;12(1):R17

hyperalgesia, tactile allodynia, and exaggerated pain behavior in animal models of diabetic neuropathy.[78,79]

9. <u>Low plasma levels of L-tryptophan seen in fibromyalgia patients can be caused by degradation of dietary tryptophan by the bacterial enzyme tryptophanase</u>: Patients with fibromyalgia have low blood levels of the amino acid L-tryptophan[80], which is used in the body to make serotonin (important for mood maintenance and pain alleviation) and melatonin (important for normal sleep and for support of mitochondrial function and anti-oxidation). Bacteria such as *Escherichia coli, Proteus vulgaris,* and *Bacteroides* produce the enzyme tryptophanase[81] which destroys L-tryptophan in the gut before it is absorbed from foods; bacterial overgrowth of the small intestine would be expected to exacerbate this phenomenon. In patients with fibromyalgia, higher tryptophan levels correlate positively with serotonin levels and with less pain and better sleep, while lower tryptophan levels are associated with sleep impairment, reduced serotonin levels, and higher levels of substance P, a neurotransmitter that promotes inflammation and pain perception.[82] Fibromyalgia patients produce 31% less melatonin than do healthy controls, and "this may contribute to impaired sleep at night, fatigue during the day, and changed pain perception."[83]

10. <u>The therapies that help fibromyalgia share mechanisms of action consistent with the model presented here</u>: As will be reviewed below under *Therapeutic Interventions*, essentially all of the most successful therapies for fibromyalgia have effects on intestinal flora, muscle perfusion/contractility, or mitochondrial bioenergetics. This is true for vegetarian diets (which favorably alter gut flora), supplementation with tryptophan/melatonin (which preserve mitochondrial function during LPS exposure), physical treatments such as acupuncture (which restore tissue perfusion), and the use of nutrients such as magnesium, acetyl-L-carnitine, D-ribose, creatine, and coenzyme Q-10 (which optimize mitochondrial function).

11. <u>Restless leg syndrome and fibromyalgia commonly co-exist, and restless leg syndrome can be alleviated by eradication of SIBO</u>: Restless leg syndrome (RLS) occurs in approximately 30% of fibromyalgia patients and can be effectively treated by addressing SIBO with a combination of antibiotics and probiotics.[84]

12. <u>Antimicrobial treatment alleviates fibromyalgia in most FM patients</u>: Finally and most importantly, **antimicrobial therapy alleviates FM (and IBS) symptoms in direct proportion to the success of bacterial overgrowth eradication**, thus adding strong evidence in support of SIBO as a main cause of FM.[85,86] Recent clinical trials have shown that treatment of the fibromyalgia-related conditions IBS and SIBO by use of the nonabsorbed oral antibiotic rifaximin results in significant diminution of IBS-SIBO symptomatology with benefits lasting after the discontinuation of therapy.[87,88]

   ▫ <u>Clinical trial: Rifaximin therapy for patients with irritable bowel syndrome without constipation (*New England Journal of Medicine* 2011 Jan[89])</u>: Authors of this study evaluated rifaximin, a

[78] Wang ZQ, Porreca F, Cuzzocrea S, Galen K, Lightfoot R, Masini E, Muscoli C, Mollace V, Ndengele M, Ischiropoulos H, Salvemini D. A newly identified role for superoxide in inflammatory pain. *J Pharmacol Exp Ther.* 2004 Jun;309(3):869-78

[79] Ilnytska O, Lyzogubov VV, Stevens MJ, Drel VR, Mashtalir N, Pacher P, Yorek MA, Obrosova IG. Poly(ADP-ribose) polymerase inhibition alleviates experimental diabetic sensory neuropathy. *Diabetes.* 2006 Jun;55(6):1686-94

[80] "Plasma-free tryptophan is inversely related to the severity of subjective pain in 8 patients who fulfilled criteria for a variety of non-articular rheumatism, the "fibrositis syndrome". The observation is consistent with animal and human studies suggesting a relationship between reduced brain serotonin metabolism and pain reactivity." Moldofsky H, Warsh JJ. Plasma tryptophan and musculoskeletal pain in non-articular rheumatism ("fibrositis syndrome"). *Pain.* 1978 Jun;5(1):65-71

[81] Demoss RD, Moser K. Tryptophanase in Diverse Bacterial Species. *Journal of Bacteriology* 1969; 98: 167-171

[82] "A strong negative correlation between SP and 5-HIAA (P = .000) as well as between SP and TRP (P = .009) could be demonstrated. High serum concentrations of 5-HIAA and TRP showed a significant relation to low pain scores (5-HIAA: P = .030; TRP: P = .014). Moreover, 5-HIAA was strongly related to good quality of sleep (P = .000), while SP was related to sleep disturbance (P = .005)." Schwarz MJ, Späth M, Müller-Bardorff H, Pongratz DE, Bondy B, Ackenheil M. Relationship of substance P, 5-hydroxyindole acetic acid and tryptophan in serum of fibromyalgia patients. *Neurosci Lett.* 1999 Jan 15;259(3):196-8

[83] "The FMS patients had a 31% lower MT secretion than healthy subjects during the hours of darkness... Patients with fibromyalgic syndrome have a lower melatonin secretion during the hours of darkness than healthy subjects. This may contribute to impaired sleep at night, fatigue during the day, and changed pain perception." Wikner J, Hirsch U, Wetterberg L, Röjdmark S. Fibromyalgia--a syndrome associated with decreased nocturnal melatonin secretion. *Clin Endocrinol* (Oxf). 1998 Aug;49(2):179-83

[84] Weinstock LB, Fern SE, Duntley SP. Restless Legs Syndrome in Patients with Irritable Bowel Syndrome: Response to Small Intestinal Bacterial Overgrowth Therapy. *Dig Dis Sci.* 2007 May;53(5):1252-6

[85] Wallace DJ, Hallegua DS. Fibromyalgia: the gastrointestinal link. *Curr Pain Headache Rep.*2004 Oct;8(5):364-8

[86] Pimentel M, Hallegua DS, Wallace DJ, et al.: Improvement of symptoms by eradication of small intestinal overgrowth in FM: a double-blind study. [Abstract] *Arthritis Rheum* 1999, 42:S343

[87] Pimentel M, Park S, Mirocha J, Kane SV, Kong Y. The effect of a nonabsorbed oral antibiotic (rifaximin) on the symptoms of the irritable bowel syndrome: a randomized trial. *Ann Intern Med.* 2006 Oct 17;145(8):557-63

[88] Sharara AI, Aoun E, Abdul-Baki H, Mounzer R, Sidani S, Elhajj I. A randomized double-blind placebo-controlled trial of rifaximin in patients with abdominal bloating and flatulence. *Am J Gastroenterol.* 2006 Feb;101(2):326-33

[89] Pimentel M, Lembo A, Chey WD, et al. Rifaximin therapy for patients with irritable bowel syndrome without constipation. *N Engl J Med.* 2011 Jan 6;364(1):22-32

minimally absorbed antibiotic, as treatment for IBS. Subjects were given rifaximin at a dose of 550 mg or placebo, three times daily for 2 weeks and were followed for 10 weeks thereafter. "Significantly more patients in the rifaximin group than in the placebo group had adequate relief of global IBS symptoms during the first 4 weeks after treatment (40.8% vs. 31.2%). Similarly, more patients in the rifaximin group than in the placebo group had adequate relief of bloating (39.5% vs. 28.7%). In addition, significantly more patients in the rifaximin group had a response to treatment as assessed by daily ratings of IBS symptoms, bloating, abdominal pain, and stool consistency. The incidence of adverse events was similar in the two groups." Thus, among patients who had IBS without constipation, treatment with rifaximin for 2 weeks provided significant relief of IBS symptoms, bloating, abdominal pain, and loose or watery stools. Shortcomings of the intervention used in this study include ❶ failure to use long-term treatment, which is often necessary in the treatment of chronic dysbiosis, ❷ failure to co-administer an antifungal agent to avert fungal growth in the intestines which commonly occurs as a result of antimicrobial/antibacterial drug treatment, ❸ failure to administer probiotics to re-establish beneficial flora, and ❹ failure to implement dietary modification to sustain the beneficial eradication of excess bacteria.

▫ Review of clinical trials: Rifaximin as treatment for SIBO and IBS (*Expert Opinion on Investigational Drugs* 2009 Mar[90]): A recognized expert in the treatment of SIBO-related conditions, Dr Pimentel writes, "Rifaximin is a broad-range, gastrointestinal-specific antibiotic that demonstrates no clinically relevant bacterial resistance. Therefore, rifaximin may be useful in the treatment of gastrointestinal disorders associated with altered bacterial flora, including irritable bowel syndrome (IBS) and small intestinal bacterial overgrowth (SIBO)." "Rifaximin improved global symptoms in 33 - 92% of patients and eradicated SIBO in up to 84% of patients with IBS, with results sustained up to 10 weeks post-treatment. Rifaximin caused a lower number of adverse events compared with metronidazole or levofloxacin and may have a more favorable adverse event profile than systemic antibiotics, without clinically relevant antibiotic resistance."

▫ Results of two clinical trials of antibiotics in the treatment of fibromyalgia: Fibromyalgia—the gastrointestinal link (*Current Pain and Headache Reports* 2004 Oct[91]): ❶ 96 patients with SIBO diagnosed by lactulose hydrogen breath testing (LHBT) were offered antibiotic treatment for the reduction of gastrointestinal bacteria; 25 of the 96 patients returned for a follow-up LHBT. Neomycin was the most commonly used antibiotic. Eleven of the 25 patients achieved complete transient eradication of SIBO after antibiotic treatment and experienced better improvement in more of their FM symptom scores when compared with the patients who did not achieve complete eradication. This indicates that a relationship exists between the presence of SIBO and intestinal and extraintestinal symptoms in fibromyalgia. ❷ In this double-blind trial of eradication of SIBO in fibromyalgia, 46 patients fulfilling the established criteria for FM were tested for SIBO using LHBT. Forty-two of the 46 patients (91.3%) were positive for SIBO and were randomized to receive placebo or 500 mg of liquid neomycin twice daily for 10 days. Only six of the 20 patients (30%) in the neomycin group achieved eradication (indicating inefficacy of treatment); thus, no statistically significant difference between groups was available for analysis. Thereafter, 28 patients in the double-blind study testing positive for SIBO went on to receive open-label antibiotic treatment to eradicate SIBO, and this time 17 of the 28 patients (60.7%) achieved eradication of SIBO. When these 23 patients were compared with the 15 patients who failed to eradicate or did not undergo open-label treatment, significant improvement attributable to antibiotic treatment in the FM scores was detected. **Results suggest that eradication of bacterial overgrowth results in a statistically and clinically significant alleviation of fibromyalgia symptoms.**

---

[90] Pimentel M. Review of rifaximin as treatment for SIBO and IBS. *Expert Opin Investig Drugs*. 2009 Mar;18(3):349-58
[91] Wallace DJ, Hallegua DS. Fibromyalgia: the gastrointestinal link. *Curr Pain Headache Rep*. 2004 Oct;8(5):364-8

Thus, the research literature provides compelling evidence linking SIBO with the genesis and perpetuation of fibromyalgia. Chronic low-dose exposure to **immunogens** (defined as substances which are **immune-response gen**erating) and metabolic toxins from SIBO is a plausible cause of impaired cellular energy production that results in chronic, widespread muscle fatigue and soreness and which may precipitate the clinical presentation of fibromyalgia. The individual components of this model have been substantiated by mechanistic studies in animals and/or research studies in humans. CFS also shares many epidemiological and clinical similarities with fibromyalgia, and a similar pathophysiology is highly probable.

A consistent report from many CFS and fibromyalgia patients is that of environmental intolerance (EI) and multiple chemical sensitivity (MCS). This can be explained by SIBO because bacterial LPS and other bacterial products impair hepatic cytochrome P450 detoxification enzymes, resulting in reduced drug metabolism and impaired clearance of xenobiotics.[92] Accumulation of xenobiotics in CFS patients[93] might therefore be explained in part by LPS-induced inhibition of xenobiotic clearance secondary to SIBO. Further, the metabolic and immunologic effects of LPS can also account for the immune activation, neurological dysfunction, and musculoskeletal complaints noted in patients with CFS, IBS, and FM. A simplified yet accurate model of fibromyalgia which accounts for the major clinical and objective abnormalities seen with this condition is presented in the diagram below.

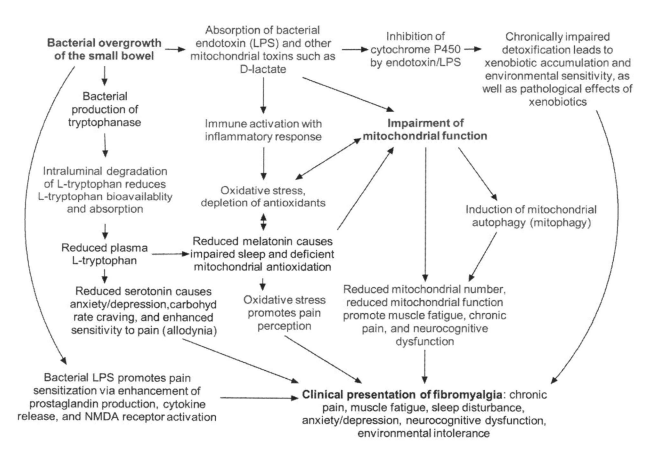

How small intestine bacterial overgrowth (SIBO) causes fibromyalgia: Bacterial overgrowth of the small bowel leads to chronic low-grade tryptophan insufficiency resulting in reduced endogenous production of serotonin (important for positive mood and relief from anxiety pain) and of melatonin (important for restful sleep and protection of mitochondria from oxidative stress). Bacterial "metabolic-mitochondrial toxins" such as endotoxin and D-lactate cause impaired mitochondrial energy production, which leads to mitophagy, muscle fatigue, pain, and cognitive impairment.

---

[92] Shedlofsky SI, Israel BC, McClain CJ, Hill DB, Blouin RA. Endotoxin administration to humans inhibits hepatic cytochrome P450-mediated drug metabolism. *J Clin Invest.* 1994 Dec;94(6):2209-14

[93] Dunstan RH, Donohoe M, Taylor W, Roberts TK, Murdoch RN, Watkins JA, McGregor NR. A preliminary investigation of chlorinated hydrocarbons and chronic fatigue syndrome. *Med J Aust.* 1995 Sep 18;163(6):294-7

Following the exclusion of diagnosable and treatable conditions that can contribute to or mimic fibromyalgia, functional medicine clinicians can design treatment plans based on the previously reviewed pathogenesis and on the therapeutic considerations detailed in the following section.

<u>**Therapeutic Interventions**</u>

- **Overview:** Clinical interventions for the treatment of SIBO include dietary carbohydrate restriction, normalization of slow gastrointestinal transit time (e.g., correction of hypothyroidism), selective use of probiotic supplements to normalize intestinal flora, support of mucosal immunity with nutrients such as vitamin A, zinc, and L-glutamine, and eradication of bacterial overgrowth with drugs such as ciprofloxacin, rifaximin, metronidazole or natural products such as berberine, artemisia, and oil of oregano, as reviewed in greater detail elsewhere by this author.[94] Failure of any monotherapeutic approach to immediately resolve all manifestations of fibromyalgia is explained by the secondary metabolic, immune, and neurophysiological effects that have generally persisted over periods ranging from years to decades for most patients. The treatment program (examples provided) must be complete in order to facilitate correction of systemic oxidative damage (broad-spectrum antioxidant consumption), resultant nutritional deficiencies (diet optimization, vitamin and mineral supplementation), immune sensitization and induction of proinflammatory cycles (anti-inflammatory nutrition), alterations in neurotransmission and membrane receptor function (amino acid and fatty acid supplementation), and the inflammation-induced disturbances in pain reception and hypothalamic-pituitary-endocrine function (assess and correct hormonal imbalances). Further, patients treated for SIBO who do not positively change their diets and lifestyles (which probably promoted the genesis and perpetuation of the disease-causing SIBO in the first place) are subject to continual recurrence until such changes are implemented and faithfully maintained.

- **Diet optimization:** The supplemented Paleo-Mediterranean Diet—the 5-part nutritional wellness protocol—as described in chapter 2 should be implemented for most fibromyalgia patients; exceptions to this general rule might include patients with renal insufficiency due to the risk for hyperkalemia due to the high content of potassium in fruits and vegetables, and the per-patient customizations and avoidances that will have to be accommodated for patients with food allergies. Otherwise, the diet should be based on fruits, vegetables, nuts, seeds, berries and lean sources of protein; atop this foundational diet are the other four components of the 5-part protocol: high-potency multivitamin and multimineral supplementation, physiologic doses of vitamin D3 to optimize serum 25-OH-D levels, combination fatty acid supplementation (with flax oil [for EPA], fish oil [for EPA and DHA], and borage oil [for GLA] with oleic acid from olive oil incorporated into the diet), and probiotics. The diet should emphasize strict avoidance of grains in general and gluten-containing grains in particular. This diet is essential for the provision of sufficient protein, fiber, phytonutrients, and alkalinization to promote restoration of homeodynamic balance and the restoration of nutritional status and hence normalization of physiologic function. The diet should be low in carbohydrates to reduce fermentable substrate to intestinal bacteria. The most important books for patients to read in support of this diet are *The Paleo Diet* by Dr Loren Cordain and *Breaking the Vicious Cycle* by Elaine Gottschall; an open-access summary of the diet plan is available at OptimalHealthResearch.com/spmd.html.

  o **Vegetarian diet:** Diets high in fruits, vegetables, nuts, berries, and seeds provide ample fiber to promote laxation and can be useful as adjunctive treatment for gastrointestinal dysbiosis in general and SIBO in particular (i.e., *quantitative* reduction in GI dysbiosis). Perhaps more importantly, plant-based diets result in *qualitative* benefits by changing microbial behavior and reducing production of irritants, toxins, and bacterial metabolites, including the bioenergetic-mitochondrial poisons D-lactate and hydrogen sulfide. Fibromyalgia patients who consume a mostly vegetarian diet have experienced significant improvements in function and reductions in fibromyalgia symptomatology.[95] Poorly designed dietary interventions that

---

[94] Vasquez A. Reducing Pain and Inflammation Naturally. Part 6: Nutritional and Botanical Treatments Against "Silent Infections" and Gastrointestinal Dysbiosis, Commonly Overlooked Causes of Neuromusculoskeletal Inflammation and Chronic Health Problems. *Nutr Perspect* 2006; Jan: 5-21. For more updated information, see: Vasquez A. *Integrative Rheumatology: Second Edition 2007*. Fort Worth, Texas; Integrative and Biological Medicine Research and Consulting, 2007.

[95] Donaldson MS, Speight N, Loomis S. Fibromyalgia syndrome improved using a mostly raw vegetarian diet: an observational study. *BMC Complement Altern Med.* 2001;1:7 http://www.biomedcentral.com/1472-6882/1/7

allow abundant intake of whole-grain bread, pasta, rice, and fruit juice[96] would be expected to fail because such high-carbohydrate diets feed intestinal bacteria with an abundance of substrate and would therefore be expected to sustain or exacerbate SIBO.

- **Coenzyme Q10 (CoQ-10):** An endogenous antioxidant and essential component of the mitochondrial electron transport chain, oral supplementation with CoQ-10 has been used therapeutically in numerous studies for the successful treatment of migraine, heart failure, hypertension, and renal failure. Additional data have shown immunomodulatory roles for CoQ-10, and many clinicians employ it as adjunctive treatment for viral infections, cancer, and allergies.[97,98] CoQ-10 levels are 40% lower in blood cells of patients with FM compared with levels in healthy persons, and reduced levels of CoQ-10 correlate with markers associated with expedited destruction of mitochondria (mitophagy).[99] In an open trial of 23 fibromyalgia patients, the combination of 200 mg CoQ-10 and 200 mg *Ginkgo biloba* (for a total dose of 48 mg flavone glycosides and 12 mg terpene lactones) daily for 84 days was shown to provide clinical benefit in 64% of patients.[100]

  o *Clinical investigation: Mitochondrial dysfunction and mitophagy activation in blood mononuclear cells of fibromyalgia patients* (*Arthritis Res Ther* 2010 Jan[101]): The authors studied 2 male and 18 female FM patients and 10 healthy controls. They evaluated mitochondrial function in blood mononuclear cells from FM patients measuring coenzyme Q10 (CoQ-10) levels with high-performance liquid chromatography (HPLC) and mitochondrial membrane potential with flow cytometry. Oxidative stress was determined by measuring mitochondrial superoxide production and lipid peroxidation in blood mononuclear cells and plasma from fibromyalgia patients. Autophagy activation was evaluated in blood mononuclear cells; mitophagy was confirmed by measuring citrate synthase activity and electron microscopy examination of blood mononuclear cells. The authors found reduced levels of CoQ-10, decreased mitochondrial membrane potential, increased levels of mitochondrial superoxide in blood mononuclear cells (indicating increased oxidative stress and reduced antioxidant defense), and increased levels of lipid peroxidation in both blood mononuclear cells and plasma from fibromyalgia patients. Importantly, the authors note that "mitochondrial dysfunction was also associated with increased expression of autophagic genes and the elimination of dysfunctional mitochondria with mitophagy"; what this means practically is that the **biochemical aberrations that cause mitochondrial dysfunction lead to destruction of mitochondria via "mitophagy"** which literally means "mitochondrial consumption", a process by which dysfunctional mitochondria are eliminated by degradative processes.

- **Tryptophan and 5-hydroxytryptophan (5-HTP):** Tryptophan is the amino acid precursor to the neurotransmitter serotonin, which has antidepressant, anti-anxiety, and analgesic properties. Patients with fibromyalgia are known to have low blood levels (i.e., functional nutritional insufficiency) of tryptophan, and the severity of the deficiency correlates with the severity of pain.[102,103,104] Blood levels of serotonin are often below normal in fibromyalgia patients.[105] The accepted medical use of selective serotonin reuptake inhibitors (SSRIs) to treat the pain, depression, and anxiety associated with fibromyalgia supports the use of 5-HTP to raise serotonin levels naturally by correcting the underlying nutritional insufficiency. As an over-the-counter nutritional supplement, the 5-hydroxylated form of tryptophan (5-HTP) has been used clinically and in numerous research studies. Supplementation with 5-HTP has been shown to significantly alleviate symptoms of fibromyalgia.[106] An open 90-day study in 50 fibromyalgia patients showed significant improvement in all measured parameters (number of tender points, anxiety, pain intensity, quality of sleep, fatigue) after

[96] Michalsen A, Riegert M, Lüdtke R, Bäcker M, Langhorst J, Schwickert M, Dobos GJ. Mediterranean diet or extended fasting's influence on changing the intestinal microflora, immunoglobulin A secretion and clinical outcome in patients with rheumatoid arthritis and fibromyalgia: an observational study. *BMC Complement Altern Med.* 2005 Dec 22;5:22
[97] Gaby AR. The role of Coenzyme Q10 in clinical medicine: Part 1. *Altern Med Rev* 1996;1:11-17
[98] Gaby AR. The role of Coenzyme Q10 in clinical medicine: Part 2. *Altern Med Rev* 1996;1: 168-175
[99] Cordero MD, De Miguel M, Moreno Fernández AM, et al. Mitochondrial dysfunction and mitophagy activation in blood mononuclear cells of fibromyalgia patients: implications in the pathogenesis of the disease. *Arthritis Res Ther.* 2010;12(1):R17. Epub 2010 Jan 28.
[100] Lister RE. An open, pilot study to evaluate the potential benefits of coenzyme Q10 combined with Ginkgo biloba extract in fibromyalgia syndrome. *J Int Med Res.* 2002 Mar-Apr;30(2):195-9
[101] Cordero MD, De Miguel M, Moreno Fernández AM, Carmona López IM, Garrido Maraver J, Cotán D, Gómez Izquierdo L, Bonal P, Campa F, Bullon P, Navas P, Sánchez Alcázar JA. Mitochondrial dysfunction and mitophagy activation in blood mononuclear cells of fibromyalgia patients: implications in the pathogenesis of the disease. *Arthritis Res Ther.* 2010;12(1):R17. Epub 2010 Jan 28.
[102] Moldofsky H, Warsh JJ. Plasma tryptophan and musculoskeletal pain in non-articular rheumatism ("fibrositis syndrome"). *Pain.* 1978 Jun;5(1):65-71
[103] Yunus MB, Dailey JW, Aldag JC, Masi AT, Jobe PC. Plasma tryptophan and other amino acids in primary fibromyalgia: a controlled study. *J Rheumatol.* 1992 Jan;19(1):90-4
[104] Russell IJ, Michalek JE, Vipraio GA, Fletcher EM, Wall K. Serum amino acids in fibrositis/fibromyalgia syndrome. *J Rheumatol* Suppl. 1989 Nov;19:158-63
[105] Wolfe F, Russell IJ, Vipraio G, Ross K, Anderson J. Serotonin levels, pain threshold, and fibromyalgia symptoms in the general population. J Rheumatol. 1997;24(3):555-9
[106] Caruso I, Sarzi Puttini P, Cazzola M, Azzolini V. Double-blind study of 5-hydroxytryptophan versus placebo in the treatment of primary fibromyalgia syndrome. *J Int Med Res.* 1990 May-Jun;18(3):201-9

treatment with 5-HTP; global clinical improvement assessed by the patient and the investigator indicated a "good" or "fair" response in nearly 50% of the patients during the treatment period.[107] A double-blind, placebo-controlled study using 5-HTP in 50 fibromyalgia patients showed significant improvement in all measured parameters, with only mild and transient side effects.[108] Commonly used doses range from 50 to 300 mg/d, with larger doses divided throughout the day. If tryptophan rather than 5-HTP is used, results are improved when taken on an empty stomach with carbohydrate to induce insulin secretion, which preferentially promotes uptake of tryptophan into the brain. Magnesium deficiency impairs conversion of 5-HTP into serotonin, and the interventional program must ensure nutritional supra-sufficiency.

- **Melatonin:** Patients with fibromyalgia show decreased nocturnal secretion of melatonin.[109] Melatonin benefits fibromyalgia patients through a wide range of mechanisms, including promotion of restful sleep and reduction in LPS-induced mitochondrial impairment. As a powerful antioxidant, melatonin scavenges oxygen and nitrogen-based reactants generated in mitochondria and thereby limits the loss of intramitochondrial glutathione; this prevents damage to mitochondrial protein and DNA. **Melatonin increases the activity of Complexes 1 and 4 of the mitochondrial electron transport chain, improving mitochondrial respiration and increasing ATP synthesis** under various physiological and experimental conditions.[110] Melatonin (3–6 mg per night, administered orally 1 hour before bedtime) has been reported to normalize sleep, alleviate pain and fatigue, and alleviate many clinical manifestations of fibromyalgia.[111] Successful treatment with melatonin or its precursor tryptophan/5-HTP should not deter the clinician from addressing other contributing or causative problems such as vitamin D deficiency, gastrointestinal dysbiosis including SIBO, magnesium deficiency, and chronic psychoemotional stress. The adult physiologic dose which mimics endogenous production is approximately 200-500 mcg [micrograms] nightly. In adults, supplementation with melatonin has a wide therapeutic index and has been used safely and effectively in doses up to 20 to 40 mg [milligrams] nightly.

- **Magnesium:** Magnesium deficiency is epidemic in industrialized societies due to insufficient dietary intake (e.g., from mineral water and leafy green vegetables) and concomitant urinary acidosis, which increases urinary magnesium loss.[112,113] Additional causes of magnesium deficiency in fibromyalgia patients include vitamin D deficiency, malabsorption due to SIBO, and the stress of chronic illness. Magnesium deficiency exacerbates the symptoms of fibromyalgia by contributing to impairment of energy (ATP) production in skeletal muscle, increased muscle tone and spasms (hypomagnesemic tetany), and anxiety and hyperalgesia via NMDA receptor overstimulation and neurocortical hyperexcitability. Magnesium deficiency also promotes constipation and intestinal stasis, which exacerbates SIBO. Magnesium supplementation (600 mg/d or to bowel tolerance) should be used routinely in fibromyalgia patients; the primary cautions with magnesium use are renal insufficiency and the use of magnesium-sparing drugs such as the diuretic drug spironolactone. Modest benefits demonstrated in clinical trials with magnesium and malic acid[114] can easily be exceeded with concomitant interventions to address vitamin D deficiency, SIBO, and mitochondrial dysfunction.

- **Acetyl L-carnitine (ALC):** A large study with 102 patients showed that ALC (administered by oral and parenteral routes, 1500 mg/d) was beneficial in patients with fibromyalgia.[115] Given the role of ALC in supporting and improving mitochondrial function, this supplement probably benefits fibromyalgia patients by compensating for LPS-induced skeletal muscle dysfunction.

---

[107] Sarzi Puttini P, Caruso I. Primary fibromyalgia syndrome and 5-hydroxy-L-tryptophan: a 90-day open study. *J Int Med Res*. 1992 Apr;20(2):182-9

[108] Caruso I, Sarzi Puttini P, Cazzola M, Azzolini V. Double-blind study of 5-hydroxytryptophan versus placebo in the treatment of primary fibromyalgia syndrome. *J Int Med Res*. 1990 May-Jun;18(3):201-9

[109] Wikner J, Hirsch U, Wetterberg L, Röjdmark S. Fibromyalgia--a syndrome associated with decreased nocturnal melatonin secretion. *Clin Endocrinol* (Oxf). 1998 Aug;49(2):179-83

[110] León J, Acuña-Castroviejo D, Escames G, Tan DX, Reiter RJ. Melatonin mitigates mitochondrial malfunction. *J Pineal Res*. 2005 Jan;38(1):1-9

[111] Acuna-Castroviejo D, Escames G, Reiter RJ. Melatonin therapy in fibromyalgia. *J Pineal Res*. 2006 Jan;40(1):98-9

[112] Cordain L, Eaton SB, Sebastian A, Mann N, Lindeberg S, Watkins BA, O'Keefe JH, Brand-Miller J. Origins and evolution of the Western diet: health implications for the 21st century. *Am J Clin Nutr*. 2005 Feb;81(2):341-54

[113] Rylander R, Remer T, Berkemeyer S, Vormann J. Acid-base status affects renal magnesium losses in healthy, elderly persons. *J Nutr*. 2006 Sep;136(9):2374-7

[114] Russell IJ, Michalek JE, Flechas JD, Abraham GE. Treatment of fibromyalgia syndrome with Super Malic: a randomized, double blind, placebo controlled, crossover pilot study. *J Rheumatol*. 1995 May;22(5):953-8

[115] Rossini M, Di Munno O, Valentini G, Bianchi G, Biasi G, Cacace E, Malesci D, La Montagna G, Viapiana O, Adami S. Double-blind, multicenter trial comparing acetyl l-carnitine with placebo in the treatment of fibromyalgia patients. *Clin Exp Rheumatol*. 2007 Mar-Apr;25(2):182-8

- **D-ribose:** D-ribose is a naturally occurring pentose carbohydrate available as a dietary supplement. When administered orally (5 g thrice daily), it provides safe and effective benefit to fibromyalgia patients, according to a recent pilot study with 41 patients.[116] Improvements are seen in energy, sleep, mental clarity, pain intensity, and well-being, as well as global assessment. Among its beneficial mechanisms of action is enhancement of mitochondrial ATP production. Thus, the benefits of D-ribose supplementation may be mediated by restoration or preservation of mitochondrial impairment caused by LPS in fibromyalgia patients.

- **Creatine monohydrate:** Skeletal muscle levels of phosphocreatine and ATP are reduced in patients with fibromyalgia compared with normal controls; thus, oral supplementation with creatine would appear to be an obvious intervention to restore these depressed levels to normal. Although no formal trials have been conducted, Artimal et al[117] reported that a patient with severe refractory fibromyalgia attained sustained alleviation of depression and pain, as well as improvements in sleep and quality of life, following oral administration of creatine monohydrate for 4 weeks (3 grams daily in the first week, then 5 grams daily). Creatine supplementation has been shown to improve ATP production and oxygen utilization in brain and skeletal muscle in humans.[118]

- *Ginkgo biloba* **extract:** This extract is an extensively researched botanical medicine with a long history of safe and effective clinical use for various conditions, especially those associated with reduced blood flow and impaired mitochondrial function. *Ginkgo biloba* provides antioxidant, anti-inflammatory, vasodilatory, and mitochondrial-protective benefits. Given these therapeutic benefits, *Ginkgo* would appear to be a reasonable therapeutic agent to address the secondary pathophysiology in fibromyalgia. As cited below, a recent clinical trial using a 2-component treatment that included *Ginkgo* showed benefit in fibromyalgia patients. *Ginkgo biloba* products are generally standardized for the content of flavone glycosides (approximately 24%) and terpene lactones (approximately 6%) with adult doses ranging from 60-240 mg/d and generally 120 mg/d.

- **Physical modalities (chiropractic, acupuncture, osteopathic manipulation, qigong, balneotherapy):** Chiropractic treatment (including spinal manipulation, stretching, soft tissue treatments, and therapeutic ultrasound) has shown benefit in several fibromyalgia case series and clinical trials.[119,120] Acupuncture (including traditional, nontraditional, and electrical stimulation) also has been found beneficial for fibromyalgia patients.[121,122,123] Acupuncture may relieve fibromyalgia pain by improving regional blood flow, in addition to other mechanisms.[124,125] Because specific needle placement does not appear to be important[126], the conclusion that true acupuncture is ineffective because it may not differ markedly from the results obtained by sham acupuncture[127] may not be logical. A similar conundrum is seen in other clinical trials involving physical interventions such as manual osseous manipulation, wherein authentic treatments and sham treatments may both be effective by virtue of common physiological responses.[128] A short-term trial showed that osteopathic manipulative therapy with standard medical care was superior to medical care alone for fibromyalgia patients.[129] Qigong was found helpful for 10 fibromyalgia patients, and benefits were still apparent at 3 months' follow-up.[130] In a randomized, controlled clinical trial among 24 female fibromyalgia

[116] Teitelbaum JE, Johnson C, St Cyr J. The use of D-ribose in chronic fatigue syndrome and fibromyalgia: a pilot study. *J Altern Complement Med*. 2006 Nov;12(9):857-62

[117] Amital D, Vishne T, Rubinow A, Levine J. Observed effects of creatine monohydrate in a patient with depression and fibromyalgia. *Am J Psychiatry*. 2006 Oct;163(10):1840-1

[118] Watanabe A, Kato N, Kato T. Effects of creatine on mental fatigue and cerebral hemoglobin oxygenation. *Neurosci Res*. 2002 Apr;42(4):279-85

[119] Citak-Karakaya I, Akbayrak T, Demirturk F, Ekici G, Bakar Y. Short and long-term results of connective tissue manipulation and combined ultrasound therapy in patients with fibromyalgia. *J Manipulative Physiol Ther*. 2006 Sep;29(7):524-8

[120] Blunt KL, Rajwani MH, Guerriero RC. The effectiveness of chiropractic management of fibromyalgia patients: a pilot study. *J Manipulative Physiol Ther*. 1997 Jul-Aug;20(6):389-99

[121] Martin DP, Sletten CD, Williams BA, Berger IH. Improvement in fibromyalgia symptoms with acupuncture: results of a randomized controlled trial. *Mayo Clin Proc*. 2006 Jun;81(6):749-57

[122] Singh BB, Wu WS, Hwang SH, Khorsan R, Der-Martirosian C, Vinjamury SP, Wang CN, Lin SY. Effectiveness of acupuncture in the treatment of fibromyalgia. *Altern Ther Health Med*. 2006 Mar-Apr;12(2):34-41

[123] Deluze C, Bosia L, Zirbs A, Chantraine A, Vischer TL.Electroacupuncture in fibromyalgia: results of a controlled trial. *BMJ*. 1992 Nov 21;305(6864):1249-52

[124] Sandberg M, Larsson B, Lindberg LG, Gerdle B.Different patterns of blood flow response in the trapezius muscle following needle stimulation (acupuncture) between healthy subjects and patients with fibromyalgia and work-related trapezius myalgia. *Eur J Pain*. 2005 Oct;9(5):497-510

[125] Sandberg M, Lindberg LG, Gerdle B. Peripheral effects of needle stimulation (acupuncture) on skin and muscle blood flow in fibromyalgia. *Eur J Pain*. 2004 Apr;8(2):163-71

[126] Harris RE, Tian X, Williams DA, Tian TX, Cupps TR, Petzke F, Groner KH, Biswas P, Gracely RH, Clauw DJ. Treatment of fibromyalgia with formula acupuncture: investigation of needle placement, needle stimulation, and treatment frequency. *J Altern Complement Med*. 2005 Aug;11(4):663-71

[127] Assefi NP, Sherman KJ, Jacobsen C, Goldberg J, Smith WR, Buchwald D.A randomized clinical trial of acupuncture compared with sham acupuncture in fibromyalgia. *Ann Intern Med*. 2005 Jul 5;143(1):10-9

[128] Mein EA, Greenman PE, McMillin DL, Richards DG, Nelson CD. Manual medicine diversity: research pitfalls and the emerging medical paradigm. *J Am Osteopath Assoc*. 2001 Aug;101(8):441-4

[129] Gamber RG, Shores JH, Russo DP, Jimenez C, Rubin BR. Osteopathic manipulative treatment in conjunction with medication relieves pain associated with fibromyalgia syndrome: results of a randomized clinical pilot project. *J Am Osteopath Assoc*. 2002 Jun;102(6):321-5

[130] Chen KW, Hassett AL, Hou F, Staller J, Lichtbroun AS.A pilot study of external qigong therapy for patients with fibromyalgia. *J Altern Complement Med*. 2006 Nov;12(9):851-6

patients, balneotherapy (bath therapy) in daily 20-minute sessions 5 days per week for 3 weeks (total of 15 sessions; water temperature: 96.8°F = 36°C), resulted in statistically significant reductions in measured inflammatory mediators (PGE2, interleukin-1, LTB4) and amelioration of clinical symptoms among treated patients.[131] The symptomatic benefits of balneotherapy for fibromyalgia patients have been corroborated in other trials.[132,133,134]

- **S-adenosylmethionine (SAMe):** Studies using oral or intravenous administration of the nutritional supplement SAMe have reported conflicting results; however, the overall trend seems to indicate that SAMe (800 mg/d orally) is safe and beneficial in the treatment of fibromyalgia.[135] SAMe helps maintain mitochondrial function by preserving glutathione, and its contribution of methyl groups is important for the regulation of gene expression and neurotransmitter synthesis.

- *Chlorella*: *Chlorella pyrenoidosa* is a unicellular green alga that grows in fresh water. It is a dense source of nutrients, particularly vitamin D (500 IU vitamin D per 1.35 g *Chlorella*). *Chlorella* may have value in treating some fibromyalgia patients, but overall the efficacy is low.[136] Thus, *Chlorella* should not be used as monotherapy for fibromyalgia, although it may be a useful adjunct either as a source of vitamin D, as a means to help modify gut flora, or as an aid in the detoxification of xenobiotics due to its ability to bind ingested and bile-excreted toxins and prevent their absorption and reabsorption in a manner similar to that of cholestyramine.[137,138,139] This detoxifying effect of *Chlorella* in humans is supported by 2 clinical trials showing that nursing mothers who supplement with *Chlorella* during lactation transfer less dioxin in their breast milk compared to nursing mothers who do not consume *Chlorella*.[140,141]

- **Probiotics:** Probiotics are beneficial bacteria that can be consumed in foods or as nutritional supplements to populate the gut, particularly following antibiotic use or long-term dietary neglect. In addition to their availability in capsules and powders, probiotics are widely consumed in the form of yogurt, kefir, and other cultured foods, and they have an excellent record of safety. Probiotic supplements are available in different strengths (quantity), potencies (viability), and combinations of bacteria (diversity). Some probiotics also contain fermentable carbohydrates (prebiotics) such as fructooligosaccharides and inulin, which are substrates to nourish the beneficial bacteria. From a practical clinical perspective, the clinician can choose probiotic foods and supplements and instruct the patient to use these on an ongoing, periodic, or rotational basis. Probiotics (i.e., bacteria only) may have a therapeutic advantage over prebiotics or synbiotics (probiotics+prebiotics) when treating SIBO because the fermentable carbohydrate in prebiotics and synbiotics may exacerbate the preexisting bacterial overgrowth by providing already overpopulated bacteria with additional substrate. The benefits of probiotic supplementation have been demonstrated in patients with IBS,[142,143] rotavirus infection[144], eczema and increased intestinal permeability,[145] and SIBO associated with renal failure.[146] To date, no studies using probiotics in the treatment of fibromyalgia have been published.

[131] Ardiç F, Ozgen M, Aybek H, Rota S, Cubukçu D, Gökgöz A. Effects of balneotherapy on serum IL-1, PGE2 and LTB4 levels in fibromyalgia patients. *Rheumatol Int.* 2007 Mar;27(5):441-6

[132] Evcik D, Kizilay B, Gökçen E. The effects of balneotherapy on fibromyalgia patients. *Rheumatol Int.* 2002 Jun;22(2):56-9

[133] Fioravanti A, Perpignano G, Tirri G, Cardinale G, Gianniti C, Lanza CE, Loi A, Tirri E, Sfriso P, Cozzi F. Effects of mud-bath treatment on fibromyalgia patients: a randomized clinical trial. *Rheumatol Int.* 2007 Oct;27(12):1157-61

[134] Dönmez A, Karagülle MZ, Tercan N, Dinler M, Işsever H, Karagülle M, Turan M. SPA therapy in fibromyalgia: a randomised controlled clinic study. *Rheumatol Int.* 2005 Dec;26(2):168-72

[135] Leventhal LJ. Management of fibromyalgia. *Ann Intern Med.* 1999 Dec 7;131(11):850-8

[136] Merchant RE, Carmack CA, Wise CM. Nutritional supplementation with Chlorella pyrenoidosa for patients with fibromyalgia syndrome: a pilot study. *Phytother Res.* 2000 May;14(3):167-73

[137] Pore RS. Detoxification of chlordecone poisoned rats with chlorella and chlorella derived sporopollenin. *Drug Chem Toxicol.* 1984;7(1):57-71

[138] Morita K, Ogata M, Hasegawa T. Chlorophyll derived from Chlorella inhibits dioxin absorption from the gastrointestinal tract and accelerates dioxin excretion in rats. *Environ Health Perspect.* 2001 Mar;109(3):289-94

[139] Morita K, Matsueda T, Iida T, Hasegawa T. Chlorella accelerates dioxin excretion in rats. *J Nutr.* 1999 Sep;129(9):1731-6

[140] Nakano S, Noguchi T, Takekoshi H, Suzuki G, Nakano M. Maternal-fetal distribution and transfer of dioxins in pregnant women in Japan, and attempts to reduce maternal transfer with Chlorella (Chlorella pyrenoidosa) supplements. *Chemosphere.* 2005 Dec;61(9):1244-55

[141] Nakano S, Takekoshi H, Nakano M. Chlorella (Chlorella pyrenoidosa) supplementation decreases dioxin and increases immunoglobulin a concentrations in breast milk. *J Med Food.* 2007 Mar;10(1):134-42

[142] Quigley EM, Flourie B. Probiotics and irritable bowel syndrome: a rationale for their use and an assessment of the evidence to date. *Neurogastroenterol Motil.* 2007 Mar;19(3):166-72

[143] O'Mahony L, McCarthy J, Kelly P, Hurley G, Luo F, Chen K, O'Sullivan GC, Kiely B, Collins JK, Shanahan F, Quigley EM. Lactobacillus and bifidobacterium in irritable bowel syndrome: symptom responses and relationship to cytokine profiles. *Gastroenterology.* 2005 Mar;128(3):541-51

[144] Shornikova AV, Casas IA, Mykkänen H, Salo E, Vesikari T. Bacteriotherapy with Lactobacillus reuteri in rotavirus gastroenteritis. *Pediatr Infect Dis* J. 1997 ;16(12):1103-7

[145] Rosenfeldt V, Benfeldt E, Valerius NH, Paerregaard A, Michaelsen KF. Effect of probiotics on gastrointestinal symptoms and small intestinal permeability in children with atopic dermatitis. *J Pediatr.* 2004 Nov;145(5):612-6

[146] Simenhoff ML, Dunn SR, Zollner GP, Fitzpatrick ME, Emery SM, Sandine WE, Ayres JW. Biomodulation of the toxic and nutritional effects of small bowel bacterial overgrowth in end-stage kidney disease using freeze-dried Lactobacillus acidophilus. *Miner Electrolyte Metab.* 1996;22(1-3):92-6

Conclusions and Clinical Approach

- In sum, current research indicates that fibromyalgia may result from impairment of cellular bioenergetics and induction of pain hypersensitivity due to absorbed metabolic toxins from bacterial overgrowth of the gastrointestinal tract; this is complicated by induction of tryptophan deficiency which is most likely caused by tryptophan degradation by bacterial tryptophanase activity and which leads to serotonin and melatonin insufficiencies. Available studies have shown that SIBO is ubiquitous among fibromyalgia patients and that antimicrobial interventions—whether pharmaceutical or nutritional—are efficacious. Secondary physiological effects such as mitochondrial impairment, pain sensitization, nutritional deficiencies, oxidative stress, and reduced tissue perfusion are addressed by combined use of select therapeutics as reviewed previously. Patients presenting with widespread pain should be screened for causative underlying disease; if no other explanation can be found, then the diagnosis of fibromyalgia should be made, and the condition should be treated with the therapeutics discussed above. The first visit can include history, physical examination, and laboratory tests; preliminary interventions include dietary modification, multivitamin-multimineral supplementation (including vitamin D3 and magnesium), tryptophan/5-HTP, and CoQ10. SIBO can be treated empirically, or it can be objectively assessed with stool analysis, culture, microscopy, and parasitology. At follow-up visits, additional assessments and interventions can be used to fine-tune the diagnosis and its contributors and to maximize patient response to treatment.

Chapter 17:
Additional Concepts and Selected Therapeutics

Introduction

Additional concepts and selected therapeutics are reviewed in this chapter. Additional review of the "basics" helps these key treatments become better known to the clinician, and these basic treatments and concepts become tools that are used every week if not every day in the clinician's practice.

Topics:

- Fatty acid supplementation and modulation of eicosanoid metabolism and genetic expression
- NF-kappaB and its phytonutritional modulation
- Selected nutritional and botanical therapeutics
    - Flaxseed oil: Alpha-linolenic acid (ALA)
    - Fish oil: Eicosapentaenoic acid (EPA), Docosahexaenoic acid (DHA)
    - Gamma-linolenic acid (GLA)
    - Vitamin D3: Cholecalciferol
    - Vitamin E: Alpha-tocopherol, beta-tocopherol, delta-tocopherol, gamma-tocopherol
    - Niacinamide
    - Glucosamine sulfate and Chondroitin Sulfate
    - Pancreatin, bromelain, papain, trypsin and alpha-chymotrypsin: "proteolytic enzymes" and "pancreatic enzymes"
    - *Zingiber officinale*, Ginger
    - *Uncaria tomentosa, Uncaria guianensis*, "Cat's claw", "una de gato"
    - *Salix alba*, Willow Bark
    - *Capsicum annuum, Capsicum frutescens*, Cayenne pepper, hot chili pepper
    - *Boswellia serrata*, Frankincense, Salai guggal
    - *Harpagophytum procumbens*, Devil's claw
    - *Curcuma longa,* Turmeric
    - Avocado/soybean unsaponifiabiles
- Piezoelectric properties of the human body and clinical implications
- Physiotherapy notes: available on-line
- Review of major vitamins and minerals

Fatty Acid Supplementation and Modulation of Eicosanoid Metabolism and Genetic Expression

Despite their tremendous importance for a wide range of conditions seen in clinical practice, the basics of fatty acid metabolism are unfamiliar to many practicing clinicians. Add to this misinformation on behalf of the lay press and from researchers and professors with financial interests in inferior products and concepts and we can easily see how students and clinicians alike misunderstand and underutilize the clinical applications of fatty acid supplementation and eicosanoid modulation. An accurate and detailed understanding of fatty acid metabolism is important for the complete and effective management of many clinical conditions including mental depression, coronary artery disease, hypertension, diabetes, other inflammatory and autoimmune disorders[1] and many of the musculoskeletal conditions described in this text. The practical application of this information is relatively straightforward, and with a detailed understanding of precursors and modulators of fatty acid, prostaglandin, and leukotriene metabolism, clinicians can facilitate or restrict the production of bioactive chemicals to promote the desired clinical result.

The section that follows is compiled from the research literature and from biochemistry and nutrition textbooks. It is noteworthy that none of the primary sources[2,3] or textbooks[4,5] contained a complete description or biochemical flow diagram of the fatty acid and eicosanoid cascade. Furthermore, there were occasionally discrepancies between the information contained in well-known texts and articles from respected authorities.

[1] Simopoulos AP. Essential fatty acids in health and chronic disease. *Am J Clin Nutr*. 1999 Sep;70(3 Suppl):560S-569S
[2] Horrobin DF. Ascorbic acid and prostaglandin synthesis. *Subcell Biochem*. 1996;25:109-15
[3] Horrobin DF. Interactions between n-3 and n-6 essential fatty acids (EFAs) in the regulation of cardiovascular disorders and inflammation. *Prostaglandins Leukot Essent Fatty Acids*. 1991 Oct;44(2):127-31
[4] McGlivery RW. Biochemistry: A Functional Approach. Third Edition. Philadelphia: WB Saunders, 1983. Pages 747-750
[5] Delvin TM. Textbook of Biochemistry with Clinical Correlations. New York: Wiley-Liss, 1997. Pages 431-441

The Major Fatty Acids and End-products of Clinical Significance

The fatty acids of major importance and the ones discussed here are all polyunsaturated fatty acids, meaning that they have *several* carbon-to-carbon double bonds (i.e., C=C), which are vulnerable to oxidation, rancidification, and/or hydrogenation. Therefore, these fatty acids must be protected from oxygen, heat, light, and prolonged storage. Once structurally altered by oxygen, heat, or light, these fatty acids lose some or all of their biologic value, and they take on disease-promoting properties by interfering with fatty acid metabolism, altering cell membrane dynamics, and/or by having direct/indirect inflammatory and carcinogenic actions.

Fatty acids serve three primary biologic functions: 1) as cell membrane components that modulate membrane pliability and receptor sensitivity, 2) as precursors to potent biologic regulators such as prostaglandins and leukotrienes, and 3) as modulators of gene expression. Each fatty acid must be either provided by diet or manufactured from enzymatic conversion of its predecessor in order to carry out its physiologic role. Deficiency of any fatty acid results in impairment of physiologic function. These impairments begin subtly and often go unrecognized by clinicians who may then erroneously employ pharmacologic and surgical interventions to alleviate *diseases* that originate from *deficiencies* of fatty acids and other nutrients.

Polyunsaturated fatty acids (PUFA) are categorized based on the location of the first carbon-to-carbon double bond from the methyl group, which is located at the opposite end from the carboxyl carbon.[6] The major categories from a biological and nutritional standpoint are the omega-3 fatty acids (having the first carbon-to-carbon double bond starting at the third carbon from the methyl group) and the omega-6 fatty acids (having the first carbon-to-carbon double bond starting at the sixth carbon from the methyl group). The most commonly known member of the omega-9 group is oleic acid from olive oil; but it is of lesser biologic importance than the omega-3 and omega-6 fatty acids, which are the key determinants of the biologically powerful thromboxanes, leukotrienes, prostaglandins, and isoprostanes. The term "omega" is commonly represented as either "Ω" or "w" or "ω" or "n". For the sake of consistency and readability, I will use either the word "omega" or the symbol "n" in this text.

The general term "eicosanoids" is used to describe the various metabolic end products of 20-carbon fatty acid metabolism, including thromboxanes (TX), leukotrienes (LT), and prostaglandins (PG). Produced in minute quantities of approximately 1 milligram per day[7], prostaglandins are produced by nearly all mammalian cells; their production is not confined to leukocytes even though they are often associated with immune activation. Since they are produced and act locally at the site of metabolic activation, they are autocrine and paracrine rather than endocrine.[8] These chemicals have short half-lives, with thromboxanes existing only for a few seconds after production[9] while leukotrienes persist for as long as four hours.[10] While specific enzymes transform one fatty acid into another (within the same family, n-3 or n-6, respectively), the production of eicosanoids is *initiated by enzymes* but often *completed by non-specific, random interactions* dependent on free radicals and/or random conformational changes in enzymes and substrates.[11]

The two main families of bioactive fatty acids are the omega-3 and omega-6 families. These families have generally *opposing* effects to each other and therefore the quantitative balance of these fatty acids serves to dictate the body's ability to establish and retain homeostasis with regard to the modulation of cellular function in general and the production of thromboxanes, leukotrienes, and prostaglandins in particular.[12] With an excess of n-6 fatty acids and a deficiency of n-3 fatty acids, the human body fails to function optimally and the clinical result is an increase in the prevalence and severity of clinical diseases associated with imbalanced gene expression, cell membrane function, and eicosanoid production—namely cancer, heart disease, diabetes, arthritis, allergy, autoimmune diseases, depression, bipolar disorder, schizophrenia, and the long list of "diseases of Western civilization."[13]

---

[6] Erasmus U. Fats that heal, fats that kill. British Columbia Canada: Alive Books, 1993 Page 15-16
[7] Delvin TM. Textbook of Biochemistry with Clinical Correlations. New York: Wiley-Liss, 1997. Pages 431-441
[8] McGlivery RW. Biochemistry: A Functional Approach. Third Edition. Philadelphia: WB Saunders, 1983. Pages 747-750
[9] McGlivery RW. Biochemistry: A Functional Approach. Third Edition. Philadelphia: WB Saunders, 1983. Pages 747-750
[10] Delvin TM. Textbook of Biochemistry with Clinical Correlations. New York: Wiley-Liss, 1997. Pages 431-441
[11] Thuresson ED, Lakkides KM, Smith WL. Different catalytically competent arrangements of arachidonic acid within the cyclooxygenase active site of prostaglandin endoperoxide H synthase-1 lead to the formation of different oxygenated products. *J Biol Chem.* 2000 Mar 24;275(12):8501-7 Available on-line at http://www.jbc.org/cgi/reprint/275/12/8501 as of December 28, 2003.
[12] Tapiero H, Ba GN, Couvreur P, Tew KD. Polyunsaturated fatty acids (PUFA) and eicosanoids in human health and pathologies. *Biomed Pharmacother.* 2002;56(5):215-22
[13] Price WA. Nutrition and Physical Degeneration. Santa Monica: Price-Pottinger Nutrition Foundation, 1945

<u>Omega-3 fatty acids:</u>

- **<u>General properties</u>**
    - o The first double bond is at third carbon from the methyl group
    - o **Primarily from flax seed and cold-water aquatic animals ("antifreeze" for deep water fish, seal, whale) and game animals, also from some leafy green vegetables in small amounts**
    - o Maintain cell membrane fluidity and tissue flexibility and elasticity due to markedly curved structure (maintains space between molecules) compared to saturated fatty acids (straight molecules are closely packed with less room for motion)
    - o N-3 fatty acids consistently lower serum triglycerides levels in contrast to n-6 fatty acids, which generally cause serum triglycerides to increase.[14]
    - o **Causes of n-3 deficiency include:**
        1. Low-fat diets (in general)
        2. Decreased intake of omega-3 (specifically)
        3. Increased intake of omega-6 (such as "to lower cholesterol")
        4. Intake of unnatural *trans*-fatty acids versus natural *cis*-fatty acids. *Trans*-fatty acids are found in hydrogenated oils (hydrogenation makes oil thicker, prevents oxidation, and "improves" taste), fried foods. *Trans*-PUFA increase LDL and reduce HDL.[15]
        5. Alteration of feed for farm animals (substitution of grasses, plants, insects with grains, which are high in n-6 FA), this is why wild game animals have more n-3
        6. High-fat diets if fats are imbalanced with excess of n-6 and trans-FA's
        7. Maldigestion and/or malabsorption
        8. Primary or secondary defects in enzyme function for the conversion of dietary precursors to the end-stage biologically-active fatty acids
    - o **Clinical manifestations of deficiency of omega-3 fats are far more subtle than those associated with omega-6 deficiency: (in animal studies) reduced learning, impaired vision, polydypsia.** Given the importance of n-3 fatty acids in health and disease and the relative deficiency state which is the norm in America, we could also argue that deficiency of n-3 fatty acids predispose to the chronic degenerative diseases of cancer, diabetes, cardiovascular disease and to the more subtle functional problems of dermatitis and the epidemic of neurocognitive and neuropsychiatric disorders.
    - o **Tissue levels are measurably changed within one week of supplementation and are restored to constant levels in 12 weeks of supplementation (in monkeys).** Not all manifestations of deficiency are corrected with supplementation, indicating that fatty acid deficiencies may leave permanent residual effects, particularly if deficiency occurs early in life during the time of rapid growth and development, especially of the brain.
- **<u>Alpha-linolenic acid, linolenic acid, ALA, α-LNA, ALNA, 18:3n3</u>**
    - o **Essential fatty acid:** ALA is the parent fatty acid of the omega-3 class; it is the "first in line."
    - o Sources include **flax seed oil** (57% ALA) and canola (rape seed) oil (9% ALA), soy oil, breast milk, English/black walnuts, soybeans, pine nuts, green vegetables, and beans.
    - o ALA may theoretically be converted to EPA and DHA but this should not be expected to occur sufficiently in all patients at all times due to interindividual variations in enzyme activity and inadequate nutritional/cofactor status. To attain a measurable increase in EPA from ALA supplementation, approximately eleven-times (11x) the amount of ALA must be consumed to achieve a proportional response to that which can be achieved with direct supplementation of EPA.[16] No increase in DHA has been observed in humans after supplementation of ALA; in fact, supplementation with flax seed oil has actually been shown to reduce DHA levels in humans.[17,18]

[14] Simopoulos AP. Essential fatty acids in health and chronic disease. *Am J Clin Nutr*. 1999 Sep;70(3 Suppl):560S-569S

[15] Tapiero H, Ba GN, Couvreur P, Tew KD. Polyunsaturated fatty acids (PUFA) and eicosanoids in human health and pathologies. *Biomed Pharmacother*. 2002;56(5):215-22

[16] "Indu and Ghafoorunissa showed that while keeping the amount of dietary LA constant, 3.7 g ALA appears to have biological effects similar to those of 0.3 g long-chain n-3 PUFA with conversion of 11 g ALA to 1 g long-chain n-3 PUFA." Simopoulos AP. Essential fatty acids in health and chronic disease. *Am J Clin Nutr*. 1999 Sep;70(3 Suppl):560S-569S

[17] Saldeen T. <u>Health Effects of Fish Oil with a Focus on Natural, Stable, Fish Oil</u>. Buxton Road, New Mills, High Peak: Nutri Ltd. [Date unknown] page 33

[18] "Linear relationships were found between dietary alpha-LA and EPA in plasma fractions and in cellular phospholipids. ... There was an inverse relationship between dietary alpha-LA and docosahexaenoic acid concentrations in the phospholipids of plasma, neutrophils, mononuclear cells, and platelets." Mantzioris E, James MJ, Gibson RA, Cleland LG. Differences exist in the relationships between dietary linoleic and alpha-linolenic acids and their respective long-chain metabolites. *Am J Clin Nutr*. 1995 Feb;61(2):320-4

- Lipid-lowering effects are not seen with ALA supplementation and are only attained with the use of EPA and DHA; however ALA can reduce blood pressure.[19]
- **ALA has potent anti-inflammatory benefits independent of its conversion to EPA or DHA.**[20] The mechanism of action appears to be downregulation of NF-KappaB rather than the direct modulation of eicosanoid biosynthesis. One study using flax oil as a source of ALA to treat rheumatoid arthritis found no clinical or biochemical benefit (i.e., no change in Hgb, CRP, ESR).[21]

- **Stearidonic acid, 18:4n3, octadecatetraenoic acid**
  - Small amount found in black currant oil
  - Human studies have found that stearidonic acid increases EPA 2x more efficiently than does ALA but does not increase DHA.[22]
  - Inhibits 5-lipoxygenase.[23]

- **N-3 Eicosatetraenoic acid, 20:4n3**
  - 20:4n-3 is eicosatetraenoic acid.[24,25]
  - The term "eicosatetraenoic acid" applies to both 20:4n6 (arachidonic acid) of the omega-6 fatty acid family[26] and 20:4n3 of the omega-3 fatty acid family.[27,28] Therefore, to avoid the confusion that would result from the use of the term "eicosatetraenoic acid" by itself, "n-6 eicosatetraenoic acid" should be used when referring to 20:4n6 (arachidonic acid) and "n-3 eicosatetraenoic acid" should be used when referring to 20:4n3.

- **Eicosapentaenoic acid, EPA, 20:5n3**
  - Effectively absent in vegan diets; the major dietary source is fish oil.
  - EPA can decrease production of DGLA.[29]
  - EPA doses of at least 4 grams per day are needed to increase bleeding time.[30]
  - EPA–derived eicosanoids have anti-inflammatory properties, including a reduction in the production of pro-inflammatory eicosanoids such as LT-B4, PAFs, and cytokines such as TNF-alpha and IL-1, and a large reduction in PG-E2 and TX-B2.[31]
  - Animal studies suggest that vitamin B-6 deficiency can reduce the function of delta-6-desaturase by 64% and lead to a reduction in EPA and DHA.[32]
  - Children with allergies show altered fatty acid metabolism[33] that is not caused by impaired delta-6-desaturase activity and which results reduced EPA levels.[34]
  - N-6 fatty acids facilitate elongation of EPA to n-3 DPA.[35] Thus, anti-inflammatory EPA is depleted by consumption of proinflammatory n-6 fatty acids.
  - Evidence suggests that EPA must be incorporated into cell membrane phospholipids for its beneficial effects on eicosanoid metabolism to be realized. Administration of n-6 fatty acids removes EPA from cell membranes and relocates EPA from phospholipids into triacylglycerols. Therefore the benefits of EPA are mitigated by n-6 fatty acids, and thus

[19] Simopoulos AP. Essential fatty acids in health and chronic disease. *Am J Clin Nutr.* 1999 Sep;70(3 Suppl):560S-569S

[20] "CONCLUSIONS: Dietary supplementation with ALA for 3 months decreases significantly CRP, SAA and IL-6 levels in dyslipidaemic patients. This anti-inflammatory effect may provide a possible additional mechanism for the beneficial effect of plant n-3 polyunsaturated fatty acids in primary and secondary prevention of coronary artery disease." Rallidis LS, Paschos G, Liakos GK, Velissaridou AH, Anastasiadis G, Zampelas A. Dietary alpha-linolenic acid decreases C-reactive protein, serum amyloid A and interleukin-6 in dyslipidaemic patients. *Atherosclerosis.* 2003 Apr;167(2):237-42

[21] "Thus, 3-month's supplementation with alpha-LNA did not prove to be beneficial in rheumatoid arthritis." Nordstrom DC, Honkanen VE, Nasu Y, Antila E, Friman C, Konttinen YT. Alpha-linolenic acid in the treatment of rheumatoid arthritis. A double-blind, placebo-controlled and randomized study: flaxseed vs. safflower seed. *Rheumatol Int.* 1995;14(6):231-4

[22] "RESULTS: Dietary SDA increased EPA and docosapentaenoic acid concentrations but not DHA concentrations in erythrocyte and in plasma phospholipids. The relative effectiveness of the tested dietary fatty acids in increasing tissue EPA was 1:0.3:0.07 for EPA:SDA:ALA." James MJ, Ursin VM, Cleland LG. Metabolism of stearidonic acid in human subjects: comparison with the metabolism of other n-3 fatty acids. *Am J Clin Nutr.* 2003 May;77(5):1140-5

[23] Guichardant M, Traitler H, Spielmann D, Sprecher H, Finot PA. Stearidonic acid, an inhibitor of the 5-lipoxygenase pathway. A comparison with timnodonic and dihomogammalinolenic acid. *Lipids.* 1993 Apr;28(4):321-4

[24] Tapiero H, Ba GN, Couvreur P, Tew KD. Polyunsaturated fatty acids (PUFA) and eicosanoids in human health and pathologies. *Biomed Pharmacother.* 2002;56(5):215-22

[25] Erasmus U. Fats that heal, fats that kill. British Columbia Canada: Alive Books, 1993 Page 276

[26] "5,8,11,14-eicosatetraenoic (20:4(n-6))" Mimouni V, Christiansen EN, Blond JP, Ulmann L, Poisson JP, Bezard J. Elongation and desaturation of arachidonic and eicosapentaenoic acids in rat liver. Effect of clofibrate feeding. *Biochim Biophys Acta.* 1991 Nov 27;1086(3):349-53

[27] Tapiero H, et al. Polyunsaturated fatty acids (PUFA) and eicosanoids in human health and pathologies. *Biomed Pharmacother.* 2002 Jul;56(5):215-22

[28] Erasmus U. Fats that heal, fats that kill. British Columbia Canada: Alive Books, 1993 Page 276

[29] Horrobin DF. Interactions between n-3 and n-6 essential fatty acids (EFAs) in the regulation of cardiovascular disorders and inflammation. *Prostaglandins Leukot Essent Fatty Acids.* 1991 Oct;44(2):127-31

[30] "A dose of 1.8 g EPA/d did not result in any prolongation in bleeding time, but 4 g/d increased bleeding time and decreased platelet count with no adverse effects. In human studies, there has never been a case of clinical bleeding..." Simopoulos AP. Essential fatty acids in health and chronic disease. *Am J Clin Nutr.* 1999 Sep;70(3 Suppl):560S-569S

[31] Tapiero H, et al. Polyunsaturated fatty acids (PUFA) and eicosanoids in human health and pathologies. *Biomed Pharmacother.* 2002 Jul;56(5):215-22

[32] Tsuge H, Hotta N, Hayakawa T. Effects of vitamin B-6 on (n-3) polyunsaturated fatty acid metabolism. *J Nutr.* 2000 Feb;130(2S Suppl):333S-334S

[33] Yu G, Bjorksten B. Serum levels of phospholipid fatty acids in mothers and their babies in relation to allergic disease. *Eur J Pediatr.* 1998 Apr;157(4):298-303

[34] Yu G, Bjorksten B. Polyunsaturated fatty acids in school children in relation to allergy and serum IgE levels. *Pediatr Allergy Immunol.* 1998 Aug;9(3):133-8

[35] "The major findings of this study were: 1) n-6 fatty acids markedly stimulated the elongation of EPA to 22:5..." Rubin D, Laposata M. Cellular interactions between n-6 and n-3 fatty acids: a mass analysis of fatty acid elongation/desaturation, distribution among complex lipids, and conversion to eicosanoids. *J Lipid Res.* 1992 Oct;33(10):1431-40

"…dietary therapies designed to increase the EPA content of tissue phospholipids may need to focus on limiting n-6 fatty acid intake in addition to increasing EPA intake."[36]

- **DPA: n-3 docosapentaenoic acid, 22:5n3**
  - Production is increased slightly with consumption of the n-3 precursor ALA.[37]
  - Production can be increased with consumption of n-6 fatty acids.[38] The clinical implications of this finding are significant, because it implies that concomitant administration of n-6 fatty acids such as ALA and arachidonate with EPA would preferentially shuttle EPA to DPA, and therefore the formation of the beneficial EPA-derived eicosanoids would be reduced.
  - The term "docosapentaenoic acid" can apply to both 22:5n3 of the omega-3 fatty acid family[39,40] and 22:5n6 of the omega-6 fatty acid family.[41,42,43] Because to use the term "docosapentaenoic acid" may be ambiguous, the terms "n-3 docosapentaenoic acid" should be used when discussing 22:5n3 and "n-6 docosapentaenoic acid" should be used when discussing 22:5n6.

- **DHA: docosahexaenoic acid, 22:6n-3**
  - Found only in plants of the sea, phytoplankton/microalgae, and consumers of microalgae (such as fish)
  - Essential for neural function, effectively absent in vegan diets, present in breast milk (low in vegetarians); major n-3 in tissues; component of phosphatidylethanolamine and phosphatidylserine; deficiency is associated with inadequate intake of DHA and/or deficient conversion from ALA or EPA.
  - Animal studies have shown that induction of DHA deficiency causes memory deficits and a reduction in hippocampal cell size.[44]
  - DHA is an important component of cell membranes and generally appears to improve cell membrane function via improving receptor function and signal transduction.
  - DHA levels are reduced by ethanol consumption.[45]
  - Animal studies suggest that vitamin B-6 deficiency can reduce the function of delta-6-desaturase by 64% and lead to a reduction in EPA and DHA.[46]
  - Supplementation with EPA+DHA is generally safe and reduces all-cause mortality.[47]
  - In late 2003, bioactive metabolites of DHA were discovered. Previous to the publication of this research, production of bioactive metabolites of DHA via lipoxygenase and cyclooxygenase was unsuspected and/or unproved, and the anti-inflammatory biochemical and clinical effects of DHA were mostly thought to be due to alterations in membrane/receptor function and retroconversion to EPA. We now know that DHA is converted by several mechanisms (lipoxygenase, cyclooxygenase, random reactions, and cell-to-cell interactions) into docosatrienes and resolvins, which are described below.[48]

[36] Rubin D, Laposata M. Cellular interactions between n-6 and n-3 fatty acids: a mass analysis of fatty acid elongation/desaturation, distribution among complex lipids, and conversion to eicosanoids. *J Lipid Res*. 1992 Oct;33(10):1431-40

[37] Tarpila S, Aro A, Salminen I, Tarpila A, Kleemola P, Akkila J, Adlercreutz H. The effect of flaxseed supplementation in processed foods on serum fatty acids and enterolactone. *Eur J Clin Nutr*. 2002 Feb;56(2):157-65

[38] Rubin D, Laposata M. Cellular interactions between n-6 and n-3 fatty acids: a mass analysis of fatty acid elongation/desaturation, distribution among complex lipids, and conversion to eicosanoids. *J Lipid Res*. 1992 Oct;33(10):1431-40

[39] "docosapentaenoic acid (22:5n-3)" Williard DE, Harmon SD, Kaduce TL, Preuss M, Moore SA, Robbins ME, Spector AA. Docosahexaenoic acid synthesis from n-3 polyunsaturated fatty acids in differentiated rat brain astrocytes. *J Lipid Res*. 2001 Sep;42(9):1368-76

[40] "…docosapentaenoic acid (22:5n-3)…" Takahashi R, Nassar BA, Huang YS, Begin ME, Horrobin DF. Effect of different ratios of dietary N-6 and N-3 fatty acids on fatty acid composition, prostaglandin formation and platelet aggregation in the rat. *Thromb Res*. 1987 Jul 15;47(2):135-46

[41] Retterstol K, Haugen TB, Christophersen BO. The pathway from arachidonic to docosapentaenoic acid (20:4n-6 to 22:5n-6) and from eicosapentaenoic to docosahexaenoic acid (20:5n-3 to 22:6n-3) studied in testicular cells from immature rats. *Biochim Biophys Acta*. 2000 Jan 3;1483(1):119-31

[42] "docosapentaenoic acid (DPAn-6)" Ahmad A, Murthy M, Greiner RS, Moriguchi T, Salem N Jr. A decrease in cell size accompanies a loss of docosahexaenoate in the rat hippocampus. *Nutr Neurosci*. 2002 Apr;5(2):103-13

[43] "The desaturation of adrenic acid to n-6 docosapentaenoic acid was decreased in the normo- and hyperglycemic diabetic rats." Mimouni V, Narce M, Huang YS, Horrobin DF, Poisson JP. Adrenic acid delta 4 desaturation and fatty acid composition in liver microsomes of spontaneously diabetic Wistar BB rats. *Prostaglandins Leukot Essent Fatty Acids*. 1994 Jan;50(1):43-7

[44] Ahmad A, Murthy M, Greiner RS, Moriguchi T, Salem N Jr. A decrease in cell size accompanies a loss of docosahexaenoate in the rat hippocampus. *Nutr Neurosci*. 2002 Apr;5(2):103-13

[45] Pawlosky RJ, Bacher J, Salem N Jr. Ethanol consumption alters electroretinograms and depletes neural tissues of docosahexaenoic acid in rhesus monkeys: nutritional consequences of a low n-3 fatty acid diet. *Alcohol Clin Exp Res*. 2001 Dec;25(12):1758-65

[46] Tsuge H, Hotta N, Hayakawa T. Effects of vitamin B-6 on (n-3) polyunsaturated fatty acid metabolism. *J Nutr*. 2000 Feb;130(2S Suppl):333S-334S

[47] "The recent GISSI (Gruppo Italiano per lo Studio della Sopravvivenza nell'Infarto miocardico)-Prevention study of 11,324 patients showed a 45% decrease in risk of sudden cardiac death and a 20% reduction in all-cause mortality in the group taking 850 mg/d of omega-3 fatty acids." O'Keefe JH Jr, Harris WS. From Inuit to implementation: omega-3 fatty acids come of age. *Mayo Clin Proc*. 2000 Jun;75(6):607-14

[48] "These results indicate that DHA is the precursor to potent protective mediators generated via enzymatic oxygenations to novel docosatrienes and 17S series resolvins that each regulate events of interest in inflammation and resolution." Hong S, Gronert K, Devchand PR, Moussignac RL, Serhan CN. Novel docosatrienes and 17S-resolvins generated from docosahexaenoic acid in murine brain, human blood, and glial cells. Autacoids in anti-inflammation. *J Biol Chem*. 2003 Apr 25;278(17):14677-87

Bioactive and Clinically Significant End-products of Omega-3 Fatty Acids

End-products from n-3 fatty acids generally have what are considered "health-promoting effects" which are generally weaker than and opposite to the end-products of the major n-6 fatty acid, arachidonate. Additionally, since n-3 fatty acids compete with the same metabolizing enzymes as do the n-6 family of fatty acids, a major portion of the "clinical effectiveness" of n-3 fatty acids comes not from the production of n-3 end-products but rather from the *impairment of the n-6 cascade*.

- **Prostaglandin E-3 (PG-E3)**
  - PG-E3 and EPA both reduce formation of arachidonate-derived eicosanoids[49]
- **Prostaglandin G-3 (PG-G3)**
  - Formed from EPA by cyclooxygenase (COX)
- **Prostaglandin H-3 (PG-H3)**
  - Formed from PG-G3 by peroxidase
- **Prostaglandin I-3 (PG-I3)**
  - Decreases platelet aggregation[50]
  - Causes vasodilation[51]
  - Possibly antiarrhythmic
  - Probably contributes to the hypotensive effect of fish oil[52]
- **Thromboxane A-3 (TX-A3)**
  - Biologically inert
- **Leukotriene B-5 (LT-B5)**
  - Significantly weaker than LT-B4; "functionally attenuated"[53]
  - May possess mild anti-inflammatory activity either directly or by reducing production of the more powerful arachidonate-derived LT-B4. [54]
- **Plasminogen activator inhibitor-1 (PAI-1)**
  - Increased with fish oil supplementation to maintain hemostasis
- **Docosatrienes**
  - Formed by (12-, 15-, 17-) lipoxygenase and cyclooxygenase-2 from DHA
  - Potent inhibitors of TNFa
  - Downregulate gene expression for proinflammatory IL-1
  - Reduce neutrophil entry to sites of inflammation
- **Resolvins**
  - Downregulate cytokine expression
  - Reduce neutrophil entry to sites of inflammation

---

[49] Erasmus U. Fats that heal, fats that kill. British Columbia Canada: Alive Books, 1993 Page 278

[50] Horrobin DF. Ascorbic acid and prostaglandin synthesis. *Subcell Biochem.* 1996;25:109-15

[51] Horrobin DF. Ascorbic acid and prostaglandin synthesis. *Subcell Biochem.* 1996;25:109-15

[52] Du Plooy WJ, Venter CP, Muntingh GM, Venter HL, Glatthaar II, Smith KA. The cumulative dose response effect of eicosapentaenoic and docosahexaenoic acid on blood pressure, plasma lipid profile and diet pattern in mild to moderate essential hypertensive black patients. *Prostaglandins Leukot Essent Fatty Acids* 1992 Aug;46(4):315-21

[53] Rubin D, Laposata M. Cellular interactions between n-6 and n-3 fatty acids: a mass analysis of fatty acid elongation/desaturation, distribution among complex lipids, and conversion to eicosanoids. *J Lipid Res.* 1992 Oct;33(10):1431-40

[54] Rubin D, Laposata M. Cellular interactions between n-6 and n-3 fatty acids: a mass analysis of fatty acid elongation/desaturation, distribution among complex lipids, and conversion to eicosanoids. *J Lipid Res.* 1992 Oct;33(10):1431-40

Metabolism of Omega-3 Fatty Acids and Related Eicosanoids

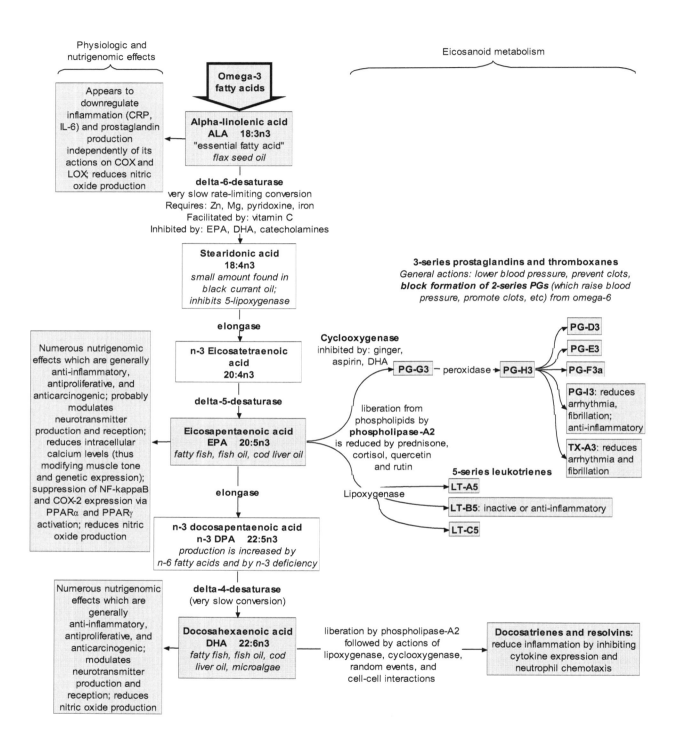

<u>OMEGA-6</u>—first double bond at 6th carbon from the methyl group

- <u>**linoleic acid, LA, 18:2n6, linoleate**</u>
  - <u>Essential fatty acid</u> from nut, seed, and vegetable oils, especially safflower oil, sunflower oil, corn oil, walnut oil, sesame seed oil, LA is the parent fatty acid of the omega-6 class,
  - EPA and DHA decrease conversion of linoleate to arachidonate; high doses of LA inhibit conversion of alpha-LNA to EPA and DHA due to competition for delta-6 desaturase
  - Hydrogenated "trans" forms are common in processed and fried foods,
  - LA favors oxidative modification of LDL cholesterol, increases platelet response to aggregation, and suppresses the immune system.[55] Adipose LA levels are positively correlated with CVD.
  - Promotes metastasis and inflammation.
  - LA is the predominant PUFA in US diets. Daily intake of linoleic acid is approximately 10 grams, only a small amount of which is converted to arachidonate.[56]
  - LA effectively lowers cholesterol, but otherwise this fatty acid is consistently associated with exacerbation of cancer and inflammation and thus should be avoided.
  - LA undergoes oxidative metabolism by 15-lipoxygenase-1 to form 13-S-HODE[57], and this is discussed in greater detail later in this section
- <u>**gamma (γ)-linolenic acid, GLA, 18:3n6, gamma-linolenate**</u>
  - Formation is increased from linoleic acid by vitamin C[58]
  - Found in evening primrose oil, borage seed oil, hemp seed oil, and black currant seed oil
  - GLA restores action of delta-6-desaturase (D6D) in aging animals, suggesting that GLA intake should increase in older rats and humans
  - Useful in eczema for improvement in skin health and in diabetes especially for improvement in nerve function
  - GLA may facilitate the conversion of ALA to EPA and perhaps to DHA.
  - In patients who respond to GLA supplementation, we can reasonably hypothesize that they have impaired D-6-Desaturase activity since most patients have adequate dietary intake of LA. Therefore, by extension, we can suppose that their conversion of ALA to EPA is likewise impaired and that they may benefit from EPA supplementation.
  - Formation of GLA from LA is inhibited by EPA and other n-3 EFAs[59]
  - Overall, the weight of the research suggests that supplementation with GLA *does* lead to modest increases in arachidonate, despite the slow conversion of DGLA to arachidonate by delta-5 desaturase. Coadministration of EPA with GLA prevents any rise in arachidonate, as discussed later in this section.
- <u>**Dihomo-gamma-linolenic acid, 20:3n6, DGLA, eicosatrienoic acid, eicosatrienoate**</u>
  - DGLA eicosanoids have benefits for the cardiovascular system and have anti-inflammatory effects
  - Generally speaking, metabolites of DGLA are fewer in number and weaker in physiologic effect than the metabolites of arachidonic acid.
  - Vitamin C "has a significant effect in stimulating the conversion of DGLA into its metabolites..." at doses which are "...clinically relevant."[60]
  - DGLA levels are 34% lower than normal in patients with magnesium deficiency.[61]
  - Production is decreased with supplementation of ALA[62] and EPA and other n-3 EFAs except when GLA is provided directly[63]

[55] Simopoulos AP. Essential fatty acids in health and chronic disease. *Am J Clin Nutr*. 1999 Sep;70(3 Suppl):560S-569S
[56] Delvin TM. <u>Textbook of Biochemistry with Clinical Correlations</u>. New York: Wiley-Liss, 1997. Pages 431-441
[57] Shureiqi I, Lippman SM. Lipoxygenase modulation to reverse carcinogenesis. *Cancer Res*. 2001 Sep 1;61(17):6307-12
[58] Horrobin DF. Ascorbic acid and prostaglandin synthesis. *Subcell Biochem* 1996;25:109-15
[59] Horrobin DF. Interactions between n-3 and n-6 essential fatty acids (EFAs) in the regulation of cardiovascular disorders and inflammation. *Prostaglandins Leukot Essent Fatty Acids* 1991 Oct;44(2):127-31
[60] Horrobin DF. Ascorbic acid and prostaglandin synthesis. *Subcell Biochem*. 1996;25:109-15
[61] "...dihomogamma linoleic acid (20:3 n-6) was 34% lower..." Galland L. Impaired essential fatty acid metabolism in latent tetany. *Magnesium* 1985;4(5-6):333-8
[62] Simopoulos AP. Essential fatty acids in health and chronic disease. *Am J Clin Nutr*. 1999 Sep;70(3 Suppl):560S-569S
[63] Horrobin DF. Interactions between n-3 and n-6 essential fatty acids (EFAs) in the regulation of cardiovascular disorders and inflammation. *Prostaglandins Leukot Essent Fatty Acids*. 1991 Oct;44(2):127-31

- o Low levels of DGLA are associated with increased risk for stroke and myocardial infarction.[64] We could speculate that low levels of DGLA may be associated with pyridoxine or magnesium deficiency, of which are associated with cardiovascular disease.
- o DGLA metabolites reduce the formation of the arachidonate-derived 2-series prostaglandins, 4-series leukotrienes and platelet-activating factor.[65]

- **Arachidonic acid, 20:4n6, n-6 eicosatetraenoic acid, AA, ARA**
  - o Arachidonic acid is the predominant fatty acid in most tissues (diet-dependent!) acted upon by cyclooxygenase (to form prostaglandins and thromboxanes) and lipoxygenase (to form leukotrienes); it is the major n-6 in cell membranes and body tissues
  - o Liberated from phospholipids by phospholipase enzymes, most notably phospholipase A2.
  - o Most end-products of arachidonate metabolism are pro-inflammatory and are "in general harmful"[66] although arachidonate itself is a necessary component of phospholipids and sphingolipids in cell membranes.
  - o Arachidonate and its metabolites are referred to as eicosanoids.[67] Arachidonic acid is the predominant fatty acid in membrane phospholipids and is the preferred substrate for eicosanoid production relative to EPA.[68] Given that arachidonate's eicosanoids are biologically more powerful than those of EPA, we can accurately generalize that arachidonate and its respective prostaglandins and leukotrienes dominate the fatty acid and eicosanoid playground in both *quantitative* and *qualitative* respects. Therefore, successful intervention against arachidonate metabolism must consider 1) the quantity of arachidonate, 2) the balance of n-3 to n-6, and also 3) specific measures to hinder the production of the harmful arachidonate metabolites.
  - o Arachidonic acid is the direct precursor to the isoprostanes 8-iso prostaglandin-E2 (8-iso-PG-E2) and 8-iso prostaglandin-F2-alpha (8-iso-PG-F2-alpha), mediators that possess **inflammatory and hyperalgesic** properties and which are produced by the radical-mediated non-enzymatic peroxidation of arachidonate.[69] Inhibition of cyclooxygenase and/or lipoxygenase does not decrease the inflammatory and pain-producing effects of isoprostanes. Production of 8-iso-PG-F2-alpha is increased by and is a marker of oxidative stress. Obviously, inhibition of isoprostane formation is part of the biochemical and therefore clinical justification for antioxidant therapy in the treatment of painful orthopedic and rheumatic disorders. Supplemental ascorbic acid, tocopherols, and EPA have been shown to lower isoprostane levels in humans.
  - o Formation of arachidonate from DGLA is inhibited by EPA.[70]
  - o Formation of arachidonic metabolites is not increased by vitamin C.[71]
  - o The term "eicosatetraenoic acid" can apply to both 20:4n6 (arachidonic acid) of the omega-6 fatty acid family[72] and to 20:4n3 of the omega-3 fatty acid family. [73,74] Therefore, to avoid the confusion that would result from the use of the term "eicosatetraenoic acid" by itself, "n-6 eicosatetraenoic acid" should be used when referring to 20:4n6 (arachidonic acid) and "n-3 eicosatetraenoic acid" should be used when referring to 20:4n3.
  - o Liberation of arachidonic acid from membrane phospholipids phosphatidylcholine and phosphatidylinositol is increased by contact with IgE.[75] This finding presumably helps explain why inflammatory conditions are generally exacerbated by allergen exposure and why

---

[64] Horrobin DF. Interactions between n-3 and n-6 essential fatty acids (EFAs) in the regulation of cardiovascular disorders and inflammation. *Prostaglandins Leukot Essent Fatty Acids* 1991 Oct;44(2):127-31

[65] Fan YY, Chapkin RS. Importance of dietary gamma-linolenic acid in human health and nutrition. *J Nutr.* 1998 Sep;128(9):1411-4

[66] Horrobin DF. Ascorbic acid and prostaglandin synthesis. *Subcell Biochem.* 1996;25:109-15

[67] Delvin TM. Textbook of Biochemistry with Clinical Correlations. New York: Wiley-Liss, 1997. Pages 431-441

[68] Rubin D, Laposata M. Cellular interactions between n-6 and n-3 fatty acids: a mass analysis of fatty acid elongation/desaturation, distribution among complex lipids, and conversion to eicosanoids. *J Lipid Res.* 1992 Oct;33(10):1431-40

[69] Evans AR, Junger H, Southall MD, Nicol GD, Sorkin LS, Broome JT, Bailey TW, Vasko MR. Isoprostanes, novel eicosanoids that produce nociception and sensitize rat sensory neurons. *J Pharmacol Exp Ther.* 2000 Jun;293(3):912-20

[70] Horrobin DF. Interactions between n-3 and n-6 essential fatty acids (EFAs) in the regulation of cardiovascular disorders and inflammation. *Prostaglandins Leukot Essent Fatty Acids* 1991 Oct;44(2):127-31

[71] Horrobin DF. Ascorbic acid and prostaglandin synthesis. *Subcell Biochem.* 1996;25:109-15

[72] "5,8,11,14-eicosatetraenoic (20:4(n-6))" Mimouni V, Christiansen EN, Blond JP, Ulmann L, Poisson JP, Bezard J. Elongation and desaturation of arachidonic and eicosapentaenoic acids in rat liver. Effect of clofibrate feeding. *Biochim Biophys Acta.* 1991 Nov 27;1086(3):349-53

[73] Tapiero H, Ba GN, Couvreur P, Tew KD. Polyunsaturated fatty acids (PUFA) and eicosanoids in human health and pathologies. *Biomed Pharmacother.* 2002 Jul;56(5):215-22

[74] Erasmus U. Fats that heal, fats that kill. British Columbia Canada: Alive Books, 1993 Page 276

[75] McGlivery RW. Biochemistry: A Functional Approach, Third Edition. Philadelphia: WB Saunders, 1983. Pages 747-750

allergy elimination and anti-allergy immunomodulatory treatments result in a reduction in pain and inflammation.

- o Elevated ARA may lead to altered binding of hormones, growth factors, neurotransmitters, and common food antigen peptides.
- o Dietary ARA works synergistically with proinflammatory genotypes such as the variant 5-lipoxygenase alleles which are common in the general population: Africans (24%), Asians and Pacific Islanders (19.4%), other racial/ethnic groups (18.2%), Hispanics (3.6%), whites (3.1%), and the atherogenic effect of dietary arachidonic acid in these patients can be mitigated by dietary EPA.[76]

- **Adrenic acid, 22:4n6, docosatetraenoic acid**
  - o Little is known about this fatty acid.
  - o Concentrated in and may have a regulatory role in the adrenal glands.[77]
- **N-6 docosapentaenoic acid, 22:5n6**
  - o 22:5n6 is increased by n-3 fatty acid deficiency, especially in the brain cortex.[78]
  - o The term "docosapentaenoic acid" can apply to both 22:5n3 of the omega-3 fatty acid family[79,80] and to 22:5n6 of the omega-6 fatty acid family.[81,82,83] Therefore, because to use the term "docosapentaenoic acid" may be ambiguous, the terms "n-3 docosapentaenoic acid" should be used when discussing 22:5n3 and "n-6 docosapentaenoic acid" should be used when discussing 22:5n6.

DGLA metabolites formed by cyclooxygenase

- **Prostaglandin E-1 (PG-E1)**
  - o The main metabolite from DGLA.[84]
  - o Production is increased by vitamin C.[85]
  - o Decreases platelet aggregation.[86]
  - o Causes vasodilation.[87]
  - o Lowers blood pressure.[88]
  - o Inhibits cholesterol biosynthesis and lowers cholesterol levels in animals.[89]
  - o "A potent anti-inflammatory agent."[90]
  - o Probably the most potent PG with respect to bronchodilation.[91]
  - o Production is decreased by n-3 fatty acids.[92]
  - o May have a mood elevating effect insofar as levels are elevated in patients with mania, reduced in patients with depression, and are elevated by ethanol intake.[93]
  - o Certain biological properties of PG-E1 are 20 times stronger than those of PG-E2.[94]
  - o PG-E1 inhibits vascular smooth muscle cell proliferation in vitro.[95]

[76] Dwyer JH, Allayee H, Dwyer KM, Fan J, Wu H, Mar R, Lusis AJ, Mehrabian M. Arachidonate 5-lipoxygenase promoter genotype, dietary arachidonic acid, and atherosclerosis. *N Engl J Med.* 2004 Jan 1;350(1):29-37
[77] Horrobin DF. Ascorbic acid and prostaglandin synthesis. *Subcell Biochem.* 1996;25:109-15
[78] Retterstol K, Woldseth B, Christophersen BO. The metabolism of 22:5(-6) and of docosahexaenoic acid [22:6(-3)] compared in rat hepatocytes. *Biochim Biophys Acta.* 1996 Oct 18;1303(3):180-6
[79] "docosapentaenoic acid (22:5n-3)" Williard DE, Harmon SD, Kaduce TL, Preuss M, Moore SA, Robbins ME, Spector AA. Docosahexaenoic acid synthesis from n-3 polyunsaturated fatty acids in differentiated rat brain astrocytes. *J Lipid Res.* 2001 Sep;42(9):1368-76
[80] "…docosapentaenoic acid (22:5n-3)…" Takahashi R, Nassar BA, Huang YS, Begin ME, Horrobin DF. Effect of different ratios of dietary N-6 and N-3 fatty acids on fatty acid composition, prostaglandin formation and platelet aggregation in the rat. *Thromb Res.* 1987 Jul 15;47(2):135-46
[81] Retterstol K, Haugen TB, Christophersen BO. The pathway from arachidonic to docosapentaenoic acid (20:4n-6 to 22:5n-6) and from eicosapentaenoic to docosahexaenoic acid (20:5n-3 to 22:6n-3) studied in testicular cells from immature rats. *Biochim Biophys Acta.* 2000 Jan 3;1483(1):119-31
[82] "docosapentaenoic acid (DPAn-6)" Ahmad A, Murthy M, Greiner RS, Moriguchi T, Salem N Jr. A decrease in cell size accompanies a loss of docosahexaenoate in the rat hippocampus. *Nutr Neurosci.* 2002 Apr;5(2):103-13
[83] "The desaturation of adrenic acid to n-6 docosapentaenoic acid was decreased in the normo- and hyperglycemic diabetic rats." Mimouni V, Narce M, Huang YS, Horrobin DF, Poisson JP. Adrenic acid delta 4 desaturation and fatty acid composition in liver microsomes of spontaneously diabetic Wistar BB rats. *Prostaglandins Leukot Essent Fatty Acids.* 1994 Jan;50(1):43-7
[84] Horrobin DF. Ascorbic acid and prostaglandin synthesis. *Subcell Biochem* 1996;25:109-15
[85] Horrobin DF. Ascorbic acid and prostaglandin synthesis. *Subcell Biochem.* 1996;25:109-15
[86] Horrobin DF. Interactions between n-3 and n-6 essential fatty acids (EFAs) in the regulation of cardiovascular disorders and inflammation. *Prostaglandins Leukot Essent Fatty Acids* 1991 Oct;44(2):127-31
[87] Tapiero H, Ba GN, Couvreur P, Tew KD. Polyunsaturated fatty acids (PUFA) and eicosanoids in human health and pathologies. *Biomed Pharmacother.* 2002 Jul;56(5):215-22
[88] Horrobin DF. Interactions between n-3 and n-6 essential fatty acids (EFAs) in the regulation of cardiovascular disorders and inflammation. *Prostaglandins Leukot Essent Fatty Acids* 1991 Oct;44(2):127-31
[89] Horrobin DF. Interactions between n-3 and n-6 essential fatty acids (EFAs) in the regulation of cardiovascular disorders and inflammation. *Prostaglandins Leukot Essent Fatty Acids* 1991 Oct;44(2):127-31
[90] Horrobin DF. Ascorbic acid and prostaglandin synthesis. *Subcell Biochem.* 1996;25:109-15
[91] Horrobin DF. Ascorbic acid and prostaglandin synthesis. *Subcell Biochem.* 1996;25:109-15
[92] Rubin D, Laposata M. Cellular interactions between n-6 and n-3 fatty acids: a mass analysis of fatty acid elongation/desaturation, distribution among complex lipids, and conversion to eicosanoids. *J Lipid Res.* 1992 Oct;33(10):1431-40
[93] Horrobin DF, Manku MS. Possible role of prostaglandin E1 in the affective disorders and in alcoholism. *Br Med J.* 1980 Jun 7;280(6228):1363-6
[94] Fan YY, Chapkin RS. Importance of dietary gamma-linolenic acid in human health and nutrition. *J Nutr.* 1998 Sep;128(9):1411-4
[95] Fan YY, Chapkin RS. Importance of dietary gamma-linolenic acid in human health and nutrition. *J Nutr.* 1998 Sep;128(9):1411-4

DGLA metabolites formed by 15-lipoxygenase

- **15-hydroxy-eicosatrienoic acid, 15-OH-DGLA, 15-OH-20:3n-6, 15-HETrE**
  - Potent anti-inflammatory action and inhibition of arachidonic acid cascade via inhibition of 5-lipoxygenase and 12-lipoxygenase.[96,97]

Arachidonic acid metabolites formed by cyclooxygenase

- **Thromboxane A-2 (TX-A2)**
  - Causes platelet aggregation[98] and vasoconstriction.[99]
  - Promotes cardiac arrhythmias and hypertension.
  - Considered much more powerful than the thromboxanes derived from EPA and DGLA.
  - Precursor to TX-B2.
- **Thromboxane B2**
  - Inactive[100]
- **Prostaglandin I2,PG-I2, prostacyclin**
  - Commonly considered one of the only desirable/beneficial end-products of arachidonic acid metabolism[101] despite the little known fact that increases nociception and thus promotes hyperalgesia.[102]
  - Production is increased by vitamin C.[103]
  - Decreases platelet aggregation.
  - Causes vasodilation[104] and lowers blood pressure.[105,106]
  - Formed from PG-H2 via prostacyclin synthase.[107]
- **Prostaglandin D2, PG-D2**
  - Causes bronchoconstriction, smooth muscle contraction, and hypotension and is the major arachidonate-cyclooxygenase product produced in mast cells.[108]
  - Accentuates production of histamine and can trigger release of histamine from mast cells in the absence of IgE binding.
- **Prostaglandin E2, PG-E2**
  - Produced from arachidonic acid by cyclooxygenase. PG-E2 increases expression of cyclooxygenase and IL-6; thus inflammation manifested by an increase in PG-E2 leads to additive expression of cyclooxygenase, which further increases inflammation.[109]
  - Suppresses lymphocyte proliferation and natural killer cell activity[110]; appears to cause stimulation of "suppressor cells"
  - Released by tumor cells and suppressor cells
  - Promotes chemotaxis
  - Increases platelet aggregation
  - Causes relaxation of bronchus and uterus smooth muscle in nonpregnant animals and uterine contractions in pregnant animals[111]
  - PG-E2 causes pain and also but increases the intensity and duration of pain sensations that are mediated by other triggers such as histamine and bradykinin[112]
  - Increases IgE production[113]

---

[96] Horrobin DF. Interactions between n-3 and n-6 essential fatty acids (EFAs) in the regulation of cardiovascular disorders and inflammation. *Prostaglandins Leukot Essent Fatty Acids* 1991 Oct;44(2):127-31

[97] Fan YY, Chapkin RS. Importance of dietary gamma-linolenic acid in human health and nutrition. *J Nutr.* 1998 Sep;128(9):1411-4

[98] Delvin TM. Textbook of Biochemistry with Clinical Correlations. New York: Wiley-Liss, 1997. Pages 431-441

[99] Horrobin DF. Ascorbic acid and prostaglandin synthesis. *Subcell Biochem* 1996;25:109-15

[100] Delvin TM. Textbook of Biochemistry with Clinical Correlations. New York: Wiley-Liss, 1997. Pages 431-441

[101] Horrobin DF. Ascorbic acid and prostaglandin synthesis. *Subcell Biochem.* 1996;25:109-15

[102] Evans AR, Junger H, Southall MD, Nicol GD, Sorkin LS, Broome JT, Bailey TW, Vasko MR. Isoprostanes, novel eicosanoids that produce nociception and sensitize rat sensory neurons. *J Pharmacol Exp Ther.* 2000 Jun;293(3):912-20

[103] Horrobin DF. Ascorbic acid and prostaglandin synthesis. *Subcell Biochem.* 1996;25:109-15

[104] Horrobin DF. Ascorbic acid and prostaglandin synthesis. *Subcell Biochem.* 1996;25:109-15

[105] Delvin TM. Textbook of Biochemistry with Clinical Correlations. New York: Wiley-Liss, 1997. Pages 431-441

[106] Tapiero H, Ba GN, Couvreur P, Tew KD. Polyunsaturated fatty acids (PUFA) and eicosanoids in human health and pathologies. *Biomed Pharmacother.* 2002 Jul;56(5):215-22

[107] "Prostacyclin synthase catalyzes an intramolecular redox reaction in which prostaglandin endoperoxide, PGH2, is converted to prostacyclin." http://www.oxfordbiomed.com/pg61prossyn.html on September 6, 2006

[108] Peters SP, Schleimer RP, Kagey-Sobotka A, Naclerio RM, MacGlashan DW Jr, Schulman ES, Adkinson NF Jr, Lichtenstein LM. The role of prostaglandin D2 in IgE-mediated reactions in man. *Trans Assoc Am Physicians.* 1982;95:221-8

[109] Bagga D, Wang L, Farias-Eisner R, Glaspy JA, Reddy ST. Differential effects of prostaglandin derived from omega-6 and omega-3 polyunsaturated fatty acids on COX-2 expression and IL-6 secretion. *Proc Natl Acad Sci U S A.* 2003 Feb 18;100(4):1751-6. Available at http://www.pnas.org/cgi/reprint/100/4/1751.pdf

[110] Calder PC. Long-chain n-3 fatty acids and inflammation: potential application in surgical and trauma patients. *Braz J Med Biol Res.* 2003 Apr;36(4):433-46

[111] McGlivery RW. Biochemistry: A Functional Approach. Third Edition. Philadelphia: WB Saunders, 1983. Pages 747-750

[112] Calder PC. Long-chain n-3 fatty acids and inflammation: potential application in surgical and trauma patients. *Braz J Med Biol Res.* 2003 Apr;36(4):433-46

[113] Calder PC. Long-chain n-3 fatty acids and inflammation: potential application in surgical and trauma patients. *Braz J Med Biol Res.* 2003 Apr;36(4):433-46

- o   Increases vascular permeability and vasodilation thus enhancing edema[114]
- o   Promotes action of epidermal growth factor[115]
- o   Production is decreased by n-3 fatty acids[116]
- **Prostaglandin F2-alpha, PG-F2a, PG-F2α**
    - o   Promotes bronchoconstriction and uterine contractions
    - o   Increased levels associated with dysmenorrhea
    - o   Increased production with vitamin C deficiency, formation is reduced by vitamin C, and low levels of vitamin C are seen in women with dysmenorrhea.[117]
    - o   Promotes formation of MMP-2 and other collagenases that promote joint destruction in various types of arthritis and are required by metastasizing cancer cells to penetrate basement membranes
- **Prostaglandin G2 (PG-G2)**
    - o   Induces rapid and irreversible platelet aggregation[118]
- **Prostaglandin H2 (PG-H2)**
    - o   Induces rapid and irreversible platelet aggregation[119]

Linoleic acid metabolites formed by lipoxygenases
- **13-S-HODE, 13-S-hydroxyoctadecadienoic acid**
    - o   13-S-HODE is formed from linolenic acid by 15-LOX-1 and is generally considered to have anticancer actions[120]
    - o   13-S-HODE inhibits ornithine decarboxylase[121]

Arachidonic acid metabolites formed by lipoxygenases
- **5-hydroperoxyeicosatetraenoic acid, 5-HPETE**
    - o   HPETEs are converted to their respective HETEs either spontaneously or by peroxidases.[122]
    - o   5-hydroxyeicosatetraenoic acid is known to reduce the depolarization threshold of primary afferent neurons and may thus lead to pain
    - o   Reinforces activation of 5-lipoxygenase
    - o   May be directly cytotoxic
    - o   Necessary for the formation of MMP-2 and other collagenases that promote joint destruction in various types of arthritis and are required by metastasizing cancer cells to penetrate basement membranes; formation is inhibited by the lipoxygenase inhibitors esculetin and caffeic acid[123]
    - o   5-HPETE is the major lipoxygenase product in inflamed tissues and promotes chemotaxis and neutrophil degranulation of lysosomal hydrolytic enzymes[124]
    - o   5-HPETE is considered to have pro-cancer actions and facilitates production of proteolytic enzymes that promote joint destruction and tumor invasiveness[125]
- **5-HETE, 5-S-HETE**
    - o   5-HETE is considered to have pro-cancer actions by blocking apoptosis in cancer cells and promoting tumor growth[126]
- **8-S-HETE**
    - o   8-S-HETE is genotoxic and promotes cancer development[127]
- **12-HPETE, 12-hydroperoxyeicosatetraenoic acid, 12-hydroperoxyeicosatetraenoate,**

---

[114] Calder PC. Long-chain n-3 fatty acids and inflammation: potential application in surgical and trauma patients. *Braz J Med Biol Res.* 2003 Apr;36(4):433-46
[115] Tapiero H, Ba GN, Couvreur P, Tew KD. Polyunsaturated fatty acids (PUFA) and eicosanoids in human health and pathologies. *Biomed Pharmacother.* 2002;56(5):215-22
[116] Rubin D, Laposata M. Cellular interactions between n-6 and n-3 fatty acids: a mass analysis of fatty acid elongation/desaturation, distribution among complex lipids, and conversion to eicosanoids. *J Lipid Res.* 1992 Oct;33(10):1431-40
[117] Horrobin DF. Ascorbic acid and prostaglandin synthesis. *Subcell Biochem* 1996;25:109-15
[118] McGlivery RW. Biochemistry: A Functional Approach. Third Edition. Philadelphia: WB Saunders, 1983. Pages 747-750
[119] McGlivery RW. Biochemistry: A Functional Approach. Third Edition. Philadelphia: WB Saunders, 1983. Pages 747-750
[120] Shureiqi I, Lippman SM. Lipoxygenase modulation to reverse carcinogenesis. *Cancer Res.* 2001 Sep 1;61(17):6307-12
[121] Shureiqi I, Lippman SM. Lipoxygenase modulation to reverse carcinogenesis. *Cancer Res.* 2001 Sep 1;61(17):6307-12
[122] Delvin TM. Textbook of Biochemistry with Clinical Correlations. New York: Wiley-Liss, 1997. Pages 431-441
[123] Reich R, Martin GR. Identification of arachidonic acid pathways required for the invasive and metastatic activity of malignant tumor cells. *Prostaglandins* 1996 Jan;51(1):1-17
[124] Delvin TM. Textbook of Biochemistry with Clinical Correlations. New York: Wiley-Liss, 1997. Pages 431-441
[125] "Specific metabolites of each pathway, i.e. PGF2 alpha and 5-HPETE, are able to transcend the block and restore collagenase production, invasiveness in vitro and metastatic activity in vivo." Reich R, Martin GR. Identification of arachidonic acid pathways required for the invasive and metastatic activity of malignant tumor cells. *Prostaglandins* 1996 Jan;51(1):1-17
[126] Shureiqi I, Lippman SM. Lipoxygenase modulation to reverse carcinogenesis. *Cancer Res.* 2001 Sep 1;61(17):6307-12
[127] Shureiqi I, Lippman SM. Lipoxygenase modulation to reverse carcinogenesis. *Cancer Res.* 2001 Sep 1;61(17):6307-12

- o 12-HPETE is the major lipoxygenase product in platelets and the pancreas[128]
- **12-R-HETE**
  - o 12-R-HETE is produced by 12-R-LOX and promotes proliferation of colon cancer cells[129]
- **12-S-HETE**
  - o 12-S-HETE promotes tumor growth by several mechanisms, including 1) "up-regulating adhesion molecules and increasing the adhesion of tumor cells to the microvessel endothelium," 2) "...promoting tumor spread,"" and 3) inhibiting apoptosis[130]
  - o Expression of 12-S-LOX and presumably therefore production of 12-S-HETE is directly correlated with aggressiveness, stage, and grade in human prostate cancer[131]
- **15-hydroperoxyeicosatetraenoic acid, 15-HPETE, 15-hydroperoxyeicosatetraenoate**
  - o 15-HPETE is the major lipoxygenase product in eosinophils, T-lymphocytes, and the trachea[132]
- **15-S-HETE**
  - o 15-S-HETE is formed from arachidonic acid by the action of 15-LOX-2 and appears to have anticancer action, yet the data on this are conflicting[133]
- **Leukotriene B4: LT-B4**
  - o Promotes immunosuppression via inhibition of CD4 cells and promotion of proliferation of CD8 cells.[134]
  - o Promotes edema: increases vascular permeability, enhances local blood flow, is a potent chemotactic agent for leukocytes,
  - o Exacerbates tissue damage: induces release of lysosomal enzymes, increases production of reactive oxygen species, TNF-a, IL-1, and IL-6[135]
  - o Associated with accelerated atherosclerosis in patients with proinflammatory variants of 5-lipoxygenase[136]
  - o Production is increased by dietary arachidonic acid and production is reduced by EPA.[137]
  - o LT-B4 inhibits apoptosis in cancer cells and is generally considered procarcinogenic.[138]
- **LT-C4 and LT-D4 and LT-E4:**
  - o Promote muscle contraction, bronchoconstriction, intestinal muscle contraction,
  - o Promote increased capillary permeability which results in edema
  - o More powerful than histamine in promotion of "allergic" symptoms[139]
  - o Patients with severe asthma have elevated levels of LT-E4 that are not reduced with steroid treatment.[140]

[128] Delvin TM. Textbook of Biochemistry with Clinical Correlations. New York: Wiley-Liss, 1997. Pages 431-441
[129] Shureiqi I, Lippman SM. Lipoxygenase modulation to reverse carcinogenesis. *Cancer Res.* 2001 Sep 1;61(17):6307-12
[130] Shureiqi I, Lippman SM. Lipoxygenase modulation to reverse carcinogenesis. *Cancer Res.* 2001 Sep 1;61(17):6307-12
[131] Shureiqi I, Lippman SM. Lipoxygenase modulation to reverse carcinogenesis. *Cancer Res.* 2001 Sep 1;61(17):6307-12
[132] Delvin TM. Textbook of Biochemistry with Clinical Correlations. New York: Wiley-Liss, 1997. Pages 431-441
[133] Shureiqi I, Lippman SM. Lipoxygenase modulation to reverse carcinogenesis. *Cancer Res.* 2001 Sep 1;61(17):6307-12
[134] Delvin TM. Textbook of Biochemistry with Clinical Correlations. New York: Wiley-Liss, 1997. Pages 431-441
[135] Calder PC. Long-chain n-3 fatty acids and inflammation: potential application in surgical and trauma patients. *Braz J Med Biol Res.* 2003 Apr;36(4):433-46
[136] Dwyer JH, Allayee H, Dwyer KM, Fan J, Wu H, Mar R, Lusis AJ, Mehrabian M. Arachidonate 5-lipoxygenase promoter genotype, dietary arachidonic acid, and atherosclerosis. *N Engl J Med.* 2004 Jan 1;350(1):29-37
[137] Dwyer JH, Allayee H, Dwyer KM, Fan J, Wu H, Mar R, Lusis AJ, Mehrabian M. Arachidonate 5-lipoxygenase promoter genotype, dietary arachidonic acid, and atherosclerosis. *N Engl J Med.* 2004 Jan 1;350(1):29-37
[138] Shureiqi I, Lippman SM. Lipoxygenase modulation to reverse carcinogenesis. *Cancer Res.* 2001 Sep 1;61(17):6307-12
[139] Delvin TM. Textbook of Biochemistry with Clinical Correlations. New York: Wiley-Liss, 1997. Pages 431-441
[140] Vachier I, Kumlin M, Dahlen SE, Bousquet J, Godard P, Chanez P. High levels of urinary leukotriene E4 excretion in steroid treated patients with severe asthma. *Respir Med.* 2003 Nov;97(11):1225-9

Metabolism of Omega-6 Fatty Acids and Related Eicosanoids

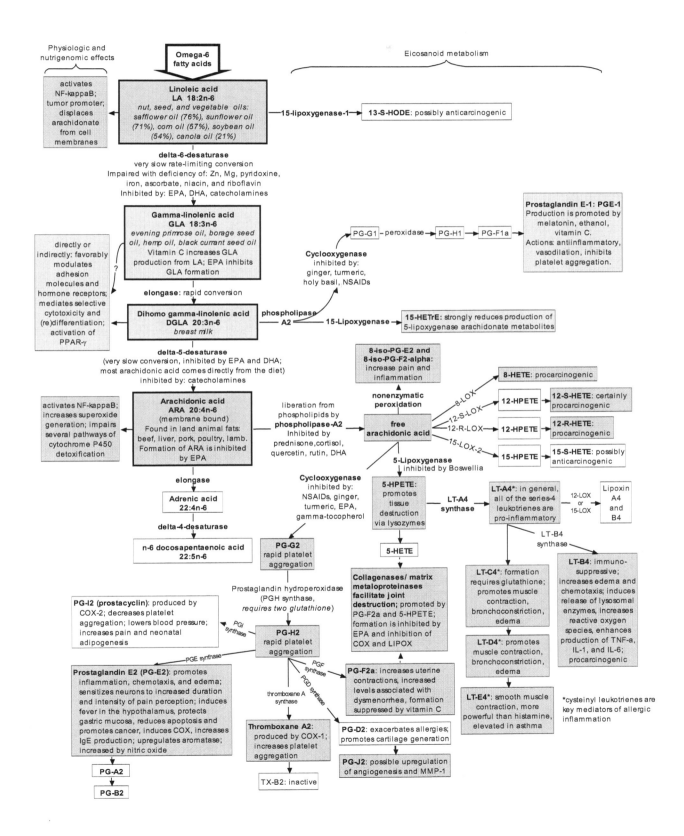

Important Enzymes in Fatty Acid Metabolism

Fatty acids are converted to other fatty acids in the same family by the desaturase and elongase enzymes. The major "direction" of these reactions is depicted in the diagrams; however these reactions, like nearly all enzymatic reactions, are reversible to a limited extent. Fatty acids are converted to biologically active end-products by enzymes such as the cyclooxygenases, lipoxygenases, cytochrome P-450 enzymes and by nonenzymatic conversion. Four important concepts need to be understood in relation to the enzymes that interconvert fatty acids:

1) **These enzymes do not work with equal efficiency**, and thus their end-products may not be produced in sufficient amounts to be biologically or clinically significant. Therefore, *on paper*, the cascade of fatty acid metabolism appears to flow easily from one fatty acid to its downstream progeny; in reality however, this process is often slow and therefore not immediately reliable when one is looking for rapid and reliable clinical results. The desaturase enzymes are slow and rate limiting, whereas the elongase enzymes function efficiently and rapidly. For example, Horrobin noted, "Because the 6-desaturation step is so rate-limiting, it is impossible to produce any significant elevation of DGLA levels in humans by increasing linoleic acid intake."[141]

2) **These enzymes are subject to significant interpatient variability** due to inherited and acquired factors that can reduce enzyme activity. For example, many patients (especially those with eczema and diabetes) have extreme reductions in the activity of delta-6-desaturase, the rate-limiting enzyme in the fatty acid cascades from ALA and LA. When delta-6-desaturase is slow to perform its conversions, synthesis of all downstream fatty acids is greatly reduced.

3) **These enzymes, like all enzymes, require cofactors.** If the patient is deficient in cofactors, the efficiency of enzymatic conversions is greatly impaired. Since micronutrient deficiencies are common even in developed countries, and since people can have clinically significant micronutrient deficiencies (i.e., "marginal malnutrition"[142]) yet still be "apparently healthy", a wise clinical strategy is to ensure that the patient's micronutrient status is adequate by encouraging the patient to consume a nutritious organic[143] whole foods diet along with a high-potency broad-spectrum multivitamin and multimineral supplement. Patients with magnesium deficiency show impaired fatty acid metabolism because desaturase enzymes are unable to function properly without sufficient magnesium.[144] Animal studies suggest that vitamin B-6 deficiency can reduce the function of delta-6-desaturase by 64% and lead to a reduction in EPA and DHA.[145]

4) **Substrates compete for enzymatic conversion.** In several instances, the same enzyme must act upon two different fatty acids in two different omega families. For example, delta-6-desaturase converts the omega-3 linolenic acid to stearidonic acid, yet this same enzyme also converts the omega-6 linoleic acid to gamma-linolenic acid. If the diet contains an absolute or relative excess of linoleic acid, then on a molecular and functional level, this excess linoleic acid will disproportionately utilize delta-6-desaturase and conversion of available linoleic acid to gamma-linolenic acid will be reduced. As reviewed by Dupont[146], "A competitive interaction between fatty acids exists so that those of the [alpha-linolenic acid, omega-3] family suppress the metabolism of those of the [linoleic acid, omega-6] family, and the [linoleic acid, omega-6] family suppress metabolism of the [linolenic acid, omega-3] family although less strongly. Both the [linoleic acid, omega-6] and [alpha-linolenic acid, omega-3] fatty acids suppress metabolism of the [oleic acid, omega-9] fatty acids." Stated more plainly by Pizzorno[147], "...a relative excess of one fatty acid will tend to hog an enzyme system, resulting in decreased conversion of the other fatty acids." In reviewing clinical evidence that EPA

---

[141] Horrobin DF. Interactions between n-3 and n-6 essential fatty acids (EFAs) in the regulation of cardiovascular disorders and inflammation. *Prostaglandins Leukot Essent Fatty Acids*. 1991 Oct;44(2):127-31

[142] Allen LH. The nutrition CRSP: what is marginal malnutrition, and does it affect human function? *Nutr Rev*. 1993 Sep;51(9):255-67

[143] Bob Smith. *Journal of Applied Nutrition* 1993; 45: 35-39

[144] Galland L. Impaired essential fatty acid metabolism in latent tetany. *Magnesium*. 1985;4(5-6):333-8

[145] Tsuge H, Hotta N, Hayakawa T. Effects of vitamin B-6 on (n-3) polyunsaturated fatty acid metabolism. *J Nutr*. 2000 Feb;130(2S Suppl):333S-334S

[146] Dupont J. Lipids. In: Brown ML (ed). Present Knowledge in Nutrition. Sixth Edition. Washington DC: International Life Sciences Institute Nutrition Foundation;1990page 62

[147] Pizzorno JE. Total Wellness. Rocklin: Prima; 1996 page 170

supplementation leads to significant reductions (50%) in DGLA levels, Horrobin[148] noted, "However, the n-3 EFAs are much more effective in inhibiting n-6 EFA metabolism than vice versa." A practical example: in a patient who is deficient in both omega-3 and omega-6 fatty acids, supplementation exclusively with flax oil will exacerbate the deficiency of gamma-linolenic acid.

- **Delta-6-desaturase (D6D):**
  - o In omega-3 fatty acid metabolism, D6D converts linolenic acid to stearidonic acid. In omega-6 fatty acid metabolism, D6D converts linoleic acid to gamma-linolenic acid. D6D is the rate-limiting enzyme in fatty acid metabolism, meaning that it is the slowest functioning enzyme in the cascade of fatty acid conversions. Recall that in biochemistry the first enzyme in a series of biochemical reactions tends to be the rate-limiting enzyme for the sake of avoiding unnecessary downstream conversions. D6D is inhibited by trans fatty acids.[149] Action of this enzyme is increased during essential fatty acid deficiency.[150] Patients with eczema and diabetes have been noted to have defects in the function of D6D.[151]
  - o Efficient function of D6D requires iron, magnesium, zinc, pyridoxine, niacin, and riboflavin. Administration of supraphysiologic doses of enzyme cofactors can improve function of defective or mutated enzymes.[152]
  - o The catecholamines epinephrine and norepinephrine inhibit D5D and D6D.[153]
- **Delta-5-desaturase (D5D):**
  - o In omega-6 fatty acid metabolism, D5D converts DGLA to arachidonic acid. However, this enzyme is slow, so that virtually all arachidonic acid found in body tissues originated from the consumption of land animal fats/meats[154] such as beef, liver, pork, lamb, and poultry. Additionally, some people (such as those with X-linked retinitis pigmentosa[155]) have reduced action of D5D and therefore have low levels of DHA. D5D is inhibited by EPA.[156] Released in increased amounts during stress and anxiety, the catecholamines epinephrine and norepinephrine inhibit D5D and D6D.[157]
- **Delta-4-desaturase**
  - o Action of this enzyme is increased during essential fatty acid deficiency.[158]
- **Elongase**: These enzymes efficiently add carbon groups to the fatty acid chain.
- **Prostaglandin synthase complex (PGS)**: This is the major enzyme system that is responsible for prostaglandin biosynthesis. PGS includes phospholipase A2 and cyclooxygenase.[159]
- **Phospholipase-A2**
  - o Crucial to the arachidonic acid cascade since cyclooxygenase can act only on free arachidonate (i.e., after arachidonate has been liberated from membrane phospholipids); this is the rate-limiting step in the formation of arachidonate-derived prostaglandins.[160]
  - o Contact of IgE with mast cells stimulates the release of arachidonate, which must occur via phospholipase A2[161]
  - o Inhibited by adrenal steroids (cortisol) and prednisone

[148] Horrobin DF. Interactions between n-3 and n-6 essential fatty acids (EFAs) in the regulation of cardiovascular disorders and inflammation. *Prostaglandins Leukot Essent Fatty Acids*. 1991 Oct;44(2):127-31
[149] Simopoulos AP. Essential fatty acids in health and chronic disease. *Am J Clin Nutr*. 1999 Sep;70(3 Suppl):560S-569S
[150] "The delta 4 desaturase activity is increased in essential fatty acid deficiency similar to delta 6 desaturase." Christophersen BO, Hagve TA, Christensen E, Johansen Y, Tverdal S. Eicosapentaenoic- and arachidonic acid metabolism in isolated liver cells. *Scand J Clin Lab Invest Suppl*. 1986;184:55-60
[151] "This concept is illustrated by atopic eczema and diabetes, which may represent inherited and acquired examples of inadequate delta-6-desaturation." Horrobin DF. Fatty acid metabolism in health and disease: the role of delta-6-desaturase. *Am J Clin Nutr*. 1993 May;57(5 Suppl):732S-736S
[152] Ames BN, Elson-Schwab I, Silver EA. High-dose vitamin therapy stimulates variant enzymes with decreased coenzyme binding affinity (increased K(m)): relevance to genetic disease and polymorphisms. *Am J Clin Nutr*. 2002 Apr;75(4):616-58
[153] Mamalakis G, Kafatos A, Tornaritis M, Alevizos B. Anxiety and adipose essential fatty acid precursors for prostaglandin E1 and E2. *J Am Coll Nutr*. 1998 Jun;17(3):239-43
[154] Pizzorno JE. *Total Wellness*. Rocklin: Prima; 1996 page 169
[155] Hoffman DR, DeMar JC, Heird WC, Birch DG, Anderson RE. Impaired synthesis of DHA in patients with X-linked retinitis pigmentosa. *J Lipid Res* 2001 Sep;42(9):1395-401 This article is available on-line at http://www.jlr.org/cgi/reprint/42/9/1395.pdf as of December 26, 2003
[156] Barham JB, Edens MB, Fonteh AN, Johnson MM, Easter L, Chilton FH. Addition of eicosapentaenoic acid to gamma-linolenic acid-supplemented diets prevents serum arachidonic acid accumulation in humans. *J Nutr*. 2000 Aug;130(8):1925-31
[157] Mamalakis G, Kafatos A, Tornaritis M, Alevizos B. Anxiety and adipose essential fatty acid precursors for prostaglandin E1 and E2. *J Am Coll Nutr*. 1998 Jun;17(3):239-43
[158] "The delta 4 desaturase activity is increased in essential fatty acid deficiency similar to delta 6 desaturase." Christophersen BO, Hagve TA, Christensen E, Johansen Y, Tverdal S. Eicosapentaenoic- and arachidonic acid metabolism in isolated liver cells. *Scand J Clin Lab Invest Suppl*. 1986;184:55-60
[159] Delvin TM. *Textbook of Biochemistry with Clinical Correlations*. New York: Wiley-Liss, 1997. Pages 431-441
[160] Delvin TM. *Textbook of Biochemistry with Clinical Correlations*. New York: Wiley-Liss, 1997. Pages 431-441
[161] McGlivery RW. *Biochemistry: A Functional Approach. Third Edition*. Philadelphia: WB Saunders, 1983. Pages 747-750

- **Cyclooxygenase (COX) (also called "prostaglandin synthase" or "PGS" or "prostaglandin endoperoxide synthase")**
  - COX-1 is "constitutive" and is found in all cells, while COX-2 is inducible by stimulation from monocytes/macrophages following stimulation by PAF, IL-1, or bacterial lipopolysaccharide; its induction is inhibited by glucocorticoids.[162]
  - COX is irreversibly inhibited following acetylation by aspirin.
  - The expression of COX is inhibited by glucocorticoids,[163] which also inhibit phospholipase A2.
  - **COX forms TXs and PGs, while LIPOX form LTs.**
  - The COX metabolite PG-F2alpha is necessary for the formation of matrix metalloproteinase-2 and other collagenases which are utilized for the destruction of connective tissue[164]
  - **COX is apparently activated by either n-6 fatty acids or the oxidized metabolites of n-6 fatty acids.[165] Therefore, consumption of n-6 fatty acids alone—*without trauma or inflammatory stimuli*—is sufficient for the increased production of the harmful arachidonate-derived prostaglandins and leukotrienes.** Thus, by definition, a diet high in n-6 fatty acids may subtly yet significantly promote pain, inflammation, joint destruction, and cancer.
  - A well-established consequence of inhibiting COX is that of increasing LIPOX metabolites. Inhibiting COX will decrease COX metabolites, yet will cause an increase in LIPOX metabolites because of increased substrate levels; i.e., the liberated arachidonate that is not metabolized by COX is now available to be metabolized by LIPOX. Thus, inhibiting COX produces a "metabolic shunt" effect that increases production of inflammatory mediators such as HETE and the leukotrienes. Additionally, inhibition of COX inhibits formation of the beneficial anti-inflammatory DGLA metabolites.
  - Arachidonate metabolites from COX function for the most part to increase inflammation and pain.[166]
  - Increased expression of COX-2 increases production of PG-E2 and has been associated with increased production of anti-apoptotic proteins and a reduction in pro-apoptotic proteins in cultured rat intestinal cells.[167]
  - The activity of lipoxygenase and cyclooxygenase produces reactive oxygen species (ROS) intermediates.
  - The paradox of how a single enzyme such as cyclooxygenase can produce such a wide array of metabolites from a single substrate such as arachidonic acid is solved by recognizing that arachidonate is three-dimensionally rearranged once within the cyclooxygenase enzyme and that these random arrangements favor the production of different metabolites by the preferential molecular modification of the original arachidonate.[168] Additionally, cyclooxygenase may become slightly rearranged as well, thus further promoting the heterogeneity of progeny.
- **Lipoxygenases**: a family of enzymes that form leukotrienes
  - Corneal lipoxygenase is inhibited by vitamin C[169]
  - The activity of lipoxygenase and cyclooxygenase produce ROS intermediates
  - **5-lipoxygenase, 5-LOX**

[162] Delvin TM. Textbook of Biochemistry with Clinical Correlations. New York: Wiley-Liss, 1997. Pages 431-441
[163] Tapiero H, Ba GN, Couvreur P, Tew KD. Polyunsaturated fatty acids (PUFA) and eicosanoids in human health and pathologies. *Biomed Pharmacother*. 2002;56(5):215-22
[164] "Specific metabolites of each pathway, i.e. PGF2 alpha and 5-HPETE, are able to transcend the block and restore collagenase production, invasiveness in vitro and metastatic activity in vivo." Reich R, Martin GR. Identification of arachidonic acid pathways required for the invasive and metastatic activity of malignant tumor cells. *Prostaglandins* 1996 Jan;51(1):1-17
[165] "...due to activation of cyclooxygenase either by oxygenated metabolites of n-6 fatty acids or by the n-6 fatty acids themselves." Rubin D, Laposata M. Cellular interactions between n-6 and n-3 fatty acids: a mass analysis of fatty acid elongation/desaturation, distribution among complex lipids, and conversion to eicosanoids. *J Lipid Res*. 1992 Oct;33(10):1431-40
[166] Tapiero H, Ba GN, Couvreur P, Tew KD. Polyunsaturated fatty acids (PUFA) and eicosanoids in human health and pathologies. *Biomed Pharmacother*. 2002;56(5):215-22
[167] Tapiero H, Ba GN, Couvreur P, Tew KD. Polyunsaturated fatty acids (PUFA) and eicosanoids in human health and pathologies. *Biomed Pharmacother*. 2002;56(5):215-22
[168] Thuresson ED, Lakkides KM, Smith WL. Different catalytically competent arrangements of arachidonic acid within the cyclooxygenase active site of prostaglandin endoperoxide H synthase-1 lead to the formation of different oxygenated products. *J Biol Chem*. 2000 Mar 24;275(12):8501-7 Available on-line at http://www.jbc.org/cgi/reprint/275/12/8501 on March 16, 2004
[169] Horrobin DF. Ascorbic acid and prostaglandin synthesis. *Subcell Biochem* 1996;25:109-15

- This is a pro-inflammatory enzyme that has different basal levels of activity in different people and in different disease conditions. Proinflammatory variances of this enzyme are seen in Africans (24%), Asians and Pacific Islanders (19.4%), other racial/ethnic groups (18.2%), Hispanics (3.6%) and whites (3.1%) and are associated with accelerated atherosclerosis and elevations in CRP especially when the diet is high in arachidonic acid and low in EPA.[170]
- 5-LOX has been described as "procarcinogenic" due to its role in producing LT-B4 which has mitogenic and anti-apoptotic actions[171]
- The 5-LOX metabolite 5-HPETE is necessary for the formation of matrix metalloproteinase-2 and other collagenases which are utilized for the destruction of connective tissue[172]

- **8-lipoxygenase, 8-LOX**
  - 8-LOX is upregulated in animal models of cancer and has been described as "procarcinogenic" due to its role in producing 8-HETE, which has genotoxic effects and which is found in humans[173]
- **12-R-lipoxygenase, 12-R-LOX**
  - 12-R-LOX has been described as "procarcinogenic" due to its role in producing 12-R-HETE[174]
- **12-S-lipoxygenase, 12-S-LOX**
  - 12-S-LOX has been described as "procarcinogenic" due to its role in producing 12-S-HETE[175]
  - Expression of 12-S-LOX is directly correlated with aggressiveness, stage, and grade in human prostate cancer[176]
- **15-lipoxygenase-1, 15-LOX-1**
  - 15-LOX-1 metabolizes n-6 linoleic acid into 13-S-HODE, which appears to have *anti*cancer actions[177]
- **15-lipoxygenase-2, 15-LOX-2**
  - 15-LOX-2 metabolizes n-6 arachidonic acid into 15-S-HETE, which appears to have *anti*cancer actions[178]

Notes:

_____

_____

_____

_____

_____

_____

_____

_____

_____

_____

[170] Dwyer JH, Allayee H, Dwyer KM, Fan J, Wu H, Mar R, Lusis AJ, Mehrabian M. Arachidonate 5-lipoxygenase promoter genotype, dietary arachidonic acid, and atherosclerosis. *N Engl J Med*. 2004 Jan 1;350(1):29-37

[171] "These targets include procarcinogenic lipoxygenases (LOXs), including 5-, 8-, and 12-LOX, and anticarcinogenic LOXs, including 15-LOX-1 and possibly 15-LOX-2." Shureiqi I, Lippman SM. Lipoxygenase modulation to reverse carcinogenesis. *Cancer Res*. 2001 Sep 1;61(17):6307-12

[172] "Specific metabolites of each pathway, i.e. PGF2 alpha and 5-HPETE, are able to transcend the block and restore collagenase production, invasiveness in vitro and metastatic activity in vivo." Reich R, Martin GR. Identification of arachidonic acid pathways required for the invasive and metastatic activity of malignant tumor cells. *Prostaglandins* 1996 Jan;51(1):1-17

[173] Shureiqi I, Lippman SM. Lipoxygenase modulation to reverse carcinogenesis. *Cancer Res*. 2001 Sep 1;61(17):6307-12

[174] Shureiqi I, Lippman SM. Lipoxygenase modulation to reverse carcinogenesis. *Cancer Res*. 2001 Sep 1;61(17):6307-12

[175] Shureiqi I, Lippman SM. Lipoxygenase modulation to reverse carcinogenesis. *Cancer Res*. 2001 Sep 1;61(17):6307-12

[176] Reich R, Martin GR. Identification of arachidonic acid pathways required for the invasive and metastatic activity of malignant tumor cells. *Prostaglandins* 1996 Jan;51(1):1-17

[177] Shureiqi I, Lippman SM. Lipoxygenase modulation to reverse carcinogenesis. *Cancer Res*. 2001 Sep 1;61(17):6307-12

[178] Shureiqi I, Lippman SM. Lipoxygenase modulation to reverse carcinogenesis. *Cancer Res*. 2001 Sep 1;61(17):6307-12

NF-kappaB and Its Phytonutritional Modulation

Nuclear transcription factor kappaB (NF-kappaB) is one of several transcription factors which act as "facilitators" for the elaboration and amplification of specific gene products. In the case of NF-kappaB, most of the genes that appear to be influenced are those that increase the production of pro-inflammatory mediators such as IL-2 (which increases production of collagen-digesting proteases), IL-6 (which then increases production of C-reactive protein), cyclooxygenase-2 (which then increases production of prostaglandins), lipoxygenase (which produces leukotrienes), and inducible nitric oxide synthase (for the production of nitric oxide), etc. Inhibition of NF-kappaB is increasingly considered a major therapeutic goal in the treatment and prevention of a wide range of illnesses, including cancer, arthritis, autoimmune diseases, neurologic illnesses such as Alzheimer's and Parkinson's disease, and other "inflammatory" diseases.[179] [180] While we as holistic clinicians work to address the underlying cause of the problem in a given patient, I believe that some degree of "suppression" of NF-kappaB is therapeutically appropriate for at least two reasons: 1) it helps to limit tissue damage and to improve patient outcomes, and 2) suppression of NF-kappaB helps to *break the vicious cycle* of positive feedback wherein *inflammation promotes more inflammation* by the NF-kappaB stimulating effect of several of the products of NF-kappaB activation: NF-kappaB increases the production of IL-1, PG-E2, oxidative stress, TNF-a, and CRP—all of which work additively and synergistically to increase activation of NF-kappaB. Therefore, regardless of the underlying cause, which may have already been addressed and eradicated, it is conceivable that some patients will suffer from inflammatory disorders simply because of the positive feedback that mediators have on the activation of NF-kappaB, which then promotes more inflammation.

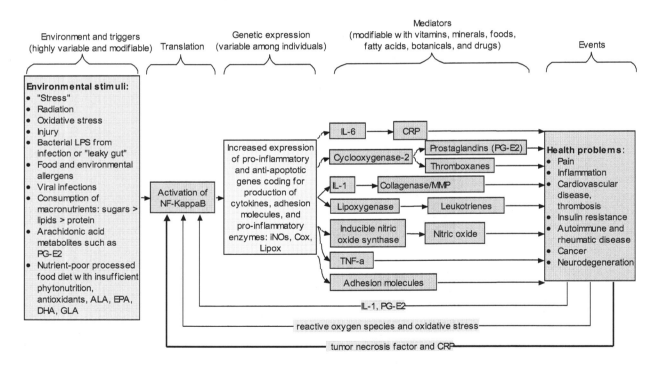

Pharmaceutical companies are currently scrambling to develop clinically useful synthetic inhibitors of NF-kappaB. These companies will eventually be successful in this endeavor, and we can also confidently predict that the pharmaceutical version of NF-kappaB suppression will arrive with a plethora of adverse effects, most likely <u>because of</u> the potency and specificity of the drug. NF-kappaB plays an important role in a wide range of normal, healthy physiologic processes, including the immune response to infectious diseases. We should therefore seek to *modulate* its function rather than sophomorically *suppress* its function. Fortunately, we can do

[179] D'Acquisto F, May MJ, Ghosh S. Inhibition of Nuclear Factor Kappa B (NF-B): An Emerging Theme in Anti-Inflammatory Therapies. *Mol Interv*. 2002 Feb;2(1):22-35 http://molinterv.aspetjournals.org/cgi/content/full/2/1/22
[180] Tak PP, Firestein GS. NF-kappaB: a key role in inflammatory diseases. *J Clin Invest*. 2001 Jan;107(1):7-11 http://www.jci.org/cgi/content/full/107/1/7

this with several natural interventions, not the least of which are vitamin D[181,182], curcumin[183] (requires piperine for absorption[184]), lipoic acid[185], green tea[186], rosemary[187], grape seed extract[188], propolis[189], zinc[190], high-dose selenium[191], indole-3-carbinol[192,193], N-acetyl-L-cysteine[194], and resveratrol.[195,196] Other nutrients such as isohumulones from *Humulus lupulus*[197] and fatty acids inhibit NF-kappaB *indirectly* via activation of peroxisome proliferator-activated receptors alpha (PPAR-α) and gamma (PPAR-γ). GLA activates PPAR-gamma and thereby inhibits NF-kappaB[198], while (oxidized) EPA activates PPAR-alpha and thus inhibits NF-kappaB[199]; these latter findings reflect a quantum leap in our understanding of the mechanisms of diet-induced anti-inflammation (i.e., anti-inflammatory nutrigenomics, or anti-inflammatory immunonutrigenomics) since they show that food constituents modify human physiology and phenotype at the genetic/pre-transcriptional level and not only at the metabolic/post-transcriptional level as was previously thought.[200]

I believe that future research will elucidate that the proposed anti-inflammatory benefits of plant-based diets[201] are partially resultant from the downregulation of NF-kappaB by dietary phytonutrients, of which more than 5,000 exist.[202] Notice that the above-mentioned suppressors of NF-kappaB are mostly phenolic compounds that are naturally occurring in fruits, vegetables, herbs, and spices. A diet based upon fruits and vegetables would be naturally high in these compounds and would be likely to provide an anti-inflammatory influence on genetic expression. Indeed, this dietary and phytonutritional environment would be consistent with that in which human physiology evolved, to which it adapted, and upon which it thereby became dependent.[203,204] Relatedly, our epidemic of vitamin D deficiency[205] resultant from our artificial, indoor, clothed lifestyles unquestionably contributes to our modern pro-inflammatory tendency, and vitamin D supplementation has already proven to be immunomodulating and anti-inflammatory in human clinical trials.[206,207,208]

---

[181] "1Alpha,25-dihydroxyvitamin D3 (1,25-(OH)2-D3), **the active metabolite of vitamin D, can inhibit NF-kappaB activity** in human MRC-5 fibroblasts, targeting DNA binding of NF-kappaB but not translocation of its subunits p50 and p65." Harant H, Wolff B, Lindley IJ. 1Alpha,25-dihydroxyvitamin D3 decreases DNA binding of nuclear factor-kappaB in human fibroblasts. *FEBS Lett*. 1998 Oct 9;436(3):329-34

[182] "Thus, 1,25$(OH)_2D_3$ may negatively regulate IL-12 production by downregulation of NF-kB activation and binding to the p40-kB sequence." D'Ambrosio D, Cippitelli M, Cocciolo MG, Mazzeo D, Di Lucia P, Lang R, Sinigaglia F, Panina-Bordignon P. Inhibition of IL-12 production by 1,25-dihydroxyvitamin D3. Involvement of NF-kappaB downregulation in transcriptional repression of the p40 gene. *J Clin Invest*. 1998 Jan 1;101(1):252-62

[183] "Curcumin, EGCG and resveratrol have been shown to suppress activation of NF-kappa B." Surh YJ, Chun KS, Cha HH, Han SS, Keum YS, Park KK, Lee SS. Molecular mechanisms underlying chemopreventive activities of anti-inflammatory phytochemicals: down-regulation of COX-2 and iNOS through suppression of NF-kappa B activation. *Mutat Res*. 2001 Sep 1;480-481:243-68

[184] Shoba G, Joy D, Joseph T, Majeed M, Rajendran R, Srinivas PS. Influence of piperine on the pharmacokinetics of curcumin in animals and human volunteers. *Planta Med*. 1998 May;64(4):353-6

[185] "ALA reduced the TNF-alpha-stimulated ICAM-1 expression in a dose-dependent manner, to levels observed in unstimulated cells. Alpha-lipoic acid also reduced NF-kappaB activity in these cells in a dose-dependent manner." Lee HA, Hughes DA.Alpha-lipoic acid modulates NF-kappaB activity in human monocytic cells by direct interaction with DNA. *Exp Gerontol*. 2002 Jan-Mar;37(2-3):401-10

[186] "In conclusion, EGCG is an effective inhibitor of IKK activity. This may explain, at least in part, some of the reported anti-inflammatory and anticancer effects of green tea." Yang F, Oz HS, Barve S, de Villiers WJ, McClain CJ, Varilek GW. The green tea polyphenol (-)-epigallocatechin-3-gallate blocks nuclear factor-kappa B activation by inhibiting I kappa B kinase activity in the intestinal epithelial cell line IEC-6. *Mol Pharmacol*. 2001 Sep;60(3):528-33

[187] "These results suggest that carnosol suppresses the NO production and iNOS gene expression by inhibiting NF-kappaB activation, and provide possible mechanisms for its anti-inflammatory and chemopreventive action." Lo AH, Liang YC, Lin-Shiau SY, Ho CT, Lin JK. Carnosol, an antioxidant in rosemary, suppresses inducible nitric oxide synthase through down-regulating nuclear factor-kappaB in mouse macrophages. *Carcinogenesis*. 2002 Jun;23(6):983-91

[188] "Constitutive and TNFalpha-induced NF-kappaB DNA binding activity was inhibited by GSE at doses > or =50 microg/ml and treatments for > or =12 h." Dhanalakshmi S, Agarwal R, Agarwal C. Inhibition of NF-kappaB pathway in grape seed extract-induced apoptotic death of human prostate carcinoma DU145 cells. *Int J Oncol*. 2003 Sep;23(3):721-7

[189] "Caffeic acid phenethyl ester (CAPE) is an anti-inflammatory component of propolis (honeybee resin). CAPE is reportedly a specific inhibitor of nuclear factor-kappaB (NF-kappaB)." Fitzpatrick LR, Wang J, Le T. Caffeic acid phenethyl ester, an inhibitor of nuclear factor-kappaB, attenuates bacterial peptidoglycan polysaccharide-induced colitis in rats. *J Pharmacol Exp Ther*. 2001 Dec;299(3):915-20

[190] "Our results suggest that zinc supplementation may lead to downregulation of the inflammatory cytokines through upregulation of the negative feedback loop A20 to inhibit induced NF-kappaB activation." Prasad AS, Bao B, Beck FW, Kucuk O, Sarkar FH. Antioxidant effect of zinc in humans. *Free Radic Biol Med*. 2004 Oct 15;37(8):1182-90

[191] Note that the patients in this study received a very high dose of selenium: 960 micrograms per day. This is at the top—and some would say over the top—of the safe and reasonable dose for long-term supplementation. In this case, th study lasted for three months. "In patients receiving selenium supplementation, selenium NF-kappaB activity was significantly reduced, reaching the same level as the nondiabetic control group. CONCLUSION: In type 2 diabetic patients, activation of NF-kappaB measured in peripheral blood monocytes can be reduced by selenium supplementation, confirming its importance in the prevention of cardiovascular diseases." Faure P, Ramon O, Favier A, Halimi S. Selenium supplementation decreases nuclear factor-kappa B activity in peripheral blood mononuclear cells from type 2 diabetic patients. *Eur J Clin Invest*. 2004 Jul;34(7):475-81

[192] Takada Y, Andreeff M, Aggarwal BB. Indole-3-carbinol suppresses NF-{kappa}B and I{kappa}B{alpha} kinase activation causing inhibition of expression of NF-{kappa}B-regulated antiapoptotic and metastatic gene products and enhancement of apoptosis in myeloid and leukemia cells. *Blood*. 2005 Apr 5; [Epub ahead of print]

[193] "Overall, our results indicated that indole-3-carbinol inhibits NF-kappaB and NF-kappaB-regulated gene expression and that this mechanism may provide the molecular basis for its ability to suppress tumorigenesis." Takada Y, Andreeff M, Aggarwal BB. Indole-3-carbinol suppresses NF-kappaB and IkappaBalpha kinase activation, causing inhibition of expression of NF-kappaB-regulated antiapoptotic and metastatic gene products and enhancement of apoptosis in myeloid and leukemia cells. *Blood*. 2005 Jul 15;106(2):641-9. Epub 2005 Apr 5.

[194] "CONCLUSIONS: Administration of N-acetylcysteine results in decreased nuclear factor-kappa B activation in patients with sepsis, associated with decreases in interleukin-8 but not interleukin-6 or soluble intercellular adhesion molecule-1. These pilot data suggest that antioxidant therapy with N-acetylcysteine may be useful in blunting the inflammatory response to sepsis." Paterson RL, Galley HF, Webster NR. The effect of N-acetylcysteine on nuclear factor-kappa B activation, interleukin-6, interleukin-8, and intercellular adhesion molecule-1 expression in patients with sepsis. *Crit Care Med*. 2003 Nov;31(11):2574-8

[195] "Resveratrol's anticarcinogenic, anti-inflammatory, and growth-modulatory effects may thus be partially ascribed to the inhibition of activation of NF-kappaB and AP-1 and the associated kinases." Manna SK, Mukhopadhyay A, Aggarwal BB. Resveratrol suppresses TNF-induced activation of nuclear transcription factors NF-kappa B, activator protein-1, and apoptosis: potential role of reactive oxygen intermediates and lipid peroxidation. *J Immunol*. 2000 Jun 15;164(12):6509-19

[196] "Both resveratrol and quercetin inhibited NF-kappaB-, AP-1- and CREB-dependent transcription to a greater extent than the glucocorticosteroid, dexamethasone." Donnelly LE, Newton R, Kennedy GE, Fenwick PS, Leung RH, Ito K, Russell RE, Barnes PJ.Anti-inflammatory Effects of Resveratrol in Lung Epithelial Cells: Molecular Mechanisms. *Am J Physiol Lung Cell Mol Physiol*. 2004 Jun 4 [Epub ahead of print]

[197] Yajima H, Ikeshima E, Shiraki M, Kanaya T, Fujiwara D, Odai H, Tsuboyama-Kasaoka N, Ezaki O, Oikawa S, Kondo K. Isohumulones, bitter acids derived from hops, activate both peroxisome proliferator-activated receptor alpha and gamma and reduce insulin resistance. *J Biol Chem*. 2004 Aug 6;279(32):33456-62. Epub 2004 Jun 3. http://www.jbc.org/cgi/content/full/279/32/33456

[198] "Thus, PPAR gamma serves as the receptor for GLA in the regulation of gene expression in breast cancer cells. " Jiang WG, Redfern A, Bryce RP, Mansel RE. Peroxisome proliferator activated receptor-gamma (PPAR-gamma) mediates the action of gamma linolenic acid in breast cancer cells. *Prostaglandins Leukot Essent Fatty Acids*. 2000 Feb;62(2):119-27

[199] "...EPA requires PPARalpha for its inhibitory effects on NF-kappaB." Mishra A, Chaudhary A, Sethi S. Oxidized omega-3 fatty acids inhibit NF-kappaB activation via a PPARalpha-dependent pathway. *Arterioscler Thromb Vasc Biol*. 2004 Sep;24(9):1621-7. Epub 2004 Jul 1. http://atvb.ahajournals.org/cgi/content/full/24/9/1621

[200] "Indeed, the previous view that nutrients only interact with human physiology at the metabolic/post-transcriptional level must be updated in light of current research showing that nutrients can, in fact, modify human physiology and phenotype at the genetic/pre-transcriptional level." Vasquez A. Reducing pain and inflammation naturally - part 4: nutritional and botanical inhibition of NF-kappaB, the major intracellular amplifier of the inflammatory cascade. A practical clinical strategy exemplifying anti-inflammatory nutrigenomics. *Nutritional Perspectives*, July 2005:5-12. www.OptimalHealthResearch.com/part4

[201] Seaman DR. The diet-induced proinflammatory state: a cause of chronic pain and other degenerative diseases? *J Manipulative Physiol Ther*. 2002;25(3):168-79

[202] "We propose that the additive and synergistic effects of phytochemicals in fruit and vegetables are responsible for their potent antioxidant and anticancer activities, and that the benefit of a diet rich in fruit and vegetables is attributed to the complex mixture of phytochemicals present in whole foods." Liu RH. Health benefits of fruit and vegetables are from additive and synergistic combinations of phytochemicals. *Am J Clin Nutr*. 2003 Sep;78(3 Suppl):517S-520S

[203] **Heaney RP. Long-latency deficiency disease: insights from calcium and vitamin D. *Am J Clin Nutr*. 2003 Nov;78(5):912-9**

[204] **O'Keefe JH Jr, Cordain L. Cardiovascular disease resulting from a diet and lifestyle at odds with our Paleolithic genome: how to become a 21st-century hunter-gatherer. *Mayo Clin Proc*. 2004 Jan;79(1):101-8**

[205] Thomas MK, Lloyd-Jones DM, Thadhani RI, Shaw AC, Deraska DJ, Kitch BT, Vamvakas EC, Dick IM, Prince RL, Finkelstein JS. Hypovitaminosis D in medical inpatients. *N Engl J Med*. 1998 Mar 19;338(12):777-83

[206] Van den Berghe G, Van Roosbroeck D, Vanhove P, Wouters PJ, De Pourcq L, Bouillon R. Bone turnover in prolonged critical illness: effect of vitamin D. *J Clin Endocrinol Metab*. 2003 Oct;88(10):4623-32

[207] Hypponen E, Laara E, Reunanen A, Jarvelin MR, Virtanen SM. Intake of vitamin D and risk of type 1 diabetes: a birth-cohort study. *Lancet*. 2001 Nov 3;358(9292):1500-3

Basic Physiology of NF-kappaB: A Simplified Conceptual Model

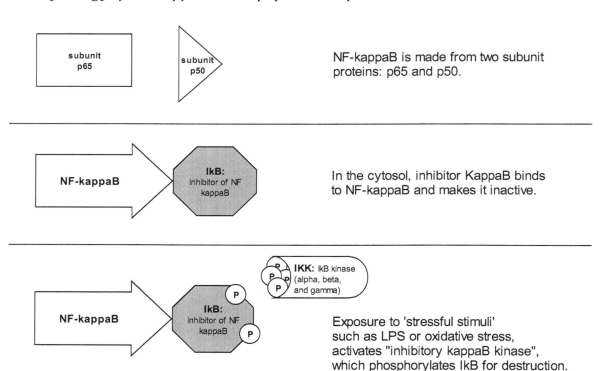

NF-kappaB is made from two subunit proteins: p65 and p50.

In the cytosol, inhibitor KappaB binds to NF-kappaB and makes it inactive.

Exposure to 'stressful stimuli' such as LPS or oxidative stress, activates "inhibitory kappaB kinase", which phosphorylates IkB for destruction.

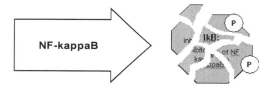

Once IkB is destroyed, then NF-kappaB is free to enter the nucleus and bind with DNA.

NF-kappaB enters the nucleus and binds with DNA to activate genes which encode for the increased production of inflammatory mediators.

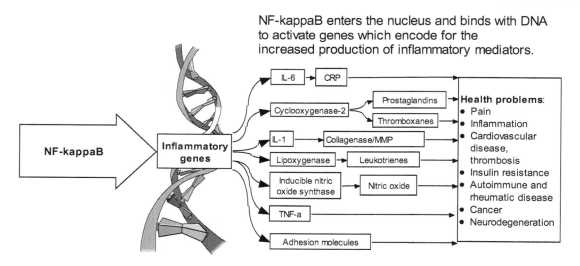

Increased production of inflammatory mediators - such as cytokines, prostaglandins, leukotrienes - promotes cellular dysfunction and tissue destruction.

[208] Mahon BD, Gordon SA, Cruz J, Cosman F, Cantorna MT. Cytokine profile in patients with multiple sclerosis following vitamin D supplementation. *J Neuroimmunol*. 2003;134(1-2):128-32

Selected Nutritional and Botanical Therapeutics: Brief Clinical Monographs

The following pages emphasize clinically relevant concise reviews of **selected nutritional and botanical therapeutics** that are commonly considered in the treatment of musculoskeletal pain and for the promotion of tissue healing. Future editions of this book will contain a broader compendium. However, the power of natural medicine lies not in the size of our pharmacopoeia; it is rather to be found in the completeness of our approach and in the conceptual and philosophical underpinnings which support our assessments and interventions.

By now, the concept of "holistic treatment" as advocated in this text should be clear to the reader. While the medical model of disease treatment continues to seek a single "silver bullet" to treat each disease, the advantage of holistic medicine is that we consider and address a wide range of therapeutics—each of which addresses a particular aspect of the patient's complex pathophysiologic phenomena. For example, in the treatment of low-back pain, rather than relying on a single treatment/drug to effect 100% benefit (100% "cure" is almost never attained with single interventions, especially with drugs), we seek a 20% improvement from EPA+DHA supplementation, 40% improvement from proprioceptive retraining and exercise, 30% improvement with anti-inflammatory botanical medicines, and at least another 10% improvement with vitamin C. In the end, my experience in using this style of *multiple intervention therapy* is that the majority of patients are not only effectively "cured" of their former health problem(s), but that they enjoy a higher level of overall health as a result of dietary improvements, nutritional supplementation, exercise, and the other biochemical and behavioral modifications that I have prescribed, such as described in this text.

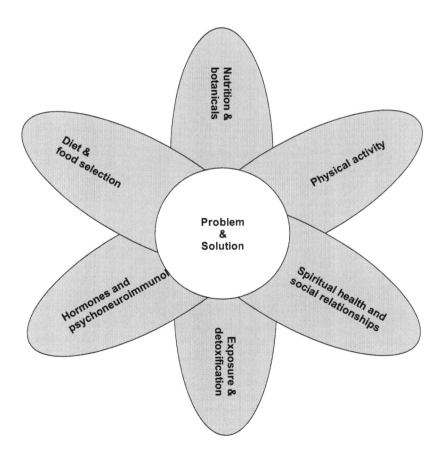

Nutrient:	*Alpha-linolenic acid (ALA)*
Common name:	**Flaxseed oil (57% ALA)**

Applications and mechanisms of action:

- Anti-inflammatory, modulation of gene transcription, and several other benefits: ALA clearly has anti-inflammatory benefits as consistently demonstrated in human studies. In a study of men with metabolic syndrome, ALA was shown to have anti-inflammatory benefits independent of its conversion to EPA or DHA.[209] The mechanism of action appears to be downregulation of NF-KappaB (the main "amplifier" for the expression of proinflammatory gene products[210]) rather than the direct modulation of eicosanoid biosynthesis. One study using flaxseed oil as a source of ALA to treat rheumatoid arthritis found no clinical or biochemical benefit (i.e., no change in Hgb, CRP, ESR)[211]; however, the poor results of this study may have been due to the inferior quality of the flaxseed oil product that was used which only supplied 32% ALA compared with the much higher concentration of 57% found in most products. **Moderate intakes of ALA from flaxseed oil profoundly reduce production of proinflammatory prostaglandins (e.g., PG-E2, measured by urinary excretion) by 52% to 85% in humans.**[212] This level of prostaglandin inhibition is greater than the 42% reduction induced by rofecoxib/Vioxx.[213] However, since the reduction in prostaglandin formation by ALA is more generalized (rather than specific for the Cox-2 enzyme), the anti-inflammatory benefit occurs without adverse cardiovascular effects caused by Cox-2 inhibitors.

Toxicity and contraindications:

- None that are generally known.
- Overconsumption or imbalanced intake of ALA is known to cause reductions in DHA, and this reduction would be expected to have adverse effects on neurological performance, cognition, and vision.

Dosage and administration:

- One to two tablespoons of flaxseed oil contain 6,200 mg or 12,400 mg of ALA, respectively.
- Fatty acids should always be supplemented in balanced combination rather than in isolation.[214]

Additional information:

- Conversion of ALA to the more biologically active EPA and DHA does not reliably or efficiently occur in humans.[215] No increase in DHA has been consistently observed in humans after supplementation of ALA[216]; in fact, supplementation with flax seed oil has actually been shown to reduce DHA levels in humans.[217]

[209] "CONCLUSIONS: Dietary supplementation with ALA for 3 months decreases significantly CRP, SAA and IL-6 levels in dyslipidaemic patients. This anti-inflammatory effect may provide a possible additional mechanism for the beneficial effect of plant n-3 polyunsaturated fatty acids in primary and secondary prevention of coronary artery disease." Rallidis LS, Paschos G, Liakos GK, Velissaridou AH, Anastasiadis G, Zampelas A. Dietary alpha-linolenic acid decreases C-reactive protein, serum amyloid A and interleukin-6 in dyslipidaemic patients. *Atherosclerosis*. 2003 Apr;167(2):237-42

[210] Tak PP, Firestein GS. NF-kappaB: a key role in inflammatory diseases. *J Clin Invest*. 2001 Jan;107(1):7-11

[211] "Thus, 3-month's supplementation with alpha-LNA did not prove to be beneficial in rheumatoid arthritis." Nordstrom DC, Honkanen VE, Nasu Y, Antila E, Friman C, Konttinen YT. Alpha-linolenic acid in the treatment of rheumatoid arthritis. A double-blind, placebo-controlled and randomized study: flaxseed vs. safflower seed. *Rheumatol Int*. 1995;14(6):231-4

[212] Adam O, Wolfram G, Zollner N. Effect of alpha-linolenic acid in the human diet on linoleic acid metabolism and prostaglandin biosynthesis. *J Lipid Res*. 1986 Apr;27(4):421-6

[213] Van Hecken A, Schwartz JI, Depre M, De Lepeleire I, Dallob A, Tanaka W, Wynants K, Buntinx A, Arnout J, Wong PH, Ebel DL, Gertz BJ, De Schepper PJ. Comparative inhibitory activity of rofecoxib, meloxicam, diclofenac, ibuprofen, and naproxen on COX-2 versus COX-1 in healthy volunteers. *J Clin Pharmacol*. 2000 Oct;40(10):1109-20

[214] **Vasquez A. Reducing Pain and Inflammation Naturally. Part 2: New Insights into Fatty Acid Supplementation and Its Effect on Eicosanoid Production and Genetic Expression.** *Nutritional Perspectives* **2005; January: 5-16** www.optimalhealthresearch.com/part2

[215] "Indu and Ghafoorunissa showed that while keeping the amount of dietary LA constant, 3.7 g ALA appears to have biological effects similar to those of 0.3 g long-chain n-3 PUFA with conversion of 11 g ALA to 1 g long-chain n-3 PUFA." Simopoulos AP. Essential fatty acids in health and chronic disease. *Am J Clin Nutr*. 1999 Sep;70(3 Suppl):560S-569S

[216] Francois CA, Connor SL, Bolewicz LC, Connor WE. Supplementing lactating women with flaxseed oil does not increase docosahexaenoic acid in their milk. *Am J Clin Nutr*. 2003 Jan;77(1):226-33

[217] "Linear relationships were found between dietary alpha-LA and EPA in plasma fractions and in cellular phospholipids. ... There was an inverse relationship between dietary alpha-LA and docosahexaenoic acid concentrations in the phospholipids of plasma, neutrophils, mononuclear cells, and platelets." Mantzioris E, James MJ, Gibson RA, Cleland LG. Differences exist in the relationships between dietary linoleic and alpha-linolenic acids and their respective long-chain metabolites. *Am J Clin Nutr*. 1995 Feb;61(2):320-4

Nutrients:	*Eicosapentaenoic acid (EPA)*
	Docosahexaenoic acid (DHA)
Common name:	**Fish oil**

Applications and mechanisms of action:

- **Anti-inflammatory, modulation of gene transcription, and many other benefits**: Fish oil has a wide range of applications, proven effectiveness, and record of safety that is second to none; no other single treatment is as effective for such a wide range of conditions. Positive results have been documented in clinical trials in patients with hypertension, hypercholesterolemia, various types of joint pain, mental depression, diabetes, bipolar illness, ulcerative colitis, Crohn's disease, schizophrenia and various other conditions, particularly inflammatory and neurologic diseases. Rather than being specific for any one disease, the provision of EPA and DHA via supplementation with fish oil quite simply *makes the body work better* by supplying the long-chain omega-3 fatty acids that are necessary for proper physiologic function but which are commonly deficient in our modern diets. Benefits include reduction in harmful 2-series pro-inflammatory and pain-enhancing eicosanoids, increased production of 3-series eicosanoids, modulation of gene transcription, and enhancement of cell membranes with the general result of increased receptor sensitivity and thus improved intercellular communication and improved efficiency of cell membrane signal transduction.

- **Clinical benefits: EPA supplementation has proven beneficial for patients with lupus,[218] cancer[219], borderline personality disorder[220], mental depression[221,222,223], schizophrenia[224], and osteoporosis (when used with GLA).[225]** DHA appears essential for optimal cognitive function in infants and adults, and DHA in fish oil provides some protection against thrombosis, arrhythmia, cardiovascular death, Alzheimer's disease[226], otitis media (when used with nutritional supplementation[227]), and coronary restenosis following angioplasty.[228] Supplementation with DHA (often in the form of fish oil, which includes EPA) has been shown to benefit patients with bipolar disorder[229], Crohn's disease[230], rheumatoid arthritis[231,232,233], lupus[234], cardiovascular disease[235], psoriasis[236], and cancer.[237] DHA appears to have an "anti-stress" benefit manifested by 30%

[218] Duffy EM, Meenagh GK, McMillan SA, Strain JJ, Hannigan BM, Bell AL. The clinical effect of dietary supplementation with omega-3 fish oils and/or copper in systemic lupus erythematosus. *J Rheumatol*. 2004 Aug;31(8):1551-6

[219] Wigmore SJ, Barber MD, Ross JA, Tisdale MJ, Fearon KC. Effect of oral eicosapentaenoic acid on weight loss in patients with pancreatic cancer. *Nutr Cancer*. 2000;36(2):177-84

[220] Zanarini MC, Frankenburg FR. omega-3 Fatty acid treatment of women with borderline personality disorder: a double-blind, placebo-controlled pilot study. *Am J Psychiatry*. 2003 Jan;160(1):167-9

[221] Nemets B, Stahl Z, Belmaker RH. Addition of omega-3 fatty acid to maintenance medication treatment for recurrent unipolar depressive disorder. *Am J Psychiatry*. 2002 Mar;159(3):477-9

[222] Puri BK, Counsell SJ, Hamilton G, Richardson AJ, Horrobin DF.Eicosapentaenoic acid in treatment-resistant depression associated with symptom remission, structural brain changes and reduced neuronal phospholipid turnover. *Int J Clin Pract*. 2001 Oct;55(8):560-3

[223] Peet M, Horrobin DF.A dose-ranging study of the effects of ethyl-eicosapentaenoate in patients with ongoing depression despite apparently adequate treatment with standard drugs. *Arch Gen Psychiatry*. 2002 Oct;59(10):913-9

[224] Emsley R, Myburgh C, Oosthuizen P, van Rensburg SJ. Randomized, placebo-controlled study of ethyl-eicosapentaenoic acid as supplemental treatment in schizophrenia. *Am J Psychiatry*. 2002 Sep;159(9):1596-8

[225] Kruger MC, Coetzer H, de Winter R, Gericke G, van Papendorp DH. Calcium, gamma-linolenic acid and eicosapentaenoic acid supplementation in senile osteoporosis. *Aging* (Milano). 1998 Oct;10(5):385-94

[226] Horrocks LA, Yeo YK. Health benefits of docosahexaenoic acid (DHA). *Pharmacol Res*. 1999 Sep;40(3):211-25

[227] Linday LA, Dolitsky JN, Shindledecker RD, Pippenger CE. Lemon-flavored cod liver oil and a multivitamin-mineral supplement for the secondary prevention of otitis media in young children: pilot research. *Ann Otol Rhinol Laryngol*. 2002 Jul;111(7 Pt 1):642-52

[228] Bairati I, Roy L, Meyer F. Double-blind, randomized, controlled trial of fish oil supplements in prevention of recurrence of stenosis after coronary angioplasty. *Circulation*. 1992 Mar;85(3):950-6

[229] Stoll AL, Severus WE, Freeman MP, Rueter S, Zboyan HA, Diamond E, Cress KK, Marangell LB. Omega 3 fatty acids in bipolar disorder: a preliminary double-blind, placebo-controlled trial. *Arch Gen Psychiatry*. 1999 May;56(5):407-12

[230] Belluzzi A, Brignola C, Campieri M, Pera A, Boschi S, Miglioli M. Effect of an enteric-coated fish-oil preparation on relapses in Crohn's disease. *N Engl J Med*. 1996 Jun 13;334(24):1557-60

[231] Adam O, Beringer C, Kless T, Lemmen C, Adam A, Wiseman M, Adam P, Klimmek R, Forth W. Anti-inflammatory effects of a low arachidonic acid diet and fish oil in patients with rheumatoid arthritis. *Rheumatol Int*. 2003 Jan;23(1):27-36

[232] Lau CS, Morley KD, Belch JJ. Effects of fish oil supplementation on non-steroidal anti-inflammatory drug requirement in patients with mild rheumatoid arthritis--a double-blind placebo controlled study. *Br J Rheumatol*. 1993 Nov;32(11):982-9

[233] Kremer JM, Jubiz W, Michalek A, Rynes RI, Bartholomew LE, Bigaouette J, Timchalk M, Beeler D, Lininger L. Fish-oil fatty acid supplementation in active rheumatoid arthritis. A double-blinded, controlled, crossover study. *Ann Intern Med*. 1987 Apr;106(4):497-503

[234] Walton AJ, Snaith ML, Locniskar M, Cumberland AG, Morrow WJ, Isenberg DA. Dietary fish oil and the severity of symptoms in patients with systemic lupus erythematosus. *Ann Rheum Dis*. 1991 Jul;50(7):463-6

[235] "The recent GISSI (Gruppo Italiano per lo Studio della Sopravvivenza nell'Infarto miocardico)-Prevention study of 11,324 patients showed a 45% decrease in risk of sudden cardiac death and a 20% reduction in all-cause mortality in the group taking 850 mg/d of omega-3 fatty acids." O'Keefe JH Jr, Harris WS. From Inuit to implementation: omega-3 fatty acids come of age. *Mayo Clin Proc*. 2000 Jun;75(6):607-14

[236] Bittner SB, Tucker WF, Cartwright I, Bleehen SS. A double-blind, randomised, placebo-controlled trial of fish oil in psoriasis. *Lancet*. 1988;1(8582):378-80

[237] Gogos CA, Ginopoulos P, Salsa B, Apostolidou E, Zoumbos NC, Kalfarentzos F. Dietary omega-3 polyunsaturated fatty acids plus vitamin E restore immunodeficiency and prolong survival for severely ill patients with generalized malignancy: a randomized control trial. *Cancer*. 1998 Jan 15;82(2):395-402

reductions in norepinephrine and improved resilience to psychoemotional stress.[238,239] Supplementation with EPA+DHA in fish oil is extremely safe and reduces all-cause mortality.[240]

Toxicity and contraindications:

- EPA and DHA have been used in relatively high doses with little or no evidence of adverse effects. In one study, 10,000 mg per day of EPA did not cause adverse effects[241]; this dose is equivalent to approximately 6-7 tablespoons of cod-liver oil per day—much more than is commonly prescribed for long-term use. Another study found that administration of 13.1 g of eicosapentaenoic acid + docosahexaenoic acid resulted only in gastrointestinal effects such as diarrhea and abdominal discomfort.[242]

- Anticoagulant medications, surgery, and bleeding: Although EPA+DHA doses of at least 4 grams per day may be necessary to increase bleeding time[243], I routinely recommend dose reduction or discontinuation of EPA+DHA supplementation for patients who are thrombocytopenic or otherwise at risk for hemorrhage due to illness or upcoming surgery. Fish oil can potentate anticoagulant medication such as warfarin/coumadin.[244]

- Vitamin D: High doses of cod-liver oil—4 tablespoons per day (one-quarter cup)—provide approximately 6,000 IU of vitamin D, an amount which is much less than the 10,000 IU of vitamin D that is synthesized following a few minutes of full-body sun exposure and which appears safe according to the extensive review by Vieth.[245] For patients consuming cod-liver oil at one tablespoon per day (long-term use) or up to one-quarter cup (four tablespoons per day for short-term use), the risk of vitamin D toxicity appears to be nonexistent. Interestingly, vitamin D *deficiency* appears to be endemic among people with persistent, nonspecific musculoskeletal pain.[246]

- Vitamin A: Cod-liver oil typically contains up to 1,250 IU of vitamin A per teaspoon, which is 3,750 IU per tablespoon. **Thus, a quarter-cup of cod-liver oil contains 15,000 IU vitamin A—this is a safe dose for several months of supplementation in most adult patients**, but this modest dose is too high for women who are pregnant or might become pregnant because of the theoretical and controversial association between birth defects and vitamin A intakes greater than 10,000 IU per day. Other brands of liquid fish oil contain 1,950 IU vitamin A per teaspoon, or 5,850 IU vitamin A per tablespoon, which totals 23,400 IU per quarter cup of oil—this dose is too high for multi-year consumption, but is safe for short-term use in most patients. Vitamin A toxicity is seen with chronic ingestion of therapeutic doses (for example: **25,000 IU per day for 6 years**, or 100,000 IU per day for 2.5 years[247]). Manifestations of vitamin A toxicity (hypervitaminosis A) include dry skin, chapped or split lips, skin rash

[238] Hamazaki T, Itomura M, Sawazaki S, Nagao Y. Anti-stress effects of DHA. *Biofactors.* 2000;13(1-4):41-5

[239] Sawazaki S, Hamazaki T, Yazawa K, Kobayashi M. The effect of docosahexaenoic acid on plasma catecholamine concentrations and glucose tolerance during long-lasting psychological stress: a double-blind placebo-controlled study. *J Nutr Sci Vitaminol* (Tokyo). 1999 Oct;45(5):655-65

[240] O'Keefe JH Jr, Harris WS. From Inuit to implementation: omega-3 fatty acids come of age. *Mayo Clin Proc.* 2000 Jun;75(6):607-14

[241] " eicosapentaenoic acid (EPA) and docosahexaenoic acid (DHA) were given in a cumulative manner, every 6 weeks, starting with 10 mg, then 100 mg, 1000 mg and 10,000 mg EPA daily to mild to moderate essential hypertensive black patients. The corresponding DHA doses were 3, 33, 333 and 3333 mg." Du Plooy WJ, Venter CP, Muntingh GM, Venter HL, Glatthaar II, Smith KA. The cumulative dose response effect of eicosapentaenoic and docosahexaenoic acid on blood pressure, plasma lipid profile and diet pattern in mild to moderate essential hypertensive black patients. *Prostaglandins Leukot Essent Fatty Acids* 1992 Aug;46(4):315-21

[242] "This means that a 70-kg patient can generally tolerate up to 21 1-g capsules/day containing 13.1 g of eicosapentaenoic acid + docosahexaenoic acid, the two major omega-3 fatty acids" Burns CP, Halabi S, Clamon GH, Hars V, Wagner BA, Hohl RJ, Lester E, Kirshner JJ, Vinciguerra V, Paskett E. Phase I clinical study of fish oil fatty acid capsules for patients with cancer cachexia: cancer and leukemia group B study 9473. *Clin Cancer Res.* 1999 Dec;5(12):3942-7

[243] "... EPA/d ... 4 g/d increased bleeding time and decreased platelet count with no adverse effects. In human studies, there has never been a case of clinical bleeding, even in patients undergoing angioplasty, while the patients were taking fish oil supplements." Simopoulos AP. Essential fatty acids in health and chronic disease. *Am J Clin Nutr.* 1999;70(3 Suppl):560S-569S

[244] "Although controversial, this case report illustrates that fish oil can provide additive anticoagulant effects when given with warfarin. CONCLUSIONS: This case reveals a significant rise in INR after the dose of concomitant fish oil was doubled." Buckley MS, Goff AD, Knapp WE. Fish oil interaction with warfarin. *Ann Pharmacother.* 2004 Jan;38(1):50-2

[245] "Total-body sun exposure easily provides the equivalent of 250 microg (10,000 IU) vitamin D/d. ...Published cases of vitamin D toxicity ...all involve intake of > or = 1000 microg (40000 IU)/d. ... no observed adverse effect limit of 50 microg (2000 IU)/d is too low by at least 5-fold." Vieth R. Vitamin D supplementation, 25-hydroxyvitamin D concentrations, and safety. *Am J Clin Nutr* 1999 May;69(5):842-56

[246] "CONCLUSION: All patients with persistent, nonspecific musculoskeletal pain are at high risk for the consequences of unrecognized and untreated severe hypovitaminosis D. This risk extends to those considered at low risk for vitamin D deficiency: nonelderly, nonhousebound, or nonimmigrant persons of either sex." Plotnikoff GA, Quigley JM. Prevalence of severe hypovitaminosis D in patients with persistent, nonspecific musculoskeletal pain. *Mayo Clin Proc.* 2003 Dec;78(12):1463-70

[247] Geubel AP, De Galocsy C, Alves N, Rahier J, Dive C. Liver damage caused by therapeutic vitamin A administration: estimate of dose-related toxicity in 41 cases. *Gastroenterology.* 1991 Jun;100(6):1701-9

(erythematous dermatitis), hair loss, joint pain, bone pain, headaches (pseudotumor cerebri), anorexia (loss of appetite), fatigue, elevated liver enzymes, and increased serum calcium. Women who are pregnant or might become pregnant and who are planning to carry the baby to full term delivery should not ingest more than 10,000 IU of vitamin A per day. Most patients should probably not consume more than 20,000 IU of vitamin A per day for more than 2 months without express supervision by a healthcare provider. **Vitamin A is present in some multivitamin supplements, in cod-liver oil, and in other supplements—patients and doctors are advised to read labels to ensure that the total daily intake is not greater than 20,000 IU per day for long-term use unless it is being used for a specific indication**

Dosage and administration:

- In my clinical practice, **I routinely recommend one tablespoon of cod-liver oil per day for essentially all adult patients**. One tablespoon of fish oil provides 3,000 mg of EPA+DHA, which is consistent with the amounts used in the research literature to provide clinical benefit.[248] Further justification for this recommendation is found in the literature documenting that the provision of EPA and DHA reduces the risk of death and "all-cause mortality" particularly cardiovascular disease, that these two fatty acids have health-promoting and anti-inflammatory effects, and that the risk for adverse effects is minimal to clinically nonexistent. The dose of vitamin A per tablespoon of cod-liver oil is 3,750 IU per day—clearly this is safe for long-term use. Vitamin D at 1,500 IU per day is safe and appears to have antidepressant, immunomodulatory, and anticancer effects.

- Periodically, I start patients at one-quarter cup of fish oil per day for five to ten days, and then reduce the dose to one tablespoon per day thereafter for maintenance. This technique can provide clinical benefit even for patients whom have supplemented fish oil at lower doses for long periods of time without benefit. The probable mechanism of action is primarily the more rapid exchange of fatty acids in cell membranes, with the resultant benefits in eicosanoid production and cell membrane receptor function.

Dosage and administration:

Clinical application	*Approximate daily dosage range for combined EPA and DHA (i.e., mg of EPA + mg of DHA)*
General preventive medicine for adults and dosage for children	1,000 mg
Therapeutic dose and assertive prevention	3,000 mg
High-dose supplementation (adult dose for short-term or aggressive therapy only)	Up to approximately 12,000 mg

---

[248] "…clinical benefits of the n-3 fatty acids were not apparent until they were consumed for > or =12 wk. It appears that a minimum daily dose of 3 g eicosapentaenoic and docosahexaenoic acids is necessary to derive the expected benefits [in patients with rheumatoid arthritis]." Kremer JM. n-3 fatty acid supplements in rheumatoid arthritis. *Am J Clin Nutr*. 2000 Jan;71(1 Suppl):349S-51S

Dosage and administration (continued):	▪ <u>Coadminister GLA when using fish oil</u>: Since EPA and other n-3 EFAs inhibit formation of GLA from LA[249] [250] and since administration of GLA will increase levels of arachidonic acid unless EPA is coadministered[251], **the most reasonable clinical approach to improving eicosanoid metabolism in favor of reducing inflammation is to always combine GLA supplementation with EPA/DHA supplementation**. Coadministration of EPA or fish oil will prevent the rise in arachidonate that might occur with supplementation with GLA alone[252], and using GLA when using fish oil and EPA will prevent the reduction in GLA that occurs with administration of EPA alone.[253]
Additional information:	▪ Given the low cost, high safety, and tremendous benefits of omega-3 fats in general and EPA and DHA in particular, I believe that all adult patients should supplement with one teaspoon to one tablespoon of fish oil per day, providing that they do not have disturbances of hemostasis or of vitamin D or vitamin A metabolism. Failure to address the underlying fatty acid imbalances in the majority of patients is one of the main reasons why otherwise appropriate treatment plans fail.
	▪ Liquid fish oil supplements are easily consumed in a morning smoothie, mixed in tomato or orange juice, or taken straight from the bottle. Liquid supplements are much less expensive per dose than are capsule supplements. To obtain an equivalent dose of EPA and DHA found in one tablespoon of cod-liver oil would require the consumption of 6-21 capsules, depending on the brand and concentration of the capsule fish oil supplement.
	▪ Although the data are inconclusive on the need for vitamin E supplementation to prevent the depletion of antioxidants induced by consumption of polyunsaturated fatty acids, I generally recommend 800-1,200 IU of vitamin E taken as mixed tocopherols with an emphasis on high concentrations of gamma-tocopherol, which has biologic benefits beyond its antioxidant function. For patients with cancer however, I do not use tocopherols because they have consistently been shown to abrogate the anticancer benefits of polyunsaturated fatty acids.[254]

[249] Horrobin DF. Interactions between n-3 and n-6 essential fatty acids (EFAs) in the regulation of cardiovascular disorders and inflammation. *Prostaglandins Leukot Essent Fatty Acids* 1991 Oct;44(2):127-31

[250] Rubin D, Laposata M. Cellular interactions between n-6 and n-3 fatty acids: a mass analysis of fatty acid elongation/desaturation, distribution among complex lipids, and conversion to eicosanoids. *J Lipid Res.* 1992 Oct;33(10):1431-40

[251] "The decrease in serum eicosapentaenoic acid and the increase in arachidonic acid concentrations induced by evening primrose oil may not be favourable effects in patients with rheumatoid arthritis in the light of the roles of these fatty acids as precursors of eicosanoids." Jantti J, Nikkari T, Solakivi T, Vapaatalo H, Isomaki H. Evening primrose oil in rheumatoid arthritis: changes in serum lipids and fatty acids. *Ann Rheum Dis.* 1989 Feb;48(2):124-7

[252] "This study revealed that a GLA and EPA supplement combination may be utilized to reduce the synthesis of proinflammatory AA metabolites, and importantly, not induce potentially harmful increases in serum AA levels." Barham JB, Edens MB, Fonteh AN, Johnson MM, Easter L, Chilton FH. Addition of eicosapentaenoic acid to gamma-linolenic acid-supplemented diets prevents serum arachidonic acid accumulation in humans. *J Nutr.* 2000 Aug;130(8):1925-31

[253] "...intake of fish oil caused a significant depression in the content of DGLA... Since DGLA is the precursor of PGE1, which has been shown to be anti-inflammatory, our findings suggest that the anti-inflammatory effects of fish oil consumption could be mitigated by an associated reduction in DGLA." Cleland LG, Gibson RA, Neumann M, French JK. The effect of dietary fish oil supplement upon the content of dihomo-gammalinolenic acid in human plasma phospholipids. *Prostaglandins Leukot Essent Fatty Acids.* 1990 May;40(1):9-12

[254] See my forthcoming ***The Scientific Basis for the Natural Treatment of Cancer in Humans*** for information on natural cancer treatments:OptimalHealthResearch.com

Nutrient:	**Gamma-linolenic acid**
Common name:	**GLA**

Applications and mechanisms of action:

- <u>Anti-inflammatory effects</u>: As described previously in the section detailing fatty acid metabolism, GLA is efficiently converted to DGLA and is then preferentially converted to the anti-inflammatory prostaglandin PG-E1. While GLA/DGLA have manifold effects, most of the benefits appear to be attributable to increased production of PG-E1. DGLA helps reduce the formation of the arachidonate-derived 2-series prostaglandins, 4-series leukotrienes and platelet-activating factor.[255] GLA is proven to be clinically effective in reducing inflammation and manifestations of disease activity in patients with **rheumatoid arthritis**[256,257,258], eczema[259], and respiratory distress syndrome (when used with EPA)[260]

- <u>Additional clinical benefits</u>: GLA supplementation benefits patients with breast cancer (when used with tamoxifen[261]), premenstrual syndrome[262], diabetic neuropathy[263], and migraine headaches (when used with ALA[264])

Toxicity and contraindications:

- <u>GLA is very safe</u>: In general, no toxicity has been noted using GLA in doses up to 4 grams per day in several long-term studies. Remarkably, one study used 3 grams (3,000 mg per day) of GLA in infants of age < 12 months and found no adverse effects[265] thus testifying to the non-existent toxicity of GLA. As with all dietary oils, some patients note belching and loose stools[266] but this is not an indication of toxicity

- <u>Temporal lobe epilepsy</u>: According to a small trial, GLA administration appears to worsen temporal lobe epilepsy[267]

Dosage and administration:

- <u>Approximately 500 mg per day is the common anti-inflammatory dose</u>: Studies have used 540 mg per day[268] and up to 2.8 grams per day in rheumatoid arthritis[269]

- <u>Coadminister ascorbate</u>: The conversion of DGLA to its bioactive metabolites is expedited by coadministration of vitamin C[270]

[255] Fan YY, Chapkin RS. Importance of dietary gamma-linolenic acid in human health and nutrition. *J Nutr*. 1998 Sep;128(9):1411-4

[256] "CONCLUSION: GLA at doses used in this study is a well-tolerated and effective treatment for active RA." Zurier RB, Rossetti RG, Jacobson EW, DeMarco DM, Liu NY, Temming JE, White BM, Laposata M. gamma-Linolenic acid treatment of rheumatoid arthritis. A randomized, placebo-controlled trial. *Arthritis Rheum*. 1996 Nov;39(11):1808-17

[257] "GLA treatment is associated with clinical improvement in patients with RA, as evaluated by duration of morning stiffness, joint pain and swelling, and ability to reduce other medications." Rothman D, DeLuca P, Zurier RB. Botanical lipids: effects on inflammation, immune responses, and rheumatoid arthritis. *Semin Arthritis Rheum*. 1995 Oct;25(2):87-96

[258] "Forty patients with rheumatoid arthritis and upper gastrointestinal lesions due to non-steroidal anti-inflammatory drugs entered a prospective 6-month double-blind placebo controlled study of dietary supplementation with gamma-linolenic acid 540 mg/day... Other results showed a significant reduction in morning stiffness with gamma-linolenic acid at 3 months..." Brzeski M, Madhok R, Capell HA. Evening primrose oil in patients with rheumatoid arthritis and side-effects of non-steroidal anti-inflammatory drugs. *Br J Rheumatol*. 1991 Oct;30(5):370-2

[259] Fiocchi A, Sala M, Signoroni P, Banderali G, Agostoni C, Riva E. The efficacy and safety of gamma-linolenic acid in the treatment of infantile atopic dermatitis. *J Int Med Res*. 1994 Jan-Feb;22(1):24-32

[260] Pacht ER, DeMichele SJ, Nelson JL, Hart J, Wennberg AK, Gadek JE. Enteral nutrition with eicosapentaenoic acid, gamma-linolenic acid, and antioxidants reduces alveolar inflammatory mediators and protein influx in patients with acute respiratory distress syndrome. *Crit Care Med*. 2003 Feb;31(2):491-500

[261] Kenny FS, Pinder SE, Ellis IO, Gee JM, Nicholson RI, Bryce RP, Robertson JF. Gamma linolenic acid with tamoxifen as primary therapy in breast cancer. *Int J Cancer*. 2000 Mar 1;85(5):643-8

[262] Puolakka J, Makarainen L, Viinikka L, Ylikorkala O. Biochemical and clinical effects of treating the premenstrual syndrome with prostaglandin synthesis precursors. *J Reprod Med*. 1985 Mar;30(3):149-53

[263] Jamal GA, Carmichael H. The effect of gamma-linolenic acid on human diabetic peripheral neuropathy: a double-blind placebo-controlled trial. *Diabet Med*. 1990 May;7(4):319-23

[264] Wagner W, Nootbaar-Wagner U. Prophylactic treatment of migraine with gamma-linolenic and alpha-linolenic acids. *Cephalalgia*. 1997 Apr;17(2):127-30

[265] "The children (mean age, 11.4 months) with atopic dermatitis (mean duration, 8.56 months) were openly treated with 3 g/day gamma-linolenic acid, for 28 days... A gradual improvement in erythema, excoriations and lichenification was seen; .... No side-effects were recorded." Fiocchi A, Sala M, Signoroni P, Banderali G, Agostoni C, Riva E. The efficacy and safety of gamma-linolenic acid in the treatment of infantile atopic dermatitis. *J Int Med Res*. 1994 Jan-Feb;22(1):24-32

[266] "With regard to safety, dietary sources of GLA appear to be completely nontoxic. Although limited cases of soft stools, belching and abdominal bloating have been reported ... long-term GLA administration may be feasible." Fan YY, Chapkin RS. Importance of dietary gamma-linolenic acid in human health and nutrition. J Nutr. 1998 Sep;128(9):1411-4

[267] "Three long-stay, hospitalised schizophrenics who had failed to respond adequately to conventional drug therapy were treated with gamma-linolenic acid and linoleic acid in the form of evening primrose oil. They became substantially worse and electroencephalographic features of temporal lobe epilepsy became apparent." Vaddadi KS. The use of gamma-linolenic acid and linoleic acid to differentiate between temporal lobe epilepsy and schizophrenia. *Prostaglandins Med*. 1981 Apr;6(4):375-9

[268] "Forty patients with rheumatoid arthritis and upper gastrointestinal lesions due to non-steroidal anti-inflammatory drugs entered a prospective 6-month double-blind placebo controlled study of dietary supplementation with gamma-linolenic acid 540 mg/day..." Brzeski M, Madhok R, Capell HA. Evening primrose oil in patients with rheumatoid arthritis and side-effects of non-steroidal anti-inflammatory drugs. *Br J Rheumatol*. 1991 Oct;30(5):370-2

[269] Zurier RB, Rossetti RG, Jacobson EW, DeMarco DM, Liu NY, Temming JE, White BM, Laposata M. gamma-Linolenic acid treatment of rheumatoid arthritis. A randomized, placebo-controlled trial. *Arthritis Rheum*. 1996 Nov;39(11):1808-17

[270] Horrobin DF. Ascorbic acid and prostaglandin synthesis. *Subcell Biochem*. 1996;25:109-15

- Coadminister fish oil (EPA) and GLA: Since EPA and other n-3 EFAs inhibit formation of GLA from LA[271][272] and since administration of GLA will probably increase levels of arachidonic acid unless EPA is coadministered[273], **the most reasonable clinical approach to improving eicosanoid metabolism in favor of reducing inflammation is to always combine GLA supplementation with EPA/DHA supplementation.** Coadministration of EPA or fish oil will prevent the rise in arachidonate that might occur with supplementation with GLA alone[274], and using GLA when using fish oil and EPA will prevent the reduction in GLA that occurs with administration of EPA alone[275]

Additional information:

- In my clinical practice, I only recommend GLA when I am already using fish oil. No patient has ever noted adverse effects even with doses as high as 4 grams per day of GLA for periods of months or years

Notes:

_____

_____

_____

_____

_____

_____

_____

_____

_____

_____

_____

_____

_____

_____

_____

_____

_____

_____

_____

_____

_____

_____

[271] Horrobin DF. Interactions between n-3 and n-6 essential fatty acids (EFAs) in the regulation of cardiovascular disorders and inflammation. *Prostaglandins Leukot Essent Fatty Acids* 1991 Oct;44(2):127-31

[272] Rubin D, Laposata M. Cellular interactions between n-6 and n-3 fatty acids: a mass analysis of fatty acid elongation/desaturation, distribution among complex lipids, and conversion to eicosanoids. *J Lipid Res.* 1992 Oct;33(10):1431-40

[273] "The decrease in serum eicosapentaenoic acid and the increase in arachidonic acid concentrations induced by evening primrose oil may not be favourable effects in patients with rheumatoid arthritis in the light of the roles of these fatty acids as precursors of eicosanoids." Jantti J, Nikkari T, Solakivi T, Vapaatalo H, Isomaki H. Evening primrose oil in rheumatoid arthritis: changes in serum lipids and fatty acids. *Ann Rheum Dis.* 1989 Feb;48(2):124-7

[274] "This study revealed that a GLA and EPA supplement combination may be utilized to reduce the synthesis of proinflammatory AA metabolites, and importantly, not induce potentially harmful increases in serum AA levels." Barham JB, Edens MB, Fonteh AN, Johnson MM, Easter L, Chilton FH. Addition of eicosapentaenoic acid to gamma-linolenic acid-supplemented diets prevents serum arachidonic acid accumulation in humans. *J Nutr.* 2000 Aug;130(8):1925-31

[275] "...intake of fish oil caused a significant depression in the content of DGLA... Since DGLA is the precursor of PGE1, which has been shown to be anti-inflammatory, our findings suggest that the anti-inflammatory effects of fish oil consumption could be mitigated by an associated reduction in DGLA." Cleland LG, Gibson RA, Neumann M, French JK. The effect of dietary fish oil supplement upon the content of dihomo-gammalinolenic acid in human plasma phospholipids. *Prostaglandins Leukot Essent Fatty Acids.* 1990 May;40(1):9-12

Vitamin:	**Vitamin D3**
Common name:	**Vitamin D, Cholecalciferol**

Applications and mechanisms of action:

- <u>Musculoskeletal Pain</u>: Vitamin D deficiency causes dull, achy musculoskeletal pain that is incompletely responsive to both pharmacologic and manual treatments. The pain may be widespread or confined to a particular area, most commonly the low-back and lumbar spine. The mechanism by which this pain is produced has been clearly elucidated by Holick[276]: 1) vitamin D deficiency causes a reduction in calcium absorption, 2) production of parathyroid hormone (PTH) is increased to maintain blood calcium levels, 3) PTH results in increased urinary excretion of phosphorus, which leads to hypophosphatemia, 4) insufficient calcium phosphate results in deposition of unmineralized collagen matrix on the endosteal (inside) and periosteal (outside) of bones, 5) when the collagen matrix hydrates and swells, it causes pressure on the sensory-innervated periosteum resulting in pain. Several clinical investigations have recently shown that vitamin D deficiency is particularly common among people with musculoskeletal pain.[277,278,279] Most importantly, the finding that musculoskeletal pain can be eliminated in a high proportion (>95%) of patients with vitamin D deficiency proves the cause-and-effect relationship between vitamin D deficiency and musculoskeletal pain; among patients who are deficient in vitamin D, their pain levels can be tremendously reduced within 3 months of high-dose vitamin D supplementation[280,281]

- **Anti-inflammatory effect**: Vitamin D has shown a modest anti-inflammatory benefit in two recent studies that used insufficient doses of vitamin D for insufficient durations[282,283]

Toxicity and contraindications:

- Vitamin D has a wide range of safety according to an extensive review of the literature performed by Vieth.[284]
- Doses of 2,000 IU per day of vitamin D3 have been given to children starting at one year of age and were not associated with toxicity but lead to a reduction in the incidence of type 1 diabetes by 80%.[285]
- **Vitamin D hypersensitivity syndromes are seen with primary hyperparathyroidism, granulomatous diseases (such as sarcoidosis, Crohn's disease, and tuberculosis), adrenal insufficiency, hyperthyroidism, hypothyroidism, various forms of cancer, as well as adverse drug effects, particularly with thiazide diuretics. When these patients require vitamin D supplementation, additional vigilance must be employed—1) starting with a lower dose of supplementation, and 2) more frequent monitoring of serum calcium.**
- Thiazide diuretics are known to potentiate hypercalcemia.

Dosage and administration:

- **Vitamin D deficiency and sufficiency are defined by analysis of serum 25(OH) vitamin D levels.** Serum 25(OH)D levels must be above 40 ng/mL (100 nmol/L) in order to sufficiently suppress any rise in PTH levels according to Zittermann[286], Dawson-Hughes et al[287] and Kinyamu et al[288]. Based on the current literature, in our recent review

[276] Holick MF. Vitamin D deficiency: what a pain it is. *Mayo Clin Proc*. 2003 Dec;78(12):1457-9
[277] Al Faraj S, Al Mutairi K. Vitamin D deficiency and chronic low back pain in Saudi Arabia. *Spine*. 2003 Jan 15;28(2):177-9
[278] Plotnikoff GA, Quigley JM. Prevalence of severe hypovitaminosis D in patients with persistent, nonspecific musculoskeletal pain. *Mayo Clin Proc*. 2003 Dec;78(12):1463-70
[279] Masood H, Narang AP, Bhat IA, Shah GN. Persistent limb pain and raised serum alkaline phosphatase the earliest markers of subclinical hypovitaminosis D in Kashmir. *Indian J Physiol Pharmacol*. 1989 Oct-Dec;33(4):259-61
[280] Al Faraj S, Al Mutairi K. Vitamin D deficiency and chronic low back pain in Saudi Arabia. *Spine*. 2003 Jan 15;28(2):177-9
[281] Masood H, Narang AP, Bhat IA, Shah GN. Persistent limb pain and raised serum alkaline phosphatase the earliest markers of subclinical hypovitaminosis D in Kashmir. *Indian J Physiol Pharmacol*. 1989 Oct-Dec;33(4):259-61
[282] Mahon BD, Gordon SA, Cruz J, Cosman F, Cantorna MT. Cytokine profile in patients with multiple sclerosis following vitamin D supplementation. *J Neuroimmunol*. 2003;134(1-2):128-32
[283] Van den Berghe G, et al. Bone turnover in prolonged critical illness: effect of vitamin D. *J Clin Endocrinol Metab*. 2003 Oct;88(10):4623-32
[284] Vieth R. Vitamin D supplementation, 25-hydroxyvitamin D concentrations, and safety. *Am J Clin Nutr*. 1999 May;69(5):842-56
[285] Hypponen E, Laara E, Reunanen A, Jarvelin MR, Virtanen SM. Intake of vitamin D and risk of type 1 diabetes: a birth-cohort study. *Lancet*. 2001 Nov 3;358(9292):1500-3
[286] Zittermann A. Vitamin D in preventive medicine: are we ignoring the evidence? *Br J Nutr*. 2003 May;89(5):552-72
[287] Dawson-Hughes B, Harris SS, Dallal GE. Plasma calcidiol, season, and serum parathyroid hormone concentrations in healthy elderly men and women. *Am J Clin Nutr*. 1997 Jan;65(1):67-71
[288] Kinyamu HK, Gallagher JC, Rafferty KA, Balhorn KE. Dietary calcium and vitamin D intake in elderly women: effect on serum parathyroid hormone and vitamin D metabolites. *Am J Clin Nutr*. 1998 Feb;67(2):342-8

of the literature[289], we proposed that **optimal vitamin D status is defined as 40 – 65 ng/mL (100 - 160 nmol/L).** This proposed optimal range is compatible with other published recommendations: Zittermann[290] states that serum levels of 40 - 80 ng/mL (100 - 200 nmol/L) are "adequate", and Mahon *et al*[291] recently advocated an optimal range of 40 - 100 ng/mL (100 - 250 nmol/L) for patients with multiple sclerosis. There are no acute or subacute risks associated with the 25(OH)D levels suggested here. Conversely, there is clear evidence of long-term danger associated with vitamin D levels that are *insufficient*.

- In our recent review article[292], we concluded, "Until proven otherwise, the balance of the research clearly indicates that oral supplementation in the range of 1,000 IU per day for infants, 2,000 IU per day for children and 4,000 IU per day for adults is safe and reasonable to meet physiologic requirements, to promote optimal health, and to reduce the risk of several serious diseases. Safety and effectiveness of supplementation are assured by periodic monitoring of serum 25(OH)D and serum calcium."

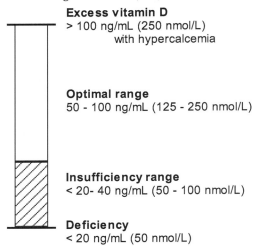

Excess vitamin D
> 100 ng/mL (250 nmol/L)
   with hypercalcemia

Optimal range
50 - 100 ng/mL (125 - 250 nmol/L)

Insufficiency range
< 20- 40 ng/mL (50 - 100 nmol/L)

Deficiency
< 20 ng/mL (50 nmol/L)

Interpretation of serum 25(OH) vitamin D levels.
Modified from Vasquez et al, *Alternative Therapies in Health and Medicine* 2004 and Vasquez A. *Musculoskeletal Pain: Expanded Clinical Strategies* (Institute for Functional Medicine) 2008.

Additional information:

- Exposure to sunlight can produce the equivalent of more than 10,000 IU vitamin D3 per day and can produce serum levels of 25(OH)D greater than 80 ng/mL (200 nmol/L).[293,294] No one has ever become vitamin D toxic from sun exposure.
- Patients with hypercalcemia should discontinue vitamin D supplementation and receive a thorough diagnostic evaluation to determine the cause of the problem.
- **Summary: vitamin D supplementation in the doses recommended here is generally very safe. However, safety *in a particular patient* is determined by periodic monitoring of serum calcium (perhaps weekly at first, then monthly until a steady state and confidence are attained). Routine vitamin D supplementation and testing for vitamin D insufficiency should become standard, day-to-day components of patient care. Caution must be used in patients predisposed to hypercalcemia ("vitamin D hypersensitivity syndromes") and patients taking drugs that affect calcium metabolism.**
- For additional research on the importance and safety of vitamin D, see the articles by Vieth[295], Heaney et al[296], Holick[297], and Vasquez, Manso, and Cannell.[298]

[289] Vasquez A, Manso G, Cannell J. The Clinical Importance of Vitamin D (Cholecalciferol): A Paradigm Shift with Implications for All Healthcare Providers. *Alternative Therapies in Health and Medicine* 2004; 10: 28-37. Also published in *Integrative Medicine: A Clinician's Journal* 2004; 3: 44-54. See optimalhealthresearch.com/monograph04
[290] Zittermann A. Vitamin D in preventive medicine: are we ignoring the evidence? *Br J Nutr*. 2003 May;89(5):552-72
[291] Mahon BD, Gordon SA, Cruz J, Cosman F, Cantorna MT. Cytokine profile in patients with multiple sclerosis following vitamin D supplementation. *J Neuroimmunol*. 2003;134(1-2):128-32
[292] Vasquez A, Manso G, Cannell J. The Clinical Importance of Vitamin D (Cholecalciferol): A Paradigm Shift with Implications for All Healthcare Providers. *Alternative Therapies in Health and Medicine* 2004; 10: 28-37. Also published in *Integrative Medicine: A Clinician's Journal* 2004; 3: 44-54. See optimalhealthresearch.com/monograph04
[293] Vieth R. Vitamin D supplementation, 25-hydroxyvitamin D concentrations, and safety. *Am J Clin Nutr*. 1999 May;69(5):842-56
[294] Holick MF. Calcium and Vitamin D. Diagnostics and Therapeutics. *Clin Lab Med*. 2000 Sep;20(3):569-90
[295] Vieth R. Vitamin D supplementation, 25-hydroxyvitamin D concentrations, and safety. *Am J Clin Nutr*. 1999 May;69(5):842-56

THE LANCET.com

May 6, 2005

Subphysiologic Doses of Vitamin D are Subtherapeutic: Comment on the Study by The Record Trial Group

Dear Editor,

Based on recently published research, it is clear that the study by The Record Trial Group [1] on vitamin D and calcium in the prevention of fractures suffered from at least four important shortcomings which negatively skewed their results.

First, and most important, the dose of vitamin D used in their study (800 IU/d) is subphysiologic and would therefore not be expected to produce a clinically meaningful effect. The physiologic requirement for vitamin D was determined scientifically in a recent study by Heaney and colleagues [2], who showed that healthy men utilize 3,000 to 5,000 IU of cholecalciferol per day, and several recent clinical trials have been published documenting the safety and effectiveness of administering vitamin D in physiologic doses of at least 4,000 IU per day.[3-5] In fact, studies have shown a dose-response relationship with vitamin D supplementation [6], and low doses (e.g., 600 IU) are clearly less effective than higher doses in the physiologic range (e.g., 4,000 IU).[5] It is important to note that the commonly used dose of vitamin D at 800 IU per day was not determined scientifically; rather this amount was determined arbitrarily before sufficient scientific methodology was available.[2,7] Given that the commonly recommended daily intake of vitamin D in the range of 200-800 IU is not sufficient for maintaining adequate serum levels of vitamin D [8], it is therefore incumbent upon modern researchers and clinicians to use doses of vitamin D that are consistent with the physiologic requirement as established in current research.

Second, the authors recognize that patient compliance in their study population was quite poor. This poor compliance obviously contributed to the purported lack of treatment efficacy.

Third, and consistent with recent data published elsewhere [8], virtually all of their patients were still vitamin D deficient at the end of one year of treatment, thereby affirming the inadequacy of the treatment dose. Vitamin D deficiency is common in industrialized nations, particularly those of northern latitudes [9-11], including the UK, where this study was performed. By modern criteria for serum vitamin D levels [12], virtually all of the patients in this study were vitamin D deficient at the beginning of the study, and the insufficient treatment dose of 800 IU/d failed to correct this deficiency even after 1 year of treatment. Given that vitamin D levels must be raised to approximately 40 ng/mL (100 nmol/L) in order to maximally reduce parathyroid hormone levels and bone resorption [13,14], supplementation that does not accomplish the goal of raising serum vitamin D levels into the optimal physiologic range cannot be considered adequate therapy.[12]

Fourth, and finally, there is reason to question the bioavailability of their vitamin D3 supplement, as the authors note that their dose-response was generally lower than that seen in other studies. Bioavailability is a prerequisite for treatment efficacy, and the elderly have higher likeliness of comorbid conditions that impair digestion and absorption of nutrients. Specifically, it is well documented that vitamin D absorption is decreased in elderly patients compared to younger controls [15,16], and this is complicated by an age-related reduction in renal calcitriol production [17,18] and intestinal vitamin D receptors [19], thereby further impairing vitamin D metabolism and calcium absorption. Since emulsification of fat soluble vitamins is required for their absorption [20], and since pre-emulsification of nutrients has been shown to increase absorption and dose-responsiveness of the fat-soluble nutrient coenzyme Q [21, 22], it seems apparent that attention to the form (not merely the dose) of nutrient supplementation is clinically important, particularly when working with elderly patients.

---

[296] Heaney RP, Davies KM, Chen TC, Holick MF, Barger-Lux MJ. Human serum 25-hydroxycholecalciferol response to extended oral dosing with cholecalciferol. *Am J Clin Nutr*. 2003 Jan;77(1):204-10

[297] Holick MF. Vitamin D: importance in the prevention of cancers, type 1 diabetes, heart disease, and osteoporosis. *Am J Clin Nutr*. 2004 Mar;79(3):362-71

[298] Vasquez A, Manso G, Cannell J. The Clinical Importance of Vitamin D (Cholecalciferol): A Paradigm Shift with Implications for All Healthcare Providers. *Alternative Therapies in Health and Medicine* 2004; 10: 28-37. Also published in *Integrative Medicine: A Clinician's Journal* 2004; 3: 44-54. See optimalhealthresearch.com/monograph04

These shortcomings, when combined, could have lead to an additive or synergistic reduction in treatment potency that skewed their results toward a conclusion of inefficacy. In order to produce more meaningful results in clinical trials, our group published guidelines [12] recommending that future studies 1) ensure patient compliance, 2) use physiologic doses of vitamin D (e.g., 4,000 IU per day), and 3) ensure that serum levels are raised to a minimum of 40 ng/mL (100 nmol/L), since levels below this threshold are associated with increased parathyroid hormone levels, increased bone resorption, and recalcitrance to bone-building interventions.[23,24]

Alex Vasquez
Biotics Research Corporation
Rosenberg, Texas, USA 77471

Competing Interests: Dr. Vasquez is a researcher at Biotics Research Corporation, an FDA-licensed drug manufacturing facility in the USA.

References:

1. Record Trial Group. Oral vitamin D3 and calcium for secondary prevention of low-trauma fractures in elderly people (Randomised Evaluation of Calcium Or vitamin D, RECORD): a randomised placebo-controlled trial. *Lancet* (Early Online Publication), 28 April 2005

2. Heaney RP, Davies KM, Chen TC, Holick MF, Barger-Lux MJ. Human serum 25-hydroxycholecalciferol response to extended oral dosing with cholecalciferol. *Am J Clin Nutr* 2003;77:204-10

3. Vieth R, Chan PC, MacFarlane GD. Efficacy and safety of vitamin D3 intake exceeding the lowest observed adverse effect level. *Am J Clin Nutr*. 2001;73:288-94

4. Al Faraj S, Al Mutairi K. Vitamin D deficiency and chronic low back pain in Saudi Arabia. *Spine*. 2003;28:177-9

5. Vieth R, Kimball S, Hu A, Walfish PG. Randomized comparison of the effects of the vitamin D3 adequate intake versus 100 mcg (4000 IU) per day on biochemical responses and the wellbeing of patients. *Nutr J*. 2004 Jul 19;3(1):8 http://www.nutritionj.com/content/pdf/1475-2891-3-8.pdf

6. Van den Berghe G, Van Roosbroeck D, Vanhove P, Wouters PJ, De Pourcq L, Bouillon R. Bone turnover in prolonged critical illness: effect of vitamin D. *J Clin Endocrinol Metab*. 2003;88:4623-32

7. Vieth R. Vitamin D supplementation, 25-hydroxyvitamin D concentrations, and safety. *Am J Clin Nutr*. 1999;69:842-56 http://www.ajcn.org/cgi/reprint/69/5/842.pdf

8. Glerup H, Mikkelsen K, Poulsen L, Hass E, Overbeck S, Thomsen J, Charles P, Eriksen EF. Commonly recommended daily intake of vitamin D is not sufficient if sunlight exposure is limited. *J Intern Med*. 2000;247:260-8

9. Thomas MK, Lloyd-Jones DM, Thadhani RI, Shaw AC, Deraska DJ, Kitch BT, Vamvakas EC, Dick IM, Prince RL, Finkelstein JS. Hypovitaminosis D in medical inpatients. *N Engl J Med* 1998;338:777-83

10. Dubbelman R, Jonxis JH, Muskiet FA, Saleh AE. Age-dependent vitamin D status and vertebral condition of white women living in Curacao (The Netherlands Antilles) as compared with their counterparts in The Netherlands. *Am J Clin Nutr* 1993;58:106-9

11. Kauppinen-Makelin R, Tahtela R, Loyttyniemi E, Karkkainen J, Valimaki MJ. A high prevalence of hypovitaminosis D in Finnish medical in- and outpatients. *J Intern Med*. 2001;249:559-63

12. Vasquez A, Manso G, Cannell J. The clinical importance of vitamin D (cholecalciferol): a paradigm shift with implications for all healthcare providers. *Altern Ther Health Med*. 2004;10:28-36; quiz 37, 94

13. Kinyamu HK, Gallagher JC, Rafferty KA, Balhorn KE. Dietary calcium and vitamin D intake in elderly women: effect on serum parathyroid hormone and vitamin D metabolites. *Am J Clin Nutr* 1998;67:342-8

14. Dawson-Hughes B, Harris SS, Dallal GE. Plasma calcidiol, season, and serum parathyroid hormone concentrations in healthy elderly men and women. *Am J Clin Nutr* 1997;65:67-71

15. Harris SS, Dawson-Hughes B, Perrone GA. Plasma 25-hydroxyvitamin D responses of younger and older men to three weeks of supplementation with 1800 IU/day of vitamin D. *J Am Coll Nutr*. 1999;18:470-4

16. Barragry JM, France MW, Corless D, Gupta SP, Switala S, Boucher BJ, Cohen RD. Intestinal cholecalciferol absorption in the elderly and in younger adults. *Clin Sci Mol Med*. 1978;55:213-20

17. Tsai KS, Heath H 3rd, Kumar R, Riggs BL. Impaired vitamin D metabolism with aging in women. Possible role in pathogenesis of senile osteoporosis. *J Clin Invest*. 1984;73:1668-72

18. Gallagher JC, Riggs BL, Eisman J, Hamstra A, Arnaud SB, DeLuca HF. Intestinal calcium absorption and serum vitamin D metabolites in normal subjects and osteoporotic patients: effect of age and dietary calcium. *J Clin Invest*. 1979;64:729-36

19. Ebeling PR, Sandgren ME, DiMagno EP, Lane AW, DeLuca HF, Riggs BL. Evidence of an age-related decrease in intestinal responsiveness to vitamin D: relationship between serum 1,25-dihydroxyvitamin D3 and intestinal vitamin D receptor concentrations in normal women. *J Clin Endocrinol Metab*. 1992;75:176-82

20. Gallo-Torres HE. Obligatory role of bile for the intestinal absorption of vitamin E. *Lipids*. 1970;5:379-84

21. Bucci LR, Pillors M, Medlin R, Henderson R, Stiles JC, Robol HJ, Sparks WS. Enhanced uptake in humans of coenzyme Q10 from an emulsified form. *Third International Congress of Biomedical Gerontology*; Acapulco, Mexico: June 1989

22. Bucci LR, Pillors M, Medlin R, Klenda B, Robol H, Stiles JC, Sparks WS. Enhanced blood levels of coenzyme Q-10 from an emulsified oral form. In Faruqui SR and Ansari MS (editors). *Second Symposium on Nutrition and Chiropractic Proceedings*. April 15-16, 1989 in Davenport, Iowa

23. Stepan JJ, Burckhardt P, Hana V. The effects of three-month intravenous ibandronate on bone mineral density and bone remodeling in Klinefelter's syndrome: the influence of vitamin D deficiency and hormonal status. *Bone* 2003;33:589-596

24. Vasquez A. Health care for our bones: a practical nutritional approach to preventing osteoporosis. [letter] *J Manipulative* Physiol Ther. 2005;28:213

Citation: Vasquez A. Subphysiologic Doses of Vitamin D are Subtherapeutic: Comment on the Study by The Record Trial Group. *Lancet* 2005 published online May 6

Internet: http://www.thelancet.com/journals/lancet/article/PIIS0140673605630139/comments

Vitamin: *Alpha-tocopherol, beta-tocopherol, delta-tocopherol, gamma-tocopherol*

Common name: **Vitamin E**

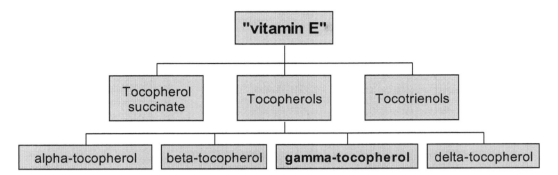

Applications and mechanisms of action:

- Antioxidant: vitamin E is a tremendously important fat-soluble antioxidant vitamin that is generally non-toxic in doses up to 3,200 IU per day.[299] Given that increased oxidative stress is associated with nearly every known disease including the aging process itself, common sense provides us with sufficient justification for the use of vitamin E as a matter of course in nearly all patients, including those who are asymptomatic.

- Anti-inflammatory and analgesic: The gamma form of vitamin E inhibits cyclooxygenase and thus has anti-inflammatory activity.[300] Patients with **rheumatoid arthritis** treated with methotrexate, oral sulfasalazine, and indomethacin show significant subjective and objective improvements when antioxidants and vitamin E are added to the treatment plan.[301] Another study of patients with RA showed no biochemical evidence of improvement, but patients reported a reduction in pain.[302] An abstract from the foreign medical research found that patients with **spondylosis and back pain** had lower levels of vitamin E than did the control group, and that administration of vitamin E lead to "complete pain relief" and "cure" of spondylosis.[303] German research abstracts state that vitamin E is able to reduce the pain and swelling associated with **osteoarthritis**[304] and that higher serum levels of vitamin E following supplementation correlated with improved clinical outcome.[305] Indeed the majority of research suggests a mild-moderate analgesic and anti-inflammatory effect of vitamin E in patients with arthritis.[306] The noteworthy research by Ayres and Mihan[307] has suggested that vitamin E may have efficacy in the treatment of **autoimmune diseases** via its antioxidant and membrane-stabilizing effects; the authors state, "Among the diseases that were successfully controlled were a number in the autoimmune category, including **scleroderma**, **discoid lupus erythematosus**[308], **porphyria cutanea tarda**, several types of **vasculitis**, and **polymyositis**.[309] Since vitamin E is a physiologic stabilizer of cellular and lysosomal membranes, and since some autoimmune diseases respond to vitamin E, we suggest that a relative deficiency

[299] Meydani M. Vitamin E. *Lancet.* 1995 Jan 21;345(8943):170-5
[300] Jiang Q, Christen S, Shigenaga MK, Ames BN. gamma-tocopherol, the major form of vitamin E in the US diet, deserves more attention. *Am J Clin Nutr* 2001;74(6):714-22
[301] Helmy M, Shohayeb M, Helmy MH, el-Bassiouni EA. Antioxidants as adjuvant therapy in rheumatoid disease. A preliminary study. *Arzneimittelforschung.* 2001;51(4):293-8
[302] Edmonds SE, Winyard PG, Guo R, Kidd B, Merry P, Langrish-Smith A, Hansen C, Ramm S, Blake DR. Putative analgesic activity of repeated oral doses of vitamin E in the treatment of rheumatoid arthritis. Results of a prospective placebo controlled double blind trial. *Ann Rheum Dis.* 1997 Nov;56(11):649-55
[303] Mahmud Z, Ali SM. Role of vitamin A and E in spondylosis. *Bangladesh Med Res Counc Bull.* 1992 Apr;18(1):47-59
[304] Blankenhorn G. [Clinical effectiveness of Spondyvit (vitamin E) in activated arthroses. A multicenter placebo-controlled double-blind study] [Article in German] *Z Orthop Ihre Grenzgeb.* 1986 May-Jun;124(3):340-3
[305] Scherak O, Kolarz G, Schodl C, Blankenhorn G. [High dosage vitamin E therapy in patients with activated arthrosis] [Article in German] Z Rheumatol. 1990 Nov-Dec;49(6):369-73
[306] Machtey I, Ouaknine L. Tocopherol in Osteoarthritis: a controlled pilot study. *J Am Geriatr Soc.* 1978 Jul;26(7):328-30
[307] Ayres S Jr, Mihan R. Is vitamin E involved in the autoimmune mechanism? *Cutis.* 1978 Mar;21(3):321-5
[308] Ayres S Jr, Mihan R. Lupus erythematosus and vitamin E: an effective and nontoxic therapy. *Cutis.* 1979 Jan;23(1):49-52, 54
[309] Killeen RN, Ayres S Jr, Mihan R. Polymyositis: response to vitamin E. *South Med J.* 1976 Oct;69(10):1372-4

of vitamin E damages lysosomal membranes, thus initiating the autoimmune process."

- *Other uses*: In dialysis patients who suffer from leg cramps, vitamin E is just as effective but less toxic that quinine.[310]

Toxicity and contraindications:

- <u>Anticoagulant medications, surgery, and bleeding</u>: Vitamin E has some weak ability to impair coagulation. Therefore it should be used advisedly in patients taking other "blood thinners" such as aspirin, fish oil, and ginkgo. Particular care and attention are needed when coadministering vitamin E with coumadin/warfarin. Any clinically significant increase in bleeding or bruising associated with vitamin E supplementation indicates the need for dosage reduction.

Dosage and administration:

- <u>400 IU BID-TID</u>: "Vitamin E" should be administered in a mixed tocopherol combination that provides a high percentage (i.e., ~40%) of gamma-tocopherol. Common doses are 400 IU BID-TID. While consumption of sesame seeds raises gamma-tocopherol levels[311], all researchers agree that consumption of vitamin E supplements is necessary to obtain the high doses necessary to achieve clinical benefit in severe illnesses.

Additional information:

- The term "vitamin E" applies to several different chemicals, each with its own biochemical and clinical effects. Generally speaking, regarding the tocopherols, alpha- and gamma- are the most important, with gamma-appearing to provide the greatest degree of benefit. Most multivitamin products contain only the alpha-form of the vitamin, which unfavorably impairs gamma-tocopherol function and creates the illusion that one is obtaining sufficient vitamin E supplementation despite the lack of the most important form of vitamin E: gamma-tocopherol.
- The "dl" forms of vitamin E are synthetic and should be avoided; adverse effects from this type of vitamin E include transient hypertension and headache.
- Many of the clinical trials with vitamin E, especially those reporting negative effects have used either 1) the synthetic "dl" form of the vitamin, 2) exclusively alpha-tocopherol, rather than the blend of all tocopherols, or 3) have used insufficient doses to achieve clinical benefit. Thus the "failure of vitamin E" in these studies is directly related to the failure by these researchers to understand the basic pharmacodynamics of the agent they were testing, namely that vitamin E comes in different forms with different effects and that the commonly used alpha-tocopherol does not possess the stronger anti-inflammatory, antiproliferative, and analgesic effects of gamma-tocopherol. Furthermore, in conditions such as rheumatoid arthritis and other inflammatory conditions that are characterized by greatly increased oxidative stress, low doses of antioxidant supplementation are barely sufficient for creating a state of *normal* redox potential and are thus unable to provide clinical "supranutritional" or pharmacologic benefit.

[310] Roca AO, Jarjoura D, Blend D, Cugino A, Rutecki GW, Nuchikat PS, Whittier FC. Dialysis leg cramps. Efficacy of quinine versus vitamin E. *ASAIO J.* 1992 Jul-Sep;38(3):M481-5
[311] Cooney RV, Custer LJ, Okinaka L, Franke AA. Effects of dietary sesame seeds on plasma tocopherol levels. *Nutr Cancer.* 2001;39(1):66-71

Vitamin:	## Niacinamide
Common name:	## Niacinamide, Nicotinamide, Vitamin B3

Applications and mechanisms of action:	▪ <u>Joint pain and inflammation</u>: The credit for discovering the effectiveness of niacinamide in the treatment of arthritis goes to Kaufman, whose studies published in 1949 documented the safety and efficacy in hundreds of patients with **rheumatoid arthritis** and **osteoarthritis**. While the mechanism of action is probably multifaceted, inhibition of joint-destroying nitric oxide appears to be an important benefit.[312] A recent double-blind placebo-controlled study found that niacinamide therapy improved joint mobility, reduced objective inflammation as assessed by ESR, reduced the impact of the arthritis on the activities of daily living, and allowed a reduction in medication use.[313]
Toxicity and contraindications:	▪ The treatment is generally safe ▪ <u>Liver damage</u>: Given that a small risk for liver damage exists, liver enzymes should be assessed before and after the first month of treatment and periodically thereafter in patients receiving more than 2,000 mg per day. Patients are advised to discontinue treatment with the onset of abdominal pain, jaundice or nausea.
Dosage and administration:	▪ <u>Doses have ranged from 1,000 mg per day to 4,000 mg per day. 500 mg 4-6 times per day is a common dosing regimen</u>. ▪ The most important clinical pearl for improving the effectiveness of niacinamide in the treatment of osteoarthritis is found in the timing and distribution of the dosing. The treatment must be administered several times per day in small doses rather than a few times per day in large doses. As Gaby and Wright[314] point out, "500 mg taken 3 times a day is about half as effective as 250 mg taken every 3 hours for 6 doses, even though the total daily dose is the same." ▪ Treatment must be maintained for a minimum of 4 weeks before beneficial subjective and objective improvements can be expected. The general trend is rapid improvement in joint mobility and a reduction in pain in the first 1-2 months followed by slower improvement which may continue for the next 1-3 years. ▪ Improved results may be seen with concomitant administration of other vitamins, particularly thiamine and riboflavin.
Additional information:	▪ To refer to niacinamide as "vitamin B-3" is accurate, but to refer to "vitamin B-3" as niacinamide is somewhat incomplete since vitamin B-3 represents a family of related compounds including 1) niacinamide, 2) NADH, 2) plain niacin, 3) time-released niacin (hepatotoxic), 4) prescription strength sustained-release niacin ("Niaspan"), and 5) inositol hexaniacinate. Each form of niacin has its form, function, clinical applications, risk and safety.

---

[312] McCarty MF, Russell AL. Niacinamide therapy for osteoarthritis--does it inhibit nitric oxide synthase induction by interleukin 1 in chondrocytes? *Med Hypotheses*. 1999 Oct;53(4):350-60
[313] Jonas WB, Rapoza CP, Blair WF. The effect of niacinamide on osteoarthritis: a pilot study. *Inflamm Res* 1996 Jul;45(7):330-4
[314] Gaby AR, Wright JV. <u>Nutritional therapy in medical practice. Reference manual and study guide. 1996 edition</u>. Wright/Gaby Seminars 1996. page 102

Nutrient:	## Glucosamine Sulfate ## Chondroitin Sulfate

Applications and mechanisms of action:

- <u>Promotion of cartilage regeneration</u>: Glucosamine and chondroitin stimulate the synthesis of glycosaminoglycan, proteoglycan and hyaluronic acid, which are the "building blocks" of joint cartilage. The goal with supplementation with glucosamine/chondroitin is to shift the anabolic:catabolic ratio in favor of cartilage formation rather than cartilage destruction. Thus, the classic application for glucosamine/chondroitin is the treatment of joint degeneration and joint pain seen with osteoarthritis.[315,316,317] A recent study showed that glucosamine sulfate 500 mg TID was nearly as effective as and much safer than ibuprofen 400 mg TID for the relief of knee pain.[318] Glucosamine sulfate 500 mg TID is superior to ibuprofen 400 mg TID for the treatment of TMJ osteoarthritis.[319]

Toxicity and contraindications:

- <u>Allergy</u>: Immediate allergy to glucosamine sulfate has been reported, as has another case involving exacerbation of asthma in a patient following supplementation with glucosamine and chondroitin.[320] Since glucosamine is commonly sourced from shells of shrimp, crab, or lobster, it is conceivable that people with **hypersensitivity to shellfish or seafood** might have an allergic response to the ingestion of glucosamine. Such people should either avoid glucosamine supplementation or use glucosamine from a synthetic/hypoallergenic source.
- Glucosamine is safe in patients with diabetes, as it does not alter blood glucose or HgbA1c levels.[321]

Dosage and administration:

- <u>Glucosamine 1500 mg and/or chondroitin 1000-1,500 mg in divided doses</u>: Can be taken with or without food.
- Treatment must be continued for at least eight weeks before significant results can be expected. Long-term treatment for several years is both safe and effective in treating joint pain and reducing progression of joint destruction.[322]

Additional information:

- To improve results, glucosamine can be coadministered with niacinamide and botanical antiinflammatories, particularly *Uncaria.*
- Chondroitin sulfate is cardioprotective and ameliorates atherosclerosis.[323,324,325,326]

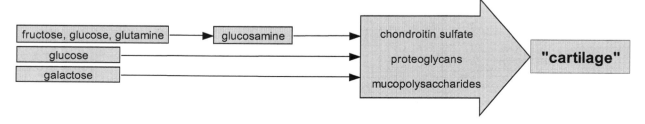

[315] Braham R, Dawson B, Goodman C. The effect of glucosamine supplementation on people experiencing regular knee pain. *Br J Sports Med.* 2003;37(1):45-9

[316] Nguyen P, Mohamed SE, Gardiner D, Salinas T. A randomized double-blind clinical trial of the effect of chondroitin sulfate and glucosamine hydrochloride on temporomandibular joint disorders: a pilot study. *Cranio.* 2001 Apr;19(2):130-9

[317] "...oral glucosamine therapy achieved a significantly greater improvement in articular pain score than ibuprofen, and the investigators rated treatment efficacy as 'good' in a significantly greater proportion of glucosamine than ibuprofen recipients. In comparison with piroxicam, glucosamine significantly improved arthritic symptoms after 12 weeks of therapy..." Matheson AJ, Perry CM. Glucosamine: a review of its use in the management of osteoarthritis. *Drugs Aging.* 2003; 20(14): 1041-60

[318] Muller-Fassbender H, Bach GL, Haase W, Rovati LC, Setnikar I. Glucosamine sulfate compared to ibuprofen in osteoarthritis of the knee. *Osteoarthritis Cartilage.* 1994 Mar;2(1):61-9

[319] "...patients taking GS had a significantly greater decrease in TMJ pain with function, effect of pain, and acetaminophen used between Day 90 and 120 compared with patients taking ibuprofen." Thie NM, Prasad NG, Major PW. Evaluation of glucosamine sulfate compared to ibuprofen for the treatment of temporomandibular joint osteoarthritis: a randomized double blind controlled 3 month clinical trial. *J Rheumatol.* 2001 Jun;28(6):1347-55

[320] Tallia AF, Cardone DA. Asthma exacerbation associated with glucosamine-chondroitin supplement. J Am Board Fam Pract. 2002 Nov-Dec;15(6):481-4 Available at http://www.jabfp.org/cgi/reprint/15/6/481.pdf on March 21, 2004

[321] Scroggie DA, Albright A, Harris MD. The effect of glucosamine-chondroitin supplementation on glycosylated hemoglobin levels in patients with type 2 diabetes mellitus: a placebo-controlled, double-blinded, randomized clinical trial. *Arch Intern Med.* 2003 Jul 14;163(13):1587-90

[322] "Long-term treatment with glucosamine sulfate retarded the progression of knee osteoarthritis, possibly determining disease modification." Pavelka K, Gatterova J, Olejarova M, Machacek S, Giacovelli G, Rovati LC. Glucosamine sulfate use and delay of progression of knee osteoarthritis: a 3-year, randomized, placebo-controlled, double-blind study. *Arch Intern Med.* 2002 Oct 14;162(18):2113-23

[323] Morrison LM. Treatment of coronary arteriosclerotic heart disease with chondroitin sulfate-A: preliminary report. *J Am Geriatr Soc.* 1968;16(7):779-85

[324] Morrison LM, Branwood AW, Ershoff BH, Murata K, Quilligan JJ Jr, Schjeide OA, Patek P, Bernick S, Freeman L, Dunn OJ, Rucker P. The prevention of coronary arteriosclerotic heart disease with chondroitin sulfate A: preliminary report. *Exp Med Surg.* 1969;27(3):278-89

[325] Morrison LM, Bajwa GS. Absence of naturally occurring coronary atherosclerosis in squirrel monkeys (Saimiri sciurea) treated with chondroitin sulfate A. *Experientia.* 1972 Dec 15;28(12):1410-1

[326] Morrison LM, Enrick N. Coronary heart disease: reduction of death rate by chondroitin sulfate A. *Angiology.* 1973 May;24(5):269-87

Nutrients:	**Pancreatin, bromelain, papain, trypsin and alpha-chymotrypsin**
Common name:	**"Proteolytic enzymes" "Pancreatic enzymes"**

Applications and mechanisms of action:

- Actions and mechanisms: Orally administered proteolytic enzymes are well absorbed from the gastrointestinal tract into the systemic circulation[327,328] and that the anti-tumor, anti-metastatic, anti-infectious, anti-inflammatory , analgesic, and anti-edematous actions result from synergism between a variety of mechanisms of action, including the dose-dependent stimulation of reactive oxygen species production and anti-cancer cytotoxicity in human neutrophils[329], a pro-differentiative effect[330], reduction in PG-E2 production[331], reduction in substance P production[332], modulation of adhesion molecules and cytokine levels[333], fibrinolytic effects and a anti-thrombotic effect mediated at least in part by a reduction in 2-series thromboxanes.[334]

- Acute injuries: Reporting from the Tulane University Health Service Center, Trickett[335] reported that a papain-containing preparation benefited 40 patients with various injuries (e.g., contusions, sprains, lacerations, strains, fracture, surgical repair, and muscle tears); no adverse effects were seen. Bromelain also attenuates experimental contraction-induced skeletal muscle injury[336] and reduces production of hyperalgesic PG-E2 and substance P[337],

- Osteoarthritis: Walker et al[338] found a dose-dependent reduction in pain and disability as well as a significant improvement in psychological well-being in patients consuming bromelain orally. Most of the bromelain studies reviewed by Brien et al[339] were suggestive of a positive benefit in patients with knee osteoarthritis, but inadequate dosing clearly prohibited the attainment of optimal results.

- Sinusitis: In a double-blind placebo-controlled trial with 59 patients, Taub[340] documented that oral administration of bromelain significantly promoted the resolution of congestion, inflammation, and edema in patients with acute and chronic refractory sinusitis; no adverse effects were seen in any patient.

- Anti-cancer benefit: One of the first experimental studies was published by Beard in 1906 in the *British Medical Journal* wherein he showed that proteolytic enzymes significantly inhibited tumor growth in mice with implanted tumors[341], and a year later in that same journal, Cutfield[342] reported tumor regression and other objective improvements in a patient treated with proteolytic enzymes. In the American research literature, anti-cancer effects of proteolytic enzymes were reported during this same time in the *Journal of the American Medical Association* in anecdotal case reports of patients with fibrosarcoma[343], breast cancer[344], and head and neck malignancy[345]—all

[327] Gotze H, Rothman SS. Enteropancreatic circulation of digestive enzymes as a conservative mechanism. *Nature* 1975; 257(5527): 607-609
[328] Liebow C, Rothman SS. Enteropancreatic Circulation of Digestive Enzymes. *Science* 1975; 189(4201): 472-474
[329] Zavadova E, Desser L, Mohr T. Stimulation of reactive oxygen species production and cytotoxicity in human neutrophils in vitro and after oral administration of a polyenzyme preparation. *Cancer Biother.* 1995;10(2):147-52
[330] Maurer HR, Hozumi M, Honma Y, Okabe-Kado J. Bromelain induces the differentiation of leukemic cells in vitro: an explanation for its cytostatic effects? *Planta Med.* 1988;54(5):377-81
[331] Brien S, Lewith G, Walker A, Hicks SM, Middleton D. Bromelain as a Treatment for Osteoarthritis: a Review of Clinical Studies. *Evidence-based Complementary and Alternative Medicine.* 2004;1(3)251–257
[332] Gaspani L, Limiroli E, Ferrario P, Bianchi M. In vivo and in vitro effects of bromelain on PGE(2) and SP concentrations in the inflammatory exudate in rats. *Pharmacology.* 2002;65(2):83-6
[333] Leipner J, Saller R. Systemic enzyme therapy in oncology: effect and mode of action. *Drugs.* 2000 Apr;59(4):769-80
[334] Vellini M, Desideri D, Milanese A, Omini C, Daffonchio L, Hernandez A, Brunelli G. Possible involvement of eicosanoids in the pharmacological action of bromelain. *Arzneimittelforschung.* 1986;36(1):110-2
[335] Trickett P. Proteolytic enzymes in treatment of athletic injuries. *Appl Ther.* 1964;30:647-52
[336] Walker JA, Cerny FJ, Cotter JR, Burton HW. Attenuation of contraction-induced skeletal muscle injury by bromelain. *Med Sci Sports Exerc.* 1992 Jan;24(1):20-5
[337] Gaspani L, Limiroli E, Ferrario P, Bianchi M. In vivo and in vitro effects of bromelain on PGE(2) and SP concentrations in the inflammatory exudate in rats. *Pharmacology.* 2002;65(2):83-6
[338] Walker AF, Bundy R, Hicks SM, Middleton RW. Bromelain reduces mild acute knee pain and improves well-being in a dose-dependent fashion in an open study of otherwise healthy adults.*Phytomedicine.*2002;9:681-6
[339] Brien S, Lewith G, Walker A, Hicks SM, Middleton D. Bromelain as a Treatment for Osteoarthritis: a Review of Clinical Studies. *Evidence-based Complementary and Alternative Medicine.* 2004;1(3)251–257
[340] Taub SJ. The use of bromelains in sinusitis: a double-blind clinical evaluation. Eye Ear Nose Throat Mon. 1967 Mar;46(3):361-5
[341] Beard J. The action of trypsin upon the living cells of Jensen's mouse-tumour. *Br Med J* 1906; 4 (Jan 20): 140-1
[342] Cutfield A. Trypsin Treatment in Malignant Disease. *Br Med J.* 1907; 5: 525
[343] Wiggin FH. Case of Multiple Fibrosarcoma of the Tongue, With Remarks on the Use of Trypsin and Amylopsin in the Treatment of Malignant Disease." *Journal of the American Medical Association* 1906; 47: 2003-8
[344] Goeth RA. Pancreatic treatment of cancer, with report of a cure. *Journal of the American Medical Association* 1907; (March 23) 48: 1030
[345] Campbell JT. Trypsin Treatment of a Case of Malignant Disease. *Journal of the American Medical Association* 1907; 48: 225-226

of whom responded positively to the administration of proteolytic enzymes; no adverse effects were seen. Nearly a century would pass before Beard's study and results were replicated with modern techniques[346,347], and modern controlled clinical trials in cancer patients have established the value of enzyme therapy, which produces important clinical benefit (e.g., symptom reduction and prolonged survival) for little cost and with negligible adverse effects.[348,349,350]

Toxicity and contraindications:

- Allergy: As with all treatments—dietary, nutritional, botanical, and pharmaceutical— allergy is generally a manifestation of immune dysfunction which requires specific and personalized treatment. In the meanwhile, or when normalization of immune function is not achieved, then of course the "offending agent" should be avoided. Allergy to proteolytic enzymes is rare; but some patients manifest allergy as rectal itching following the oral administration of enzymes, particularly bromelain.

- Theoretical contraindications: Most doctors are aware of a potential anticoagulant effect and therefore proceed cautiously when using proteolytic enzymes in patients on anticoagulant medications. It is reasonable to discontinue supplements that have an anticoagulant effect for at least one week before any surgical procedures. Likewise, since safety during pregnancy has not been conclusively demonstrated, doctors would be wise to avoid use in patients who are pregnant; lactation is probably not a legitimate reason to withhold use of proteolytic/pancreatic enzymes.

Dosage and administration:

- Although bromelain may be used in isolation, enzyme therapy is generally delivered in the form of polyenzyme preparations containing pancreatin, bromelain, papain, amylase, lipase, trypsin and alpha-chymotrypsin.

- Dosage is determined per product and obviously tailored per patient. The therapeutic margin is exceedingly large, and therefore overdose/toxicity is unlikely with any reasonable dosage regimen.

Additional information:

- Most of the early studies in humans were done with a German-made formulation called "Wobenzym" which no longer exists and which is commonly confused with a product called "Wobenzym-N" which is not chemically or clinically identical to the original formulation. The closest formulation to the original "Wobenzym" is "Intenzyme Forte" from Biotics Research Corporation. I commonly use 8 tablets 3 times per day in patients with cancer, marked inflammation, or infection since the effectiveness of proteolytic/pancreatic enzymes is dose-dependent[351] up to approximately the dose I have described here. Since each tablet contains 50 mg of bromelain, then only 4 tablets per day would be required to produce relief from osteoarthritis according to the study by Walker et al[352] even if there were no other components in the product.

- The anticancer benefits of proteolytic/pancreatic enzymes are augmented by the use of thymus extract. Some studies that emphasize the use of "oral enzymes" in their title and abstract actually use enzymes *with thymus extract* according to the details in the methodology section of the printed paper.[353] Proteolytic/pancreatic enzymes by themselves have anticancer benefits, and thymus extract is immunosupportive — indeed immunostimulatory — especially in elderly and severely ill patients.

[346] Saruc M, Standop S, Standop J, Nozawa F, Itami A, Pandey KK, Batra SK, Gonzalez NJ, Guesry P, Pour PM. Pancreatic enzyme extract improves survival in murine pancreatic cancer. *Pancreas.* 2004;28(4):401-12
[347] Batkin S, Taussig SJ, Szekerezes J. Antimetastatic effect of bromelain with or without its proteolytic and anticoagulant activity. *J Cancer Res Clin Oncol.* 1988;114(5):507-8
[348] Gonzalez NJ, Isaacs LL. Evaluation of pancreatic proteolytic enzyme treatment of adenocarcinoma of the pancreas, with nutrition and detoxification support. *Nutr Cancer.* 1999;33(2):117-24
[349] Sakalova A, Bock PR, Dedik L, Hanisch J, Schiess W, Gazova S, Chabronova I, Holomanova D, Mistrik M, Hrubisko M. Retrolective cohort study of an additive therapy with an oral enzyme preparation in patients with multiple myeloma. *Cancer Chemother Pharmacol.* 2001 Jul;47 Suppl:S38-44
[350] Popiela T, Kulig J, Hanisch J, Bock PR. Influence of a complementary treatment with oral enzymes on patients with colorectal cancers--an epidemiological retrolective cohort study. *Cancer Chemother Pharmacol.* 2001;47 Suppl:S55-63
[351] Zavadova E, Desser L, Mohr T. Stimulation of reactive oxygen species production and cytotoxicity in human neutrophils in vitro and after oral administration of a polyenzyme preparation. *Cancer Biother.* 1995 Summer;10(2):147-52
[352] Walker AF, Bundy R, Hicks SM, Middleton RW. Bromelain reduces mild acute knee pain and improves well-being in a dose-dependent fashion in an open study of otherwise healthy adults.*Phytomedicine.*2002;9:681-6
[353] Sakalova A, Bock PR, Dedik L, Hanisch J, Schiess W, Gazova S, Chabronova I, Holomanova D, Mistrik M, Hrubisko M. Retrolective cohort study of an additive therapy with an oral enzyme preparation in patients with multiple myeloma. *Cancer Chemother Pharmacol.* 2001 Jul;47 Suppl:S38-44

Botanical Medicine:	***Zingiber officinale***
Common name:	**Ginger**

Applications and mechanisms of action:

- <u>Anti-inflammatory and analgesic actions:</u> Ginger is a well known spice and food with a long history of use as an anti-inflammatory, anti-nausea, and gastroprotective agent.[354] Components of ginger have been shown to reduce production of the leukotriene LTB4 by inhibiting 5-lipoxygenase and to reduce production of the prostaglandin PG-E2 by inhibiting cyclooxygenase.[355,356] With its dual reduction in the formation of inflammation-promoting prostaglandins and leukotrienes, ginger has been shown to safely reduce **musculoskeletal pain in general**[357,358] and to provide relief from **osteoarthritis** of the knees[359] and **migraine headaches**.[360]

Toxicity and contraindications:

- Doses up to one gram of ginger per day have been safely used during pregnancy to reduce the nausea and vomiting of pregnancy[361] and the more severe hyperemesis gravidarum.[362]
- The pungent principles of ginger often create a warm or burning sensation in the stomach that is mild, reducible with food consumption, and not indicative of tissue irritation.

Additional information:

- Ginger can be consumed as a root or in capsule or powder form. Most capsules are standardized for the concentration of gingerols.

Notes:

_____

_____

_____

_____

_____

_____

_____

_____

_____

_____

_____

_____

_____

_____

_____

_____

_____

_____

_____

[354] Langner E, Greifenberg S, Gruenwald J. Ginger: history and use. *Adv Ther* 1998 Jan-Feb;15(1):25-44
[355] Kiuchi F, Iwakami S, Shibuya M, Hanaoka F, Sankawa U. Inhibition of prostaglandin and leukotriene biosynthesis by gingerols and diarylheptanoids. *Chem Pharm Bull* (Tokyo) 1992 Feb;40(2):387-91
[356] Tjendraputra E, Tran VH, Liu-Brennan D, Roufogalis BD, Duke CC. Effect of ginger constituents and synthetic analogues on cyclooxygenase-2 enzyme in intact cells. *Bioorg Chem* 2001 Jun;29(3):156-63
[357] Srivastava KC, Mustafa T. Ginger (Zingiber officinale) in rheumatism and musculoskeletal disorders. *Med Hypotheses*. 1992 Dec;39(4):342-8
[358] Srivastava KC, Mustafa T. Ginger (Zingiber officinale) and rheumatic disorders. *Med Hypotheses*. 1989 May;29(1):25-8
[359] Altman RD, Marcussen KC. Effects of a ginger extract on knee pain in patients with osteoarthritis. *Arthritis Rheum*. 2001 Nov;44(11):2531-8
[360] Mustafa T, Srivastava KC. Ginger (Zingiber officinale) in migraine headache. *J Ethnopharmacol*. 1990 Jul;29(3):267-73
[361] Vutyavanich T, Kraisarin T, Ruangsri R. Ginger for nausea and vomiting in pregnancy: randomized, double-masked, placebo-controlled trial. *Obstet Gynecol* 2001 Apr;97(4):577-82
[362] Fischer-Rasmussen W, Kjaer SK, Dahl C, Asping U. Ginger treatment of hyperemesis gravidarum. *Eur J Obstet Gynecol Reprod Biol*. 1991 Jan 4;38(1):19-24

Botanical Medicine:	## *Uncaria tomentosa, Uncaria guianensis*
Common names:	## "Cat's claw" "una de gato"

Applications and mechanisms of action:

- Osteoarthritis: 30 patients with osteoarthritis of the knees benefited from highly-concentrated freeze-dried aqueous extraction of *U. guianensis* dosed at 1 capsule of 100 mg daily. Reduction in pain was approximately 36% at 4 weeks. No major adverse effects were noted; however headache and dizziness were more common in the treatment group. *Uncaria* inhibits NF-κB, TNFα, COX-2, and thus PGE-2 production.[363]
- Rheumatoid arthritis: A year-long study of patients with active rheumatoid arthritis (RA) treated with sulfasalazine or hydroxychloroquine showed "relative safety and modest benefit" of *Uncaria tomentosa* (UT).[364]

Toxicity and contraindications:

- No major adverse effects were noted; however headache and dizziness were more common in the treatment group.
- This herb should probably not be used during pregnancy based on its historical use as a contraceptive.

Dosage and administration:

- High-quality extractions from reputable manufacturers used according to directions are recommended. Most products contain between 250-500 mg and are standardized to 3.0% alkaloids and 15% total polyphenols; QD-TID po dosing should be sufficient as *part* of a comprehensive plan.

Additional information:

- Other studies with *Uncaria tomentosa* have shown enhancement of post-vaccination immunity[365] and enhancement of DNA repair in humans.[366] Traditional uses have included the use of the herb as a contraceptive and as treatment for gastrointestinal ulcers.

Notes:

_____
_____
_____
_____
_____
_____
_____
_____
_____
_____
_____
_____
_____

[363] Piscoya J, Rodriguez Z, Bustamante SA, Okuhama NN, Miller MJ, Sandoval M.Efficacy and safety of freeze-dried cat's claw in osteoarthritis of the knee: mechanisms of action of the species Uncaria guianensis. *Inflamm Res.* 2001 Sep;50(9):442-8

[364] "This small preliminary study demonstrates relative safety and modest benefit to the tender joint count of a highly purified extract from the pentacyclic chemotype of UT in patients with active RA taking sulfasalazine or hydroxychloroquine." Mur E, Hartig F, Eibl G, Schirmer M. Randomized double blind trial of an extract from the pentacyclic alkaloid-chemotype of uncaria tomentosa for the treatment of rheumatoid arthritis. *J Rheumatol.* 2002 Apr;29(4):678-81

[365] "C-Med-100 is a novel nutraceutical extract from the South American plant Uncaria tomentosa or Cat's Claw which is known to possess immune enhancing and antiinflammatory properties in animals. However, statistically significant immune enhancement for the individuals on C-Med-100 supplement was observed..." Lamm S, Sheng Y, Pero RW. Persistent response to pneumococcal vaccine in individuals supplemented with a novel water soluble extract of Uncaria tomentosa, C-Med-100. *Phytomedicine.* 2001 Jul;8(4):267-74

[366] "There was a statistically significant decrease of DNA damage and a concomitant increase of DNA repair in the supplement groups (250 and 350 mg/day) when compared with non-supplemented controls (p < 0.05)." Sheng Y, Li L, Holmgren K, Pero RW. DNA repair enhancement of aqueous extracts of Uncaria tomentosa in a human volunteer study. *Phytomedicine.* 2001 Jul;8(4):275-82

| *Botanical Medicine:* | ***Salix alba, Salix* species** |
| *Common names:* | **"Willow bark"** |

| *Applications and mechanisms of action:* | • Musculoskeletal pain, osteoarthritis, low-back pain: Clinical studies in humans with musculoskeletal pain have consistently demonstrated safety and effectiveness of willow bark. In a double-blind placebo-controlled clinical trial in 210 patients with moderate/severe low-back pain (20% of patients had positive straight-leg raising test), extract of willow bark showed a dose-dependent analgesic effect with benefits beginning in the first week of treatment.[367] In a head-to-head study of 228 patients comparing willow bark (standardized for 240 mg salicin) with Vioxx (rofecoxib), treatments were equally effective yet willow bark was safer and 40% less expensive.[368] Because willow bark's salicylates were the original source for the chemical manufacture of acetylsalicylic acid (aspirin), researchers and clinicians have erroneously mistaken willow bark to be synonymous with aspirin; this is certainly inaccurate and therefore clarification of willow's mechanism of action will be provided here. Aspirin has two primary effects via three primary mechanisms of action: 1) anticoagulant effects mediated by the acetylation and permanent inactivation of thromboxane-A synthase, which is the enzyme that makes the powerful proaggregatory thromboxane-A2; 2) antiprostaglandin action via acetylation of both isoforms of cyclooxygenase (COX-1 inhibition 25-166x more than COX-2) with widespread inhibition of prostaglandin formation, and 3) antiprostaglandin formation via "retroconversion" of acetylsalicylate into salicylic acid which then inhibits cyclooxygenase-2 gene transcription.[369] Notice that the acetylation reactions are specific to aspirin and thus actions #1 and #2 are not seen with willow bark; whereas #3—inhibition of COX-2 transcription by salicylates—appears to be the major mechanism of action of willow bark extract. Proof of this principle is supported by the lack of adverse effects associated with willow bark in the research literature. If willow bark were pharmacodynamically synonymous with aspirin, then we would expect case reports of gastric ulceration, hemorrhage, and Reye's syndrome to permeate the research literature; this is not the case and therefore—with the exception of possible allergic reactions in patients previously allergic to aspirin and salicylates—extensive "warnings" on willow bark products[370] are unnecessary.[371] Salicylates are widely present in fruits, vegetables, herbs and spices and are partly responsible for the anti-cancer, anti-inflammatory, and health-promoting benefits of plant consumption.[372,373] |

| *Toxicity and contraindications:* | • Allergy: There is one single case report of serious anaphylaxis following use of willow bark in a patient previously sensitized to aspirin.[374] |

| *Dosage and administration:* | • The daily dose should not exceed 240 mg of salicin, and products should include other components of the whole plant. Of course, we would expect that lower doses will be effective in our clinical practices because we always use willow bark with other anti-inflammatory diet and nutritional interventions, particularly EPA/DHA and ALA—each of which has been shown to lower prostaglandin formation. |

[367] Chrubasik S, Eisenberg E, Balan E, Weinberger T, Luzzati R, Conradt C. Treatment of low-back pain exacerbations with willow bark extract: a randomized double-blind study. *Am J Med.* 2000;109:9-14

[368] Chrubasik S, Kunzel O, Model A, Conradt C, Black A. Treatment of low-back pain with a herbal or synthetic anti-rheumatic: a randomized controlled study. Willow bark extract for low-back pain. *Rheumatology* (Oxford). 2001;40:1388-93

[369] Hare LG, Woodside JV, Young IS. Dietary salicylates. *J Clin Pathol* 2003 Sep;56(9):649-50

[370] Clauson KA, Santamarina ML, Buettner CM, Cauffield JS. Evaluation of Presence of Aspirin-Related Warnings with Willow Bark (July/August). *Ann Pharmacother.* 2005 May 31; [Epub ahead of print]

[371] **Vasquez A, Muanza DN. Evaluation of Presence of Aspirin-Related Warnings with Willow Bark: Comment on the Article by Clauson et al. *Ann Pharmacotherapy* 2005 Oct;39(10):1763**

[372] Lawrence JR, Peter R, Baxter GJ, Robson J, Graham AB, Paterson JR. Urinary excretion of salicyluric and salicylic acids by non-vegetarians, vegetarians, and patients taking low dose aspirin. *J Clin Pathol.* 2003 Sep;56(9):651-3

[373] Paterson JR, Lawrence JR. Salicylic acid: a link between aspirin, diet and the prevention of colorectal cancer. *QJM.* 2001 Aug;94(8):445-8

[374] Boullata JI, McDonnell PJ, Oliva CD. Anaphylactic reaction to a dietary supplement containing willow bark. *Ann Pharmacother.* 2003 Jun;37(6):832-3

Botanical Medicine:	## *Capsicum annuum, Capsicum frutescens*
Common names:	## **Cayenne pepper, hot chili pepper**

Applications and mechanisms of action:

- <u>Pain relief</u>: Controlled clinical trials have conclusively demonstrated capsaicin's ability deplete sensory fibers of the neuropeptide substance P to thus reduce pain. Capsaicin also blocks transport and de-novo synthesis of substance P. Topical capsaicin is proven effective in relieving the pain associated with **diabetic neuropathy**[375], **chronic low back pain**[376], **chronic neck pain**[377], **osteoarthritis**[378], **rheumatoid arthritis**[379], **notalgia paresthetica**[380], **reflex sympathetic dystrophy** and **cluster headache** (intranasal application).[381] Surprisingly, capsaicin was shown to be ineffective in the treatment of pain associated with temporomandibular dysfunction.[382]

Toxicity and contraindications:

- Do not get into eyes.
- Transient burning, sneezing, and coughing are common following intranasal application.
- Topical application of capsaicin during pregnancy has not been evaluated but is almost certain to be safe.

Dosage and administration:

- Capsaicin creams are available OTC at strengths of 0.025% and 0.075%. The stronger creams have a more powerful analgesic effect but result in more initial burning, which abates with continued use. The cream is generally not applied to areas of skin that are broken or bleeding.

Additional information:

- Since the cream reduces sensitivity to pain, patients should not use a heating pad at the site where the capsaicin is applied, as the capsaicin may induce insensitivity to local overheating.

Notes:

_____

_____

_____

_____

_____

_____

_____

_____

_____

_____

_____

_____

_____

[375] Treatment of painful diabetic neuropathy with topical capsaicin. A multicenter, double-blind, vehicle-controlled study. The Capsaicin Study Group. [No authors listed] *Arch Intern Med.* 1991 Nov;151(11):2225-9

[376] Keitel W, Frerick H, Kuhn U, Schmidt U, Kuhlmann M, Bredehorst A. Capsicum pain plaster in chronic non-specific low back pain. *Arzneimittelforschung.* 2001 Nov;51(11):896-903

[377] Mathias BJ, Dillingham TR, Zeigler DN, Chang AS, Belandres PV. Topical capsaicin for chronic neck pain. A pilot study. *Am J Phys Med Rehabil* 1995 Jan-Feb;74(1):39-44

[378] McCarthy GM, McCarty DJ. Effect of topical capsaicin in the therapy of painful osteoarthritis of the hands. *J Rheumatol.* 1992;19(4):604-7

[379] Deal CL, Schnitzer TJ, Lipstein E, Seibold JR, Stevens RM, Levy MD, Albert D, Renold F. Treatment of arthritis with topical capsaicin: a double-blind trial. *Clin Ther.* 1991 May-Jun;13(3):383-95

[380] Leibsohn E. Treatment of notalgia paresthetica with capsaicin. *Cutis* 1992 May;49(5):335-6

[381] Hautkappe M, Roizen MF, Toledano A, Roth S, Jeffries JA, Ostermeier AM. Review of the effectiveness of capsaicin for painful cutaneous disorders and neural dysfunction. *Clin J Pain* 1998 Jun;14(2):97-106

[382] Winocur E, Gavish A, Halachmi M, Eli I, Gazit E. Topical application of capsaicin for the treatment of localized pain in the temporomandibular joint area. *J Orofac Pain.* 2000 Winter;14(1):31-6

Botanical Medicine:	### *Boswellia serrata*
Common names:	### **Frankincense, Salai guggal**

Applications and mechanisms of action:

- Anti-inflammatory, via inhibition of 5-lipoxygenase[383] with no apparent effect on cyclooxygenase[384]: A recent clinical study showed that *Boswellia* was able to reduce pain and swelling while increasing joint flexion and walking distance in patients with **osteoarthritis of the knees**.[385] While reports from clinical trials published in English are relatively rare, a recent abstract from the German medical research[386] stated, "In clinical trials promising results were observed in patients with rheumatoid arthritis, chronic colitis, ulcerative colitis, Crohn's disease, bronchial asthma and peritumoral brains edemas." Additional recent studies have confirmed the effectiveness of *Boswellia* in the treatment of **asthma**[387] and **ulcerative colitis**.[388] A German study showing that *Boswellia* was ineffective for rheumatoid arthritis[389] was poorly conducted, with inadequate follow-up, inadequate controls, and abnormal dosing of the herb.

Toxicity:

- Minor gastrointestinal upset has been reported.

Dosage and administration:

- Products are generally standardized to contain 37.5–65% boswellic acids, which are currently considered the active constituents with clinical benefit. The target dose is approximately 150 mg of boswellic acids TID; dose and number of capsules/tablets will vary depending upon the concentration found in differing products.

Additional information:

- Even though *Boswellia* is an effective anti-inflammatory, its use should not preclude searching for and addressing the underlying cause of the inflammatory problem.

Notes:

_____

_____

_____

_____

_____

_____

_____

_____

_____

_____

[383] Wildfeuer A, Neu IS, Safayhi H, Metzger G, Wehrmann M, Vogel U, Ammon HP. Effects of boswellic acids extracted from a herbal medicine on the biosynthesis of leukotrienes and the course of experimental autoimmune encephalomyelitis. *Arzneimittelforschung* 1998 Jun;48(6):668-74

[384] Safayhi H, Mack T, Sabieraj J, Anazodo MI, Subramanian LR, Ammon HP. Boswellic acids: novel, specific, nonredox inhibitors of 5-lipoxygenase. *J Pharmacol Exp Ther* 1992 Jun;261(3):1143-6

[385] Kimmatkar N, Thawani V, Hingorani L, Khiyani R. Efficacy and tolerability of Boswellia serrata extract in treatment of osteoarthritis of knee--a randomized double blind placebo controlled trial. *Phytomedicine*. 2003 Jan;10(1):3-7

[386] Ammon HP. [Boswellic acids (components of frankincense) as the active principle in treatment of chronic inflammatory diseases] [Article in German] *Wien Med Wochenschr*. 2002;152(15-16):373-8

[387] Gupta I, Gupta V, Parihar A, Gupta S, Ludtke R, Safayhi H, Ammon HP. Effects of Boswellia serrata gum resin in patients with bronchial asthma: results of a double-blind, placebo-controlled, 6-week clinical study. *Eur J Med Res*. 1998 Nov 17;3(11):511-4

[388] Gupta I, Parihar A, Malhotra P, Singh GB, Ludtke R, Safayhi H, Ammon HP. Effects of Boswellia serrata gum resin in patients with ulcerative colitis. *Eur J Med Res*. 1997 Jan;2(1):37-43

[389] Sander O, Herborn G, Rau R. [Is H15 (resin extract of Boswellia serrata, "incense") a useful supplement to established drug therapy of chronic polyarthritis? Results of a double-blind pilot study] [Article in German] *Z Rheumatol*. 1998 Feb;57(1):11-6

Botanical Medicine:	*Harpagophytum procumbens*
Common name:	*Devil's claw*

Applications and mechanisms of action:

- Analgesic and weak anti-inflammatory: Safety and moderate effectiveness of *Harpagophytum* has been demonstrated in patients with **hip pain, low back pain**, and **knee pain**.[390] An abstract from the German research literature showed that *Harpagophytum* is safe and effective for the treatment of **muscle pain and muscle tension of the low back, shoulders, and neck**.[391] In a study of patients with **osteoarthritis of the hip and knee**, *Harpagophytum* was found to be just as effective yet safer and better tolerated than the drug diacerhein.[392,393] While anti-inflammatory effects have been reported, the anti-inflammatory effects are weak[394] and appear secondary to the analgesic benefits. Administration of *Harpagophytum* to healthy volunteers does not alter eicosanoid production.[395] In a study involving 183 patients with low back pain, *Harpagophytum* was found to be safe and moderately effective in patients with **"severe and unbearable pain" and radiating pain with neurologic deficit**.[396] Most recently, *Harpagophytum* was studied in a head-to-head clinical trial with the popular but dangerous selective Cox-2 inhibitor Vioxx (rofecoxib); the data clearly indicate that *Harpagophytum* was safer and at least as effective.[397]

Toxicity and contraindication:

- Treatment is generally considered very safe. About 8% of patients may experience diarrhea or other mild gastrointestinal effects. A few patients may experience dizziness. Long-term multi-year safety data is not available.

Dosage and administration:

- Treatment should be continued for at least 4 weeks, and many patients will continue to improve after 8 weeks from the initiation of treatment.[398]
- Products are generally standardized for the content of harpagosides, with a target dose of 60 mg harpagoside per day.[399] However, the whole plant is considered to contain effective constituents, not only the iridoid glycosides.
- The results of one laboratory study suggest that the active components are reduced following exposure to acid[400], and therefore the product might be consumed between meals, perhaps with Alka Seltzer or sodium bicarbonate.

Additional information:

- Immediately before the revision of this monograph in August 2004, I was in communication with Dr. Sigrun Chrubasik who shared with me her most recent article[401] in which she reviewed the clinical trials to date. In her 2004 review published in *Phytotherapy Research*, she states that while *Harpagophytum* appears to be safe and moderately effective for the treatment musculoskeletal pain, different proprietary products show significant variances in potency and clinical effectiveness. She states that additional research is necessary before the clinical value of *Harpagophytum* can be firmly established. However, if one reviews the data presented in Table 1 of her 2003 review article published in *Phytomedicine*[402], then one is entitled to conclude that *Harpagophytum* does indeed consistently show clinical benefit that is better than no treatment (open trials), better than placebo (placebo-controlled trials), and at least as good as the pharmaceutical drugs diacerhein and rofecoxib (head-to-head comparisons). Since therapeutic efficacy of *Harpagophytum* is at least as good as commonly used NSAIDs, *Harpagophytum* should be clinically preferred over NSAIDs due to its lower cost and apparently greater safety.[403]

[390] Chrubasik S, Thanner J, Kunzel O, Conradt C, Black A, Pollak S. Comparison of outcome measures during treatment with the proprietary Harpagophytum extract doloteffin in patients with pain in the lower back, knee or hip. *Phytomedicine* 2002 Apr;9(3):181-94

[391] Gobel H, Heinze A, Ingwersen M, Niederberger U, Gerber D. [Effects of Harpagophytum procumbens LI 174 (devil's claw) on sensory, motor und vascular muscle reagibility in the treatment of unspecific back pain] [Article in German] *Schmerz* 2001 Feb;15(1):10-8

[392] Chantre P, Cappelaere A, Leblan D, Guedon D, Vandermander J, Fournie B. Efficacy and tolerance of Harpagophytum procumbens versus diacerhein in treatment of osteoarthritis. *Phytomedicine* 2000 Jun;7(3):177-83

[393] Leblan D, Chantre P, Fournie B. Harpagophytum procumbens in the treatment of knee and hip osteoarthritis. Four-month results of a prospective, multicenter, double-blind trial versus diacerhein. *Joint Bone Spine* 2000;67(5):462-7

[394] Whitehouse LW, Znamirowska M, Paul CJ. Devil's Claw (Harpagophytum procumbens): no evidence for anti-inflammatory activity in the treatment of arthritic disease. *Can Med Assoc J* 1983 Aug 1;129(3):249-51

[395] Moussard C, Alber D, Toubin MM, Thevenon N, Henry JC. A drug used in traditional medicine, harpagophytum procumbens: no evidence for NSAID-like effect on whole blood eicosanoid production in human. *Prostaglandins Leukot Essent Fatty Acids* 1992 Aug;46(4):283-6

[396] "...subgroup analyses suggested that the effect was confined to patients with more severe and radiating pain accompanied by neurological deficit. ...a slightly different picture, with the benefits seeming, if anything, to be greatest in the H600 group and in patients without more severe pain, radiation or neurological deficit." Chrubasik S, Junck H, Breitschwerdt H, Conradt C, Zappe H. Effectiveness of Harpagophytum extract WS 1531 in the treatment of exacerbation of low back pain: a randomized, placebo-controlled, double-blind study. *Eur J Anaesthesiol* 1999 Feb;16(2):118-29

[397] Chrubasik S, Model A, Black A, Pollak S. A randomized double-blind pilot study comparing Doloteffin and Vioxx in the treatment of low back pain. *Rheumatology* (Oxford). 2003 Jan;42(1):141-8

[398] Chrubasik S, Thanner J, Kunzel O, Conradt C, Black A, Pollak S. Comparison of outcome measures during treatment with the proprietary Harpagophytum extract doloteffin in patients with pain in the lower back, knee or hip. *Phytomedicine* 2002 Apr;9(3):181-94

[399] "They took an 8-week course of Doloteffin at a dose providing 60 mg harpagoside per day... Doloteffin is well worth considering for osteoarthritic knee and hip pain and nonspecific low back pain." Chrubasik S, Thanner J, Kunzel O, Conradt C, Black A, Pollak S. Comparison of outcome measures during treatment with the proprietary Harpagophytum extract doloteffin in patients with pain in the lower back, knee or hip. *Phytomedicine* 2002 Apr;9(3):181-94

[400] Lanhers MC, Fleurentin J, Mortier F, Vinche A, Younos C. Anti-inflammatory and analgesic effects of an aqueous extract of Harpagophytum procumbens. *Planta Med* 1992 Apr;58(2):117-23

[401] Chrubasik S, Conradt C, Roufogalis BD. Effectiveness of Harpagophytum extracts and clinical efficacy. *Phytother Res.* 2004 Feb;18(2):187-9

[402] Chrubasik S, Conradt C, Black A. The quality of clinical trials with Harpagophytum procumbens. *Phytomedicine*. 2003;10(6-7):613-23

[403] Chrubasik S, Junck H, Breitschwerdt H, Conradt C, Zappe H. Effectiveness of Harpagophytum extract WS 1531 in the treatment of exacerbation of low back pain: a randomized, placebo-controlled, double-blind study. *Eur J Anaesthesiol* 1999 Feb;16(2):118-29

Botanical Medicine:	## *Curcuma longa*
Common names:	## **Turmeric**

Applications and mechanisms of action:

- <u>Anti-inflammatory *in vitro*</u>: Turmeric is a common spice and food additive, providing foods with antioxidant/preservative benefit, as well as the characteristic golden yellow color which is characteristic of curry and mustard. The anti-inflammatory effects of turmeric have been well established in many *in vitro* studies and studies in animals involving *intraperitoneal* administration. Many researchers and supplement companies have interpreted this to mean that turmeric would also have strong clinical effectiveness in humans with conditions such as arthritis, and thus turmeric is marketed as an anti-inflammatory botanical medicine. The problem with this approach is that the active components of turmeric are only minimally absorbed from oral dosing and therefore the systemic and intraarticular concentrations of the active components are only minimally increased or not increased at all with oral dosing in humans.[404] Nearly all studies that show potential relevance for clinical use of turmeric in treating arthritis, cancer, and other human illnesses have been performed either *in vitro* or *in vivo with intraperitoneal administration* to achieve cellular levels of the active constituents that could never be achieved with oral administration. However, a single report that turmeric administered as a hydroalcoholic extract could reduce the serum levels of the acute phase reactant fibrinogen does suggest that turmeric, when processed or coadministered with alcohol, might be absorbed and possess a systemic anti-inflammatory effect.[405] **To my knowledge, no human studies exist showing that pure curcumin/turmeric when used alone (i.e., not with other herbs, drugs, or piperine) has effectiveness in the treatment of joint pain or inflammation in humans following oral administration.[406]**

Toxicity and contraindications:

- Turmeric is generally considered non-toxic
- No drug interactions are commonly known

Dosage and administration:

- Doses of up to eight grams per day have been used with moderate clinical effectiveness on local oral and gastrointestinal tissues with no evidence of toxicity[407]
- Coadministration with 10 of piperine increases bioavailability of curcuminoids to humans by 2,000%[408]—thus, coadministration of curcumin with piperine appears to be the best and perhaps the only way to increase bioavailability of the active components of the spice and obtain systemic benefits

Notes:

_____

_____

_____

_____

_____

---

[404] "…curcumin is absorbed poorly by the gastrointestinal tract and/or underlies presystemic transformation. Systemic effects therefore seem to be questionable after oral application except that they occur at very low concentrations of curcumin. This does not exclude a local action in the gastrointestinal tract." Ammon HP, Wahl MA. Pharmacology of Curcuma longa. *Planta Med* 1991 Feb;57(1):1-7

[405] Ramirez Bosca A, Soler A, Carrion-Gutierrez MA, Pamies Mira D, Pardo Zapata J, Diaz-Alperi J, Bernd A, Quintanilla Almagro E, Miquel J. An hydroalcoholic extract of Curcuma longa lowers the abnormally high values of human-plasma fibrinogen. *Mech Ageing Dev.* 2000 Apr 14;114(3):207-10

[406] **Vasquez A, Muanza DN. Accolades and Addenda for "Use of Botanicals in Osteoarthritis and Rheumatoid Arthritis": Comment on Article by Ahmed et al. *Evidence-based Complementary and Alternative Medicine.* 2005 published on-line December 15** http://ecam.oxfordjournals.org/cgi/eletters/2/3/301#19

[407] "In conclusion, this study demonstrated that curcumin is not toxic to humans up to 8,000 mg/day when taken by mouth for 3 months." Cheng AL, Hsu CH, Lin JK, Hsu MM, Ho YF, Shen TS, Ko JY, Lin JT, Lin BR, Ming-Shiang W, Yu HS, Jee SH, Chen GS, Chen TM, Chen CA, Lai MK, Pu YS, Pan MH, Wang YJ, Tsai CC, Hsieh CY. Phase I clinical trial of curcumin, a chemopreventive agent, in patients with high-risk or pre-malignant lesions. *Anticancer Res.* 2001 Jul-Aug;21(4B):2895-900

[408] Shoba G, Joy D, Joseph T, Majeed M, Rajendran R, Srinivas PS. Influence of piperine on the pharmacokinetics of curcumin in animals and human volunteers. *Planta Med.* 1998;64(4):353-6

Botanical Medicine:	## *Avocado/soybean unsaponifiables*
Common name:	## **ASU**

Applications and mechanisms of action:

- Osteoarthritis: The use of avocado/soybean unsaponifiables (ASU) has been shown to improve joint function and reduce the need for NSAIDs/analgesic medication in patients with osteoarthritis.[409,410] A study of patients with **hip osteoarthritis** suggested that ASU may retard the progression of joint space narrowing.[411] A study of patients with **knee osteoarthritis** showed that patients receiving ASU were able to reduce the use of NSAIDs and analgesics by 60% compared to only a 36% reduction by the patients receiving placebo.[412] The mechanism of action of ASU appears to be the stimulation of collagen/cartilage synthesis in addition to a modest anti-inflammatory effect via reduction in nitric oxide, PG-E2, and other mediators.[413]

Toxicity:

- None known.

Dosage and administration:

- Common doses are 300 mg per day or 600 mg per day, with a slight increase in efficacy with the 600 mg per day dose, according to a study of patients with knee osteoarthritis.[414]

Additional information:

- ASU products are generally not available in the United States.
- Due to the reduced clinical efficacy of ASU compared to other natural therapeutics as reported in the research, I would consider ASU a "last resort" treatment for osteoarthritis after using glucosamine sulfate, fish oil, vitamin E, niacinamide, and *Uncaria* and *Boswellia*.
- Be sure to rule out iron overload in any patient with osteoarthritis, especially osteoarthritis that is polyarticular or resistant to treatment.[415]
- The unsaponifiable fraction of vegetable oils includes plant sterols, or phytosterols, which have documented benefit in hypercholesterolemia and prostate hyperplasia.

Notes: _____

_____

_____

_____

_____

_____

_____

_____

_____

_____

_____

_____

[409] Blotman F, Maheu E, Wulwik A, Caspard H, Lopez A. Efficacy and safety of avocado/soybean unsaponifiables in the treatment of symptomatic osteoarthritis of the knee and hip. A prospective, multicenter, three-month, randomized, double-blind, placebo-controlled trial. *Rev Rhum Engl Ed.* 1997 Dec;64(12):825-34

[410] Maheu E, Mazieres B, Valat JP, Loyau G, Le Loet X, Bourgeois P, Grouin JM, Rozenberg S. Symptomatic efficacy of avocado/soybean unsaponifiables in the treatment of osteoarthritis of the knee and hip: a prospective, randomized, double-blind, placebo-controlled, multicenter clinical trial with a six-month treatment period and a two-month followup demonstrating a persistent effect. *Arthritis Rheum.* 1998;41(1):81-91

[411] Lequesne M, Maheu E, Cadet C, Dreiser RL. Structural effect of avocado/soybean unsaponifiables on joint space loss in osteoarthritis of the hip. *Arthritis Rheum.* 2002 Feb;47(1):50-8

[412] Appelboom T, Schuermans J, Verbruggen G, Henrotin Y, Reginster JY. Symptoms modifying effect of avocado/soybean unsaponifiables (ASU) in knee osteoarthritis. A double blind, prospective, placebo-controlled study. *Scand J Rheumatol.* 2001;30(4):242-7

[413] Henrotin YE, Sanchez C, Deberg MA, Piccardi N, Guillou GB, Msika P, Reginster JY. Avocado/soybean unsaponifiables increase aggrecan synthesis and reduce catabolic and proinflammatory mediator production by human osteoarthritic chondrocytes. *J Rheumatol.* 2003 Aug;30(8):1825-34

[414] Appelboom T, Schuermans J, Verbruggen G, Henrotin Y, Reginster JY. Symptoms modifying effect of avocado/soybean unsaponifiables (ASU) in knee osteoarthritis. A double blind, prospective, placebo-controlled study. *Scand J Rheumatol.* 2001;30(4):242-7

[415] Vasquez A. Musculoskeletal disorders and iron overload disease: comment on the American College of Rheumatology guidelines for the initial evaluation of the adult patient with acute musculoskeletal symptoms. *Arthritis Rheum* 1996;39: 1767-8

Piezoelectric Properties of the Human Body and Clinical Implications

"…pyroelectric [and piezoelectric] behavior constitutes a basic physical property of all living organisms." [416]

Piezoelectricity has been defined as "the generation of electricity or of electric polarity in dielectric crystals subjected to mechanical stress, or the generation of stress in such crystals subjected to an applied voltage."[417] When we are discussing the piezoelectric properties of the human body, we are discussing the translation/transformation of mechanical energy into and out of electric energy. Relatedly, **pyroelectricity is defined as "the electrical potential created in certain materials when they are heated."**[418] Therefore, we can schematize a relationship between the tissues of living organisms (plants, animals, humans), mechanical stress, electrical energy, and heat. Clinically relevant questions/issues then become those of qualifying/quantifying these pyroelectric and piezoelectric properties of the human body, and determining whether and/or how these are clinically relevant.

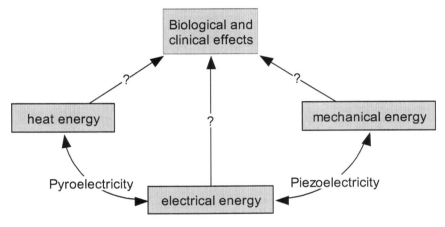

All living tissue—namely plant and animal tissues—have both pyroelectric and piezoelectric properties. Since these properties are seen in the tissues, they are of course seen in the organisms themselves. With regard to physical medicine in general and spinal manipulation in particular, we note that bone, collagen, and the spinal cord are notably pyroelectric/piezoelectric, as detailed in the *Annals of the New York Academy of Sciences* monograph by Athenstaedt in 1974. Other tissues and molecules with pyroelectric/piezoelectric and "semiconductive" properties include wood, silk, skin, nucleic acids, fibrin, hyaluronic acid, actin and myosin.[419] This electrophysiologic property is based not on the inherent "electrical" and ionic properties of the nervous system or the cell membranes, but rather upon the alignment of the molecules within the tissues. **When linear, organic molecules of varying length are aligned in parallel along a longitudinal axis, the resultant microscopic and therefore macroscopic structure will have a permanent dipole moment.** [420]

Indeed, as Athenstaedt notes in *American Journal of Physiology*[421], "The existence of an inherent electric dipole moment has been established throughout the entire length of the spinal cord of humans, horses, and cows." This is illustrated in the diagram to the right.

Clinical relevance: In 1977, Lipiski from Tufts University School of Medicine[422] summarized the current research of the day and speculated on the effects of spinal manipulation, osteopathic manipulation, yoga, and acupuncture as mediated via the body's inherent pyroelectric and piezoelectric properties. Lipinski's literature

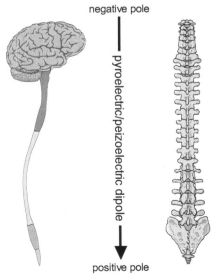

---

416 Athenstaedt H. Pyroelectric and piezoelectric properties of vertebrates. *Ann N Y Acad Sci*. 1974;238:68-94
417 American Heritage Dictionary
418 http://www.free-definition.com/Pyroelectricity.html on October 3, 2004
419 Lipinski B. Biological significance of piezoelectricity in relation to acupuncture, Hatha Yoga, osteopathic medicine and action of air ions. *Med Hypotheses*. 1977 Jan-Feb;3(1):9-12
420 Athenstaedt H. Pyroelectric and piezoelectric properties of vertebrates. *Ann N Y Acad Sci*. 1974;238:68-94
421 Athenstaedt H. "Functional polarity" of the spinal cord caused by its longitudinal electric dipole moment. *Am J Physiol*. 1984 Sep;247(3 Pt 2):R482-7
422 Lipinski B. Biological significance of piezoelectricity in relation to acupuncture, Hatha Yoga, osteopathic medicine and action of air ions. *Med Hypotheses*. 1977 Jan-Feb;3(1):9-12

review (particularly including the work of Bassett[423]) suggests that **"…piezoelectricity present in many biological systems may theoretically control cell nutrition, local pH, enzyme activation and inhibition, orientation of intra-and extra-cellular macromolecules, migratory and proliferative activity of cells, contractility of permeability of cell membranes, and energy transfer."** With these concepts and possibilities considered, we can construct a conceptual model that allows an understanding of the interconnectedness of *mechanical stimuli* **such as massage, manipulation, stretching/exercise, and yoga** with *"energetic" stimuli* **such as acupuncture, meditation, "prayer" and intentionality** with their possible biochemical/physiological effects which then translate into clinical effects. This integrated model helps to explain the nonbiochemical nonpharmacologic effects of "energetic" therapeutics such as moxibustion, acupuncture, and yoga that may be mediated by nonlinear/nonbiochemical physiologic mechanisms. This model also helps us to understand the observed but hitherto unexplainable clinical effects of phenomena such as the well-reported sensitivity that some people display in relation to changes in the weather and the positioning of their bodies in relation to electromagnetic fields of the planet and electrical equipment and power lines, the effect of "distance healing" via prayer[424,425] and intentionality[426], and the clinical benefits of grounding/earthing the human body for the resultant improvements in sleep, normalization of cortisol rhythms, and reduction in somatic pain.[427]

Speculative model for the interconnectedness and biologic effects of heat, mechanical and electrician energies and their clinical effects as mediated physiologically and biochemically via the pyroelectric-piezoelectric and "superconductive" properties of body tissues and organ systems: modified from the discussion by Lipinski[428]

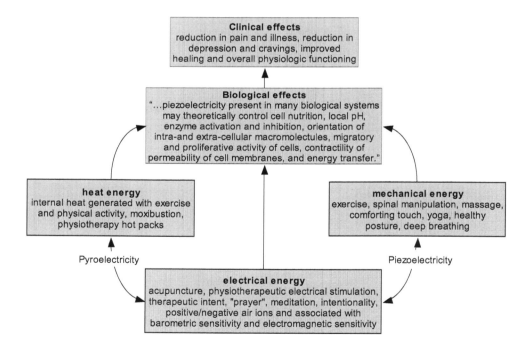

[423] Bassett CA. Biologic significance of piezoelectricity. *Calcif Tissue Res.* 1968 Mar;1(4):252-72

[424] "The control patients required ventilatory assistance, antibiotics, and diuretics more frequently than patients in the IP group. These data suggest that intercessory prayer to the Judeo-Christian God has a beneficial therapeutic effect in patients admitted to a CCU." Byrd RC. Positive therapeutic effects of intercessory prayer in a coronary care unit population. *South Med J.* 1988 Jul;81(7):826-9

[425] "CONCLUSIONS: In-person intercessory prayer may be a useful adjunct to standard medical care for certain patients with rheumatoid arthritis. Supplemental, distant intercessory prayer offers no additional benefits." Matthews DA, Marlowe SM, MacNutt FS. Effects of intercessory prayer on patients with rheumatoid arthritis. *South Med J.* 2000 Dec;93(12):1177-86

[426] "CONCLUSIONS: Remote, intercessory prayer was associated with lower CCU course scores. This result suggests that prayer may be an effective adjunct to standard medical care." Harris WS, Gowda M, Kolb JW, Strychacz CP, Vacek JL, Jones PG, Forker A, O'Keefe JH, McCallister BD. A randomized, controlled trial of the effects of remote, intercessory prayer on outcomes in patients admitted to the coronary care unit. *Arch Intern Med.* 1999 Oct 25;159(19):2273-8

[427] "Results indicate that grounding the human body to earth ("earthing") during sleep reduces night-time levels of cortisol and resynchronizes cortisol hormone secretion … Furthermore, subjective reporting indicates that grounding the human body to earth during sleep improves sleep and reduces pain and stress." Ghaly M, Teplitz D. The biologic effects of grounding the human body during sleep as measured by cortisol levels and subjective reporting of sleep, pain, and stress. *J Altern Complement Med.* 2004 Oct;10(5):767-76

[428] Lipinski B. Biological significance of piezoelectricity in relation to acupuncture, Hatha Yoga, osteopathic medicine and action of air ions. *Med Hypotheses.* 1977 Jan-Feb;3(1):9-12

Physiotherapy—notes available on-line

Commonly utilized physiotherapeutic interventions include the following:

1. **Constitutional Hydrotherapy**
2. **Ultrasound**
3. **Contrast hydrotherapy**
4. **Heating compress,**
5. **Wet sock treatments**
6. **Cold friction rub**
7. **Immersion bath**
8. **Cold compress**
9. **Hyperthermia**
10. **Hot pack**
11. **Ice pack**
12. **Interferential**
13. **Tens—transcutaneous electrical nerve stimulation**
14. **Infrared**
15. **Electrical muscle stimulation**
16. **Bipolar for muscle contraction (using interferential machine)**
17. **Ionophoresis, ion transfer**
18. **Uni/mono-polar motor point stimulation of denervated muscle with electrical muscle stimulation**
19. **Short wave diathermy**

Since I do not consider this an area that I specialize in nor necessarily advocate, I have provided a draft of my physiotherapy notes at the website where you can download and print 20 pages of notes for free by accessing the page at http://OptimalHealthResearch.com/physiotherapy. One of the main reasons I've decided to forgo detailing these treatments here is particularly relevant to the use of the physiotherapy electronic equipment: with so many different brands and machines, detailing the settings and use for each type of machine would prove impossible. See the notes for general concepts and ideas.

Appendix A: Brief Overview of Clinical Considerations of Vitamins and Minerals

Nutrients	Physiology, toxicity, and contraindications	Clinical applications (adult doses)
Vitamin A	♦ Vitamin A comes in different forms with different characteristics; of these, all-*trans* retinol is the most common, and retinol palmitate is one of the least toxic. The richest dietary source of vitamin A is liver. Vitamin A has little or no antioxidant activity; rather, the antioxidant action commonly attributed to vitamin A is more accurately ascribed to its carotenoid precursor. Vitamin A is necessary for proper immune function, vision, and cell growth and differentiation (especially in epithelial tissue). Insufficiency of vitamin A causes epithelial tissue to produce excess keratin; hence the keratinization of the eye and skin in patients with vitamin A deficiency. ♦ Because of the risks of toxicity even with modest doses in the range of 25,000 IU per day[429] , most patients should consume <10,000-20,000 IU per day unless they are aware of the warning signs of toxicity and/or are under the care of a nutrition-knowledgeable doctor. This is particularly true for women who might get pregnant while supplementing with vitamin A, as an association between an increased risk of birth defects in association with daily intake ≥10,000 has been published and generally accepted, controversy notwithstanding. ♦ Vitamin A is present in some multivitamins, in cod liver oil, and in other supplements—read labels to ensure that the total daily intake is not greater than 10,000-20,000 IU per day. Approximately 200 cases of vitamin A toxicity are reported worldwide each year. ♦ Manifestations of vitamin A deficiency are "night blindness" (more properly termed "flash blindness" since vitamin A deficiency impairs ability of photoreceptors to recover following light exposure), follicular hyperkeratosis, frequent infections, and poor wound healing. Tissue damage (i.e., burns and trauma) and infections greatly increase the requirement for and tolerability of vitamin A supplementation.	♦ Short-term (few days) prescription of 100,000 – 200,000 IU per day is common for children and adults, especially during acute viral infections and the initial treatment of acne. ♦ Vitamin A toxicity is seen with chronic ingestion of therapeutic doses, for example: 25,000 IU per day for 6 years, or 100,000 IU per day for 2.5 years.[430] Because of the possible increased risk of hepatotoxicity, do not administer high doses of vitamin A to patients on numerous medications or with liver disease. ♦ Doses of vitamin A ≥ 10,000 IU are controversially associated with an increased risk for birth defects; therefore women who are pregnant or might soon become pregnant should keep their daily intake of vitamin A below 10,000 IU from all sources. ♦ **Clinical applications for supraphysiologic doses in the range of 100,000-300,000 IU per day of vitamin A include: adult acne, menorrhagia, and viral infections, especially measles.** ♦ **Medicolegal considerations: Any time high-dose vitamin A (i.e., greater than 25,000-50,000 IU per day) is used, the doctor must clearly define the time limit of this treatment *in writing* so that the patient will not mistakenly continue taking the vitamin and end up with vitamin A toxicity.** ♦ Patients must be advised of limited duration of use (e.g., 1-4 weeks) and to reduce or stop supplementation if signs of toxicity occur such as skin problems (dry skin, flaking skin, chapped or split lips, red skin rash, hair loss), joint pain, bone pain, headaches, anorexia (loss of appetite), edema (water retention, weight gain, swollen ankles, difficulty breathing), fatigue, and/or liver damage.

---

[429] "At 25,000 IU vitamin A per day, although elevated liver enzymes may be seen, hepatotoxicity is rare. We report a case of severe hepatotoxicity associated with the habitual daily ingestion of 25,000 IU of vitamin A bought as an over-the-counter dietary supplement." Kowalski TE, Falestiny M, Furth E, Malet PF. Vitamin A hepatotoxicity: a cautionary note regarding 25,000 IU supplements. *Am J Med*. 1994 Dec;97(6):523-8

[430] Geubel AP, De Galocsy C, Alves N, Rahier J, Dive C. Liver damage caused by therapeutic vitamin A administration: estimate of dose-related toxicity in 41 cases. *Gastroenterology*. 1991 Jun;100(6):1701-9

Appendix A: Clinical and Physiologic Considerations of Vitamins and Minerals—*continued*

Nutrients	Physiology, toxicity, and contraindications	Clinical applications (adult doses)
Carotenoids	♦ Carotenoids are antioxidants and have additional specific functions. Fewer than 10% of carotenoids can serve as precursors to vitamin A; of these, beta-, alpha-, and gamma-carotene are the most efficient. Provitamin carotenoids are converted to all-*trans* retinal which is then converted to retinyl ester. ♦ Carotenoids are generally administered in microgram doses and should be delivered in a broad-spectrum combination including: beta carotene, alpha carotene, zeaxanthin, cryptoxanthin, and lutein. Due to competitive absorption, the use of high doses of a single carotenoid will tend to induce a deficiency of the other carotenoids; this mechanism probably explains the adverse effects associated with long-term high dose supplementation with beta-carotene, especially when the synthetic ♦ Virtually non-toxic when administered in rational doses from natural sources and in balanced combination. Conversion of carotenes to vitamin A is impaired in patients with diabetes and hypothyroidism.	♦ **Antioxidant** ♦ **Immunosupportive (e.g., in HIV)** ♦ **Eye protection (especially lutein)** ♦ **Prostate protection (especially lycopene)**
Vitamin E	♦ Deficiency of vitamin E is rarely recognized but can present as ataxia and neurologic dysfunction, especially in patients with malabsorption. Best dietary sources are seed and nut oils, especially sesame seeds, almonds, sunflower seeds, and wheat germ oil. ♦ A reasonable preventive dose is 200-800 IU per day. Doses up to 3,200 IU per day are generally considered nontoxic.[431] ♦ Vitamin E is commonly described as a "chain breaking antioxidant" with special importance in protecting cell membranes and lipoproteins from oxidative damage.	♦ "Vitamin E" is a family of related chemicals including: ▪ DL-tocopherol: This is synthetic and should not be used clinically; can cause headache and hypertension. ▪ Alpha-tocopherol: commonly used but it depletes the body of the more important gamma-tocopherol.[432] ▪ Beta-tocopherol: ▪ Delta-tocopherol: ▪ Gamma-tocopherol: this is the most important form of vitamin E and should be provided at approximately 40% when "mixed tocopherols" are consumed. ▪ Tocopherol succinate: specific for improving mitochondrial function and for its anti-cancer effect.[433] ▪ Tocotrienols: appear protective against breast cancer

[431] Meydani M. Vitamin E. *Lancet*. 1995 Jan 21;345(8943):170-5
[432] Jiang Q, Christen S, Shigenaga MK, Ames BN. gamma-tocopherol, the major form of vitamin E in the US diet, deserves more attention. *Am J Clin Nutr*. 2001 Dec;74(6):714-22
[433] Prasad KN, Kumar B, Yan XD, Hanson AJ, Cole WC. Alpha-tocopheryl succinate, the most effective form of vitamin E for adjuvant cancer treatment: a review. *J Am Coll Nutr*. 2003 Apr;22(2):108-17

Nutrients	Physiology, toxicity, and contraindications	Clinical applications (adult doses)
Vitamin D3 (cholecalciferol)	◆ Vitamin D deficiency is well documented to be extremely common: ~40% of the general population and >90% of patients with musculoskeletal pain. ◆ The physiologic requirement for vitamin D3 is approximately 4,000 IU per day in adult men. [Data not yet collected in women; but is probably about the same, and higher during pregnancy and lactation.] Clinical guidelines for supplementation are as follows: 1,000 – 2,000 IU for infants; 2,000 IU for children and adolescents; 2,000-4,000 IU for adults, may go up to 10,000 IU per day for adults for up to 6 months and/or with periodic laboratory supervision (starting weekly). Dietary sources of vitamin D are insufficient to meet physiologic needs — vitamin D needs can only be met by sun exposure (full-body, without sunscreen, less than latitude 35 degrees from the equator, near noon, for 15-45 minutes) or by high-dose vitamin D supplementation. ◆ Physiologic doses are non-toxic except in patients with vitamin D hypersensitivity or those taking certain medications that induce hypercalcemia. ◆ The thiazide class of diuretics (including hydrochlorothiazide) can induce hypercalcemia. Correction of underlying hypovitaminosis D may precipitate hypercalcemia. ◆ "Vitamin D hypersensitivity" is seen in granulomatous diseases including tuberculosis, sarcoidosis, Crohn's disease, and some types of cancer; also adrenal failure, hypothyroidism and hyperthyroidism.	◆ Implement vitamin D replacement in all patients unless contraindicated. Vitamin D assessment and administration is becoming the standard of care and failure to implement vitamin D therapy when clinically indicated may be grounds for malpractice.[434] ◆ **Assess vitamin D status with serum 25-OH-vitamin D.** ◆ **Monitor for vitamin D toxicity by measuring serum calcium.** **<u>Conditions Associated with Vitamin D Deficiency:</u>** ◆ Rickets (children) and osteomalacia (adults) ◆ Osteoporosis ◆ Diabetes mellitus ◆ Osteoarthritis ◆ **Hypertension** ◆ Cardiovascular disease ◆ **Metabolic syndrome** ◆ **Depression** ◆ Multiple sclerosis ◆ Rheumatoid arthritis ◆ Grave's disease ◆ Ankylosing spondylitis ◆ Systemic lupus erythematosus ◆ Cancers of the breast, prostate, and colon ◆ Polycystic ovary syndrome ◆ **Musculoskeletal pain**[435] ◆ Epilepsy ◆ Migraine headaches ◆ **Chronic low-back pain** ◆ **Inflammation**

---

[434] Heaney RP. Vitamin D, nutritional deficiency, and the medical paradigm. *J Clin Endocrinol Metab.* 2003 Nov;88(11):5107-8
[435] Al Faraj S, Al Mutairi K. Vitamin D deficiency and chronic low back pain in Saudi Arabia. *Spine.* 2003 Jan 15;28(2):177-9

Appendix A: Clinical and Physiologic Considerations of Vitamins and Minerals—*continued*

Nutrients	Physiology, toxicity, and contraindications	Clinical applications (adult doses)
Vitamin K1 (phylloquinone): from plants **Vitamin K2 (menaquinone):** from animals and bacteria **Vitamin K3 (menadione):** synthetic	♦ **Vitamin K1 (phylloquinone)**—this is the form of vitamin K found in plants ♦ **Vitamin K2 (menaquinone)**—found in animal tissues and synthesized by bacteria ♦ **Vitamin K3 (menadione)**—synthetic form that must be alkylated in the body prior to use; this form of vitamin K is difficult to obtain and is generally not used for nutritional supplementation. ♦ 500-1000 mcg is a common supplemental dose. ♦ Vitamin K must not be taken by patients needing anticoagulation and taking coumadin-warfarin-heparin. Vitamin K is necessary for the production of clotting factors: factor II (prothrombin), factor VII, factor IX, and factor X. ♦ Vitamin K is also necessary for the formation of osteocalcin—a calcium-binding protein in bone	♦ Vitamin K is necessary for bone formation and blood clotting, thus obvious clinical applications include osteoporosis/osteopenia and menorrhagia/ecchymosis. ♦ **Vitamin K1 (phylloquinone)**—doses of at least 1,000 IU per day of K1 are needed in order to optimize carboxylation of osteocalcin.[436] ♦ **Vitamin K2 (menaquinone)**—A recent study with 21 patients in the treatment group published in JAMA used 45 mg/d (forty five milligrams per day = 45,000 mcg per day) of vitamin K2 for an 80% reduction in liver cancer in patients with viral cirrhosis: *"Compliance with vitamin K2 in the treatment group was good; no patient had adverse reactions or dropped out of the study."*[437]
B-1 (thiamine)	♦ Classic deficiency is dry beriberi (central and peripheral neurologic dysfunction, dementia, psychosis, weakness, neuropathy) and wet beriberi (congestive heart failure). The classic CNS manifestations of thiamine/magnesium deficiency seen in alcoholics is Wernecke-Korsakoff syndrome. ♦ Conversion from the inactive form to the active form of the vitamin requires magnesium. ♦ Functions include: enzyme cofactor, aldehyde transfer, modulates chloride ion channels in the CNS, energy production in hexose monophosphate shunt, phagocytic respiratory burst, neurotransmitter synthesis and release. ♦ Anaphylaxis to parenteral thiamine has been reported	♦ 20-100 mg is a common supplemental dose; one study used 5,000 mg to find evidence of a cholinergic effect.[438] The densest food source of thiamine is brewer's yeast. ♦ Thiamine insufficiency is common in patients with **cardiomyopathy**.[439,440] Alleviates congestive heart failure in some patients, especially when used with CoQ10 and magnesium.[441] ♦ Deficiency is common in the demented elderly; alleviates "Alzheimer's disease" in some patients
B-2 (riboflavin)	♦ Classic deficiency: angular stomatitis ♦ 20-200 mg is a common supplemental dose. The richest dietary sources are yeast and liver. ♦ Several studies have used 400 mg per day in patients with migraine and have not reported any serious adverse effects. ♦ Functions include: enzyme cofactor (especially for energy production as FAD in the electron transport chain), drug/xenobiotic detoxification via support of Cy-P450, antioxidant functions via glutathione reductase.	♦ 400 mg per morning is safe and effective for the alleviation of **migraine**.[442]

[436] Binkley NC, Krueger DC, Kawahara TN, Engelke JA, Chappell RJ, Suttie JW. A high phylloquinone intake is required to achieve maximal osteocalcin gamma-carboxylation. *Am J Clin Nutr.* 2002 Nov;76(5):1055-60

[437] Habu D, Shiomi S, Tamori A, Takeda T, Tanaka T, Kubo S, Nishiguchi S. Role of vitamin K2 in the development of hepatocellular carcinoma in women with viral cirrhosis of the liver. *JAMA.* 2004 Jul 21;292(3):358-61

[438] Meador KJ, Nichols ME, Franke P, Durkin MW, Oberzan RL, Moore EE, Loring DW. Evidence for a central cholinergic effect of high-dose thiamine. *Ann Neurol.* 1993 Nov;34(5):724-6

[439] da Cunha S, Albanesi Filho FM, da Cunha Bastos VL, Antelo DS, Souza MM. Thiamin, selenium, and copper levels in patients with idiopathic dilated cardiomyopathy taking diuretics. *Arq Bras Cardiol.* 2002 Nov;79(5):454-65

[440] Wohl MG, Brody M, Shuman CR, Turner R, Brody J. Thiamine and cocarboxylase concentration in heart, liver and kidney, of patients with heart failure. *J Clin Invest.* 1954;33(11):1580-6

[441] Shimon I, Almog S, Vered Z, Seligmann H, Shefi M, Peleg E, Rosenthal T, Motro M, Halkin H, Ezra D. Improved left ventricular function after thiamine supplementation in patients with congestive heart failure receiving long-term furosemide therapy. *Am J Med.* 1995 May;98(5):485-90

[442] Boehnke C, Reuter U, Flach U, Schuh-Hofer S, Einhaupl KM, Arnold G. High-dose riboflavin treatment is efficacious in migraine prophylaxis: an open study in a tertiary care centre. *Eur J Neurol.* 2004 Jul;11(7):475-7

Nutrients	*Physiology, toxicity, contraindications*	*Clinical applications (adult doses)*
Vitamin B-3: niacin	◆ Classic deficiency is pellagra: depression, dermatitis, dementia, diarrhea, death. Endogenous production requires 60 mg tryptophan to make 1 mg niacin. Richest dietary sources are yeast, rice bran, wheat bran, liver, and poultry breast meat. ◆ 20-100 mg is a common supplemental dose; doses up to 2,000 mg per day in divided doses are used for the treatment of hypercholesterolemia and must be monitored with lab tests to assess for possible liver dysfunction. Up to 6 grams (6,000 mg) per day in divided doses has been used safely. ◆ Liver damage has been seen with doses > 2,000 mg per day. Patients on high doses must be monitored with periodic measurements of liver enzymes; not to be used in patients with liver disease. "Time-release niacin" is the most hepatotoxic form of niacin.	◆ **Dyslipidemia**: Niacin at 2000-3000 mg per day in divided doses can lower total and LDL cholesterol, fibrinogen, triglyceride levels, and raise HDL. In a head-to-head study 2,000 mg niacin was more powerful than 1,200 mg gemfibrozil for favorably modifying lipids.[443]
B-3: niacinamide	◆ 20-100 mg is a common supplemental dose. ◆ 500 mg 4-6 times per day for 2,000 – 3,000 mg per day is safe and effective for osteoarthritis. ◆ Toxicity is rare; however monitoring liver enzymes at 1 and 4 months and yearly thereafter is encouraged when doses ≥ 2000 mg are used.	◆ anti-aging (reversal of aging phenotypes via histone acetylation) ◆ **osteoarthritis**
B-3: inositol hexaniacinate ("no-flush niacin")	◆ This is a slow release form of vitamin B3 that allows supplementation with niacin at high doses without the flushing and hepatotoxicity seen with plain niacin. However, despite one enthusiastic article stating that this is the preferred form of B3 for treating lipid disorders, inositol hexaniacinate appears clinically ineffective for the treatment of dyslipidemia.	◆ 2000 mg per day in divided doses of 500-1000 mg each is common. ◆ 4,000 mg per day safely improves circulation in patients with **Raynaud's phenomenon**[444]
B-5 (pantothenic acid)	◆ Deficiency is generally unrecognized, but may include depression, acne, anemia, and weight gain; richest dietary sources are yeast and liver. ◆ Main physiologic functions include its structural role in the formation of the Coenzyme A molecule.	◆ 20-100 mg is a common supplemental dose, and doses of 10,000 mg calcium pantothenate have been used safely; it is virtually non-toxic. ◆ May help alleviate **fatigue** in some patients. ◆ May alleviate **acne** in some patients.

[443] Sprecher DL. Raising high-density lipoprotein cholesterol with niacin and fibrates: a comparative review. *Am J Cardiol*. 2000 Dec 21;86(12A):46L-50L
[444] Sunderland GT, Belch JJ, Sturrock RD, Forbes CD, McKay AJ. A double blind randomised placebo controlled trial of hexopal in primary Raynaud's disease. *Clin Rheumatol*. 1988 Mar;7(1):46-9

Appendix A: Clinical and Physiologic Considerations of Vitamins and Minerals—*continued*

Nutrients	Physiology, toxicity, and contraindications	Clinical applications (adult doses)
Vitamin B-6 Pyridoxine	♦ Deficiency can cause widespread—subtle or severe—problems and manifestations since this cofactor is used in more than 100 enzymatic reactions. Modest dietary sources are yeast, sunflower seeds, and wheat germ. Deficiency of B6 can be induced by the drug Isoniazid. ♦ 20-100 mg is a common supplemental dose; 250 mg per day with breakfast is safe and reasonable when higher doses are needed; this should be co-administered with a multivitamin/multimineral supplement that supplies other vitamins and minerals, especially replacement doses (200-600 mg) of magnesium. Very high doses of vitamin B6 (600-900 mg) are supported by the literature for the treatment of specific conditions, and doses ≤ 1,000 mg per day have been used safely with doctor supervision.[445] ♦ Peripheral sensory (and motor) neuropathy has been reported in patients taking gram doses for several years. Most of these reports appear associated with synthetic pyridoxine HCl and the toxicity is likely due to untreated magnesium deficiency which impairs conversion of neurotoxic pyridoxine HCl into the safe and active pyridoxal 5' phosphate. Doses of B6 greater than 150 mg may suppress prolactin and lactation.	♦ Pyridoxine HCl is synthetic and somewhat neurotoxic until it is converted to pyridoxal 5' phosphate which requires magnesium. Pyridoxine HCl must always be coadministered with magnesium. ♦ **Clinical applications: carpal tunnel syndrome, autism, epilepsy, PMS, calcium oxalate nephrolithiasis, nausea/vomiting of pregnancy.** ♦ Vitamin B6 is commonly used to promote various forms of detoxification; however high doses may paradoxically inhibit the sulfotransferase aspect of detoxification.
B-12 (cobalamin) "Active" and biologically useful forms of this vitamin: ♦ Hydroxy-cobalamin also called hydroxo-cobalamin ♦ Adenosyl-cobalamin ♦ Methyl-cobalamin ♦ Cyanocobala min contains cyanide, which is poisonous at high doses[446]	♦ Classic deficiency manifests as megaloblastic anemia, dorsal column lesions (i.e., loss of pedal vibration and proprioception), mental depression, fatigue, peripheral neuropathy. "Pernicious anemia" is a type of B12 deficiency caused by autoimmune atrophic gastritis wherein parietal cells are destroyed, leaving the host without intrinsic factor. Best dietary sources are liver, clams, and kidneys—vegetarian diets are notoriously deficient in B12. ♦ 100 – 2,000 mcg is a common supplemental dose; at least 2,000 mcg per day is required to increase blood levels in patients with B12 deficiency and malabsorption ♦ essentially non-toxic ♦ cyanocobalamin contains cyanide and should be avoided; anaphylaxis to parenteral b12 has been reported	♦ Cyanocobalamin contains cyanide and should be avoided as it can contribute to chronic cyanide toxicity and loss of vision (tobacco-alcohol amblyopia)—the treatment for the latter problem is administration of nutrients with an emphasis on hydroxocobalamin ♦ "active" forms include methylcobalamin and hydroxocobalamin ♦ At least 2,000 mcg per day is required to increase blood levels in patients with B12 deficiency to the same levels that can be obtained with standard regimens of parenteral/intramuscular administration.[447] ♦ **Vitamin B12 in high doses appears to help alleviate low-back pain[448]: this study used intramuscular administration, but high-dose oral supplementation should be superior if doses >2,000 mcg are used.** ♦ Can alleviate fatigue, especially neurogenic fatigue in patients with chronic infections.

[445] Ames BN, Elson-Schwab I, Silver EA. High-dose vitamin therapy stimulates variant enzymes with decreased coenzyme binding affinity (increased K(m)): relevance to genetic disease and polymorphisms. *Am J Clin Nutr*. 2002 Apr;75(4):616-58

[446] Reidenberg MM. Cyanocobalamin--a case for withdrawal. *J R Soc Med*. 1993 May;86(5):309

[447] Kuzminski AM, Del Giacco EJ, Allen RH, Stabler SP, Lindenbaum J. Effective treatment of cobalamin deficiency with oral cobalamin. *Blood*. 1998 Aug 15;92(4):1191-8

[448] Mauro GL, Martorana U, Cataldo P, Brancato G, Letizia G. Vitamin B12 in low back pain: a randomised, double-blind, placebo-controlled study. *Eur Rev Med Pharmacol Sci*. 2000 May-Jun;4:53-8

Nutrients	Physiology, toxicity, and contraindications	Clinical applications (adult doses)
Biotin	◆ Necessary for fatty acid metabolism and mitochondrial function. Deficiency can include hyperlactatemia, ataxia, seizures, hypotonia, seborrheic dermatitis, and hair loss. Richest dietary source is brewer's yeast. Deficiency is uncommon in the general population however it is commonly seen in patients taking inadequate parenteral nutrition. ◆ **Virtually non-toxic:** In 2001, the Food and Nutrition Board (FNB) reported that no adverse effects had been documented due to either dietary or supplemental consumption of biotin, and this document was still presented as accurate/current as of September 2005.[449] ◆ Avidin in raw egg whites irreversibly binds to biotin and prevents absorption	◆ 50 – 3,000 mcg is a common supplemental dose. ◆ **May provide benefit to diabetics, especially for the treatment/prevention of peripheral neuropathy**[450] ◆ **Biotin deficiency during pregnancy is common may result in birth defects; supplementation of pregnant women with ~300 mcg is warranted**[451]
Folic acid	◆ Found in low doses in foliage. Numerous functions include the transfer of methyl groups, necessary for the formation of myelin, neurotransmitters, and for the protection of DNA. Brewer's yeast is clearly the densest dietary source of folic acid. Deficiency causes macrocytic anemia, fatigue, depression, and hyperhomocysteinemia. B12 and folic acid should be coadministered. ◆ 800 mcg is a reasonable supplemental dose and should be considered the minimal supplemental dose. Doses of 5, 10, and 20 mg (i.e., up to 20,000 mcg) are commonly used and are generally safe. ◆ Use folic acid cautiously in patients with a history of seizure or those who are taking anti-seizure medications. Anti-seizure medications induce deficiency of folate, and if folate is replaced, then anti-seizure protection may be lost.	◆ Always use with B-12 and other B-vitamins ◆ **Potentiates antidepressants by addressing the previously undiagnosed folic acid deficiency** ◆ **Improves efficacy and reduces toxicity of methotrexate** ◆ **Lowers homocysteine levels, may also require B12, B6, NAC, etc.**
Vitamin C **Ascorbic acid**	◆ Classic deficiency is scurvy: bleeding gums, subcutaneous bleeding (ecchymoses, petechiae), weak and friable skin and mucus membranes, reduced immunity, corkscrew hairs, and follicular hyperkeratosis. Vitamin C has some function as an antioxidant, in immune support, and in (dopaminergic) neurotransmission. The best dietary sources are fresh fruits and vegetables, which also contain the phytochemicals necessary to optimize the function of vitamin C. ◆ 500-1,000 mg is a reasonable daily dosage for preventive healthcare; ◆ High doses cause benign loose stools; this varies from patient to patient and time to time; some patients get loose stools with 500 mg while others can tolerate 10,000 mg with no problems. ◆ Intravenous ascorbate can induce hemolysis in patients with G6PD deficiency ◆ Oral supplementation can exacerbate cardiac complications of iron overload[452]	◆ **Anti-allergy benefits in high doses due to mechanisms including ~40% reductions in serum histamine** ◆ **6,000 mg/d in divided doses has been shown to have anti-stress benefits.**[453] ◆ **Anticancer effects may require bowel-tolerance dosing or intravenous administration.** ◆ **High doses benefit autistic children via a dopaminergic mechanism**[454]

[449] Food and Nutrition Board (FNB). Dietary Reference Intakes-Vitamins. http://www.nal.usda.gov/fnic/etext/000105.html http://www.iom.edu/Object.File/Master/7/296/0.pdf Sept 6, 2005
[450] Koutsikos D, Agroyannis B, Tzanatos-Exarchou H. Biotin for diabetic peripheral neuropathy. *Biomed Pharmacother*. 1990;44(10):511-4
[451] Mock DM, Quirk JG, Mock NI. Marginal biotin deficiency during normal pregnancy. *Am J Clin Nutr*. 2002 Feb;75(2):295-9
[452] McLaran CJ, Bett JH, Nye JA, Halliday JW. Congestive cardiomyopathy and haemochromatosis--rapid progression possibly accelerated by excessive ingestion of ascorbic acid. *Aust N Z J Med*. 1982 Apr;12(2):187-8
[453] Brody S, Preut R, Schommer K, Schurmeyer TH. A randomized controlled trial of high dose ascorbic acid for reduction of blood pressure, cortisol, and subjective responses to psychological stress. *Psychopharmacology* (Berl). 2002 Jan;159(3):319-24
[454] Dolske MC, Spollen J, McKay S, Lancashire E, Tolbert L. A preliminary trial of ascorbic acid as supplemental therapy for autism. *Prog Neuropsychopharmacol Biol Psychiatry*. 1993 Sep;17(5):765-74

Appendix A: Clinical and Physiologic Considerations of Vitamins and Minerals—*continued*

Nutrients	Physiology, toxicity, and contraindications	Clinical applications (adult doses)
Calcium	◆ 500 - 1,500 mg is the common supplemental dose ◆ 1,000 - 1,500 mg is the recommended supplemental dose in patients with osteopenia ◆ may promote constipation, especially if not balanced with magnesium, supplementation should provide a 1:2 to 1:1 ratio of calcium to magnesium ◆ Do not administer with certain medications, especially antibiotics such as tetracycline, due to the binding effect which renders the drug systemically unavailable and can result in death in patients with life-threatening infections like pneumonia	◆ **can promote constipation** ◆ **always use with magnesium** ◆ **alleviates bruxism** ◆ **alleviates PMS** ◆ **significantly lowers blood pressure in hypertensive patients when used with vitamin D**
Magnesium	◆ Magnesium deficiency is clearly one of the most common nutritional deficiencies in all populations. ◆ 200 -800 mg is a common supplemental dose; high doses cause loose stools. ◆ Do not administer high doses to patients with severe constipation or with renal failure due to potential for hypermagnesemia. ◆ Do not administer with certain medications, especially antibiotics such as tetracycline, due to the binding effect; spironolactone is a magnesium-sparing diuretic that can potentiate hypermagnesemia	◆ **alleviates bruxism** ◆ **alleviates PMS** ◆ **alleviates migraine headaches** ◆ **alleviates constipation** ◆ **alleviates muscle spasm and hypertonicity** ◆ **helps with asthma, hypertension, insomnia, irritability, anxiety, detoxification,**
Zinc	◆ 10 – 25 mg per day is common in supplements; ◆ Doses up to 150 mg can be used therapeutically, preferably for short-term only or balanced with 2-4 mg copper ◆ Excess or imbalanced zinc supplementation can promote copper deficiency by competition for absorption ◆ Do not use high-dose zinc in patients with Alzheimer's disease[455] ◆ Must be administered with food in order to avoid stomach irritation	◆ **Improves mucosal integrity in patients with Crohn's disease when used at 150 mg per day** ◆ **Promotes tissue healing: trauma, diabetic ulcers**
Copper	◆ 2 mg is the most common supplemental dose ◆ Excess or imbalanced copper supplementation can promote zinc deficiency by competition for absorption ◆ Wilson's disease is a type of copper toxicity associated with liver disease and neuropsychiatric disorder	◆ **A good multivitamin should have enough so that you don't have to use a separate supplement.** ◆ **up to 4 mg per day can be used in patients with connective tissue disorders such as Marfan's syndrome and/or to promote healing**

---

[455] Vasquez A. A brief review of two potential adverse effects of zinc supplementation: cognitive deterioration in patients with Alzheimer's disease, and copper deficiency. *Nutritional Perspectives* 1995; 18: 11, 19

Nutrients	Physiology and contraindications	Clinical applications (adult doses)
Chromium	♦ Appears to have a homeostatic effect on glucose-insulin metabolism ♦ may potentiate diabetic medications; start slowly and with 6x daily glucose monitoring in severe diabetics	♦ 200 mcg is the most common supplemental dose ♦ 500 mcg is commonly used in diabetics ♦ doses up to 1,000 mcg have been used safely in diabetics ♦ Quality multivitamin-multimineral supplements will contain at least 200 mcg of chromium ♦ Can alleviate diabetes mellitus and hypoglycemia
Iodide & Iodine	♦ Necessary for the formation of thyroid hormone ♦ May beneficially modulate estrogen metabolism in women ♦ Thins mucus ♦ May have antimicrobial benefits, especially in the stomach and upper intestine ♦ Iodine is the natural elemental diatomic form of this element, consisting of two iodide molecules; **both iodine and iodine have beneficial properties and one does not necessarily substitute for the other—supplementation should include both forms** ♦ A few patients appear allergic to iodine-iodide and should avoid supplementation until their immune function is normalized	♦ **Several experts in iodine/iodide nutrition—namely Wright, Abraham, and Brownstein—are now advocating iodine-iodide supplementation with daily doses of 12 milligrams (12,000 micrograms) since these doses provide benefit, are without acute toxicity, and are very comparable to the average daily Japanese intake at 13.8 milligrams per day**[456] ♦ High doses of iodine 3-6 mg per day can reduce breast pain during 6 months of treatment[457] ♦ Lecithin-bound iodine modulates cytokine release and may improve symptoms in patients with asthma[458] ♦ Daily doses greater than 750 mcg iodide can contribute to exacerbation of hypothyroidism in patients with *pre-existing* thyroid disorders or borderline thyroid function[459]; the combination of iodine-iodide may actually improve thyroid function in patients with thyroid disease[460] ♦ Abraham[461] has advocated the use of high-dose iodine supplementation ("orthoiodosupplementation") and has used short-term doses as high as 50 mg per day (fifty milligrams per day). He reports that the toxicity associated with iodine-containing drugs (Amiodarone: antiarrhythmic) is due to the drug itself and not the iodine. Rationale for "high dose" iodine supplementation is suggested by the increased prevalence of halogenated/brominated pesticides/herbicides and other pollutants in our environment which are known to have adverse health effects
Potassium	♦ Get potassium from fruits and vegetables, not from supplements ♦ High-normal intake of potassium from fruits and vegetables can cause fatal hyperkalemia in patients with renal failure such as due to diabetes	♦ lowers blood pressure ♦ reduces risk of stroke independently from its ability to lower blood pressure ♦ promotes urinary alkalinization, which is important for mineral retention and increased excretion of most xenobiotics
Selenium	♦ 200 mcg is considered the standard supplemental and therapeutic dose ♦ Daily doses should be kept below 800-1,000 mcg, and high doses are generally used for a limited time only, such as a few days to a maximum of 3 months at a time	♦ antioxidant ♦ protects against cancer and heart disease ♦ immunosupportive; powerfully inhibits risk of serious infection in patients with HIV ♦ highly effective for relieving lymphedema

[456] Wright JV. Why you need 83 times more of this essential, cancer-fighting nutrient than the 'experts' say you do. *Nutrition and Healing* 2005; 12: 1
[457] "Patients recorded statistically significant decreases in pain by month 3 in the 3.0 and 6.0 mg/day treatment groups, but not the 1.5 mg/day or placebo group; more than 50% of the 6.0 mg/day treatment group recorded a clinically significant reduction in overall pain. All doses were associated with an acceptable safety profile." Kessler JH. The effect of supraphysiologic levels of iodine on patients with cyclic mastalgia. *Breast J.* 2004 Jul-Aug;10(4):328-36
[458] "Also, a longer course of treatment with LBI may markedly improve the clinical conditions of the asthmatic children, because even a period of just 8 weeks LBI therapy improved the cough and reduced the severity of the asthmatic attacks in two out of the nine patients enrolled in this study." Kawano Y, Saeki T, Noma T. Effect of lecithin-bound iodine on the patients with bronchial asthma. *Int Immunopharmacol.* 2005 Apr;5(4):805-10
[459] Chow CC, Phillips DI, Lazarus JH, Parkes AB. Effect of low dose iodide supplementation on thyroid function in potentially susceptible subjects: are dietary iodide levels in Britain acceptable? *Clin Endocrinol* (Oxf.) 1991 May;34(5):413-6
[460] Brownstein D. Clinical Experience with Inorganic Non-radioactive Iodine/Iodide. http://www.optimox.com/pics/Iodine/IOD-09/IOD_09.htm Accessed January 15, 2007
[461] Abraham GE. Serum inorganic iodide levels following ingestion of a tablet form of Lugol solution: evidence for an enterohepatic circulation of iodine. *The Original Internist.* 2004; 11: 29-35

Appendix A: Clinical and Physiologic Considerations of Vitamins and Minerals—*continued*

Nutrients	Physiology, toxicity, and contraindications	Clinical applications (adult doses)
Iron	◆ Iron supplementation should not be used in patients unless their iron levels are low, and this is determined by measuring serum ferritin—not by performing a CBC which can show anemia that is unrelated to iron deficiency and which may be associated with iron overload. ◆ The finding of iron deficiency in any adult patient requires that the patient be referred to a gastroenterologist for endoscopic evaluation. Failure to make a timely referral for any adult patient with iron deficiency is grounds for malpractice litigation. ◆ Iron promotes the formation of "free radicals" and is thus implicated in several diseases, such as infections, cancer, liver disease, diabetes, and cardiovascular disease. Iron supplements should not be consumed except by people who have been definitively diagnosed with iron deficiency by measurement of serum ferritin. For a simplistic review, see http://vix.com/menmag/alexiron.htm	◆ **Never use iron supplementation without first testing serum ferritin.**[462,463] ◆ **Replacement dose for iron deficiency is 60-180 mg of iron per day. 40-60 mg 3x per day is reasonable for correcting iron deficiency; may promote constipation and stomach upset; consume with food, especially meat;** ◆ <u>**All adult patients with iron deficiency have a gastrointestinal lesion such as cancer until proven otherwise.**</u> **CLINICIANS MUST REFER THESE PATIENTS TO A GASTROENTEROLOGIST.**[464]

Screen asymptomatic patients.	**Follow-up abnormal laboratory results.** (high serum iron, elevated liver enzymes, high blood glucose, etc.)	**Screen high-risk and symptomatic patients.**

Assess iron status with transferrin saturation and serum ferritin. Use fasting morning specimen.

IRON-DEFICIENCY serum ferritin:<10-15 in women, <20 in men, transferrin saturation:<16%

"HEALTHY IRON STATUS" transferrin saturation:25-30% serum ferritin: 30-70

"MODERATE IRON OVERLOAD" transferrin saturation: >33-45% serum ferritin: 80-160

POSSIBLE SEVERE IRON OVERLOAD transferrin saturation: >40% and/or serum ferritin: >160 in women; >200 in men

In adults with no obvious cause of blood loss: Assume pathologic gastrointestinal bleeding until proven otherwise. Simply testing for occult blood in the stool is insufficient. **Refer for complete (endoscopic) evaluation.**

Periodically assess iron status as part of routine health assessment. Consider assessment for impending iron deficiency. Consider periodic blood donation and low-iron diet to maintain healthy iron status.

No treatment is mandatory. Periodically assess iron status as part of routine health assessment. Consider low-iron diet and regular blood donation to reduce risk of cancer and myocardial infarction.

Repeat tests with fasting morning specimen. Consider other causes of elevated transferrin saturation or elevated serum ferritin.*

Second assessment suggests "healthy iron status" or "moderate iron overload": Average results and/or reassess within 1 month, or periodically assess iron status as part of routine health assessment.

PROBABLE SEVERE IRON OVERLOAD Ferritin >200 in women, or Ferritin >300 in men. **Confirm with diagnostic phlebotomy, or liver biopsy, or MRI.**

***Factors that alter iron assessment tests**: **False elevations of transferrin saturation:** cancer, liver disease, inflammation, infection, excess alcohol consumption, non-fasting specimens. **False elevations of ferritin:** inflammation, infection, cancer, excess alcohol consumption, liver disease, early pregnancy, hyperthyroidism, tissue necrosis, hyperferremia-cataract syndrome and other rare genetic/congenital syndromes.

Refer as needed (usually gastroenterologist, hematologist, or internist) for phlebotomy therapy and/or deferoxamine chelation.

---

[462] Vasquez A. <u>Integrative Orthopedics: Concepts, Algorithms, and Therapeutics. The art of creating wellness while effectively managing acute and chronic musculoskeletal disorders</u>. Natural Health Consulting Corporation: www.OptimalHealthResearch.com 2004, Revised edition August 2004

[463] Hollan S, Johansen KS. Adequate iron stores and the 'Nil nocere' principle. *Haematologia* (Budap). 1993;25(2):69-84

[464] Green BT, Rockey DC. Gastrointestinal endoscopic evaluation of premenopausal women with iron deficiency anemia. *J Clin Gastroenterol*. 2004 Feb;38(2):104-9

Core Competencies and Standards of Clinical Excellence:

1) You must know how to diagnose developmental dysplasia of the hip in a newborn.
2) What is the proper management of stress fractures of the proximal femur?
3) Define atlantoaxial instability and os odontoidium and list their presentations, complications and management.
4) How do you diagnose and manage slipped capital femoral epiphysis, avascular necrosis, and septic arthritis?
5) How do you differentially diagnose and manage meralgia paresthetica from femoral neuropathy?
6) Since differentiation based on physical examination and history is impossible, you must know which lab tests are used to distinguish hip osteoarthritis from hemochromatoic arthropathy and how the tests are correlatively interpreted.
7) You must know how to diagnose by cauda equina syndrome *by history and physical examination alone* (e.g., without CT or MRI results).
8) You must know how to diagnose and manage vertebral osteomyelitis and infectious discitis.
9) Be able to explain the mechanism by which vitamin D deficiency causes low back pain; know the indications, contraindications, dosing, and monitoring involved with vitamin D supplementation.
10) Name five inflammatory disorders that can affect the lumbar spine and sacroiliac joints. Provide the diagnostic criteria and management strategy of each.
11) List at least five ways to improve proprioceptive/sensorimotor function in patients with low-back pain.
12) Differentially diagnose a bladder infection from a kidney infection; describe appropriate management strategies for both problems.
13) Be able to explain why "fibromyalgia" is an overused diagnosis and be able to provide a list of treatable conditions that are often misdiagnosed as fibromyalgia.
14) Name the proper angle for obtaining an anteroposterior radiograph of the knee to demonstrate osteoarthritis.
15) List the characteristics of migraine headaches and the proper administration of six nutritional treatments.
16) Differentiate a benign headache from one that is potentially life-threatening.
17) Name the two best and most commonly used tests for assessing the anterior cruciate ligament. Which test is better and why?
18) McMurray's test is one of the most commonly used tests for assessing menisci. How is the test performed, and what is the sensitivity and specificity of a positive finding?
19) You must know how to identify and manage acute compartment syndrome.
20) If you think your patient may have a meniscus injury, how do you decide for or against ordering an MRI?
21) Describe the clinical manifestations of spinal cord compression.
22) Your patient is a cyclist and presents with knee pain under the patella on the lateral aspect. What is the most likely diagnosis and your treatment?
23) Why must you examine the *hip* of an adolescent patient who presents with *knee* pain? Provide the specific anatomic basis.
24) You must know how to distinguish *benign* sacroiliac and pelvic pain from that which results from rheumatic diseases such as the spondyloarthropathies and infections.
25) You must know the wrist/hand manifestations of hemochromatosis and how to differentiate this potentially life-threatening condition from benign osteoarthritis. Compare and contrast the physical examination, laboratory, and treatment differences.
26) You must know how to differentially diagnose and treat rheumatoid arthritis, osteoarthritis, and hemochromatosis.
27) You must know how to properly administer high-dose pyridoxine as a component of the treatment plan for a patient with carpal tunnel syndrome.
28) You must know how to diagnose and manage fracture of the scaphoid.
29) You must know how to manage a hand/bone injury that has been contaminated with human saliva, such as a hand injury resulting from a fist fight.
30) You must know how to diagnose and manage supracondylar fractures of the humerus.
31) You must know how to diagnose and manage lateral epicondylitis.
32) Differentially diagnose and treat rotator cuff tendonitis from proximal biceps tendonitis.
33) Differentially diagnose overuse bursitis from septic bursitis.
34) Differentiate thoracic outlet syndrome from fibromyalgia and the musculoskeletal manifestations of hypothyroidism.
35) You must know how to grade reflexes and muscle strength and know the implications and management of abnormal findings

36) You must know how to rapidly diagnose and effectively manage the following musculoskeletal emergencies: Neuropsychiatric lupus, Giant cell arteritis, Temporal arteritis, Acute red eye, including acute iritis and scleritis, Atlantoaxial subluxation & instability, Myelopathy, spinal cord compression, Cauda equina syndrome, Septic arthritis, Osteomyelitis, Acute nontraumatic monoarthritis

37) Following a joint aspiration for acute monoarthritis, which analyses are used to differentiate septic arthritis from inflammatory arthritis and gout?

38) Demonstrate competency in the interpretation and correlative interpretation of the following commonly performed tests: CRP, ESR, CBC, Chemistry/metabolic panel, Ferritin, Serum 25(OH)-vitamin D, TSH, ANA, CCP.

39) For example, what is the important difference between "elevated CRP with a normal ferritin" and "elevated CRP with elevated ferritin."

40) *Bonus*: If the lactulose-mannitol assay is abnormal (elevated lactulose-to-mannitol ratio) and the comprehensive stool analysis and comprehensive parasitology results are normal, what are the two most likely diagnoses, assuming that your patient does not overconsume alcohol or NSAIDs.

41) If your patient's serum 25(OH)-vitamin D is low but the serum calcium level is elevated, what are three possible underlying diseases and what single blood test is most indicated?

42) Describe how to clinically distinguish fibromyalgia from polymyalgia rheumatica.

43) How are nondisplaced clavicle fractures managed?

44) Provide one example from each letter of the "p.r.i.c.e. a. t.u.r.n." and "b.e.n.d. s.t.e.m.s." mnemonic acronyms for holistic acute care for musculoskeletal injuries.

45) List the two most common clinical findings associated with myofascial trigger points and describe appropriate physical/manual and nutritional treatments.

46) Describe a plan for proproceptive retraining/rehabilitation for a patient who has no exercise equipment.

47) Describe the effects of stereotypic NSAIDs on chrondrocyte metabolism and the long-term effects on joint structure.

48) Name four biochemical/physiologic mechanisms by which COX-2 inhibiting drugs predispose to cardiovascular death.

49) Name the only absolute contraindication to the use of willow bark extract.

50) In a patient with fever and focal back pain exacerbated by spinal percussion, what is the most likely diagnosis?

51) How do you differentiate chest/back pain resulting from a "benign" musculoskeletal condition from pain that is a manifestation of intrathoracic pathology?

52) Briefly and generally describe how to administer the following relative to the treatment of musculoskeletal pain; you must know the treatments by their commonly used names and abbreviations: ALA, EPA, DHA, GLA, D3, Niacinamide, Glucosamine sulfate and Chondroitin Sulfate, proteolytic enzymes, *Zingiber*, Cat's claw, *Salix*, topical *Capsicum annuum*, *Boswellia*, Devil's claw, *Curcuma longa*

The following questions are derived from the midterm and final exam questions that I created when I taught Orthopedics at Bastyr University in 2000. The emphasis of the exam is on clinical synthesis—combining history, physical examination, lab and imaging, along with basic knowledge of therapeutics such as manipulation, botanical medicine, nutrition, physiotherapy, and other subjects taught and tested in other courses. "Core competencies" represent the information that every student and doctor must know; missing even one of these questions meant failure for the entire examination. An answered version of first edition of this assessment is available on-line at: www.OptimalHealthResearch.com/tests/**musculoskeletal**. Questions in **bold** were added in March 2007.

PART ONE

List and provide one example of the **4 general categories** that need to be assessed during the history and physical when a patient presents with a musculoskeletal complaint:
1. Example:
2. Example:
3. Example:
4. Example:

Your patient presents with a complex history and examination picture that suggests the possibility of organic disease as a cause of his/her complaints, but you are not sure what disease might be present. **List the combination of lab tests that represent a safe and reasonably inexpensive means of laboratory investigation that allows you to objectively screen for several different diseases:**
1. (essential)
2. (essential)
3. (essential)
4. (optional)
5. (optional)

What percentage range of "trauma-related" injuries
are actually associated with organic disease? _____

A 50-year-old woman presents with generalized stiffness and pain in the shoulder for 2 months duration; she recalls no trauma. On examination she exhibits severe loss of internal and external rotation and abduction at the shoulder.

What is the most likely diagnosis?_____

What two endocrine conditions must she be assessed for with a blood test? _____

A 60-year-old man presents with diffuse pain in the left shoulder region for 4-weeks duration; he recalls no trauma and notes that the pain is worse at night. His health history reveals that he follows a typical American diet, walks for exercise, is right-handed, is a house painter by profession, and that he no longer smokes. Physical examination reveals the following:
- Shoulder ROM is full and generally painless except for what you consider to be mild age-related stiffness that is symmetric
- Provocative maneuvers are negative
- He is afebrile, and blood pressure, pulse, and peripheral capillary refill are normal
- Lab tests performed by his MD last week show slight anemia, normal ferritin, and slightly elevated Hgb-A1c

What condition should he be assessed for?_____

What additional physical examination procedures should be performed? _____

If the above test is positive, what is your next step? _____

Mark the 1 (one) best answer for each of the following questions.

1) Which of the following are characteristics of "cancer pain:"
   A. Vague, diffuse pain
   B. Worse at night
   C. Increasing severity
   D. Unrelieved by rest, unresponsive to standard musculoskeletal treatment
   E. All of the above.

2) Your patient is over age 50 and has back pain, which he cannot ascribe to any recent injury, motions, or positions. The ESR is 40 and ferritin is 8. Which of the following is the best next step?
   A. High-dose proteolytic enzymes
   B. *Boswellia* tincture dosed per body weight
   C. Topical capsaicin
   D. Radiographs
   E. A 2-week trial of spinal manipulation

3) Your 55-year-old patient presents with left-sided shoulder pain, wrist weakness, miosis, ptosis of the left eyelid, and anhidrosis (decreased sweating) of the left side of the face. The condition for which you must assess is:
   A. Cauda equina syndrome
   B. Thoracic outlet syndrome
   C. Pancoast syndrome
   D. Chronic fatigue syndrome
   E. Frozen shoulder syndrome

4) Which of the following are causes of shoulder pain:
   A. Apical lung tumor
   B. Cervical radiculopathy
   C. Impingement syndrome
   D. Biceps tendonitis
   E. All of the above

5) Your 25-year-old patient presents to you following a car accident that occurred earlier that morning. He has neck pain, and requests that you treat him homeopathically and with herbs for the tingling he now has in his arms and legs. You should:
   A. Immediately perform the Sotto-Hall neck-flexion test to assess him for cervical instability.
   B. Take a complete homeopathic history and send him home with a remedy after telling him to avoid coffee and mint. Follow-up visit is scheduled for 2 weeks.
   C. Prescribe high-dose bromelain.
   D. Perform a cautious physical examination to determine which is more appropriate: radiographs or hospital referral.
   E. Begin treatment with manipulation.

6) Your 42-year-old patient presents with "shoulder pain" and "insomnia." History reveals that she has difficulty getting to sleep due to the shoulder pain. During physical examination, you find that ROM is full and does not exacerbate her pain, and that there is slight swelling in the supraclavicular fossa. The best choice from the selection below is:
   A. Order radiographs or CT scan
   B. Request a diet diary
   C. Request a urinalysis
   D. Recommend that she get a new pillow
   E. Valerian tincture to help her sleep

7) Your new 20-year-old patient presents with chief complaints of "back pain" and "the flu." The onset of both complaints was yesterday with a slight fever and now the back pain is rated 7 on a scale of 1-10 with 10 being severe pain. Lungs are clear to auscultation, and the lower back is stiff and painful to percussion. Your main concern is:
   A. Pancoast syndrome
   B. Myofascial trigger points
   C. Costochondritis
   D. Osteomyelitis
   E. Pneumonia

8) **Your diabetic adult male patient has CRP of 5, ESR of 5, and ferritin of 600. He is asymptomatic. The most likely cause to explain these findings is:**
   A. **Diabetes mellitus**
   B. **Osteochondritis**
   C. **Behcet's disease**
   D. **Hepatitis**
   E. **Hemochromatosis**

9) Rust's sign, whereby the patient needs to support head/neck during normal motions and positions to prevent pain, is considered indicative of:
   A. Cervical instability
   B. Cervical radiculopathy
   C. Tietze's syndrome
   D. Myofascial trigger points in the sternocleidomastoid
   E. Impingement syndrome

10) **Your elderly adult female patient presents with subacute back pain and has ESR of 40, CRP of 28, and ferritin of 5. She is afebrile and has no cardiac or intestinal complaints. Your next action is:**
    A. **Referral to a rheumatologist for immunosuppression**
    B. **Lumbar radiographs**
    C. **Referral to a gastroenterologist**
    D. **Joint aspiration**
    E. **Treat conservatively and repeat labs in 2 months**

11) Cervical radiculopathy is characterized by:
    A. Babinski reflex
    B. Upper extremity motor deficits with dermatomal sensory abnormalities
    C. Lower extremity hyperreflexia
    D. Bowel and bladder dysfunction
    E. Delayed Achilles' reflex return

12) In a patient with neck pain and dermatomal sensory changes in the arm, associated onset of which of the following suggests the need for additional investigation and/or referral to a surgeon?
    A. Asymmetric biceps weakness
    B. Babinski reflex
    C. Lower extremity clonus
    D. Incontinence
    E. All of the above

13) Recent trauma-related onset of myelopathy indicates the need for treatment, specifically with methylprednisolone, within:
    A. 8 hours
    B. 10 days
    C. 12 weeks
    D. The first 30 days of treatment

14) Which of the following are causes of torticollis?
    A. Cancer
    B. Infection
    C. Injury at birth
    D. Neuromuscular disease
    E. All of the above

15) **Your patient was in a severe car accident 2 days ago. Now she feels sleepy during the day, despite sleeping 10 hours each night, and has recent onset clonus. Proper management for this patient includes:**
    A. **Adrenergic agonist treatment, either with drugs or amino acid therapy**
    B. **Dopamine agonist, either with drugs or botanical medicines**
    C. **Laboratory assessment for anti-myelin antibodies**
    D. **CT scan**
    E. **Sotto-Hall test**

16) Pain in the C5 dermatome, with biceps strength +5
  A. Bicipital tendonitis—conservative treatment, no need for referral
  B. Cervical myelopathy—urgent referral
  C. Cervical radiculitis—conservative treatment, no need for referral
  D. Cervical radiculopathy—conservative treatment, no need for referral
  E. Supraspinatus tendonitis—conservative treatment, no need for referral

17) Pain in the C5 dermatome, with biceps strength +3
  A. Bicipital tendonitis—consider conservative treatment, PAR
  B. Cervical myelopathy—urgent referral
  C. Cervical radiculitis—consider conservative treatment, PAR
  D. Cervical radiculopathy—consider conservative treatment, PAR, recommend referral
  E. Supraspinatus tendonitis—consider conservative treatment, no need for referral

18) Pain in the C5 dermatome, lower extremity weakness, patellar and Achilles reflexes +4
  A. Bicipital tendonitis—conservative treatment, PAR
  B. Cervical myelopathy—urgent referral
  C. Cervical radiculitis—conservative treatment, PAR
  D. Cervical radiculopathy—conservative treatment, PAR, recommend referral
  E. Supraspinatus tendonitis—conservative treatment, no need for referral

19) Positive Speed's test and Yergason's test, sensory testing WNL, with biceps strength +4
  A. Bicipital tendonitis—conservative treatment, no need for referral
  B. Cervical myelopathy—urgent referral
  C. Cervical radiculitis—conservative treatment
  D. Cervical radiculopathy—recommend referral
  E. Supraspinatus tendonitis—conservative treatment, no need for referral

20) Pain with 90° shoulder abduction and internal rotation, pain with "empty can" test
  A. Bicipital tendonitis—conservative treatment, no need for referral
  B. Cervical myelopathy—urgent referral
  C. Cervical radiculitis—conservative treatment
  D. Cervical radiculopathy—recommend referral
  E. Supraspinatus tendonitis—conservative treatment, no need for referral

21) Your patient presents with neck pain following trauma. Your clinical assessment needs to evaluate for which of the following:
  A. Myelopathy
  B. Radiculopathy
  C. Fracture
  D. Instability
  E. All of the above

22) Tom is a 47-year-old right-handed male who presents to your office with a chief complaint of "chest pain" on the right that he first noticed this morning when he was finishing a tennis match with his son. He has anterior peristernal chest pain with point tenderness, increased pain with hyperabduction of the ipsilateral arm, increased pain with deep inspiration, increased pain with palpation-provocation of the peristernal structures. Cardiopulmonary assessments are WNL. Tom most likely has:
  A. Costochondritis
  B. Pancoast syndrome
  C. Horner's syndrome
  D. Intercostal neuralgia
  E. Cardiovascular disease

23) Bob is a 47-year-old right-handed male who presents to your office with a chief complaint of "chest pain" on the left that he first noticed this morning when he was finishing a tennis match with his son. He experienced anterior peristernal chest pain with diffuse tenderness, and your clinical assessment finds no increased pain with hyperabduction of the ipsilateral arm, no increased pain with deep inspiration, and no increased pain with palpation-provocation of the thoracic structures. Bob most likely has:
  A. Costochondritis (Tietze's syndrome)
  B. Pancoast syndrome
  C. Horner's syndrome
  D. Intercostal strain
  E. Cardiovascular disease

24) Mary is a 47-year-old right-handed female who presents to your office with a chief complaint of "chest pain" on the right that she first noticed this morning when she was finishing a tennis match with her son. She experienced anterior-lateral chest pain with sharp tenderness, and your clinical assessment finds increased pain with hyperabduction of the ipsilateral arm, increased pain with deep inspiration, and increased pain with deep palpation of the space between her 8th and 9th ribs. Mary most likely has:
   A. Costochondritis (Tietze's syndrome)
   B. Pancoast syndrome
   C. Horner's syndrome
   D. Intercostal muscle strain
   E. Cardiovascular disease

25) Suggested by signs of myelopathy with flexion and diagnosed with lateral radiographs demonstrating dens abnormities or increased atlantodental interval; may be seen in a patient with rheumatoid arthritis or ankylosing spondylitis:
   A. Atlantoaxial instability
   B. Cervical radiculitis
   C. Cervical radiculopathy
   D. Supraspinatus tendonitis
   E. De Quervain's syndrome

26) Common in patients with Down's syndrome, contraindication to cervical spine manipulation
   A. Atlantoaxial instability
   B. Foraminal encroachment
   C. Cervical radiculopathy
   D. Supraspinatus tendonitis
   E. Lesion of the subscapularis

27) Inability of the patient to lift the dorsum of the hand from the sacrum
   A. Atlantoaxial instability
   B. Bicipital tendonitis
   C. Cervical myelopathy
   D. Supraspinatus tendonitis
   E. Lesion of the subscapularis

28) Any patient diagnosed with adhesive capsulitis (and/or frozen shoulder) needs to be assessed with which of the following tests:
   A. Phalen's test
   B. Serum glucose
   C. Adson's test
   D. Soto-Hall test
   E. Serum CK-Mb

29) Elbow extended or flexed, forearm pronated, wrist extended, patient resists wrist flexion force by doctor
   A. Speed's test
   B. Lift-off test
   C. Codman's test
   D. Yergason's test
   E. Cozen's test

30) Elbow extended, passive wrist flexion to stretch the wrist extensors
   A. Phalen's test
   B. Mill's test
   C. Adson's test
   D. Soto-Hall test
   E. Varus testing

31) Inability to elevate the dorsum of the hand from the sacrum
   A. "Empty can" test, supraspinatus isolation test—supraspinatus tendonitis
   B. Speed's test—biceps tendonitis
   C. Lift-off test—subscapularis lesion
   D. Codman's test, arm drop test—supraspinatus tendonitis
   E. Yergason's test—biceps tendonitis

32) Weakness and pain when patient resists downward force applied to the distal forearm when shoulder is 90° abducted, internally rotated, with the arm in the scapular plane, with the elbow extended.
   A.   "Empty can" test, supraspinatus isolation test—supraspinatus tendonitis
   B.   Speed's test—biceps tendonitis
   C.   Lift-off test—subscapularis pathology
   D.   Codman's test, arm drop test—supraspinatus tendonitis
   E.   Yergason's test—biceps tendonitis

33) Which of the following problems is potentially serious and requires immediate assessment for neurovascular injury?
   A.   Supracondylar fracture of the humerus
   B.   Carpal tunnel syndrome
   C.   Rotator cuff tear
   D.   Costochondritis
   E.   De Quervain's syndrome

34) Following trauma or overuse of the brachioradialis or the wrist extensors; positive Cozen's test, positive Mill's test
   A.   Supraspinatus tendonitis
   B.   Lateral epicondylitis
   C.   Medial epicondylitis
   D.   Lesion of the subscapularis
   E.   De Quervain's syndrome

35) Positive Finkelstein's test
   A.   Pancoast syndrome
   B.   Lateral epicondylitis
   C.   Medial epicondylitis
   D.   Lesion of the subscapularis
   E.   De Quervain's syndrome

36) Reproduction of carpal tunnel syndrome manifestations with forced wrist flexion, may be held for 1 minute
   A.   Phalen's test
   B.   Mill's test
   C.   Codman's test
   D.   Yergason's test
   E.   Cozen's test

37) Your patient presents with pain at the "anatomic snuff box" following a fall on the palm with an extended wrist. While your evaluation should include assessment of neighboring regions, which condition is most likely in this patient:
   A.   Fracture of the dens
   B.   Medial epicondylitis
   C.   Fracture of the scaphoid
   D.   Supraspinatus tendonitis
   E.   Supracondylar fracture of the humerus

38) Flexion deformities of the fingers, usually 3rd and 4th fingers and/or a tender nodule in the ulnar palm suggests which of the following problems:
   A.   De Quervain's
   B.   Dupuytren's
   C.   Finkelstein's
   D.   Phalen's
   E.   Normal finding—no need for additional investigation

39) Spinal percussion causes deep dull pain that disappears slowly. Choose the best single answer.
   A.   Atlantoaxial instability
   B.   Spinal fracture
   C.   Bilateral pneumothorax
   D.   Spinal tumor or vertebral osteomyelitis
   E.   Normal finding—no need for additional investigation

40) Spinal percussion causes acute pain that rapidly subsides
    A. Desiccated intervertebral disc
    B. Recent joint or ligament injury
    C. Normal finding—no need for additional investigation
    D. Supracondylar fracture
    E. Acute compartment syndrome

41) **Your patient is a 15-yo male with progressive scoliosis for the past 6 months. Which of the following is inconsistent with early benign idiopathic scoliosis?**
    A. Platelet abnormalities
    B. Morphologic changes in the cerebellum
    C. Pain
    D. Proprioceptive defects
    E. Compensatory lateral curvature of the spine

42) **Your patient presents with ESR of 30, CRP of 25, negative rheumatoid factor, negative HLA-B27, ferritin of 150, and positive cyclic citrullinated peptide antibodies. What is this patient's clinical status?**
    A. Early iron overload
    B. Severe lupus
    C. Probable early rheumatoid arthritis
    D. Seronegative spondyloarthropathy
    E. Klippel-Feil syndrome

43) **Which of the following is consistent with occult gastrointestinal dysbiosis?**
    A. Increased lactulose-mannitol ratio
    B. Upregulated phase 1 of detoxification/biotransformation
    C. Inhibited phase 1 of detoxification/biotransformation
    D. Systemic immune activation
    E. All of the above

44) Which of the following characteristics places a patient in a higher risk category when associated with musculoskeletal pain and suggests the need for additional assessment?
    A. Age greater than 50 years, or diabetes
    B. Drug or alcohol use
    C. Low-grade fever
    D. Elevated WBC, ESR, or CRP; anemia
    E. All of the above.

45) Your 12-year-old gymnast patient presents with non-traumatic elbow pain in her dominant arm associated with stiffness, locking, and crepitus. Cozen's and Mill's tests are negative, and neurologic screening examination is normal. Regional assessments of neighboring regions are unremarkable. Your clinical concern and means of assessment are:
    A. Fracture of the olecranon—radiographs
    B. Supracondylar fracture of the humerus—radiographs
    C. Osteochondritis dissecans or osteochondrosis—radiographs
    D. Dislocation of the ulna—radiographs
    E. Fracture of the scaphoid—radiographs

46) Your 55-year-old patient presents with left-sided shoulder pain, wrist weakness, miosis, ptosis of the left eyelid, and anhidrosis on the left side of the face. The condition for which you must assess is:
    A. Cauda equina syndrome
    B. Thoracic outlet syndrome
    C. Pancoast syndrome
    D. Chronic fatigue syndrome
    E. Frozen shoulder syndrome

47) Which of the following are causes of shoulder pain:
    A. Apical lung tumor
    B. Cervical radiculopathy
    C. Impingement syndrome
    D. Biceps tendonitis
    E. All of the above

48) Your new 20-year-old patient presents with chief complaints of "back pain" and "the flu." The onset of both complaints was yesterday with a slight fever and now the back pain is rated 7 on a scale of 1-10 with 10 being severe pain. Lungs are clear to auscultation, and the lower back is stiff and painful to percussion. Your main concern is:
    A. Pancoast syndrome
    B. Myofascial trigger points
    C. Costochondritis
    D. Osteomyelitis
    E. Pneumonia

49) **Elevated ferritin with elevated CRP correlates with:**
    A. Cancer
    B. Iron overload
    C. Systemic inflammation
    D. Acute infection
    E. All of the above

50) Acute onset of pain in the C5 dermatome, lower extremity strength +3, patellar and Achilles reflexes +4
    A. Bicipital tendonitis—conservative treatment, PAR
    B. Cervical myelopathy—urgent referral
    C. Cervical radiculitis—conservative treatment, PAR
    D. Cervical radiculopathy—conservative treatment, PAR, recommend referral
    E. Supraspinatus tendonitis—conservative treatment, no need for referral

51) Positive Speed's test and Yergason's test, sensory testing WNL, with biceps strength +4
    A. Bicipital tendonitis—conservative treatment, no need for referral
    B. Cervical myelopathy—urgent referral
    C. Cervical radiculitis—conservative treatment
    D. Cervical radiculopathy—recommend referral
    E. Supraspinatus tendonitis—conservative treatment, no need for referral

52) Billy Bob is a 51-year-old right-handed male who presents to your office with a chief complaint of "chest pain" on the right that he first noticed this morning when he was finishing a tennis match with his daughter. He has anterior peristernal chest pain with point tenderness, increased pain with hyperabduction of the ipsilateral arm, increased pain with deep inspiration, increased pain with palpation-provocation of the peristernal structures. Heart and lung auscultation are WNL. Billy Bob most likely has:
    A. Costochondritis
    B. Pancoast syndrome
    C. Horner's syndrome
    D. Intercostal neuralgia
    E. Cardiovascular disease

53) Your patient presents with pain at the "anatomic snuff box" following trauma. Which condition is most likely in this patient?
    A. Fracture of the dens
    B. Medial epicondylitis
    C. Fracture of the scaphoid
    D. Supraspinatus tendonitis
    E. Supracondylar fracture of the humerus

54) Which of the following conditions can predispose your patient to atlantoaxial instability?
    A. Down syndrome
    B. Inflammatory arthropathy, such as rheumatoid arthritis
    C. Congenital agenesis of the dens, os odontoidium
    D. Trauma
    E. All of the above

55) Patient seated with flexion of spine, patient then extends knee; a test for lumbar discogenic radiculopathy:
    A. Bechterew's test
    B. Sotto-Hall test
    C. Empty can test
    D. Kemp's test
    E. Cozen's test

56) Patient seated, then lumbar spine is passively moved into rotation, extension, lateral flexion:
    A. Bechterew's test
    B. Braggard's test
    C. Empty can test
    D. Kemp's test
    E. Cozen's test

57) Dorsiflexion of ankle with straight leg raising, confirms the radicular nature of a positive straight leg raising test
    A. Bechterew's test
    B. Braggard's test
    C. Empty can test
    D. Kemp's test
    E. Cozen's test

58) Your patient is a 60-year-old male who presents with back pain and slight nausea of 1-month duration. During your comprehensive low back examination, your abdominal examination reveals a large midline pulsatile abdominal mass, and the femoral and dorsalis pedis pulses are weak. Your main concern and method of assessment are:
    A. Ovarian cancer—assess with ultrasound
    B. Aneurysm of the abdominal aorta—assess with ultrasound
    C. Lymphoma—assess with CBC
    D. Testicular torsion—assess with palpation and transillumination
    E. Meralgia paresthetica—assess with MRI

59) Which of the following are general categories of causes of low back pain:
    A. Serious organic diseases
    B. Serious musculoskeletal disorders requiring immediate attention
    C. Psychogenic
    D. Benign musculoskeletal disorders requiring conservative treatment and monitoring
    E. All of the above

60) Patient age 30-50 years with a history of chronic/recurrent low back pain notices an exacerbation of low back pain or the onset of leg pain associated with a bending and/or twisting motion; leg pain predominates over the severity of the low back pain. This is the classic presentation for:
    A. Atlantoaxial instability
    B. Meralgia paresthetica
    C. Osteochondrosis dissecans
    D. Lumbar disc herniation
    E. De Quervain's syndrome

61) Low back and leg pain exacerbated by spinal extension and relieved by flexion suggests which of the following differential diagnoses:
    A. Lumbar disc herniation or De Quervain's syndrome
    B. Meralgia paresthetica or cauda equina syndrome
    C. Sacroiliac joint dysfunction or scoliosis
    D. Spinal stenosis or facet syndrome
    E. Atlantoaxial instability or Tietze's syndrome

62) Results from rupture/laxity of the soft tissues at the symphysis pubis; associated with pregnancy and/or vaginal delivery in women or repetitive overuse in men; conservative management with a trochanteric-SIJ support belt is appropriate:
    A. Symphysis pubis diastasis or osteitis pubis
    B. SIJ sprain
    C. SIJ functional subluxation and/or dysfunction
    D. SIJ infection
    E. All of the above

63) Supine infant with flexed and abducted hip, the physician gently pulls the femur anteriorly while palpating at the trochanter for hints of anterior glide/dislocation
   A. Ortolani test
   B. Barlow test
   C. Allis's sign
   D. Thomas test
   E. Ober's test

64) Supine infant with flexed and adducted hip; physician gently pushes the femur posteriorly while palpating at the gluteus maximus for hints of posterior glide/dislocation
   A. Ortolani test
   B. Barlow test
   C. Allis's sign
   D. Thomas test
   E. Ober's test

65) Management of infants with congenital hip dysplasia minimally includes:
   A. Antiinflammatories
   B. Calcium supplementation
   C. Bromelain
   D. Manipulation
   E. Orthopedic referral

66) Children and adolescents with afebrile hip pain are evaluated by which of the following:
   A. Applied kinesiology
   B. Urinalysis
   C. Food allergy elimination and provocation
   D. Radiographs
   E. Assessing response to a 3-week trail of manipulation

67) Which of the following are causes of hip pain in children?
   A. Avascular necrosis of the femoral head
   B. Apophysitis
   C. Slipped capital femoral epiphysis
   D. Transient synovitis
   E. All of the above

68) In your office, what procedure(s) allows you do you differentiate septic arthritis from transient synovitis (assume classic location and presentation)?
   A. Observation and "vitals"
   B. Patrick's test
   C. Lift-off test confirmed by active internal rotation
   D. Sotto-Hall test
   E. Spinal percussion and lung auscultation

69) Your patient is a 40-year-old woman who presents with pain of the right hip. She recalls no trauma; and the onset of pain and limited motion has been gradual over the past week. She is obese, diabetic, smokes, and drinks a 6-pack of beer per day. Except for her prednisone to treat her asthma, she is not on any other medications. Physical examination of her right hip reveals painful limited ROM, and pain with compressive circumduction. Otherwise, she is in no acute distress, and vitals are normal, except for hypertension of 150/95. This patient most likely has:
   A. Transient synovitis
   B. Slipped femoral capital epiphysis
   C. Avascular necrosis of the femoral head
   D. Septic arthritis
   E. Meralgia paresthetica

70) Your management of the above patient includes:
   A. Radiographs of the hip
   B. Immediate referral for joint aspiration
   C. Immediate referral to the emergency room
   D. Urinalysis
   E. Ultrasound of the abdomen

71) You are a student clinician at the Bastyr clinic, and your supervising doctor assesses the 35-year-old patient with osteoarthritis of both hips and knees. Since you are well educated and since you care enough about your patient to ensure that he/she gets a proper evaluation, you tactfully remind your clinician that this patient needs to be assessed with which of the following lab tests?
   A. Lipoprotein(a)
   B. Urinalysis
   C. Blood pH
   D. Creatine phosphokinase
   E. Serum ferritin

72) Positive McMurray's test, positive bounce test, pain and limited motion with waddling, negative Lachman's test, negative patellar ballottement test, negative patellar grinding test:
   A. Joint effusion
   B. Meniscus injury
   C. Patellofemoral arthralgia
   D. Meralgia paresthetica
   E. None of the above

73) Which of the following suggest the need for knee radiographs following trauma:
   A. Local tenderness at the head of fibula or patella
   B. Inability to flex the knee to 90°
   C. Inability to walk >4 steps
   D. Blunt trauma or fall with one of the following: Age <12 years or >50 years
   E. All of the above

74) Your 14-year-old overweight male patient presents with knee pain and a limp. Clinical assessment reveals the following: negative McMurray's test, negative bounce test, negative Lachman's test, negative patellar ballottement test, negative patellar grinding test, and pain and hesitancy with the following assessments: Patrick's (FABER) test, Thomas test, circumduction. He is afebrile. This patient most likely has _____ and needs to be assessed with _____.
   A. Meniscus injury—MRI of the knee
   B. Congenital hip dysplasia—ultrasound of both hips
   C. Slipped femoral capital epiphysis—radiographs of both hips
   D. Osteochondritis dissecans of the knee—radiographs of both knee
   E. Osteoarthritis--radiographs

75) **Which of the following is the most consistent finding associated with compartment syndrome?**
   A. Elevated troponin and positive Rovsing's sign
   B. Painful passive stretch and elevated serum haptoglobin
   C. Proximal pallor, arterial hypotension, low TSH
   D. Pulselessness with elevated urobilinogen
   E. Sensory deficit, distal pulselessness, elevated CK

76) Which of the following are nerve root tension tests for the assessment of lumbar radiculopathy?
   A. Straight leg raising
   B. Bechterew's test
   C. Braggard's test
   D. All of the above
   E. Only two of the above answers (A, B, or C) are correct

77) Regarding the management of what appears to be mechanical low back pain, failure to produce significant resolution of pain and symptoms after _____ indicates the need for additional evaluation, imaging, and/or referral to a specialist.
   A. 2 days
   B. 1 week
   C. 2 weeks
   D. 4 weeks
   E. 10 weeks

78) **Leg weakness, bladder/bowel incontinence, and perineal numbness suggests:**
   A. **Klippel-Feil syndrome**
   B. **Turner syndrome**
   C. **Acute compartment syndrome**
   D. **Cauda equina syndrome**
   E. **Pelvic inflammatory disease**

79) **Your patient is an overweight 55-year-old woman who presents to your office after a recent diagnosis of meralgia paresthetica. A doctor at her HMO, who saw her for 5 minutes and performed essentially no physical examination, made the diagnosis. She would like you to treat her for this condition, and to help her modify her lifestyle so that she can loose weight, get off her blood pressure meds, stop smoking, and reduce her risk for ovarian cancer, which was the cause of death in her mother and sister. After your physical examination confirms that she has meralgia paresthetica and excludes radiculopathy, which of the following should you perform?**
   A. **Hemoglobin A1c**
   B. **Lumbosacral radiographs**
   C. **Diagnostic ultrasound**
   D. **Electromyography**
   E. **Joint aspiration**

Match the following.
   A. Tibial stress fracture
   B. Shin splints
   C. Compressive compartment syndrome
   D. Jones fracture
   E. Metatarsal stress fracture
   E. Metatarsalgia

80) Overuse strain of the compartmentalized muscles of the lower leg and/or inflammation of the tibial periosteum

81) Localized leg pain in an endurance or overtrained athlete; exacerbation of pain with static weight-bearing

82) Diffuse pain in a novice overtrained athlete; clinical findings include: painful passive stretch, pallor, pulselessness

83) Pain at the 2nd or 3rd metatarsal head in a runner or obese patient;

84) Pain at the middle inferior lateral aspect of the foot following a "twisted ankle"; exacerbation of pain with weight-bearing and walking

85) Pain in the metatarsal shaft in a runner or obese patient

Mark "A" for true and "B" for false for the remaining questions.

86) Generally speaking, any patient with a history of cancer who presents with a complaint of pain or loss of function needs to be carefully clinically evaluated for metastatic disease and should be assessed with laboratory tests (e.g., ESR, CRP, alk phos) and imaged with radiographs, ultrasound, CT, or MRI, as indicated.

87) Trauma to the thoracolumbar region mandates a urinalysis to assess for kidney damage.

88) Any patient with a recent head injury who demonstrates depressed sensorium must be evaluated with CT to assess for possible subdural hematoma or other intracranial pathology.

89) Any woman over the age of 40 who presents with chronic or recalcitrant neck, chest, shoulder, or arm pain which is not definitively ascribed to another condition must be assessed for breast cancer: history, family history, physical examination (breast exam, lymph nodes, regional exam, and mammography if appropriate).

90) Patients with recent trauma and the possibility of serious bleeding such as subdural hematoma or internal bleeding are not treated with medications/nutrients/botanicals that significantly impair coagulation.

91) Physical examination of a painful region also requires examination of neighboring regions and organs.

92) Differentiating viscerosomatic referral from mechanical causes of musculoskeletal pain, depends upon 1) the doctor's taking a complete patient history, 2) the doctor's performing a complete examination, 3) the doctor's obtaining proper laboratory tests, 4) the doctor's effective and appropriate use of imaging studies.

93) "Osteoarthritis" is a diagnosis of exclusion, and one of the diseases that must be ruled out before osteoarthritis can be diagnosed is hemochromatosis, which must be screened for with the laboratory tests serum ferritin and transferrin saturation.

Provide the standard grading and description of MUSCLE STRENGTH.

Grade	Description

Provide the standard grading and description of REFLEXES.

Grade	Description

Verbal assessment for myelopathy, cauda equina syndrome, and radiculopathy includes the following:

1) _____

2) _____

3) _____

List the **4 general categories** that need to be assessed during the history and physical when a patient presents with **any musculoskeletal complaint**:

1.	2.
3.	4.

5.   Describe the clinical management of the patient with cauda equina syndrome—be specific with regard to <u>what you will do</u> and <u>what the patient will do</u>:

_____

_____

_____

Your patient presents with a complex history and examination picture that suggests the possibility of organic disease as a cause of his/her complaints. A safe and reasonably inexpensive means of laboratory investigation that allows you to objectively screen for several different diseases includes (essential tests only):

6.	7.	8.

9. Your patient is sick and presents with recent onset of severe back pain, a rigid back, fever, and a raised WBC and sedimentation rate. The most likely diagnosis and your method for managing this patient are: _____

_____

Your patient is a 46-year-old woman whom you have been treating for various complaints including low back and neck pain, which she has had for several years following two car accidents. Today she presents to you with some concern because her low-back pain is worse, and she mentions that she has recently noticed a decrease in sensitivity of the regions around her anus and genitals. She denies pain or sensory changes in her legs and arms. Vital signs and routine neurologic examination of the upper and lower extremities are normal.

10. What is the most serious and likely diagnosis that you must consider? _____

11. What key question must you ask? _____

12. If your clinical suspicion of #10 is high, and #11 is positive/abnormal, how will you manage this patient? What needs to happen? _____

_____

_____

13. What is the approximate time frame for implementing the management plan that you have described in #12?_____

Two causes of knee joint locking:

14.	15.

4 musculoskeletal conditions that can typically cause low back pain with thigh pain:

16.	17.
18.	19.

20. Proper method of evaluation for **acute febrile non-traumatic monoarthritis** is (provide at least 3 specific answers, at least one of which must be the "gold standard"): _____

_____

_____

_____

Phrases coined by the author during the development of this text and other recent projects:

- **Antibiologic:** Although I am not the first to use this word (as of January 2006, only eight international websites used this word), I am the first to use it "medically" since the term is not listed in Medline (as of January 2006). My use of the word describes misused pharmaceutical drugs—most of which are enzyme *inhibitors* and thus work *against* physiology—and/or drugs which are used to mask an underlying problem that could have been identified and addressed to provide the patient an opportunity for *cure* rather than *codependence* upon lifelong medicalization. Most pharmaceutical drugs can be accurately described as antibiologic (against the logic of life) because they interfere with normal *eu*biologic functions or because they serve as a detour away from effective intervention. For example, as generally used, HMG-CoA reductase cholesterol-lowering drugs are antibiologic to the extent that they dysfunctionally enable patients to continue their destructive lifestyles by continuing to overeat and underexercise. Such a co-dependent enabling of dysfunctional behavior is **anti-health**, even if it does prolong life for patients unable to self-regulate. Proof of the superfluous overutilization of these drugs was demonstrated by O'Keefe, Cordain, et al[1] in their article noting that in healthy and active cultures, the average serum cholesterol level is approximately 100-150 mg/dL whereas in so-called industrialized nations such as the US the average serum cholesterol level is > 205 mg/dL, a level which "requires" drug intervention according to the pharmaceutical model. A more glaring example of the antibiologic use of drugs is the overuse of so-called antidepressant medications, which detour patients away from dealing with their internal emotional issues thanks to a corporate-driven "healthcare" paradigm that pushes medications for problems that *originate emotionally* and then later *manifest biochemically*.[2] Admittedly, some enzyme inhibitors such as Anastrozole (Arimidex®) clearly do have a place in healthcare and medicine, since for many patients this drug provides the only means by which to effectively lower their estrogen levels. Similarly, a statin HMG-CoA reductase inhibiting drug might be eubiologic in a patient with hypercholesterolemia who has already optimized diet and lifestyle but continues to have hypercholesterolemia. Thus, "antibiologic" relates more to the use of a given drug or treatment, rather than the treatment or drug itself. Forcing a patient to use a drug rather than empowering the patient toward disease resolution when available is against the inherent logic of life and can thus be described as antibiologic. Using that same drug to prolong life and maximize function in a patient who has earnestly exhausted other natural *primary* interventions could very well be eubiologic. Obviously, analyzing an intervention as *antibiologic* or *eubiologic* is best performed within a framework that appreciates the importance of a "hierarchy of therapeutics" such as outlined in Chapter 1 in the section on Naturopathic Medicine.

- **Anticausative:** Anticausative is a word used in the field of linguistics to describe "an intransitive verb that shows an event affecting its subject, while giving no semantic or syntactic indication of the cause of the event.[3] My use of the word implies **treatments that intentionally avoid addressing the underlying cause of the disease so that the patient experiences incomplete improvement yet must continue using the treatment (generally a drug) in order to avoid complications from the disease**. In other words, **anticausative treatments are detours** *away from effective healthcare* **under the guise of "healthcare."** Hypercholesterolemic drugs are the best example, since they are so often used to mask the cause of the problem (unhealthy diet and lifestyle) by addressing the manifestation of the problem (hypercholesterolemia) while the real metabolic problem (nutritional deficiencies, sarcopenia, insulin resistance) are left unaddressed.

- **Antidysbiotic:** (*adjective*) Describes anything that counteracts dysbiosis by elimination of microbes.

- **Dietary haptenization:** The binding of dietary moieties to body tissues for the formation of an immunogenic neoantigen.

- **Disease identification:** When a patient uses his/her disease as a source of personal identity.

- **Dysbiotic arthropathy, dysbiotic autoimmunity:** Arthritis, arthropathy, systemic inflammation, and "autoimmunity" that results from unifocal or multifocal dysbiosis.

- **Envirosociogenomics:** The phenomenon by which our social, economic, and political environments shape our biology by shaping our lifestyles and experiences for the induction of a specific phenotype. A recent example is the epidemic of diabetic obesity triggered by the impoverishment of the populace due to political manipulations that enrich the few at the expense of the many. America's trend toward increased concentration of wealth—rather than equitable and democratic distribution of resources—is a nonmedical contributor to the problems of hypertension, depression, insulin resistance, and obesity. See the recent article by McCarthy[4] for an excellent and concise review.

- **Idiopathicization:** The intentional action of attempting to convince doctors and patients that a disease or group of diseases are "of unknown origin" and that therefore—since the cause of the disease is not known and cannot therefore be treated—both doctor and patient must turn their hopes *away from health* and *toward medicalization in general and pharmaceuticalization in particular*. The cause(s) of many diseases is known and can be treated; however, those who benefit from *selling drugs* and from *keeping the population dependent on drugs* work to convince us that nutrition is ineffective, that proactive strategies are futile, and that drugs and surgery are the best answers to our problems, even

[1] O'Keefe JH, Cordain L, Harris, WH, Moe RM, Vogel R. Optimal low-density lipoprotein is 50 to 70 mg/dl. Lower is better and physiologically normal. *J Am Coll Cardiol* 2004;43: 2142-6 http://www.thepaleodiet.com/published_research/
[2] Miller A. The truth will set you free: overcoming emotional blindness and finding your true adult self. [Translated from German]. New York: Basic Books; 2001
[3] http://en.wikipedia.org/wiki/Anticausative_verb
[4] McCarthy M. The economics of obesity. *Lancet.* 2004 Dec 18-31;364(9452):2169-70

those within our control which are easily addressed with intentional action.[5] See my 2006 Editorial for further explication: http://www.naturopathydigest.com/archives/2006/mar/idiopathic.php

- **Immunonutrigenomics**: The phenomenon by which nutrients influence genetic expression to modulate immune function either toward or away from inflammation, toward or away from immune dysfunction.

- **Intracellular hypercalcinosis**: I coined this phrase in 2004 following the publication of my vitamin D monograph[6] and reading a brief but very important paper in which Fujita[7] noted, in essence, that vitamin D deficiency and/or calcium deficiency resulted in a secondary hyperparathyroidism which essentially drove excess calcium into the intracellular compartment. Since excess intracellular calcium acts to stimulate and disrupt a wide range of intracellular *and therefore systemic* processes, this condition, which I have labeled as "intracellular hypercalcinosis" appears, as suggested by Fujita, to contribute to the development of hypertension, arteriosclerosis, diabetes mellitus, neurodegenerative diseases, malignancy, and degenerative joint disease. Beyond deficiencies of 1) vitamin D and 2) calcium (both of which increase intracellular calcium by stimulating release of parathyroid hormone), other nutritional and lifestyle contributors to this phenomenon are likely to include 3) the epidemic of magnesium deficiency, 4) the Western style of eating which promotes loss of magnesium and calcium in the urine to due the net acid load placed on the kidneys[8,9] and consumption of foods and beverages with 5) caffeine, 6) sugar, and/or 7) alcohol/ethanol, and 6) fatty acid imbalances — namely insufficient intake of the omega-3 fatty acids in general and EPA in particular, particularly in a setting of excess arachidonic acid.[10] No doubt that 8) psychoemotional/physical stress also plays a role here due to the induced renal hyperexcretion of calcium and/or magnesium occurs following stressful events.[11] The concept of intracellular hypercalcinosis is supported by the medical use of "calcium channel blocking drugs" for example in the treatment of hypertension, which also responds to 1) vitamin D supplementation, 2) calcium supplementation, 3) magnesium supplementation, 4) an un-Western style of eating which promotes alkalinization, 5) caffeine avoidance, 6) sugar avoidance, 7) alcohol/ethanol avoidance, 6) n-3 fatty acid supplementation, and 8) stress reduction. For further discussion, please see http://www.naturopathydigest.com/archives/2006/sep/vasquez.php

- **Multifocal dysbiosis**: Dysbiosis occurring in more than one location at the same time in the same patient. Each locus may be subtle and "subclinical" however the effects are at least **additive** and are more often **synergistic.** See the most current edition of *Integrative Rheumatology* for details, clinical implications, and interventions; for a superficial overview, see my article on-line: http://www.naturopathydigest.com/archives/2006/jun/vasquez.php

- **Multifocal polydysbiosis**: See *polydysbiosis* below.

- **Myalgenic**: (adjective) Producing muscle pain.

- **NeoHeroic Medicine**: I coined this phrase in November 2006 to connote the similarities between the *passé* Heroic medicine and modern allopathic medicine

- **Naturogenomics**: I coined this phrase on October 29, 2006 while writing the third part of an Editorial for *Naturopathy Digest*—see http://www.naturopathydigest.com/archives/2006/dec/editor.php. I define it as the study and clinical application of the modulation of gene expression with "naturopathic" and "natural" interventions such as diet, nutritional supplementation, botanical medicines, spinal and musculoskeletal manipulation, exercise, and other non-surgical non-pharmacologic interventions.

- **Orthoendocrinology**: Optimization of hormonal status by assessing and correcting levels of all major hormones, particularly those with inflammatory/anti-inflammatory actions—thyroid, prolactin, Cortisol, DHEA, estrogen(s), testosterone. This is detailed in *Integrative Rheumatology*.

- **Pharmacopathic**: Disease caused by drugs; pharmaceutical iatrogenesis

- **Pharmacoeconomic**: Describes the link between drugs and money, such as the financial interests that push drugs on the American people.

- **Polydysbiosis**: I coined this term in May 2006 during a discussion on the IFM Forum (FunctionalMedicine.org) to connote that gastrointestinal dysbiosis is generally multi-/poly-microbial in nature, rather than due to a single dysbiotic microbe. Thus, the probability is that many dysbiotic patients have **multifocal polydysbiosis**—dysbiosis in more than one location caused by the presence of more than one dysbiotic microbe or overgrowth of otherwise benign microbes.

[5] van der Steen WJ, Ho VK. Drugs versus diets: disillusions with Dutch health care. *Acta Biotheor.* 2001;49(2):125-40

[6] Vasquez A, Manso G, Cannell J. The Clinical Importance of Vitamin D (Cholecalciferol): A Paradigm Shift with Implications for All Healthcare Providers. *Alternative Therapies in Health and Medicine* 2004; 10: 28-37 http://www.optimalhealthresearch.com/monograph04

[7] "Such intracellular paradoxical Ca overload as a consequence of nutritional calcium deficiency may give rise to a number of diseases common in old age: hypertension, arteriosclerosis, diabetes mellitus, neurodegenerative diseases, malignancy, and degenerative joint disease." Fujita T. Calcium paradox: consequences of calcium deficiency manifested by a wide variety of diseases. *J Bone Miner Metab.* 2000;18(4):234-6

[8] Maurer M, Riesen W, Muser J, Hulter HN, Krapf R. Neutralization of Western diet inhibits bone resorption independently of K intake and reduces cortisol secretion in humans. *Am J Physiol Renal Physiol.* 2003 Jan;284(1):F32-40 http://ajprenal.physiology.org/cgi/content/full/284/1/F32

[9] "Acid loading resulted in massive calciuria in both groups, with significantly higher urinary calcium excretion rates in the stone-formers compared to the healthy subjects. ... Acid loading (i.e. protein ingestion) may contribute to disturbed bone metabolism in idiopathic calcium nephrolithiasis as well as calcium stone formation." Osther PJ. Effect of acute acid loading on acid-base and calcium metabolism. *Scand J Urol Nephrol.* 2006;40(1):35-44

[10] "The Ca(2+) influx rate varied from 0.5 to 3 nM Ca(2+)/s in the presence of AA and from 0.9 to 1.7 nM Ca(2+)/s with EPA." Soldati L, Lombardi C, Adamo D, Terranegra A, Bianchin C, Bianchi G, Vezzoli G. Arachidonic acid increases intracellular calcium in erythrocytes. *Biochem Biophys Res Commun.* 2002 May 10;293(3):974-8

[11] "Our study shows that noise induces significant increases of serum calcium and magnesium, with a borderline increase of serum phosphorus; this in turn is reflected in a significantly increased urinary excretion of magnesium and phosphate after exposure, which lasts for the following 2 days." Mocci F, Canalis P, Tomasi PA, Casu F, Pettinato S. The effect of noise on serum and urinary magnesium and catecholamines in humans. *Occup Med* (Lond). 2001 Feb;51(1):56-61 http://occmed.oxfordjournals.org/cgi/reprint/51/1/56

12630217R10324